CANCER DRUG DESIGN AND DISCOVERY

CANCER DRUG DESIGN AND DISCOVERY

SECOND EDITION

STEPHEN NEIDLE

School of Pharmacy, University College London, UK

AMSTERDAM • BOSTON • HEIDELBERG • LONDON
NEW YORK • OXFORD • PARIS • SAN DIEGO
SAN FRANCISCO • SINGAPORE • SYDNEY • TOKYO
Academic Press is an imprint of Elsevier

Academic Press is an imprint of Elsevier
32 Jamestown Road, London NW1 7BY, UK
225 Wyman Street, Waltham, MA 02451, USA
525 B Street, Suite 1800, San Diego, CA 92101-4495, USA

Second edition

Notice
No responsibility is assumed by the publisher for any injury and/or damage to persons or property as
a matter of products liability, negligence or otherwise, or from any use or operation of any methods,
products, instructions or ideas contained in the material herein. Because of rapid advances in the
medical sciences, in particular, independent verification of diagnoses and drug dosages should be made

British Library Cataloguing-in-Publication Data
A catalogue record for this book is available from the British Library

Library of Congress Cataloging-in-Publication Data
A catalog record for this book is available from the Library of Congress

Cover graphic: A view of the crystal structure (Protein Data Bank entry 3RUK) of the prostate cancer
drug abiraterone bound in the active site of the human cytochrome P450 17A1 enzyme (NM DeVore
and EE Scott, Nature 2012, 482, 116-119).

ISBN: 978-0-12-396521-9

For information on all Academic Press publications
visit our website at www.store.elsevier.com

Typeset by TNQ Books and Journals
www.tnq.co.in

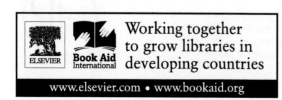

Contents

I

BASIC PRINCIPLES AND METHODOLOGY

1. Modern Cancer Drug Discovery: Integrating Targets, Technologies, and Treatments for Personalized Medicine

PAUL WORKMAN, IAN COLLINS

2. Pharmacogenomics and Personalized Medicines in Cancer Treatment

WEI-PENG YONG, ROSS SOO, FEDERICO INNOCENTI

3. Natural Product Chemistry and Cancer Drug Discovery

DONNA M. HURYN, PETER WIPF

II

DRUGS IN THE LABORATORY
AND CLINIC

10. Inhibitors of Tumor Angiogenesis

ADRIAN L. HARRIS, DANIELE GENERALI

11. The Renaissance of CYP17 Inhibitors for the Treatment of Prostate Cancer

QINGZHONG HU, ROLF W. HARTMANN

12. Apoptosis in Cancer: Mechanisms, Deregulation, and Therapeutic Targeting

ZAHID H. SIDDIK

13. Targeting the MDM2–p53 Protein–Protein Interaction: Design, Discovery, and Development of Novel Anticancer Agents

IAN R. HARDCASTLE

14. Targeting Altered Metabolism—Emerging Cancer Therapeutic Strategies

MINSUH SEO, ROBERT BLAKE CROCHET, YONG-HWAN LEE

15. Inhibitors of the Phosphatidylinositol 3-Kinase Pathway

WILLIAM A. DENNY, GORDON W. REWCASTLE

III

THE REALITY OF CANCER DRUGS IN THE CLINIC

Introduction

In my introduction to the 1st edition of this book in 2008, I wrote that "The public, and the biomedical community, have an insatiable appetite for new anticancer drugs". This is even more the case now. Even though the past five years have been a period of unprecedented turmoil in the pharmaceutical industry, the number of new anticancer therapies that are being invented and developed shows no sign of diminishing, and the number of phase I clinical trials of new agents and combinations continues to run into many hundreds each year. The trends that were apparent in 2008 are even more marked in 2013, with advances in our basic understanding of the molecular (and, increasingly, genetic) basis of human cancers being translated into new therapeutic agents. Perhaps the best example of this is in malignant melanoma, where the identification of oncogenic mutations in the *B-raf* gene has led to the development of effective inhibitors, some of which have shown remarkable effectiveness in clinical use, although the rapid onset of resistance is currently a significant challenge. Another major clinical advance is in the treatment of chemo-resistant prostate cancer, where the hitherto bleak outlook for many men is being transformed with the accelerated approval for clinical use of the hormonal pathway inhibitor compound abiraterone (Zytiga™). This drug is one of the great success stories of academic cancer drug discovery; it is unsurprising that one of the major trends in the field over the past five years has been the increase in drug discovery activities in academic environments. These are often staffed and led by ex-industry chemists and biologists, ensuring that their unique expertise is not lost. However, most new drugs continue to come from industry, and even the best-resourced academic initiative will at some stage need to link in with an industrial partner. So the authorship of the chapters in this book reflects this diversity of institutions where cancer drug discovery takes place and flourishes, with contributors from small and big pharma, universities, and research institutes.

The 1st edition had its origins in my time at the Institute of Cancer Research UK from 1986 to 2002, when I was privileged to come into contact with a number of visionary clinicians and scientists, especially Tim McElwain, Tom Connors, and Ken Harrap. They were instrumental in the development of cancer therapeutics as a discipline, and most importantly in the translation of science from the bench to the bedside for patient benefit. In this spirit, I hope that the 2nd edition continues to play a role in fostering the interplay of fundamental and translational aspects of cancer drug discovery. Its central aim continues to be the provision of detailed accounts of the twenty-first-century cancer drug discovery process, from target identification and validation, through lead discovery and optimization, to pharmacological evaluation and eventual clinical trial and registration, so that the reader emerges with a broad overall view, and most importantly understanding, of the key issues and complexities involved. The book continues to be divided into five sections: "Basic Principles", "Methodology", "Drugs in the Clinic", "New Agents", and "The Reality of Cancer Drugs in the Clinic".

Some chapters are updates of previous ones, especially where there have been significant advances; others are new and reflect the increasing importance of particular topics. The fundamentals of cancer biology are not described since the reader is already well served by a number of excellent books. Case histories of particular drugs continue to feature in a number of chapters throughout the book, and some also conclude with questions that can be used in a classroom setting. It is to be hoped that this book will play a role in training future generations of cancer scientists and clinicians, not least to meet the challenges of those many cancers that are still hard to treat.

I thank all the contributors, not only for their hard work and dedication to this project, but also for their cooperation in meeting challenging deadlines. I am also very grateful to my colleague Hilary Calvert for very kindly agreeing to write the Foreword from the expert perspective of a clinician who not only has been instrumental in the clinical trials of several of the most important cancer drugs in current use, but also has a profound understanding of the underlying science. The staff of Elsevier/Academic Press in the USA and the UK has been enormously skillful and professional in ensuring the success of this project, and I am especially grateful to Andy Albrecht and Kristine Jones for their involvement and expertise. Last, but not least, many thanks to my wife Andrea for her unwavering support, wise advice, and patience.

Stephen Neidle
School of Pharmacy
University College London, UK

Foreword

In 1972, as a newly appointed junior doctor at the Royal Marsden Hospital in London, I was asked to give a patient 'platinum'. The patient vomited profusely and went into renal failure, but her ovarian cancer melted away. She was one of the first patients with ovarian cancer to respond to cis-diamminedichloro-platinum II. This was not the first directly cytotoxic anticancer drug. It had taken medicine 25 years to reach this point since Goodman and Gilman had published their finding of tumor shrinkage in patients treated with nitrogen mustard. Stemming from the observation that troops exposed to mustard gas in the First World War suffered from suppression of the white cell count, Goodman and Gilman developed a series of water-soluble analogs and finally published their results in 1946. Soon after this discovery, a large number of additional bifunctional alkylating agents were developed, several of which are still in use today.

Cisplatin was discovered by a serendipitous observation made by Rosenberg, when he found that passing electrical currents through cultures of bacteria led to the formation of cisplatin by dissolution of the electrodes. Cisplatin and the subsequently discovered analogs carboplatin and oxaliplatin act in a similar way to the alkylating agents by forming adducts on, and cross-linking, DNA. The platinum analogs significantly expanded the role of anticancer drugs, particularly in the curative treatment of germ cell tumors of the testis and ovary, significant extension of life in ovarian cancer, the adjuvant treatment of colorectal cancer, and palliation of lung cancer.

Also in the late 1940s, Sydney Farber in Boston, United States, noted that children with acute leukemia had low folic acid levels in their blood. Giving folate supplements, rather than slowing the disease, caused an 'acceleration effect' on the leukemia. This led to the development of the first targeted anticancer agent, methotrexate, which interferes with folate metabolism and prevents dividing cells from synthesizing thymidine and purine bases, essential for DNA synthesis. Further antifolates were developed—in particular, pemetrexed is now a major drug in the treatment of mesothelioma and lung cancer. Pemetrexed is distinguished from methotrexate in that it acts directly on thymidylate synthase. This enzyme is responsible for the conversion of deoxyuridine monophosphate to thymidine, which, in turn, is exclusively used for DNA synthesis.

A number of natural products were also identified during the next few decades. The most important of these are drugs acting on tubulin (vinca alkaloids and taxanes). Vinca alkaloids were discovered by the Eli Lilly Company during investigations of the therapeutic properties of the periwinkle plant. Vincas in combination with other drugs, including methotrexate and 6-mercaptopurine, allowed the development of curative regimens for childhood leukemia. A second class of tubulin-binding drugs, the taxanes, was discovered in the bark of yew trees in the 1980s. These drugs (paclitaxel and docetaxel) act by binding to, and stabilizing, tubulin and thereby preventing mitosis. They continue to have major roles in the treatment of many cancers, including breast cancer, lung cancer, and ovarian cancer. A further group of natural products act by inhibiting topoisomerase enzymes. Anthracyclines such as doxorubicin bind to DNA and prevent topoisomerase II religation of the DNA strands, thus causing DNA fragmentation. Podophyllotoxins such as etoposide also inhibit topoisomerase II. Camptothecin analogs (topotecan and irinotecan) act by inhibiting topoisomerase I. All of these agents have found applications in the treatment of common cancers.

The agents described here, along with hormonal agents for breast and prostate cancers, formed the basis of the arsenal available for systemic cancer treatment until the 1990s. Their impact on the cancer problem was significant, if not overwhelming. Many leukemias and hematological tumors were cured. Use of drug combinations as adjuvant therapy following surgery increased the survival rate in several common cancers, particularly breast cancer and colorectal cancer. In other instances, such as ovarian cancer, survival was substantially prolonged, although a cure was not achieved. Notably, all of the cytotoxic agents (meaning nonhormonal agents) are toxic to proliferating cells. This action is responsible not only for their anticancer activity but also for many toxicities to other proliferating tissues, including the bone marrow, hair follicles, and gastrointestinal mucosa. It is surprising that any cancer cures and improvements in survival were achieved at all with such nonspecific therapies.

By the early 1990s, there was a general belief that further progress could be made only by devising better targeted drugs. Advances in biology had begun to elucidate cell-signaling pathways and define the role of cell surface receptors for growth factors and the mechanisms by which their activation transmitted signals to the nucleus to initiate cell division. Mutations in these pathways that caused their constitutive activation led to the identification of oncogenes, elucidating

the genetic cause of some cancers. Advances in medicinal chemistry and structural biology made it possible to discover 'designer' drugs to inhibit specifically these pathways. Most pharmaceutical companies and academic institutions abandoned their research programs on new cytotoxic drugs in favor of developing 'targeted' agents aimed at the cell-signaling pathways. By far, the majority of putative new anticancer drugs that have undergone clinical evaluation in the last 20 years have been such targeted agents. Some of these targeted agents have made a dramatic impact on a particular type of cancer, but overall the results of this effort have been disappointing. Toxic side effects have been dose limiting, and the use of combinations of targeted agents has been particularly problematic.

The initial trials of epidermal growth factor receptor (EGFR) tyrosine kinase inhibitors in combination with chemotherapy for lung cancer showed no improvement in survival (in fact, a statistically nonsignificant reduction was documented). Further trials of single-agent treatment in chemoresistant patients showed a significant, but modest, improvement in survival of a few months. Targeted agents have been licensed for renal cell cancer and hepatocellular carcinoma, but, again, these produce modest survival improvements but not cures.

One possible reason for the many disappointing results is that these drugs, although 'targeted' to a biochemical pathway, are not targeted to the cancer itself. Indeed, the signal transduction pathways are responsible for homeostasis in a wide range of normal tissues, including many vital organs, whether they are proliferating or not. The old-fashioned cytotoxic agents may be more targeted in that their side effects are in principle limited to proliferating tissues.

As mentioned, there have been some dramatic successes with some targeted agents.

In each successful case, there is evidence that that drug target is both unique to the tumor and essential to its survival. Imatinib has transformed the prognosis for chronic myeloid leukemia. It targets the Bcr–Abl fusion protein that is a result of the chromosomal translocation (Philadelphia chromosome) that is causative for the leukemia. EGFR kinase inhibitors do work well in the small proportion of lung cancer patients in whom there is an activating mutation in EGFR. Activating mutations occur almost exclusively in nonsmokers, suggesting that this mutation is responsible for their cancer. Another subgroup of lung cancers in nonsmokers have a translocation including the *ALK* gene, and an inhibitor aimed directly at this has remarkable activity. Another example, covered in this book, is a result of systematic genomic studies in cancer cells. The *BRAF* gene was found to have a specific activating mutation in the tumor in about 50% of patients with malignant melanoma. *BRAF* inhibitors now provide hope for patients with this previously refractory tumor.

We should now focus on developing new drugs that are tumor specific rather than targeting a general pathway that the tumor may rely on along with normal tissues. This book illustrates several such approaches.

Since patients and their tumors are very heterogeneous, a personalized approach to treatment is beginning to look essential. The increasing availability and the decreasing cost of whole-genome sequencing will be important in making this feasible. The role of DNA repair defects in oncogenesis makes tumor-selective treatment possible by exploiting the concept of 'synthetic lethality' using specific DNA repair inhibitors. It is sometimes possible to target otherwise nonspecific drugs to the tumor using antibodies, and it may also be possible to exploit specific mutations in the energy pathways of intermediary metabolism.

Finally, we need to expedite the final stage—clinical development. The regulatory environment has become increasingly stringent in recent years, adding to the time and cost of performing essential clinical evaluations. Current clinical methodologies are poorly designed to detect activity in a small genetic subset of patients, while the drugs we are developing are likely to be active only in a small subset. These issues are covered in the final part of the book.

Hilary Calvert
UCL Cancer Institute
University College London

Editor Biography

Stephen Neidle is professor of chemical biology at the School of Pharmacy, University College London, where he directs a multidisciplinary group working on cancer drug discovery, focusing on novel approaches to pancreatic and other cancers with unmet clinical need. His work has been recognized by the Sosnovsky and Interdisciplinary Awards of the Royal Society of Chemistry and the Aventis Prize in Medicinal Chemistry of the French Societé de Chimie Thérapeutique. He was chair of the Chemistry in Cancer Research Working Group of the American Association for Cancer Research for 2011–2012 and is European editor of the journal Bioorganic and Medicinal Chemistry Letters.

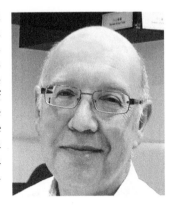

Contributors

Paola B. Arimondo Institut de Recherche Pierre Fabre, Centre de Recherche et Développement, Toulouse, France

Christian Bailly Institut de Recherche Pierre Fabre, Centre de Recherche et Développement, Toulouse, France

Tracy M. Bryan Children's Medical Research Institute, Westmead, NSW, Australia; University of Sydney, Sydney, NSW, Australia

Silvia Chioato Pfizer Srl, Milan, Italy

Scott B. Cohen Children's Medical Research Institute, Westmead, NSW, Australia; University of Sydney, Sydney, NSW, Australia

Ian Collins Cancer Research UK Cancer Therapeutics Unit, The Institute of Cancer Research, London, UK

Robert Blake Crochet Department of Biological Sciences, Louisiana State University, Baton Rouge, LA, USA

Nicola J. Curtin Newcastle Cancer Centre, Northern Institute for Cancer Research, Newcastle University, Newcastle upon Tyne, UK

William A. Denny Auckland Cancer Society Research Centre, School of Medical Sciences, University of Auckland, New Zealand

Erling Donnelly Pfizer Inc, Cambridge, MA, USA

Daniele Generali U.O. Multidisciplinare di Patologia Mammaria, U.S. di Terapia Molecolare e Farmacogenomica, Az. Istituti Ospitalieri di Cremona, Cremona, Italy

Nicolas Guilbaud Institut de Recherche Pierre Fabre, Centre de Recherche et Développement, Toulouse, France

Ian R. Hardcastle Newcastle Cancer Centre, Northern Institute for Cancer Research, Newcastle University, Newcastle upon Tyne, UK

Adrian L. Harris Molecular Oncology Laboratory, Cancer Research UK, Weatherall Institute of Molecular Medicine, John Radcliffe Hospital, Oxford, UK

Philip A. Harris GlaxoSmithKline, Collegeville, PA, USA

John A. Hartley Cancer Research UK Drug-DNA Interactions Research Group, UCL Cancer Institute, London, UK

Rolf W. Hartmann Pharmaceutical & Medicinal Chemistry, Saarland University, Saarbrücken, Germany; Helmholtz Institute for Pharmaceutical Research Saarland (HIPS), Saarbrücken, Germany

Qingzhong Hu Pharmaceutical & Medicinal Chemistry, Saarland University, Saarbrücken, Germany

Donna M. Huryn Center for Chemical Methodologies and Library Development (UPCMLD), University of Pittsburgh, Pittsburgh, PA, USA

Federico Innocenti Eshelman School of Pharmacy, Institute for Pharmacogenomics and Individualized Therapy, University of North Carolina, Chapel Hill, NC, USA; Linerberger Comprehensive Cancer Center, School of Medicine, University of North Carolina, Chapel Hill, NC, USA

Harren Jhoti Astex Therapeutics, Cambridge, UK

Keith Jones Cancer Research UK Cancer Therapeutics Unit, The Institute of Cancer Research, London, UK

Yong-Hwan Lee Department of Biological Sciences, Louisiana State University, Baton Rouge, LA, USA

David Norton Astex Therapeutics, Cambridge, UK

Puja Pathuri Astex Therapeutics, Cambridge, UK

Gordon W. Rewcastle Auckland Cancer Society Research Centre, School of Medical Sciences, University of Auckland, New Zealand

Minsuh Seo Department of Biological Sciences, Louisiana State University, Baton Rouge, LA, USA

Swee Sharp Cancer Research UK Cancer Therapeutics Unit, The Institute of Cancer Research, London, UK

Zahid H. Siddik Department of Experimental Therapeutics, The University of Texas MD Anderson Cancer Center, Houston, TX, USA

Christopher A. Slapak Lilly Research Laboratories, Eli Lilly and Company, Indianapolis, IN, USA

Ross Soo Department of Hematology–Oncology, National University Health System, Singapore; Cancer Science Institute of Singapore, Singapore

Malcolm F.G. Stevens Centre for Biomolecular Sciences, University of Nottingham, Nottingham, UK

David Taylor UCL School of Pharmacy, London, UK

Dominic Tisi Astex Therapeutics, Cambridge, UK

Christopher G. Tomlinson Children's Medical Research Institute, Westmead, NSW, Australia; University of Sydney, Sydney, NSW, Australia

Stephany Veuger Newcastle Cancer Centre, Northern Institute for Cancer Research, Newcastle University, Newcastle upon Tyne, UK

Richard A. Walgren Lilly Research Laboratories, Eli Lilly and Company, Indianapolis, IN, USA

Henriette Willems Astex Therapeutics, Cambridge, UK

Peter Wipf Center for Chemical Methodologies and Library Development (UPCMLD), University of Pittsburgh, Pittsburgh, PA, USA

Paul Workman Cancer Research UK Cancer Therapeutics Unit, The Institute of Cancer Research, London, UK

Wei-Peng Yong Department of Hematology–Oncology, National University Health System, Singapore; Cancer Science Institute of Singapore, Singapore

PART I

BASIC PRINCIPLES
AND METHODOLOGY

Modern Cancer Drug Discovery: Integrating Targets, Technologies, and Treatments for Personalized Medicine

Paul Workman, Ian Collins

Cancer Research UK Cancer Therapeutics Unit, The Institute of Cancer Research, London, UK

INTRODUCTION: CHANGING TIMES

Cancer drug discovery has undergone a remarkable series of changes over the last 15 years. So what has changed so much? First, the molecular *targets* of contemporary cancer drug discovery projects are very different. Current targets reflect our increasing understanding of the genetic and epigenetic changes that are responsible for the initiation and malignant progression of cancer through the dysregulation of cell biochemistry and signaling networks [1,2]. Second, the integrated application of a range of powerful drug discovery *technologies* has had a major impact [3]. Third, many new *treatments* have emerged over the last 15 years based on this paradigm that are firmly established in the clinic [4]. The present volume brings together many of the important aspects of the discovery and design of new cancer drugs, emphasizing small molecules. In this chapter, we provide a scene-setting introduction to, and overview of, modern small-molecule cancer drug discovery. We will argue that success is dependent on the close integration of the three major themes: *targets*, *treatments*, and *technologies*. In this regard, cancer drugs are leading the way in the development of personalized medicine. On the other hand, it is clear that drug resistance is just as much a problem with molecularly targeted agents as it has been with cytotoxic drugs.

First, however, it is useful to assess at the overview level what progress has been made and what the current limitations are. This provides a firm foundation for understanding what needs to be done to move the field forward. Following this, we will review the drug discovery process in detail from the identification of the molecular target through to selection of a drug candidate. Specific examples and case histories will be provided. We end the chapter by drawing some conclusions and taking a look into the future, including the potential for combinatorial therapies to overcome the problem of drug resistance.

SUCCESSES AND LIMITATIONS

Cytotoxic Agents

The first generation of cancer drugs, originating since the 1950s, were almost all cytotoxic agents. These frequently act by damaging DNA, inhibiting its synthesis or interfering with the mechanics of cell division, for example, by blocking topoisomerases or binding to micro-tubules [5,6]. Many of these agents were discovered by screening for chemical compounds that were able to kill cancer cells, as with a natural product like the microtubule inhibitor paclitaxel [7]. DNA-alkylating agents, originally based on sulfur and nitrogen mustards, were structurally modified so as to control their rates of chemical reactivity, leading to drugs like cyclophosphamide and ifosfamide [8]. Drugs developed in this first, cytotoxic era of cancer drug development were not designed to take advantage of our current knowledge of the genetic and molecular basis of cancer. Nevertheless, many of them were "molecularly tar-geted", as in the case of the antifolate thymidylate synthase inhibitors, in the sense that they were designed according to the principles of contemporary medicinal chemistry and in some cases involved the application of structure–activity relationships and X-ray crystallography to a single, defined molecular target [9].

There have been many notable successes with cytotoxic drug treatments for cancer. The dis-ease exists in a large number of forms, as defined anatomically under the light microscope and, more recently, at the molecular level. The effectiveness of drug treatment varies across these dif-ferent anatomical, histological, and molecular types. Major improvements have been achieved in the treatment of leukemias, lymphomas, testicular cancer, and children's malignancies with cytotoxic drugs, leading to marked increases in survival (www.cancer.org/acs/groups/content/@epidemiologysurveilance/documents/document/acspc-031941.pdf). On the other hand, progress has been modest at best in the common adult epithelial tumors, although suc-cessful exceptions have included adjuvant cytotoxic chemotherapy in breast and prostate can-cers. Despite some advances, cancer remains the second most frequent cause of death in the United States (http://www.cdc.gov/nchs/data/nvsr/nvsr61/nvsr61_06.pdf). Furthermore, despite a decrease in incidence for many cancers, incidence rates for other cancers are increasing, including human papillomavirus-related oropharyngeal cancer; melanoma; and cancers of the pancreas, liver, and kidney. The worldwide increase in cancer burden in part reflects the chang-ing demography of both developed and developing countries, where older age groups with the highest cancer risk are increasing in size [10]. Together with tremendous opportunities afforded by the availability of new targets and technologies, the major unmet need for cancer treatment continues to drive the extensive contemporary efforts in cancer drug discovery.

New Molecular Cancer Therapeutics

From the late 1990s onward, it became clear that major gains in survival were unlikely to be made by fine-tuning the classical cytotoxic agents. Antiestrogen and antiandrogen therapies in breast and prostate cancers, respectively, continued to lead to improved outcomes in specific cancer subtypes, as exemplified by the recent approval of abiraterone (Zytiga) for the treatment of metastatic castration-resistant prostate cancer [11] (see Chapter 11), but new approaches were needed to tackle the wider forms of the disease. This view coincided with the arrival of new molecular target opportunities emerging from basic cancer research and large-scale genomics. Consistent with common usage, we will use the term "molecular cancer therapeutics" to refer to mechanism-based agents acting on drug targets involved in the molecular causation of cancer. Success with the new molecularly targeted approach is evidenced by the approval by the US Food and Drug Administration (FDA) of many innovative drugs, both antibodies and small molecules, since the introduction of trastuzumab (Herceptin) in 1998 (Table 1.1; and see http://www.centerwatch.com/patient/drugs/druglist.html).

As the first example of a modern, targeted molecular cancer therapeutic, the humanized monoclonal antibody trastuzumab showed substantial therapeutic activity in patients with breast cancers that overexpress the ERBB2/HER2 oncoprotein as a result of DNA amplification [12]. This population represents about 30% of patients with node-positive breast cancer, and they benefited from a 50% decrease in disease recurrence over a 20-month period. Since its first approval in 1998, trastuzumab has become part of the standard of care in treating metastatic ERBB2/HER2-positive breast cancer and exemplifies the potential of individualized treatment based on a molecular biomarker to stratify the patient population [13].

The first successful small-molecule targeted cancer therapeutic was the tyrosine kinase inhibitor (TKI) imatinib (Gleevec; see Fig. 1.1 for the chemical structures of this and other small molecules discussed in this chapter). Imatinib is often considered a prototype for drugs targeting oncogenic signal transduction proteins [14], although the extent to which it is atypical and represents a "significant outlier" rather than a "poster child" has been debated [15,16]. The primary target of imatinib is the Abelson tyrosine kinase (ABL), which is activated by a chromosomal translocation that occurs in chronic myeloid leukemia (CML), creating the BCR–ABL fusion protein. The molecular abnormality generates a unique dependence on the ABL kinase. This explains why imatinib is so impressively effective in chronic-phase CML. The median overall survival was 88% at 30 months [17]. Equally important, ABL does not seem to be very critical for normal tissues, which probably explains why the drug is so well tolerated, even during chronic treatment. Imatinib has become the first-line therapy for CML, and has been followed by multiple second-generation BCR–ABL inhibitors such as dasatinib (Table 1.1) [18]. In part, the development of new BCR–ABL inhibitors has been driven by the need to address the development of imatinib resistance in patients (discussed in this chapter).

The first small-molecule inhibitors of epidermal growth factor receptor (EGFR) tyrosine kinase, gefitinib (Iressa) and erlotinib (Tarceva), showed activity in patients with non-small-cell lung cancer (NSCLC). A survival advantage was seen with patients receiving erlotinib plus chemotherapy compared to those receiving chemotherapy alone [19]. Gefitinib showed activity in only a small subset of NSCLC patients in initial trials, subsequently identified as carrying activating mutations in EGFR [20]. While the links between EGFR mutations and sensitivity to the TKIs were initially disputed, mainly due to the low frequency of the mutations in the early trial populations and a low accrual of tumor tissue samples, multiple prospective trials in NSCLC since 2005 have confirmed the effectiveness of the agents in EGFR-mutant NSCLC [21]. More recent EGFR inhibitors in development

TABLE 1.1   Examples of Targeted Molecular Cancer Therapeutics Receiving Marketing Approval by the US Food and Drug Administration (FDA), 1998–2012[1]

Year	Therapeutic	Drug type	Disease indication	Primary molecular target(s)
2012	Enzalutamide	Small molecule	Metastatic castration-resistant prostate cancer	Androgen receptor
	Pazopanib	Small molecule	Soft tissue sarcoma	VEGFR1, 2, 3
	Regorafenib	Small molecule	Metastatic colorectal cancer[2]	Multikinase
	Pertuzumab	Antibody	Metastatic breast cancer[3]	ERBB2
	Carfilzomib	Small molecule	Multiple myeloma[4]	26S proteasome
	Axitinib	Small molecule	Renal cancer[5]	VEGFR1, 2, 3
	Vismodegib	Small molecule	Basal cell carcinoma	Hedgehog signaling pathway
	Bosutinib	Small molecule	Chronic myelogenous leukemia	BCR–ABL, SRC
	Everolimus	Small molecule	ER-positive, HER2-negative breast cancer	mTOR
2011	Abiraterone	Small molecule	Metastatic castration-resistant prostate cancer[6]	CYP17
	Vemurafenib	Small molecule	Unresectable or metastatic BRAFV600E-positive melanoma[7]	BRAFV600E
	Ipilimumab	Antibody	Unresectable or metastatic melanoma	CTLA-4
	Crizotinob	Small molecule	EML4–ALK-positive non-small-cell lung cancer[8]	ALK, c-MET
	Vandetanib	Small molecule	Thyroid cancer	VEGFR, EGFR
	Sunitinib	Small molecule	Pancreatic neuroendocrine tumors[9]	Multikinase
	Brentuximab vedotin	Antibody–cytotoxic conjugate[10]	Hodgkin lymphoma and anaplastic large-cell lymphoma	CD30
	Everolimus	Small molecule	Pancreatic neuroendocrine tumors[9]	mTOR
2010	Trastuzumab	Antibody	Gastric cancer[11]	ERBB2
2009	Pazopanib	Small molecule	Renal cancer	VEGFR1, 2, 3
	Romedepsin	Small molecule	Cutaneous T-cell lymphoma	HDAC
	Bevacizumab	Antibody	Renal cancer[12]	VEGF
	Ofatumumab	Antibody	B-cell chronic lymphocytic leukemia	CD20
	Everolimus	Small molecule	Renal cancer	mTOR
2007	Lapatinib	Small molecule	Metastatic breast cancer[13]	EGFR, ERBB2
	Temsirolimus	Small molecule	Renal cancer	mTOR
	Nilotinib	Small molecule	Chronic myeloid leukemia	BCR–ABL,c-KIT, PDGFR

TABLE 1.1 Examples of Targeted Molecular Cancer Therapeutics Receiving Marketing Approval by the US Food and Drug Administration (FDA), 1998–2012[1] (*cont'd*)

Year	Therapeutic	Drug type	Disease indication	Primary molecular target(s)
2006	Dasatinib	Small molecule	Imatinib-resistant chronic myeloid leukemia	BCR–ABL, SRC
	Sunitinib	Small molecule	Renal cancer and gastrointestinal stromal tumor	Multikinase including PDGFR, VEGFR, c-KIT
	Panitumumab	Antibody	Colorectal cancer	EGFR
	Vorinostat	Small molecule	Cutaneous T-cell lymphoma	HDAC
2005	Sorafenib	Small molecule	Renal cell carcinoma	VEGFR, C-RAF, PDGFR
2004	Bevacizumab	Antibody	Metastatic colorectal carcinoma	VEGF
	Cetuximab	Antibody	EGFR-expressing metastatic colorectal cancer	EGFR
	Erlotinib	Small molecule	Metastatic non-small-cell lung cancer	EGFR
2003	Gefitinib	Small molecule	Metastatic non-small-cell lung cancer[14]	EGFR
	Bortezomib	Small molecule	Multiple myeloma[15]	26S Proteasome
2002	Imatinib	Small molecule	Gastrointestinal stromal tumor	c-KIT, PDGFR
	90Y-ibritumomab tiuxetan	Radiolabeled antibody	Non-Hodgkin's lymphoma	CD20
2001	Alemtuzumab	Antibody	B-cell chronic lymphocytic leukemia	CD52
	Letrozole	Small molecule	Metastatic breast cancer[16]	Aromatase
	Imatinib	Small molecule	Chronic myeloid leukemia	BCR–ABL
1999	Exemestane	Small molecule	Metastatic breast cancer[17]	Aromatase
1998	Trastuzumab	Antibody	HER2-positive metastatic breast cancer[18]	ERBB2

[1] *See www.centerwatch.com.*

[2] *Patients who have been previously treated with multiple lines of therapy.*

[3] *In combination with trastuzumab and docetaxel.*

[4] *Patients who have received at least two prior therapies, including bortezomib and an immunomodulatory agent, and have demonstrated disease progression.*

[5] *After failure of one prior systemic therapy.*

[6] *In combination with prednisone.*

[7] *FDA-approved companion diagnostic test for the presence of BRAFV600E mutation.*

[8] *FDA-approved companion diagnostic test for the presence of ALK rearrangement.*

[9] *Unresectable locally advanced or metastatic disease.*

[10] *CD30-targeting antibody cleavably conjugated to monomethyl auristatin E.*

[11] *In combination with cisplatin and a fluoropyrimidine.*

[12] *In combination with interferon alpha 2a.*

[13] *In combination with capecitibine.*

[14] *Second-line treatment.*

[15] *Patients who have received at least two prior therapies.*

[16] *First-line therapy for postmenopausal women with locally advanced or metastatic breast cancer.*

[17] *Advanced breast cancer in postmenopausal women whose disease has progressed following therapy with tamoxifen.*

[18] *Second- or third-line therapy.*

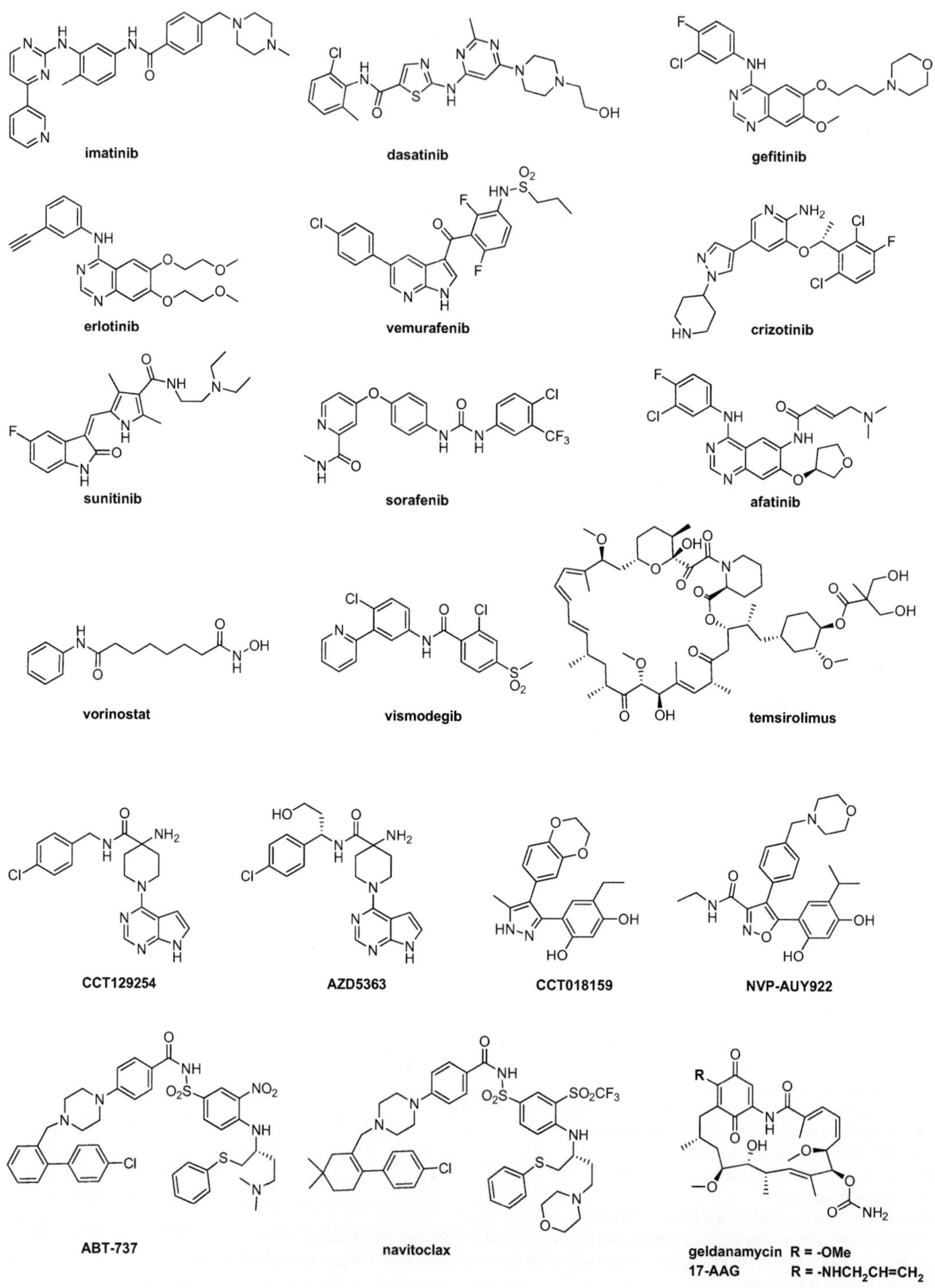

FIGURE 1.1 Chemical structures of selected small molecules described in the text.

include irreversible agents such as afatinib, which binds covalently to both the wild-type EGFR and the T790M kinase gatekeeper mutant that shows reduced binding of the first-generation inhibitors [22].

Two other recently approved signal transduction kinase inhibitors illustrate the progress that has been made in the discovery of targeted therapeutics. In 2002, mutation of the serine/threonine-protein kinase B-Raf (BRAF), particularly the V600E variant, was identified as an oncogenic driver of many different cancers, with especially high prevalence (ca. 50%) in malignant melanoma [23]. The inhibitor vemurafenib (Zelboraf) showed exceptional activity against V600E BRAF melanoma in early clinical trials [24], and was approved as the first targeted agent for the treatment of metastatic melanoma in 2011 [25]. As with imatinib in BCR–ABL-dependent CML, vemurafenib targets an essential driver oncogene in the V600E BRAF patient population, and dramatic effects on tumor response and patient survival were achieved. Importantly, a companion diagnostic using RT-PCR to detect the mutant V600E BRAF allele in patients' tumors prior to treatment was developed in parallel with the clinical development, which fortuitously also detected the V600D and V600K oncogenic variants, allowing for a truly targeted treatment strategy.

The approval of crizotinib (Xalkori) in 2011 for the treatment of EML4–ALK-positive NSCLC further exemplifies the practice-changing potential of targeted therapeutics when the appropriate combinations of molecular target, inhibitor, and companion diagnostic are brought together [26]. Approximately 5% of NSCLC result from the formation of a fusion protein between the receptor tyrosine kinase ALK and the EML4 protein, resulting in constitutive ALK activation. The identification of the rearranged oncogene in 2007 [27] was followed by the first reports of dramatic clinical activity in advanced NSCLC only three years later [28]. This rapid development was made possible in part by the repurposing of crizotinib, which was already in development as an inhibitor of hepatocyte growth factor receptor tyrosine kinase (MET) and was found to inhibit ALK as well [29]. The development of crizotinib also shows how previous experience with molecularly targeted therapy for receptor tyrosine kinases, such as gefitinib and erlotinib, can be brought to bear to accelerate the development of new agents of this type. As with vemurafenib, a companion diagnostic was developed, this time using fluorescent in situ hybridization technology to identify the ALK rearrangement [30]. The test was applied in the pivotal clinical trials of crizotinib and was approved by the FDA in parallel to the drug.

Despite certain caveats, the clinical activity with the agents discussed here is consistent with the concept of "oncogene addiction", whereby cancers develop dependence upon, or become "addicted to", activated oncogenes [31–33]. This idea reconciles the observation that despite the activation of several oncogenes being necessary to initiate and sustain the hallmark properties of malignant cells, inhibition of the action of just one may have significant therapeutic effect. The agents discussed in this section and in Table 1.1 also provide proof of the concept that clinically useful therapeutic activity and patient benefit can be achieved with drugs that inhibit oncogenic signal transduction.

In addition to targeting oncogenic signaling pathways, the approach of mechanism-based inhibition of angiogenesis has also been validated by both small-molecule kinase inhibitors and antibodies. New blood vessel formation is required to support the growth of solid tumors, and this process of angiogenesis is therefore a logical target for therapeutic modulation. Bevacizumab (Avastin) is a monoclonal antibody that binds vascular endothelial growth factor (VEGF), which is an important driver of the proliferation and functions of the endothelial cells responsible for angiogenesis. Activity has been seen in various solid cancers [34]. When used in combination with cytotoxic agents, bevacizumab offers an extension of survival by a few months in advanced disease, as in the case of colorectal cancer [35]. The activity of the small-molecule kinase inhibitors sunitinib (Sutent) and sorafenib (Nexovar) in renal cell cancer may well be due, at least in part, to inhibition of the tyrosine kinase activity associated with the membrane receptors for VEGF and another angiogenic growth factor, platelet-derived growth factor (PDGF). However, these drugs inhibit a range of kinases and are members of a growing class of "multitargeted" kinase inhibitors [36]. The attribution of action through any one molecular target is difficult for such agents, and the polypharmacology may be essential for maximizing their effects.

The approval of vorinostat (Zolinza) in 2006 for the treatment of cutaneous T-cell lymphoma represented the first entry of an agent targeting chromatin-modifying enzymes into clinical use [37]. Histone acetyl transferases (HATs) and deacetylases (HDACs) contribute to the regulation of gene expression through acetylation of residues in the histone proteins that act as the core scaffolds for DNA in nucleosomes. In turn, the conformational changes associated with the histone functionalization determine the accessibility of the DNA toward transcription factors. Mutation, overexpression, translocation, and amplification of genes encoding HATs have been observed in various cancers. HDACs cooperate with oncogenic protein products to determine their effect, acting as posttranslational modifiers of the onco-gene function. The mechanism of action of vorinostat likely involves both altering gene expression through changing histone and transcription factor acetylation, and also altering the function of cell cycle proteins through inhibiting their deacetylation [38]. In a pivotal phase IIb trial in cutaneous T-cell lymphoma, vorinostat showed an overall response rate of 30% in heavily pretreated patients with persistent, progressive, or refractory disease [39].

The challenges encountered with molecular targeted therapies

There is no doubt that the agents discussed in this section are quite distinct from those from the cytotoxic era in that they target the precise molecular mechanisms that are responsible for the initiation and progression of cancer, often to the level of a single, specific protein target. They clearly have sufficient therapeutic activity to warrant regulatory approval. On the other hand, a range of complications and limitations have emerged [4,40]. These are particularly concerned with uncertainties over the clinically relevant mechanism of action, unexpected toxicities, and, most importantly, the development of resistance to the new agents [41]. As an example of the first point, it is likely that at least part of the activity of trastuzumab is due to antibody-directed cellular cytotoxicity, and the precise role of the effects on receptor signaling is still unclear. In addition, the combination of trastuzumab with anthracycline-based chemotherapy causes an increase in cardiac toxicity.

In the case of imatinib, responses in accelerated-phase and blast-crisis CML are less dramatic than those in the chronic phase, potentially due to the involvement of additional oncogenic drivers in the more advanced forms of the disease. Resistance to imatinib is common and is associated with mutations that lead to an impairment of binding to the adenosine triphosphate (ATP) site of the kinase [42], or with the activation of BCR–ABL-independent pathways such as signaling through SRC-family of non-receptor tyrosine kinases [43]. On the other hand, sensitivity of many of the mutant forms can be maintained to nilotinib (Tasigna), dasatinib (Sprycel), and bosutinib (Bosulif), which also inhibit SRC-family kinases [43,44]. Although these agents effectively tackle a spectrum of imatinib-resistant BCR–ABL mutants with modifications to the kinase domain P-loop, the T315I mutation remains intractable with currently approved agents [45].

Kinase domain mutations are likewise responsible for secondary resistance to gefitinib and erlotinib in NSCLC, particularly the T790M mutation on exon 20 of EGFR. Thus, responses to gefitinib and erlotinib have often proved to be of limited duration, and acquired resistance to current TKI therapy appears unavoidable in NSCLC [46]. Once again, alternative inhibitors are being developed to overcome this, with the irreversible EGFR, ERBB2, and ERBB4 kinase inhibitor afatinib one of the most advanced agents that has potent activity against mutant as well as wild-type EGFR [47]. Regardless of EGFR mutational status, amplification of the MET gene and/or activation of MET signaling has been observed in up to 20% of tumor samples following gefitinib or erlotinib treatment and provides another mechanism of resistance to the drugs [48], in this case treatable with crizotinib. Here, combination therapy with MET inhibitors is one means to counter the resistance. Other tractable resistance mechanisms to EGFR inhibitors have been described [49]. There are also indications that a so-called vertical blockade of EGFR signaling by combining an intracellular receptor tyrosine kinase inhibitor with an extracellular antibody therapy to the same EGFR target may offer increased prospects for disease control [50]. Kinase domain mutations also underlie resistance to crizotinib [51].

In the case of vemurafenib, resistance does not appear to result from further mutations in V600E BRAF, although splice variants of V600E BRAF that are resistant to the drug are known [52]. Instead, mechanisms that lead to retention of mitogen-activated protein kinase (MAPK) pathway signaling in a V600E BRAF-independent manner, including activation of EGFR and potentially other receptor tyrosine kinases, upregulation of RAF proto-oncogene serine/threonine-protein kinase (CRAF) expression, a pathway switch to serine/threonine-protein kinase A-Raf (ARAF) or CRAF signaling, and oncogenic activation of neuroblastoma RAS viral oncogene homolog (NRAS), are important [25,53]. Another problem is that while ATP-competitive inhibitors such as vemurafenib inhibit extracellular-signal-regulated kinase (ERK) signaling in cells with mutant V600E BRAF, paradoxical activation of signaling is seen in cells with wild-type BRAF. Several mechanistic rationales have been advanced based on the formation of homodimers and heterodimers for transactivation of wild-type BRAF and related proteins such as CRAF, ARAF, or kinase suppressor of Ras 1 (KSR), whereby binding of the kinase inhibitor to one component of the dimer inhibits that enzyme but stabilizes the dimer and promotes activation of the other component [54]. In contrast, mutant V600E BRAF is active as a monomer. A consequence of this paradoxical transactivation of wild-type BRAF signaling is a distinctive toxicity of V600E BRAF inhibitors, with the emergence of cutaneous squamous cell carcinomas and benign keratoacanthomas associated with activating RAS mutations in wild-type BRAF cells in patients treated with vemurafenib [55]. Although the superficial keratoacanthomas can be removed surgically, there are concerns about the potential for malignant progression of cells with mutant RAS in deep-seated organs such as the lung and colon [56]. Combination treatments to tackle the activation of these bypass signaling pathways have been proposed, particularly the combination of BRAF and MAPK kinase (MEK) inhibitors.

Turning to multitargeted inhibitors like sorafenib and sunitinib, understanding their mechanism of action is somewhat confounded by their multitargeted nature, and reasons for differences in the therapeutic activity of the various small molecules and antibodies targeted to the VEGF–VEGF receptor axis are unclear [57]. While bevacizumab was approved by the FDA in 2008 for treating metastatic breast cancer, approval for this indication was withdrawn in the United States in 2011. Although the agent was shown to slow disease progression, there was insufficient evidence of extension of life or improvement in quality of life to support continued approval when balanced against the adverse effects of treatment [58]. The clinical experience with bevacizumab in breast cancer exemplifies two limitations now recognized with molecularly targeted agents. First, molecularly targeted agents do not always lack significant side effects, despite the targeting of cancer-specific processes, and the side effects of each drug or antibody treatment must still be considered relative to the benefit of the treatment and the severity of the disease [59]. Of note in this regard has been the potential for cardiotoxicity observed with some receptor tyrosine kinase inhibitors, which may be mechanism based or due to off-target kinase inhibition depending on the agent [60,61].

Another limitation of molecularly targeted agents illustrated by bevacizumab in breast cancer is that the targeted mechanism may not translate across cancer tissue types as generally as originally expected. A further example of this is provided by the V600E BRAF inhibitor vemurafenib, which did not show efficacy as a single agent in the treatment of V600E BRAF colorectal cancer despite the presence of the specific mutation in the disease [62]. The lack of sensitivity was associated with feedback activation of EGFR in colon cancer cells, whereas melanoma cells express low levels of EGFR and remain sensitive to V600E BRAF inhibition. Thus, the biological context in which an oncogenic mutation occurs is important in determining the response to therapeutic interventions targeting the abnormality. On the other hand, the data in Table 1.1 very clearly show the extension of use of a number of approved molecularly targeted agents across multiple tumor tissue types, emphasizing that the targeting of underlying molecular lesions common to different tumor types remains a valid concept, exploitable for increased patient benefit.

Rising to the Current Challenges of Oncology Drug Discovery and Development

The preceding section shows that overall the results with the new molecular therapeutics have been mixed. With respect to small-molecule drug development, it is notable that many of the agents are directed to the same small set of molecular targets. While this repetition reflects the established importance of certain targets in cancer, and a choice between several drugs for a given target can be desirable in clinical practice, there are notable absences in the current selection of approved molecularly targeted agents. For example, despite significant and sustained preclinical research, there is as yet no approved small molecule directed toward a cell cycle or mitotic kinase [63]. While upstream receptor tyrosine kinases are extensively drugged, inhibitors acting at downstream nodes in mitogenic signaling pathways remain restricted to BRAF and mammalian target of rapamycin (mTOR) inhibitors. However, given current late-stage clinical trial activities, it would be expected that inhibitors of phosphatidylinositide 3-kinase (PI3K), protein Kinase B (PKB, otherwise known as AKT), MEK, and checkpoint kinase 1 (CHK1), among others, may appear in the near future to address these gaps [4].

Assessments of the overall success rates for oncology drug development illustrate how challenging an activity it is [15,64,65]. A frequently cited analysis showed that failure rates for cancer drugs in clinical trials during the period from 1990 to 2000 were worse than for most other therapeutic areas [64]. Only 5% of oncology drugs entering the clinic went on to gain regulatory approval for marketing, while 95% failed. This is compared with an 11% success rate—more than double—for other diseases. A subsequent study looking at the extended period of 1990–2006 showed a similarly low US approval success rate (8%) for oncology drugs [65]. An analysis of the economics of new drug development found that oncology drugs benefit from a disproportionally high share of FDA priority review ratings, orphan drug designations at approval, and inclusion in the FDA's expedited access programs [66]. Those authors also found that clinical approval rates were in fact similar for oncology versus other drugs, but that a greater proportion of cancer drug candidates were abandoned in advanced-stage clinical evaluation, where failures are very expensive. This study also showed that clinical oncology drug development timelines were longer than for other therapeutic areas, probably due to evaluation in a greater number of indications. In a more recent analysis, the mean development time for oncology drugs over the period 2000–2009 was determined as 6.9 years, with only central nervous system drugs taking longer on average [67]. However, the authors also noted that the numbers of approved new anticancer drugs increased steadily and significantly each decade from the 1980s through the decade 2000–2009. Data on contemporary kinase inhibitor development suggest that they have markedly better prospects (odds of one in two) for successfully completing clinical development from phase I trial initiation to new drug approval than oncology drugs as a whole [68]. However, consistent with the earlier analysis of Kola and Landis, the greatest attrition was seen at the transition from phase II to phase III, suggesting that the attainment of sufficient therapeutic activity remains the major challenge in cancer drug development. Such late-stage failures contribute in a major way to the estimated fully capitalized cost of US$1000 million or more per approved new drug [69,70].

Clearly, we would like to see the success rates for cancer drugs to be higher, development times shortened, and failing drugs to be identified earlier. It is very instructive to understand the reasons for the attrition of oncology drugs in the clinic, since this allows us to focus attention on the areas that are most problematic. Metrics show that the reasons for failure have changed with time [64]. In the early 1990s, poor pharmacokinetics and limited bioavailability were the major problems. Recognition of this led to the use of predictive assays for absorption, distribution, metabolism, and excretion (ADME) properties [71]. Implementation of these assays to weed out compounds with ADME liabilities led to a fall in the clinical failure rate due to this cause from 40% to 10% by the year 2000 [64]. As a result, the principal causes of attrition in clinical development became insufficient therapeutic efficacy (30%) and unacceptable toxicity (30%). A more recent analysis across multiple disease indications showed that lack of efficacy (51%) and toxicity (19%) continue to be the dominant reasons for failure in phase II development [72]. Particular attention therefore needs to be paid to reducing failure due to these factors.

The risk of failure because of inadequate therapeutic activity could be reduced by better selection of molecular targets [4,15,73]. For target selection and validation, perspectives on the best targets have changed as a result of clinical experiences with the first generation of molecularly targeted agents [40]. First, there is a greater understanding of the inherent differences between genetic target validation technologies, such as RNA interference (RNAi) methods, and the use of pharmacological inhibitors to probe target biology [74,75], and of the limitations of both techniques. As a result, there is increased emphasis on the validation of new targets using multiple approaches. This has led to a more explicit focus on the qualities of preclinical small molecules that will make them "fit for purpose" chemical probes for target validation [76]. The integrated approach to the discovery and refinement of drug candidates (discussed later in this chapter) is invaluable to the discovery and credentialing of chemical probes for specific biologies. In parallel to the better use of target validation technologies, there is also an increased understanding of what comprises a validated target and, importantly, the accompanying genetic or epigenetic backgrounds that may be required for modulation of a given target to achieve a therapeutic outcome [77]. Increased use of functional genomics technologies, such as RNAi and compound screens in panels of genetically well-characterized cancer cells, is allowing a more systematic approach to defining the right combinations of targets and the accompanying contexts in which they function [78]. The range of potential targets has also expanded to include survival pathways that may remain critical for cancer cell survival in response to the stress caused by multiple underlying genetic or epigenetic changes, and thus may operate over wider genetic contexts [79]. These include protein quality control mechanisms and DNA damage detection and repair processes [80,81].

Of note is that while the genetic understanding of many cancers and the discovery of cancer genes and potential molecular targets have increased dramatically in the era of genomic sequencing [82], the selection of targets has remained largely ad hoc. Patel et al. [83] have recently published a systematic and objective, multifaceted computational approach to assessing and prioritizing potential targets, including an estimation of the "druggability" of a given target based on prior structural biology and pharmacological data. A point to stress is the importance of the reproducibility of the preclinical data, whether biochemical, cellular, or in animal models, on which preclinical target validation assessments are made and drug discovery projects are launched [84].

The success rate of clinical development can also be improved by identifying animal models of human cancer that have better predictive power [85–88]. Molecularly characterized human tumor xenografts in immunosuppressed mice remain useful for drug discovery, with increasing emphasis placed on orthotopic implantation and early-passage patient-derived xenografts [89]. The use of genetically engineered mouse models (GEMMs) in the validation of proposed cancer target biology offers one approach to achieving better animal models [90,91]. For example, mice that conditionally express endogenous mutant Kirsten rat sarcoma viral oncogene homolog (KRAS) and p53 alleles in their pancreatic cells develop pancreatic tumors with pathophysiological and molecular features resembling those of human pancreatic ductal adenocarcinoma. This model has been used to understand the marked resistance to chemotherapy of pancreatic cancer, and to validate new targets for intervention [92,93].

The risk of attrition due to unacceptable side effects can be mitigated by developing improved methods for predicting on-target and off-target toxicity [94]. First-in-class drugs acting on previously unprecedented molecular targets carry a higher level of risk compared to those that work on targets that are well precedented in the clinic [95]—but, at the same time, these high-risk drugs also have more potential to be truly innovative. An analysis by DiMasi and Grabowski [66] indicated that oncology drugs had the highest rate of first-in-class introductions. In addition to judicious target validation and selection and the use of more predictive models for efficacy and toxicity, late-stage failure can also be minimized by the careful use of biomarkers to identify the most responsive patients and to provide proof of concept for the proposed molecular mechanism, especially in phase I and II clinical trials [14,96–98]. The success of this approach has been demonstrated in the development of vemurafenib and crizotinib and their accompanying diagnostic tests as detailed in this chapter. Later in this chapter, we will advocate the use of patient selection biomarkers together with pharmacokinetic–pharmacodynamic endpoints as part of the "pharmacological audit trail" concept designed to aid decision making in clinical development [97,99–102].

The often rapid emergence of resistance mechanisms to molecularly targeted agents compromises the effectiveness of drugs that have been successfully developed. To address this, research into possible resistance mechanisms is being brought forward into the preclinical discovery phase of new molecularly targeted agents [41,78]. New molecular targets can be considered along with companion targets that may modulate resistance mechanisms, and may need to be inhibited in combination to maximize the effectiveness of a new targeted drug. The genetic backgrounds where a specific targeted agent will have maximal effect can also be defined using synthetic lethality approaches [103,104]. The need for combination therapies of targeted agents has encouraged the realization of commercial mechanisms for first-in-human clinical trials of drugs in combination, which might otherwise be developed separately due to distinct proprietary interests [105]. There is also renewed interest in intrinsic multitargeted small-molecule drugs, sometimes referred to as "selective nonselective inhibitors" [36], where a controlled polypharmacology is engineered into a single chemical agent. However, combinations of multiple specific inhibitors may give more flexibility for longitudinal adaptive therapy to target the changing genotypes' underlying resistance.

Recent sequencing studies have shown the extent of genetic heterogeneity within individual patients' tumors [106]. These indicate that patients presenting with multiple sites of disease are likely to harbor tumors with multiple, different molecular lesions, and therefore different sensitivities to treatments. For example, in a study of renal clear cell carcinoma, the somatic mutations present differed between regions of the anatomically defined primary tumor, as well as between the primary site and distant metastases [107]. In a recent study of BRAF-inhibitor-resistant melanoma, molecular heterogeneity was observed at the intralesional level, with two distinct subclones populating a single metastasis site [108]. The concept of personalized cancer medicine is changing to tackle the issues of resistance to targeted agents and tumor heterogeneity. The likely presence of multiple genotypes within an individual patient's tumor burden is reinforcing research into combining new molecular-targeted agents to increase treatment effectiveness [41,78]. Observations that the clonal constitution of tumors also changes in response to the selection pressure of treatment, as exemplified in recent longitudinal case studies in multiple myeloma [109,110], suggests that individualized iterative diagnostic and treatment sequences will be necessary to mitigate the evolution of tumor genetics in response to therapies.

INTEGRATED SMALL-MOLECULE DRUG DISCOVERY AND DEVELOPMENT

The successful discovery and development of small-molecule cancer drugs are highly dependent upon the creative interplay between many disciplines: these include genetics, genomics, and bioinformatics; cell and molecular biology; structural biology; tumor biology; pharmacology; pharmacokinetics and metabolism; medicinal chemistry; and experimental medicine. The application of a wide range of powerful technologies has had a major impact. Examples include high-throughput genomic approaches for discovering new targets and identifying molecular biomarkers [78,111], and the use of biochemical or cell-based high-throughput screening (HTS) to discover chemical starting points for drug discovery [112,113]. Structure-based drug design using X-ray crystallography has had a profound influence [114], not least in the application of fragment-based technologies for the discovery of chemical starting points [115]. Bioinformatic and chemoinformatic approaches have become indispensable for analyzing the large amounts of data generated by the high-throughput genomic and chemical screening approaches [116,117], while in silico chemistry methods are widely and routinely applied in the generation and optimization of chemical leads [4].

Preclinical small-molecule drug development is commonly portrayed as a linear process, progressing from molecular target, to early chemical "hits" and leads, to highly optimized lead compounds, to preclinical development candidates, and finally to drug candidates for clinical evaluation. Although this is a useful and not wholly inaccurate depiction, the more holistic view illustrated in Fig. 1.2 captures the integrated and iterative way in which modern drug discovery often occurs [3]. According to this model, structural biology and the various approaches collectively referred to as chemical biology play central roles in accelerating the path to the clinic and in linking the multiple elements of the drug discovery endeavor. For example, small-molecule chemical probes can be used as tools for target validation and to help determine the best biological models for guiding drug development, to anticipate potential pharmacological outcomes, and to identify possible biomarkers [76]. They can also act as pathfinders to help define potential hurdles and ways to overcome them later in

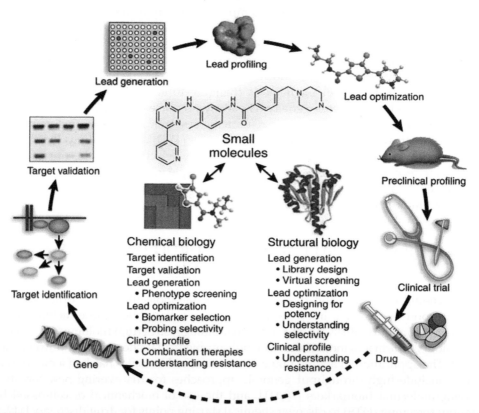

FIGURE 1.2 The integrated and nonlinear way in which modern drug discovery often occurs. Structural biology and the various approaches collectively referred to as "chemical biology" link together the multiple elements of the drug discovery process. (This figure is reproduced in color in the color plate section.) *Reproduced with permission from [3].*

the drug discovery project. The visualization of the process as a circle rather than the usual straight line is particularly useful in emphasizing how the different elements can be closely connected, with opportunities for feed-forward and feedback between the various stages. As an example, observations that are made preclinically in basic and translational research can often now have an immediate impact on clinical development. Equally, feedback of information on disease response, resistance mechanisms, and biomarker changes from the clinic to the laboratory can often lead rapidly to innovation in the selection of targets or the refinement of inhibitors. Thus, the lab–clinic interaction in drug discovery and development, as in other areas of contemporary translational research, is a two-way street.

While many individual approaches and technologies can have a profound influence on a particular drug discovery project, it is the integrated application of these that is particularly important in enhancing the quality and robustness of the innovative cancer drugs that enter the clinic—and also in shortening the time and reducing the cost to progress from a new molecular target to an approved drug.

NEW MOLECULAR TARGETS: THE DRUGGABLE CANCER GENOME AND EPIGENOME

The selection of the best possible molecular targets is clearly crucial to the success of a drug discovery and development project [4,15,73]. A number of factors influence the choice of target, including, in particular, (1) the involvement of the target in the initiation and progression of cancer, and (2) the technical feasibility or "druggability" of the target. With the mapping of the human genome sequence, the concept of the "druggable genome" has become popular and useful [83,118,119]. Since cancer is above all else a disease of aberrant genetics and epigenetics, and particularly with our burgeoning understanding of the differences between the genomes of cancer versus normal cells, the notion of "drugging the cancer genome" has been used to embrace the contemporary approach [1–3,6,120].

There are various ways in which identifying and then validating new targets can be considered. Ultimate validation can be achieved in the clinic only with the provision of evidence of therapeutic activity via the intended mechanism of action. However, projects aimed at drugging novel targets inevitably have to be initiated with less secure credentials. Figure 1.3(A) depicts the various classes of genes that are involved in malignancy and illustrates how targets can be selected so as to modulate the multiple biochemical pathways that are hijacked by cancer genes and also to act upon the resulting multiple hallmark traits of cancer, as articulated by Hanahan and Weinberg [121,122]. These include increased proliferation, inappropriate survival and decreased apoptosis, immortalization, invasion, angiogenesis, and the metastasis or spreading to distant sites around the body that is the usual cause of death from solid tumors. The introduction of reprogramming of energy metabolism pathways and evasion of immune surveillance, as additional hallmark features of cancer, has expanded the opportunities for new targeted treatments [122]. The approval of the cytotoxic T-lymphocyte-associated antigen 4 (CTLA-4) antibody ipilimumab (Yervoy) for the treatment of metastatic melanoma demonstrates the potential of targeting immune activation in cancer therapy [123].

Targeting different types of genes, pathways, and hallmark traits provides the basis with which to attack cancer in multiple ways and at distinct levels, either with single agents or,

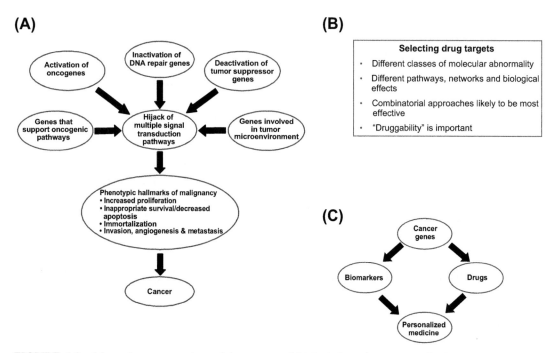

FIGURE 1.3 Schematic representations of the genes and biological mechanisms involved in cancer and their exploitation in the development of new treatments. (A) The classes of genes that are involved in cancer and are potential targets for drug discovery. (B) A portfolio of new drug discovery projects can be built by selecting targets in the different categories that affect different biochemical effects and phenotypic traits of cancer. Due attention should also be paid to druggability (see text of this chapter). (C) The translation of new cancer genes into drugs and biomarkers. The integrated use of biomarkers is essential for traditional drug development leading to personalized medicine. (For color version of this figure, the reader is referred to the online version of this book.)

more likely, with combinations of agents to achieve greater clinical effectiveness. From the point of view of commercial pharmaceutical research, selection of different targets from the various classes provides a means to "spread risk" rather than have all the drug discovery eggs in one basket. The importance of druggability is also highlighted (see Fig. 1.3(B) and later in this chapter). Figure 1.3(C) emphasizes the considerable value of discovering and developing molecular biomarkers alongside molecular cancer therapeutics so that the two can be used together in a progressive move toward personalized or individualized cancer medicine. It is hard to understand why a modern drug discovery project would be initiated without a plan to produce one or more biomarkers for patient selection and target engagement (see Ref. [97] and later in this chapter). This is particularly important given our current understanding of the inherent high genetic heterogeneity of many tumors and the envisioned need to regularly reassess the matching of targeted treatment to tumor genetics during a treatment sequence [78].

At the heart of the contemporary approach to cancer drug discovery is the identification of the aberrant genes or epigenetic abnormalities that are responsible for various cancers by hijacking cellular signaling networks [124,125], and hence lead to the characteristic hallmark traits or phenotypic features of cancer. The molecular comprehension of malignancy can be traced back to the study of cancer-causing animal viruses in the 1960s and 1970s, the discovery of oncogenes and tumor suppressor genes during the 1970s and 1980s, and the understanding of how cancer genes subvert cellular processes in the 1990s [126,127]. Although our increasing understanding of cancer as a disease of abnormal genes and signaling pathways is not new, it is only over the past 15 years or so that molecular oncology has been embraced by the drug development community as a rich source of targets for cancer drug discovery. This has required cultural evolution as well as technological and scientific advances.

It seems obvious that the best targets for the development of cancer drugs with minimal side effects will be those that are responsible for major differences between cancer and healthy cells. In retrospect, the antiproliferative toxicities associated with cytotoxic agents are unsurprising, since many important normal tissues also contain rapidly proliferating cells and are affected by agents targeting the rapid DNA synthesis and cell division of tumor cells. The development of molecular cancer therapeutics seeks to avoid the more damaging toxicities associated with cytotoxic drugs through targeting processes that are more specific to cancer cells. Although significant side effects are perhaps inevitably seen with drugs that interfere with biochemical pathways and biological processes that play a key role in normal cells, the potential to achieve a therapeutic window is clear.

Kamb et al. [15] have suggested that there is a fundamental distinction between those cancer drug targets that have an essential function in at least one normal cell type in the body and those that have nonessential functions in normal cells. They proposed, not unreasonably, that drugs acting on essential functions would have a narrower therapeutic index than those that interfere with nonessential functions in normal cells. Imatinib (discussed in this chapter) is an excellent example of a drug acting on a target that does not appear to be essential in normal cells (i.e., the ABL kinase). Although Kamb et al. [15] did not rule out the development of drugs acting on targets with essential functions in normal cells, the narrower therapeutic index likely to be seen with such agents led them to describe such agents as "neocytotoxics".

Referring again to Fig. 1.3(A), cancer genes—and potential drug targets—can be categorized as (1) activated oncogenes (e.g. *RAS*, *RAF*, and *PIK3CA*); (2) deactivated tumor suppressor genes (e.g., *p53* and *PTEN*); (3) genes that, when inactivated, lead to DNA repair defects (e.g., *BRCA1* and *BRCA2*); (4) genes that support oncogenic pathways, for example those encoding the molecular chaperone heat shock protein 90 (HSP90) and the histone deacetylases, which are involved in posttranslational modification of proteins, chromatin modification, and the control of gene expression; and (5) genes controlling the tumor microenvironment, including cancer–host interactions.

Another way of considering various cancer gene targets is a classification based on four different categories of "dependency" [73]. The first category, "genetic dependency", relates to the concept of oncogene addiction outlined in this chapter. Examples cited by the authors include the use of imatinib in leukemias driven by the *BRC–ABL* translocation and of MEK 1/2 inhibitors in *BRAF*-mutated melanoma models [128]. The second category, "synergy dependency", is founded on the notion of synthetic lethality, in which genetic loss of a particular function predisposes the cancer cell to respond to pharmacological modulation of a second function [103], and is exemplified by the preferential killing of *BRCA*-defective breast cancer cells by poly(ADP-ribose) polymerase (PARP) inhibitors [129]. The third category, "lineage dependency", refers to cancers that originate from a certain tissue or cell and have multiple features in common, some of which can constitute an addiction based on the cell lineage. This is exemplified by antihormonal drugs that target the sex hormone dependency of breast and prostate cancers, which is shared with the normal tissue of origin. The identification of the differentiation regulator *MITF* (micropthalemia-associated transcription factor) as an amplified oncogene in melanoma [130] and the dependence of certain lung adenocarcinomas on the developmental regulator *TTF1* (thyroid transcription factor-1) [131] are further examples. The final category made by Benson et al. [73] is "host dependency". This is based on the recognition that physiological factors involved in the tumor microenvironment, including tumor–host cell interactions, are vitally important for malignant progression. Examples of drugs acting on such targets are the antibodies (e.g., bevacizumab) and small molecules (e.g., sorafenib and sunitinib) that inhibit the VEGF–VEGF receptor axis. Drugs blocking the functions of hypoxia-inducible factor (*HIF*), which is upregulated in tumor hypoxia—as well as following loss of the *VHL* tumor suppressor—would also fall into this category, as would drugs acting on invasion and metastasis.

Maintaining the constantly replicative malignant state is highly stressful to the cell. Pathways that are activated in response to cope with this stress have emerged as an important set of targets for therapeutic intervention. These are mechanisms that are present and useful in nonmalignant cells in response to short-term stress, but that are chronically activated in cancer cells and have become essential for survival [79]. Two key examples that are the focus of current drug discovery efforts are the proteostasis functions of molecular chaperones such as heat shock protein 90 (HSP90) [81], and the DNA damage response pathways that monitor and direct repair of damaged DNA [80]. Another example would be the switch from mitochondrial oxidative phosphorylation to aerobic glycolysis for the production of ATP that takes place in cancer cells, first noted by Warburg over 80 years ago [132]. These examples of "non-oncogene addiction" are of increasing interest since they may represent points of convergence for the effects of multiple underlying oncogenic or epigenetic events. Agents targeted to the critical elements in these pathways may operate over wider genetic contexts than agents targeted at the specific oncogenes.

In a matter of a few years, we have progressed from a situation in which there was a perceived lack of targets for the development of new cancer drugs to one in which there is a considerable excess. The ongoing survey from the Wellcome Trust Cancer Genome Project (http://www.sanger.ac.uk/genetics/CGP/Census) tallies the human genes that are causally implicated in cancer via mutation, with more than 450 implicated by somatic mutation alone [83]. Moreover, new cancer genes continue to be identified. Whereas cancer gene discovery previously arose from painstaking hypothesis-driven cell and molecular biology research, it is now increasingly driven by genome-wide high-throughput systematic screening technologies, including gene copy number analysis, gene expression profiling, gene resequencing, and profiling of epigenetic markers [82]. Array-based DNA copy number and gene expression profiling can be used to identify amplified and overexpressed genes and provide complementary approaches to high-throughput mutation analysis. The application of high-throughput RNAi technology is also used extensively for gene and target discovery [133].

The discovery of *BRAF* as a bona fide oncogene in melanoma and other cancers was the first example of the power of high-throughput cancer genome mutation detection analysis

[23]. Since then, the number of oncogenes identified through high-throughput genome sequencing for mutations has burgeoned rapidly and includes *EFGR* in lung cancer, *JAK2* in myeloproliferative disorders, *FGFR2* in endometrial cancer, and *ALK* in neuroblastoma [134]. High-resolution copy number profiling has identified, among many others, *MITF* as an oncogene in melanoma [130] and *CDK8* as an oncogene in colorectal cancer [135]. The improvements in throughput and the reduced cost of second-generation DNA-sequencing technologies, where individual DNA molecules are amplified on solid-phase arrays or beads before massively parallel sequence generation, have enabled the complete sequencing of entire genomes. As a result, the amount of cancer genetic information will continue to increase hugely in the future, supported by multinational efforts such as the International Cancer Genome Consortium (ICGC) [136].

The studies outlined here show that a large number of cancer genes are involved in human malignancies. Moreover, the involvement of any one of these genes across human cancers is commonly very low (e.g., compared to *BRAF*), and many cancers harbor a large number of potential oncogenes. This reinforces the value of high-throughput cancer genome resequencing for the detection of cancer genes. However, the findings suggest challenges for drug development with respect to the potentially small number of patients being suitable for a given drug targeted to a specific driver mutation, and also to the choice of which target to go after in a cancer with many mutations. However, there is the possibility that many mutations may occur in genes that lie on a particular pathway, which could be drugged at a common downstream locus, or that the mutations lead to a reliance on common survival mechanisms through "non-oncogene dependence" [79].

While all of the high-throughput, genome-wide technologies described in this chapter are invaluable for gene discovery, they do not particularly help us to validate or prioritize a potentially new target for cancer drug discovery, particularly when the number of candidate targets is very high. A prioritization has to be made. How can we do this? There is no checklist for cancer target validation and prioritization, but some rules of thumb have emerged from more than a decade of work on targeted molecular cancer therapeutics, including proposals for a systematic approach [83]. A combination of human genetics and genomics with functional analysis involving overexpression, mutation, and knockdown by RNAi, together with the use of genetically modified mouse cancer models or other model organisms, has proved effective [4,73].

Taking the example of an oncogene, high priority is likely to be given to a gene that is mutated in human cancers (ideally at a high frequency); that lies on a pathway in which other genetic or epigenetic abnormalities are found; that, when overexpressed or mutated, recapitulates the relevant cancer phenotype; that, when knocked down, leads to the reciprocal loss of the cancer phenotype; and for which the oncogenic activity can be recapitulated in an animal model. The extent of the unmet medical need will often be influential, particularly to pharmaceutical and biotechnology companies for which the potential market size is an inevitable consideration. This is, however, notoriously difficult to predict. It is well-known in the field that the imatinib development project was nearly dropped because of concerns about the size of commercial revenues, yet imatinib became a highly effective, multibillion US dollar drug. Academic and other not-for-profit drug discovery groups can be less constrained by commercial considerations, allowing potential therapies for rare cancers, such as pediatric malignancies, to be explored. Furthermore, the direction of personalized cancer medicine is to better and more narrowly define patient populations for treatment with agents targeting specific mechanisms. This fragmentation of the cancer patient population for well-targeted drugs reduces the size of potential markets. It has been suggested that new economic models for drug discovery and development will be essential to accommodate the personalized medicine paradigm [137]. This is likely to include a greater emphasis on partnerships between academic, commercial, and not-for-profit drug discovery research scientists, to gain the benefits of a more collaborative, "open-source" approach to target validation [138].

In addition to the factors described here that give credence to the genetic validation of a target, higher priority will usually be given to more druggable targets for which the technical feasibility of finding a drug is more likely [118]. Receptors for small endogenous molecules, enzymes with well-defined active sites (e.g., kinases), and protein–protein interactions involving small domains are all accepted as druggable with the technology that is currently available to us. On the other hand, large-domain protein–protein interactions remain very difficult, although the experience with inhibitors of the interaction of the tumour suppressor p53 and its regulator HDM2, or between the apoptosis regulators BCL and BAK shows that the boundaries of druggability are expanding [139]. Phosphatases are also challenging targets. Despite progress in identifying potent inhibitors of several phosphatase enzymes, including the progression of compounds to early-phase trials, achieving cell permeability and selectivity is still a challenge [140]. Many other potentially important targets remain stubbornly undruggable. For example, no drugs have yet emerged that are able to directly inhibit the mutant RAS G protein or the myelocytomatosis viral oncogene homolog (MYC) oncoprotein, or to reactivate mutant p53.

In situations where a particular target of interest is not druggable, knowledge of the biochemical pathway may allow a downstream target to be selected. As an example, although RAS itself cannot be inhibited, the downstream MEK 1/2 kinases proved tractable with small-molecule inhibitors, interestingly of an allosteric nature [128]. Recent clinical data show a benefit to progression-free survival of combining MEK inhibition with V600E BRAF kinase inhibition, to counter the reactivation of the MAPK signaling pathway associated with selective V600E BRAF inhibition [141]. Inhibition of RAS prenylation, which blocks the essential membrane localization of the oncoprotein, has proved technically feasible, although the clinical significance of RAS prenylation inhibitors is still unclear [142].

While one of the most classically druggable family of targets, the G protein-coupled receptors (GPCRs), did not feature significantly as cancer genes in an early census [143], there is growing evidence of links between GPCRs and the initiation and progression of cancer [144]. As well as overexpression of GPCRs in certain cancers, the extensive cross-talk between GPCRs and growth factor receptors also argues for a role for GPCRs in the development of aberrant cancer-signaling networks. The manipulation of a GPCR-like protein to treat cancer has been proven with the approval of the smoothened (SMO) receptor ligand vismodegib (Erivedge) for the treatment of basal cell carcinoma [145]. Vismodegib binds to SMO, a seven-transmembrane-helix receptor, and prevents activation of Hedgehog (Hh) pathway signaling through the receptor, inhibiting the action of the Hh transcription factors Gli1 and Gli2. Interestingly, vismodegib was discovered by a phenotypic pathway screen in murine fibroblasts, using a luciferase reporter under the control of Gli transcription factor binding to identify inhibitors of signaling elicited by sonic hedgehog (Shh) ligand [146].

The examples given here illustrate how a good target must pass the dual test of relevance to disease mechanisms and potential for druggability. At the same time it is important to not be overly conservative, but to seek creative solutions to expand the druggable cancer genome. It is not very long ago that kinases were regarded as high-risk targets, yet they now lie second in frequency only to GPCRs in the druggable genome [118]. A target's druggability is often estimated by placing it within known gene families that have been shown by past precedent to be technically feasible. Publicly available databases such as canSAR (http://cansar.icr.ac.uk), developed in our drug discovery unit, can be very helpful in assessing the protein sequence or structural homology of a new target to known cancer drug targets, and also in identifying published chemical compounds that modulate targets in a given class [117]. De novo prediction of protein druggability based on structure or structural homology is commonly attempted using a variety of computational tools that in essence seek out and enumerate potential pockets for small-molecule binding on the surface of the protein [83,147].

Alongside all of the factors discussed in this chapter that concern both disease involvement and technical feasibility, it is very valuable to have a hypothesis as to why a drug acting on a potential new target would be expected to give a therapeutic differential between cancer and normal cells [15]. This can be based on one or more of the cancer dependencies discussed in this chapter, such as exploitation of oncogene addiction or prospects for synthetic lethality— where inhibition of a target is effective only when combined with a specific genetic defect, with neither therapeutic agent nor genetic defect producing an effect on its own. Useful information can be gained from genetically modified mouse models, but it should be realized that genetic manipulation does not always produce the same outcome as a small-molecule modulator [74,75]. A suitably potent and selective small-molecule compound, either a natural product or a synthetic agent, can be very useful in target validation [76].

Despite oncogene addiction and other cancer dependencies, mechanism-based toxicity to normal tissues clearly does still occur [59]. An example is the skin rash seen with EGFR inhibitors [148] or the hyperlipidemia and hyperglycemia associated with inhibitors of the PI3 kinase–AKT–mTOR pathway [149]. Although it can be useful to investigate possible on-target and indeed potential off-target effects in tissue culture or in model organisms, the therapeutic index is probably still best evaluated in animal models once chemical compounds with adequate potency, selectivity, and pharmacokinetic properties have been produced.

A final comment on the important topic of target validation is that at the end of the day, the selection of a drug target is a matter of judgment based on science, experience, and practicality. There will always be a risk of failure. This risk can be managed by judicious target selection based on more systematic, multifaceted analysis, coupled with careful selection of a balanced portfolio of projects featuring different types of biology and varying types of biological and technical risk (Fig. 1.3).

FROM DRUG TARGET TO DEVELOPMENT CANDIDATE

The Overall Approach to Drug Discovery

Success in discovering a drug requires a creative interplay between the essential disciplines of biology, pharmacology, and medicinal chemistry. The stages involved in small-molecule drug discovery are illustrated in Fig. 1.4(A). Following target validation and selection (see preceding section), one or more chemical starting points must be generated. These are normally produced by some type of screening activity that generates "hits" with preliminary

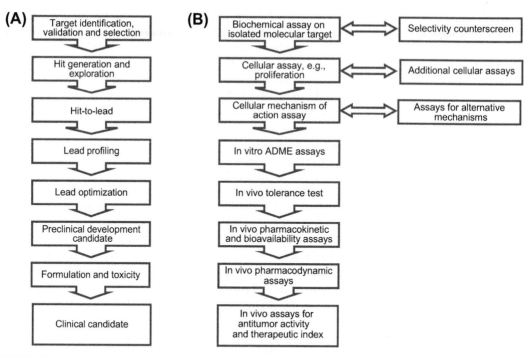

FIGURE 1.4 Schematic depiction of (A) the stages of drug discovery from target identification to clinical candidate; and (B) a typical biological test cascade. (For color version of this figure, the reader is referred to the online version of this book.)

biological activity against the target. Hit compounds are then evaluated in a hit exploration phase. Following this, selected hits are converted into more robust chemical entities according to preestablished criteria (see next section in this chapter) in the hit-to-lead phase. Leads are often then assessed during a lead-profiling stage, and selected chemical series are improved in the lead optimization phase, so that one or more compounds can be chosen for preclinical development. Following successful formulation and toxicology studies, a candidate molecule will be ready to begin clinical trials.

The engine of small-molecule drug discovery consists of iterative cycles of chemical synthesis and biological evaluation. At each cycle, hypotheses are generated, determining which new chemical entities are designed, made, and tested. Modern lead optimization focuses on the simultaneous optimization of multiple parameters, including in particular potency, selectivity, and the set of parameters collectively known as ADMET (absorption, distribution, metabolism, excretion, and toxicology) or DMPK (drug metabolism and pharmacokinetics).

A set of assays must be put in place that allows the biological properties of test compounds to be evaluated. This is commonly referred to as a "biological test cascade" (Fig. 1.4(B)). The test cascade is a sequence of appropriate assays, predictive of the intended therapeutic mechanism and effect, that allows compounds to be selected for further evaluation or structural modification. After many rounds of structural refinement, leading to improvements in the biological profile of the compounds, candidates for preclinical and clinical development are selected. Care must be taken that the biological assays accurately reflect the biological properties required in the final drug, including on-target and on-pathway biomarker modulation.

The timescale from target identification to regulatory approval of oncology drugs has typically taken up to 10–15 years, with preclinical discovery commonly requiring 5–10 years [26,67]. If the assessment of success or failure to improve biological properties through compound structural refinement can be done more quickly, as is now the case, this allows more opportunities to be evaluated in any given time period.

Hit and Lead Generation

After target selection, the next critical step in small-molecule drug discovery is the generation of lead compounds. Apart from natural products, which have commonly been "optimized" for compatibility with biological systems over the millennia by the selective forces of evolution [150], small-molecule compounds that are identified initially in a drug discovery project only very rarely turn out to be the clinical candidate. Instead, they represent chemical starting points that need considerable structural modification and refinement of biological properties before a drug can be generated.

The chemical starting points that are required for small-molecular drug discovery may be derived from the structures of endogenous biological ligands, existing drugs, or biologically active natural products. Alternatively, they may come from high-throughput or focused screening of compound collections or, increasingly more common, may originate from design and screening using information on the structural biology of the target [4]. Bioactive natural products have historically been the origin of important cytotoxic chemotherapies for cancer, such as the taxane or *Vinca* alkaloid families of microtubule poisons, the mitomycin DNA-alkylating agents, or derivatives of the alkaloid camptothecin as topoisomerase inhibitors. However, natural products may also be inhibitors of specific molecular targets, as exemplified by the clinically approved mTOR inhibitors temsirolimus and everolimus, which are analogs of the natural product rapamycin [151].

Biochemical high-throughput screening (HTS) of large libraries of chemically diverse small molecules has been very effective in generating leads against isolated molecular cancer targets, usually recombinant proteins [113]. Notable examples are enzymes such as kinases [152,153] and the molecular chaperone HSP90 [154,155]. HTS has typically been carried out with libraries from around 100,000 up to 1 or 2 million compounds. For enzyme superfamilies with closely related three-dimensional (3D) structures in their active sites, such as the enzymes comprising the human kinome, it has also proved productive to screen smaller compound libraries that are restricted to a number of "privileged" chemical scaffolds matching the common 3D structure of the targets [156,157]. The concatenation of several enzymes in a signaling cascade into a single biochemical screen has also been demonstrated, for example to find inhibitors of the RAS–MEK–ERK pathway [158].

However, many interesting targets cannot be screened as isolated components in a biochemical assay. For these systems, specific phenotypic screens conducted in whole cells or simple model organisms, such as zebrafish or nematode worms, may be appropriate [112]. This approach also offers the opportunity to probe several targets simultaneously, and by necessity identifies only cell or tissue penetrant hit compounds. For example, compounds modulating cellular protein acetylation and others inhibiting HSP90 molecular chaperone function were identified simultaneously in an efficient duplexed cell-based screen; the different compounds identified were shown to have a variety of molecular mechanisms, not all of which were precisely defined [159].

Identification of the precise locus of action of the compounds identified in cell-based screens is not always straightforward, but can be tackled with a number of chemical biology technologies such as gene expression and protein array profiling, affinity chromatography of cell lysates, or yeast chemical genetic screens [160,161]. Increasingly, high-content screening technologies provide a means to shortcut the mechanistic deconvolution typically associated with phenotypic screening [162]. For example, by using imaging-based screens, very specific phenotypic effects elucidated by small molecules within cells can be probed, such that a narrower range of molecular targets is examined in situ. Such screens have identified AKT kinase inhibitors through examining the inhibition of recruitment of labeled protein to the cell membrane [163], while following the translocation of FOXO1a picked-out inhibitors of both the PI3K–AKT pathway and the nuclear protein transport machinery [164]. Mechanistic cell-based screens for specific pathways, often using a luciferase reporter as the measured readout, are highly useful for identifying druggable targets and accompanying hit matter in pathways associated with technically difficult targets. An example is the identification of vismodegib, discussed in this chapter, from a luciferase reporter assay for inhibitors of the Hh signaling pathway [146]. In another example, a luciferase reporter assay was used to screen for inhibitors of the Wnt signaling pathway, and identified the enzymes tankyrase 1 and 2 as novel, druggable targets in a system previously intractable to small-molecule inhibition [165].

The first approach to more systematic, large-scale cancer cell–based screening was the use of the "NCI 60 human tumor cell panel" developed under the auspices of the US National Cancer Institute (NCI; [166–168]; see http://dtp.nci.nih.gov/docs/compare/compare_intro. html). Extensive screening of drug and compound sensitivity, together with the cataloging of multiple genetic and molecular features, has generated a large, publicly available database that can be used as part of chemical biology and drug discovery investigations. For example, the database can be queried for compounds that act on cell lines with a particular abnormality or for which activity parallels that of a known inhibitor of a drug target. In a related "connectivity map" approach, compounds can be sought that mimic a particular, desired gene expression profile related to a disease or small-molecule perturbation [169]. In an even larger scale extension of cancer cell line screening, a publicly available endeavor established by the Wellcome Trust and Massachusetts General Hospital Cancer Center is the Genomics of Drug Sensitivity in Cancer Project, which seeks to identify the molecular features of cancers that can predict response to anticancer drugs [170] (see http://www.cancerrxgene.org). The project is screening a wide range of anticancer therapeutics, both drug candidates and well-characterized chemical probes, against >1000 genetically characterized human cancer cell lines that provide a much better representation of the genetic diversity of human cancers. The sensitivity patterns of the cell lines can be correlated with genomic and expression data to identify genetic features that are predictive of sensitivity. Likewise, the Cancer Cell Line Encyclopedia compiles gene expression, chromosomal copy number, sequencing and compound sensitivity data from 947 cancer cell lines [171].

Increasingly, the generation of small-molecule leads involves the use of powerful biophysical technologies for measuring and characterizing the binding of the compounds to the biological target. Screening platforms based on nuclear magnetic resonance (NMR), X-ray crystallography, or surface-plasmon resonance are capable of detecting the weak interactions between proteins and low-molecular-weight chemical compounds, referred to as "fragments". In particular, fragment-based screening using NMR or X-ray crystallography has proved valuable in finding new chemical leads [115,172] (see Chapter 4 for a detailed discussion of this topic). As an example from our own work, 7-azaindole was identified by virtual and crystallographic screening as a fragment binding to the ATP site of AKT [173]. A chimeric AKT–PKA (protein kinase A) protein was used to guide the structure-based elaboration of the fragment into a larger, more potent and selective AKT inhibitor CCT129254 with oral activity in vivo [174,175] (Fig. 1.6(A)). The lead compound from this series was developed into the clinical candidate AZD5363 [176]. The value of structural details from ligand–target complexes in directing the improvement of the initial leads through structure-based design is also seen in our development of the pyrazole-resorcinol HSP90 inhibitor CCT018159 into the clinical candidate NVP-AUY922 ([155,178] Fig. 1.6(B) and the "Examples of Case Histories" section).

The physicochemical and structural features of lead chemical compounds are of paramount importance in determining the likely success of their progression to clinical candidates. Some problematic chemical functionalities are best avoided, particularly those associated with frequent nonspecific activity or toxicity due to chemical reactivity, or that interfere with common bioassay readouts [180–182]. Several empirically derived definitions of drug-like and lead-like chemical space have been described, made up of easily calculated properties such as molecular weight, lipophilicity, hydrogen-bonding capacity and surface polarity, and molecular flexibility [183–186]. These definitions are not proscriptive rules, but rather use the cumulative experience of drug discovery science thus far to define areas of chemical space with a higher probability of generating molecules able to function in whole organisms as effective therapeutics. A drug must not only demonstrate effective action at its molecular target, but also have a balance of aqueous and nonaqueous solubilities to allow sufficient distribution between the aqueous and nonaqueous pharmacokinetic compartments of the body. A discrimination is made between the properties of leads and drugs to account for the usual increase in molecular size and complexity that accompanies the optimization of a lead into a candidate drug [187]. The application of lead-like and drug-like parameters to select appropriate small molecules is applied both to the establishment of screening collections and also to the choice of elaborated molecules made during lead optimization [188] (Table 1.2). Increasingly, similar considerations are applied in the refinement of chemical probes or tool compounds for nonclinical use, leading to the concept of "fitness factors" for such materials [76]. As with any probabilistic guideline, there are exceptions, and the optimization of ABT-737 to the orally active clinical candidate navitoclax (which violates three of Lipinski's five guidelines for achieving oral absorption) shows that the boundaries of drug-like chemical space are not rigidly defined [189] (see "Examples of Case Histories" section).

Computational technologies can contribute to the generation of lead compounds. In silico screening examines the ability of compounds to fit within 3D models of the binding site that may be generated from structure–activity relationships of known ligands or from protein inhibitor co-crystal structures [190,191]. Subsequent biochemical screening of the "virtual

TABLE 1.2 Typical Physicochemical and Biological Properties of Fragments, Leads, and Drugs

Property	Fragment	Lead	Drug
Molecular weight (MF)	<300	<400	<500
Lipophilicity (LogP)	<3	<4	<5
H-bond donor atoms (OH, NH)	≤3	≤4–5	≤5
H-bond acceptor atoms (N,O)	≤3	≤8–9	≤10
Polar surface area (PSA)	n.a.	n.a.	$\leq 140\text{--}150\,\text{A}^2$
Rotatable bonds (nRot)	n.a.	≤8	≤10
Chemically reactive groups	n.a.	None present	None present
Target activity (IC$_{50}$ or K_i)	$>>10^{-5}\text{--}10^{-6}\,\text{M}$	$10^{-6}\text{--}10^{-7}\,\text{M}$	$10^{-8}\text{--}10^{-9}\,\text{M}$
Structure–activity Relationship (SAR)	NMR or X-ray data	Useful SAR established	Full SAR understood

n.a. = not assessed.

hits" found in this way is still required to find and confirm valid biologically active compounds, but virtual screening can reduce the number of compounds that need to be assayed, as shown for inhibitors of checkpoint kinase 1 (CHK1) [192,193].

The most appropriate strategy for finding small-molecule leads is dependent on the nature of the molecular target and the associated biology. In cases where little is known about the chemical biology or 3D structure of the target, but robust biochemical assays are available, then high-throughput screening of large, diverse compound libraries is often effective. Alternatively, when the target belongs to a well-characterized family of proteins, or a number of small molecule ligands are already known, then screening of more focused libraries, in which the compounds have a pedigree for interaction with the target class, may be more appropriate. This strategy has been particularly successful for discovering inhibitors of kinases [156,157], although a caveat is the increased likelihood that the lead compounds will show cross-reactivity with other members of the target class. However, such cross-reactivity can also be exploited to generate new leads, as exemplified in the discovery of imatinib (see "Examples of Case Histories" section). In such cases, the introduction of selectivity for the target becomes an important objective in the medicinal chemistry optimization of the lead series. Lead generation using fragment-based screening is usually dependent on the target biomolecule having experimentally tractable structural biology by NMR or crystallography. However, the similarity of protein structures within enzyme superfamilies can again be turned to advantage, through the use of surrogate or chimeric proteins, as demonstrated in the search for inhibitors of AKT by crystallographic fragment screening using an AKT–PKA chimera [173].

Lead Profiling and Multiparameter Lead Optimization

The chemical compounds that are generated at the start of a small-molecule drug discovery program usually require extensive modification to optimize them before a clinical candidate is identified. This typically entails improvements in key parameters that include potency and specificity for the mechanism of action on the target biomolecule and in cells; pharmaceutical properties, such that the compounds are compatible with the proposed route of administration and will distribute effectively to the target tissues and cells for sustained periods; relevant pharmacodynamic effects in vivo that recapitulate the cellular effects seen in vitro and confirm the action of the drug on its target; and, most importantly, tolerability and efficacy against tumors in appropriate in vivo models. Achievement of the appropriate preclinical therapeutic profile is critical to give confidence that the compound is "fit for purpose" to progress to a hypothesis-testing clinical trial. This is particularly the case when a first-in-class agent is considered because molecular targets, and the methodologies used to discover drugs for them, are not completely validated until a pharmacological agent has been shown to have therapeutic utility in clinical studies—and where the predominant mechanism of action can be convincingly ascribed to modulation of the molecular target [3].

Prospective lead series will be profiled for their potential to deliver the properties described here before selecting one or a small number of series for lead optimization. In addition to potency for the target, ligand efficiency has proved to be a useful measure of how effectively the chemical structure interacts with its locus of action [194]. The establishment of productive structure–activity relationships (SARs) is essential to relate changes in chemical structure to the target and cell potencies, informed by mechanistic biomarkers, and the range of other properties that need to be optimized [195]. Medicinal chemists have one main tool with which to engineer the desired multiparameter profile of a small-molecule drug: the molecular structure of the compound. Multiple SARs define the way in which these properties respond to changes in compound structure. As mentioned in this chapter, in carrying out the optimization from hit-to-lead to clinical candidate, the compounds are assessed in a biological test cascade, comprising a hierarchy of assays of increasing complexity (Fig. 1.4(B)). Driving the process is the iterative medicinal chemistry cycle of compound design, synthesis, biological evaluation, and interpretation. Each assay provides feedback to inform the design of new compounds aimed at improving the properties of the compounds (Fig. 1.5). The assays will have associated thresholds, tied to the desired therapeutic profile, which act as gatekeepers regulating whether further assessment of a compound is merited. However, it should be noted that the model in Fig. 1.5 is illustrative rather than prescriptive. In many cases, it is helpful to push early, unoptimized compounds further through the assay cascade to help validate the assays themselves and anticipate future challenges for a given chemical series. For new molecular targets, the early stage of the discovery process is often as much concerned with validating the assay cascade as it is with using it to discover a drug molecule. It is important that the multiple, iterative cycles remain closely coupled, so that the design of new compounds for synthesis benefits from as much biological information across the multiple parameters as possible.

The SAR for any one property may be complementary, partially aligned, or antagonistic to that of another. Thus, the clinical candidate will sit at an acceptable intersection of the multiple SARs, but may not be fully optimized for any one of these. The exact therapeutic profile aimed for may evolve as the science develops and more is learned about the

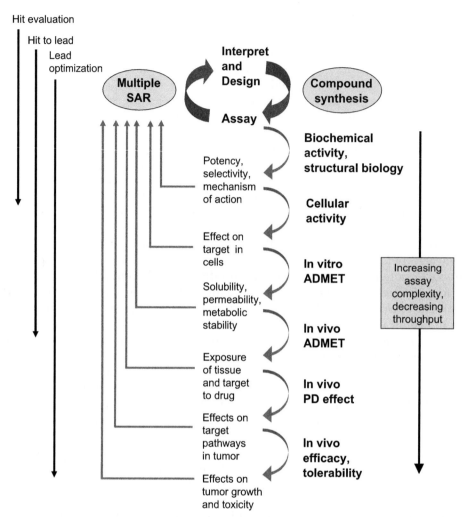

FIGURE 1.5 Drug discovery is a series of linked iterative cycles of compound design, synthesis, and evaluation. As the compound biological profile becomes more sophisticated, the complexity and number of assays required for evaluation also increase. (For color version of this figure, the reader is referred to the online version of this book.)

pharmacology of the drug molecules. Therefore, although outwardly a systematic process, expert judgment is needed to navigate through the various stages of lead optimization and candidate selection. Naturally, the choice of a clinical candidate compound will be driven more heavily by the assays considered to be most relevant to the totality of clinical performance, such as in vivo efficacy, pharmacodynamic, pharmacokinetic, and tolerability studies. Fortunately, key structural determinants of different SARs may well occur in distinct regions of the molecule. For example, the structures of the receptor tyrosine kinase inhibitors imatinib, dasatinib, gefitinib, and erlotinib contain pendant groups

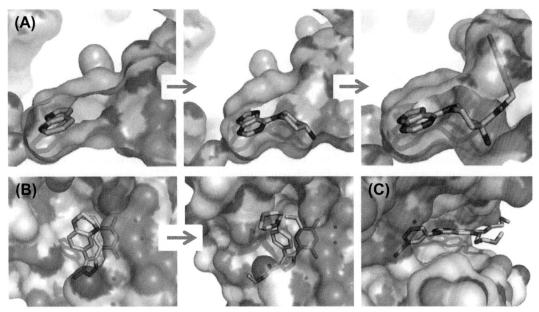

FIGURE 1.6 Structure-based design in the discovery of new targeted treatments. Ligands are shown as stick models colored according to atom type (carbon = green). Proteins are shown as transparent surfaces colored according to atom type (carbon = gray). (A) Sequence showing the X-ray crystal structure of the fragment 7-azaindole bound to the adenosine triphosphate (ATP) site of a chimeric PKA–PKB protein (adapted from PDB 2UVX [173]), its elaboration by fragment growing into a more potent and selective pyrrolopyrimidine PKB inhibitor (adapted from PDB 2VNY [174]), and subsequently into the orally active inhibitor CCT129254 (adapted from PDB 2X39 [175]). (B) Sequence showing the X-ray crystal structure of CCT018159 bound to the HSP90 ATPase domain (adapted from PDB 2BRC [177]) and its elaboration into the clinical candidate NVP-AUY922 bound to the HSP90 ATPase domain (adapted from PDB 2VCI [178]). The resorcinol group in CCT018159 that interacts with protein-bound water molecules is retained, while additional potency is gained from new interactions to the additional amide substituent. The morpholine group that modulates pharmacokinetic behavior extends out into solvent. (C) Detail of the X-ray crystal structure of erlotinib bound to the EGFR kinase domain (adapted from PDB 1M17 [179]) showing the separation of the functionality that mediates target binding, buried in the binding pocket, and the group that modulates solubility and pharmacokinetic properties, which is exposed to solvent. (This figure is reproduced in color in the color plate section.)

associated predominantly with effects on pharmacokinetic properties rather than target potency. Structures of the ligand–protein complexes shows that these areas are oriented away from the kinase domain and into solvent [120] (Fig. 1.6(C)). Similar considerations can be applied prospectively using structure-based design to identify regions of a hit compound that can be modified to separately target either potency or physicochemical properties, as demonstrated in the evolution of the resorcinylic isoxazole inhibitor of HSP90, NVP-AUY922 [155,196] (Fig. 1.6(B)). In other circumstances, it may prove more difficult to manipulate multiple SARs concurrently, as is sometimes encountered when trying to avoid toxic hERG ion channel inhibition with compounds where a basic, highly lipophilic structure is associated with optimal target activity [196]. An inability to find an acceptable combination of the multiple properties in a single structure would prevent a candidate drug from being identified in that chemical series. For this reason, it is beneficial to consider many structurally diverse hits as chemical starting points in the early stages of a drug discovery project.

In contemporary drug discovery, importance is placed on beginning the multiparameter optimization as early as possible [197]. This includes careful choice of the types of compounds that enter into hit generation according to the empirical definitions of drug-likeness and lead-likeness, to enhance the probability of successful progression from hits to candidates [3]. During the initial stages of hit evaluation and hit-to-lead, emphasis will naturally fall on assessment of compounds in vitro in biochemical and cellular assays. It is also essential that versatile and reliable organic synthesis routes are developed early in the program. Nevertheless, evaluating the pharmacokinetic (ADMET) behavior of the nascent leads at an early stage is vital, and has been shown to significantly decrease the probability of failure due to inadequate pharmacokinetic properties of compounds at later stages in discovery or clinical development [64]. While high-throughput assays to assess the in vitro behavior of compounds are well established, capacity is limited for measuring the in vivo properties of large numbers of compounds. Thus, the time taken to feed back the results of biological experiments becomes increasingly rate limiting as compound optimization progresses. For pharmacokinetics, the use of cassette-dosing protocols to appraise multiple compounds simultaneously may be a solution to increasing capacity for some chemotypes [198,199]. Alternatively, limited time-point sampling protocols to compare compounds within a series can reduce the in vivo experimental burden, as demonstrated for the recent discovery of orally bioavailable CHK1 inhibitors [200].

Assessment of efficacy, such as xenograft tumor growth inhibition over a 3–4 week dosing period, is inherently time-consuming and limits the number of iterative cycles that can be achieved in a reasonable time. For molecular-targeted agents, a preliminary in vivo assessment of short-term target modulation and downstream pharmacodynamic effects (typically, a 2–24 h time course) can serve as a way of quickly selecting compounds that reach and modulate the intended molecular target. This is also an important part of establishing the "pharmacological audit trail" that gives confidence in the mechanism of action and the appropriateness for clinical use of a targeted molecular therapeutic [97,201].

EXAMPLES OF CASE HISTORIES FOR MOLECULARLY TARGETED CANCER THERAPEUTICS

The development of selected molecularly targeted agents illustrates the various strategies and technologies that are applied in small-molecule lead optimization. The feedback of information from clinical studies back into the early drug discovery process has proved important in several cases and is emphasized in this section.

Imatinib and Dasatinib

Highly selective BCR–ABL kinase inhibitors were generated from a series of anilinopyrimidine protein kinase C inhibitors by a simple adjustment of the 3D conformation of the lead molecule, an example of "target hopping" where chemical leads developed against one target are adapted to serve as starting points for inhibiting another within the same protein superfamily. Lead optimization to give imatinib focused on improving pharmacokinetic properties through the introduction of solubilizing groups (Scheme 1.1(A)) [202]. The success of imatinib in clinical trials for CML provided an important proof of concept for the development of molecularly targeted small-molecule drugs in oncology. The observation that imatinib inhibits a limited number of other kinases, notably the oncoprotein c-KIT, led to successful clinical trials of the drug for the treatment of gastrointestinal stromal tumor, which is often driven by a mutant KIT kinase [203]. The emergence of imatinib-resistant kinase mutants in CML patients prompted the development of second-generation inhibitors, such as dasatinib, which targets the more conserved active form of the kinase and inhibits many of the imatinib-resistant mutants, as well as other cancer targets such as SRC [43,44].

Sorafenib

Sorafenib exemplifies the use of combinatorial chemistry for lead generation and optimization from a privileged structure, the diarylurea (Scheme 1.1(B)) [204]. Although developed as a targeted CRAF inhibitor, sorafenib was subsequently recognized as exhibiting useful receptor tyrosine kinase polypharmacology, particularly inhibition of VEGF receptors, PDGF receptors, and c-KIT and FLT3 kinases, leading to drug approval for the treatment of renal cell cancers [205]. Single-agent activity was not, however, seen in melanoma, despite the fact that sorafenib has activity against RAF isoforms.

Vemurafenib

Selectively targeting oncogenic BRAF became a major goal following the identification of the importance of the V600E BRAF mutation in the development of melanoma [23]. The discovery of the first-in-class V600E BRAF inhibitor vemurafenib illustrates how protein structure information can be used at the outset of a drug discovery project to generate new lead chemical structures, and demonstrates the power of fragment-based technologies for identifying inhibitor scaffolds (Scheme 1.1(C)) [25]. This started with a very broad approach to finding inhibitors of the kinase target class. A library of 20,000 fragments (MW 150–350 Da) was screened at high concentration (200 µM) against multiple kinases to identify a set of 238 compounds, including 7-azaindole, with measurable activity against at least three kinases and crystallographic evidence of binding in the ATP site [206]. Simple elaboration of the 7-azaindole scaffold generated the monosubstituted 3-anilino-7-azaindole, which had a well-defined crystallographic binding mode in the kinase Pim-1 (Pim1 $IC_{50} \sim 100$ µM). On the basis of these data, further elaboration led to a 3-benzyl-7-azaindole analog, which now displayed interactions to the kinase aspartate-phenylalanine-glycine (DFG) motif when crystallized in FGFR1, and increased potency (FGFR1 $IC_{50} \sim 2$ µM). Libraries of mono- and disubstituted 7-azaindoles were prepared based around this motif and screened against multiple kinases, from which a subset of compounds bearing a specific difluorophenylsulfonamide substituent were identified with high potency for V600E BRAF. Co-crystallization in mutant and wild-type BRAF proteins was used to enable structure-guided optimization of the inhibitors toward this specific molecular target, leading ultimately to vemurafenib [207].

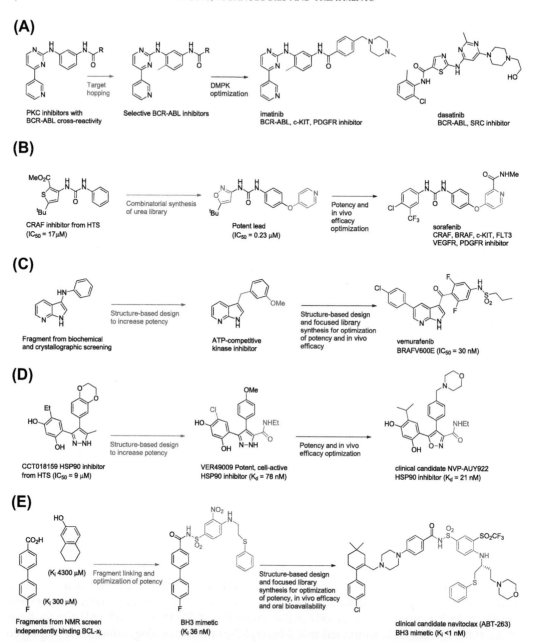

SCHEME 1.1 Selected case histories of lead generation and lead optimization for small-molecule targeted molecular cancer therapeutics. (A) The phenylaminopyrimidine core of imatinib emerged from screening of protein kinase C inhibitors and was rendered selective for BCR–ABL by addition of a single methyl substituent (red). Lead optimization focused on improving DMPK properties (blue). The second-generation BCR–ABL inhibitor dasatinib has activity against some imatinib-resistant BCR–ABL mutant kinases. (B) The starting point for the discovery of the multitargeted kinase inhibitor sorafenib came from high-throughput screening (HTS) of a large compound collection against CRAF. Combinatorial variation of the two substituents on the central urea generated a potent lead (red).

HSP90 Inhibitors 17-AAG and NVP-AUY922

The search for small-molecule inhibitors of the molecular chaperone HSP90 was given impetus by successful proof-of-concept clinical trials with the clinical path-finding drug 17-AAG [208]. This derivative of the natural product geldanamycin [154] showed the molecular signature of target inhibition in tumor tissue and evidence of activity in melanoma patients, but has solubility, formulation, and metabolic liabilities [208,209]. The optimization of the 3-(2,4-dihydroxyphenyl)-pyrazole HTS hit CCT018159 [177] exemplifies the use of protein structural information to guide the choice and positioning of extra functionality to improve inhibitor affinity for the nucleotide binding site of the HSP90 ATPase. This initially led to the amidopyrazole VER-49009, with significantly increased potency reflecting additional hydrogen bonding to the protein surface in the ATP pocket (Scheme 1.1(D)) [210]. Isothermal titration calorimetry used together with the analysis of binding mode by protein–ligand crystallography provided a powerful means to elucidate in detail the thermodynamics of the inhibitor–protein interactions. Further lead optimization concentrated on increasing inhibitor affinity while improving pharmacokinetic properties and in vivo efficacy, leading to the isoxazole clinical candidate NVP-AUY922 (Fig. 1.6) [178,211,212].

ABT-737 and Navitoclax

The discovery of the BCL-2 homology domain 3 (BH3) mimetic ABT-737 illustrates how a fragment-based approach can be applied to tackle molecular targets seen as being on the edge of druggable space (Scheme 1.1(E)) [213]. The heterodimerization of antiapoptotic BCL-2 family proteins and proapoptotic proteins with a BH3 domain suppresses the functions of the proapoptotic partner [214]. A particular feature of this protein–protein interaction is the docking of a hydrophobic alpha-helix in the BH3 domain into a corresponding deep hydrophobic groove in the BCL-2 proteins. Such helix-docked protein–protein interaction sites are now recognized as a general motif, potentially tractable with small molecules due to the relatively enclosed and rigid nature of the binding site [215]. NMR-based biophysical screening identified fragments that bound weakly to two separate sites in the hydrophobic groove of BCL-X_L [216]. Pairs of fragments were joined in a variety of ways, leading to the identification of linked molecules that could occupy both subsites at the same time. The optimization of potency through

---

Lead optimization focused on improving potency and in vivo antitumor activity (blue). (C) The 3-anilino-7-azaindole core of vemurafenib was identified as a low-molecular-weight drug fragment binding to the ATP-binding site of kinases, including BRAF, by a combined biochemical and crystallographic screening approach. Elaboration of the fragment generated more active 3-benzyl-7-azaindole inhibitors (red). A focused library approach combined with structure-based design led to the optimized compound vemurafenib (PLX4720) (blue). (D) HTS against the HSP90 ATPase identified the novel resorcinylic pyrazole inhibitor CCT018159, which was co-crystallized with the enzyme. Structure-based design guided the positioning of extra lipophilic and hydrogen-bonding functional groups to generate the potent cell active inhibitor VER-49009 (red). Further optimization of potency and of pharmacokinetic and pharmacodynamic properties (blue) gave the isoxazole clinical candidate NVP-AUY922. (E) Screening using NMR identified fragments binding weakly to two adjacent subsites on the BCL-X_L protein. Linking of the fragments to retain their orientations and further substitution gave a potent inhibitor of BH3 binding to BCl-X_L that occupies the whole binding site (red). Structure-based design to optimize potency and in vivo efficacy, and subsequently oral pharmacokinetic properties, led to the clinical candidate navitoclax (blue). (This figure is reproduced in color in the color plate section.)

focused library synthesis, guided by NMR structural studies, gave highly potent inhibitors of the BCL-X_L–BH3 interaction, which were further optimized for in vivo efficacy to ABT-737 [213]. Although potent and effective in vivo, ABT-737 lacked oral bioavailability. Therefore, further optimization was carried out to peripheral groups in the molecule to improve cellular activity and in vivo pharmacokinetics, generating the oral agent navitoclax (ABT-263) [189]. The discoveries of ABT-737 and navitoclax exemplify the application of new technologies in contemporary drug design to extend the boundaries of what is regarded as classically druggable space. It is also interesting to note that navitoclax challenges dogma on the definition of small-molecule "drug-likeness" in terms of limits on size and hydrophobicity [183].

BIOMARKERS, THE PHARMACOLOGICAL AUDIT TRAIL, AND CLINICAL DEVELOPMENT

An extremely important element of the development of any new cancer drug is the application of biomarkers for patient selection together with pharmacokinetic–pharmacodynamic endpoints [97,99–101,111,201]. Indeed, such markers are required during the preclinical stage as well as the clinical phase. We consider biomarkers to be so informative and important that in our own drug discovery center, we apply the rule "No biomarker, no project."

Molecular diagnostics are needed to select animal models and patients that are the most appropriate for assessing the activity of the particular agent. Molecular biomarkers are also absolutely essential to determine proof of mechanism for modulation of the desired target and to help determine what is the optimal dose and administration schedule. It seems obvious that biomarkers are required to make clinical trials more intelligent and informative and also to make decision making throughout the preclinical and clinical phases more rational and effective [250]. However, their use in early clinical trials of cancer drugs has taken some time to become widely established [98,217].

As mentioned earlier, the concept of the "pharmacological audit trail" has been advocated [97–101,201] as a rational and practical framework for assessing the performance of lead compounds in preclinical discovery and then of the drug candidate during early clinical trials. In addition, the pharmacological audit trail can be used as a tool for estimating the likelihood of drug failure at the various stages of development and for making the critical "go or no go" decisions (i.e. whether to proceed to the next stage or abandon the drug).

The use of the pharmacologic audit trail involves addressing a series of important questions (Fig. 1.7):

- How is the status of the target relevant to the tumor to be treated?
- What predictive assay can be used for the molecular aberration, to identify suitable patient populations?
- Are active drug levels achieved in the plasma and in tumor tissues?
- Is the molecular target of interest inhibited?
- Is the biochemical pathway in which the target operates modulated?
- Are the intended biological processes also affected, for example one or more of the various hallmark traits of cancer?
- Do the above parameters relate to or explain any therapeutic or toxic effects?

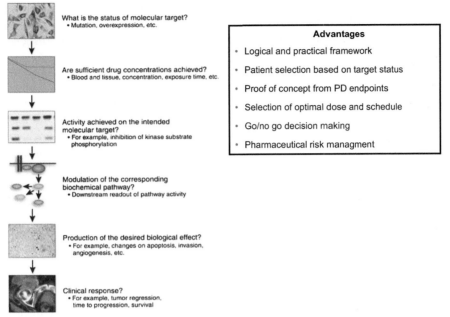

What is the status of molecular target?
• Mutation, overexpression, etc.

Are sufficient drug concentrations achieved?
• Blood and tissue, concentration, exposure time, etc.

Activity achieved on the intended molecular target?
• For example, inhibition of kinase substrate phosphorylation

Modulation of the corresponding biochemical pathway?
• Downstream readout of pathway activity

Production of the desired biological effect?
• For example, changes on apoptosis, invasion, angiogenesis, etc.

Clinical response?
• For example, tumor regression, time to progression, survival

Advantages

- Logical and practical framework
- Patient selection based on target status
- Proof of concept from PD endpoints
- Selection of optimal dose and schedule
- Go/no go decision making
- Pharmaceutical risk managment

FIGURE 1.7 Schematic illustrating the pharmacological audit trail. This hierarchical set of parameters provides a conceptual and practical framework to aid decision making in preclinical and clinical drug development. The audit trail links the status of the molecular target (through pharmacokinetic exposures and pharmacodynamic effects on the target), pathway, and biological effect to therapeutic and toxic responses. It is also useful to help select the optimal drug dose and schedule. (This figure is reproduced in color in the color plate section.) *Modified with permission from Ref. [3].*

- Can intermediate endpoints of clinical response (e.g., tumor markers, circulating tumor cells, or functional imaging) be used to test the hypothesis that modulating the target is of benefit?
- What are the molecular alterations occurring at disease progression (e.g., potential resistance mechanisms)?
- What alternative therapy or appropriate combination can address the resistance mechanisms?

Ideally, data should be collected at each individual stage of the audit trail illustrated in Fig. 1.7. Failure to achieve appropriate drug exposure or modulation of the desired target, pathway, or biological effect means that the project may be at risk. A solution to the problem may simply require altering the dose or schedule of drug administration. Alternatively, it may involve refining the compound or drug structure. Most seriously, if the desired endpoints cannot be met, a "no go" decision may be made leading to termination of the project. Thus, by using the audit trail, the serious problem of late-stage attrition can be minimized. It is also important to emphasize that this approach supports the development of molecular cancer therapeutics in hypothesis-testing clinical trials. In situations where the outcome is successful in that the target is modulated and the drug is therapeutically active, the audit trail allows the results to be interpreted in a mechanistic and informed fashion. On the other hand, where target modulation is seen but no therapeutic effects are observed, this is likely to indicate that the molecular target is not valid in the human cancer under study. If the target is not inhibited, then no mechanistic conclusions may be drawn until a better drug candidate is produced.

Prognostic, mechanism-of-action, or pharmacodynamic biomarkers may become readily apparent from a prior understanding of the molecular target and cognate pathway. Alternatively, the unbiased discovery of biomarkers can be facilitated by the use of high-throughput genomic and proteomic methods [78,111]. Western blotting and ELISA-based immunoassays are often used, the latter having the advantage of accurate quantitation. This is extremely important as knowledge of the extent and duration of target modulation is often lacking. It is especially useful if these assays can operate in multiplex mode. In this way, the effects on multiple molecular targets or several pathways, including both on-target and off-target changes, can be determined. Immunohistochemistry is used quite extensively in clinical trials, as in the case of kinase inhibitors [218]. However, considerable care is required to check that the antibodies used have the necessary specificity, to ensure that the stability of the epitope is maintained (especially for protein phosphorylation endpoints) and to guarantee optimal, robust, and reproducible assay conditions [219]. Biomarkers clearly need to undergo rigorous validation, not only in terms of their scientific suitability but also from the point of view of accuracy, reproducibility, and robustness, and taking into account the regulatory approval perspective.

Barriers to the use of biomarker endpoints for decision making in early clinical trials of cancer drugs may result from ethical and logistic reasons [98,217]. In particular, the need for pre- and post-treatment biopsies for pharmacodynamic biomarkers is very demanding and may limit recruitment to trials. Surrogate tissues such as skin, hair follicles, and peripheral blood mononuclear cells may provide a useful guide but do not necessarily behave in the same way as the cancer. Circulating tumor cells can be used for biomarker studies [220]. Soluble, secreted biomarkers can also be assessed in the plasma. The development of minimally invasive endpoints that use technologies such as positron emission tomography and nuclear magnetic spectroscopy or imaging is very important [102]. The availability of minimally invasive biosensor technology has exciting potential for the future [221].

It is already clear that the selection of the most appropriate patients to enter clinical trials for a particular drug, based on biomarkers showing the presence and status of the molecular target, can dramatically enhance the clinical development process. This is evidenced by the rapid approvals of vemurafenib and crizotinib, along with their companion diagnostic tests, for well-defined patient populations where the drugs offer significant benefits [25,26]. It is expected that the use of biomarkers will grow and that pharmacokinetic–pharmacodynamic relationships will inform clinical trial activities.

There will be continuing developments in other aspects of clinical trial design, for both early- and late-phase trials [98,222–224]. There are significant differences between phase I trial designs for cytotoxic agents versus the new molecularly targeted agents. Escalation to the maximum tolerated dose may not always be appropriate with the new targeted drugs. Although tumor shrinkage can be seen with some molecular cancer therapeutics, they tend to be cytostatic rather than cytotoxic. Hence, the use of response rates by RECIST criteria (Response Evaluation Criteria in Solid Tumors) in the phase II setting may not always be optimal. Randomized discontinuation trials have proved informative in some cases. In addition to differences in assessing the tumor, it is also clear that different side effects are seen with the new molecular therapeutic agents compared to the old cytotoxics, often involving nonproliferating tissues [225]. Another key area for clinical trials will be to address drug combinations. Better computational and laboratory methods to predict effective combinations are needed, as are more creative ways to run the trials [41].

CONCLUSIONS AND OUTLOOK: TOWARD INDIVIDUALIZED MOLECULAR CANCER MEDICINE

Small-molecule targeted cancer drugs like imatinib, gefitinib, erlotinib, vemurafenib, crizotinib, and others discussed in this chapter provide clear proof of concept that clinical benefit can be obtained by developing drugs that act on particular oncogenic abnormalities. Over the past 15 years, we have moved from a concentration on cytotoxic agents that damage DNA and block proliferation in other ways that generally do not confer selectivity toward malignant cells to a new focus on molecular targets linked to the genetic and epigenetic abnormalities that propel cells into and through the process of malignant transformation and progression [1,3,6]. Drugging the cancer genome is now a reality, albeit that we are still in the early stages. The growing pharmacopeia of molecularly targeted agents, listed in Table 1.1, is without doubt benefiting patients through extending lives and improving quality of life. On the other hand, although the importance and usefulness of the molecularly targeted approach are now well established, cancer is still a formidably complicated disease, the treatments are far from optimal, and many obstacles remain to be overcome—particularly drug resistance due to clonal heterogeneity and biochemical feedback loops [41].

There is ongoing debate over the effectiveness of the molecularly targeted approach, and how the paradigm can be improved to meet the major challenges, whether scientific or economic, of the future [40,226,227]. The underpinning feature that enables the development of the hallmark traits of cancer cells is genetic instability [121]. Given this, in retrospect it may seem naïve to have expected that precisely targeting singular genetic changes would lead to lasting effects on the disease. The genetic abnormalities driving the progression of cancer are unlikely to remain constant over time in a given patient. The picture is therefore one of groups of moving targets—both as part of the natural history of untreated disease and in response to therapeutic intervention.

One way forward in the face of this complex reality is already apparent and involves a more adaptive view of the design, discovery, and delivery of targeted treatments [41,77]. By understanding and anticipating the routes to resistance that genetic instability, clonal heterogeneity, and clonal evolution provide for cancer cells, we may seek to develop diagnostic and treatment regimes that can tackle the complexity and mutability of the underlying drivers of the disease. It is also obvious that the development of molecularly targeted therapies does not take place in isolation. Drugs with systemic distribution are essential for treating disseminated and metastatic cancer, and new-targeted agents are often first approved in patients with advanced disease where several lines of prior therapy have failed (see footnotes to Table 1.1). However, earlier, more localized disease is often highly controllable and even curable through surgery and radiotherapy. Combinations of targeted agents with these modes of treatment, either simultaneously or as adjuvants in a therapeutic regime, may further enhance the treatment of a wide range of cancers [228,229].

It is clear that new molecular targets will continue to emerge from the increasingly high-throughput analysis of human cancers and model organisms. A particular challenge is the recognition that there are many molecular abnormalities that occur in relatively small numbers of cancers, and a second challenge is that many of these abnormalities, as well as the more common ones, are often found in multiples together within the same cancer [230]. Moreover, a deeper understanding of the clonal evolutionary processes in cancer has shown how diverse the molecular characteristics may be in a single patient's tumor burden across both the primary and metastatic sites, and how they change over time and in response to therapeutic intervention [78,106]. It remains unclear the extent to which many of these targets will need to be drugged individually or the degree to which the diverse genetics of human cancers will converge on a smaller number of druggable pathways. Certainly, decisions will need to be made about priorities, and in this chapter we have described various ways of looking at this issue. Whereas in the discovery of the first wave of molecular cancer therapeutics, the selection of molecular targets, inevitably, followed the genes and pathways of current interest (and fashion) that were championed in the scientific community, the technologies now available for molecular profiling make it possible to run very large unbiased screens. The application of these high-throughput methodologies will accelerate the elucidation of all of the potential targets, and the improved technologies will empower the molecular detection, classification, monitoring, treatment, and potentially prevention of cancer.

With respect to functional classes of target, drugging the cancer kinome in terms of single kinases or groups of closely related kinase isoforms is now quite readily achievable [231]. The next challenge will be to improve the selection of rational combinations of kinase inhibitors to prevent the emergence of resistant disease, or to refine the sequential application of kinase inhibitors in a treatment regime to prolong the time before untreatable resistance arises [41,232]. A large number of drugs targeting the PI3K signaling pathway or the HSP90 molecular chaperone are in late-phase clinical trials and show potential for the near future [233,234]. Progress into the clinic has been made with drugs against epigenetic targets such as HDACs and DNA methyl transferases, while inhibitors of histone methyl transferases and of the chromatin-reading bromodomain 4 (BRD4) have been identified [124].

However, certain other target types, especially many protein–protein interactions and certain enzymes such as phosphatases, have thus far remained difficult or intractable with existing technologies. Nevertheless, certain small-domain protein–protein interactions have been rendered druggable, as exemplified by the success with BH3 mimetics such as ABT-737 and navitoclax [213] and with nutlin MDM2-binding agents [235]. Phosphatase inhibitors have also been identified [140]. Difficult-to-drug transcription factor pathways, such as the Wnt/alpha-catenin pathway, have succumbed to the identification of new targets involved in the network, such as the tankyrase enzymes that offer more likelihood of successful small-molecule inhibition [165].

As the list of cancer genes and targets continues to grow, we must develop improved methods for their validation and prioritization, since better target selection should lead to better drugs [83]. The use of high-throughput RNAi methods is clearly proving to be very powerful for target discovery and validation. However, removal of the target does not necessarily give the same effect as inhibition by a small molecule, whereas dominant negative constructs and pharmacological inhibition with probe compounds may have advantages [74,76]. Genetically modified mouse models can be very valuable. Although these do not always mimic precisely the human disease, continuing refinements are improving their predictive power. Exploiting oncogene dependence and addiction will continue to be important, but greater emphasis on achieving synthetic lethal effects, as seen with PARP inhibitors in cancer cells and patients with *BRCA* gene defects [129], or on targeting non-oncogene addiction to stress survival pathways [79], is clearly warranted. In order that cancer can be attacked at the level of all of its malignant phenotypic manifestations, drugs acting on targets that regulate each of these traits are needed. Mechanism-based antiangiogenic small molecules and antibodies are now well established. Mechanism-based apoptosis-inducing drugs have entered clinical trials [214]. Telomerase inhibitors show potential for blocking immortalization [236]. However, there are still relatively few approaches to specifically block invasion and metastasis, and this area warrants greater investment. The identification of the premetastatic niche and the conditioning of the host stromal environment to facilitate the establishment of new sites of tumor growth have provided new suggestions for pathways and receptors to target in order to inhibit metastasis and invasion [237]. However, clinical endpoints for such agents are problematic. Matrix metalloproteinase inhibitors were developed clinically without sufficient consideration of their mechanism of action and biological effects on invasion, and this may explain, at least in part, their poor performance [238]. Clinical evaluation of targeted antimetastasic agents is even more challenging as the trials needed to demonstrate efficacy would have a very long timescale. A way forward is needed to trial such agents, as metastasis is the major cause of death from cancer.

Turning to developments in medicinal chemistry, there is no doubt that the quality of the chemical leads that are now identified for optimization against new targets has improved very much as a result of the recognition of drug-like and lead-like chemical characteristics. The use of high-throughput, multiparameter profiling now allows us to anticipate potential issues, such as metabolism and toxicity, that can then be addressed earlier in the lead optimization process than was the case in the past. A more "holistic" view of preclinical discovery increases success in the extremely sophisticated task of seeking to optimize a large number of different pharmaceutical properties and biological activities into a single molecular entity. The use of chemical biology methods, X-ray crystallography, and NMR to assist this aim is particularly noteworthy.

As highlighted throughout this chapter, a major challenge to medicinal chemists, biologists, and clinicians alike is that we now know for sure that resistance is still going to be a problem even with our new signaling inhibitors. We also know that there are likely to be several cancer genes or pathways operating within a given cancer. Given these two things, it is clear that combination therapy will be needed for optimal therapeutic effect. Combinations of highly targeted agents can be put together in a logical way, based on the detailed genetic and epigenetic makeup of the individual malignancy, on the spectrum of genotypes identified within the tumor tissue, and on an understanding of the potential mechanisms for resistance to any specific targeted treatment. Such hypothesis-driven approaches are complemented by unbiased large-scale combinatorial screening [41,77]. One challenge for future drug discovery will be to develop very well-tolerated single agents, so that combination with multiple other agents is possible without compromising the therapeutic index. It is clear that multitargeted kinase inhibitors like sorafenib and sunitinib can be useful drugs, probably as a result of hitting several targets. The development of general methods to engineer controlled polypharmacology within a single drug molecule [239] would be highly desirable to address the twin issues of combinatorial target inhibition and tolerability of multicomponent combinations. In addition, agents that modulate specific nodes in pathways that influence multiple downstream targets have considerable potential, most notably the molecular chaperone HSP90 inhibitors [81] or inhibitors of chromatin-modifying enzymes controlling the histone code [124].

It has been argued that the potential of the human genome sequence will best be realized by focusing on signaling pathways, networks, and systems [240]. As we begin to understand more about the complex networks in which cancer genes operate, it seems clear that systems biology approaches will be required, not only to fully understand how these networks function in terms of kinetics, outputs, pathway intersections, feedback and feed-forward loops, and so on, but also to figure out where best to perturb them for maximal therapeutic benefit [241]. Systems engineering logic tells us once again that combinatorial approaches are likely to be needed to overcome network robustness [242]. The computational power and bioinformatics resources required to implement a serious and broad-based systems biology approach to drug discovery [240,241] will be considerably greater than the already extensive use of high-throughput "electronic biology" for data mining [243].

As additional areas to be addressed in more detail in the future, a topic of considerable interest is the presence of tumor stem cells, which are potentially capable of repopulating the whole tumor [244]. Recent data on the clonal heterogeneity of tumors have shown that in addition to the competing subclones that make up the bulk of the tumor, each is derived from a genetically distinct cancer stem cell population. Because of this, it will clearly be important, as the stem cells are defined and characterized molecularly, to identify therapeutic targets specific to these cells as well [245]. One of the challenges will be to discover agents that ideally would act on the tumor stem cells without unduly affecting normal stem cells.

Although there are tremendous challenges ahead, we have the privilege to be working in cancer drug discovery during what surely must be its most exciting era. It has been proposed that it should be an achievable scientific goal to identify a chemical probe for every protein encoded by the genome [246]. The therapeutic equivalent of that goal in cancer is to develop a molecularly targeted drug for each of the individual oncogenic proteins that are encoded by the cancer genome, or at least for all of the key oncogenic pathways. These molecular cancer therapeutics can then be combined to deliver personalized therapies based on the genomic and molecular makeup of individual cancers, and adapted for each patient to respond to changes in the genetic drivers over time and in response to treatment. As this present chapter has emphasized, we increasingly have at our disposal the targets and technologies, and we are beginning to build up the treatments. The ability to sequence a human genome for less than US$1 million was reported in 2007 [247], and by 2010 the $3 \times 10^{9^9}$ base pairs of the whole human genome could be sequenced for less than US$50,000 [248]. By 2012, the cost had reduced to approximately US$7700 (less than 10 cents per megabase of sequence) (see http://www.genome.gov/sequencingcosts) [249]; and the $1000 genome is clearly within sight, bringing the prospects for bespoke treatments and prevention based on genome sequencing a step closer.

The integrated application of all the information and tools that are available for drug discovery, development, and clinical use is crucial for success. Teamwork is also an essential and potentially the most important ingredient. The challenges ahead for cancer drug discovery—technical, clinical, and societal (in the case of the last, e.g., the questions of who pays for the expensive development process for cancer drugs, how do drugs get developed for rare cancers, and how to bridge the gap between scientific innovation and translation to the clinic)—will require coordinated action by academia, government, and industry so that patients can benefit fully from the potential benefits of exploiting the cancer genome for personalized cancer medicine.

DISCLOSURE

The authors have, or have had, collaborative or commercial relationships with Antisoma, Astex Pharmaceuticals, AstraZeneca, Caliper Life Sciences, Cancer Research Technology Ltd, Chroma Therapeutics, Cyclacel Pharmaceuticals, Genentech, Merck Serono, Nextech Invest, Novartis, Piramed Pharma (acquired by Roche), Sareum Ltd, Vernalis Ltd, and Yamanouchi (now Astellas).

Acknowledgments

The authors' work in the Cancer Research UK Cancer Therapeutic Unit (http://www.icr.ac.uk/research/research_divisions/Cancer_Therapeutics/index.shtml) is supported primarily by Cancer Research UK program grant number C309/A11566 and by The Institute of Cancer Research. Paul Workman is a Cancer Research UK Life Fellow. We thank our colleagues in the Unit and The Institute of Cancer Research and our many external collaborators for valuable discussions.

References

[1] Workman P. Drugging the cancer kinome: progress and challenges in developing personalised molecular cancer therapeutics. Cold Spring Harb Symp Quant Biol 2005;70:499–515.

[2] Yap TA, Workman P. Exploiting the cancer genome: strategies for the discovery and clinical development of targeted molecular therapeutics. Annu Rev Pharmacol Toxicol 2012;52:549–73.

[3] Collins I, Workman P. New approaches to molecular cancer therapeutics. Nat Chem Biol 2006;2:689–700.

[4] Hoelder S, Clark PA, Workman P. Discovery of small molecule cancer drugs: successes, challenges and opportunities. Mol Oncol 2012;6:155–76.

[5] Chabner BA, Roberts TG. Chemotherapy and the war on cancer. Nat Rev Cancer 2005;5:65–72.

[6] Workman P. Genomics and the second golden era of cancer drug development. Mol BioSyst 2005;1:17–26.

[7] Rowinsky EK, Onetto N, Canetta RM, Arbuck SG. Taxol: the first of the taxanes, an important new class of antitumour agents. Semin Oncol 1992;19:646–92.

[8] Colvin OM. An overview of cyclophosphamide development and clinical applications. Curr Pharm Des 1999;5:555–60.

[9] Marsham PR, Wardleworth JM, Boyle FT, Hennequin LF, Kimbell R, Brown M, et al. Design and synthesis of potent non-polyglutamatable quinazoline antifolate thymidylate synthase inhibitors. J Med Chem 1999;42:3809–20.

[10] Varmus H, Trimble EL. Integrating cancer control into global health. Sci Transl Med 2011;3:101cm28.

[11] Pezaro CJ, Mukherji D, De Bono JS. Abiraterone acetate: redefining hormone treatment for advanced prostate cancer. Drug Discov Today 2012;17:221–6.

[12] Pegram MD, Pienkowski T, Northfelt DW, Eiermann W, Patel R, Fumoleau P, et al. Results of two open-label, multicenter phase II studies of docetaxel, platinum salts, and trastuzumab in HER2-positive advanced breast cancer. J Natl Cancer Inst 2004;96:759–69.

[13] Stern HM. Improving treatment of HER2-positive cancers: opportunities and challenges. Sci Transl Med 2012;4:127rv2.

[14] Sawyers CL. Opportunities and challenges in the development of kinase inhibitor therapy for cancer. Genes Dev 2003;17:2998–3010.

[15] Kamb A, Wee S, Lengauer C. Why is cancer drug discovery so difficult? Nat Rev Drug Discov 2007;6:115–20.

[16] Kaelin W G Jr. Gleevec: prototype or outlier? Sci STKE 2004;12:225.

[17] Lahaye T, Riehm B, Berger U, Paschka P, Muller MC, Kreil S, et al. Response and resistance in 300 patients with BCR-ABL-positive leukemias treated with imatinib in a single center: a 4.5-year follow-up. Cancer 2005;103:1659–69.

[18] Bixby D, Talpaz M. Seeking the causes and solutions to imatinib-resistance in chronic myeloid leukaemia. Leukaemia 2011;25:7–22.

[19] Eberhard DA, Johnson BE, Amler LC, Goddard AD, Heldens SL, Herbst RS, et al. Mutations in the epidermal growth factor receptor and in KRAS are predictive and prognostic indicators in patients with non-small-cell lung cancer treated with chemotherapy alone and in combination with erlotinib. J Clin Oncol 2005;23:5900–9.

[20] Lynch TJ, Bell DW, Sordella R, Gurubhagavatula S, Okimoto RA, Brannigan BW, et al. Activating mutations in the epidermal growth factor receptor underlying responsiveness of non-small-cell lung cancer to gefitinib. N Engl J Med 2004;350:2129–39.

[21] Pao W, Chmieleck J. Rational, biologically based treatment of EGFR-mutant non-small-cell lung cancer. Nat Rev Cancer 2010;10:760–74.

[22] Solca F, Dahl G, Zoephel A, Bader G, Sanderson M, Klein C, et al. Target binding properties and cellular activity of afatinib (BIBW 2992), an irreversible ErbB family blocker. J Pharmacol Exp Ther 2012;343:342–50.

[23] Davies H, Bignell GR, Cox C, Stephens P, Edkins S, Clegg S, et al. Mutations of the BRAF gene in human cancer. Nature 2002;417:949–54.

[24] Flaherty KT, Puzanov I, Kim KB, Ribas A, McArthur GA, Sosman JA, et al. Inhibition of mutated, activated BRAF in metastatic melanoma. N Engl J Med 2010;363:809–19.

[25] Bollag G, Tsai J, Zhang J, Zhang C, Ibrahim P, Nolop K, et al. Vemurafenib: the first drug approved for BRAF-mutant cancer. Nat Rev Drug Discov 2012;11:873–86.

[26] Gerber DE, Minna JD. ALK inhibition for non-small cell lung cancer: from discovery to therapy in record time. Cancer Cell 2010;18:548–51.

[27] Soda M, Choi YL, Enomoto M, Takada S, Yamashita Y, Ishikawa S, et al. Identification of the transforming EML4-ALK fusion gene in non-small-cell lung cancer. Nature 2007;448:561–6.

[28] Kwak EL, Bang YJ, Camidge DR, Shaw AT, Solomon B, Maki RG, et al. Anaplastic lymphoma kinase inhibition in non-small-cell lung cancer. N Engl J Med 2010;363:1693–703.

[29] Christensen JG, Zou HY, Arango ME, Li Q, Lee JH, McDonnell SR, et al. Cytoreductive antitumor activity of PF-2341066, a novel inhibitor of anaplastic lymphoma kinase and c-Met, in experimental models of anaplastic large-cell lymphoma. Mol Cancer Ther 2007;6:3314–22.

[30] Shaw AT, Solomon B, Kenudson MM. Crizotinib and testing for ALK. J Natl Compr Canc Netw 2011;9:1335–41.

[31] Felsher DW. Oncogene addiction versus oncogene amnesia: perhaps more than just a bad habit? Cancer Res 2008;68:3081–6.

[32] Weinstein IB. Cancer. Addiction to oncogenes—the Achilles heel of cancer. Science 2002;297:63–4.

[33] Weinstein IB, Joe AK. Oncogene addiction. Cancer Res 2008;68:3077–80.

[34] Ellis LM. Bevacizumab. Nat Rev Drug Discov 2005(Suppl.):S8–9.

[35] Kabbinavar FF, Hambleton J, Mass RD, Hurwitz HI, Bergsland E, Sarkar S. Combined analysis of efficacy: the addition of bevacizumab to fluorouracil/leucovorin improves survival for patients with metastatic colorectal cancer. J Clin Oncol 2005;23:3706–12.

[36] Morphy R. Selectively nonselective kinase inhibition: striking the right balance. J Med Chem 2010;53:1413–37.

[37] Richon VM, Garcia-Vargas J, Hardwick JS. Development of vorinostat: current applications and future perspectives for cancer therapy. Cancer Lett 2009;280:201–10.

[38] Marks PA, Breslow R. Dimethylsulfoxide to vorinostat: development of this histone deacetylase inhibitor as an anticancer drug. Nat Biotechnol 2007;25:84–90.

[39] Olsen EA, Kim YH, Kuzel TM, Pacheco TR, Foss FM, Parker S, et al. Phase IIb multicenter trial of vorinostat in patients with persistent, progressive, or treatment refractory cutaneous T-cell lymphoma. J Clin Oncol 2007;25:3109–15.

[40] Bates S, Amiri-Kordestani L, Giaccone G. Drug development: portals of discovery. Clin Cancer Res 2012;18:23–32.

[41] Al-Lazikani B, Banerji U, Workman P. Combinatorial drug therapy for cancer in the post-genomic age. Nat Biotechnol 2012;30:1–3.

[42] Shah NP, Sawyers CL. Mechanisms of resistance to STI571 in Philadelphia chromosome-associated leukemias. Oncogene 2003;22:7389–7395.

[43] Kujawski L, Talpaz M. Strategies for overcoming imatinib resistance in chronic myeloid leukemia. Leuk Lymphoma 2007;48:2310–22.

[44] Shah NP, Tran C, Lee FY, Chen P, Norris D, Sawyers CL. Overriding imatinib resistance with a novel ABL kinase inhibitor. Science 2004;305:399–401.

[45] Quintas-Cardama A, Kantarjian H, Cortes J. Bosutinib for the treatment of chronic myeloid leukemia in chronic phase. Drugs Today 2012;48:177–88.

[46] Brugger W, Thomas M. EGFR-TKI resistant non-small cell lung cancer (NSCLC): new developments and implications for future treatment. Lung Cancer 2012;77:2–8.

[47] Miller VA, Hirsh V, Cadranel J, Chen YM, Park K, Kim SW, et al. Afatinib versus placebo for patients with advanced, metastatic non-small-cell lung cancer after failure of erlotinib, gefitinib, or both, and one or two lines of chemotherapy (LUX-Lung 1): a phase 2b/3 randomised trial. Lancet Oncol 2012;13:528–38.

[48] Nguyen KS, Kobayashi S, Costa DB. Acquired resistance to epidermal growth factor receptor tyrosine kinase inhibitors in non-small-cell lung cancers dependent on the epidermal growth factor receptor pathway. N Engl J Med 2009;10:281–9.

[49] De Castro DG, Clarke PA, Al-Lazikani B, Workman P. Personalized cancer medicine: molecular diagnostics, predictive biomarkers and drug resistance. Clin Pharmacol Ther 2013;93:252–9.

[50] Regales L, Gong Y, Shen R, de Stanchina E, Vivanco I, Goel A, et al. Dual targeting of EGFR can overcome a major drug resistance mutation in mouse models of EGFR mutant lung cancer. J Clin Invest 2009;119:3000–10.

[51] Choi YL, Soda M, Yamashita Y, Ueno T, Takashima J, Nakajima T, et al. EML4-ALK mutations in lung cancer that confer resistance to ALK inhibitors. N Engl J Med 2010;363:1734–9.

[52] Poulikakos PI, Persaud Y, Janakiraman M, Kong X, Ng C, Moriceau G, et al. RAF inhibitor resistance is mediated by dimerization of aberrantly spliced BRAF (V600E). Nature 2011;480:387–90.

[53] Alcala AM, Flaherty KT. BRAF inhibitors for the treatment of metastatic melanoma: clinical trials and mechanisms of resistance. Clin Cancer Res 2012;18:33–9.

[54] Poulikakaos PI, Rosen N. Mutant BRAF melanomas – dependence and resistance. Cancer Cell 2011;19:11–5.

[55] Su F, Viros A, Milagre C, Trunzer K, Bollag G, Spleiss O, et al. RAS mutations in cutaneous squamous-cell carcinomas in patients treated with BRAF inhibitors. N Engl J Med 2012;366:207–15.

[56] Downward J. Targeting RAF: trials and tribulations. Nat Med 2011;17:286–8.

[57] Jain RK, Duda DG, Clark JW, Loeffler JS. Lessons from phase III clinical trials on anti-VEGF therapy for cancer. Nat Clin Pract Oncol 2006;3:24–40.

[58] Dienstmann R, Ades F, Saini KS, Metzger-Filho O. Benefit-risk assessment of bevacizumab in the treatment of breast cancer. Drug Saf 2012;35:15–25.

[59] Giamas G, Man YL, Hirner H, Bischof J, Kramer K, Khan K, et al. Kinases as targets in the treatment of solid tumors. Cell Signal 2010;22:984–1002.

[60] Dasanau CA, Padmanabhan P, Clark 3rd BA, Do C. Cardiovascular toxicity associated with small molecule tyrosine kinase inhibitors currently in use. Expert Opin Drug Saf 2012;11:445–57.

[61] Force T, Kolaja KL. Cardiotoxicity of kinase inhibitors: the prediction and translation of preclinical models to clinical outcomes. Nat Rev Drug Discov 2011;10:111–26.

[62] Prahallad A, Sun C, Huang S, Di Nicolantonio F, Salazar R, Zecchin D, et al. Unresponsiveness of colon cancer to BRAF(V600E) inhibition through feedback activation of EGFR. Nature 2012;483:100–3.

[63] Komlodi-Pasztor E, Sackett DL, Tito Fojo A. Inhibitors targeting mitosis: tales of how great drugs against a promising target were brought down by a flawed rationale. Clin Cancer Res 2012;18:51–63.

[64] Kola I, Landis J. Can the pharmaceutical industry reduce attrition rates? Nat Rev Drug Discov 2004;3:711–5.

[65] Reichert JM, Wenger JB. Development trends for new cancer therapeutics and vaccines. Drug Discov Today 2008;13:30–7.

[66] DiMasi JA, Grabowski HG. Economics of new drug development. J Clin Oncol 2007;25:209–16.

[67] Kaitin KI, DiMasi JA. Pharmaceutical innovation in the 21st century: new drug approvals in the first decade, 2000–2009. Clin Pharmacol Ther 2011;89:183–8.

[68] Walker I, Newell H. Do molecularly targeted agents in oncology have reduced attrition rates? Nat Rev Drug Discov 2009;8:15–6.

[69] Adams CP, Brantner VW. Estimating the cost of new drug development: is it really $802 million? J Clin Oncol 2006;21:3683–95.

[70] Vernon JA, Golec JH, DiMasi JA. Drug development costs when financial risk is measured using the Fama-French three-factor model. Health Econ 2010;19:1002–1005.

I. BASIC PRINCIPLES AND METHODOLOGY

[71] Kassel DB. Applications of high-throughput ADME in drug discovery. Curr Opin Chem Biol 2004;8:339–45.

[72] Arrowsmith J. Phase II failures: 2008–2010. Nat Rev Drug Discov 2011;10:328–9.

[73] Benson JD, Chen YN, Cornell-Kennon SA, Dorsch M, Kim S, Leszczyniecka M, et al. Validating cancer drug targets. Nature 2006;441:451–6.

[74] Kaelin WG. Use and abuse of RNAi to study mammalian gene function. Science 2012;337:412–22.

[75] Knight ZA, Shokat KM. Chemical genetics: where genetics and pharmacology meet. Cell 2007;128:425–30.

[76] Workman P, Collins I. Probing the probes: fitness factors for small molecule tools. Chem Biol 2010;17:561–77.

[77] De Palma M, Hanahan D. The biology of personalized cancer medicine: facing individual complexities underlying hallmark capabilities. Mol Oncol 2012;6:111–27.

[78] Lee AJX, Swanton C. Tumour heterogeneity and drug resistance: personalising cancer medicine through functional genomics. Biochem Pharmacol 2012;83:1013–20.

[79] Luo J, Solimini NL, Elledge SJ. Principles of cancer therapy: oncogene and non-oncogene dependence. Cell 2009;136:823–37.

[80] Basu B, Yap TA, Molife LR, de Bono JS. Targeting the DNA damage response in oncology: past, present and future perspectives. Curr Opin Oncol 2012;24:316–24.

[81] Travers J, Sharp S, Workman P. HSP90 inhibition: two-pronged exploitation of cancer dependencies. Drug Discov Today 2012;17:242–52.

[82] Lizardi PM, Forloni M, Wajapeyee N. Genome-wide approaches for cancer gene discovery. Trends Biotechnol 2011;29:558–68.

[83] Patel MN, Halling-Brown MD, Tym JE, Workman P, Al-Lazikani B. Objective assessment of cancer genes for drug discovery. Nat Rev Drug Discov 2013;12:35–50.

[84] Begley CG, Ellis LM. Drug development: raise standards for preclinical cancer research. Nature 2012;483:531–3.

[85] Becher OJ, Holland EC. Genetically engineered models have advantages over xenografts for preclinical studies. Cancer Res 2006;66:3355–9.

[86] Kamb A. What's wrong with our cancer models? Nat Rev Drug Discov 2005;4:161–5.

[87] Sausville EA, Burger AM. Contributions of human tumour xenografts to anticancer drug development. Cancer Res 2006;66:3351–4.

[88] Workman P, Aboagye EO, Balkwill F, Balmain A, Bruder G, Chaplin DJ, et al. Guidelines for the welfare and use of animals in cancer research. Br J Cancer 2010;102:1555–77.

[89] Tentler JJ, Tan AC, Weekes CD, Jimeno A, Leong S, Pitts TM, et al. Patient-derived tumour xenografts as models for oncology drug development. Nat Rev Clin Oncol 2012;9:338–50.

[90] Gopinathan A, Tuveson DA. The use of GEM models for experimental cancer therapeutics. Dis Model Mech 2008;1:83–6.

[91] Singh M, Murriel CL, Johnson L. Genetically engineered mouse models: closing the gap between preclinical data and trial outcomes. Cancer Res 2012;72:2695–700.

[92] Cook N, Frese KK, Bapiro TE, Jacobetz MA, Gopinathan A, Miller JL, et al. Gamma secretase inhibition promotes hypoxic necrosis in mouse pancreatic ductal adenocarcinoma. J Exp Med 2012;209:437–44.

[93] Olive KP, Jacobetz MA, Davidson CJ, Gopinathan A, McIntyre D, Honess D, et al. Inhibition of Hedgehog signaling enhances delivery of chemotherapy in a mouse model of pancreatic cancer. Science 2009;324:1457–61.

[94] Whitebread S, Hamon J, Bpjanic D, Urban L. In vitro safety pharmacology profiling: an essential tool for successful drug development. Drug Discov Today 2005;10:1421–33.

[95] Ma P, Zemmel R. Value of novelty? Nat Rev Drug Discov 2002;1:571–2.

[96] Roberts TG, Lynch TJ, Chabner BA. The phase III trial in the era of targeted therapy: unravelling the "go or no go" decision. J Clin Oncol 2003;21:3683–95.

[97] Sarker D, Workman P. Pharmacodynamic biomarkers for molecular cancer therapeutics. Adv Cancer Res 2007;96:213–68.

[98] Tan DW, Thomas GV, Garrett MD, Banerji U, de Bono JS, Kaye SB, et al. Biomarker-driven early clinical trials in oncology. Cancer J 2009;15:406–20.

[99] Workman P. Challenges of PK/PD measurements in modern drug development. Eur J Cancer 2002;38:2189–93.

[100] Workman P. How much gets there and what does it do? The need for better pharmacokinetic and pharmacodynamic endpoints in contemporary drug discovery and development. Curr Pharm Des 2003;9:891–902.

[101] Workman P. Auditing the pharmacological accounts for Hsp90 molecular chaperone inhibitors: unfolding the relationship between pharmacokinetics and pharmacodynamics. Mol Cancer Ther 2003;2:131–138.

[102] Workman P, Aboagye EO, Chung Y, Griifiths JR, Hart R, Leach MO, et al. Minimally invasive pharmacokinetic and pharmacodynamic technologies in hypothesis-testing clinical trials of innovative therapies. J Natl Cancer Inst 2006;98:580–98.

[103] Kaelin W G Jr. The concept of synthetic lethality in the context of anticancer therapy. Nat Rev Cancer 2005;5:689–98.

[104] Chan DA, Giaccia AJ. Harnessing synthetic lethal interactions in anticancer drug discovery. Nat Rev Drug Discov 2011;10:351–64.

[105] The Lancet Oncology. The sum is greater than the parts. Lancet Oncol 2010;11:103.

[106] Greaves M. Cancer stem cells: back to Darwin? Semin Cancer Biol 2010;20:65–70.

[107] Gerlinger M, Rowan AJ, Horswell S, Larkin J, Endesfelder D, Gronroos E, et al. Intratumor heterogeneity and branched evolution revealed by multiregion sequencing. N Engl J Med 2012;366:883–92.

[108] Wilmott JS, Tembe V, Howle JR, Sharma R, Thompson JF, Rizos H, et al. Intratumoral molecular heterogeneity in a BRAF-mutant, BRAF inhibitor-resistant melanoma: a case illustrating the challenges for personalized medicine. Mol Cancer Ther 2012;11:2704–8.

[109] Egan JB, Shi CX, Tembe W, Christoforides A, Kurdoglu A, Sinari S, et al. Whole-genome sequencing of multiple myeloma from diagnosis to plasma cell leukemia reveals genomic initiating events, evolution, and clonal tides. Blood 2012;120:1060–6.

[110] Keats JJ, Chesi M, Egan JB, Garbitt VM, Palmer SE, Braggio E, et al. Clonal competition with alternating dominance in multiple myeloma. Blood 2012;120:1067–76.

[111] Dalton WS, Friend SH. Cancer biomarkers – an invitation to the table. Science 2006;312:1165–8.

[112] Clemons PA. Complex phenotypic assays in high-throughput screening. Curr Opin Chem Biol 2004;8:334–8.

[113] Macarron R, Banks MN, Bojanic D, Burns DJ, Cirovic DA, Garyantes T, et al. Impact of high-throughput screening in biomedical research. Nat Rev Drug Discov 2011;10:188–95.

[114] Van Montfort RL, Workman P. Structure-based design of molecular cancer therapeutics. Trends Biotechnol 2009;27:315–28.

[115] Carr RA, Congreve M, Murray CW, Rees DC. Fragment-based lead discovery: leads by design. Drug Discov Today 2009;10:987–92.

[116] Gaulton A, Bellis LJ, Bento AP, Chambers J, Davies M, Hersey A, et al. ChEMBL: a large-scale bioactivity database for drug discovery. Nucleic Acids Res 2012;40:D1100–7.

[117] Halling-Brown MD, Bulusu KC, Patel M, Tym JE, Al-Lazikani B. canSAR: an integrated cancer public translational research and drug discovery resource. Nucleic Acids Res 2012;40:D947–56.

[118] Hopkins AL, Groom CR. The druggable genome. Nat Rev Drug Discov 2002;1:727–30.

[119] Overington JP, Al-Lazikani B, Hopkins AL. How many drug targets are there? Nat Rev Drug Discov 2006;5:993–6.

[120] Collins I, Workman P. Design and development of signal transduction inhibitors for cancer treatment: experience and challenges with kinase targets. Curr Signal Transduct Ther 2006;1:13–23.

[121] Hanahan D, Weinberg RA. The hallmarks of cancer. Cell 2000;100:57–70.

[122] Hanahan D, Weinberg RA. Hallmarks of cancer: the next generation. Cell 2011;144:646–74.

[123] Hodi FS, O'Day SJ, McDermott DF, Weber RW, Sosman JA, Haanen JB, et al. Improved survival with ipilimumab in patients with metastatic melanoma. N Engl J Med 2010;363:711–23.

[124] Popovic R, Licht JD. Emerging epigenetic targets and therapies in cancer medicine. Cancer Discov 2012;2:405–13.

[125] Vogelstein B, Kinzler KW. Cancer genes and the pathways they control. Nat Med 2004;10:789–99.

[126] Varmus H. The new era in cancer research. Science 2006;312:1162–5.

[127] Varmus H, Pao W, Politi K, Podsypanina K, Du YC. Oncogenes come of age. Cold Spring Harb Symp Quant Biol 2006;70:1–9.

[128] Solit DB, Garraway LA, Pratilas CA, Sawai A, Getz G, Basso A, et al. BRAF mutation predicts sensitivity to MEK inhibition. Nature 2006;439:358–62.

[129] Lord CJ, Ashworth A. Targeted therapy for cancer using PARP inhibitors. Curr Opin Pharmacol 2008;8:363–9.

[130] Garraway LA, Widlund HR, Rubin MA, Getz G, Berger AJ, Ramaswamy S, et al. Integrative genomic analyses identify MITF as a lineage survival oncogene amplified in malignant melanoma. Nature 2005;436:117–22.

[131] Tanaka H, Yanagisawa K, Shinjo K, Taguchi A, Maeno K, Tomida S, et al. Lineage-specific dependency of lung adenocarcinomas on the lung development regulator TTF-1. Cancer Res 2007;67:6007–11.

[132] Zhao Y, Liu H, Riker AI, Fodstad O, Ledoux SP, Wilson GL, et al. Emerging metabolic targets in cancer therapy. Front Biosci 2011;16:1844–1860.

[133] Chatterjee-Kishore M, Miller CP. Exploring the sounds of silence: RNAi-mediated gene silencing for target identification and validation. Drug Discov Today 2005;10:1559–65.

[134] Chin L, Hahn WC, Getz G, Meyerson M. Making sense of cancer genomic data. Genes Dev 2011;25:534–55.

[135] Firestein R, Bass AJ, Kim SY, Dunn IF, Silver SJ, Guney I, et al. CDK8 is a colorectal cancer oncogene that regulates beta-catenin activity. Nature 2008;455:547–51.

[136] ICGC, Hudson TJ, Anderson W, Artez A, Barker AD, Bell C, et al. International network of cancer genome projects. Nature 2010;464:993–8.

[137] Dixon J, England P, Lawton G, Machin P, Palmer A. Medcines in the 21st century: the case for a stakeholder corporation. Drug Discov Today 2010;15:700–3.

[138] Norman T, Edwards A, Bountra C, Friend S. The precompetitive space: time to move the yardsticks. Sci Transl Med 2011:3; 76cm10.

[139] Wilson AJ. Inhibition of protein–protein interactions using designed molecules. Chem Soc Rev 2009;38:3289–300.

[140] Barr AJ. Protein tyrosine phosphatases as drug targets: strategies and challenges of inhibitor development. Future Med Chem 2010;2:1563–76.

[141] Flaherty KT, Infante JR, Daud A, Gonzalez R, Kefford RF, Sosman J, et al. Combined BRAF and MEK inhibition in melanoma with BRAF V600 mutations. N Engl J Med 2012;367:1694–703.

[142] Tsimberidou AM, Chandhasin C, Kurzrock R. Farnesyltransferase inhibitors: where are we now? Expert Opin Investig Drugs 2010;19:1569–80.

[143] Futreal PA, Coin L, Marshall M, Down T, Hubbard T, Wooster R, et al. A census of human cancer genes. Nat Rev Cancer 2004;4:177–83.

[144] Lappano R, Maggiolini M. G protein-coupled receptors: novel targets for drug discovery in cancer. Nat Rev Drug Discov 2011;10:47–60.

[145] Sekulic A, Migden MR, Oro AE, Dirix L, Lewis KD, Hainsworth JD, et al. Efficacy and safety of vismodegib in advanced basal-cell carcinoma. N Engl J Med 2012;366:2171–9.

[146] Robarge KD, Brunton SA, Castanedo GM, Cui Y, Dina MS, Goldsmith R, et al. GDC-0449 – a potent inhibitor of the Hedgehog pathway. Bioorg Med Chem Lett 2009;19:5576–81.

[147] Fauman EB, Rai BK, Huang ES. Structure-based druggability assessment – identifying suitable targets for small molecule therapeutics. Curr Opin Chem Biol 2011;15:463–8.

[148] Li T, Perez-Soler R. Skin toxicities associated with epidermal growth factor receptor inhibitors. Targeted Oncol 2009;4:107–19.

[149] Busaidy NL, Farooki A, Dowlati A, Perentesis JP, Dancey JE, Doyle LA, et al. Management of metabolic effects associated with anticancer agents targeting the PI3K-Akt-mTOR pathway. J Clin Oncol 2012;30:2919–28.

[150] Mann J. Natural products in cancer chemotherapy: past, present and future. Nat Rev Cancer 2002;2:143–8.

[151] Hartford CM, Ratain MJ. Rapamycin: something old, something new, sometimes borrowed and now renewed. Clin Pharmacol Ther 2007;82:381–8.

[152] Goldstein DM, Gray NS, Zarrinkar PP. High-throughput kinase profiling as a platform for drug discovery. Nat Rev Drug Discov 2008;7:391–7.

[153] Wesche H, Xiao S, Young SW. High-throughput screening for protein kinase inhibitors. Comb Chem High Throughput Screen 2005;8:181–95.

[154] McDonald E, Jones K, Brough PA, Drysdale MJ, Workman P. Inhibitors of the HSP90 molecular chaperone: attacking the master regulator in cancer. Curr Top Med Chem 2006;6:1091–107.

[155] McDonald E, Jones K, Brough PA, Drysdale MJ, Workman P. Discovery and development of pyrazole-scaffold Hsp90 inhibitors. Curr Top Med Chem 2006;6:1193–203.

[156] Prien O. Target-family-oriented focused libraries for kinases – conceptual design aspects and commercial availability. ChemBioChem 2005;6:500–5.

[157] Harris CJ, Hill RD, Sheppard DW, Slater MJ, Stouten PF. The design and application of target-focused compound libraries. Comb Chem High Throughput Screen 2011;14:521–31.

[158] Newbatt Y, Burns S, Hayward R, Whittaker S, Kirk R, Marshall C, et al. Identification of inhibitors of the kinase activity of oncogenic V600E BRAF in an enzyme cascade high-throughput screen. J Biomol Screen 2006;11:145–54.

[159] Hardcastle A, Tomlin P, Norris C, Richards J, Cordwell M, Boxall K, et al. A duplexed phenotypic screen for the simultaneous detection of inhibitors of the molecular chaperone heat shock protein 90 and modulators of cellular acetylation. Mol Cancer Ther 2007;6:1112–1122.

[160] Bantscheff M, Drewes G. Chemoproteomic approaches to drug target identification and drug profiling. Bioorg Med Chem 2012;20:1973–8.

[161] Hart CP. Finding the target after screening the phenotype. Drug Discov Today 2005;10:513–9.

[162] Feng Y, Mitchison TJ, Bender A, Young DW, Tallarico JA. Multi-parameter phenotypic profiling: using cellular effects to characterize small-molecule compounds. Nat Rev Drug Discov 2009;8:567–78.

[163] Lundholt BK, Linde V, Loechel F, Pedersen HC, Moller S, Praestegaard M, et al. Identification of Akt pathway inhibitors using redistribution screening on the FLIPR and the IN cell 3000 analyzer. J Biomol Screen 2005;10:20–9.

[164] Kau TR, Schroeder F, Ramaswamy S, Wojciechowski CL, Zhao JJ, Roberts TM, et al. A chemical genetic screen identifies inhibitors of regulated nuclear export of a Forkhead transcription factor in PTEN-deficient tumor cells. Cancer Cell 2003;4:463–76.

[165] Huang SM, Mishina YM, Liu S, Cheung A, Stegmeier F, Michaud GA, et al. Tankyrase inhibition stabilizes axin and antagonizes Wnt signalling. Nature 2009;461:614–20.

[166] Boyd MR, Paull KD. Some practical considerations and applications of the National Cancer Institute in vitro anticancer drug discovery screen. Drug Discov Res 1999;34:91–109.

[167] Park ES, Rabinovsky R, Carey M, Hennessy BT, Agarwal R, Liu W, et al. Integrative analysis of proteomic signatures, mutations, and drug responsiveness in the NCI 60 cancer cell line set. Mol Cancer Ther 2010;9:257–67.

[168] Shoemaker RH. The NCI60 human cancer screen. Nat Rev Cancer 2006;6:813–23.

[169] Lamb J, Crawford ED, Peck D, Modell JW, Blat IC, Wrobel MJ, et al. The connectivity map: using gene-expression signatures to connect small molecules, genes and disease. Science 2006;313:1929–39.

[170] Garnett MJ, Edelman EJ, Heidorn SJ, Greenman CD, Dastur A, Lau KW, et al. Systematic identification of genomic markers of drug sensitivity in cancer cells. Nature 2012;483:570–5.

[171] Barretina J, Caponigro G, Stransky N, Venkatesan K, Margolin AA, Kim S, et al. The Cancer Cell Line Encyclopedia enables predictive modelling of anticancer drug sensitivity. Nature 2012;483:603–7.

[172] Hajduk PJ, Greer J. A decade of fragment-based drug design: strategic advances and lessons learned. Nat Rev Drug Discov 2007;6:211–9.

[173] Donald A, McHardy T, Rowlands MG, Hunter LK, Davies TG, Berdini V, et al. Rapid evolution of 6-phenylpurine inhibitors of protein kinase B through structure-based design. J Med Chem 2007;50:2289–92.

[174] Caldwell JJ, Davies TG, Donald A, McHardy T, Rowlands MG, Aherne GW, et al. Identification of 4-(4-aminopiperidin-1-yl)-7H-pyrrolo[2,3-d]pyrimidines as selective inhibitors of protein kinase B through fragment elaboration. J Med Chem 2008;51:2147–57.

[175] McHardy T, Caldwell JJ, Cheung KM, Hunter LJ, Taylor K, Rowlands M, et al. Discovery of 4-amino-1-(7H-pyrrolo[2,3-d]pyrimidin-4-yl)piperidine-4-carboxamides as selective, orally active inhibitors of protein kinase B (Akt). J Med Chem 2010;53:2239–49.

[176] Davies BR, Greenwood H, Dudley P, Crafter C, Yu DH, Zhang J, et al. Preclinical pharmacology of AZD5363, an inhibitor of AKT: pharmacodynamics, antitumor activity, and correlation of monotherapy activity with genetic background. Mol Cancer Ther 2012;11:873–87.

[177] Cheung KM, Matthews TP, James K, Rowlands MG, Boxall KJ, Sharp SY, et al. The identification, synthesis, protein crystal structure and in vitro biochemical evaluation of a new 3,4-diarylpyrazole class of Hsp90 inhibitors. Bioorg Med Chem Lett 2005;15:3338–43.

[178] Brough PA, Aherne W, Barril X, Borgognoni J, Boxall K, Cansfield JE, et al. 4,5-Diarylisoxazole Hsp90 chaperone inhibitors: potential therapeutic agents for the treatment of cancer. J Med Chem 2008;51:196–218.

[179] Stamos J, Sliwkowski MX, Eigenbrot C. Structure of the epidermal growth factor receptor kinase domain alone and in complex with a 4-anilinoquinazoline inhibitor. J Biol Chem 2002;277:46265–72.

[180] McGovern SL, Caselli E, Grigorieff N, Shoichet BK. A common mechanism underlying promiscuous inhibitors from virtual and high-throughput screening. J Med Chem 2002;45:1712–22.

[181] Baell JB, Holloway GA. New substructure filters for removal of pan assay interference compounds (PAINS) from screening libraries and for their exclusion in bioassays. J Med Chem 2010;53:2719–40.

[182] Rishton GM. Nonleadlikeness and leadlikeness in biochemical screening. Drug Discov Today 2003;8:86–96.

[183] Lipinski CA, Lombardo F, Dominy BW, Feeney PJ. Experimental and computational approaches to estimate solubility and permeability in drug discovery and development settings. Adv Drug Deliv Rev 2001;46:3–26.

[184] Lu JJ, Crimin K, Goodwin JT, Crivori P, Orrenius C, Xing L, et al. Influence of molecular flexibility and polar surface area metrics on oral bioavailability in the rat. J Med Chem 2004;47:6104–6107.

[185] Veber DF, Johnson SR, Cheng HY, Smith BR, Ward KW, Kopple KD. Molecular properties that influence the oral bioavailability of drug candidates. J Med Chem 2002;45:2615–23.

[186] Vieth M, Siegel MG, Higgs RE, Watson IA, Robertson DH, Savin KA, et al. Characteristic physical properties and structural fragments of marketed oral drugs. J Med Chem 2004;47:224–32.

[187] Oprea TI, Davis AM, Teague SJ, Leeson PD. Is there a difference between leads and drugs? A historical perspective. J Chem Inf Comput Sci 2001;41:1308–15.

[188] Lumley JA. Compound selection and filtering in library design. QSAR Comb Sci 2005;24:1066–75.

[189] Park C, Bruncko M, Adickes J, Bauch J, Ding H, Kunzer A, et al. Discovery of an orally bioavailable small molecule inhibitor of prosurvival B-cell lymphoma 2 proteins. J Med Chem 2008;51:6902–15.

[190] Cheng T, Li Q, Zhou Z, Wang Y, Bryant SH. Structure-based virtual screening for drug discovery: a problem-centric review. AAPS J 2012;14:133–41.

[191] Ripphausen P, Nisius B, Bajorath J. State-of-the-art in ligand-based virtual screening. Drug Discov Today 2011;16:372–6.

[192] Foloppe N, Fisher LM, Howes R, Potter A, Robertson AG, Surgenor AE. Identification of chemically diverse Chk1 inhibitors by receptor-based virtual screening. Bioorg Med Chem 2006;14:4792–802.

[193] Lyne PD, Kenny PW, Cosgrove DA, Deng C, Zabludoff S, Wendoloski JJ, et al. Identification of compounds with nanomolar binding affinity for checkpoint kinase-1 using knowledge-based virtual screening. J Med Chem 2004;47:1962–8.

[194] Hopkins AL, Groom CR, Alex A. Ligand efficiency: a useful metric for lead selection. Drug Discov Today 2004;9:430–1.

[195] Andricopulo AD, Montanari CA. Structure–activity relationships for the design of small-molecule inhibitors. Mini Rev Med Chem 2005;5:585–93.

[196] Jamieson C, Moir EM, Rankovicz Z, Wishart G. Medicinal chemistry of hERG optimizations: highlights and hang-ups. J Med Chem 2006;49:5029–46.

[197] Davis AM, Keeling DJ, Steele J, Tomkinson NP, Tinker AC. Components of successful lead generation. Curr Top Med Chem 2005;5:421–39.

[198] Smith NF, Hayes A, James K, Nutley BP, McDonald E, Henley A, et al. Preclinical pharmacokinetics and metabolism of a novel diaryl pyrazole resorcinol series of heat shock protein 90 inhibitors. Mol Cancer Ther 2006;5:1628–37.

[199] Smith NF, Raynaud FI, Workman P. The application of cassette dosing for pharmacokinetic screening in small-molecule cancer drug discovery. Mol Cancer Ther 2007;6:428–40.

[200] Lainchbury M, Matthews TP, McHardy T, Boxall KJ, Walton MI, Eve PD, et al. Discovery of 3-alkoxyamino-5-(pyridin-2-ylamino)pyrazine-2-carbonitriles as selective, orally bioavailable CHK1 inhibitors. J Med Chem 2012;55:10229–40.

[201] Yap TA, Sandhu SK, Workman P, de Bono JS. Envisioning the future of early anticancer drug development. Nat Rev Cancer 2010;10:514–23.

[202] Capdeville R, Buchdunger E, Zimmerman J, Matter A. Glivec (ST571, imatinib), a rationally developed, targeted anticancer drug. Nat Rev Drug Discov 2002;1:493–502.

[203] Judson I. Gastrointestinal stromal tumours (GIST): biology and treatment. Ann Oncol 2002;13:287–9.

[204] Lowinger TB, Riedl B, Dumas J, Smith RA. Design and discovery of small molecules targeting Raf-1 kinase. Curr Pharm Des 2002;8:2269–78.

[205] Strumberg D. Preclinical and clinical development of the oral multikinase inhibitor sorafenib in cancer. Drugs Today (Barcelona) 2005;41:773–84.

[206] Tsai J, Lee JT, Wang W, Zhang J, Cho H, Mamo S, et al. Discovery of a selective inhibitor of oncogenic B-Raf kinase with potent antimelanoma activity. Proc Natl Acad Sci U S A 2008;105:3041–6.

[207] Yang H, Higgins B, Kolinsky K, Packman K, Go Z, Iyer R, et al. RG7204 (PLX4032), a selective BRAF^{V600E} inhibitor, displays potent antitumor activity in preclinical melanoma models. Cancer Res 2010;70:5518–27; correction in 70, 9527.

[208] Banerji U, O'Donnell A, Scurr M, Pacey S, Stapleton S, Asad Y, et al. Phase I pharmacokinetic and pharmaco-dynamic study of 17-allylamino, 17-demethoxygeldanamycin in patients with advanced malignancies. J Clin Oncol 2005;23:4152–61.

[209] Banerji U, Walton M, Raynaud F, Grimshaw R, Kelland L, Valenti M, et al. Pharmacokinetic–pharmacodynamic relationships for the heat shock protein 90 molecular chaperone inhibitor 17-allylamino, 17-demethoxygeldanamycin in human ovarian cancer xenograft models. Clin Cancer Res 2005a;11:7023–7032.

[210] Dymock BW, Barril X, Brough PA, Cansfield JE, Massey A, McDonald E, et al. Novel, potent small-molecule inhibitors of the molecular chaperone Hsp90 discovered through structure-based design. J Med Chem 2005;48:4212–5.

[211] Eccles SA, Massey A, Raynaud FI, Sharp SY, Box G, Valenti M, et al. NVP-AUY922: a novel heat shock protein 90 inhibitor active against xenograft tumor growth, angiogenesis, and metastasis. Cancer Res 2008;68:2850–60.

[212] Sharp SY, Prodromou C, Boxall K, Powers MV, Holmes JL, Box G, et al. Inhibition of the heat shock protein 90 molecular chaperone in vitro and in vivo by novel, synthetic, potent resorcinylic pyrazole/isoxazole amide analogues. Mol Cancer Ther 2007;6:1198–211.

[213] Oltersdorf T, Elmore SW, Shoemaker AR, Armstrong RC, Augeri DJ, Belli BA, et al. An inhibitor of Bcl-2 family proteins induces regression of solid tumours. Nature 2005;435:677–81.

[214] Chongaile TN, Letai A. Mimicking the BH3 domain to kill cancer cells. Oncogene 2008;27:S149–57.

[215] Fry DC. Drug-like inhibitors of protein-protein interactions: a structural examination of effective protein mimicry. Curr Protein Pept Sci 2008;9:240–7.

[216] Petros AM, Dinges J, Augeri DJ, Baumeister SA, Betebenner DA, Bures MG, et al. Discovery of a potent inhibitor of the antiapoptotic protein Bcl-X_L from NMR and parallel synthesis. J Med Chem 2006;49:656–63.

[217] Parelukar WR, Eisenhauer EA. Phase I trial design for solid tumor studies of targeted, non-cytotoxic agents: theory and practice. J Natl Cancer Inst 2004;96:990–7.

[218] Baselga J, Albanell J, Ruiz A, Lluch A, Gascon P, Guillern V, et al. Phase II and tumor pharmacodynamic study of gefitinib in patients with advanced breast cancer. J Clin Oncol 2005;10:5323–33.

[219] Henson DE. Back to the drawing board on immunohistochemistry and predictive factors. J Natl Cancer Inst 2005;97:1796–7.

[220] Attard G, de Bono JS. Utilizing circulating tumor cells: challenges and pitfalls. Curr Opin Genet Dev 2011;21:50–8.

[221] Corrie SR, Fernando GJ, Crichton ML, Brunck ME, Anderson CD, Kendall MA. Surface-modified micro-projection arrays for intradermal biomarker capture, with low non-specific protein binding. Lab Chip 2010;10:2655–8.

[222] Ratain MJ, Eckhardt SG. Phase II studies of modern drugs directed against new targets: if you are fazed, too, then resist RECIST. J Clin Oncol 2004;22:4442–5.

[223] Brunetto AT, Kristeleit RS, de Bono JS. Early oncology clinical trial design in the era of molecular-targeted agents. Future Oncol 2010;6:1339–52.

[224] Scher HI, Nasso SF, Rubin EH, Simon R. Adaptive clinical trial designs for simultaneous testing of matched diagnostics and therapeutics. Clin Cancer Res 2011;17:6634–40.

[225] Molife LR, Alam S, Olmos D, Puglisi M, Shah K, Fehrmann R, et al. Defining the risk of toxicity in phase I oncology trials of novel molecularly targeted agents: a single centre experience. Ann Oncol 2012;23:968–73.

[226] Sams-Dodd F. Is poor research the cause of the declining productivity of the pharmaceutical industry? An industry in need of a paradigm shift. Drug Discov Today 201210.1016/j.drudis.2012.10.010.

[227] Swinney DC, Anthony J. How were new medicines discovered? Nat Rev Drug Discov 2011;10:507–19.

[228] Begg AC, Stewart FA, Vens C. Strategies to improve radiotherapy with targeted drugs. Nat Rev Cancer 2011;11:239–53.

[229] Boere IA, Hamberg P, Sleijfer S. It takes two to tango: combinations of conventional cytotoxics with compounds targeting the vascular endothelial growth factor-vascular endothelial growth factor receptor pathway in patients with solid malignancies. Cancer Sci 2010;101:7–15.

[230] Greenman C, Stephens P, Smith R, Dalgliesh GL, Hunter C, Bignell G, et al. Patterns of somatic mutation in human cancer genomes. Nature 2007;446:153–8.

[231] Zhang J, Yang PL, Gray NS. Targeting cancer with small molecule kinase inhibitors. Nat Rev Cancer 2009;9:28–39.

[232] Janne PA, Gray N, Settleman J. Factors underlying sensitivity of cancers to small-molecule kinase inhibitors. Nat Rev Drug Discov 2009;8:709–23.

[233] Neckers L, Workman P. Hsp90 molecular chaperone inhibitors: are we there yet? Clin Cancer Res 2012;18:64–76.

[234] Yap TA, Garrett MD, Walton MI, Raynaud F, de Bono JS, Workman P. Targeting the PI3K-AKT-mTOR pathway: progress, pitfalls, and promises. Curr Opin Pharmacol 2008;8:393–412.

[235] Vassilev LT, Vu BT, Graves B, Carvajal D, Podlaski F, Filipovic Z, et al. In vivo activation of the p 53 pathway by small-molecule antagonists of MDM2. Science 2004;303:844–88.

[236] Buseman CM, Wright WE, Shay JW. Is telomerase a viable target in cancer? Mutat Res 2012;730:90–7.

[237] Zoccoli A, Iuliani M, Pantano F, Imperatori M, Intagliata S, Vincenzi B, et al. Premetastatic niche: ready for new therapeutic interventions? Expert Opin Ther Targets 2012;16(Suppl. 2):S119–S129.

[238] Zucker S, Cao J, Chen WT. Critical appraisal of the use of matrix metalloproteinase inhibitors in cancer treatment. Oncogene 2000;19:6642–50.

[239] Koutsoukas A, Simms B, Kirchmair J, Bond PJ, Whitmore AV, Zimmer S, et al. From in silico target prediction to multi-target drug design: current databases, methods and applications. J Proteomics 2011;74:2554–74.

[240] Fishman MC, Porter JA. Pharmaceuticals: a new grammar for drug discovery. Nature 2005;437:491–3.

[241] Kitano H. A robustness-based approach to systems-oriented design. Nat Rev Drug Discov 2007;6:202–10.

[242] Fitzgerald JB, Schoeberl B, Nielsen UB, Sorger PK. Systems biology and combination therapy in the quest for clinical efficacy. Nat Chem Biol 2006;2:458–66.

[243] Loging W, Harland L, Williams-Jones B. High throughput electronic biology: mining information for drug discovery. Nat Rev Drug Discov 2007;6:220–9.

[244] Baccelli I, Trumpp A. The evolving concept of cancer and metastasis stem cells. J Cell Biol 2012;198:281–93.

[245] Maitland NJ, Collins AT. Cancer stem cells – a therapeutic target? Curr Opin Mol Ther 2010;12:662–73.

[246] Schreiber SL. Stuart Schreiber: biology from a chemist's perspective. Interview by Joanna Owens. Drug Discov Today 2004;9:299–303.

[247] Wolinsky H. The thousand-dollar genome. Genetic brinkmanship or personalized medicine? EMBO Rep 2007;8:900–3.

[248] Bonetta L. Whole-genome sequencing breaks the cost barrier. Cell 2010;141:917–9.

[249] Shendure J, Aiden EL. The expanding scope of DNA sequencing. Nat Biotechnol 2012;30:1084–94.

[250] Gelmon KA, Eisenhauer EA, Harris AL, Ratain MJ, Workman P. Anticancer agents targeting signaling molecules and the cancer cell environment: challenges for drug development? J Natl Cancer Inst 1999;91:1281–7.

Recommended Further Reading

Al-Lazikani B, Banerji U, Workman P. Combinatorial drug therapy for cancer in the post-genomic age. Nat Biotechnol 2012;30:1–3.
A review of approaches using drug combinations to tackle the problems of genetic heterogeneity and drug resistance in personalized cancer medicine.

Benson JD, Chen YN, Cornell-Kennon SA, Dorsch M, Kim S, Leszczyniecka M, et al. Validating cancer drug targets. Nature 2006;441:451–6.
A review containing a systematic categorization of cancer molecular targets and a discussion of the approaches to validating targets prior to, and during, a drug discovery project.

Collins I, Workman P. New approaches to molecular cancer therapeutics. Nat Chem Biol 2006;2:689–700
A review of the application of chemical biology to interconnect stages in the discovery and development of molecularly targeted cancer therapeutics.

Workman P, Collins I. Probing the probes: fitness factors for small molecule tools. Chem Biol 2010;17:561–77
A review of guidelines or "fitness factors" that should be considered to help determine if a particular small-molecule probe is suitable for chemical biology research to elucidate new biology.

Davis AM, Keeling DJ, Steele J, Tomkinson NP, Tinker AC. Components of successful lead generation. Curr Top Med Chem 2005;5:421–39.
A review of good medicinal chemistry practice in the discovery and development of small-molecule therapeutics from high-throughput screening.

Hart CP. Finding the target after screening the phenotype. Drug Discov Today 2005;10:513–9
A review of the experimental approaches used to identify the discrete molecular target(s) of biologically active compounds identified through whole-cell or organismal phenotypic screens.

Lee AJX, Swanton C. Tumour heterogeneity and drug resistance: personalising cancer medicine through functional genomics. Biochem Pharmacol 2012;83:1013–20.
A review of the use of functional genomics technologies in understanding drug resistance and tumor heterogeneity, and the application of this approach to personalized cancer medicine.

Patel MN, Halling-Brown MD, Tym JE, Workman P, Al-Lazikani B, Objective assessment of cancer genes for drug discovery. Nat Rev Drug Discov 2013;12:35–50.
Describes an objective, systematic computational approach to assess biological and chemical space that can be applied to human gene sets to prioritize targets for therapeutic exploration.

Sarker D, Workman P. Pharmacodynamic biomarkers for molecular cancer therapeutics. Adv Cancer Res 2007;96:213–68.

A review of the discovery, validation, and implementation of pharmacodynamic biomarkers in the development and clinical evaluation of molecular cancer therapeutics.

Useful Websites

American Cancer Society, Inc. Cancer Facts and Figures 2012, http://www.cancer.org/acs/groups/content/@epidemiologysurveilance/documents/document/acspc-031941.pdf; 2012.

A report from the American Cancer Society detailing statistical data on cancer incidence, mortality and survival.

The Institute of Cancer Research. CanSAR, https://cansar.icr.ac.uk; 2012.

Entry point to an integrated database that brings together biological, chemical, pharmacological (and eventually clinical) data, in order to help with hypothesis generation in cancer research and to support translational research.

Thompson Centerwatch. Drugs approved by FDA, http://www.centerwatch.com/patient/drugs/druglist.html; 2012.

A list of drugs approved by the US F.D.A., ordered by year and therapeutic class.

U. S. Center for Disease Control. National Vital Statistics Report, http://www.cdc.gov/nchs/data/nvsr/nvsr61/nvsr61_06.pdf; 2012.

A preliminary report of data on causes of death in the USA for 2011.

U. S. Food and Drug Administration. Drugs@FDA, http://www.accessdata.fda.gov/scripts/cder/drugsatfda/; 2012.

Entry point to Drugs@FDA, a searchable database of the approval process for small molecule and biological therapeutics, including data submitted to support regulatory approval.

U. S. National Cancer Institute. NCI-60 in vitro anticancer screen, http://dtp.nci.nih.gov/docs/compare/compare_intro.html; 2012.

Entry point to a searchable relational data base (COMPARE) on the sensitivity to >100,000 drugs and compounds that have been screened against the NCI-60 human tumor cell line panel. Also included is a wealth of genomic, molecular and biochemical data on the same panel, allowing correlations to be made with computational tools also available on these Websites.

U. S. National Human Genome Research Institute. U. S. National Institutes of Health DNA Sequencing Costs, http://www.genome.gov/sequencingcosts; 2012.

The National Human Genome Research Institute (NHGRI) tracks the costs associated with DNA sequencing performed at the sequencing centers funded by the Institute.

Wellcome Trust and Massachusetts General Hospital Cancer Center. Genomics of Drug Sensitivity in Cancer Project, http://www.cancerrxgene.org; 2012.

Compounds, including cytotoxic chemotherapeutics as well as targeted therapeutics from commercial sources, academic collaborators, and from the biotech and pharmaceutical industries, are screened against >1000 genetically characterized human cancer cell lines, and the sensitivity patterns are correlated with genomic and expression data.

Wellcome Trust Sanger Institute Cancer Genome Project. Cancer Gene Census, http://www.sanger.ac.uk/genetics/CGP/Census; 2012.

An ongoing effort to catalog those genes for which mutations have been causally implicated in cancer.

2

Pharmacogenomics and Personalized Medicines in Cancer Treatment

Wei-Peng Yong[1,2], Ross Soo[1,2], Federico Innocenti[3,4]

[1]Department of Hematology–Oncology, National University Health System, Singapore
[2]Cancer Science Institute of Singapore, Singapore [3]Eshelman School of Pharmacy, Institute for Pharmacogenomics and Individualized Therapy, University of North Carolina, Chapel Hill, NC, USA [4]Linerberger Comprehensive Cancer Center, School of Medicine, University of North Carolina, Chapel Hill, NC, USA

INTRODUCTION

We have long recognized that individuals respond differently to the same drug. In simplistic terms, for any given treatment, there are four broad therapeutic response phenotypes: responders with minimal toxicity, responders with severe toxicity, nonresponders with minimal toxicity, and nonresponders with severe toxicity. The host, tumoral, and extrinsic factors influence how an individual responds to an anticancer drug.

Pharmacogenomics seeks to identify and establish the relationship between genetic variants and drug response. Genetic alteration can occur in genes of the host (germline polymorphisms) or the tumor (somatic mutations). Genetic information from patients can provide an opportunity to individualize therapy guiding drug and dose selection so as to maximize the chance of treatment success and minimize the risk of treatment toxicity.

Genomic markers can be broadly classified as predictive or prognostic. Predictive markers are used to identify individuals most likely to (1) respond to a drug, (2) fail to respond to a drug, and (3) develop adverse events that might require dose modification or selection of an alternative drug. Prognostic markers, on the other hand, are used to predict the clinical course of a given cancer, irrespective of treatment, although they may predict the likelihood of benefiting from treatment based on the risk of cancer relapse. Examples of such prognostic markers include the array-based Mammaprint, Mammostrat, and Oncotype Dx tests that are used to prognosticate early-stage breast cancers and identify individuals whose risk of cancer recurrence is sufficiently high to warrant adjuvant chemotherapy. However, it is beyond the scope of this chapter to cover prognostic genomic markers.

MOLECULAR GENETIC BASIS FOR VARIATION IN DRUG RESPONSE

The earlier pharmacogenomic studies frequently focused primarily on inherited genetic variants of the germline DNA. Over the years, the field of pharmacogenomics has expanded to encompass somatic alterations of the DNA of cancers. The development of drugs targeting specific genomic aberrations in cancer cells has provided an opportunity for the use of genomic biomarkers to identify individuals most likely to benefit from treatment.

Germline Polymorphisms

The human genome comprises about 3×10^9 base pairs of DNA. The most common genetic variations in the human genome are single base pair differences known as single-nucleotide polymorphisms (SNPs), defined as single base variations that occur at a frequency of 1% or higher in the population. It is estimated that there are 10 million SNPs in the human genome. Other types of genetic variations – for example, copy number variations and chromosomal rearrangements (inversions and translocation) – are less common [1].

Most of the variations in the genomic DNA sequences, however, do not affect drug response. The potential impact the genomic variation depends on the location and the nature of the variation. Nonsynonymous variations occurring in the gene-coding regions (exons) that change amino acid sequence are more likely to alter the function of proteins, whereas SNPs located at the noncoding regions are less likely to affect protein function or expression unless they are located within gene splice sites and regulatory regions, respectively. Synonymous variations located in the gene-coding regions were historically thought to be silent, but increasing evidence has suggested these mutations can influence mRNA splicing, mRNA stability, protein conformation, and function [2].

Germline DNA is frequently extracted from peripheral blood monocytes or buccal mucosa cells. Germline variations that change drug response often involve genes that affect the pharmacokinetics of an anticancer drug. Clinically important pharmacogenetic gene–drug pairs include thiopurine methyltransferase (*TPMT*) with 6-mercaptopurine (6-MP), uridine 5′-diphospho-glucuronosyltransferase 1A1 (*UGT1A1*) with irinotecan, and dihydropyrimidine dehydrogenase (*DPYD*) and 5-fluorouracil (5-FU). In each example, variants conferring reduced expression or activity of the coded enzyme have been associated with severe treatment-related toxicity due to increased exposure of either the parent drug or its active metabolites. The relevance of testing these variants to personalized treatment will be discussed in this chapter.

Although germline polymorphisms more commonly influence treatment toxicity, treatment efficacy may be affected as well, either indirectly through changes in drug exposure or directly if SNP changes the function of a target or the mechanism of action of the drug (Table 2.1).

TABLE 2.1 Oncologic Drugs with Germline Pharmacogenomic Biomarkers in US Drug Labels

Drugs	Biomarkers	Responses affected	References
5-FU, capecitabine	DPYD	DPYD deficiency is associated with higher risk of severe stomatitis, diarrhea, neutropenia, and neurotoxicity.	[3]
Irinotecan	UGT1A1	Increased risk of neutropenia in UGT1A1*28/*6 homozygotes	[4–7]
6-Mercaptopurine	TPMT	Increased risk of myelosuppression in homozygous TPMT-deficiency patients. Substantial dose reduction is required. Efficacy may be influenced by 6-MP exposure.	[8–10]
Nilotinib	UGT1A1	Increased risk of hyperbilirubinemia in UGT1A1*28 homozygotes	[11]
Rasburicase	G6PD	Increased risk of hemolytic anemia in G6PD-deficient individuals, induced by hydrogen peroxide produced from the conversion of uric acid to allantoin	[12]
Thioguanine	TPMT	Increased risk of myelosuppression in homozygous-TPMT deficiency patients	[13]

The three gene–drug pairs discussed here represent examples where the genetic variation acts as a monogenic trait. It is typically manifested as a bimodal or multiple distribution of the clinical phenotype. However, most drugs exhibit a unimodal distribution in drug response phenotypes because the variations are influenced by multiple genes that encode for proteins involved in drug absorption, transport, metabolism, elimination, and mechanism of action pathways.

In addition, the drug response phenotype can also be affected by the aggregate effect of multiple polymorphisms that occur together at adjacent loci of a gene, known as a haplotype. The combination of different polymorphisms or alleles that are closely linked is frequently inherited together. Hence, a haplotype can be considered as a functional unit, and each haplotype block, across the genome, may be represented by a marker SNP. This property allows large sections of the genome to be studied using relatively fewer marker SNPs. The use of marker SNPs has enabled genome-wide interrogations of the pattern of common variations in the genome [14].

Somatic Mutation

Cancer is a disease of the genome, with each cancer cell harboring a constellation of genomic alterations. There are substantial heterogeneities in the frequency of base mutations and rearrangements across different tumor types. Heterogeneity in the cancer genome can be observed within the same tumor in the same patient. Similar to germline polymorphisms, genomic variations in cancers include single base mutations, copy number variations, and chromosomal rearrangements. However, structural variations are more extensive compared to normal tissues. Furthermore, unlike germline variations, somatic mutations are not present in normal cells, nor are they inheritable. In addition, these mutations may evolve over time through adaptation or selection. Somatic mutations may have a prognostic role, influencing the aggressiveness and metastatic potential of tumors. Somatic alterations can also have a predictive role: in these cases when such alterations are located in the oncogenes, the cancer cells are "addicted" to the function of such oncogenes, and the oncogenes are the target of therapy [15].

Somatic mutations can functionally be divided into driver and passenger mutations. Most somatic mutations are passenger mutations that do not contribute to cancer development. Embedded amongst the passenger mutations are driver mutations that confer growth or survival advantages in cancer cells [16]. Despite the complexity of the cancer genome, it is estimated that solid tumors such as breast and colon cancers may be dependent on as little as five to seven driver mutations, and the number of driver mutations may even be fewer in hematological malignancies [17,18]. The phenomenon of "oncogene addiction" where cancer cells' growth and survival are overly reliant on one or more aberrantly regulated genes or pathways can be exploited for therapeutic intervention, often achieving dramatic treatment response.

Several large-scale efforts such as the International Cancer Genome Consortium (ICGC), the Cancer Genome Atlas (TCGA), and the Cancer Genome Project (CGP) have been launched to systemically catalog the genome abnormalities in different cancer types. To date, comprehensive genomic information on several cancer types, including breast, brain, colorectal, liver, lung, ovarian, pancreatic, renal, and uterine cancers, has been released. An important goal of these initiatives is to identify genomic aberrations that are potentially targetable or associated with drug resistance, thus enabling a personalized approach to cancer therapy. Analysis of the breast cancer genome has revealed potential targets for specific molecular subtypes of breast cancer [19].

METHODOLOGIES FOR PHARMACOGENOMIC DISCOVERY, VALIDATION, AND IMPLEMENTATION

Advancements in sequencing capability have enabled the shift from studies of single genes or pathways to comprehensive genome-wide discoveries [20]. However, the discovery of genomic biomarkers is only the first step in the long and complex process of translating the pharmacogenomic knowledge into clinical practice. Further development of robust pharmacogenomic tests and demonstration of clinical benefits in relevant patient populations will be required.

Candidate Gene Association Studies

The discovery of genetic determinants of drug response phenotypes is often driven by the clinical observation of variability in drug response. A candidate gene is a gene whose variation is supposed to be associated with a clinical trait such as a drug response phenotype. The first step of a candidate gene association study involves defining the drug response phenotype to be examined. The drug response phenotype is usually a measurable or discernable pharmacodynamic trait. Survival, response rate, toxicity, and ex vivo measurements of endophenotypes (e.g., like enzyme activity) may be used as endpoints to test phenotype–genotype associations. Pharmacokinetic parameters such as drug exposure and metabolite levels are frequently used as phenotypic intermediates (other endophenotypes) for toxicity and response because they can provide intermediate proof-of-principle evidence of a genetic variant associated with a clinical phenotype. The next step in the candidate gene approach is to select the candidate gene and relevant genetic variants based on a priori knowledge of the drug pathway and the biology of the target. The effect of genetic variants can then be studied for association with the phenotype of interest. The main advantage of such a hypothesis-driven approach is that a relatively small sample size could be sufficient to establish a phenotype–genotype association. The limitation of candidate gene association studies is that a level of understanding of the drug response pathway is required in order to identify the candidate genes that may affect drug response; hence, unknown genes may potentially be missed in this approach.

Multiple candidate genes relevant to a drug pathway can be studied together to improve the chance of correctly identifying and assessing the relative predictive value of each genetic determinant of a drug response phenotype. However, the overall statistic power of the study will decrease with the increase in the number of candidate genes studied. Hence, it is important to prioritize and select candidate gene variants most likely to be associated with a drug response phenotype, particularly genetic variants that have been demonstrated to alter the protein function or expression in molecular functional studies, or that are predicted to alter the gene function according to bioinformatics analysis.

Genome-Wide Association Studies (GWASs) and Deep Sequencing

Advances in high-throughput genotyping technology have driven down the cost and time required to survey the whole genome. Unlike the candidate gene approach where prior knowledge of the biological function of a genetic variant is required, genome-wide approaches enable an unbiased screen for novel, common genomic determinant of the drug response phenotype [21].

A common genome-wide scanning method involves identification of marker SNPs across the whole genome to create an SNP map. When an SNP is found to be associated with a drug response phenotype, it does not imply causation but serves as a marker for a region of the genome where novel candidate genes might reside. This is because the SNP chips have been designed to interrogate the haplotypes of the genome, but not necessarily all the functional SNPs. Hence, additional steps have to be taken, including sequencing the locus "marked" by the associated SNP, to identify the causative genetic variant. The development of next-generation sequencing allows scanning of the exome (all the exonic regions of the genome) or the whole genome of individuals, identifying variants at low frequency in the population. GWASs and sequencing-based studies require the use of advanced bioinformatics to handle the large amount of data generated. In addition, the false-positive and false-negative rates are high even after correction for multiple comparisons because of the large number of genetic variants analyzed. A large sample size and functional assays are required to increase the confidence of identifying true causative variants. A solution to this problem is to validate the potential causative genetic variants that are generated from the initial screening sample using an independent sample [22]. Even after a potential genetic variant is identified, there is often little information on its functional implications at the molecular level [23]. It is necessary to further investigate newly discovered genetic variants for their putative effects on gene expression and to establish their functional relevance using knock-in or knock-out cellular models [24].

Clinical Implementation of Pharmacogenomic Tests

The application of pharmacogenomics to personalize treatment has been most successful in guiding the selection of patients most likely to respond to drugs. Its role in dose optimization and toxicity reduction is more limited. Despite the presence of a large body of evidence associating candidate genomic variations with variation in drug response, translation into clinical practice has often lagged behind pharmacogenomic discoveries. Several hurdles need to be overcome before clinical implementation of pharmacogenetic markers might become a reality in routine practice. The Evaluation of Genomic Applications in Practice and Prevention (EGAPP) Initiative has recommended the use of the ACCE Model Process for evaluating genetic tests (ACCE stands for **a**nalytic validity, **c**linical validity, **c**linical utility, and **e**thical, legal, and social implications) [25]. This involved establishing the analytical validity, clinical validity, and clinical relevance or benefit of a pharmacogenomic test in a population defined by the test.

Analytical validation should be performed to ensure the accuracy and reliability of a pharmacogenomic test before clinical introduction of the assay. This is crucial in biomarker-directed studies as a suboptimal or unreliable assay can confound the results of the clinical trials. Extensive analytic validation of pharmacogenomic tests would entail establishing within- and between-laboratory precision, performing replicates using positive and negative controls to ensure reproducibility, as part of a quality control program.

The association of genomic variations with drug response does not necessarily imply usefulness in the clinical setting. An important step toward clinical implementation of a genetic test is to determine its ability to accurately predict (1) the clinical sensitivity, which is the probability that the test will be positive in people who are truly positive (e.g., the percentage of responders who are correctly identified as responders); (2) the clinical specificity, which is the probability that the test will be negative in people who are truly negative (e.g., the percentage of nonresponders who are correctly identified as nonresponders); (3) the positive predictive value, which is the proportion of true positive status in people who tested positive; and (4) the negative predictive value, which is the proportion of true negative status in people who tested negative [25]. Unlike sensitivity and specificity, the positive and negative predictive values of a biomarker are affected by the prevalence of the drug response phenotype it tests.

Ultimately, any pharmacogenomic marker must demonstrate clinical utility in terms of improving treatment outcome before clinical implementation. Ideally, pharmacogenomic biomarkers should be identified and validated prospectively in randomized controlled clinical trials. Unfortunately, it is often not feasible to confirm clinical utility prospectively in a randomized fashion. The validation of the *KRAS* mutation as a negative predictive marker for the efficacy of anti-EGFR (epidermal growth factor receptor) antibodies (cetuximab and panitumumab) was performed retrospectively using banked tumor tissues from completed phase III clinical trials [26,27]. This approach provides an alternative way of establishing the clinical utility of pharmacogenomic markers compared to a new randomized clinical trial. The clinical relevance of pharmacogenomic testing should also be assessed in the context of the target population and its ethnicity, especially when applying data generated from a different population. The allelic frequencies of pharmacogenomic markers can vary substantially among different ethnic populations (see the section on irinotecan and *UGT1A1*). Prospective studies should therefore be performed to determine the performance of the genetic test in populations of different ethnic backgrounds.

Development of Companion Diagnostics

The use of pharmacogenomic biomarkers has triggered a paradigm change in drug development that not all patients will benefit from an investigational drug, and a larger magnitude-of-treatment benefit can be demonstrated using a smaller population enriched by using an appropriate predictive biomarker. Codevelopment of new therapeutics with companion pharmacogenomic biomarkers allowed the accelerated development and approval of crizotinib for *ALK* (anaplastic lymphoma kinase) gene fusion–driven lung cancer and vemurafenib for *BRAF* mutation–positive melanoma together with the corresponding diagnostic tests.

However, the simultaneous approval of new anticancer drugs and companion biomarkers is still in its infancy. Codevelopment of drugs and predictive biomarkers would require that candidate biomarkers be available fairly early in the development of the drug. The appropriate biomarker can come to light only at a late stage of clinical drug development. In such a scenario, bridging studies or retrospective analysis of a predictive biomarker would be required. Using *KRAS* as an example, in 2009 at the US Food and Drug Administration's (FDA) Industry In Vitro Diagnostic (IVD)/Companion Diagnostic Drug Roundtable Meeting, it was proposed that retrospective analysis of pharmacogenomic markers might be considered when the following criteria were met: (1) an adequate, well-conducted, controlled trial or trials; (2) a large sample size that approximates random allocation; (3) genomic status ascertained in a large proportion of randomized subjects; (4) an assay with acceptable analytical performance; and (5) an acceptable, prespecified, powered analysis plan.

CLINICALLY IMPORTANT PHARMACOGENOMIC MARKERS FOR TREATMENT RESPONSE

Clinically Important Germline Markers for Treatment Response

The FDA has approved the inclusion of pharmacogenetic information on the drug label for several anticancer drugs linking germline genomic biomarkers and drug toxicity [28]. Although *CYP2D6* testing has not been included on the tamoxifen drug label, the FDA Advisory Committee had recommended its inclusion in 2006. In this section, we will discuss in detail a few clinically relevant germline pharmacogenomic markers and corresponding anticancer drugs from Table 2.1, including tamoxifen.

6-Mercaptopurine and Thiopurine Methyltransferase

6-MP is an antimetabolite used primarily in the maintenance treatment of childhood acute lymphocytic leukemia. It interferes with DNA and RNA synthesis by inhibiting purine metabolism. The conversion of 6-MP into its inactive metabolites is mediated by TPMT (Fig. 2.1), xanthine oxidase and dehydrogenase, and aldehyde oxidase 1. TPMT is the major inactivating enzyme of 6-MP in hematopoietic tissues where xanthine oxidase activity is negligible.

Red blood cell TPMT activity exhibits a trimodal distribution typical of a monogenic trait and conforms to the Hardy–Weinberg prediction for autosomal codominant inheritance [29]. It is estimated that one in 300 Caucasians and African Americans have two copies of nonfunctional *TPMT* alleles and almost no detectable TPMT activity. Approximately one in 10 will harbor a copy of nonfunctional alleles and has intermediate TPMT activity. Patients with TPMT deficiency accumulate excessive active 6-thioguanine nucleotides when treated with a standard dose of 6-MP and are more likely to develop life-threatening toxicity [8–10]. In homozygous TPMT-deficient patients, a 90% reduction of the standard 6-MP dose is necessary to prevent life-threatening treatment-related toxicity. The treatment efficacy of patients with TPMT deficiency does not appear to be compromised with dose reduction [30]. Conversely, patients with higher TPMT activity are associated with lower 6-thioguanine nucleotide exposure and have a higher risk of relapse [31].

At least 28 *TPMT* polymorphisms have been identified, and many of them have reduced TPMT activity [32]. However, genotyping of the three commonest haplotypes—*TPMT*2* (238G>CA, P240A), *TPMT*3A* (460G>A, A154C, 719A>G, C240Y), and *TPMT*3C* (719A>G, C240Y)—detects about 95% of individuals with low TPMT activity [33]. TPMT protein variants from these haplotypes are prone to enzymatic degradation, resulting in lower catalytic activity [34]. *TPMT*2* and *3* correlated well with red blood cell TPMT activity, with

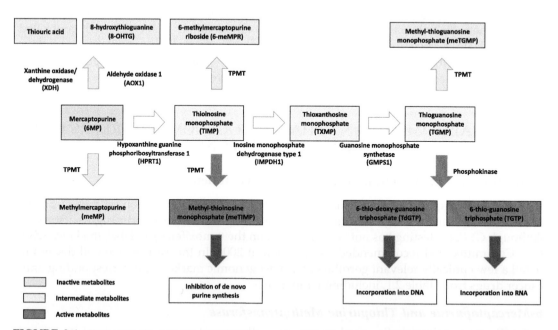

FIGURE 2.1 The metabolic pathways of 6-MP in humans. (This figure is reproduced in color in the color plate section.)

positive and negative predictive values of 94% and 99%, respectively [33]. The benefit of *TPMT* genotyping compared to the measurement of red blood cell *TPMT* activity is that it is not influenced by coadministration of drugs such as nonsteroidal anti-inflammatory drugs (NSAIDs) and diuretics, or recent blood transfusions.

There are significant interethnic variations in the frequencies of the *TPMT* variants. *TPMT*3A* is the most common *TPMT* haplotype (3–6%) in Caucasians. In the East Asian and African populations, *TPMT*3C* is most prevalent (2–8%) [35]. In some Sub-Saharan African populations, *TPMT*8*, a rare nonfunctional allele in Caucasians that is not routinely screened for, is common and accounts for a significant proportion of nonfunctional alleles [36]. This difference highlights that understanding ethnic diversity regarding the frequency of occurrence of *TPMT* variants is crucial for clinical implementation of genotype-based testing in different ethnic populations.

The benefit of using *TPMT* genotyping to customize the starting dose of maintenance 6-MP in leukemia has yet to be demonstrated in a randomized clinical trial. In addition, it is uncertain if the risk of secondary cancers associated with 6-MP in TPMT-deficient patients can be reduced with dose modification [37,38]. Nevertheless, based on the strength of preclinical mechanistic studies and retrospective clinical data, the Clinical Pharmacogenetics Implementation Consortium (CPIC) (http://www.pharmgkb.org/gene/PA356) and the Royal Dutch Pharmacists Association–Pharmacogenetics Working Group have recommended a 90% and 50% reduction in the starting dose of 6-MP in homozygotes and heterozygotes for the inactive alleles, respectively [39].

Irinotecan and Uridine 5′-Diphospho-glucuronosyltransferase 1A1

Irinotecan (CPT-11), a synthetic camptothecin derivative, is commonly used for the treatment of metastatic colorectal and lung cancer. Irinotecan and its active metabolite, SN-38, interfere with the function of topoisomerase I, an enzyme catalyzing single DNA strand breaks and reannealing of DNA strands, allowing the relief of DNA torsion for replication and repair. The binding of irinotecan and SN38 to the topoisomerase I–DNA complex prevents reannealing of DNA, leading to double DNA break and cell death. SN-38 is 100–1000 times more potent than irinotecan [40].

After intravenous administration, irinotecan is inactivated by cytochrome P450 (CYP) enzymes (predominantly CYP3A4) to form 7-ethyl-10-[4-*N*-(5-aminopentanoic acid)-1-piperidino]-carbonyloxy-camptothecin (APC), 7-ethyl-10-(4-amino-1-piperidino)-carbonyloxy-camptothecin (NPC), and four minor metabolites (M1–4) (Fig. 2.2) [41]. The conversion to SN-38 from irinotecan and NPC is mediated by plasma carboxylesterase isoforms (hCE1 and hCE2) [42–44]. SN-38 is inactivated by glucuronidation to form SN-38 glucuronide (SN-38G), rendering it more soluble for elimination via biliary and urinary excretion. UGT1A1 is the major enzyme responsible for the glucuronidation of SN-38 [45], whereas *UGT1A7* and *UGT1A9* play minor roles in the inactivation of SN-38 [46]. SN-38G may be converted back to SN-38 gut flora within the intestinal lumen and recirculated into the bloodstream.

Interindividual variation in SN-38 glucuronidation has been associated with irinotecan-related toxicities, particularly neutropenia and/or diarrhea [4,47]. *UGT1A1*28* is the commonest *UGT1A1* polymorphism in Caucasian and African populations with allelic frequencies over 30% and 50% reported, respectively [5,48]. The polymorphism is a variable number thymine–adenine (TA) tandem repeat located within the promoter region of

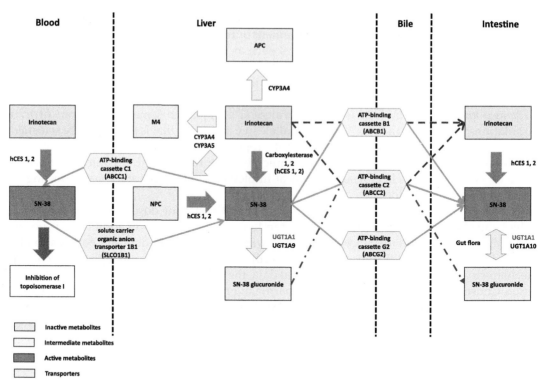

FIGURE 2.2   The metabolic pathways of irinotecan in humans. (This figure is reproduced in color in the color plate section.)

the *UGT1A1* gene. The wild-type allele (*UGT1A1*1*) has six TA repeats, and *UGT1A1*28* has seven TA repeats. The efficiency of gene transcription correlates inversely with the number of TA repeats. The resulting reduction in UGT1A1 enzyme activity in *UGT1A1*28* leads to accumulation of SN-38 and increased irinotecan toxicity [4–7,49–51]. *UGT1A1*28* also manifests as a hereditary hyperbilirubinemia or Gilbert syndrome because bilirubin is a substrate for *UGT1A1* [52,53].

In 2005, the FDA amended irinotecan labeling to indicate that *UGT1A1*28* homozygosity is a genetic risk factor increasing the risk of severe neutropenia. In the same year, the Invader® *UGT1A1* molecular assay (Third Wave Technologies) for the detection of *UGT1A1*28* was approved by the FDA. The severity of irinotecan toxicity may differ with the dosing schedule of irinotecan and may partially explain the lack of association reported in a study using a lower dose of irinotecan [54]. A meta-analysis had suggested that higher incidence of neutropenia was observed in regimens using >150 mg/m^2 of irinotecan as compared to 100–125 mg/m^2 [55]. In contrast, patients who are *UGT1A1* wild type appeared to tolerate the FOLFIRI regimen (comprising **fol**inic acid, 5-fluorouracil, and **iri**notecan) at up to twice the recommended dose for irinotecan (370 mg/m^2) [56,57].

Homozygosity for *UGT1A1*28* occurs in approximately 10% of Caucasian populations but in less than 5% of East Asian populations [58,59]. In East Asians, *UGT1A1*6* (211G>A, G71R) is the predominant functional polymorphism with a reported allelic frequency of 13–23% and is absent in Caucasians [58,60]. *UGT1A1*6* has been associated with increased risk of severe irinotecan toxicity [61,62]. Testing for *UGT1A1*28* alone would have missed a substantial proportion of individuals at risk for irinotecan toxicity in East Asian populations, and should be used in combination with *UGT1A1*6* to identify the population at risk of increased irinotecan toxicity [63,64].

Apart from *UGT1A1*28*, other variants in *UGT1As*, including *UGT1A9*1b* (−118T9>10) and *UGT1A7*3* (387T>G, 391C>A, 392G>A, 622T>C), have been associated with irinotecan toxicity [65–67]. To add to the complexity, there is a plethora of studies reporting genotype–phenotype association from genetic variants of carboxylesterases, CYP3As, adenosine triphosphate binding cassette (ABC) transporters and solute carriers, and irinotecan [68]. Examination of over 40 genetic variants relevant to the irinotecan pathway revealed that almost 50% of the variation of the neutrophil count at the nadir after irinotecan monotherapy could be explained by a combination of genetic variations in *UGT1A1*, *ABCC1*, *SLCO1B1*, ANC baseline neutrophil counts, sex, and race [69]. Although one may argue that an explanation with 50% interindividual variability is far from ideal, the current method of calculating the irinotecan dose using estimated body surface area (BSA) has never demonstrated a reduction in the variability of irinotecan or SN-38 exposure [70]. A randomized study comparing a pharmacokinetic model-based dosing using CYP3A4 phenotyping with the probe drug midazolam, height, and γ-glutamyltransferase with BSA normalized dosing led to a greater than fourfold decrease in severe neutropenia [71]. Further prospective studies are warranted to further refine the optimal dosing strategy to individualize irinotecan dosing.

5-Fluorouracil and DPYD

5-FU is an intravenous pyrimidine analog used in colorectal, gastric, breast, biliary tract, and head and neck cancer. 5-FU is converted to three main active metabolites (Fig. 2.3): fluorodeoxyuridine monophosphate (FdUMP), fluorodeoxyuridine triphosphate (FdUTP), and fluorouridine triphosphate (FUTP). The main mechanism of 5-FU cytotoxicity is mediated by FdUMP inhibition of thymidylate synthase (TS), thereby interfering with the formation of thymidine, a nucleoside essential for DNA replication. In addition, FdUTP and FUTP are incorporated into DNA and RNA, respectively, preventing the incorporation of pyrimidine bases leading to cancer cell death.

Dihydropyrimidine dehydrogenase (DPD) is a saturable rate-limiting enzyme in the catabolism of pyrimidines. 5-FU is metabolized to its inactive form, 5,6-dihydro-5-fluorouracil, by DPD [72]. Over 85% of 5-FU administered is metabolized rapidly in the liver. Decreased DPD activity can lead to the accumulation of 5-FU and severe toxicities, including mucositis, neutropenia, neurological symptoms, and death [73].

Approximately 3–5% of the population is heterozygous and 0.1% is homozygous for alleles with impaired DPD function [74]. The poor metabolizer (PM) phenotype has two copies of a nonfunctional or reduced-function *DPYD* (the gene coding for DPD) allele. The intermediate metabolizer (IM) phenotype is heterozygous for a nonfunctional or reduced-function *DPYD* allele. *DPYD*1*, *4*, *5*, *6*, and *9A* have normal DPD activity. *DPYD*9B* and *10* have reduced DPD activity, and *DPYD *2A*, *3*, *7*, *8*, *11*, *12*, *13*, 496A>G, IVS10-15T>C, 1156G>T, and 1845G>T produce nonfunctional DPD. Nonfunctional *DPYD*2A* is caused by a 5′ splice site mutation at intron 14 1G>A, resulting in the formation of a truncated protein [75].

Several studies including a large prospective cohort study evaluating 685 colorectal cancer patients treated with 5-FU monotherapy has found that *DPYD* genotyping had very low sensitivity (5.5%) and low positive predictive value (46%) for 5-FU–related severe leucopenia, diarrhea, and mucositis [76]. In another large randomized study (the FOCUS trial) examining the optimal sequencing of 5-FU–based palliative chemotherapy, 757 patients were genotyped for *DPYD*2A*. The frequency of *DPYD*2A* was less than 1%, and no significant genotype–phenotype association was observed [77]. These studies suggested that most patients who experienced treatment toxicity do not have a molecular basis for DPD deficiency. Furthermore, no study has yet addressed the appropriate dosing strategy for the IM phenotype.

FdUMP forms a stable ternary complex with TS and a folate cofactor, 5,10 methylenetetrahydrofolate. As such, tissue levels of TS are thought to be important determinants of 5-FU response. Overexpression of TS is associated with 5-FU resistance and inferior survival in advanced and localized colorectal cancer [78]. A 28 base pair variable-number tandem-repeat (VNTR) polymorphism is located at the 5′-flanking untranslated enhancer region (UTR) of the *TYMS* gene coding for TS. The number of tandem repeats varies from two to nine copies in different ethnic groups [79]. The translational efficiency of the *TYMS* gene is correlated

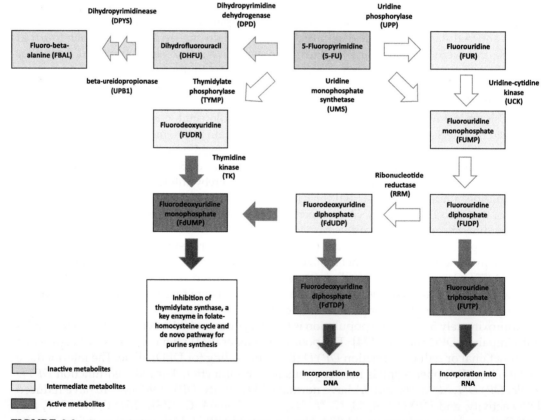

FIGURE 2.3 The metabolic pathways of 5-FU in humans. (This figure is reproduced in color in the color plate section.)

positively with the number of tandem repeats. A single G-to-C substitution located at the 12th nucleotide of the second tandem repeat of *3R*, known as *3RC*, also leads to a reduction in translational efficiency of the *TYMS* gene [80]. Two other reduced-function variants include a further G-to-C substitution in the first repeat of the *TYMS 2R* allele [81], and a six base pair deletion in the 3′UTR (1494del) [82]. For methylenetetrahydrofolate reductase, 677C>T and 1298A>C result in splice variants with reduced activity [83].

The VNTR 3R/3R genotype of *TYMS* was initially reported to be associated with less 5-FU toxicity but poorer treatment response [76,84–87]. Similarly, the *TYMS* 1494del/del has been associated with inferior 5-FU treatment response [88,89]. Differences in the 5-FU schedule, regimen, and study endpoints (response rate vs. survival) make it difficult to compare results among trials. Generally, the *TYMS* variants have low sensitivity, specificity, and predictive values across several cohort studies. In the absence of a prospective study demonstrating improvement of the outcome (efficacy and toxicity) of 5-FU, routine testing of *DPYD* and *TYMS* variants is not recommended.

Tamoxifen and *CYP2D6*

Tamoxifen is a selective estrogen receptor modulator used in the adjuvant and palliative treatment of hormone receptor–positive breast cancer and as a chemopreventive agent for patients with a high risk of developing breast cancer. After oral administration, tamoxifen is metabolized extensively by the CYP pathway to form several metabolites (Fig. 2.4). Tamoxifen is converted predominantly to *N*-desmethyl-tamoxifen by CYP3A4/5 and, to a lesser extent, to 4-OH tamoxifen by CYP2D6 [90]. Oxidation of *N*-desmethyl-tamoxifen and 4-OH tamoxifen,

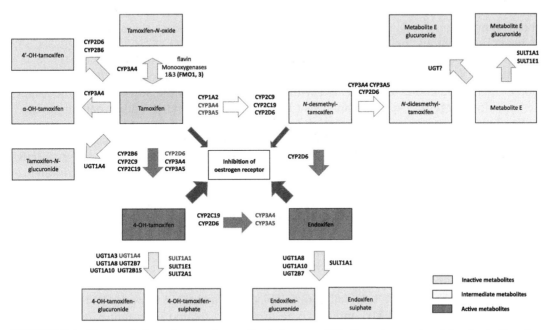

FIGURE 2.4 The metabolic pathways of tamoxifen in humans. (This figure is reproduced in color in the color plate section.)

predominantly by CYP2D6 and CYP3A4/5, respectively, forms a secondary metabolite, 4-hydroxy-N-desmethyl-tamoxifen (endoxifen). These intermediate metabolites undergo further sulphation and glucuronidation by cytosolic sulphotransferases and microsomal uridine 5'-diphospho-glucuronosyltransferases (UDP-glucuronosyltransferases, or UGTs), respectively, to form inactive metabolites [91]. Both endoxifen and 4-OH tamoxifen are 30–100 times more potent than tamoxifen. However, endoxifen is thought to be largely responsible for the therapeutic effect of tamoxifen because its plasma concentration is significantly higher than that of 4-OH tamoxifen [92].

CYP2D6 plays a key role in the formation of endoxifen [92]. Many nonfunctional, reduced-function, and hyperfunctional CYP2D6 variants have been described. A tetra-modal distribution CYP2D6 phenotype is observed in the general population comprising poor metabolizers (PMs), intermediate metabolizers (IMs), extensive metabolizers (EMs), and ultrarapid metabolizers (UMs). PMs carry two nonfunctional CYP2D6 alleles; IMs carry either two reduced-function alleles or one copy of a reduced- or normal-function allele and one nonfunctional allele; EMs carry either two copies of normal-function alleles or one copy each of a normal-function and a reduced-function allele; and UMs carry at least one ultrarapid metabolizer (UM) allele with gene duplication and multiplication of normal-function alleles. The frequencies of PM, IM, and UM in Caucasians are 7%, 12%, and 6%, respectively [93–96]. The most common nonfunctional variants in Caucasians are CYP2D6*3, *4, *5, and *6 [97]. Together, they constitute approximately 97% of the PM phenotype. The *4 allele (1934G>A) introduces a splicing defect at the junction of intron 3 and exon 4 [98]. *5 is a gene deletion, whereas *3 and *6 are a single base deletion (2637A and 1795T, respectively) causing a frame shift producing a premature stop codon and a truncated protein [99–101]. The endoxifen level in patients homozygous for these nonfunctional variants is fourfold lower than in those homozygous for wild-type alleles after 4 months of tamoxifen therapy [102]. Similarly, patients homozygous for the IM alleles such as *10 (100C>T, 4180G>C) and *41 (2850C>T, 2988G>A, 4180G>C) had twofold lower endoxifen levels compared to EMs [103,104].

There are several studies suggesting that women with decreased CYP2D6 activity had poorer clinical outcomes when treated with tamoxifen, in both the adjuvant and metastatic settings. In a large retrospective analysis ($n = 1325$), the recurrence rate in patients treated with adjuvant tamoxifen is twice as high in the PMs (defined in this study as homozygous or compound heterozygous for CYP2D6*3, *4, or *5 alleles) compared to EMs (29% vs 14.9%) [105]. Both event-free survival (HR, 1.33; 95% CI, 1.06–1.68) and disease-free survival (HR, 1.29; 95% CI, 1.03–1.61) were worse in PMs, although there was no significance difference in overall survival (OS). Poorer outcome with adjuvant tamoxifen in PMs was reported in at least six studies as compared to EMs [106–111]. In East Asians, where the frequency of *10 is over 40%, a worse survival rate was observed in IMs receiving tamoxifen in the adjuvant [104,112] and metastatic settings compared to EMs [103]. The median time to progression may differ as much as fourfold for patients with metastatic disease (5.0 vs 21.8 months, $P = 0.0032$). Several studies have reported conflicting results [113–116]. Retrospective analyses of over 6000 patients from two adjuvant breast cancer trials, ATAC (Arimidex, Tamoxifen, Alone or in Combination) and BIG1-98, failed to establish a relationship between CYP2D6 phenotypes (PMs compared to EMs) and outcome in patients treated with tamoxifen, although hot flushes were higher in IMs and PMs [117,118]. It is worth noting that these studies used tumor DNA to genotype germline CYP2D6 variants, resulting in large deviation from the

Hardy–Weinberg equilibrium in both studies [119–121]. Hence, the results from these two studies are at the moment inconclusive. Analysis of Eastern Cooperative Oncology Group 3108 (NCT01124695) and European CYPTAMBRUT-2 (NCT00965939) trials comparing outcome of tamoxifen treatment in EMs, IMs, and PMs will hopefully shed light on the role of *CYP2D6* as a predictive marker of tamoxifen efficacy. Despite the uncertainty surrounding the benefit of *CYP2D6* genotyping, it is clear that endoxifen exposure in IMs can be increased to levels similar to those in EMs with higher doses of tamoxifen (30–40 mg/day instead 20 mg/day) [122,123], but the resulting effects on efficacy are not known at this point in time.

Clinically Important Somatic Markers for Treatment Response

An improvement in the understanding of the molecular events involved in oncogenesis in solid tumors has led to the development of rational, molecularly directed targeted therapies resulting in an improvement in efficacy as the patients with the appropriate genetic aberrations are targeted and the number of patients who are unlikely to benefit reduced. The successes of imatinib and all-trans retinoic acid in hematological malignancies such as chronic myeloid leukemia [124,125] and acute promyelocytic leukemia [126,127], respectively, have paved the way for the development of treatment targeting genomic aberrations in solid tumors. This approach has been especially effective in gastrointestinal stromal tumors (GISTs), breast cancer, colorectal cancer, non-small-cell lung cancer (NSCLC), and melanoma (Table 2.2). Genetic aberrations can also be used as negative predictors of response as in the case of *KRAS* mutation and anti-EGFR antibody resistance in colorectal cancer [26,128–131]. In this section, we will discuss key somatic genetic aberrations in solid tumors and the use of targeted therapy with a focus on clinical efficacy data from key studies.

Gastrointestinal Stromal Tumors

Before the era of targeted therapy, the prognosis for patients with advanced-stage GISTs was dismal due to its inherent resistance to chemotherapy and radiotherapy [180]. The modern management of GISTs has served as an important and successful model of molecularly targeted therapy in solid tumors. GISTs are characterized by the expression of KIT (CD117), a transmembrane tyrosine kinase that acts as a receptor for the ligand stem cell factor (SCF). The binding of SCF to *KIT* results in receptor homodimerization and subsequent activation of tyrosine kinase activity and downstream phosphorylation of intracellular signal transduction pathways [181,182]. Activating mutations of *KIT* in GISTs are oncogenic and result in ligand-independent kinase activation [163]. About 75–80% of GISTs harbor *KIT* mutations, and these mutations lead to the constitutive activation of the *KIT* tyrosine kinase domain. Importantly, the mutant KIT receptor is a therapeutic target for inhibitors such as imatinib and nilotinib. *KIT* exon 11 mutations (deletions, insertions, or single base substitutions) are the most common somatic alterations, occurring in about 70% of GISTs. *KIT* exon 9 mutations (extracellular domain) occur in about 10% of GISTs, whilst mutations in exon 13 (kinase domain) and exon 17 (activation loop) are rare (about 1% for each) [181–183]. About 5–8% of GISTs harbor mutations in the platelet-derived growth factor receptor-α (*PDGFRA*) gene, and, similar to the *KIT* mutations in GISTs, tumors with mutant *PDGFRA* have constitutive kinase activity in the absence of the ligand *PDGFRA* [172]. The remaining 10–15% of GISTs do not have detectable mutations of *KIT* or *PDGFRA* ("wild-type" GISTs) but have KIT activation

TABLE 2.2   Selected Actionable Genetic Aberrations in Solid Tumors

Gene	Mechanism of dysregulation	Tumor	Targeted agent used or under clinical evaluation
ALK	Amplification	Ovarian cancer [132]	Crizotinib
ALK	Mutation	Neuroblastoma [133–136]	Crizotinib
AKT1	Mutation	Breast [137], melanoma [138], and non-small-cell lung cancer (NSCLC)	MK-2206
BCR–ABL	Translocation	Chronic myeloid leukemia [124,139–141] and acute lymphoblastic leukemia [142–144]	Bosutinib, dasatinib, imatinib, and nilotinib
BRAF	Mutation	Colorectal (CRC), melanoma, NSCLC, and ovarian cancer [145]	GSK2188436 and vemurafenib
CCDC6–RET	Fusion	NSCLC [146,147]	Regorafenib, sorafenib, sunitinib, and vandetanib
DDR2	Mutation	NSCLC [148]	Dasatinib and nilotinib
EGFR	Mutation	NSCLC [149,150]	Afatinib, dacomitinib, erlotinib, and gefitinib
EML–ALK	Fusion	Breast, CRC [151], and NSCLC [152]	AP26113, BKM 378, CH5424802, crizotinib, and LDK378
FGFR1	Amplification	Bladder [153], breast [154], NSCLC [155], and ovarian cancer [156]	AZD4547, BGJ398, brivanib, ponatinib, and regorafenib
HER-2	Mutation	NSCLC [157]	Afatinib and dacomitinib
HER-2	Amplification	Breast [158], endometrial, gastric, and gastroesophageal cancer [157,159]	Lapatinib, neratinib, pertuzumab, TDM-1, and trastuzumab
JAK2	Mutation	Myeloproliferative neoplasm [160]	Ruxolitinib
KIF5B–ALK	Fusion	NSCLC [146]	Crizotinib
KIF5B–RET	Fusion	CRC [161] and NSCLC [146,161,162]	Regorafenib sorafenib, sunitinib, and vandetanib
KIT	Mutation	Gastrointestinal stromal tumor (GIST) [163] and melanoma [164]	Dasatinib, imatinib, nilotinib, pazopanib, and regorafenib
KRAS	Mutation	CRC, NSCLC, and pancreatic cancer [165]	Tivantinib + erlotinib Docetaxel +/− AZD6244 GSK1120212
MEK1		Melanoma [166] and NSCLC [167]	AZD6244, GSK1120212, and PD0325901
MET	Amplification	Gastric [168] and NSCLC [169]	Crizotinib, MetMab, and Tivantinib
MET	Mutations	Head and neck cancer, melanoma, NSCLC, and renal cell carcinoma (RCC) [170]	

TABLE 2.2 Selected Actionable Genetic Aberrations in Solid Tumors   *(cont'd)*

Gene	Mechanism of dysregulation	Tumor	Targeted agent used or under clinical evaluation
NPM–ALK	Fusion	Anaplastic large-cell lymphoma [171]	AP26113 and crizotinib
NRAS	Mutation	Melanoma [164]	R115777
PDGFRA	Mutation	GIST [172]	Crenolanib, imatinib, nilotinib, and pazopanib
PI3K	Mutation	Breast [137], CRC, and endometrial cancer [173]	GDC-0941, GDC-0980, BKM120, and CH5132799
PML–RAR	Translocation	Acute promyelocytic leukemia [174]	All-trans retinoic acid, and arsenic trioxide
PTEN	Mutation	Breast [137], CRC, endometrial, gliomas, NSCLC [162], and prostate cancer [175]	
RET	Mutation	Medullary thyroid carcinoma [176]	Cabozantinib, sorafenib, sunitinib, and vandetanib
ROS1	Fusion	NSCLC [146,177]	AP26113 and crizotinib
TPM3–ALK TPM4–ALK	Fusion	Anaplastic large-cell lymphoma [178] and inflammatory myofibroblastic tumors [179]	AP26113 and crizotinib

due to downstream effectors [184]. Recent studies in this group of "wild-type" GISTs have reported the presence of oncogenic mutations, including *BRAF, HRAS*, and *NRAS* [183].

Imatinib, a small-molecule inhibitor of the tyrosine kinase domains of KIT and PDGFRA, has revolutionized the management of GISTs. In multiple clinical studies, 75–90% of patients with advanced GISTs treated with imatinib at 400 mg or 800 mg daily experienced a clinical benefit (stable disease, or complete or partial objective response) and a median progression-free survival (PFS) of 20–24 months [185–188]. This is in marked contrast with the effect of chemotherapy, where the overall response rate (ORR) was <10% and the median OS was approximately 18 months [189]. The success of imatinib was also demonstrated in adjuvant settings in patients with a moderate or high risk of recurrence after surgery [189,190].

The response to imatinib varies according to the type of primary mutations present in GISTs. GISTs harboring exon 11 mutations exhibit the greatest sensitivity to imatinib, followed by exon 9 and wild types. This is reflected in a longer PFS and OS in patients with exon 11 mutations compared with exon 9 or wild types [191]. In patients with exon 9 mutations, imatinib at 800 mg daily resulted in a longer PFS [192] and higher ORR [191]. A meta-analysis confirmed that patients with exon 9 mutations treated with imatinib 800 mg daily had a longer PFS and higher response rate compared with those treated with imatinib 400 mg daily, although OS was not statistically different [188]. Thus, National Comprehensive Cancer Network (NCCN) guidelines suggested that patients with documented exon 9 mutations might benefit from a starting dose of imatinib at 800 mg depending on their tolerance (*NCCN Clinical Practice Guidelines in Oncology Soft Tissue Sarcoma*, version 3.2012). The ORR of *KIT* wild-type GISTs does not appear to be affected by imatinib doses [191]. Other than the *KIT* exon 9 mutations, *PDGFRA* exon 18 D842V is the most common primary mutation that confers primary resistance to GIST [192]. In *PDGFRA*-mutant GISTs treated with imatinib, no clinical benefit was observed in patients with the D842V, whereas the median OS was not reached at 46 months of follow-up in non-D842V mutants [193].

Acquired (or secondary) resistance inevitably occurs in all patients after either an objective response or stable disease, and develops at a median time of 18–24 months. Mutations of either *KIT* or *PDGFRA* are the commonest causes of acquired resistance to imatinib. Acquired *KIT* mutations are mainly located in exons 13 and 14 (encoding the ATP binding pocket) and on exons 17 and 18. *PDGFRA* D842V is the only *PDGFRA* mutation conferring acquired resistance to imatinib [183]. Secondary mutations are more common when the tumor harbors a primary *KIT* exon 11 mutation [194–198]. Other identified molecular alterations leading to acquired resistance include *KIT* amplification [199,200], altered activity of drug transporters, and induction of *CYP3A4* [201].

Several new drugs have been developed for resistant GISTs progressing after treatment. Regorafenib is a multitarget tyrosine kinase inhibitor (TKI) with a high affinity for *KIT* and *PDGFRA* tyrosine kinases. A phase III study (GRID, or GIST–Regorafenib in Progressive Disease) compared regorafenib versus placebo in patients with advanced GISTs following progression after imatinib and sunitinib. Results showed that regorafenib significantly improved PFS (HR 0.27; 95% CI, 0.18–0.39) and that, in an exploratory analysis, regorafenib was effective in all molecular subtypes, including GISTs with *KIT* exon 9 and exon 11 mutations [202]. In addition, crenolanib, a potent inhibitor of PDGFRA, is currently investigated in GISTs with the *PDGFRA* D842V mutation.

Breast Cancer

The transmembrane receptor HER-2 is a member of the EGFR family (EGFR/HER-1, HER-2, HER-3, and HER-4) and is involved in regulating cell survival, proliferation, and differentiation. The extracellular domain of HER-2 can adopt a fixed conformation resembling a ligand-activated state, permitting it to dimerize in the absence of a ligand. The overexpression of HER-2 results in the constitutive activation of downstream signaling pathways, including PI3K–AKT and RAS–RAF–MAPK [203]. In breast cancer, HER-2 is overexpressed in 20–30% of tumors and is associated with an increased risk of recurrence and a poorer prognosis [204]. *HER-2* amplification is detected by fluorescence in situ hybridization (FISH), whereas *HER*-2 overexpression is detected using immunohistochemistry (IHC) [158]. A positive HER-2 result is an IHC staining of 3 (uniform, intense membrane staining of 30% of invasive tumor cells), a FISH result of >6 *HER*-2 gene copies per nucleus, or a FISH ratio (*HER*-2 gene signals to chromosome 17 signals) of >2.2 [205]. HER-2 is an important and validated molecular target in breast cancer. The American Society of Clinical Oncology (ASCO) and the College of American Pathologists recommend that HER-2 status should be determined for all invasive breast cancers by either using IHC or measuring the number of gene copies using FISH [205].

Trastuzumab, a humanized monoclonal antibody against HER-2, mediates its antitumor activity through several mechanisms, including antibody-dependent cell mediated cytotoxicity (ADCC), prevention of HER-2 dimerization, inhibition of shedding of the extracellular domain, inhibition of downstream signaling, angiogenesis and DNA repair, and increased apoptosis [206,207]. Trastuzumab as monotherapy was initially shown to be active in metastatic HER-2–positive breast cancer [208,209]. In a pivotal phase III study in patients with untreated advanced-stage HER-2–positive breast cancer, an improvement in time to progression, ORR, and median duration of response was seen in patients receiving trastuzumab chemotherapy compared with chemotherapy alone [210].

In multiple randomized adjuvant trials, the addition of trastuzumab has shown to be effective in improving PFS and OS [211–218].

A recent comprehensive molecular study of breast cancers revealed novel mutated genes such as *TBX3*, *RUNX1*, *CBFB*, *AFF2*, *PIK3R1*, *PTPN22*, *PTPRD*, *NF1*, *SF3B1*, and *CCND3*. Further research is required to determine their relevance as druggable targets [19].

Non-small-cell Lung Cancer

NSCLC is divided into three main histological subtypes, adenocarcinoma, squamous cell carcinoma, and large-cell carcinoma. It is now recognized that in NSCLC, the detection of driver oncogenes can potentially be inhibited by molecularly targeted therapy. Targetable alterations in oncogenes that are common in lung adenocarcinoma include mutations of *EGFR*, *BRAF*, *KRAS*, and *HER-2*; gene fusion of *EML4-ALK*, *ROS1*, and *RET*, and amplification of *HER-2* and *MET*. Targetable driver oncogenes in lung squamous cell carcinoma include *FGFR1* amplification, *DDR2* and *BRAF* mutations, and *MET* amplification [219,220]. The matching of a driver oncogene with its appropriate inhibitor has resulted in improvements in ORR and prolonged PFS as compared to standard chemotherapy. Such an approach has shown improved clinical outcome in the treatment of patients with NSCLC harboring activated *EGFR* mutations or the fusion gene *EML4-ALK*. This section will focus on markers that are used to guide treatment in NSCLC, namely, *EGFR* mutations and *EML4-ALK*.

ACTIVATING *EGFR* MUTATIONS

The EGFR (HER-1) signaling pathway plays a pivotal role in lung carcinogenesis. Dimerization of EGFR occurs after stimulation by a ligand such as epidermal growth factor (EGF), transforming growth factor-alpha (TGF-α), epiregulin, or amphiregulin; it results in autophosphorylation and the downstream activation signaling pathways, including the mitogen-activated protein kinase (MAPK) pathway, the phosphatidylinositol 3′ kinase (PI3K)–AKT pathway, and the STAT pathway, resulting in increased cell proliferation, inhibition of apoptosis, increased invasion, and metastasis [221]. EGFR TKIs inhibit the intracellular tyrosine kinase domain of EGFR and therefore block the signal transduction pathways implicated in the proliferation and survival of cancer cells.

The initial use of small-molecule EGFR TKIs such as gefitinib and erlotinib in heavily pretreated unselected patients with advanced-stage NSCLC yielded a very modest ORR of 9–10% of patients (in the BR21 and Iressa Survival Evaluation in Lung Cancer (ISEL) trials; see Refs [222,223]). The identification of activating somatic mutations in exons 18 to 21 of *EGFR* as a molecular predictor of sensitivity to gefitinib and erlotinib [149,150,224] has revolutionized targeted therapy for NSCLC. Kinase domain mutations in *EGFR* are known as activating mutations as they result in a ligand-independent activation of tyrosine kinase (TK) activity. In patients selected for sensitizing *EGFR* mutations, treatment with EGFR TKIs has resulted in a dramatic improvement in the clinical outcome (discussed in detail in this chapter). Such mutations are present predominantly in patients of female sex, adenocarcinoma histology, East Asian ethnicity, and a history of never or light smoking [225].

Activating mutations of *EGFR* are commonly found in exons 18–21 of the TK domain. *EGFR* mutations resulting in increased sensitivity to EGFR TKIs are said to be sensitizing

EGFR mutations. The majority of *EGFR* TKI-sensitizing mutations are in-frame deletions in exon 19, usually involving the amino acid residues leucine-747 to glutamic acid-749 *EGFR Del (746–750)*, and account for about 44% of all *EGFR* TK mutations. The predominant single base mutation is L858R in exon 21, accounting for about 41% of all *EGFR* TK-activating mutations [225,226].

A consequence of *EGFR* mutations is an increase in kinase activity, resulting in selective growth and survival [227]. Kinetic analysis of the intracellular domains of EGFR *L858R* and *EGFR Del (746–750)* has shown both mutants are active but show a higher KM for ATP and a lower Ki for erlotinib, relative to wild-type *EGFR* [228]. Thus, mutant kinases have a reduced affinity for ATP, providing a molecular basis for their increased sensitivity to erlotinib and gefitinib [228].

As *EGFR* mutations are associated with greater sensitivity to EGFR TKIs, phase III studies were conducted to compare the efficacy of first-line EGFR TKI monotherapy vs platinum doublet chemotherapy in this molecularly selected patient group.

Two phase III studies on a patient population enriched for *EGFR* mutations have been reported. In the First-SIGNAL study, previously untreated patients (never-smokers with adenocarcinoma) were randomized to first-line gefitinib or chemotherapy. A comparison between patients with activating *EGFR* mutations (in exons 18–21) versus *EGFR* wild type showed a superior ORR and PFS in patients with *EGFR* mutations (HR 0.377; 95% CI, 0.210 to 0.674; $P < 0.001$) [229]. In the IRESSA Pan-Asia Study (IPASS), patients (East Asians, never or light smokers, with adenocarcinoma) were randomized to gefitinib or chemotherapy [230]. Patients on gefitinib had a longer PFS (HR 0.74; 95% CI, 0.65–0.85), higher ORR (43% vs 32.2%), better quality of life [231], and similar OS [232]. In a preplanned subset analysis, patients with *EGFR* mutations had a longer PFS when treated with gefitinib compared with chemotherapy, whilst patients without *EGFR* mutations had a shorter PFS when treated with gefitinib (HR 2.85; 95% CI, 2.05–3.98). Patients were considered positive for *EGFR* mutations if at least one of 29 mutations were detected in exons 18–21. In patients treated with gefitinib, the median OS in the *EGFR* mutation-positive subgroup, the HR was 0.78 (95% CI, 0.50–1.20); and in the mutation-negative subgroup, the HR was 1.38 (95% CI, 0.92–2.09). The ORRs for *EGFR* mutation-positive and -negative patients were 71.7% and 1.1%, respectively. These results highlight the importance of a predictive biomarker in selecting a molecularly targeted therapy where the absence of the predictive biomarker was associated with a markedly poorer clinical outcome. A post-hoc analysis of *EGFR* gene copy number by FISH was also performed. A high gene copy number (defined as high polysomy, or four copies in 40% of cells; or gene amplification, which is the presence of tight *EGFR* gene clusters and a ratio of gene–chromosome per cell ≥2, or ≥15 copies of *EGFR* per cell in ≥10% of analyzed cells) was associated with an improved PFS (HR 0.66; 95% CI 0.50–0.88) and ORR with gefitinib (OR 1.79; 95% CI, 1.08–2.96) compared with chemotherapy. These findings suggest that the predictive value of *EGFR* gene copy number for PFS benefit with gefitinib was driven by the coexistence of *EGFR* mutation [232].

Results from IPASS showed *EGFR* mutation status is a more powerful predictor of sensitivity with gefitinib than clinical factors (smoking status, sex, and adenocarcinoma histology), and these results have provided the basis for the rational selection of treatment based on molecularly defined criteria in the treatment of patients with advanced NSCLC (discussed in the "*EML–ALK*" section of this chapter).

In the WJTOG3405 study, chemo-naïve patients with advanced-stage NSCLC or postoperative recurrence with an *EGFR* mutation (exon 19 deletion or L858R point mutation) were randomized to gefitinib or chemotherapy. Patients receiving gefitinib had a better PFS and a higher ORR [233], whereas no difference in OS was seen [234]. In the NEJ002 study, chemonaïve patients with sensitizing *EGFR* mutations were randomized to gefitinib or chemotherapy. Similarly, patients treated with gefitinib had a superior ORR and PFS, although OS was similar [235,236].

Two phase III studies, OPTIMAL and the European Randomised Trial of Tarceva versus Chemotherapy (EURTAC), compared first-line erlotinib monotherapy versus platinum chemotherapy in advanced-stage NSCLC patients with *EGFR* mutations. In both studies, patients treated with erlotinib had a superior ORR and PFS [237,238]. Similar to the previous phase III gefitinib studies, erlotinib did not improve OS. The lack of OS benefit with an EGFR TKI is most likely due to the high rate of patient crossover from a chemotherapy arm to an EGFR TKI at the time of disease progression.

Taken together, the evidence supports the use of first-line EGFR TKI monotherapy in patients with advanced-stage NSCLC harboring activating *EGFR* mutations given the higher ORR, longer PFS, and better quality of life when compared with cytotoxic chemotherapy. Furthermore, the presence of activating *EGFR* mutations and not the clinical characteristics determine benefit to EGFR TKI. As such, the ASCO guidelines suggest that patients with NSCLC being considered for first-line EGFR TKI therapy should have their tumor tested for *EGFR* mutations [239].

EML–ALK

EML4–ALK is a fusion gene with potent oncogenic activity that arises from an inversion of chromosome 2p [Inv(2) (p21p23)]. The chromosomal inversion joins exons 1–13 of echinoderm microtubule-associated protein-like 4 (*EML4*) to exons 20–29 of *ALK* [152]. *EML4–ALK* contains an N terminus from *EML4* and a C terminus that contains the entire intracellular tyrosine kinase domain of *ALK*. The fusion partner mediates ligand-independent dimerization of ALK, resulting in constitutive kinase activity with the downstream activation of the RAS–MAPK–ERK, JAK3-signal transducers and activators of transcription-3, and PI3K–AKT signaling pathways [240,241]. Other *ALK* fusion variants have been reported in NSCLC but are rare (Table 2.2).

The break-apart FISH assay is the companion diagnostic test approved by the FDA to detect *ALK*-rearranged NSCLC. *EML4–ALK* fusion in NSCLC is uncommon, with a frequency of 3.8%, and is generally mutually exclusive of *EGFR* or *KRAS* mutations. Patients with NSCLC bearing *EML4–ALK* tend to present at a younger age, have never smoked or are light smokers, and have adenocarcinoma [242–244]. The efficacy of crizotinib, a potent, selective, ATP-competitive, small-molecule ALK inhibitor, has been reported. In a phase I study of crizotinib in *EML4–ALK*–positive advanced-stage NSCLC patients, the ORR rate was 57% [245], similar to that in patients bearing *EGFR* mutations treated with EGFR TKIs. NCCN guidelines have suggested crizotinib as a first-line therapy in patients who are *ALK*-positive (*NCCN Clinical Practice Guidelines in Oncology: Non-small-cell Lung Cancer*, version 2.2013). In a phase II study in patients with *ALK*-rearranged NSCLC who had failed more than two lines of chemotherapy (PROFILE 1005), the ORR was 50% [246]. In a phase III study conducted in the second-line setting (PROFILE 1007) in *ALK*-positive patients, crizotinib was significantly superior to standard single-agent second-line chemotherapy (pemetrexed or docetaxel) in terms of quality of life, ORR, and PFS (HR 0.49; 95% CI, 0.37–0.64; $p < 0.0001$) [247].

Next-generation sequencing platforms have enabled a comprehensive molecular characterization of adenocarcinoma and squamous cell carcinoma of the lung with the identification of potential new targets such as *DACH1, CFTR, RELN, ABCB5, CDKN2A, NOTCH1, U2AF1, RBM10,* and *ARID1A* [248–250]. The validation of these targets and the development of inhibitors for newly identified targets are greatly anticipated.

Melanoma

Malignant melanoma has traditionally been classified according to pathologic features and anatomic site of origin. More recently, subsets of melanoma have been classified at the molecular level by recurrent driver mutations. The identification of multiple oncogenes involved in melanomagenesis has led to a dramatic improvement in clinical outcome. Several highly recurrent genetic aberrations implicated in melanomagenesis include genes encoding kinases, signaling factors, transcription factors, and tumor suppressors.

Activating *BRAF* mutations are present in 50% of melanomas. *BRAF* mutations occur mainly on exons 11 and 15, which encode for the kinase domain. T1796A results in a V600E substitution, accounting for approximately 90% of all *BRAF* mutations, and has recently been shown to be a valid therapeutic target in malignant melanoma [251].

In a phase III study, vemurafenib, a potent and highly selective BRAF inhibitor, was compared to dacarbazine in patients with untreated metastatic melanoma harboring *BRAF* V600E mutations. The ORR (48% and 5%), PFS (HR 0.26; 95% CI, 0.20–0.33), and 6-month OS (HR 0.37; 95% CI, 0.26–0.55) favored vemurafenib [251]. NCCN guidelines have recommended vemurafenib for patients with *BRAF* V600 mutations (*NCCN Clinical Practice Guidelines in Oncology: Melanoma,* version 2.2013).

In a recent study, whole-genome sequencing of malignant melanoma identified *PREX2* as a novel gene with recurrent mutations [252]. Further characterization of *PREX2* as a relevant therapeutic target is required.

Colorectal Cancer

EGFR is frequently upregulated in colorectal cancers, and cetuximab and panitumumab are antibodies that bind to EGFR and competitively inhibit EGF ligand activation of downstream signaling pathways such as PI3K–Akt–mTOR and RAS–RAF–MAPK that promote colorectal cancer survival and proliferation. About 30–50% of colorectal cancers harbor *KRAS* mutations at codons 12 and 13 of exon 2 [27,253]. These mutations result in constitutive activation of the KRAS-associated signaling cascade independent of EGF ligand activation.

The approval of cetuximab in refractory colorectal cancer is based on demonstration of superior response rate and PFS in EGFR-expressing colorectal cancer when compared to best supportive care [254]. However, initial analysis of a large phase III study (cetuximab combined with irinotecan in first-line therapy for metastatic colorectal cancer, or CRYSTAL) had failed to demonstrate the clinical benefit of cetuximab when added to standard irinotecan-based chemotherapy in EGFR-expressing colorectal cancer [27]. With growing evidence that *KRAS* mutations predicted resistance to antibodies targeting EGFR [128,253,255], *KRAS* mutational analysis was performed in about half of the study population with available tumor tissues. In subgroup analysis, the benefit of cetuximab was observed in wild-type *KRAS* but not mutant

KRAS patients (respectively, HR 0.80; 95% CI, 0.67 to 0.95 vs HR 1.04; 95% CI, 0.83 to 1.28) [131]. Similarly, the benefit of panitumumab can be observed only in wild-type *KRAS* colorectal cancer when combined with second-line irinotecan-based chemotherapy [26,256] or as a single agent in chemotherapy-refractory disease [128].

It appears that the positive predictive value of different *KRAS* mutations for anti-EGFR therapy resistance may differ substantially. Retrospective pooled analysis of 579 patients with chemotherapy-refractory colorectal cancer treated with cetuximab suggested that the survival of individuals with codon 13 mutation (G13D) was higher than that of those with other *KRAS* mutations such as G12A, G12C, G12D, G12R, G12S, G12V, G13C, and G13V (HR 0.50; 95% CI, 0.31–0.81) [257]. The clinical finding is supported by an in vitro cetuximab sensitivity assay comparing G13D- to G12V-mutated cancer cells in the same study. Another retrospective analysis of G13D-mutated metastatic colorectal cancer in the first-line setting also showed that relative treatment effects of cetuximab appeared similar to those of patients with wild-type *KRAS* tumors (OS, HR 0.80; 95% CI, 0.49–1.3 vs 0.81; 95% CI, 0.69–0.94), although the absolute benefit was smaller [258]. ASCO has recommended all patients with metastatic colorectal carcinoma who are candidates for anti-EGFR antibody therapy should have their tumor tested for *KRAS* mutations (codon 12 or 13), and anti-EGFR antibody therapy should not be used if *KRAS* mutations are detected [259].

Microsatellite instability (MSI) is caused by defect in the DNA repair mechanism resulting in abnormal lengthening or shortening of the sequence of DNA repeats (microsatellites). In colorectal cancer, it is associated with hereditary nonpolyposis colorectal cancer syndrome [260] but is also present in 15% of sporadic colon cancers due to somatic or epigenetic silencing of mismatch repair (MMR) genes [261,262]. Five markers (*BAT25*, *BAT26*, *D5S346*, *D2S123*, and *D17S250*) are recommended by the National Cancer Institute to quantify instability [263]. The presence of two or more markers with instability indicates a high frequency of MSI (MSI-H).

There is substantial evidence supporting MSI-H tumors having favorable prognosis when compared to MSI-low (MSI-L) or MSI-stable (MSS) stage II colorectal cancer [264–266]. The role of MSI status as a predictive marker for adjuvant 5-FU is more controversial. In a retrospective analysis of patients who received adjuvant 5-FU, survival benefit was observed in patients with MSS or MSI-L (HR, 0.72; 95% CI, 0.53–0.99), but not in patients with MSI-H [264]. Pooled analysis of these patients together with 457 new colorectal patients who were previously randomly assigned to adjuvant FU-based therapy confirmed that survival benefit from treatment was observed in stage III MSS and MSI-L patients [265]. In fact, treatment of stage II MSI-H patients with 5-FU may even be harmful (HR, 2.30; 95% CI, 0.85–6.24). However, these findings were not replicated in two other studies investigating the predictive value of defective MMR (biologically equivalent to MSI-H), where defective MMR did not predict survival benefit of adjuvant 5-FU [267] or irinotecan with bolus 5-FU [268]. Adding to the complexity, another pooled analysis of stage II and III colon cancer treated with 5-FU–based therapy reported that the disease-free survival benefit was restricted to patients with germline MSI-H tumors (HR, 0.29; 95% CI, 0.11–0.72) and not in sporadic MSI-H tumors with an epigenetic origin [269].

Comprehensive genome-scale analysis has revealed at least two distinct molecular subtypes of colorectal cancer, 84% nonhypermutated and 16% hypermutated tumors [270]. The majority of these tumors had a deregulated WNT-signaling pathway. The therapeutic implication is that these tumors can be targeted using WNT-signaling inhibitors and small-molecule β-catenin inhibitors. The study also discovered potentially targetable *ERBB2* and *IGF2* amplifications in colorectal cancers.

CONCLUSIONS

A better understanding of the genetic aberrations and molecular pathways involved in carcinogenesis and drug disposition has resulted in the rational development of personalized therapy. Personalized cancer treatment has become increasingly available over the past few years. The successful development of targeted drugs and their companion pharmacogenomic biomarkers has changed the traditional paradigm in drug development, promising a more cost-effective approach through the selection of patients most likely to benefit from the treatment. However, many questions need to be answered, including appropriate dosing strategy, acquired resistance, prospective validation of pharmacogenomic markers, and optimal clinical-study design as we move into the new era of personalized cancer treatment.

References

[1] Feuk L, Carson AR, Scherer SW. Structural variation in the human genome. Nat Rev Genet 2006;7(2):85–97.

[2] Sauna ZE, Kimchi-Sarfaty C. Understanding the contribution of synonymous mutations to human disease. Nat Rev Genet 2011;12(10):683–91.

[3] Raida M, Schwabe W, Hausler P, Van Kuilenburg AB, Van Gennip AH, Behnke D, et al. Prevalence of a common point mutation in the dihydropyrimidine dehydrogenase (DPD) gene within the 5'-splice donor site of intron 14 in patients with severe 5-fluorouracil (5-FU)-related toxicity compared with controls. Clin Cancer Res 2001;7(9):2832–9.

[4] Iyer L, Das S, Janisch L, Wen M, Ramirez J, Karrison T, et al. UGT1A1*28 polymorphism as a determinant of irinotecan disposition and toxicity. Pharmacogenomics J 2002;2(1):43–7.

[5] Beutler E, Gelbart T, Demina A. Racial variability in the UDP-glucuronosyltransferase 1 (UGT1A1) promoter: a balanced polymorphism for regulation of bilirubin metabolism? Proc Natl Acad Sci U S A 1998;95(14):8170–4.

[6] Innocenti F, Undevia SD, Iyer L, Chen PX, Das S, Kocherginsky M, et al. Genetic variants in the UDP-glucuronosyltransferase 1A1 gene predict the risk of severe neutropenia of irinotecan. J Clin Oncol 2004;22(8):1382–8.

[7] Ando Y, Saka H, Ando M, Sawa T, Muro K, Ueoka H, et al. Polymorphisms of UDP-glucuronosyltransferase gene and irinotecan toxicity: a pharmacogenetic analysis. Cancer Res 2000;60(24):6921–6.

[8] Evans WE, Horner M, Chu YQ, Kalwinsky D, Roberts WM. Altered mercaptopurine metabolism, toxic effects, and dosage requirement in a thiopurine methyltransferase-deficient child with acute lymphocytic leukemia. J Pediatr 1991;119(6):985–9.

[9] Relling MV, Hancock ML, Rivera GK, Sandlund JT, Ribeiro RC, Krynetski EY, et al. Mercaptopurine therapy intolerance and heterozygosity at the thiopurine S-methyltransferase gene locus. J Natl Cancer Inst 1999;91(23):2001–8.

[10] Lennard L, Van Loon JA, Lilleyman JS, Weinshilboum RM. Thiopurine pharmacogenetics in leukemia: correlation of erythrocyte thiopurine methyltransferase activity and 6-thioguanine nucleotide concentrations. Clin Pharmacol Ther 1987;41(1):18–25.

[11] Singer JB, Shou Y, Giles F, Kantarjian HM, Hsu Y, Robeva AS, et al. UGT1A1 promoter polymorphism increases risk of nilotinib-induced hyperbilirubinemia. Leukemia 2007;21(11):2311–5.

[12] Browning LA, Kruse JA. Hemolysis and methemoglobinemia secondary to rasburicase administration. Ann Pharmacother 2005;39(11):1932–5.

[13] Tai HL, Krynetski EY, Yates CR, Loennechen T, Fessing MY, Krynetskaia NF, et al. Thiopurine S-methyltransferase deficiency: two nucleotide transitions define the most prevalent mutant allele associated with loss of catalytic activity in Caucasians. Am J Hum Genet 1996;58(4):694–702.

[14] Daly AK. Genome-wide association studies in pharmacogenomics. Nat Rev Genet 2010;11(4):241–6.

[15] Innocenti F, Schilsky RL. Translating the cancer genome into clinically useful tools and strategies. Dis Model Mech 2009;2(9–10):426–9.

[16] Druker BJ, Guilhot F, O'Brien SG, Gathmann I, Kantarjian H, Gattermann N, et al. Five-year follow-up of patients receiving imatinib for chronic myeloid leukemia. N Engl J Med 2006;355(23):2408–17.

[17] Schinzel AC, Hahn WC. Oncogenic transformation and experimental models of human cancer. Front Biosci 2008;13:71–84.

[18] Stratton MR, Campbell PJ, Futreal PA. The cancer genome. Nature 2009;458(7239):719–24.

[19] The Cancer Genome Atlas Network. Comprehensive molecular portraits of human breast tumours. Nature 2012;490(7418):61–70.

[20] Madian AG, Wheeler HE, Jones RB, Dolan EM. Relating human genetic variation to variation in drug responses. Trends Genet 2012;28(10):487–95.

[21] Innocenti F, Cox NJ, Dolan ME. The use of genomic information to optimize cancer chemotherapy. Semin Oncol 2011;38(2):186–95.

[22] Pearson TA, Manolio TA. How to interpret a genome-wide association study. JAMA 2008;299(11):1335–44.

[23] Glubb DM, Innocenti F. Architecture of pharmacogenomic associations: structures with functional foundations or castles made of sand? Pharmacogenomics 2013;14(1):1–4.

[24] Glubb DM, Innocenti F. Mechanisms of genetic regulation in gene expression: examples from drug metabolizing enzymes and transporters. Wiley Interdiscip Rev Syst Biol Med 2011;3(3):299–313.

[25] Teutsch SM, Bradley LA, Palomaki GE, Haddow JE, Piper M, Calonge N, et al. The evaluation of genomic applications in practice and prevention (EGAPP) initiative: methods of the EGAPP working group. Genet Med 2009;11(1):3–14.

[26] Peeters M, Price TJ, Cervantes A, Sobrero AF, Ducreux M, Hotko Y, et al. Randomized phase III study of panitumumab with fluorouracil, leucovorin, and irinotecan (FOLFIRI) compared with FOLFIRI alone as second-line treatment in patients with metastatic colorectal cancer. J Clin Oncol 2010;28(31):4706–13.

[27] Van Cutsem E, Kohne CH, Hitre E, Zaluski J, Chang Chien CR, Makhson A, et al. Cetuximab and chemotherapy as initial treatment for metastatic colorectal cancer. N Engl J Med 2009;360(14):1408–17.

[28] Crona D, Innocenti F. Can knowledge of germline markers of toxicity optimize dosing and efficacy of cancer therapy? Biomark Med 2012;6(3):349–62.

[29] Weinshilboum RM, Sladek SL. Mercaptopurine pharmacogenetics: monogenic inheritance of erythrocyte thiopurine methyltransferase activity. Am J Hum Genet 1980;32(5):651–62.

[30] Relling MV, Hancock ML, Boyett JM, Pui CH, Evans WE. Prognostic importance of 6-mercaptopurine dose intensity in acute lymphoblastic leukemia. Blood 1999;93(9):2817–23.

[31] Koren G, Ferrazini G, Sulh H, Langevin AM, Kapelushnik J, Klein J, et al. Systemic exposure to mercaptopurine as a prognostic factor in acute lymphocytic leukemia in children. N Engl J Med 1990;323(1):17–21.

[32] Garat A, Cauffiez C, Renault N, Lo-Guidice JM, Allorge D, Chevalier D, et al. Characterisation of novel defective thiopurine S-methyltransferase allelic variants. Biochem Pharmacol 2008;76(3):404–15.

[33] Schaeffeler E, Fischer C, Brockmeier D, Wernet D, Moerike K, Eichelbaum M, et al. Comprehensive analysis of thiopurine S-methyltransferase phenotype-genotype correlation in a large population of German-Caucasians and identification of novel TPMT variants. Pharmacogenetics 2004;14(7):407–17.

[34] Tai HL, Fessing MY, Bonten EJ, Yanishevsky Y, d'Azzo A, Krynetski EY, et al. Enhanced proteasomal degradation of mutant human thiopurine S-methyltransferase (TPMT) in mammalian cells: mechanism for TPMT protein deficiency inherited by TPMT*2, TPMT*3A, TPMT*3B or TPMT*3C. Pharmacogenetics 1999;9(5):641–50.

[35] McLeod HL, Siva C. The thiopurine S-methyltransferase gene locus – implications for clinical pharmacogenomics. Pharmacogenomics 2002;3(1):89–98.

[36] Oliveira E, Quental S, Alves S, Amorim A, Prata MJ. Do the distribution patterns of polymorphisms at the thiopurine S-methyltransferase locus in sub-Saharan populations need revision? Hints from Cabinda and Mozambique. Eur J Clin Pharmacol 2007;63(7):703–6.

[37] Relling MV, Rubnitz JE, Rivera GK, Boyett JM, Hancock ML, Felix CA, et al. High incidence of secondary brain tumours after radiotherapy and antimetabolites. Lancet 1999;354(9172):34–9.

[38] Relling MV, Yanishevski Y, Nemec J, Evans WE, Boyett JM, Behm FG, et al. Etoposide and antimetabolite pharmacology in patients who develop secondary acute myeloid leukemia. Leukemia 1998;12(3):346–352.

[39] Relling MV, Gardner EE, Sandborn WJ, Schmiegelow K, Pui CH, Yee SW, et al. Clinical Pharmacogenetics Implementation Consortium guidelines for thiopurine methyltransferase genotype and thiopurine dosing. Clin Pharmacol Ther 2011;89(3):387–91.

[40] Chabot GG. Clinical pharmacokinetics of irinotecan. Clin Pharmacokinet 1997;33(4):245–59.

[41] Santos A, Zanetta S, Cresteil T, Deroussent A, Pein F, Raymond E, et al. Metabolism of irinotecan (CPT-11) by CYP3A4 and CYP3A5 in humans. Clin Cancer Res 2000;6(5):2012–20.

[42] Hatfield MJ, Tsurkan L, Garrett M, Shaver TM, Hyatt JL, Edwards CC, et al. Organ-specific carboxylesterase profiling identifies the small intestine and kidney as major contributors of activation of the anticancer prodrug CPT-11. Biochem Pharmacol 2011;81(1):24–31.

[43] Danks MK, Morton CL, Krull EJ, Cheshire PJ, Richmond LB, Naeve CW, et al. Comparison of activation of CPT-11 by rabbit and human carboxylesterases for use in enzyme/prodrug therapy. Clin Cancer Res 1999;5(4):917–24.

[44] Humerickhouse R, Lohrbach K, Li L, Bosron WF, Dolan ME. Characterization of CPT-11 hydrolysis by human liver carboxylesterase isoforms hCE-1 and hCE-2. Cancer Res 2000;60(5):1189–92.

[45] Iyer L, King CD, Whitington PF, Green MD, Roy SK, Tephly TR, et al. Genetic predisposition to the metabolism of irinotecan (CPT-11): role of uridine diphosphate glucuronosyltransferase isoform 1A1 in the glucuronidation of its active metabolite (SN-38) in human liver microsomes. J Clin Invest 1998;101(4):847–54.

[46] Gagne JF, Montminy V, Belanger P, Journault K, Gaucher G, Guillemette C. Common human UGT1A polymorphisms and the altered metabolism of irinotecan active metabolite 7-ethyl-10-hydroxycamptothecin (SN-38). Mol Pharmacol 2002;62(3):608–17.

[47] Shulman K, Cohen I, Barnett-Griness O, Kuten A, Gruber SB, Lejbkowicz F, et al. Clinical implications of UGT1A1*28 genotype testing in colorectal cancer patients. Cancer 2011;117(14):3156–62.

[48] Hall D, Ybazeta G, Destro-Bisol G, Petzl-Erler ML, Di Rienzo A. Variability at the uridine diphosphate glucuronosyltransferase 1A1 promoter in human populations and primates. Pharmacogenetics 1999;9(5):591–9.

[49] Marcuello E, Altes A, Menoyo A, Del Rio E, Gomez-Pardo M, Baiget M. UGT1A1 gene variations and irinotecan treatment in patients with metastatic colorectal cancer. Br J Cancer 2004;91(4):678–82.

[50] Rouits E, Boisdron-Celle M, Dumont A, Guerin O, Morel A, Gamelin E. Relevance of different UGT1A1 polymorphisms in irinotecan-induced toxicity: a molecular and clinical study of 75 patients. Clin Cancer Res 2004;10(15):5151–9.

[51] Massacesi C, Terrazzino S, Marcucci F, Rocchi MB, Lippe P, Bisonni R, et al. Uridine diphosphate glucuronosyl transferase 1A1 promoter polymorphism predicts the risk of gastrointestinal toxicity and fatigue induced by irinotecan-based chemotherapy. Cancer 2006;106(5):1007–16.

[52] Monaghan G, Ryan M, Seddon R, Hume R, Burchell B. Genetic variation in bilirubin UPD-glucuronosyltransferase gene promoter and Gilbert's syndrome. Lancet 1996;347(9001):578–81.

[53] Bosma PJ, Goldhoorn B, Oude Elferink RP, Sinaasappel M, Oostra BA, Jansen PL. A mutation in bilirubin uridine 5'-diphosphate-glucuronosyltransferase isoform 1 causing Crigler-Najjar syndrome type II. Gastroenterology 1993;105(1):216–20.

[54] Bomgaars LR, Bernstein M, Krailo M, Kadota R, Das S, Chen Z, et al. Phase II trial of irinotecan in children with refractory solid tumors: a Children's Oncology Group Study. J Clin Oncol 2007;25(29):4622–7.

[55] Hoskins JM, Goldberg RM, Qu P, Ibrahim JG, McLeod HL. UGT1A1*28 genotype and irinotecan-induced neutropenia: dose matters. J Natl Cancer Inst 2007;99(17):1290–5.

[56] Toffoli G, Cecchin E, Gasparini G, D'Andrea M, Azzarello G, Basso U, et al. Genotype-driven phase I study of irinotecan administered in combination with fluorouracil/leucovorin in patients with metastatic colorectal cancer. J Clin Oncol 2010;28(5):866–71.

[57] Marcuello E, Paez D, Pare L, Salazar J, Sebio A, del Rio E, et al. A genotype-directed phase I-IV dose-finding study of irinotecan in combination with fluorouracil/leucovorin as first-line treatment in advanced colorectal cancer. Br J Cancer 2011;105(1):53–7.

[58] Akaba K, Kimura T, Sasaki A, Tanabe S, Ikegami T, Hashimoto M, et al. Neonatal hyperbilirubinemia and mutation of the bilirubin uridine diphosphate-glucuronosyltransferase gene: a common missense mutation among Japanese, Koreans and Chinese. Biochem Mol Biol Int 1998;46(1):21–6.

[59] Yong WP, Innocenti F, Ratain MJ. The role of pharmacogenetics in cancer therapeutics. Br J Clin Pharmacol 2006;62(1):35–46.

[60] Sai K, Saeki M, Saito Y, Ozawa S, Katori N, Jinno H, et al. UGT1A1 haplotypes associated with reduced glucuronidation and increased serum bilirubin in irinotecan-administered Japanese patients with cancer. Clin Pharmacol Ther 2004;75(6):501–515.

[61] Han JY, Lim HS, Park YH, Lee SY, Lee JS. Integrated pharmacogenetic prediction of irinotecan pharmacokinetics and toxicity in patients with advanced non-small cell lung cancer. Lung Cancer 2009;63(1):115–20.

[62] Jada SR, Lim R, Wong CI, Shu X, Lee SC, Zhou Q, et al. Role of UGT1A1*6, UGT1A1*28 and ABCG2 c.421C>A polymorphisms in irinotecan-induced neutropenia in Asian cancer patients. Cancer Sci 2007;98(9):1461–7.

[63] Minami H, Sai K, Saeki M, Saito Y, Ozawa S, Suzuki K, et al. Irinotecan pharmacokinetics/pharmacodynamics and UGT1A genetic polymorphisms in Japanese: roles of UGT1A1*6 and *28. Pharmacogenet Genomics 2007;17(7):497–504.

[64] Yamamoto N, Takahashi T, Kunikane H, Masuda N, Eguchi K, Shibuya M, et al. Phase I/II pharmacokinetic and pharmacogenomic study of UGT1A1 polymorphism in elderly patients with advanced non-small cell lung cancer treated with irinotecan. Clin Pharmacol Ther 2009;85(2):149–54.

[65] Cecchin E, Innocenti F, D'Andrea M, Corona G, De Mattia E, Biason P, et al. Predictive role of the UGT1A1, UGT1A7, and UGT1A9 genetic variants and their haplotypes on the outcome of metastatic colorectal cancer patients treated with fluorouracil, leucovorin, and irinotecan. J Clin Oncol 2009;27(15):2457–65.

[66] Martinez-Balibrea E, Abad A, Martinez-Cardus A, Gines A, Valladares M, Navarro M, et al. UGT1A and TYMS genetic variants predict toxicity and response of colorectal cancer patients treated with first-line irinotecan and fluorouracil combination therapy. Br J Cancer 2010;103(4):581–9.

[67] Lankisch TO, Schulz C, Zwingers T, Erichsen TJ, Manns MP, Heinemann V, et al. Gilbert's syndrome and irinotecan toxicity: combination with UDP-glucuronosyltransferase 1A7 variants increases risk. Cancer Epidemiol Biomarkers Prev 2008;17(3):695–701.

[68] Di Paolo A, Bocci G, Polillo M, Del Re M, Di Desidero T, Lastella M, et al. Pharmacokinetic and pharmacogenetic predictive markers of irinotecan activity and toxicity. Curr Drug Metab 2011;12(10):932–43.

[69] Innocenti F, Kroetz DL, Schuetz E, Dolan ME, Ramirez J, Relling M, et al. Comprehensive pharmacogenetic analysis of irinotecan neutropenia and pharmacokinetics. J Clin Oncol 2009;27(16):2604–14.

[70] Mathijssen RH, Verweij J, de Jonge MJ, Nooter K, Stoter G, Sparreboom A. Impact of body-size measures on irinotecan clearance: alternative dosing recommendations. J Clin Oncol 2002;20(1):81–7.

[71] van der Bol JM, Mathijssen RH, Creemers GJ, Planting AS, Loos WJ, Wiemer EA, et al. A CYP3A4 phenotype-based dosing algorithm for individualized treatment of irinotecan. Clin Cancer Res 2010;16(2):736–42.

[72] Diasio RB, Harris BE. Clinical pharmacology of 5-fluorouracil. Clin Pharmacokinet 1989;16(4):215–37.

[73] Diasio RB. Clinical implications of dihydropyrimidine dehydrogenase on 5-FU pharmacology. Oncology (Williston Park) 2001;15(1 Suppl. 2):21–6; discussion 27.

[74] Ridge SA, Sludden J, Wei X, Sapone A, Brown O, Hardy S, et al. Dihydropyrimidine dehydrogenase pharmacogenetics in patients with colorectal cancer. Br J Cancer 1998;77(3):497–500.

[75] Wei X, McLeod HL, McMurrough J, Gonzalez FJ, Fernandez-Salguero P. Molecular basis of the human dihydropyrimidine dehydrogenase deficiency and 5-fluorouracil toxicity. J Clin Invest 1996;98(3):610–5.

[76] Schwab M, Zanger UM, Marx C, Schaeffeler E, Klein K, Dippon J, et al. Role of genetic and nongenetic factors for fluorouracil treatment-related severe toxicity: a prospective clinical trial by the German 5-FU Toxicity Study Group. J Clin Oncol 2008;26(13):2131–8.

[77] Braun MS, Richman SD, Thompson L, Daly CL, Meade AM, Adlard JW, et al. Association of molecular markers with toxicity outcomes in a randomized trial of chemotherapy for advanced colorectal cancer: the FOCUS trial. J Clin Oncol 2009;27(33):5519–28.

[78] Popat S, Matakidou A, Houlston RS. Thymidylate synthase expression and prognosis in colorectal cancer: a systematic review and meta-analysis. J Clin Oncol 2004;22(3):529–36.

[79] Shimoyama S. Pharmacogenetics of fluoropyrimidine and cisplatin: a future application to gastric cancer treatment. J Gastroenterol Hepatol 2009;24(6):970–81.

[80] Mandola MV, Stoehlmacher J, Muller-Weeks S, Cesarone G, Yu MC, Lenz HJ, et al. A novel single nucleotide polymorphism within the 5' tandem repeat polymorphism of the thymidylate synthase gene abolishes USF-1 binding and alters transcriptional activity. Cancer Res 2003;63(11):2898–904.

[81] Lincz LF, Scorgie FE, Garg MB, Ackland SP. Identification of a novel single nucleotide polymorphism in the first tandem repeat sequence of the thymidylate synthase 2R allele. Int J Cancer 2007;120(9):1930–4.

[82] Mandola MV, Stoehlmacher J, Zhang W, Groshen S, Yu MC, Iqbal S, et al. A 6 bp polymorphism in the thymidylate synthase gene causes message instability and is associated with decreased intratumoral TS mRNA levels. Pharmacogenetics 2004;14(5):319–27.

[83] Ulrich CM, Robien K, Sparks R. Pharmacogenetics and folate metabolism – a promising direction. Pharmacogenomics 2002;3(3):299–313.

[84] Pullarkat ST, Stoehlmacher J, Ghaderi V, Xiong YP, Ingles SA, Sherrod A, et al. Thymidylate synthase gene polymorphism determines response and toxicity of 5-FU chemotherapy. Pharmacogenomics J 2001;1(1):65–70.

[85] Lecomte T, Ferraz JM, Zinzindohoue F, Loriot MA, Tregouet DA, Landi B, et al. Thymidylate synthase gene polymorphism predicts toxicity in colorectal cancer patients receiving 5-fluorouracil-based chemotherapy. Clin Cancer Res 2004;10(17):5880–8.

[86] Afzal S, Gusella M, Jensen SA, Vainer B, Vogel U, Andersen JT, et al. The association of polymorphisms in 5-fluorouracil metabolism genes with outcome in adjuvant treatment of colorectal cancer. Pharmacogenomics 2011;12(9):1257–67.

[87] Ichikawa W, Takahashi T, Suto K, Sasaki Y, Hirayama R. Orotate phosphoribosyltransferase gene polymorphism predicts toxicity in patients treated with bolus 5-fluorouracil regimen. Clin Cancer Res 2006;12(13):3928–34.

[88] Ruzzo A, Graziano F, Loupakis F, Santini D, Catalano V, Bisonni R, et al. Pharmacogenetic profiling in patients with advanced colorectal cancer treated with first-line FOLFIRI chemotherapy. Pharmacogenomics J 2008;8(4):278–88.

[89] Etienne-Grimaldi MC, Milano G, Maindrault-Goebel F, Chibaudel B, Formento JL, Francoual M, et al. Methylenetetrahydrofolate reductase (MTHFR) gene polymorphisms and FOLFOX response in colorectal cancer patients. Br J Clin Pharmacol 2010;69(1):58–66.

[90] Desta Z, Ward BA, Soukhova NV, Flockhart DA. Comprehensive evaluation of tamoxifen sequential biotransformation by the human cytochrome P450 system in vitro: prominent roles for CYP3A and CYP2D6. J Pharmacol Exp Ther 2004;310(3):1062–75.

[91] Nishiyama T, Ogura K, Nakano H, Ohnuma T, Kaku T, Hiratsuka A, et al. Reverse geometrical selectivity in glucuronidation and sulfation of cis- and trans-4-hydroxytamoxifens by human liver UDP-glucuronosyltransferases and sulfotransferases. Biochem Pharmacol 2002;63(10):1817–30.

[92] Stearns V, Johnson MD, Rae JM, Morocho A, Novielli A, Bhargava P, et al. Active tamoxifen metabolite plasma concentrations after coadministration of tamoxifen and the selective serotonin reuptake inhibitor paroxetine. J Natl Cancer Inst 2003;95(23):1758–64.

[93] Lennard MS. Genetic polymorphism of sparteine/debrisoquine oxidation: a reappraisal. Pharmacol Toxicol 1990;67(4):273–83.

[94] Ingelman-Sundberg M, Oscarson M, McLellan RA. Polymorphic human cytochrome P450 enzymes: an opportunity for individualized drug treatment. Trends Pharmacol Sci 1999;20(8):342–9.

[95] London SJ, Daly AK, Leathart JB, Navidi WC, Carpenter CC, Idle JR. Genetic polymorphism of CYP2D6 and lung cancer risk in African-Americans and Caucasians in Los Angeles County. Carcinogenesis 1997;18(6):1203–14.

[96] Serin A, Canan H, Alper B, Gulmen M. The frequencies of mutated alleles of CYP2D6 gene in a Turkish population. Forensic Sci Int 2012;222(1–3):332–4.

[97] Bradford LD. CYP2D6 allele frequency in European Caucasians, Asians, Africans and their descendants. Pharmacogenomics 2002;3(2):229–43.

[98] Sachse C, Brockmoller J, Bauer S, Roots I. Cytochrome P450 2D6 variants in a Caucasian population: allele frequencies and phenotypic consequences. Am J Hum Genet 1997;60(2):284–95.

[99] Kagimoto M, Heim M, Kagimoto K, Zeugin T, Meyer UA. Multiple mutations of the human cytochrome P450IID6 gene (CYP2D6) in poor metabolizers of debrisoquine: study of the functional significance of individual mutations by expression of chimeric genes. J Biol Chem 1990;265(28):17209–14.

[100] Gaedigk A, Blum M, Gaedigk R, Eichelbaum M, Meyer UA. Deletion of the entire cytochrome P450 CYP2D6 gene as a cause of impaired drug metabolism in poor metabolizers of the debrisoquine/sparteine polymorphism. Am J Hum Genet 1991;48(5):943–50.

[101] Marez D, Legrand M, Sabbagh N, Lo Guidice JM, Spire C, Lafitte JJ, et al. Polymorphism of the cytochrome P450 CYP2D6 gene in a European population: characterization of 48 mutations and 53 alleles, their frequencies and evolution. Pharmacogenetics 1997;7(3):193–202.

[102] Jin Y, Desta Z, Stearns V, Ward B, Ho H, Lee KH, et al. CYP2D6 genotype, antidepressant use, and tamoxifen metabolism during adjuvant breast cancer treatment. J Natl Cancer Inst 2005;97(1):30–9.

[103] Lim HS, Ju Lee H, Seok Lee K, Sook Lee E, Jang IJ, Ro J. Clinical implications of CYP2D6 genotypes predictive of tamoxifen pharmacokinetics in metastatic breast cancer. J Clin Oncol 2007;25(25):3837–45.

[104] Kiyotani K, Mushiroda T, Imamura CK, Hosono N, Tsunoda T, Kubo M, et al. Significant effect of polymorphisms in CYP2D6 and ABCC2 on clinical outcomes of adjuvant tamoxifen therapy for breast cancer patients. J Clin Oncol 2010;28(8):1287–1293.

[105] Schroth W, Goetz MP, Hamann U, Fasching PA, Schmidt M, Winter S, et al. Association between CYP2D6 polymorphisms and outcomes among women with early stage breast cancer treated with tamoxifen. JAMA 2009;302(13):1429–36.

[106] Goetz MP, Rae JM, Suman VJ, Safgren SL, Ames MM, Visscher DW, et al. Pharmacogenetics of tamoxifen bio-transformation is associated with clinical outcomes of efficacy and hot flashes. J Clin Oncol 2005;23(36):9312–8.

[107] Stingl JC, Parmar S, Huber-Wechselberger A, Kainz A, Renner W, Seeringer A, et al. Impact of CYP2D6*4 genotype on progression free survival in tamoxifen breast cancer treatment. Curr Med Res Opin 2010;26(11):2535–42.

[108] Bijl MJ, van Schaik RH, Lammers LA, Hofman A, Vulto AG, van Gelder T, et al. The CYP2D6*4 polymorphism affects breast cancer survival in tamoxifen users. Breast Cancer Res Treat 2009;118(1):125–30.

[109] Abraham JE, Maranian MJ, Driver KE, Platte R, Kalmyrzaev B, Baynes C, et al. CYP2D6 gene variants: association with breast cancer specific survival in a cohort of breast cancer patients from the United Kingdom treated with adjuvant tamoxifen. Breast Cancer Res 2010;12(4):R64.

[110] Ramon y, Cajal T, Altes A, Pare L, del Rio E, Alonso C, et al. Impact of CYP2D6 polymorphisms in tamoxifen adjuvant breast cancer treatment. Breast Cancer Res Treat 2010;119(1):33–8.

[111] Newman WG, Hadfield KD, Latif A, Roberts SA, Shenton A, McHague C, et al. Impaired tamoxifen metabolism reduces survival in familial breast cancer patients. Clin Cancer Res 2008;14(18):5913–8.

[112] Xu Y, Sun Y, Yao L, Shi L, Wu Y, Ouyang T, et al. Association between CYP2D6 *10 genotype and survival of breast cancer patients receiving tamoxifen treatment. Ann Oncol 2008;19(8):1423–9.

[113] Okishiro M, Taguchi T, Jin Kim S, Shimazu K, Tamaki Y, Noguchi S. Genetic polymorphisms of CYP2D6 10 and CYP2C19 2, 3 are not associated with prognosis, endometrial thickness, or bone mineral density in Japanese breast cancer patients treated with adjuvant tamoxifen. Cancer 2009;115(5):952–61.

[114] Wegman P, Vainikka L, Stal O, Nordenskjold B, Skoog L, Rutqvist LE, et al. Genotype of metabolic enzymes and the benefit of tamoxifen in postmenopausal breast cancer patients. Breast Cancer Res 2005;7(3):R284–90.

[115] Wegman P, Elingarami S, Carstensen J, Stal O, Nordenskjold B, Wingren S. Genetic variants of CYP3A5, CYP2D6, SULT1A1, UGT2B15 and tamoxifen response in postmenopausal patients with breast cancer. Breast Cancer Res 2007;9(1):R7.

[116] Nowell SA, Ahn J, Rae JM, Scheys JO, Trovato A, Sweeney C, et al. Association of genetic variation in tamoxifen-metabolizing enzymes with overall survival and recurrence of disease in breast cancer patients. Breast Cancer Res Treat 2005;91(3):249–58.

[117] Regan MM, Leyland-Jones B, Bouzyk M, Pagani O, Tang W, Kammler R, et al. CYP2D6 genotype and tamoxifen response in postmenopausal women with endocrine-responsive breast cancer: the breast international group 1-98 trial. J Natl Cancer Inst 2012;104(6):441–51.

[118] Rae JM, Drury S, Hayes DF, Stearns V, Thibert JN, Haynes BP, et al. CYP2D6 and UGT2B7 genotype and risk of recurrence in tamoxifen-treated breast cancer patients. J Natl Cancer Inst 2012;104(6):452–60.

[119] Nakamura Y, Ratain MJ, Cox NJ, Mcleod HL, Kroetz DL, Flockhart DA. Re: CYP2D6 genotype and tamoxifen response in postmenopausal women with endocrine-responsive breast cancer: the Breast International Group 1-98 Trial. J Natl Cancer Inst 2012;104:1264.

[120] Pharoah PDP, Abraham J, Caldas C. Re: CYP2D6 genotype and tamoxifen response in postmenopausal women with endocrine-responsive breast cancer: the Breast International Group 1-98 Trial and Re: CYP2D6 and UGT2B7 genotype and risk of recurrence in tamoxifen-treated breast cancer patients. J Natl Cancer Inst 2012;104:1263–4.

[121] Regan MM, Bouzyk M, Rae JM, Viale G, Leyland-Jones B. Response. J Natl Cancer Inst 2012;104:1266–7.

[122] Kiyotani K, Mushiroda T, Imamura CK, Tanigawara Y, Hosono N, Kubo M, et al. Dose-adjustment study of tamoxifen based on CYP2D6 genotypes in Japanese breast cancer patients. Breast Cancer Res Treat 2012;131(1):137–45.

[123] Irvin Jr WJ, Walko CM, Weck KE, Ibrahim JG, Chiu WK, Dees EC, et al. Genotype-guided tamoxifen dosing increases active metabolite exposure in women with reduced CYP2D6 metabolism: a multicenter study. J Clin Oncol 2011;29(24):3232–9.

[124] O'Brien SG, Guilhot F, Larson RA, Gathmann I, Baccarani M, Cervantes F, et al. Imatinib compared with interferon and low-dose cytarabine for newly diagnosed chronic-phase chronic myeloid leukemia. N Engl J Med 2003;348(11):994–1004.

[125] Bisen A, Claxton DF. Tyrosine kinase targeted treatment of chronic myelogenous leukemia and other myeloproliferative neoplasms. Adv Exp Med Biol 2013;779:179–196.

[126] Tallman MS, Andersen JW, Schiffer CA, Appelbaum FR, Feusner JH, Ogden A, et al. All-trans-retinoic acid in acute promyelocytic leukemia. N Engl J Med 1997;337(15):1021–8.

[127] Kuhnl A, Grimwade D. Molecular markers in acute myeloid leukaemia. Int J Hematol 2012;96(2):153–63.

[128] Amado RG, Wolf M, Peeters M, Van Cutsem E, Siena S, Freeman DJ, et al. Wild-type KRAS is required for panitumumab efficacy in patients with metastatic colorectal cancer. J Clin Oncol 2008;26(10):1626–34.

[129] Douillard JY, Siena S, Cassidy J, Tabernero J, Burkes R, Barugel M, et al. Randomized, phase III trial of pani-tumumab with infusional fluorouracil, leucovorin, and oxaliplatin (FOLFOX4) versus FOLFOX4 alone as first-line treatment in patients with previously untreated metastatic colorectal cancer: the PRIME study. J Clin Oncol 2010;28(31):4697–705.

[130] Bokemeyer C, Bondarenko I, Hartmann JT, de Braud F, Schuch G, Zubel A, et al. Efficacy according to bio-marker status of cetuximab plus FOLFOX-4 as first-line treatment for metastatic colorectal cancer: the OPUS study. Ann Oncol 2011;22(7):1535–46.

[131] Van Cutsem E, Kohne CH, Lang I, Folprecht G, Nowacki MP, Cascinu S, et al. Cetuximab plus irinotecan, fluorouracil, and leucovorin as first-line treatment for metastatic colorectal cancer: updated analysis of overall survival according to tumor KRAS and BRAF mutation status. J Clin Oncol 2011;29(15):2011–9.

[132] Ren H, Tan ZP, Zhu X, Crosby K, Haack H, Ren JM, et al. Identification of anaplastic lymphoma kinase as a potential therapeutic target in ovarian cancer. Cancer Res 2012;72(13):3312–23.

[133] Mosse YP, Laudenslager M, Longo L, Cole KA, Wood A, Attiyeh EF, et al. Identification of ALK as a major familial neuroblastoma predisposition gene. Nature 2008;455(7215):930–5.

[134] Chen Y, Takita J, Choi YL, Kato M, Ohira M, Sanada M, et al. Oncogenic mutations of ALK kinase in neuroblas-toma. Nature 2008;455(7215):971–4.

[135] George RE, Sanda T, Hanna M, Frohling S, Luther 2nd W, Zhang J, et al. Activating mutations in ALK provide a therapeutic target in neuroblastoma. Nature 2008;455(7215):975–8.

[136] Janoueix-Lerosey I, Lequin D, Brugieres L, Ribeiro A, de Pontual L, Combaret V, et al. Somatic and germline activating mutations of the ALK kinase receptor in neuroblastoma. Nature 2008;455(7215):967–70.

[137] O'Brien C, Wallin JJ, Sampath D, GuhaThakurta D, Savage H, Punnoose EA, et al. Predictive biomarkers of sensitivity to the phosphatidylinositol 3' kinase inhibitor GDC-0941 in breast cancer preclinical models. Clin Cancer Res 2011;16(14):3670–83.

[138] Bastian BC, LeBoit PE, Hamm H, Brocker EB, Pinkel D. Chromosomal gains and losses in primary cutaneous melanomas detected by comparative genomic hybridization. Cancer Res 1998;58(10):2170–5.

[139] Kantarjian H, Shah NP, Hochhaus A, Cortes J, Shah S, Ayala M, et al. Dasatinib versus imatinib in newly diag-nosed chronic-phase chronic myeloid leukemia. N Engl J Med 2010;362(24):2260–70.

[140] Saglio G, Kim DW, Issaragrisil S, le Coutre P, Etienne G, Lobo C, et al. Nilotinib versus imatinib for newly diagnosed chronic myeloid leukemia. N Engl J Med 2010;362(24):2251–9.

[141] Cortes JE, Kim DW, Kantarjian HM, Brummendorf TH, Dyagil I, Griskevicius L, et al. Bosutinib versus ima-tinib in newly diagnosed chronic-phase chronic myeloid leukemia: results from the BELA trial. J Clin Oncol 2012;30(28):3486–92.

[142] Vignetti M, Fazi P, Cimino G, Martinelli G, Di Raimondo F, Ferrara F, et al. Imatinib plus steroids induces complete remissions and prolonged survival in elderly philadelphia chromosome-positive patients with acute lymphoblastic leukemia without additional chemotherapy: results of the Gruppo Italiano Malattie Emato-logiche dell'Adulto (GIMEMA) LAL0201-B protocol. Blood 2007;109(9):3676–8.

[143] Foa R, Vitale A, Vignetti M, Meloni G, Guarini A, De Propris MS, et al. Dasatinib as first-line treatment for adult patients with philadelphia chromosome-positive acute lymphoblastic leukemia. Blood 2011;118(25):6521–8.

[144] Tiribelli M, Sperotto A, Candoni A, Simeone E, Buttignol S, Fanin R. Nilotinib and donor lymphocyte infusion in the treatment of philadelphia-positive acute lymphoblastic leukemia (Ph+ ALL) relapsing after allogeneic stem cell transplantation and resistant to imatinib. Leuk Res 2009;33(1):174–7.

[145] Davies H, Bignell GR, Cox C, Stephens P, Edkins S, Clegg S, et al. Mutations of the BRAF gene in human cancer. Nature 2002;417(6892):949–54.

[146] Takeuchi K, Soda M, Togashi Y, Suzuki R, Sakata S, Hatano S, et al. RET, ROS1 and ALK fusions in lung cancer. Nat Med 2012;18(3):378–81.

[147] Matsubara D, Kanai Y, Ishikawa S, Ohara S, Yoshimoto T, Sakatani T, et al. Identification of CCDC6-RET fusion in the human lung adenocarcinoma cell line, LC-2/ad. J Thorac Oncol 2012;7(12):1872–6.

[148] Hammerman PS, Sos ML, Ramos AH, Xu C, Dutt A, Zhou W, et al. Mutations in the DDR2 kinase gene identify a novel therapeutic target in squamous cell lung cancer. Cancer Discov 2011;1(1):78–89.

[149] Lynch TJ, Bell DW, Sordella R, Gurubhagavatula S, Okimoto RA, Brannigan BW, et al. Activating mutations in the epidermal growth factor receptor underlying responsiveness of non-small-cell lung cancer to gefitinib. N Engl J Med 2004;350(21):2129–39.

[150] Paez JG, Janne PA, Lee JC, Tracy S, Greulich H, Gabriel S, et al. EGFR mutations in lung cancer: correlation with clinical response to gefitinib therapy. Science 2004;304(5676):1497–500.

[151] Lin E, Li L, Guan Y, Soriano R, Rivers CS, Mohan S, et al. Exon array profiling detects EML4-ALK fusion in breast, colorectal, and non-small cell lung cancers. Mol Cancer Res 2009;7(9):1466–76.

[152] Soda M, Choi YL, Enomoto M, Takada S, Yamashita Y, Ishikawa S, et al. Identification of the transforming EML4-ALK fusion gene in non-small-cell lung cancer. Nature 2007;448(7153):561–6.

[153] Simon R, Richter J, Wagner U, Fijan A, Bruderer J, Schmid U, et al. High-throughput tissue microarray analysis of 3p.25 (RAF1) and 8p.12 (FGFR1) copy number alterations in urinary bladder cancer. Cancer Res 2001;61(11):4514–9.

[154] Turner N, Pearson A, Sharpe R, Lambros M, Geyer F, Lopez-Garcia MA, et al. FGFR1 amplification drives endocrine therapy resistance and is a therapeutic target in breast cancer. Cancer Res 2010;70(5):2085–94.

[155] Weiss J, Sos ML, Seidel D, Peifer M, Zander T, Heuckmann JM, et al. Frequent and focal FGFR1 amplification associates with therapeutically tractable FGFR1 dependency in squamous cell lung cancer. Sci Transl Med 2010;2(62); 62ra93.

[156] Gorringe KL, Jacobs S, Thompson ER, Sridhar A, Qiu W, Choong DY, et al. High-resolution single nucleotide polymorphism array analysis of epithelial ovarian cancer reveals numerous microdeletions and amplifications. Clin Cancer Res 2007;13(16):4731–9.

[157] Moasser MM. The oncogene HER2: its signaling and transforming functions and its role in human cancer pathogenesis. Oncogene 2007;26(45):6469–87.

[158] Slamon DJ, Clark GM, Wong SG, Levin WJ, Ullrich A, McGuire WL. Human breast cancer: correlation of relapse and survival with amplification of the HER-2/neu oncogene. Science 1987;235(4785):177–82.

[159] Tanner M, Hollmen M, Junttila TT, Kapanen AI, Tommola S, Soini Y, et al. Amplification of HER-2 in gastric carcinoma: association with topoisomerase II alpha gene amplification, intestinal type, poor prognosis and sensitivity to trastuzumab. Ann Oncol 2005;16(2):273–8.

[160] Verstovsek S, Mesa RA, Gotlib J, Levy RS, Gupta V, DiPersio JF, et al. A double-blind, placebo-controlled trial of ruxolitinib for myelofibrosis. N Engl J Med 2012;366(9):799–807.

[161] Lipson D, Capelletti M, Yelensky R, Otto G, Parker A, Jarosz M, et al. Identification of new ALK and RET gene fusions from colorectal and lung cancer biopsies. Nat Med 2012;18(3):382–4.

[162] Kohno T, Ichikawa H, Totoki Y, Yasuda K, Hiramoto M, Nammo T, et al. KIF5B-RET fusions in lung adenocarcinoma. Nat Med 2012;18(3):375–7.

[163] Hirota S, Isozaki K, Moriyama Y, Hashimoto K, Nishida T, Ishiguro S, et al. Gain-of-function mutations of c-kit in human gastrointestinal stromal tumors. Science 1998;279(5350):577–80.

[164] Curtin JA, Fridlyand J, Kageshita T, Patel HN, Busam KJ, Kutzner H, et al. Distinct sets of genetic alterations in melanoma. N Engl J Med 2005;353(20):2135–47.

[165] Schubbert S, Shannon K, Bollag G. Hyperactive Ras in developmental disorders and cancer. Nat Rev Cancer 2007;7(4):295–308.

[166] Nikolaev SI, Rimoldi D, Iseli C, Valsesia A, Robyr D, Gehrig C, et al. Exome sequencing identifies recurrent somatic MAP2K1 and MAP2K2 mutations in melanoma. Nat Genet 2011;44(2):133–9.

[167] Marks JL, Gong Y, Chitale D, Golas B, McLellan MD, Kasai Y, et al. Novel MEK1 mutation identified by mutational analysis of epidermal growth factor receptor signaling pathway genes in lung adenocarcinoma. Cancer Res 2008;68(14):5524–8.

[168] Nakajima M, Sawada H, Yamada Y, Watanabe A, Tatsumi M, Yamashita J, et al. The prognostic significance of amplification and overexpression of c-met and c-erb B-2 in human gastric carcinomas. Cancer 1999;85(9): 1894–902.

[169] Bean J, Brennan C, Shih JY, Riely G, Viale A, Wang L, et al. MET amplification occurs with or without T790M mutations in EGFR mutant lung tumors with acquired resistance to gefitinib or erlotinib. Proc Natl Acad Sci U S A 2007;104(52):20932–7.

[170] Ma PC, Tretiakova MS, MacKinnon AC, Ramnath N, Johnson C, Dietrich S, et al. Expression and mutational analysis of MET in human solid cancers. Genes Chromosomes Cancer 2008;47(12):1025–37.

[171] Morris SW, Kirstein MN, Valentine MB, Dittmer KG, Shapiro DN, Saltman DL, et al. Fusion of a kinase gene, ALK, to a nucleolar protein gene, NPM, in non-Hodgkin's lymphoma. Science 1994;263(5151):1281–1284.

[172] Heinrich MC, Corless CL, Duensing A, McGreevey L, Chen CJ, Joseph N, et al. PDGFRA activating mutations in gastrointestinal stromal tumors. Science 2003;299(5607):708–10.

[173] Samuels Y, Wang Z, Bardelli A, Silliman N, Ptak J, Szabo S, et al. High frequency of mutations of the PIK3CA gene in human cancers. Science 2004;304(5670):554.

[174] Fenaux P, Chastang C, Chevret S, Sanz M, Dombret H, Archimbaud E, et al. A randomized comparison of all transretinoic acid (ATRA) followed by chemotherapy and ATRA plus chemotherapy and the role of maintenance therapy in newly diagnosed acute promyelocytic leukemia. The European APL Group. Blood 1999;94(4):1192–200.

[175] Chalhoub N, Baker SJ. PTEN and the PI3-kinase pathway in cancer. Ann Rev Pathol 2009;4:127–50.

[176] Ciampi R, Nikiforov YE. RET/PTC rearrangements and BRAF mutations in thyroid tumorigenesis. Endocrinology 2007;148(3):936–41.

[177] Rikova K, Guo A, Zeng Q, Possemato A, Yu J, Haack H, et al. Global survey of phosphotyrosine signaling identifies oncogenic kinases in lung cancer. Cell 2007;131(6):1190–203.

[178] Tabbo F, Barreca A, Piva R, Inghirami G. ALK signaling and target therapy in anaplastic large cell lymphoma. Front Oncol 2012;2:41.

[179] Lawrence B, Perez-Atayde A, Hibbard MK, Rubin BP, Dal Cin P, Pinkus JL, et al. TPM3-ALK and TPM4-ALK oncogenes in inflammatory myofibroblastic tumors. Am J Pathol 2000;157(2):377–84.

[180] Dematteo RP, Heinrich MC, El-Rifai WM, Demetri G. Clinical management of gastrointestinal stromal tumors: before and after STI-571. Hum Pathol 2002;33(5):466–77.

[181] Tornillo L, Duchini G, Carafa V, Lugli A, Dirnhofer S, Di Vizio D, et al. Patterns of gene amplification in gastrointestinal stromal tumors (GIST). Lab Invest 2005;85(7):921–31.

[182] Corless CL, Fletcher JA, Heinrich MC. Biology of gastrointestinal stromal tumors. J Clin Oncol 2004;22(18): 3813–25.

[183] Corless CL, Barnett CM, Heinrich MC. Gastrointestinal stromal tumours: origin and molecular oncology. Nat Rev Cancer 2011;11(12):865–78.

[184] Duensing A, Joseph NE, Medeiros F, Smith F, Hornick JL, Heinrich MC, et al. Protein Kinase C theta (PKCtheta) expression and constitutive activation in gastrointestinal stromal tumors (GISTs). Cancer Res 2004;64(15):5127–31.

[185] van Oosterom AT, Judson I, Verweij J, Stroobants S, Donato di Paola E, Dimitrijevic S, et al. Safety and efficacy of imatinib (STI571) in metastatic gastrointestinal stromal tumours: a phase I study. Lancet 2001;358(9291):1421–3.

[186] Blanke CD, Rankin C, Demetri GD, Ryan CW, von Mehren M, Benjamin RS, et al. Phase III randomized, intergroup trial assessing imatinib mesylate at two dose levels in patients with unresectable or metastatic gastrointestinal stromal tumors expressing the kit receptor tyrosine kinase: S0033. J Clin Oncol 2008;26(4):626–32.

[187] Verweij J, Casali PG, Zalcberg J, LeCesne A, Reichardt P, Blay JY, et al. Progression-free survival in gastrointestinal stromal tumours with high-dose imatinib: randomised trial. Lancet 2004;364(9440):1127–34.

[188] Gastrointestinal Stromal Tumor Meta-Analysis Group (MetaGIST). Comparison of two doses of imatinib for the treatment of unresectable or metastatic gastrointestinal stromal tumors: a meta-analysis of 1,640 patients. J Clin Oncol 2010;28(7):1247–53.

[189] Dematteo RP, Ballman KV, Antonescu CR, Maki RG, Pisters PW, Demetri GD, et al. Adjuvant imatinib mesylate after resection of localised, primary gastrointestinal stromal tumour: a randomised, double-blind, placebo-controlled trial. Lancet 2009;373(9669):1097–104.

[190] Joensuu H, Eriksson M, Sundby Hall K, Hartmann JT, Pink D, Schutte J, et al. One vs three years of adjuvant imatinib for operable gastrointestinal stromal tumor: a randomized trial. JAMA 2012;307(12):1265–72.

[191] Heinrich MC, Owzar K, Corless CL, Hollis D, Borden EC, Fletcher CD, et al. Correlation of kinase genotype and clinical outcome in the North American Intergroup Phase III Trial of imatinib mesylate for treatment of advanced gastrointestinal stromal tumor: CALGB 150105 Study by Cancer and Leukemia Group B and Southwest Oncology Group. J Clin Oncol 2008;26(33):5360–7.

[192] Debiec-Rychter M, Dumez H, Judson I, Wasag B, Verweij J, Brown M, et al. Use of c-KIT/PDGFRA mutational analysis to predict the clinical response to imatinib in patients with advanced gastrointestinal stromal tumours entered on phase I and II studies of the EORTC Soft Tissue and Bone Sarcoma Group. Eur J Cancer 2004;40(5):689–95.

[193] Cassier PA, Fumagalli E, Rutkowski P, Schoffski P, Van Glabbeke M, Debiec-Rychter M, et al. Outcome of patients with platelet-derived growth factor receptor alpha-mutated gastrointestinal stromal tumors in the tyrosine kinase inhibitor era. Clin Cancer Res 2012;18(16):4458–4464.

[194] Antonescu CR, Besmer P, Guo T, Arkun K, Hom G, Koryotowski B, et al. Acquired resistance to imatinib in gastrointestinal stromal tumor occurs through secondary gene mutation. Clin Cancer Res 2005;11(11):4182–90.

[195] Heinrich MC, Corless CL, Blanke CD, Demetri GD, Joensuu H, Roberts PJ, et al. Molecular correlates of imatinib resistance in gastrointestinal stromal tumors. J Clin Oncol 2006;24(29):4764–74.

[196] Wardelmann E, Merkelbach-Bruse S, Pauls K, Thomas N, Schildhaus HU, Heinicke T, et al. Polyclonal evolution of multiple secondary KIT mutations in gastrointestinal stromal tumors under treatment with imatinib mesylate. Clin Cancer Res 2006;12(6):1743–9.

[197] Desai J, Shankar S, Heinrich MC, Fletcher JA, Fletcher CD, Manola J, et al. Clonal evolution of resistance to imatinib in patients with metastatic gastrointestinal stromal tumors. Clin Cancer Res 2007;13(18 Pt. 1):5398–405.

[198] Nishida T, Kanda T, Nishitani A, Takahashi T, Nakajima K, Ishikawa T, et al. Secondary mutations in the kinase domain of the KIT gene are predominant in imatinib-resistant gastrointestinal stromal tumor. Cancer Sci 2008;99(4):799–804.

[199] Debiec-Rychter M, Cools J, Dumez H, Sciot R, Stul M, Mentens N, et al. Mechanisms of resistance to imatinib mesylate in gastrointestinal stromal tumors and activity of the PKC412 inhibitor against imatinib-resistant mutants. Gastroenterology 2005;128(2):270–9.

[200] Miselli FC, Casieri P, Negri T, Orsenigo M, Lagonigro MS, Gronchi A, et al. c-Kit/PDGFRA gene status alterations possibly related to primary imatinib resistance in gastrointestinal stromal tumors. Clin Cancer Res 2007;13(8):2369–77.

[201] Eechoute K, Franke RM, Loos WJ, Scherkenbach LA, Boere I, Verweij J, et al. Environmental and genetic factors affecting transport of imatinib by OATP1A2. Clin Pharmacol Ther 2011;89(6):816–20.

[202] Demetri GD, Reichardt P, Kang Y-K, Blay J-Y, Joensuu H, Maki RG, et al. Randomized phase III trial of regorafenib in patients (pts) with metastatic and/or unresectable gastrointestinal stromal tumor (GIST) progressing despite prior treatment with at least imatinib (IM) and sunitinib (SU): GRID trial. J Clin Oncol 2012;30(Suppl. 18); LBA10008.

[203] Yarden Y, Sliwkowski MX. Untangling the ErbB signalling network. Nat Rev Mol Cell Biol 2001;2(2):127–37.

[204] Chia S, Norris B, Speers C, Cheang M, Gilks B, Gown AM, et al. Human epidermal growth factor receptor 2 overexpression as a prognostic factor in a large tissue microarray series of node-negative breast cancers. J Clin Oncol 2008;26(35):5697–704.

[205] Wolff AC, Hammond ME, Schwartz JN, Hagerty KL, Allred DC, Cote RJ, et al. American Society of Clinical Oncology/College of American Pathologists guideline recommendations for human epidermal growth factor receptor 2 testing in breast cancer. Arch Pathol Lab Med 2007;131(1):18–43.

[206] Spector NL, Blackwell KL. Understanding the mechanisms behind trastuzumab therapy for human epidermal growth factor receptor 2-positive breast cancer. J Clin Oncol 2009;27(34):5838–47.

[207] Hudis CA. Trastuzumab – mechanism of action and use in clinical practice. N Engl J Med 2007;357(1):39–51.

[208] Cobleigh MA, Vogel CL, Tripathy D, Robert NJ, Scholl S, Fehrenbacher L, et al. Multinational study of the efficacy and safety of humanized anti-HER2 monoclonal antibody in women who have HER2-overexpressing metastatic breast cancer that has progressed after chemotherapy for metastatic disease. J Clin Oncol 1999;17(9):2639–48.

[209] Vogel CL, Cobleigh MA, Tripathy D, Gutheil JC, Harris LN, Fehrenbacher L, et al. Efficacy and safety of trastuzumab as a single agent in first-line treatment of HER2-overexpressing metastatic breast cancer. J Clin Oncol 2002;20(3):719–26.

[210] Slamon DJ, Leyland-Jones B, Shak S, Fuchs H, Paton V, Bajamonde A, et al. Use of chemotherapy plus a monoclonal antibody against HER2 for metastatic breast cancer that overexpresses HER2. N Engl J Med 2001;344(11):783–92.

[211] Gianni L, Dafni U, Gelber RD, Azambuja E, Muehlbauer S, Goldhirsch A, et al. Treatment with trastuzumab for 1 year after adjuvant chemotherapy in patients with HER2-positive early breast cancer: a 4-year follow-up of a randomised controlled trial. Lancet Oncol 2010;12(3):236–44.

[212] Piccart-Gebhart MJ, Procter M, Leyland-Jones B, Goldhirsch A, Untch M, Smith I, et al. Trastuzumab after adjuvant chemotherapy in HER2-positive breast cancer. N Engl J Med 2005;353(16):1659–72.

[213] Perez EA, Romond EH, Suman VJ, Jeong JH, Davidson NE, Geyer Jr CE, et al. Four-year follow-up of trastuzumab plus adjuvant chemotherapy for operable human epidermal growth factor receptor 2-positive breast cancer: joint analysis of data from NCCTG N9831 and NSABP B-31. J Clin Oncol 2011;29(25):3366–73.

[214] Romond EH, Perez EA, Bryant J, Suman VJ, Geyer Jr CE, Davidson NE, et al. Trastuzumab plus adjuvant chemotherapy for operable HER2-positive breast cancer. N Engl J Med 2005;353(16):1673–1684.

[215] Joensuu H, Kellokumpu-Lehtinen PL, Bono P, Alanko T, Kataja V, Asola R, et al. Adjuvant docetaxel or vinorel-bine with or without trastuzumab for breast cancer. N Engl J Med 2006;354(8):809–20.

[216] Joensuu H, Bono P, Kataja V, Alanko T, Kokko R, Asola R, et al. Fluorouracil, epirubicin, and cyclophos-phamide with either docetaxel or vinorelbine, with or without trastuzumab, as adjuvant treatments of breast cancer: final results of the FinHer Trial. J Clin Oncol 2009;27(34):5685–92.

[217] Slamon D, Eiermann W, Robert N, Pienkowski T, Martin M, Press M, et al. Adjuvant trastuzumab in HER2-positive breast cancer. N Engl J Med 2011;365(14):1273–83.

[218] Yin W, Jiang Y, Shen Z, Shao Z, Lu J. Trastuzumab in the adjuvant treatment of HER2-positive early breast cancer patients: a meta-analysis of published randomized controlled trials. PLoS One 2011;6(6):e21030.

[219] Pao W, Girard N. New driver mutations in non-small-cell lung cancer. Lancet Oncol 2011;12(2):175–80.

[220] Perez-Moreno P, Brambilla E, Thomas R, Soria JC. Squamous cell carcinoma of the lung: molecular subtypes and therapeutic opportunities. Clin Cancer Res 2012;18(9):2443–51.

[221] Ciardiello F, Tortora G. EGFR antagonists in cancer treatment. N Engl J Med 2008;358(11):1160–74.

[222] Shepherd FA, Rodrigues Pereira J, Ciuleanu T, Tan EH, Hirsh V, Thongprasert S, et al. Erlotinib in previously treated non-small-cell lung cancer. N Engl J Med 2005;353(2):123–32.

[223] Thatcher N, Chang A, Parikh P, Rodrigues Pereira J, Ciuleanu T, von Pawel J, et al. Gefitinib plus best sup-portive care in previously treated patients with refractory advanced non-small-cell lung cancer: results from a randomised, placebo-controlled, multicentre study (Iressa Survival Evaluation in Lung Cancer). Lancet 2005;366(9496):1527–37.

[224] Pao W, Miller V, Zakowski M, Doherty J, Politi K, Sarkaria I, et al. EGF receptor gene mutations are common in lung cancers from "never smokers" and are associated with sensitivity of tumors to gefitinib and erlotinib. Proc Natl Acad Sci U S A 2004;101(36):13306–11.

[225] Shigematsu H, Lin L, Takahashi T, Nomura M, Suzuki M, Wistuba II , et al. Clinical and biological fea-tures associated with epidermal growth factor receptor gene mutations in lung cancers. J Natl Cancer Inst 2005;97(5):339–46.

[226] Riely GJ, Pao W, Pham D, Li AR, Rizvi N, Venkatraman ES, et al. Clinical course of patients with non-small cell lung cancer and epidermal growth factor receptor exon 19 and exon 21 mutations treated with gefitinib or erlotinib. Clin Cancer Res 2006;12(3 Pt. 1):839–44.

[227] Sharma SV, Bell DW, Settleman J, Haber DA. Epidermal growth factor receptor mutations in lung cancer. Nat Rev Cancer 2007;7(3):169–81.

[228] Carey KD, Garton AJ, Romero MS, Kahler J, Thomson S, Ross S, et al. Kinetic analysis of epidermal growth factor receptor somatic mutant proteins shows increased sensitivity to the epidermal growth factor receptor tyrosine kinase inhibitor, erlotinib. Cancer Res 2006;66(16):8163–71.

[229] Han JY, Park K, Kim SW, Lee DH, Kim HY, Kim HT, et al. First-SIGNAL: first-line single-agent IRESSA versus gemcitabine and cisplatin trial in never-smokers with adenocarcinoma of the lung. J Clin Oncol 2012;30(10):1122–8.

[230] Mok TS, Wu YL, Thongprasert S, Yang CH, Chu DT, Saijo N, et al. Gefitinib or carboplatin-paclitaxel in pulmo-nary adenocarcinoma. N Engl J Med 2009;361(10):947–57.

[231] Thongprasert S, Duffield E, Saijo N, Wu YL, Yang JC, Chu DT, et al. Health-related quality-of-life in a random-ized phase III first-line study of gefitinib versus carboplatin/paclitaxel in clinically selected patients from Asia with advanced NSCLC (IPASS). J Thorac Oncol 2011;6(11):1872–80.

[232] Fukuoka M, Wu YL, Thongprasert S, Sunpaweravong P, Leong SS, Sriuranpong V, et al. Biomarker analyses and final overall survival results from a phase III, randomized, open-label, first-line study of gefitinib versus carboplatin/paclitaxel in clinically selected patients with advanced non-small-cell lung cancer in Asia (IPASS). J Clin Oncol 2011;29(21):2866–74.

[233] Mitsudomi T, Morita S, Yatabe Y, Negoro S, Okamoto I, Tsurutani J, et al. Gefitinib versus cisplatin plus docetaxel in patients with non-small-cell lung cancer harbouring mutations of the epidermal growth factor receptor (WJTOG3405): an open label, randomised phase 3 trial. Lancet Oncol 2010;11(2):121–8.

[234] Mitsudomi T, Morita S, Yatabe Y, Negoro S, Okamoto I, Seto T, et al. Updated overall survival results of WJTOG 3405, a randomized phase III trial comparing gefitinib (G) with cisplatin plus docetaxel (CD) as the first-line treatment for patients with non-small cell lung cancer harboring mutations of the epidermal growth factor receptor (EGFR). J Clin Oncol 2012;30(Suppl.); abstract 7521.

[235] Maemondo M, Inoue A, Kobayashi K, Sugawara S, Oizumi S, Isobe H, et al. Gefitinib or chemotherapy for non-small-cell lung cancer with mutated EGFR. N Engl J Med 2010;362(25):2380–2388.

[236] Inoue A, Kobayashi K, Maemondo M, Sugawara S, Oizumi S, Isobe H, et al. Final overall survival results of NEJ002, a phase III trial comparing gefitinib to carboplatin (CBDCA) plus paclitaxel (TXL) as the first-line treatment for advanced non-small cell lung cancer (NSCLC) with EGFR mutations. J Clin Oncol 2011;29(Suppl); abstr. 7519.

[237] Zhou C, Wu YL, Chen G, Feng J, Liu XQ, Wang C, et al. Erlotinib versus chemotherapy as first-line treatment for patients with advanced EGFR mutation-positive non-small-cell lung cancer (OPTIMAL, CTONG-0802): a multicentre, open-label, randomised, phase 3 study. Lancet Oncol 2011;12(8):735–42.

[238] Rosell R, Carcereny E, Gervais R, Vergnenegre A, Massuti B, Felip E, et al. Erlotinib versus standard chemotherapy as first-line treatment for European patients with advanced EGFR mutation-positive non-small-cell lung cancer (EURTAC): a multicentre, open-label, randomised phase 3 trial. Lancet Oncol 2012;13(3):239–46.

[239] Keedy VL, Temin S, Somerfield MR, Beasley MB, Johnson DH, McShane LM, et al. American Society of Clinical Oncology provisional clinical opinion: epidermal growth factor receptor (EGFR) mutation testing for patients with advanced non-small-cell lung cancer considering first-line EGFR tyrosine kinase inhibitor therapy. J Clin Oncol 2011;29(15):2121–7.

[240] Chiarle R, Voena C, Ambrogio C, Piva R, Inghirami G. The anaplastic lymphoma kinase in the pathogenesis of cancer. Nat Rev Cancer 2008;8(1):11–23.

[241] Chiarle R, Simmons WJ, Cai H, Dhall G, Zamo A, Raz R, et al. STAT3 is required for ALK-mediated lymphomagenesis and provides a possible therapeutic target. Nat Med 2005;11(6):623–9.

[242] Solomon B, Varella-Garcia M, Camidge DR. ALK gene rearrangements: a new therapeutic target in a molecularly defined subset of non-small cell lung cancer. J Thorac Oncol 2009;4(12):1450–4.

[243] Shaw AT, Yeap BY, Mino-Kenudson M, Digumarthy SR, Costa DB, Heist RS, et al. Clinical features and outcome of patients with non-small-cell lung cancer who harbor EML4-ALK. J Clin Oncol 2009;27(26):4247–53.

[244] Shaw AT, Solomon B. Targeting anaplastic lymphoma kinase in lung cancer. Clin Cancer Res 2011;17(8):2081–6.

[245] Kwak EL, Bang YJ, Camidge DR, Shaw AT, Solomon B, Maki RG, et al. Anaplastic lymphoma kinase inhibition in non-small-cell lung cancer. N Engl J Med 2010;363(18):1693–703.

[246] Crinò L, Kim D, Riely GJ, Janne PA, Blackhall FH, Camidge DR, et al. Initial phase II results with crizotinib in advanced ALK-positive non-small cell lung cancer (NSCLC): PROFILE 1005. J Clin Oncol 2011;29(Suppl.); abstr. 7514.

[247] Shaw AT, Kim DW, Nakagawa K, Seto T, Crinò L, Ahn MJ, et-al. Phase III study of crizotinib versus pemetrexed or docetaxel chemotherapy in patients with advanced ALK-positive non-small cell lung cancer (PROFILE 1007). ESMO Congress, 2012: abstr. LBA1.

[248] Govindan R, Ding L, Griffith M, Subramanian J, Dees ND, Kanchi KL, et al. Genomic landscape of non-small cell lung cancer in smokers and never-smokers. Cell 2012;150(6):1121–34.

[249] Imielinski M, Berger AH, Hammerman PS, Hernandez B, Pugh TJ, Hodis E, et al. Mapping the hallmarks of lung adenocarcinoma with massively parallel sequencing. Cell 2012;150(6):1107–20.

[250] Hammerman PS, Hayes DN, Wilkerson MD, Schultz N, Bose R, Chu A, et al. Comprehensive genomic characterization of squamous cell lung cancers. Nature 2012;489(7417):519–25.

[251] Chapman PB, Hauschild A, Robert C, Haanen JB, Ascierto P, Larkin J, et al. Improved survival with vemurafenib in melanoma with BRAF V600E mutation. N Engl J Med 2011;364(26):2507–16.

[252] Berger MF, Hodis E, Heffernan TP, Deribe YL, Lawrence MS, Protopopov A, et al. Melanoma genome sequencing reveals frequent PREX2 mutations. Nature 2012;485(7399):502–6.

[253] Karapetis CS, Khambata-Ford S, Jonker DJ, O'Callaghan CJ, Tu D, Tebbutt NC, et al. K-ras mutations and benefit from cetuximab in advanced colorectal cancer. N Engl J Med 2008;359(17):1757–65.

[254] Jonker DJ, O'Callaghan CJ, Karapetis CS, Zalcberg JR, Tu D, Au HJ, et al. Cetuximab for the treatment of colorectal cancer. N Engl J Med 2007;357(20):2040–8.

[255] Lievre A, Bachet JB, Boige V, Cayre A, Le Corre D, Buc E, et al. KRAS mutations as an independent prognostic factor in patients with advanced colorectal cancer treated with cetuximab. J Clin Oncol 2008;26(3):374–9.

[256] Mitchell EP, Piperdi B, Lacouture ME, Shearer H, Iannotti N, Pillai MV, et al. The efficacy and safety of panitumumab administered concomitantly with FOLFIRI or irinotecan in second-line therapy for metastatic colorectal cancer: the secondary analysis from STEPP (Skin Toxicity Evaluation Protocol with Panitumumab) by KRAS status. Clin Colorectal Cancer 2011;10(4):333–9.

[257] De Roock W, Jonker DJ, Di Nicolantonio F, Sartore-Bianchi A, Tu D, Siena S, et al. Association of KRAS p.G13D mutation with outcome in patients with chemotherapy-refractory metastatic colorectal cancer treated with cetuximab. JAMA 2010;304(16):1812–1820.

[258] Tejpar S, Celik I, Schlichting M, Sartorius U, Bokemeyer C, Van Cutsem E. Association of KRAS G13D tumor mutations with outcome in patients with metastatic colorectal cancer treated with first-line chemotherapy with or without cetuximab. J Clin Oncol 2012;30(29):3570–7.

[259] Allegra CJ, Jessup JM, Somerfield MR, Hamilton SR, Hammond EH, Hayes DF, et al. American Society of Clinical Oncology provisional clinical opinion: testing for KRAS gene mutations in patients with metastatic colorectal carcinoma to predict response to anti-epidermal growth factor receptor monoclonal antibody therapy. J Clin Oncol 2009;27(12):2091–6.

[260] Lynch HT, de la Chapelle A. Hereditary colorectal cancer. N Engl J Med 2003;348(10):919–32.

[261] Halvarsson B, Anderson H, Domanska K, Lindmark G, Nilbert M. Clinicopathologic factors identify sporadic mismatch repair-defective colon cancers. Am J Clin Pathol 2008;129(2):238–44.

[262] Cunningham JM, Christensen ER, Tester DJ, Kim CY, Roche PC, Burgart LJ, et al. Hypermethylation of the hMLH1 promoter in colon cancer with microsatellite instability. Cancer Res 1998;58(15):3455–60.

[263] Boland CR, Thibodeau SN, Hamilton SR, Sidransky D, Eshleman JR, Burt RW, et al. A National Cancer Institute Workshop on microsatellite instability for cancer detection and familial predisposition: development of international criteria for the determination of microsatellite instability in colorectal cancer. Cancer Res 1998;58(22):5248–57.

[264] Ribic CM, Sargent DJ, Moore MJ, Thibodeau SN, French AJ, Goldberg RM, et al. Tumor microsatellite-instability status as a predictor of benefit from fluorouracil-based adjuvant chemotherapy for colon cancer. N Engl J Med 2003;349(3):247–57.

[265] Sargent DJ, Marsoni S, Monges G, Thibodeau SN, Labianca R, Hamilton SR, et al. Defective mismatch repair as a predictive marker for lack of efficacy of fluorouracil-based adjuvant therapy in colon cancer. J Clin Oncol 2010;28(20):3219–26.

[266] Tejpar S, Bosman F, Delorenzi M, Fiocca R, Yan P, Klingbiel D, et al. Microsatellite instability (MSI) in stage II and III colon cancer treated with 5FU-LV or 5FU-LV and irinotecan (PETACC 3-EORTC 40993-SAKK 60/00 trial). J Clin Oncol 2009;27(15S):4001; (May 20 Supplement).

[267] Hutchins G, Southward K, Handley K, Magill L, Beaumont C, Stahlschmidt J, et al. Value of mismatch repair, KRAS, and BRAF mutations in predicting recurrence and benefits from chemotherapy in colorectal cancer. J Clin Oncol 2011;29(10):1261–70.

[268] Bertagnolli MM, Redston M, Compton CC, Niedzwiecki D, Mayer RJ, Goldberg RM, et al. Microsatellite instability and loss of heterozygosity at chromosomal location 18q: prospective evaluation of biomarkers for stages II and III colon cancer – a study of CALGB 9581 and 89803. J Clin Oncol 2011;29(23):3153–62.

[269] Sinicrope FA, Foster NR, Thibodeau SN, Marsoni S, Monges G, Labianca R, et al. DNA mismatch repair status and colon cancer recurrence and survival in clinical trials of 5-fluorouracil-based adjuvant therapy. J Natl Cancer Inst 2011;103(11):863–75.

[270] The Cancer Genome Atlas Network. Comprehensive molecular characterization of human colon and rectal cancer. Nature 2012;487(7407):330–337.

3

Natural Product Chemistry and Cancer Drug Discovery

Donna M. Huryn, Peter Wipf

Center for Chemical Methodologies and Library Development (UPCMLD),
University of Pittsburgh, Pittsburgh, PA, USA

INTRODUCTION

The history of cancer drug discovery and development is closely linked to natural products and the pharmacology of naturally occurring substances. This is neither a surprise nor a coincidence. Chemical defense mechanisms in the plant and animal kingdoms often involve cytotoxic or cytostatic agents, and rapidly proliferating malignant cell growth represents a closely related threat to normal tissue in complex organisms. Accordingly, humans can benefit from eons of competition between prokaryotic and eukaryotic life forms, and the resulting refinements in toxins that overwhelm the similarly evolving cellular defense mechanisms. Nonetheless, the distinction between selective defense and unselective toxicity is blurred for many natural products, since potency rather than (mammalian) cell type selectivity is the overwhelming evolutionary driving force. Not surprisingly, therefore, only a small but significant fraction of cytotoxic natural products shows any utility in human therapy. Mice and rats, with their considerably more aggressive metabolism and greater direct exposure to natural toxins, often provide overly positive preliminary evaluations in traditional xenograft tumor models, whereas human clinical trials frequently fail in a late stage due to adverse side effects and unanticipated organ damage. With these caveats, it is even more impressive to consider the tremendous advancements that natural products have brought to cancer treatment. A recent study by Newman and Cragg [1] finds that within the cohort of 99 small-molecule anticancer drugs available since 1981, 79 (80%) are natural products, closely related analogs, or mimics of natural products. Furthermore, this proportion has not significantly changed in the last 70 years. Since the 1940s, the 206 anticancer drugs approved worldwide contain 131 (64%) naturally inspired agents, or 75% of 175 drugs if biologicals and vaccines are excluded. The list of nature-provided or nature-inspired anticancer agents includes major blockbuster drugs such as doxorubicin, paclitaxel, vinblastine, etoposide, irinotecan, gemcitabine, and methotrexate. After a drop in the popularity of the use of natural products in the major pharmaceutical industry during the 1990s, a (initially largely academic) renaissance in the consideration of secondary metabolites in drug discovery has resulted in a large number of reviews that have covered the historical development of this area [1–16], and therefore this chapter will focus on recent additions to the field that have just entered clinical use, are in clinical trials, or are poised to be so in the near future. The discussion also includes sources of these agents (i.e., synthesis, isolation, or microbial culture).

EXEMESTANE (AROMASIN)

Aromatase catalyzes the conversion of androgens to estrogen, a steroid hormone that regulates menstruation, among other physiological processes. Since >75% of human breast cancers are hormone-dependent and estrogen receptor (ER)-positive, it has been recognized for a while that antiestrogens or inhibitors of estrogen biosynthesis can have substantial benefits in suppressing breast tumor growth. Selective estrogen receptor modulators (SERMs) such as tamoxifene and raloxifene interfere with estrogen binding and have gained US Food and Drug Administration (FDA) approval. In contrast, aromatase inhibitors (AIs) inhibit estrogen production and were found to offer attractive alternatives to SERMs in the clinic. Among the three FDA-approved AIs, anastrozole, letrozole, and exemestane, the former two are non-steroidal modulators of the heme-binding region of aromatase. Exemestane (6-methylenandrosta-1,4-diene-3,17-dione, or Aromasin; Fig. 3.1) is a novel irreversible steroidal aromatase inhibitor used as an orally active hormonal therapeutic for postmenopausal patients with advanced breast cancer that has become refractory to standard hormonal therapies [17,18].

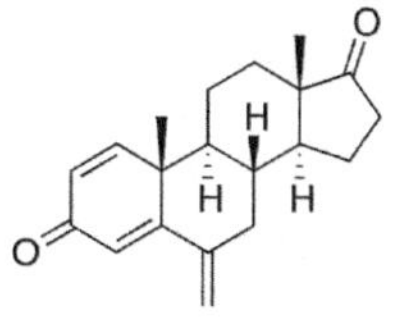

FIGURE 3.1   Structure of exemestane (aromasin).

Aromatase removes the C(19)-methyl group flanked by the A- and B-rings of androstenedione in a three-step oxidative cleavage sequence (Scheme 3.1). A modification of cytochrome P-450 mediates the specific removal of C(19) and the aromatization of the A-ring, releasing formic acid and water. In contrast to type II aromatase inhibitors, which act by reversibly binding to the enzyme and the cytochrome P-450 heme–iron group, exemestane belongs to the type I class inhibitors, which bind irreversibly. This class also includes formestane (4-hydroxyandrost-4-ene-3,17-dione), atamestane (1-methylandrosta-1,4-diene-3,17-dione), and plomestane (10H-(2-propynyl)estr-

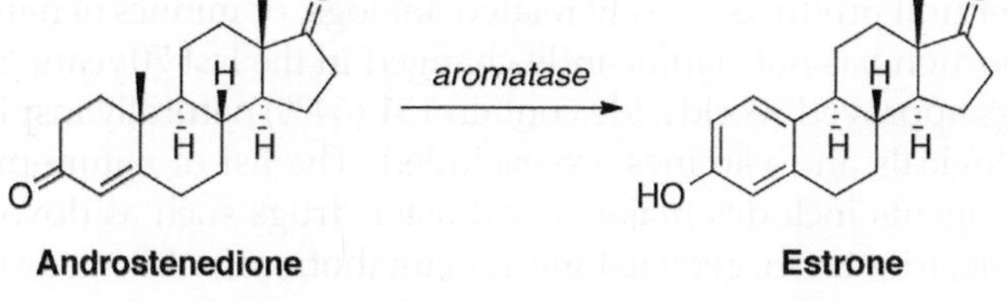

Androstenedione   **Estrone**

SCHEME 3.1   Oxidation of androstenedione by the enzyme aromatase in the biosynthesis of estrone.

4-ene-3,17-dione). These compounds mimic natural androstenedione, and the suicide inhibition of the aromatase active site requires a renewed biosynthesis of enzyme for continued turnover. A possible mechanism for the inhibition of aromatase by exemestane is shown in Scheme 3.2.

While tamoxifen still represents the gold standard for the first-line treatment of postmenopausal women with advanced breast carcinoma, the newer generation AIs such as exemestane display vastly different pharmacokinetics and effects on plasma lipids, bone, and adrenosteroidogenesis that will likely prove beneficial for the treatment of many patients [19,20].

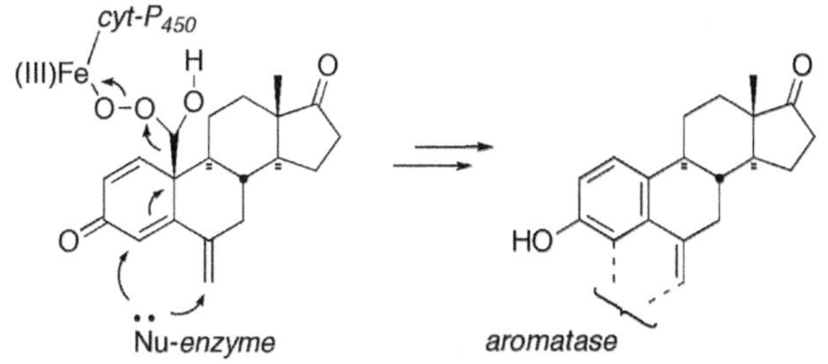

SCHEME 3.2 Possible reaction sequence for a mechanism-based inhibition of aromatase by exemestane.

FULVESTRANT (FASLODEX)

Since long-term use of tamoxifen in advanced breast cancer patients runs the risk of renewed tumorigenesis, endometrial cancer, and thromboembolic disease, third-generation AIs such as exemestane have rapidly gained market share [21]. However, these compounds also have their share of side effects, and therefore the search continues for alternative agents that can be used after tamoxifen and exemestane failures. Fulvestrant (Faslodex; ICI-182,780) is a purely antagonistic ER ligand (Fig. 3.2). When fulvestrant binds to ER monomers, it inhibits receptor dimerization, deactivates AF1 and AF2, reduces translocation of receptor to the nucleus, and accelerates ER degradation. Fulvestrant's lack of cross-resistance with other endocrine agents in phase III clinical trials has demonstrated that it is as effective as aromatase inhibitors and well tolerated in patients [22–24]. The compound appears to have little effect on sex hormone endocrinology, bone metabolism, and lipid biochemistry. It also does not appear to cause any CYP3A4-mediated drug–drug interactions [25]. A possible disadvantage is that it requires intramuscular injection in a formulation of castor oil and alcohol.

Due to the presence of the unnatural, fluorinated side chain, the synthesis of fulvestrant and analog compounds involves several steps from common steroids [26–28]. Treatment of 6,7-didehydro-19-nortestosterone (**1**) acetate with Grignard reagent **2** in the presence of CuI introduces the C_9 side chain in the correct regio- and stereochemistry (Scheme 3.3). Acidic

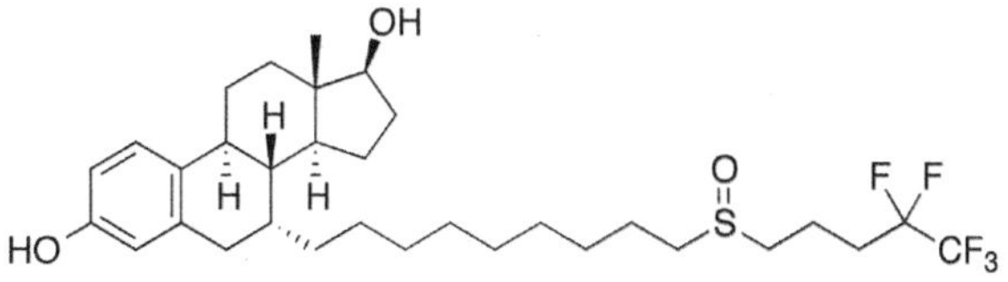

FIGURE 3.2 Structure of fulvestrant (faslodex).

I. BASIC PRINCIPLES AND METHODOLOGY

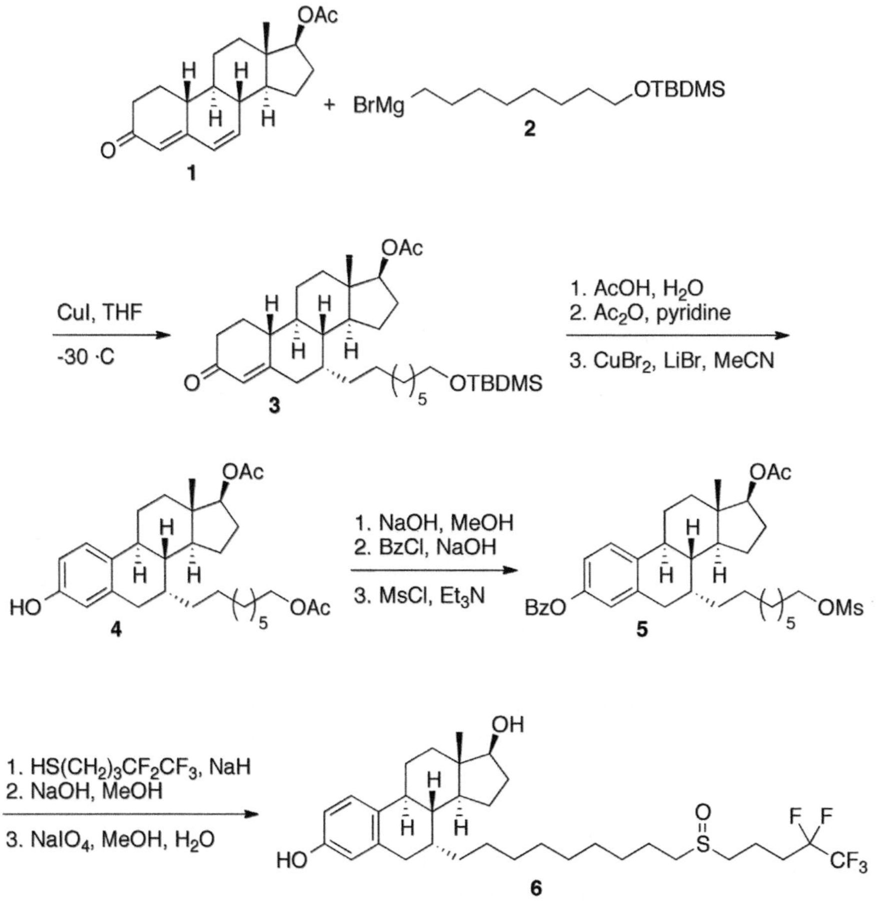

SCHEME 3.3 Synthetic approach to fulvestrant.

hydrolysis of the primary silyl ether protective group, followed by acetylation of the alcohol and Cu(II)-mediated aromatization of the A-ring enone, leads to phenol **4**. The fluorinated sulfoxide chain is now introduced by a selective saponification of the primary acetate, benzoylation of the phenol, and mesylation of the alcohol. The leaving group on **5** is displaced by the sodium salt of 4,4,5,5,5-pentafluoro-1-pentanethiol, and, after saponification of both ester functions, the thioether is converted to the sulfoxide **6** with sodium periodate.

FLAVONOIDS

The observation that many common foods appear to provide protective effects against some cancers has focused attention on flavonoids as potential anticancer agents. Flavonoids are broadly characterized by the presence of a diphenylpropane scaffold; they occur in various isomeric forms, and frequently as glycoside conjugates. They are ubiquitous in the plant kingdom, often grouped into the "phytoestrogen" class, and found in many dietary sources such as grains, legumes, fruits, vegetables, teas, and herbs. While many of these foods have been used as complementary and alternative medicine as well as traditional Eastern medicine remedies, their use as pharmaceutical agents in the West has been more limited. Complicating their study is the facile metabolism of these agents, difficulty in attributing specific biological activities to specific metabolites, and differences in nutriceutical and pharmacological doses applied. Quercetin and genistein (Fig. 3.3) are representative members of this class, and probably among the most thoroughly studied natural flavonoids [29–31].

Preclinical studies have described a wide variety of beneficial effects attributed to flavonoids, including anticancer, antiinflammatory, antioxidant, antiviral, and antiallergenic properties. As the daily dietary ingestion of flavonoids has been estimated at several hundred milligrams, the compounds are considered extremely safe. In the specific instance of cancer, flavonoids have been shown to act through a number of different mechanisms, including antioxidant properties, topoisomerase inhibition, antimitotic activity, kinase inhibition, estrogen antagonism, and modulation of multidrug resistance [32]. Based on this range of activities, and the varied structures studied, a comprehensive review of the structure–activity relationship (SAR) of this class of compounds is beyond the scope of this chapter. However, reviews of specific biochemical target activities have appeared [33–35].

Flavonoids of diverse structures and with diverse modes of action are being evaluated clinically, and some representative examples are described. Genistein is being tested in a large number of patient trials, both as a preventive agent and as a treatment agent for breast, prostate, and bladder cancers. Flavopiridol (Alvocidib; Fig. 3.4) is a semisynthetic flavonoid whose anticancer effects are attributed to inhibition of a number of cyclin-dependent kinases (CDKs), downregulation of cyclins D1 and D3, and inhibition of phosphorylation of CDKs. X-ray co-structures of flavopiridol derivatives and CDK2 confirm binding to the ATP-binding pocket. Flavopiridol induces checkpoint arrest, cell death, and apoptosis, although specific mechanisms are still unclear. Results from clinical trials as a single agent have been

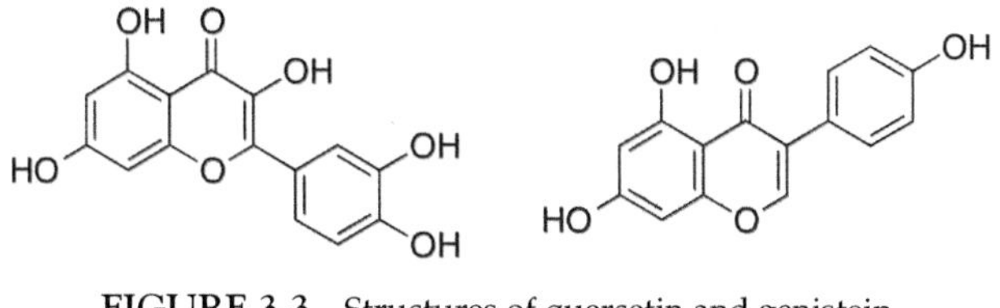

FIGURE 3.3   Structures of quercetin and genistein.

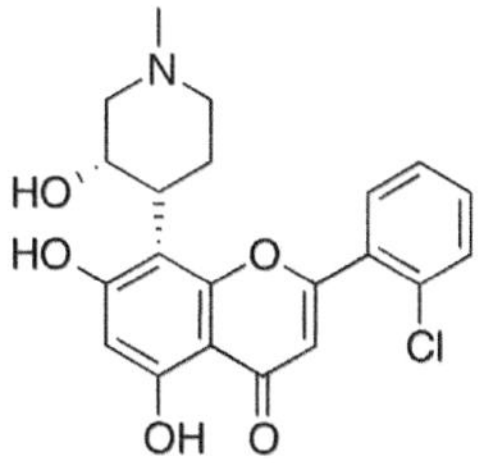

FIGURE 3.4   Structure of flavopiridol.

disappointing; its use in combination therapy has been more encouraging [34,36,37]. The multiple effects of flavonoids, their safety, and their accessibility hold promise for them as novel therapeutics for cancer treatment as well as prevention.

BEXAROTENE (TARGRETIN)

Bexarotene (Targretin; Fig. 3.5) targets an orphan nuclear receptor (NR) known as the retinoic X receptor (RXR). This receptor type is found in almost all animal species, and target gene analysis and ligand identification have raised the promise of its therapeutic utility [38]. Bexarotene is in therapeutic use for treatment of cutaneous T-cell lymphoma (CTCL) and non-small-cell lung cancer. Clinical trials and off-label use have also been extended to breast cancer, metastatic melanoma, and other indications [39].

The preparation of bexarotene employs a de novo synthetic approach [40]. A tandem Friedel–Crafts alkylation reaction with 2,5-dichloro-2.5-dimethylhexane and toluene provides the tetrahydronaphthalene 8, which is once again subjected to Friedel–Crafts acylation conditions with monomethylterephthalate (Scheme 3.4). A Wittig reaction on ketone 9 is followed by saponification and acidification to give bexarotene (10).

Interestingly, a disila-analog of bexarotene has a profile comparable to that of the parent compound in terms of its ability to activate target genes through the RXR receptor (Fig. 3.6) [41,42]. The disila-compound can be expected to have increased lipophilicity, which is likely to influence its bioavailability and tissue distribution, as well as its specificity profile for NRs.

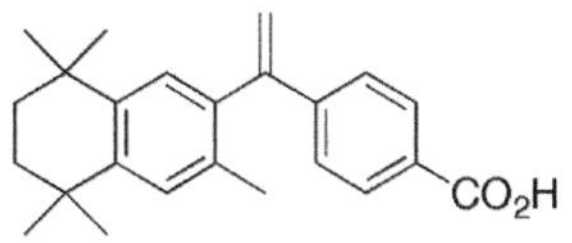

FIGURE 3.5   Structure of bexarotene (targretin).

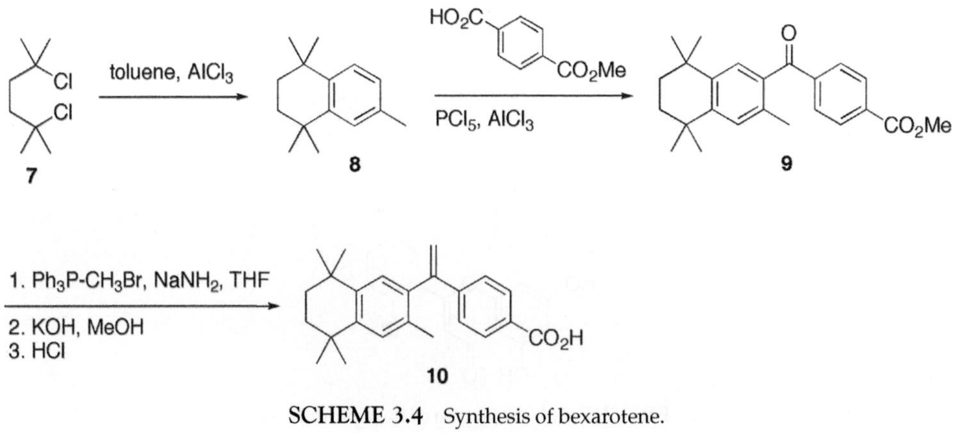

SCHEME 3.4   Synthesis of bexarotene.

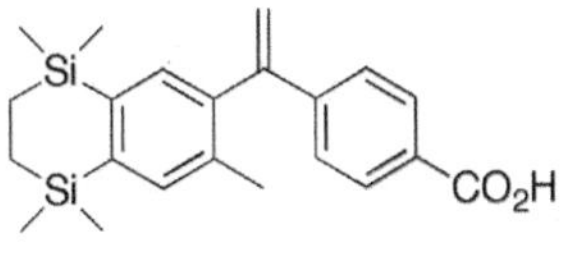

FIGURE 3.6 Structure of disila-bexarotene.

EPOTHILONES

Until the early 1990s, docetaxel and related structures were the only cytotoxic agents that worked through stabilization of microtubules (Fig. 3.7). Therefore, the scientific community welcomed the isolation of epothilones and their characterization as a second class of microtubule-stabilizing agents with considerable excitement. Epothilones A and B were isolated from a myxobacterium, *Sorangium cellulosum*, by Höfle, Reichenbach, and coworkers. These epothilones contain a 16-membered macrocyclic ring with a pendant vinyl thiazole moiety, and they differ by the substituent on the epoxide ring (Fig. 3.8; Epothilone A: R=H; Epothilone B: R=Me) [43,44]. Epothilones C and D, intermediates in the biosynthesis of epothilones A and B in which an olefin replaces the epoxide, were later isolated from the same organism in much lower yields. Epothilone B (patupilone) is in clinical trials, but the development of epothilone D (KOS-862) has been suspended [45]. The isolation of additional members of the epothilone family continues to be an active area of research [46–48].

The potent antiproliferative effects of this class of compounds were characterized by scientists at Merck, who observed the induction of tubulin polymerization and microtubule stabilization, as well as the epothilones' ability to displace docetaxel binding to microtubules [49]. Particularly exciting was the fact that epothilones, unlike docetaxel, were effective against tumor cell lines that overexpressed the efflux pump, P-glycoprotein (Pgp), and against docetaxel-resistant cell lines containing specific tubulin mutations. Furthermore, other properties of epothilones, such as their improved water solubility and relatively modest structural complexity, suggested that their advancement as anticancer agents would not suffer from the significant hurdles that plagued the development of docetaxel and its analogs (e.g., difficulties in formulation and limited supply options).

The total synthesis, semisynthesis, library synthesis (solid and solution phases), and engineered biosynthesis of epothilones have been the subject of intense research, and this topic has been covered in a number of recent reviews [50–54]. Approaches to designing improved analogs have involved simplification of the structure; modification of the macrocycle, such as constraining the ring system and incorporating heteroatoms; stabilization of the lactone; replacement and modification of the thiazole; changing the stereochemistry of the epoxide; and incorporation of functional groups designed to improve solubility and other properties. The availability of a large number of analogs has allowed for a thorough understanding of the structural requirements for activity, as well as the development of pharmacophore models of the epothilones' conformation while bound to tubulin [45,52].

Extensive reviews of the SAR have appeared, and several general trends have emerged [45,51,52]. Modification and/or replacement of the epoxide residue and the C-12,C-13-portion in epothilone B analogs is tolerated, but the epoxide often confers greater antiproliferative potency compared to the corresponding olefin. Manipulations of the lactone group are

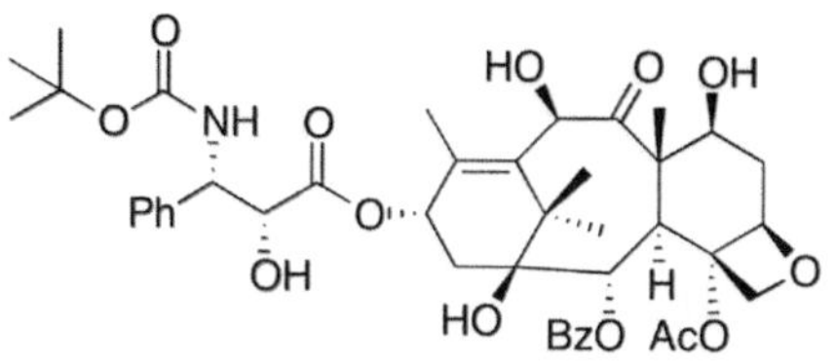

FIGURE 3.7   Structure of docetaxel.

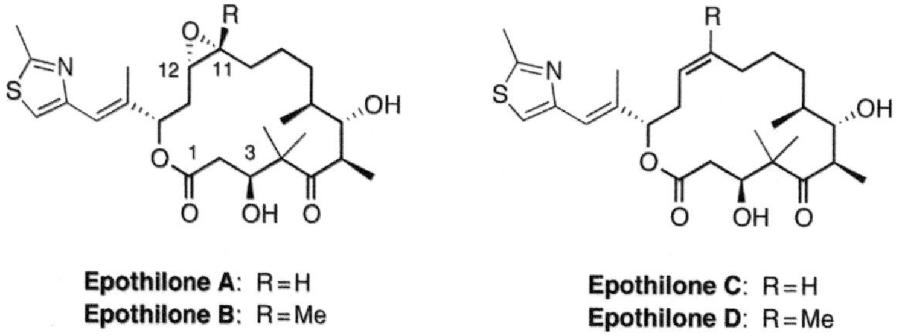

Epothilone A: R=H
Epothilone B: R=Me

Epothilone C: R=H
Epothilone D: R=Me

FIGURE 3.8   Structures of epothilones A–D.

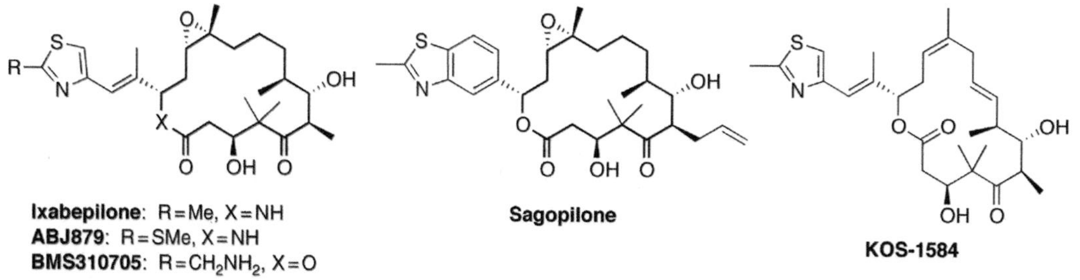

Ixabepilone: R=Me, X=NH
ABJ879: R=SMe, X=NH
BMS310705: R=CH$_2$NH$_2$, X=O

Sagopilone

KOS-1584

FIGURE 3.9   Structures of ixabepilone, ABJ879, BMS310705, sagopilone, and KOS-1584.

also tolerated, as exemplified by replacement of the lactone oxygen with a nitrogen atom in ixabepilone (BMS-247550), a compound that was approved in 2007 in combination or as single agent for the treatment of certain resistant and refractory cancers [55] (Fig. 3.9). This modification results in similar potency but improved pharmacokinetic properties, particularly stability. The pendant thiazole ring has been the subject of extensive SAR studies that indicate a requirement for a nitrogen-containing heterocycle. Three compounds containing such a modification—ABJ879, BMS310705, and the fully synthetic epothilone, sagopilone (Fig. 3.9) [56,57]—have advanced to clinical trials; however, reports suggest that only sagopilone is still being developed. An analog of epothilone D, KOS-1584 (Fig. 3.9), is also in advanced clinical trials. The ability of these compounds to act through a docetaxel-like mechanism while avoiding some of docetaxel's liabilities, such as efficient efflux by Pgp and poor solubility, holds great promise for their success.

MAYTANSINE

Maytansine, a 19-membered ring ansamacrolide, was first isolated in 1972 from the plant *Maytenus ovatus* (now known as *Maytenus serrata*) and generated considerable excitement due to its extremely potent cytotoxic effects in cell-based systems, as well as its efficacy in animal tumor models [58]. Since then, a number of maytansine analogs (termed ansamitocins when derived from microbial sources) have been isolated, most differing in the substituents on the ester group at C3 (Fig. 3.10). As the initial isolation procedures and natural sources provided only very small quantities of material, the synthesis of maytansinoids attracted considerable attention in the organic chemistry community. A number of total syntheses of maytansine have been reported and are detailed in recent reviews [59,60]. In parallel, efforts to identify higher yielding sources of material through isolation were also successful and allowed for opportunities for semisynthesis and microbial conversion to prepare new analogs [60].

The potent cytotoxic effects of maytansine have been attributed to its ability to bind to the vinca alkaloid site of β-tubulin, and inhibit microtubule assembly [61–63]. Most SAR studies on maytansines rely on correlations between structure and cytotoxic activities, rather than tubulin-binding properties. With that caveat, however, some generalizations have been reported. The C3-ester side chain is sensitive to modification. Its presence in the correct absolute configuration is essential for activity; however, the nature of the side chain can be modified. The carbinolamide moiety is proposed to be reactive, and that feature may impart biological activity, as alkylation of the hydroxyl group results in a significant reduction of potency. Neither the epoxide nor the *N*-methyl amide appear to be necessary for activity [60].

The United States' National Cancer Institute (NCI) initiated clinical trials with maytansine in 1975, and since then a number of phase I and phase II studies have been conducted [59]. Unfortunately, acceptable therapeutic indices were not realized, and the trials were terminated. Recently, however, a resurgence of interest in maytansine has developed, with a focus on antibody-targeted conjugates [59,64]. The previous efforts at understanding the structural requirements for cytotoxic activity were instrumental in designing linkers at the C3-ester that could be conjugated to cancer-specific antibodies, a number of which are undergoing clinical trials [59,64,65]. Of these, ado-trastuzumab emtansine (Kadcyla, or T-DM1) (Fig. 3.11), a Her2 antibody (Herceptin, or trastuzumab) that is linked to a maytansine analog (the cytotoxic DM1) [66], was approved in early 2013 for the treatment of HER2-positive metastatic breast cancer.

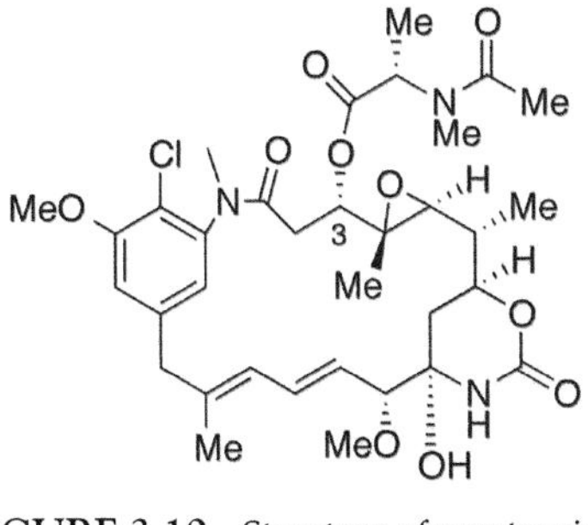

FIGURE 3.10 Structure of maytansine.

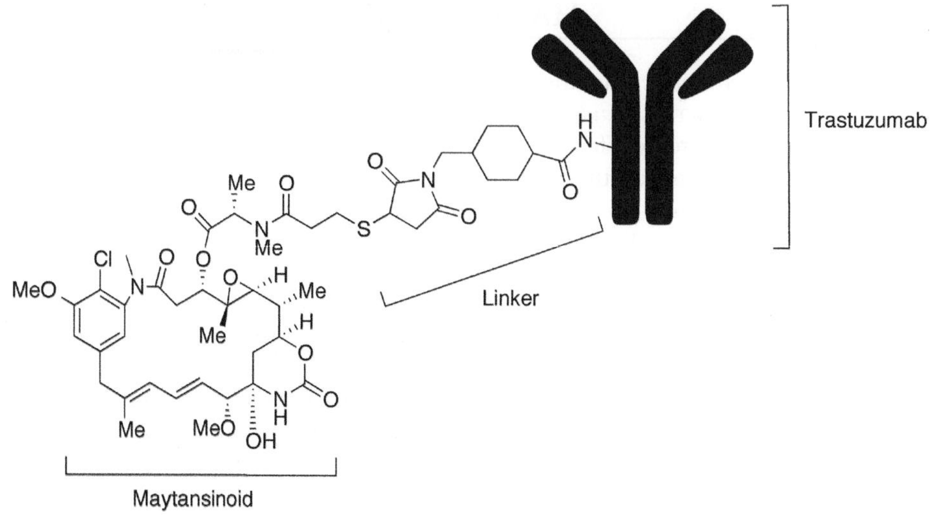

FIGURE 3.11   Structure of ado-trastuzumab emtansine.

GELDANAMYCIN

The isolation of geldanamycin, a member of the benzoquinone ansamycin family of antibiotics, was first reported in 1970 (Fig. 3.12) [67]. The natural product attracted attention because of its ability to cause transformed cells to revert to normal phenotypes, but its molecular target, heat shock protein 90 (Hsp90), was identified only in the mid-1990s [68]. Hsp's, also called "molecular chaperones", are ATP-dependent proteins that are essential for the proper folding, stability, and function of a number of proteins (see also Chapter 9 for a detailed discussion of this topic). Hsp90, in particular, is highly abundant and associates with several protein kinases, including mutated oncogenic proteins; its function is now believed to be required for malignant transformation. Geldanamycin binds to Hsp90, preventing its ATPase activity and ultimately its ability to stabilize key proteins involved in cell cycle regulation, apoptosis, oncogenesis, and cell growth, thereby resulting in a multipronged attack on cancer-causing processes. The toxicity and instability of geldanamycin precluded its clinical development; however, the related analogs 17N-allylamino-17-demethoxygeldanamycin (17-AAG, KOS-953, or tanespimycin), 17-dimethylaminoethylamino-17-demethoxygeldana-mycin (17-DMAG, or alvespimycin), IPI-493, and retaspimycin (IPI-504) were evaluated in clinical trials (Fig. 3.12). Of those, it appears that only retaspimycin trials are still ongoing (see Chapter 9).

Crystallography studies reveal that geldanamycin binds inside a deep pocket at the Hsp90 ATP-binding site. Its conformation resembles the letter "C", with the ansa ring and the benzoquinone folded on top of each other in a nearly parallel fashion, and the lactam moiety in a *cis*-conformation. The bound conformation is quite distinct from the more open conformation observed in X-ray structures of free geldanamycin [69–71]. The availability of X-ray co-crystal structures has afforded opportunities for structure-based design strategies, for example by incorporating structural features that favor the *cis*-amide bond conformation [72,73].

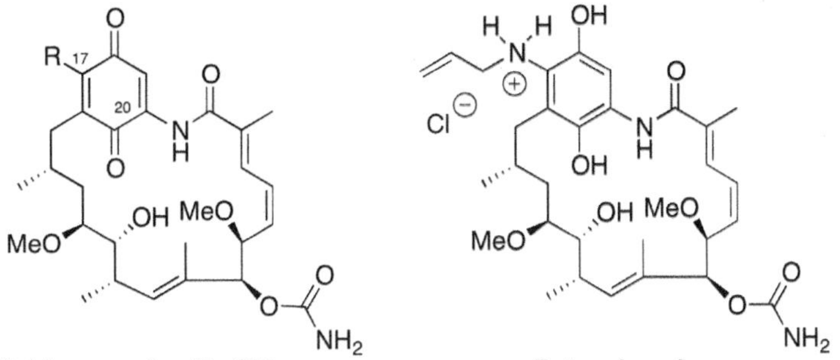

Geldanamycin: R=OMe
17-AAG: R=$NHCH_2CH{=}CH_2$
17-DMAG: R=$NHCH_2CH_2N(CH_3)_2$
IPI-493: R=NH_2

Retaspimycin

FIGURE 3.12 Structures of geldanamycin and selected analogs.

The synthesis of Hsp90 inhibitors based on geldanamycin and other ansamycin family members is an active area of research, with successes in engineered biosynthesis, total synthesis, and semisynthesis being reported [74,75]. There is a firm understanding of how the structural features of the molecule contribute to its activity, and this knowledge was applied to prepare analogs at C-17 and the C-20 amide that were used to identify Hsp90 as geldanamycin's target [76]. Furthermore, the available SAR has been used to identify improved analogs. For example, the introduction of polar groups at C-17, such as in 17-DMAG, led to improved solubility; reduction of the quinone in 17-AAG and protonation of the allylamine at C-17, as in retaspimycin, provided improved solubility and stability [77,78].

Despite the promising biological activity, geldanamycin analogs have been plagued by poor solubility and stability, as well as unacceptable toxicities. While some improvements in physical properties have been realized, many suggest that the benzoquinone moiety, inherent in all geldanamcyin analogs, is responsible for the toxicity. While this class of natural products may not find use as approved cancer agents, it has provided proof-of-concept that Hsp90 inhibition can be an effective approach to anticancer therapy, and has inspired significant efforts at identifying new compounds of distinct, nonbenzoquinone structures via design, high-throughput screening, virtual screening, and fragment-based screening [75,79].

UCN-01

UCN-01, also known as 7-hydroxy staurosporine, was isolated from *Streptomyces* and initially characterized as a selective inhibitor of protein kinase C (PKC) isoforms (Fig. 3.13) [80]. However, unlike staurosporine, another potent PKC inhibitor, UCN-01 exhibited potent antitumor effects in a number of human tumor xenograft models [81]. This inconsistency led to the realization that UCN-01's antitumor effects were the result of a number of additional effects. Specifically, UCN-01 potently inhibits checkpoint-regulating kinases chk1 and perhaps chk2, as well as phosphatidylinositide-dependent protein kinase I (PDK1). These activities help explain the myriad of effects that have been attributed to UCN-01, such as

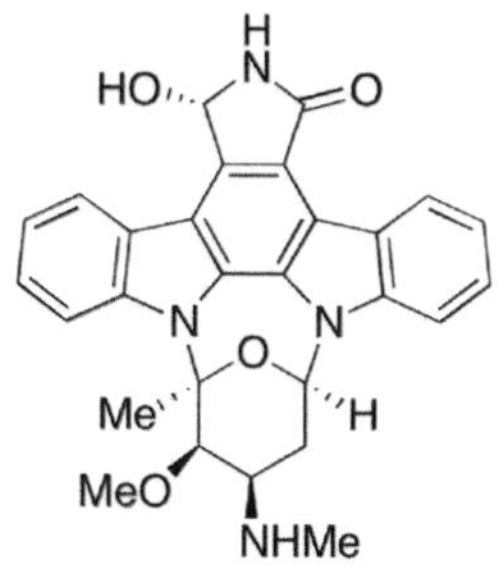

FIGURE 3.13   Structure of UCN-01.

synergistic growth inhibition when simultaneously administered with DNA-damaging agents, enhancement of the cytotoxicity of antimetabolite drugs, induction of apoptosis, and cell cycle disruption [82,83]. The complexity of its effects has made the interpretation of SAR results difficult; however, comparisons between UCN-01 and other indolocarbazoles such as staurosporine and K-252a have been reviewed [84]. UCN-01 has advanced to clinical trials but complications in its pharmacokinetic behavior and toxicities may impede its rapid development [85,86].

CAMPTOTHECIN

Camptothecin, a planar pentacyclic ring system containing a pyrrolo(3,4-b)quinoline and an α-hydroxy lactone, was isolated in the mid-1960s (Fig. 3.14) [87]. The identification of topoisomerase I as camptothecin's biological target, its unsuccessful clinical evaluation, synthetic approaches, and SAR studies to identify improved analogs have been extensively reviewed [88–94]. As a result of these efforts, three camptothecin analogs have been approved for cancer therapy: topotecan (hycamtin) is approved for the treatment of recurring ovarian cancer and small-cell lung cancer, and in combination with cisplatin for cervical cancer, and irinotecan (camptosar) is a prodrug that generates the active moiety SN-38 and is prescribed for advanced cancers of the large intestine and rectum; both are also used for glioblastomas and sarcomas. Belotecan is approved in Korea to treat small-cell lung and cervical cancers [91] (Fig. 3.15).

The availability of a number of analogs, via either total synthesis or semisynthesis; their biological activity; as well as co-crystal structures of relevant DNA–topoisomerase I complexes have contributed to an extensive understanding of the SAR of this class of compounds [92]. Notable findings include the appreciation that disruption of the planar ring system results in a substantial loss of activity, and that a variety of substitutions on the ring system, particularly at C-7, C-9, C-10, and C-11, are well tolerated. This latter finding was exploited to discover irinotecan, topotecan, and belotecan, which retain potent cytotoxic activity but exhibit enhanced water solubility. Work on the E-ring has been influenced by the understanding of the importance of the (S)-20-hydroxylactone moiety, and the significant loss of activity upon ring opening to the carboxylate, which occurs rapidly at physiological pH. Modifications of the C- and D-rings are typically detrimental to activity; however, recent studies show that specific substitution on the D-ring (e.g. compound A) is not only tolerated but also enhances the stability of the lactone function (Fig. 3.16) [95].

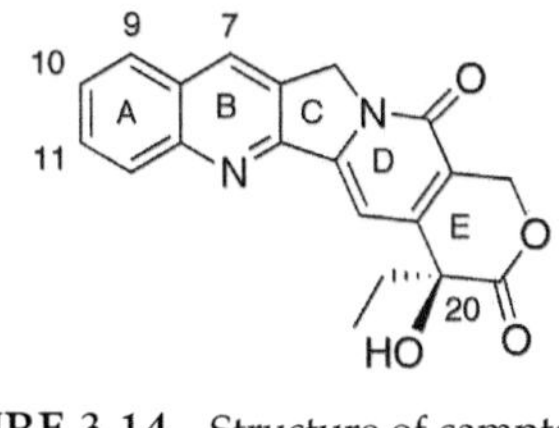

FIGURE 3.14 Structure of camptothecin.

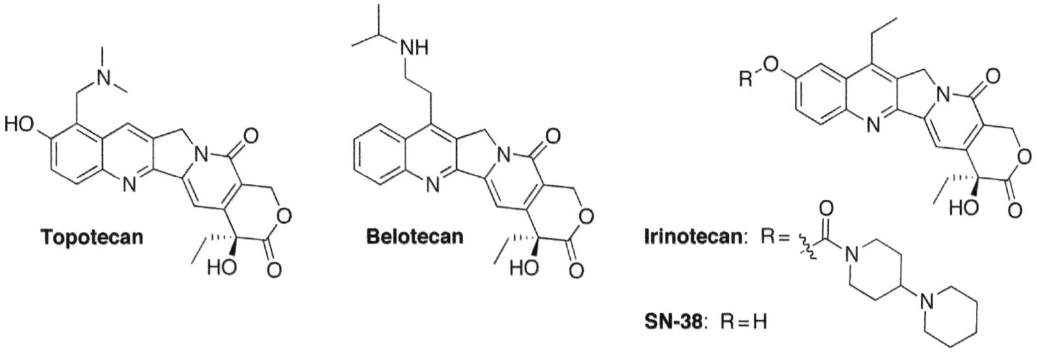

FIGURE 3.15 Structures of topotecan, belotecan, irinotecan, and SN-38.

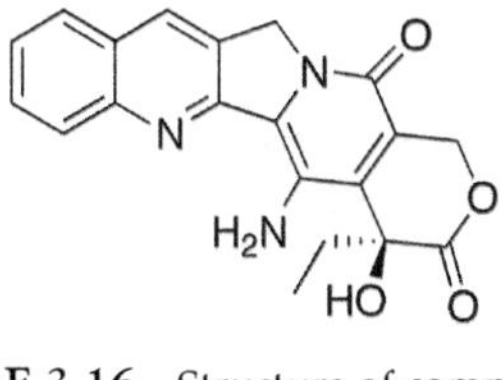

FIGURE 3.16 Structure of compound A.

Despite the clinical success of irinotecan and topotecan, these drugs exhibit some significant limitations (e.g., high plasma protein binding, limited water solubility, and instability) that have prompted additional efforts at identifying improved camptothecin derivatives. As of 2013, over 15 "tecans" are listed in the NCI thesaurus, many of which are undergoing clinical evaluation. Selected examples are shown in Fig. 3.17. Most are modified at the C-7, C-9, C-10, and/or C-11 positions; however, the specific substituents are quite diverse and include amines (e.g., exatecan), oximes (e.g., gimatecan), and silanes (e.g., silatecan) [94,96]. Approaches to stabilize the lactone ring have led to homocamptothecins such as diflomotecan (Fig. 3.17). Additional approaches for optimization have included prodrug strategies, pegylation, and immunoconjugation [88–90,94]. The promising activities of these analogs indicate that camptothecin derivatives will continue to garner significant attention, and new topoisomerase inhibitors are likely to emerge as important cancer therapeutics.

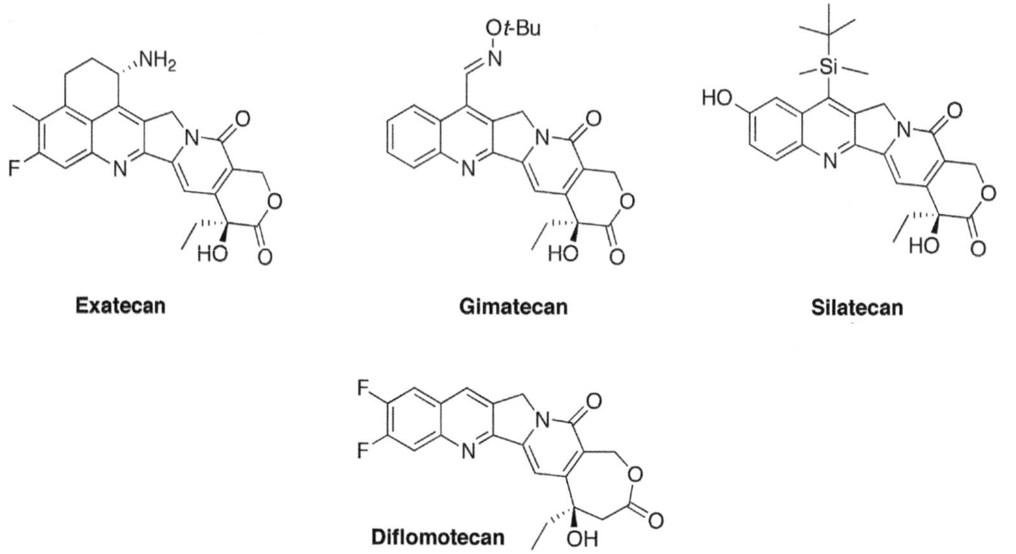

Exatecan   **Gimatecan**   **Silatecan**

Diflomotecan

FIGURE 3.17   Structures of representative tecans in clinical trials: exatecan, gimatecan, silatecan, and diflomotecan.

PRODIGIOSIN

The prodigiosin alkaloid family of natural products is characterized by a pyrrolylpyrromethene core and a deep, blood-red color. Prodigiosin is representative of the acyclic members of this family; nonylprodigiosin exemplifies the cyclic members (Fig. 3.18). The occurrence of these secondary metabolites, which are often mistaken for blood droplets in bread, has been documented for over 2000 years. Observations of prodigiosins formed the basis for the Miracle of Bolsena in 1263, the foundation of the Christian festival of Corpus Christi. Even earlier, troops of Alexander the Great ascribed its occurrence as an omen to validate the bloodshed during the siege of Tyre in 322 BC [97]. Members of this family are produced by microorganisms such as *Serratia marcescens*. They were first isolated, and their structural features characterized, in the 1930s; however, structure elucidation and total synthesis of prodigiosin were not completed until the 1960s [98,99].

Prodigiosins demonstrate potent antimicrobial, antifungal, cytotoxic, and immunosuppressive activities, although the mechanism through which these compounds act is complex and is likely to be multifactorial. Among other targets, prodigiosins are capable of uncoupling H^+/Cl^- transporters by binding to and transporting chloride ions, and thereby modulating the pH of cells. In the presence of copper, they cleave DNA, resulting in cytotoxic and apoptotic effects [97,100]. The prodigiosin derivative streptorubin B (Fig. 3.18) was found to be responsible for the activity of a natural product extract in an assay to inhibit Bcl-2's interaction with Bax, a proapoptotic protein. Structure activity studies and further optimization led to the identification of obatoclax (Fig. 3.18), one of the first Bcl-2 antagonists in clinical trials [101]. Further studies showed that obatoclax is a pan-Bcl-2 inhibitor that blocks BH3-mediated binding of Bax and Bak to their binding partners (Bcl-2, Bcl-XL, Mcl-1, and A1), thereby

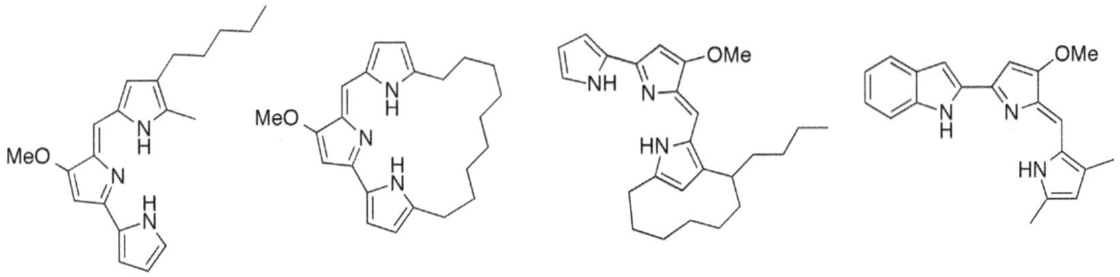

FIGURE 3.18 Structures of prodigiosin, nonylprodigiosin, streptorubin B, and obatoclax.

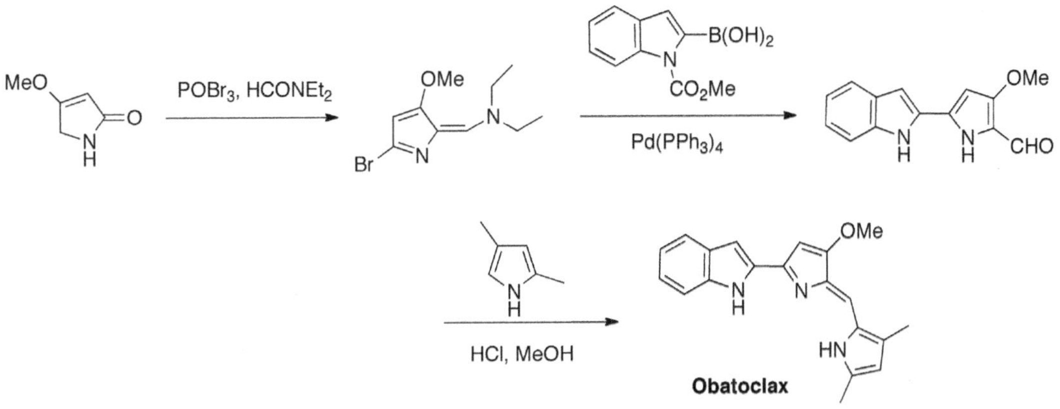

SCHEME 3.5 Synthesis of obatoclax.

resulting in the proapoptotic proteins being unopposed. Additional biological targets have also been proposed [102–104].

The synthesis of obatoclax starts with the reaction of Vilsmeier reagent with 4-methoxy-3-pyrrolin-2-one to generate the bromoenamine (Scheme 3.5). Suzuki reaction followed by hydrolysis affords the pyrrole aldehyde. Obatoclax is formed by an acid-mediated condensation with dimethylpyrrole [101].

The intriguing properties of prodigiosins and their historical significance have led to substantial efforts toward their total synthesis, and further understanding of their mechanism of action [105,106]. Furthermore, the potential of these compounds to act as inhibitors of protein–protein interactions ensures that this fascinating family of natural products will continue to garner significant interest.

AZACITIDINE

A large number of historic and current therapeutics are based on close structural mimicry of nucleotides and nucleosides. In 2004, the FDA approved the DNA methyltransferase inhibitor 5-azacitidine (Vidaza, or ladakamycin; NSC1028016; Fig. 3.19) for the treatment of myelodysplastic syndrome (MDS) [107]. In spite of its simple structure and its low molecular weight

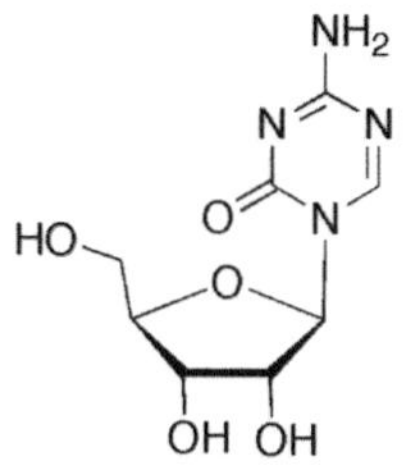

FIGURE 3.19   Structure of 5-azacytidine.

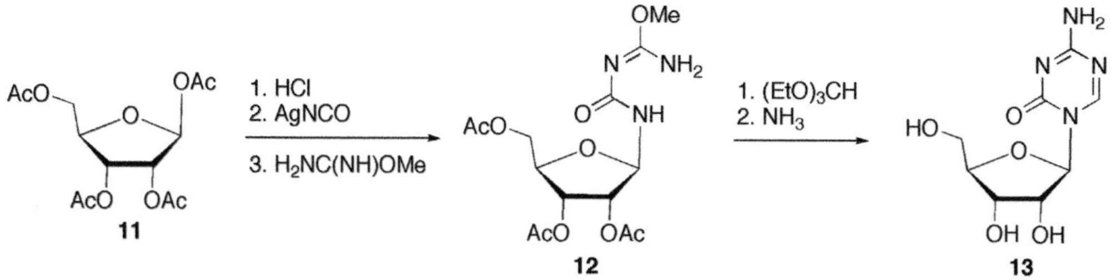

SCHEME 3.6   Synthetic approach to 5-azacytidine starting from ribofuranose.

(MW) of 244, this analog of cytidine is noteworthy for several reasons [108]. Since it was the first drug approved for MDS, it was granted orphan drug status, while in 1980 its application for approval as a cytotoxic agent was rejected by the FDA. More importantly, azacitidine is a pioneering case for counteracting epigenetic gene silencing, a mechanism that is used by cancer cells to inhibit expression of tumor suppressor genes. It is reasonable to assume that azacitidine perturbs RNA biosynthesis and causes general cytotoxic effects; its major anti-neoplastic efficacy is based on DNA hypomethylation, leading to renewed transcription of previously silenced genes [109–111].

Several efficient synthetic approaches toward azacytidine have been reported in the chemical literature [112–114]. The 1,3,5-triazine heterocycle can be installed on the ribose scaffold by selective conversion of the anomeric acetate in tetraacetate 11 to the chloride, treatment with silver isocyanate, and addition of O-methylisourea to give 12 (Scheme 3.6). Further condensation with triethylorthoformate and global deprotection with ammonia, which also converts the methoxy group to the amine substituent, complete the synthesis of 13.

Alternatively, the heterocycle can be assembled in suitably activated form before attachment to the carbohydrate moiety (Scheme 3.7). The nitrile group of N-cyanoguanidine is hydrolyzed to the carboxamide in hot formic acid, and cyclization with acetic anhydride delivers the triazinone 15. After silylation of the amino and carbonyl groups, N-glycosylation with ribose 17 occurs in the presence of Lewis acid activator to give the nucleoside 18, which is deprotected for the completion of azacytidine.

One of the shortcomings of 5-azacytidine is its lack of stability in aqueous solutions, where it provides a complex mixture of degradation product after initial ring opening to the N-formyl derivative. Reduction with borohydride leads to the more stable 5,6-dihydro-5-azacytidine, which has been suggested to act as a prodrug of 5-azacytidine (Fig. 3.20) [114].

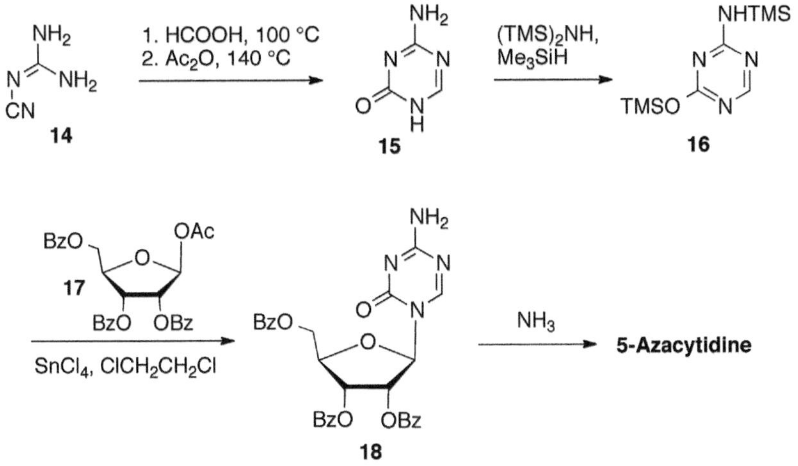

SCHEME 3.7 Alternative synthetic approach to 5-azacytidine starting from cyanoguanidine.

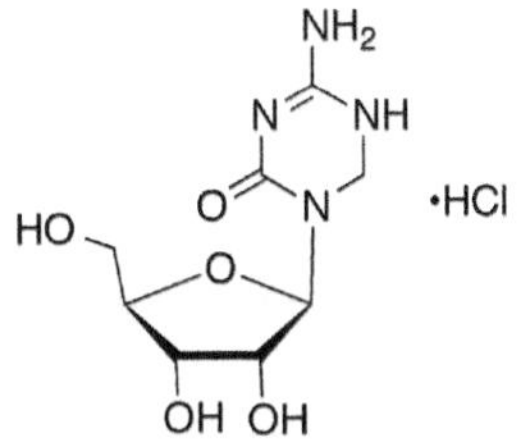

FIGURE 3.20 Structure of 5,6-dihydro-5-azacytidine hydrochloride, a more hydrolytically stable prodrug of 5-azacytidine.

FK-228

The structurally unusual bicyclic depsipeptide FK-228 (also called FR-901228, romidepsin, and Istodax; Fig. 3.21) was isolated from the culture broth of the terrestrial bacterium *Chromobacterium violaceum* using a phenotypic reversion assay of Ha-*ras*-transformed NIH-3T3 cells. Similar to other well-known natural products—such as radicicol, the tyrphostins, leptomycin B, L-739, 749, and trapoxin A—follow-up studies on FK-228 were therefore greatly encouraged by its ability to reverse the malignancy of tumorigenic cell lines. Beyond its induction of apoptosis in malignant cell lines, however, the precise molecular mechanism of action and the cellular targets of FK-228 remained obscure. A chromatin immunoprecipitation analysis revealed that FK-228 induced the accumulation of acetylated histones H3 and H4 in the peroxiredoxin 1 (Prdx1) promoter, thus activating Prdx1 expression in tumor tissues [115]. Indeed, Prdx1 suppression by RNA interference hindered the antitumor effect of FK-228. The cyclodepsipeptide is a prodrug; reduction of the disulfide bond leads to zinc-chelating thiols and blocks the activity of Zn-dependent histone deacetylase. In 2009, FK-228 received FDA approval for the treatment of CTCL, and together with SAHA (vorinostat), it is one of two histone deacetylase inhibitors (HDACIs) currently on the market [116].

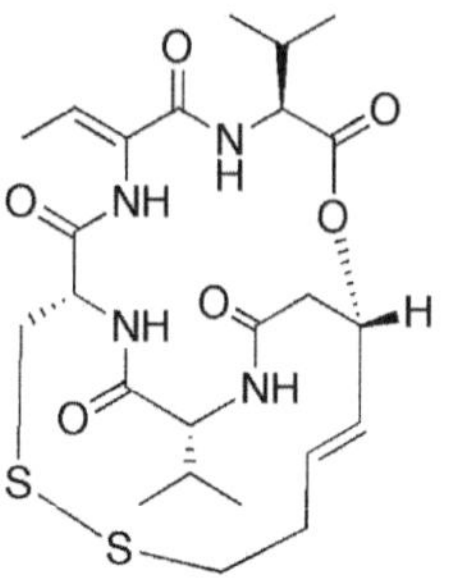

FIGURE 3.21 Structure of FK-228.

FK-228 and apicidin, another cyclotetrapeptide HDACI, represent novel antitumor agents with potential utility in multiple clinical applications. In particular, in combination with Pgp and multidrug-resistance-associated protein 1 inhibitors such as verapamil and MK-571, respectively, broad therapeutic efficacy in cancer treatment can be envisioned [116,117].

While it is possible to obtain FK-228 by fermentation, synthetic efforts have been inspired by the attempt to elucidate the role of the disulfide moiety in the depsipeptide using the tools of organic synthesis. Under physiological conditions, the disulfide is readily reduced, and the resulting dithiol represents the biologically active derivative.

Several total syntheses of FK-228 have been reported since 1996 [118]. In the earliest approach, N-acylation of valine methyl ester (19) with Fmoc-threonine provided a dipeptide that can be deprotected with diethylamine and further coupled with side chain S-tritylated D-cysteine (Scheme 3.8) [119]. Tripeptide 20 was extended with Fmoc-D-valine to give tetrapeptide 21, and subsequently the secondary alcohol was tosylated and eliminated with base. The free N-terminus was acylated with β-hydroxy acid 22 to give hydroxy ester 23, which was saponified with lithium hydroxide in methanol. While an alternative macrolactonization with the Keck modification of the Steglich esterification conditions was unsuccessful, the intramolecular Mitsunobu substitution provided 62% of the desired depsipeptide if p-toluenesulfonic acid was added to prevent elimination of the activated allylic alcohol. Finally, the disulfide was obtained by treatment of the S-tritylated derivative with iodine in dilute methanol. FR-228 (24) was thus obtained in 14 steps and in an overall yield of 18% (Scheme 3.8).

Subsequent synthetic studies addressed several shortcomings of this synthesis [118], and macrolactamization was found to be more efficient than macrolactonization (Scheme 3.9) [120].

HEMIASTERLIN

The isolation from the sponge *Hemiusterelia minor* and the structural elucidation of the three cytotoxic peptides jaspamide, geodiamolide TA, and hemiasterlin were first reported in 1994 [121–123]. Closely related cytotoxic natural peptides also include milnamide and the criamides. In the past 12 years, synthetic as well as biological studies of the structurally relatively simple but sterically congested hydrophobic tripeptide sequence of hemiasterlin have

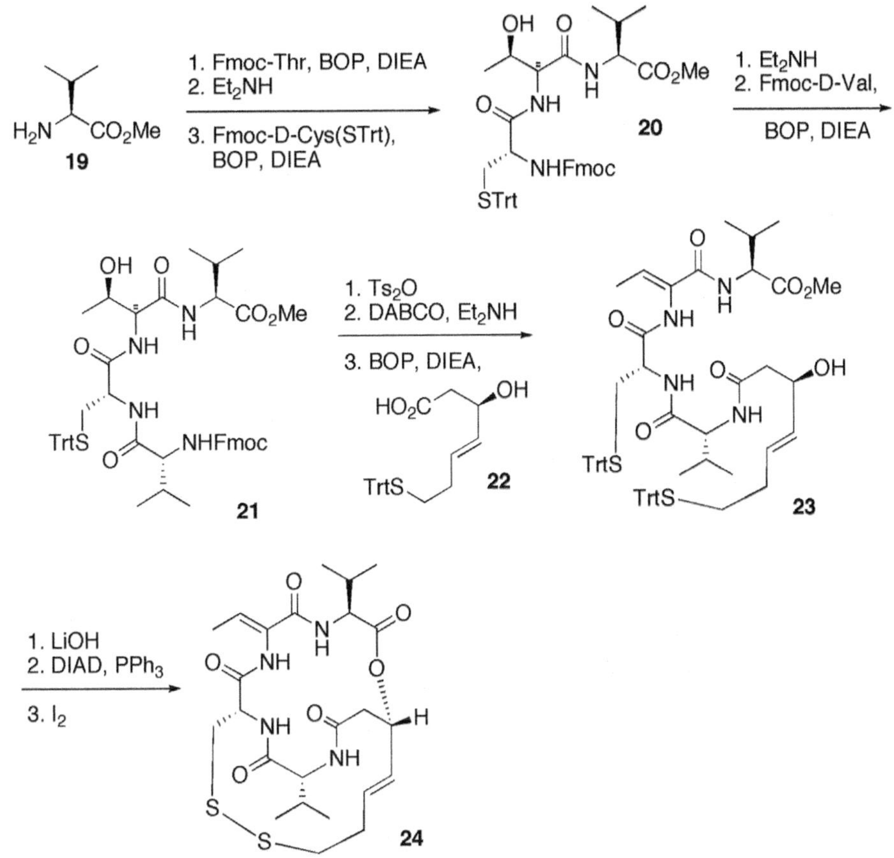

SCHEME 3.8 Total synthesis of FK-228.

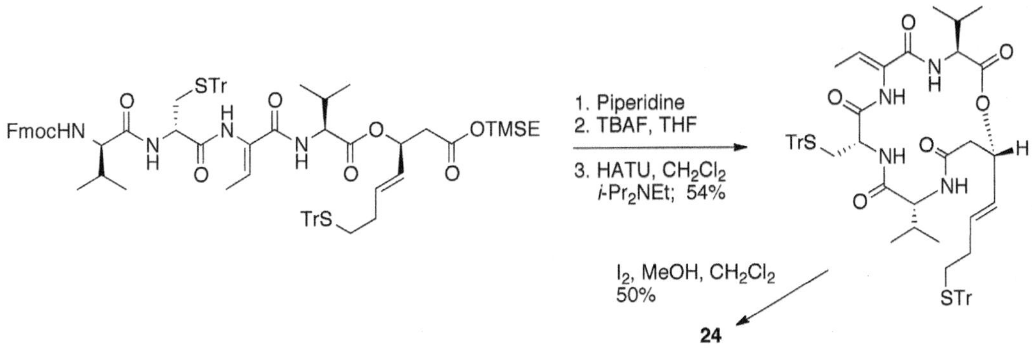

SCHEME 3.9 A macrolactamization approach to FK-228.

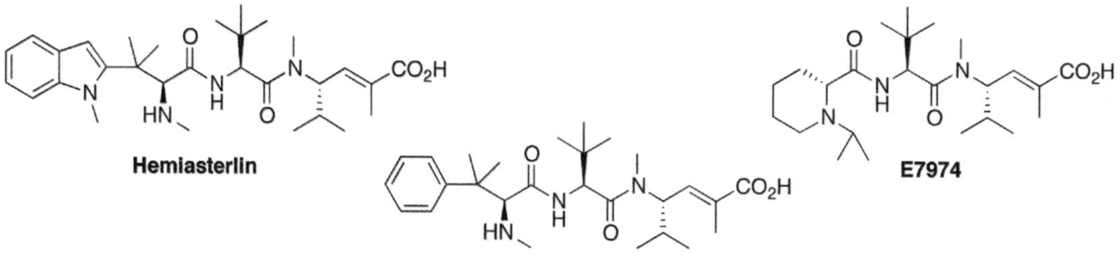

FIGURE 3.22   Structures of hemiasterlin and analogs HTI-286 and E7974.

progressed rapidly, and synthetic analogs, such as HTI-286 (taltobulin), E7974, and others, have been identified (Fig. 3.22) [124]. These compounds induce dose-dependent microtubule depolymerization and mitotic arrest, and are in early-phase clinical trials [125]. Their mechanism of action is closely related to the dolastatins, which have suffered from significant bone marrow toxicity and neuropathy, and other oligopeptide tubulin-binding agents, such as the tubulysins [126–128]. The binding site of HTI-286 was proposed to be at the tubulin dimer interface near the vinca domain, and nuclear Overhauser enhancement spectroscopy (NOESY) experiments suggested a bioactive conformation that could be extended to hemiasterlin [129].

A number of hybrid molecules of hemiasterlin and dolastatins have been explored, and the SARs of truncated analogs have been investigated [7,130,131]. HTI-286 advanced into clinical trials since it avoids rapid clearance by the G-glycoprotein transporter, a problem that hemiasterlin shares with other antimitotic agents such as paclitaxel and vincristine. Nonetheless, HTI-286-resistant tumors were obtained in cell cultures derived from ovarian carcinoma, and the source of resistance was traced back to microtubule-stabilizing mutations in β- or α-tubulin [132].

Several efficient synthetic strategies toward hemiasterlin and HTI-286 have been reported [133–135]. The synergism in the development of new synthetic methodologies, medicinal chemistry, and academic natural product synthesis is illustrated by the use of the N-benzothiazol-2-sulfonyl (Bts) protective group in the total synthesis of (−)-hemiasterlin (Scheme 3.10) [136]. Oxidation of N-Bts-(S)-valinol under Swern conditions followed by Wittig condensation gave the vinylogous amino acid 26. The Bts-protective group was removed under Fukuyama conditions with thiophenol, and the N-terminus was acylated with the acid chloride of Bts-protected tertiary leucine to give dipeptide 27. The final coupling required the preparation of the tetramethyltryptophan derivative 29, which was obtained by an asymmetric Strecker reaction from aldehyde 28. Condensation with (R)-phenylglycinol was followed by addition of cyanide into the imine, resulting in an 8:1 diastereoselectivity. Since efforts to remove the chiral auxiliary from the Strecker product under oxidative conditions failed, the nitrile was first converted to the primary amide in the presence of hydrogen peroxide, and hydrogenolysis over palladium hydroxide was used to cleave the auxiliary. Finally, treatment with BtsCl under biphasic conditions and methylation with excess methyl iodide in DMF led to the NH_2-amide, which was activated for peptide coupling by conversion to the bis-Boc derivative 29. In dichloromethane under reflux and in the presence of dimethylaminopyridine, the

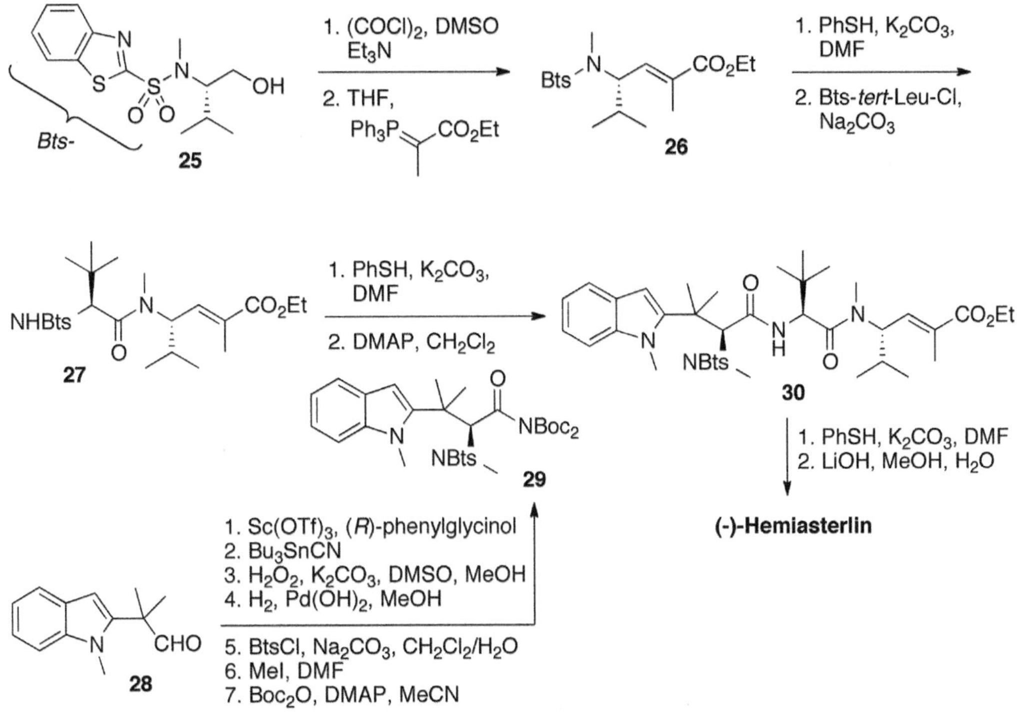

SCHEME 3.10   Total synthesis of (−)-hemiasterlin.

tripeptide **30** was obtained in excellent yield. Bts cleavage with thiophenol and ethyl ester hydrolysis with lithium hydroxide in aqueous methanol provided synthetic hemiasterlin that was identical to the natural product based on spectroscopic analysis.

HALICHONDRIN

The halichondrin family of natural products is characterized by a highly complex architecture featuring a 2,6,9-trioxatricyclo[3.3.2.0] decane core as well as exquisitely potent antiproliferative activity (minimal efficacious doses in in vivo xenograft studies are in the microgram per kilogram range). Members such as norhalichondrin and halichondrin B (Fig. 3.23) were isolated from a variety of sponges, which suggests that sponge symbiotes are the source of these highly complex molecules. Biological studies, hampered by the limited quantities of material available, showed that the halichondrins act through destabilization of tubulin, albeit through a mechanism distinct from vinca alkaloids. Importantly, activity was also observed against a variety of chemoresistant tumor types [137].

Due to the difficulty in procuring the quantities of halichondrins required for further testing from natural sources, as well as the challenge that the structure provided, the results of a number of efforts toward the total synthesis of this class of compounds have been published [137].

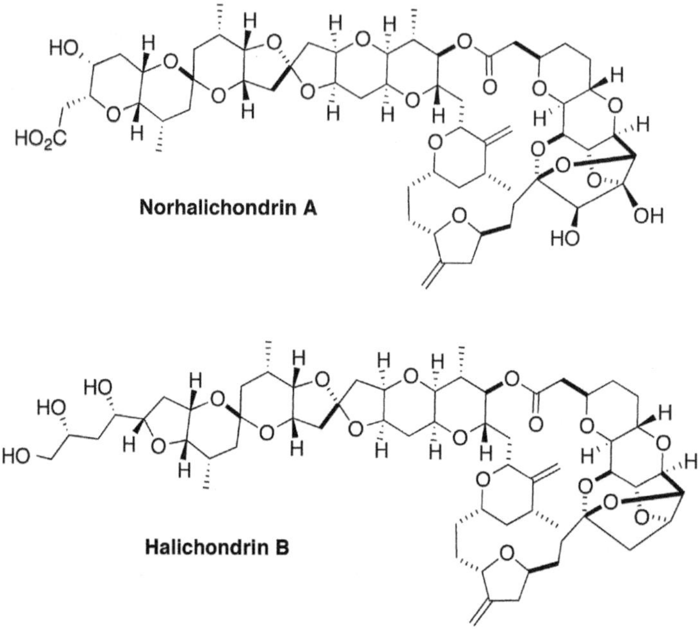

FIGURE 3.23   Structures of norhalichondrin and halichondrin B.

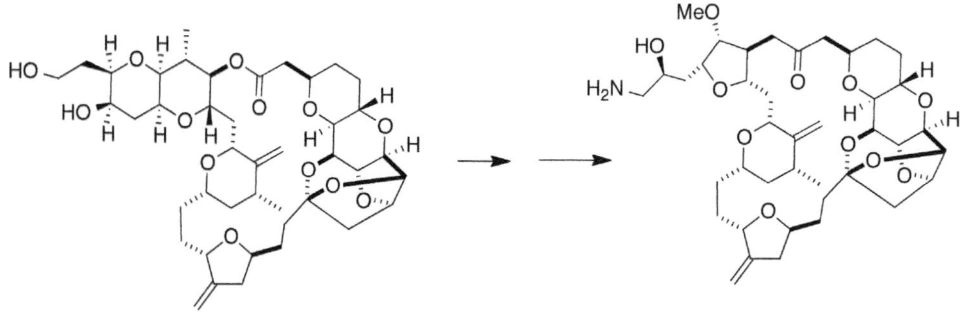

FIGURE 3.24   Structures of the minimally active halichondrin B fragment **31** and eribulin.

The Kishi lab completed the first total synthesis of halichondrin B and norhalichondrin B in 1992 through a herculean effort in which the longest linear sequence was 47 steps [138].

Testing of intermediates prepared as part of the total synthesis campaign revealed that only fragments such as **31** (Fig. 3.24) containing the right-hand macrolactone exhibited activity in cell growth inhibition assays. Further optimization efforts led to eribulin (Halaven), which exhibited excellent potency, acceptable pharmaceutical properties, and efficacy in human cancer xenograft models. Eribulin was approved for the treatment of metastatic breast cancer in 2010 [139,140]. The synthesis of simplified analogs of halichondrin B and eribulin continues to be an active area of research, with a focus on improving brain penetration and reducing interactions with Pgp efflux pumps [141,142]. The discovery of eribulin provides an excellent example of the potential of natural product total synthesis to identify novel therapeutic agents, and to overcome the supply limitations from natural sources.

TRABECTEDIN

Trabectedin (also called ET-743, ecteinascidin 743, and Yondelis) is a product of the extensive plant and marine natural product isolation and screening program pursued by the NCI in the 1960s. The tetrahydroisoquinoline alkaloid was extracted from the sea squirt *Ecteinascidia turbinata*, and its anticancer activity was discovered 15 years before its successful structure elucidation (Fig. 3.25) [143,144].

Since 2007, trabectedin has been approved for treatment of patients with soft tissue sarcoma in Europe, and it is in clinical evaluation for other cancer types, including breast, prostate, and ovarian cancer. The FDA has granted orphan drug status to this complex marine metabolite, but further clinical studies will be required before a market approval [145]. Since it is among the few marine natural products used in human therapy, trabectedin has attracted considerable interest among isolation and medicinal chemists, and its complex structure has also attracted considerable synthetic efforts, culminating in several multistep total syntheses and formal syntheses [146]. However, clinical samples are currently prepared by a bacterial fermentation in *Pseudomonas fluorescens*, which provides the cyanosafracin B starting material for the further multistep conversion to trabectedin [143]. It is questionable if the latter method would prove economical for large-scale production, in spite of the high potency of the drug.

Trabectin binds to guanines in the minor groove of DNA through an iminium species that is generated by a dehydration of the hemiaminal function. Hydrogen bond formation and van der Waals stabilization with nucleotides on the opposite strand of the DNA double helix create an equivalent to a DNA cross-link, bending the DNA backbone and interfering with the gene transcription process. Ultimately, DNA strand break and cell death result as a consequence of the malfunction of the transcription-coupled nucleotide excision repair (TC-NER)

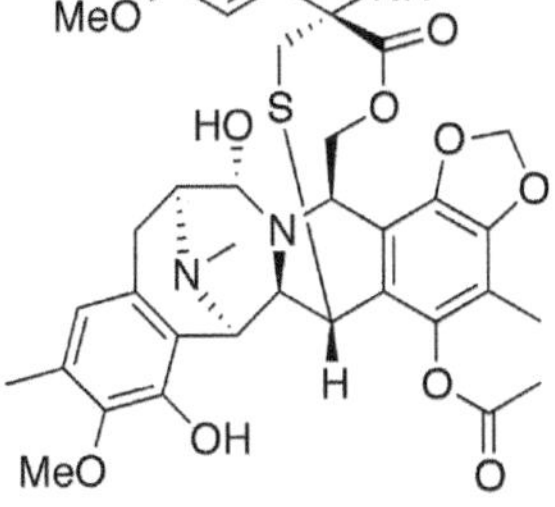

Trabectedin

FIGURE 3.25   Structure of trabectedin.

mechanism [143,147]. Other biological pathway interference and molecularly targeting processes, in particular its ability to deplete monocytes, are also important for the antitumor activity of this fascinating marine metabolite [148].

CONCLUSIONS

New therapies in oncology are increasingly evolving from the broad-spectrum profile of pure cytotoxic or cytostatic agents to the surgical strikes of enzyme inhibitors targeting signaling pathways, and agents that are preferentially absorbed by cancer cells or influence vascularization and tissue adhesion or penetration. Interestingly, natural products continue to be of great utility as biological tools for the identification and characterization of new targets and inhibitory mechanisms, as well as for use as therapeutic agents, in spite of their potential cytotoxic side effects. Moreover, the diversity of natural structures continues to impress and inspire medicinal chemistry. In many cases, synthetic modifications of natural products are necessary to gain insight into structure–activity relationships, and to improve on physicochemical features as well as biological properties. While these adjustments require dedication and talent, they are at least as likely to lead to new drugs as high-throughput screens of small-molecule libraries and traditional medicinal chemistry optimizations of unnatural lead compounds.

Acknowledgments

We gratefully acknowledge financial support for our Center for Chemical Methodologies and Library Development (UPCMLD), provided by the National Institute of General Medical Sciences (NIGMS) (P50-GM067082).

Questions

1. Use the databases referenced below to determine the structure of wortmannin, its biological targets, analogs of this natural product, and literature references on clinical studies.

2. Use the databases referenced below to identify natural products that have been reported to inhibit polo-like kinase 1.

3. Use original papers and structures from the databases referenced below as well as appropriate modeling software that you have available to investigate the binding of trabectin to DNA.

Databases: Review articles cited in this chapter and public databases, specifically PubChem (http://pubchem.ncbi.nlm.nih.gov/) and Entrez (http://www.ncbi.nlm.nih.gov/gquery/gquery.fcgi?itool=toolbar).[pbr]).

References

[1] Newman DJ, Cragg GM. Natural products as sources of new drugs over the 30 years from 1981 to 2010. J Nat Prod 2012;75:311–35.

[2] da Rocha AB, Lopes RM, Schwartsmann G. Natural products in anti-cancer therapy. Curr Opin Pharmacol 2001;1:364–9.

[3] Eldridge GR, Vervoort HC, Lee CM, Cremin PA, Williams CT, Hart SM, et al. High-throughput method for the production and analysis of large natural product libraries for drug discovery. Anal Chem 2002;74:3963–3971.

[4] Tanaka J, Trianto A, Musman M, Issa HH, Ohtani II, Ichiba T, et al. New polyoxygenated steroids exhibiting reversal of multidrug resistance from the gorgonian *Isis hippuris*. Tetrahedron 2002;58:6259–66.

[5] Newman DJ, Cragg GM. Marine natural products and related compounds in clinical and advanced preclinical trials. J Nat Prod 2004;67:1216–38.

[6] Newman DJ, Cragg GM. Advanced preclinical and clinical trials of natural products and related compounds from marine sources. Curr Med Chem 2004;11:1693–713.

[7] Nieman JA, Coleman JE, Wallace DJ, Piers E, Lim LY, Roberge M, et al. Synthesis and antimitotic/cytotoxic activity of hemiasterlin analogues. J Natural Prod 2003;66:183–99.

[8] Chang Z, Sitachitta N, Rossi JV, Roberts MA, Flatt PM, Jia J, et al. Biosynthetic pathway and gene cluster analysis of curacin A, an antitubulin natural product from the tropical marine cyanobacterium *Lyngbya majuscula*. J Natural Prod 2004;67:1356–67.

[9] Elnakady YA, Sasse F, Lunsdorf H, Reichenbach H. Disorazol A1, a highly effective antimitotic agent acting on tubulin polymerization and inducing apoptosis in mammalian cells. Biochem Pharmacol 2004;67:927–35.

[10] Kingston DG, Newman DJ. The search for novel drug leads for predominately antitumor therapies by utilizing mother nature's pharmacophoric libraries. Curr Opin Drug Discov Dev 2005;8:207–27.

[11] Rivkin A, Chou T-C, Danishefsky SJ. On the remarkable antitumor properties of fludelone: how we got there. Angew Chem Int Ed 2005;44:2838–50.

[12] Nagle A, Hur W, Gray NS. Antimitotic agents of natural origin. Curr Drug Targets 2006;7:305–26.

[13] Wilson RM, Danishefsky SJ. Small molecule natural products in the discovery of therapeutic agents: the synthesis connection. J Org Chem 2006;71:8329–51.

[14] Bailly C. Ready for a comeback of natural products in oncology. Biochem Pharmacol 2009;77:1447–57.

[15] Molinski TF, Dalisay DS, Lievens SL, Saludes JP. Drug development from marine natural products. Nat Rev Drug Discov 2009;8:69–85.

[16] Liu J, Hu Y, Waller DL, Wang J, Liu Q. Natural products as kinase inhibitors. Nat Prod Rep 2012;29:392–403.

[17] Lombardi P. Exemestane, a new steroidal aromatase inhibitor of clinical relevance. Biochim Biophys Acta Mol Basis Dis 2002;1587:326–37.

[18] DeCensi A, Dunn BK, Puntoni M, Gennari A, Ford LG. Exemestane for breast cancer prevention: a critical shift? Cancer Discov 2012;2:25–40.

[19] Buzdar AU, Robertson JFR, Eiermann W, Nabholtz J-M. An overview of the pharmacology and pharmacokinetics of the newer generation aromatase inhibitors anastrozole, letrozole, and exemestane. Cancer 2002;95:2006–16.

[20] Reimers L, Crew KD. Tamoxifen versus raloxifene versus exemestane for chemoprevention. Curr Breast Cancer Rep 2012;4:207–15.

[21] Dodwell D, Vergote I. A comparison of fulvestrant and the third-generation aromatase inhibitors in the second-line treatment of postmenopausal women with advanced breast cancer. Cancer Treat Rev 2005;31:274–82.

[22] Howell A, Abram P. Clinical development of fulvestrant ("Faslodex"). Cancer Treat Rev 2005;31:S3–9.

[23] Howell A. The future of fulvestrant ("Faslodex"). Cancer Treat Rev 2005;31:S26–33.

[24] Estevez L, Alvarez I, Tusquets I, Segui MA, Munoz M, Fernandez Y, et al. Finding the right dose of fulvestrant in breast cancer. Cancer Treat Rev 2013;39:136–41.

[25] Buzdar AU, Robertson JFR. Fulvestrant: pharmacologic profile versus existing endocrine agents for the treatment of breast cancer. Ann Pharmacother 2006;40:1572–83.

[26] Seimbille Y, Benard F, van Lier JE. Synthesis of 16α-fluoro ICI 182,780 derivatives: powerful antiestrogens to image estrogen receptor densities in breast cancer by positron emission tomography. J Chem Soc Perkin Trans 2002;1:2275–81.

[27] Jiang X-R, Walter Sowell J, Zhu BT. Synthesis of 7α-substituted derivatives of 17β-estradiol. Steroids 2006;71:334–42.

[28] Hogan PJ, Powell L, Robinson GE. Development of a catalytic cuprate 1,6-conjugate dienone addition process for the manufacture of fulvestrant EAS, a key intermediate in the synthesis of fulvestrant. Org Proc Res Dev 2010;14:1188–93.

[29] Russo M, Spagnuolo C, Tedesco I, Bilotto S, Russo GL. The flavonoid quercetin in disease prevention and therapy: facts and fancies. Biochem Pharmacol 2012;83:6–15.

[30] Dajas F. Life or death: neuroprotective and anticancer effects of quercetin. J Ethnopharmacol 2012;143:383–96.

[31] Taylor CK, Levy RM, Elliott JC, Burnett BP. The effect of genistein aglycone on cancer and cancer risk: a review of the in vitro, preclinical, and clinical studies. Nutr Rev 2009;67:398–415.

[32] Ren W, Qiao Z, Wang H, Zhu L, Zhang L. Flavonoids: promising anti-cancer agents. Med Res Rev 2003;23:519–34.

[33] Lopez-Lazaro M. Flavonoids as anticancer agents: structure–activity relationship study. Curr Med Chem Anticancer Agents 2002;2:691–714.

[34] Wang L-M, Ren D-M. Flavopiridol, the first cyclin-dependent kinase inhibitor: recent advances in combination chemotherapy. Mini Rev Med Chem 2010;10:1058–70.

[35] Nguyen TB, Lozach O, Surpateanu G, Wang Q, Retailleau P, Iorga BI, et al. Synthesis, biological evaluation and molecular modeling of natural and unnatural flavonoidal alkaloids, inhibitors of kinases. J Med Chem 2012;55:2811–9.

[36] Zhai S, Senderowicz AM, Sausville EA, Figg WD. Flavopiridol, a novel cyclin-dependent kinase inhibitor, in clinical development. Ann Pharmacother 2002;36:905–11.

[37] Dai Y, Grant S. CDK inhibitors in leukemia and lymphoma. Basic Clin Oncol 2008;35:353–77.

[38] Gong H, Xie W. Orphan nuclear receptors, PXR and LXR: new ligands and therapeutic potential. Expert Opin Ther Targets 2004;8:49–54.

[39] Qu L, Tang X. Bexarotene: a promising anticancer agent. Cancer Chemother Pharmacol 2010;65:201–5.

[40] Boehm MF, Zhang L, Badea BA, White SK, Mais DE, Berger E, et al. Synthesis and structure–activity relationships of novel retinoid X receptor-selective retinoids. J Med Chem 1994;37:2930–41.

[41] Daiss JO, Burschka C, Mills JS, Montana JG, Showell GA, Fleming I, et al. Synthesis, crystal structure analysis, and pharmacological characterization of disila-bexarotene, a disila-analogue of the RXR-selective retinoid agonist bexarotene. Organometallics 2005;24:3192–9.

[42] Bauer JB, Lippert WP, Dörrich S, Hemboldt A, Mallet JM, Sinay P, et al. Novel silicon-containing analogs of the retinoid agonist bexarotene: syntheses and biological effects on human pluripotent stem cells. Chem Med Chem 2011;6:1509–17.

[43] Gerth K, Bedorf N, Höfle G, Irschik H, Reichenbach H. Antibiotics from gliding bacteria. 74. Epothilones A and B: antifungal and cytotoxic compounds from *Sorangium cellulosum* (myxobacteria). Production, physico-chemical and biological properties. J Antibiot 1996;49:560–3.

[44] Höfle G, Bedorf N, Steinmetz H, Schomburg D, Gerth K, Reichenbach H. Epothilone A and B—novel 16-membered macrolides with cytotoxic activity: isolation, crystal structure and conformation in solution. Angew Chem Int Ed Engl 1996;35:1567–9.

[45] Krause W, Klar U. Differences and similarities of epothilones. Curr Can Ther Rev 2011;7:10–36.

[46] Hardt IH, Steinmetz H, Gerth K, Sasse F, Reichenbach H, Höfle G. New natural epothilones from *Sorangium cellulosum*, strains So ce90/B2 and So ce90/D13: isolation, structure elucidation, and SAR studies. J Nat Prod 2001;64:847–56.

[47] Wang J, Zhang H, Ying L, Wang C, Jiang N, Zhou Y, et al. Five new epothilone metabolites from *Sorangium celluosum* strain So0157-2. J Antibiot 2009;62:483–7.

[48] Wang J-D, Jiang N, Zhang H, Ying L-P, Wang C-X, Xiang W-S, et al. New epothilone congeners from *Sorangium cellulosum* strain So0157-2. Nat Prod Res 2011;25:1707–12.

[49] Bollag DM, McQueney PA, Zhu J, Hensens O, Koupal L, Liesch J, et al. Epothilones, a new class of microtubule-stabilizing agents with a taxol-like mechanism of action. Cancer Res 1995;55:2325–33.

[50] Nicolaou KC, Roschangar F, Vourloumis D. Chemical biology of epothilones. Angew Chem Int Ed 1998;37:2014–45.

[51] Altmann K-H, Flörscheimer A, O'Reilly T, Wartmann M. The natural products epothilones A and B as lead structures for anti-cancer drug discovery: chemistry, biology, and SAR studies. Prog Med Chem 2004;42:171–205.

[52] Altmann K-H. Recent developments in the chemical biology of epothilones. Curr Pharm Des 2005;11:1595–613.

[53] Watkins EB, Chittiboyina AG, Jung J-C, Avery MA. The epothilones and related analogues—a review of their syntheses and anti-cancer activities. Curr Pharm Des 2005;11:1615–53.

[54] Feyen F, Cachoux F, Gertsch J, Wartmann M, Altmann K-H. Epothilones as lead structures for the synthesis-based discovery of new chemotypes for microtubule stabilization. Acc Chem Res 2008;41:21–31.

[55] Hunt J. Discovery of ixabepilone. Mol Cancer Ther 2009;8:275–81.

[56] Klar U, Buchman B, Schwede W, Skuballa W, Hoffmann J, Lichtner RB. Total synthesis and antitumor activity of ZK-EPO: the first fully synthetic epothilone in clinical development. Angew Chem Int Ed 2006;45:7942–8.

[57] Hoffmann J, Vitale I, Buchmann B, Galluzzi L, Schwede W, Senovilla L, et al. Improved cellular pharmacokinetics and pharmacodynamics underlie the wide anticancer activity of sagopilone. Cancer Res 2008;68:5301–5308.

[58] Kupchan SM, Komoda Y, Court WA, Thomas GJ, Smith RM, Karim A, et al. Tumor inhibitors. LXXIII. Maytansine, a novel antileukemic ansa macrolide from *Maytenus ovatus*. J Am Chem Soc 1972;94:1354–6.

[59] Kirschning A, Harmrolfs K, Knobloch T. The chemistry and biology of the maytansinoid antitumor agents. C R Chim 2008;11:1523–43.

[60] Cassady JM, Chan KK, Foss HG, Leistner E. Recent developments in the maytansinoid antitumor agents. Chem Pharm Bull 2004;52:1–26.

[61] Remillard S, Rebhun LI, Howie GS, Kupchan SM. Antimitotic activity of the potent tumor inhibitor maytansine. Science 1975;189:1002–5.

[62] Wolpert-Defilippes MK, Adamson RH, Cysyk RL, Jones DG. Cytotoxic action of maytansine, a novel ansa macrolide. Biochem Pharmacol 1975;24:751–4.

[63] Hamel E. Natural products which interact with tubulin in the vinca domain: maytansine, rhizoxin, phomopsin A, dolastatins 10 and 15 and halichondrin B. Pharmacol Ther 1992;55:31–51.

[64] Chari RVJ. Targeted cancer therapy: conferring specificity to cytotoxic drugs. Acc Chem Res 2008;41:98–107.

[65] Widdison WC, Wilhelm SD, Cavanagh EE, Whiteman KR, Leece BA, Kovtun Y, et al. Semisynthetic maytansine analogues for the targeted treatment of cancer. J Med Chem 2006;49:4392–408.

[66] Burris III HA. Trastuzumab emtansine: a novel antibody-drug conjugate for HER2-positive breast cancer. Expert Opin Biol Ther 2011;11:807–19.

[67] de Boer C, Meulman PA, Wnuk RJ, R.L. Peterson DH. Geldanamycin, a new antibiotic. J Antibiot 1970;23:442–7.

[68] Whitesell ML, Mimnaugh EG, de Costa B, Myers CE, Neckers LM. Inhibition of heat shock protein HSP90-pp60^{vsrc} heteroprotein complex formation by benzoquinone ansamycins: essential role for stress proteins in oncogenic transformation. Proc Natl Acad Sci U S A 1994;91:8324–8.

[69] Stebbins CE, Russo AA, Schneider C, Rosen N, Hartl FU, Pavletich NP. Crystal structure of an Hsp90-geldanamycin complex: targeting of a protein chaperone by an antitumor agent. Cell 1997;89:239–50.

[70] Grenert JP, Sullivan WP, Fadden P, Haystead TAJ, Clark J, Mimnaugh E, et al. The amino-terminal domain of heat shock protein 90 (Hsp90) that binds geldanamycin is an ATP/ADP switch domain that regulates Hsp90 conformation. J Biol Chem 1997;272:23843–50.

[71] Roe SM, Prodromou C, O'Brien R, Ladbury JE, Piper PW, Pearl LH. Structural basis for inhibition of the HSP90 molecular chaperone by the antitumor antibiotics radicicol and geldanamycin. J Med Chem 1999;42:260–6.

[72] Jez JM, Chen JC-H, Rastelli G, Stroud RM, Santi DV. Crystal structure and molecular modeling of 17-DMAG in complex with human Hsp90. Chem Biol 2003;10:361–8.

[73] Kitson RS, Chang C-H, Xiong R, Williams HEL, Davis AL, Lewis W, et al. Synthesis of 19-substituted geldanamycins with altered conformations and their binding to heat shock protein Hsp90. Nature Chem 2013;5:307–14.

[74] Wrona IE, Agouridas V, Panek JS. Design and synthesis of ansamycin antibiotics. C R Chim 2008;11:1483–522.

[75] Taldone T, Sun W, Chiosis G. Discovery and development of heat shock protein 90 inhibitors. Bioorg Med Chem 2009;17:2225–35.

[76] Janin YL. Heat shock protein 90 inhibitors: a textbook example of medicinal chemistry? J Med Chem 2005;48:7503–12.

[77] Hollingshead M, Alley M, Burger AM, Borgel S, Pacula-Cox C, Fiebig H-H, et al. *In vivo* anti-tumor efficacy of 17-DMAG (17-dimethylaminoethylamino-17-demethoxylgeldanamycin hydrochloride), a water-soluble geldanamycin derivative. Cancer Chemother Pharmacol 2005;56:115–25.

[78] Ge J, Normant E, Porter JR, Ali JA, Dembski MS, Gao Y, et al. Design, synthesis and biological evaluation of hydroquinone derivatives of 17-amino-17-demethoxygeldanamycin as potent, water-soluble inhibitors of Hsp90. J Med Chem 2006;49:4606–15.

[79] Duerfeldt AS, Blagg BSJ. Hsp90 inhibition: elimination of shock and stress. Bioorg Med Chem Lett 2010;20:4983–7.

[80] Takahashi I, Kobayashi E, Asano K, Yoshida M, Nakano H. UCN-01, a selective inhibitor of protein kinase C from streptomyces. J Antibiot 1987;40:1782–4.

[81] Akinaga S, Gomi K, Morimoto M, Tamaoki T, Okabe M. Antitumor activity of UCN-01, a selective inhibitor of protein kinase C, in murine and human tumor models. Cancer Res 1991;51:4888–92.

[82] Sausville EA. Cyclin-dependent kinase modulators studied at the NCI: preclinical and clinical studies. Curr Med Chem Anticancer Agents 2003;3:47–56.

[83] Sausville EA. Cell cycle regulatory kinase modulators: interim progress and issues. Curr Top Med Chem 2005;5:1109–17.

[84] Prudhomme M. Staurosporines and structurally related indolocarbazoles as antitumor agents. Anticancer Agents Nat Prod 2005:499–517.

[85] Tse AN, Carvajal R, Schwartz GK. Targeting checkpoint kinase 1 in cancer therapeutics. Clin Cancer Res 2007;13:1955–60.

[86] Fuse E, Kuwabara T, Sparreboom A, Sausville EA, Figg WD. Review of UCN-01 development: a lesson in the importance of clinical pharmacology. J Clin Pharmacol 2005;45:394–403.

[87] Wall ME, Wani MC, Cooke CE, Palmer KH, McPhail AT, Sim GA. Plant antitumor agents I: the isolation and structure of camptothecin, a novel alkoloidal leukemia and tumor inhibitor from *Camptotheca acuminata*. J Am Chem Soc 1966;88:3888–90.

[88] Liew ST, Yang L-Y. Design, synthesis and development of novel camptothecin drugs. Curr Pharm Des 2008;14:1078–97.

[89] Thomas CJ, Rahier NJ, Hecht SM. Camptothecin: current perspectives. Bioorg Med Chem 2004;12:1585–604.

[90] Sriram D, Yogeeswari P, Thirumurugan R, Bal TR. Camptothecin and its analogues: a review on their chemo-therapeutic potential. Natural Prod Res 2005;19:393–412.

[91] Fontana G, Merlini L. Drug discovery from natural substances—a case study: camptothecins. In: Corrado T, editor. Bioactive Compounds from Natural Sources. 2nd ed. Natural Products as Lead Compounds in Drug Discovery. New York: CRC Press; 2011. p. 379–408.

[92] Verma RP, Hansch C. Camptothecins: a SAR/QSAR study. Chem Rev 2009;109:213–35.

[93] Pommier Y. Drugging topoisomerases: lessons and challenges. ACS Chem Biol 2013;8:82–95.

[94] Venditto VJ, Simaneck EE. Cancer therapies utilizing the camptothecins: a review of the *in vivo* literature. Mol Pharmacol 2010;7:307–49.

[95] Duan J-X, Cai X, Meng F, Sun JD, Liu Q, Jung D, et al. 14-Aminocamptothecins: their synthesis, preclinical activity, and potential use for cancer treatment. J Med Chem 2011;54:1715–23.

[96] Beretta GL, Zuco V, De Cesare M, Perego P, Zaffaroni N. Curr Med Chem 2012;19:3488–501.

[97] Fürstner A. Chemistry and biology of roseophilin and the prodigiosin alkaloids: a survey of the last 2500 years. Angew Chem Int Ed 2003;42:3582–603.

[98] Wasserman HH, McKeon JE, Smith L, Forgione P. Prodigiosin structure and partial synthesis. J Am Chem Soc 1960;82:506–7.

[99] Rapoport H, Holden KG. The synthesis of prodigiosin. J Am Chem Soc 1962;84:635–42.

[100] Perez-Tomas R, Vinas M. New insights on the antitumoral properties of prodiginines. Curr Med Chem 2010;17:2222–31.

[101] Daïri K, Yao Y, Faley M, Tripathy S, Rioux E, Billot X, et al. A scalable process for the synthesis of the Bcl inhibitor obatoclax. Org Proc Res Dev 2007;11:1051–4.

[102] Trudel S, Li ZH, Rauw J, Tiedemann RE, Wen XY, Stewart AK. Preclinical studies of the pan-Bcl inhibitor obatoclax (GX015-070) in multiple myeloma. Blood 2007;109:5430–8.

[103] Joudeh J, Claxton D. Obatoclax mesylate: pharmacology and potential for therapy of hematological neoplasms. Expert Opin Investig Drugs 2012;21:363–73.

[104] Bodur C, Basaga H. Bcl-2 inhibitors: emerging drugs in cancer therapy. Curr Med Chem 2012;19:1804–20.

[105] Espona-Fiedler M, Soto-Cerrato V, Hosseini A, Lizcano JM, Guallar V, Quesada R, et al. Identification of dual mTORC1 and mTORC2 inhibitors in melanoma cells: prodigiosin vs. obatoclax. Biochem Pharmacol 2012;83:489–96.

[106] Su J-C, Chen K-F, Chen W-L, Liu C-Y, Huang J-W, Tai W-T, et al. Synthesis and biological activity of obatoclax derivatives as novel and potent SHP-1 agonists. Eur J Med Chem 2012;56:127–33.

[107] Issa J-PJ, Kantarjian HM, Kirkpatrick P. Fresh from the pipeline: azacitidine. Nat Rev Drug Discov 2005;4:275–6.

[108] Quintas-Cardama A, Santos FPS, Garcia-Manero G. Therapy with azanucleosides for myelodysplastic syndromes. Nature Rev Clin Oncol 2010;7:433–44.

[109] Jones PA. Altering gene expression with 5-azacytidine. Cell 1985;40:485–6.

[110] Elkabani M, List AF. Management of transfusion-dependent myelodysplastic syndromes: current and emerging strategies. Am J Cancer 2006;5:71–80.

[111] Oliver SS, Denu JM. Disrupting the reader of histone language. Angew Chem Int Ed 2011;50:5801–5803.

[112] Winkley MW, Robins RK. Direct glycosylation of 1,3,5-triazinones. New approach to the synthesis of the nucleoside antibiotic 5-azacytidine (4-amino-1-β-D-ribofuranosyl-1,3,5-triazin-2-one) and related derivatives. J Org Chem 1970;35:491–5; and references cited therein.

[113] Niedballa U, Vorbrueggen H. Synthesis of nucleosides. 13. General synthesis of N-glycosides. V. Synthesis of 5-azacytidines. J Org Chem 1974;39:3672–3.

[114] Beisler JA, Abbasi MM, Kelley JA, Driscoll JS. Synthesis and antitumor activity of dihydro-5-azacytidine, a hydrolytically stable analog of 5-azacytidine. J Med Chem 1977;22:806–12.

[115] Hoshino I, Matsubara H, Hanari N, Mori M, Nishimori T, Yoneyama Y, et al. Histone deacetylase inhibitor FK228 activates tumor suppressor Prdx1 with apoptosis induction in esophageal cancer cells. Clin Cancer Res 2005;11:7945–52.

[116] Harrison SJ, Bishton M, Bates SE, Grant S, Piekarz RL, Johnstone RW, et al. A focus on the preclinical development and clinical status of the histone deacetylase inhibitor, romidepsin (depsipeptide, istodax®). Epigenomics 2012;4:571–89.

[117] Okada T, Tanaka K, Nakatani F, Sakimura R, Matsunobu T, Li X, et al. Involvement of P-glycoprotein and MRP1 in resistance to cyclic tetrapeptide subfamily of histone deacetylase inhibitors in the drug-resistant osteosarcoma and Ewing's sarcoma cells. Int J Cancer 2006;118:90–7.

[118] Stolze SC, Kaiser M. Case studies of the synthesis of bioactive cyclodepsipeptide natural products. Molecules 2013;18:1337–67.

[119] Li KW, Wu J, Xing W, Simon JA. Total synthesis of the antitumor depsipeptide FR-901,228. J Am Chem Soc 1996;118:7237–8.

[120] Wen S, Packham G, Ganesan A. Macrolactamization versus macrolactonization: total synthesis of FK228, the depsipeptide histone deacetylase inhibitor. J Org Chem 2008;73:9353–61.

[121] Talpir R, Benayahu Y, Kashman Y, Pannell L, Schleyer M. Hemiasterlin and geodiamolide TA; two new cytotoxic peptides from the marine sponge Hemiasterella-minor (Kirkpatrick). Tetrahedron Lett 1994;35:4453–6.

[122] Coleman JE, da Silva ED, Kong F, Andersen RJ, Allen TM. Cytotoxic peptides from the marine sponge Cymbastela sp. Tetrahedron 1995;51:10653–62.

[123] Gamble WR, Durso NA, Fuller RW, Westergaard CK, Johnson TR, Sackett DL, et al. Cytotoxic and tubulin-interactive hemiasterlins from Auletta sp. and Siphonochalina spp. sponges. Bioorg Med Chem 1999;7:1611–5.

[124] Hsu L-C, Durrant DE, Huang C-C, Chi N-W, Baruchello R, Rondanin R, et al. Development of hemiasterlin derivatives as potential anticancer agents that inhibit tubulin polymerization and synergize with a stilbene tubulin inhibitor. Invest New Drugs 2012;30:1379–88.

[125] Rocha-Lima CM, Bayraktar S, Macintyre J, Raez L, Flores AM, Ferrell A, et al. A phase 1 trial of E7974 administered on day 1 of a 21-day cycle in patients with advanced solid tumors. Cancer 2012;118:4262–70.

[126] Khalil MW, Sasse F, Lünsdorf H, Elnakady YA, Reichenbach H. Mechanism of action of tubulysin, an antimitotic peptide from myxobacteria. Chem Bio Chem 2006;7:678–83.

[127] Rawat DS, Joshi MC, Joshi P, Atheaya H. Marine peptides and related compounds in clinical trial. Anti Cancer Agents Med Chem 2006;6:33–40.

[128] Wang Z, McPherson PA, Raccor BS, Balachandran R, Zhu G, Day BW, et al. Structure–activity and high-content imaging analyses of novel tubulysins. Chem Biol Drug Des 2007;70:75–86.

[129] Ravi M, Zask A, Rush III TS. Structure-based identification of the binding site for the hemiasterlin analogue HTI-286 on tubulin. Biochemistry 2005;44:15871–9.

[130] Zask A, Birnberg G, Cheung K, Kaplan J, Niu Chuan, Norton E, et al. D-piece modifications of the hemiasterlin analog HTI-286 produce potent tubulin inhibitors. Bioorg Med Chem Lett 2004;14:4353–8.

[131] Zask A, Kaplan J, Musto S, Loganzo F. Hybrids of the hemiasterlin analogue taltobulin and the dolastatins are potent antimicrotubule agents. J Am Chem Soc 2005;127:17667–71.

[132] Poruchynsky MS, Kim J-H, Nogales E, Annable T, Loganzo F, Greenberger LM, et al. Tumor cells resistant to a microtubule-depolymerizing hemiasterlin analogue, HTI-286, have mutations in α- or β-tubulin and increased microtubule stability. Biochemistry 2004;43:13944–54.

[133] Andersen RJ, Coleman JE, Piers E, Wallace DJ. Total synthesis of (−)-hemiasterlin, a structurally novel tripeptide that exhibits potent cytotoxic activity. Tetrahedron Lett 1997;38:317–20.

[134] Yamashita A, Norton EB, Kaplan JA, Niu C, Loganzo F, Hernandez R, et al. Synthesis and activity of novel analogs of hemiasterlin as inhibitors of tubulin polymerization: modification of the A segment. Bioorg Med Chem Lett 2004;14:5317–5322.

[135] Simoni D, Lee RM, Durrant DE, Chi N-W, Baruchello R, Rondanin R, et al. Versatile synthesis of new cytotoxic agents structurally related to hemiasterlins. Bioorg Med Chem Lett 2010;20:3431–5.

[136] Vedejs E, Kongkittingam C. A total synthesis of (–)-hemiasterlin using *N*-Bts methodology. J Org Chem 2001;66:7355–64.

[137] Jackson KL, Henderson JA, Phillips AJ. The halichondrins and E7389. Chem Rev 2009;109:3044–79.

[138] Aicher TD, Buszek KR, Fang FG, Forsyth CJ, Jung SH, Kishi Y, et al. Total synthesis of halichondrin B and norhalichondrin B. J Amer Chem Soc 1992;114:3162–4.

[139] Yu MJ, Zheng W, Seletsky BM, Littlefield BA, Kishi Y. Case history: discovery of eribulin (HALAVEN), a halichondrin B analogue that prolongs overall survival in patients with metastatic breast cancer. Annu Rep Med Chem 2011;46:227–41.

[140] Cortes J, Montero AJ, Glück S. Eribulin mesylate, a novel microtubule inhibitor in the treatment of breast cancer. Cancer Treat Rev 2012;38:143–51.

[141] Narayan S, Carlson EM, Cheng H, Du H, Hu Y, Jiang Y, et al. Novel second generation analogs of eribulin. Part I: compounds containing a lipophilic C32 side chain overcome P-glycoprotein susceptibility. Bioorg Med Chem Lett 2011;21:1630–3.

[142] Narayan S, Carlson EM, Cheng H, Condon K, Du H, Eckley S, et al. Novel second generation analogs of eribulin. Part II: orally available and active against resistant tumors *in vivo*. Bioorg Med Chem Lett 2011;21:1634–8.

[143] Cuevas C, Francesch A. Development of Yondelis® (trabectedin, ET-743). A semisynthetic process solves the supply problem. Nat Prod Rep 2009;26:322–37.

[144] Patel RM. Trabectedin: a novel molecular therapeutic in cancer. Int J Current Pharm Res 2011;3:65–70.

[145] del Campo JM, Sessa C, Krasner CN, Vermorken JB, Colombo N, Kaye S, et al. Trabectedin as single agent in relapsed advanced ovarian cancer: results from a retrospective pooled analysis of three phase II trials. Med Oncol 2013;30:435.

[146] Imai T, Nakata H, Yokoshima S, Fukuyama T. Synthetic studies toward ecteinascidin 743 (trabectedin). Synthesis 2012;44:2743–53.

[147] D'Incalci M, Galmarini CM. A review of trabectedin (ET-743): a unique mechanism of action. Mol Cancer Ther 2010;9:2157–63.

[148] Germano G, Frapoli R, Belgiovine C, Anselmo A, Pesche S, Liguori M, et al. Role of macrophage targeting in the antitumor activity of trabectedin. Cancer Cell 2013;23:249–62.

Structural Biology and Anticancer Drug Design

Puja Pathuri, David Norton, Henriette Willems, Dominic Tisi, Harren Jhoti

Astex Therapeutics, Cambridge, UK

INTRODUCTION

Optimization of an early hit molecule can be broken into two main sections, "hits to leads" and "lead optimization". Hits to leads involves validation of the hit molecule, initially by identifying the crucial binding motif; this may require removal of some of the functionality and testing simpler molecules. Synthesis of a limited number of structurally related compounds is used to determine the broad background structure activity relationship of a compound series. With this validated set of compounds in hand, further rounds of chemical optimization will be performed to improve activity against the biological target of interest. As a series of compounds improves in activity against the biological target, other extensive in vitro testing will be carried out looking at selectivity (used to minimize off-target effects) and cellular activity (a surrogate for in vivo activity). Compounds with the required overall properties will be profiled in vivo to assess drug pharmacokinetics (effect of an organism on the compound) and pharmacodynamics (effect of the compound on an organism), before looking for the required therapeutic effect in a suitable animal model. A compound with the correct properties successfully passing through these stages may progress into preclinical and clinical development to eventually become a drug.

Historically, structural biology has had its major impact during later-stage optimization of potential drug molecules, primarily due to the length of time necessary to generate good structural data. Early hit molecules have traditionally come from medium- to high-throughput screening (HTS) of corporate compound collections. Much emphasis has been placed on making these collections "drug-like", with libraries designed to conform to Lipinski's "rule of five" [1]. Whilst this approach has undoubtedly proved successful in the past, the limitations of screening "drug-like" molecules have become apparent. Hit rates are often very low,

Cancer Drug Design and Discovery, Second Edition
http://dx.doi.org/10.1016/B978-0-12-396521-9.00004-8

and those hits that are identified are often not easily optimized. Hits that progress through optimization generally increase in molecular weight, log P, and the number of hydrogen bond donors and acceptors, reducing their original drug-like properties and therefore reducing their potential for development [2,3].

Fragment-based screening is now established as a powerful method for hit generation and continues to provide an alternative to traditional high-throughput screening [4–8].

Fragments are low-molecular-weight (MW) organic molecules (MW 100–300 Da), which typically exhibit low binding affinities (>100 μM) and are therefore difficult to detect using standard bioassay-based screening methods. However, biophysical techniques such as nuclear magnetic resonance (NMR) and X-ray crystallography have been shown to be highly suited to detecting the binding of these low-affinity fragments [9–11].

In recent years, there have been considerable advances in the use of protein crystallography at the hit generation and hit validation stages of the drug discovery process. The utility of protein crystallography at these earlier stages has been made possible by several major technological advances, some of which are discussed further in this chapter. Improvements in many areas of protein crystallography have enabled it to be used as a screening tool for hit generation in an increasingly high-throughput manner. Whilst some of these advances have been process driven, there are compelling reasons to suggest that high-throughput crystallography is a powerful screening tool. Protein crystallography is a more sensitive technique than the conventional bioassays used in HTS and can typically identify the binding of much weaker ligands (in the mM affinities compared with the μM range in bioassays). This means that less complex, lower molecular weight fragments can be screened and binding events detected that might otherwise be missed by HTS. These fragments can be combined onto a template or used as a starting point for growing out an inhibitor structure into other parts of the target protein's active site. The use of protein crystallography as a screening technique also enables the identification of all the interactions between the fragment and the protein much earlier in the drug discovery process. This key information that would previously have been available only during the lead optimization phase can now be used to drive the drug design at an earlier stage.

STRUCTURAL BIOLOGY METHODS

Protein Expression and Purification

Protein samples for crystallization need to be of the highest purity, typically >95% pure. The production of recombinant protein is a multistep process. First, the cDNA sequence encoding the gene of interest is cloned into an expression vector. There are several different established approaches for cloning that can be automated for increased throughput. These approaches include the sequence-specific restriction enzyme method, the recombination method, and the ligation-independent cloning method. The following step involves the generation of multiple expression constructs, which can be engineered to have different N- and C-terminal domain boundaries, affinity tags, and/or mutations to increase solubility, stability, or functionality of the protein. Affinity tags such as the hexa-histidine (6xHis), glutathione-S-transferase, or maltose-binding protein can be fused to the protein to facilitate protein purification and increase solubility [12].

Depending on the desired yield and application of the protein sample, protein expression can be performed in in vivo prokaryotic (bacterial), eukaryotic (yeast, baculovirus or insect, or mammalian), or cell-free systems. *Escherichia coli (E. coli)* is the most commonly used expression system for generating recombinant protein for structural studies. This is due to the rapid growth in inexpensive media, the production of high yields of recombinant protein, and its adaptability to high-throughput methods. Yeast (*Saccharomyces cerevisiae* or *Pichia pastoris*) and baculovirus or insect (Sf9, Sf21, and Hi-5) cell systems have also been used successfully by structural biology groups when proteins have failed to express in *E. coli* due to insolubility and/or lack of posttranslational modifications. Typically, mammalian in vivo expression systems and cell-free expression systems are used less frequently by structural biology groups due to the low yield, the time consumption, and the cost of protein production [13].

A large number of parameters can be varied when producing recombinant proteins. These include host cell lines, media, temperature of growth, and length of induction. Coupled with potentially numerous protein constructs under investigation, the time required to perform these experiments becomes a limiting factor. More recently, the use of small-volume microplate fermentations has enabled comprehensive expression screens to be performed more rapidly and with greater ease. The results from an expression screen could be a visible protein band on sodium dodecyl sulfate polyacrylamide gel electrophoresis (SDS-PAGE), detection of antibody binding to the protein, or a functional assay. The most promising results can be progressed to large-scale expression, purification, and crystallization. More recently, statistical methods have been employed to improve the throughput of protein expression and purification. The statistical design of experiments (DoE) approach takes the multiparameter problem that is protein expression and determines the mathematical relationship between factors affecting protein expression. From a modest set of test expressions, the key factors can be identified as well as, critically, how factors interact with each other. DoE can also give an indication of how best to optimize these key factors in order to give optimized protein expression [14]. The utilization of liquid-handling robots for gene cloning, the advances in low-volume fermentation for protein expression, and the addition of DoE modules in protein purification hardware continue to have positive impacts on the throughput of structural biology platforms [15].

Crystallization and Data Collection

The significant improvement in high-throughput methods for gene cloning and protein expression and purification has been a driving factor behind recent developments in the protein crystallization field. The miniaturization of the individual crystallization experiments and the automation of the liquid-handling steps have revolutionized protein crystallization and are fundamental to successful high-throughput protein crystallography.

The production of diffraction-quality protein crystals is a multiparameter challenge. Many different parameters can be altered to drive a protein molecule to nucleate to form protein crystals. Some of these parameters include the purity and homogeneity of the protein sample, the crystallization conditions (pH, precipitant concentration, ionic strength, temperature, detergent, and additives), and the protein concentration. These varying parameters are screened during the initial crystallization process. Crystallization experiments can be set up in several ways, for example as hanging-drop vapor diffusion, sitting-drop vapor diffusion, and microbatch methods for soluble proteins, and the lipidic cubic phase method for membrane proteins. In general, commercial crystallization screens are used to screen for initial crystallization conditions of a protein (Hampton Research, http://www.hamptonresearch.com; Qiagen, http://www.qiagen.com; Emerald Biosystems, http://www.emeraldbiosystems.com; Jena Bioscience, http://www.jenabioscience.com). The crystallization methods listed here can be utilized in high-performance liquid-handling robotic systems, which enable the accurate dispensing of protein samples and viscous crystallization solutions at the nanoliter scale in 96-well plates [16–18].

Once a set of crystallization conditions has been identified, alterations (e.g., salt, pH, temperature, and precipitant) to the initial crystallization conditions will be tested to improve the size and diffraction quality of the protein crystals. The quality of the diffraction achieved from a crystal will determine whether data can be collected on an "in-house" laboratory generator or detector or at a synchrotron radiation source. These factors relate to the packing of the protein molecules within the crystals, and the intrinsic order that is associated with this. Developments in technology for both laboratory generators and synchrotrons have provided systems with more intense X-rays to improve diffraction quality, X-ray optics giving more controllable and better collimated X-ray beams, and more sensitive detectors (e.g., Pilatus, Dectris Ltd) for high signal-to-noise ratio and quicker readout [19].

Further advances in robotic hardware and software have had a significant impact on throughput and have tackled the more inefficient manual aspects of data collection. Sample mounting, centering, crystal quality evaluation, and optimal data collection strategies are now all automated features at synchrotrons and thus require little to no human intervention [20]. The combination of automated sample changing and "intelligent" data characterization software has made a significant impact on high-throughput crystallography and has advanced the drive for fully integrated data collection considerably. Although there have been many advancements in "in-house" radiation sources, synchrotron radiation is still a necessity in order to collect data from small, weakly diffracting crystals and is essential to collect and analyze hundreds of protein–ligand structures in a high-throughput manner. Currently, there are over 130 synchrotron radiation facilities throughout the Americas, Europe, and Asia (http://biosync.sdbk.org), and several are now equipped with third-generation synchrotron sources with microfocus beams (submicron beams for small samples). Several synchrotron facilities are now offering remote-data collection or mail-in data collection, where the user does not have to be present at the beamline and can collect data remotely on shipped crystals either from their work environment or in the leisurely environment of their own home [20,21].

The emergence of X-ray free electron lasers (XFELs) as a novel and powerful X-ray source has the potential to revolutionize high-throughput data collection. The XFEL technology, whilst still in its infancy for macromolecular crystallography, can produce X-ray pulses that are a billion (i.e., a thousand million) times higher and have a 1000-fold shorter pulse length than the current X-ray sources. This will enable high-resolution data collection from microcrystals in a matter of femtoseconds [22].

Structure Determination

Determining the three-dimensional structure of a protein from its X-ray diffraction data depends on solving what is termed the "phase problem". X-ray data collected from a protein crystal consist of structure amplitudes, but the phases associated with these cannot be recorded directly. Deciphering the phases is vital to protein structure determination and can be generated in three principle ways. Techniques such as single (or multiple) isomorphous replacement (SIR or MIR, respectively) and single (or multiple) anomalous dispersion (SAD or MAD, respectively) are termed ab initio methods, as no prior structural information is required to solve the target structure. The molecular replacement (MR) method relies on having available a structurally similar model of the target protein. Ab initio methods utilize the introduction of heavy atoms or anomalous scatterers into the protein crystal and compare the structure amplitudes between this and the native protein crystal. These differences can be analyzed computationally and enable the position of the heavy atoms or anomalous scatterers to be located within the protein and an estimate of the phases calculated. The MR method uses the phase information from a previously solved structure as an estimate for the target protein. For this method to be effective, a relatively high level of structural similarity must exist between the known structure and the target protein. The Protein Data Bank (http://www.rcsb.org/pdb/home) is a global repository for solved protein structures and can be searched for existing structural motifs. With over 86,000 structures deposited, there is an ever-increasing chance that a structurally characterized homolog of the target protein exists. Advances in computer technology and software development for both ab initio methods and molecular replacement methods have accelerated the process of structure determination. With all the recent improvements, data can be collected in a matter of minutes and the structure can be determined at the synchrotron facility. In addition, automated model-building and ligand refinement programs have further reduced the time needed to rebuild structures [23,24].

Small-Angle X-ray Scattering

Over recent years, small-angle X-ray scattering (SAXS) has been used as another biophysical tool in high-throughput structural studies of proteins [25]. X-ray crystallography is used to determine a high-resolution structure in the crystalline state, and NMR is used to determine a low-molecular-weight protein at high resolution in solution. In contrast to X-ray crystallography and NMR, SAXS does not require the protein to be crystallized and is not limited by the size of the protein. SAXS is a solution-based method utilized to determine the envelope or different conformations on a wide range of small proteins or large protein complexes at low resolution under different buffer conditions or in the presence of ligands. The recent integration of automated sample preparation, data acquisition, and data analysis and the development of the microfluidic chip have made it possible to use SAXS in a high-throughput manner [26].

Nuclear Magnetic Resonance

In addition to X-ray crystallography, NMR is another powerful structural biology tool used in high-resolution three-dimensional structure determination and in hit generation. In contrast to X-ray crystallography, which provides a frozen snapshot of the protein, NMR can be used to observe the dynamics of a protein in solution at different temperatures, pH, and buffer conditions or in the presence of ligands. Recent advances in NMR probe technology, software development, and methodology have proven that NMR is an important complement to X-ray crystallography in structure-based hit generation. Due to the high sensitivity of NMR spectroscopy, ligand-based NMR screening methods are being applied to detect weak interactions between a protein target and a compound that would otherwise be missed by lower sensitivity techniques like conventional functional assays. The binding of a ligand to a protein of interest in a high-throughput manner can be observed in one-dimensional (1D) experiments or two-dimensional (2D) experiments depending on the information required. 1D experiments are performed on native recombinant protein, can estimate protein folding and stability, and can also be utilized in protein- or ligand-detected NMR (discussed further in this chapter). Isotope labeling of the protein is required for 2D experiments and involves growing *E. coli* cells in culture supplemented with stable isotopes (^{2}H, ^{13}C, and ^{15}N). 2D experiments are used in protein-detected NMR to monitor the methyl group chemical shifts under different conditions. NMR screening methods can be utilized to observe either protein-detected resonances in 1D or 2D experiments (1D-^{1}H, 2D-TOCSY, and 2D-HSQC) or ligand-detected resonances in 1D experiments (Water-LOGSY, STD, and Tr-NOE) (for detailed reviews, see Refs [27–32]). If using protein-detected methods, there is no upper limit in compound affinity (typically the mM to nM range), and the binding site and dissociation constant can be measured; however, this requires soluble and isotope-labeled protein for 2D methods. The ligand-detected resonances method does not require isotope-labeled protein, requires a shorter acquisition time, and has no upper limit in size of protein target; with this method, ligand binding can be detected using 1D methods, but it cannot be used for high-affinity ligands. Recently, these two methods for data acquisition have been combined and applied in a high-throughput manner to overcome their limitations. In addition, other developments have allowed high-throughput NMR spectroscopy to be performed on high-molecular-weight proteins (>50 kDa) and integral proteins in micelles or bicelles [33–35].

As the drug discovery field progresses, X-ray crystallography, NMR, and SAXS will play complementary and pivotal roles in the advancement of high-throughput techniques.

STRUCTURAL BIOLOGY AND STRUCTURE-BASED DRUG DESIGN

Structural biology applied to drug design has played an important role in a number of success stories in cancer research. Dihydrofolate reductase (DHFR) was the first target protein solved in complex with a cancer drug, methotrexate [36]. The three-dimensional (3D) structure has since been used to design several improved inhibitors [37]. The structure of the DNA repair enzyme poly-(ADP-ribose) polymerase forms a basis for the development of anticancer agents that are currently being evaluated in clinical studies [38]. Structural biology and structure-based drug design (SBDD) have had major impacts in the field of kinase drug discovery with the first kinase inhibitor anticancer agent, Gleevec™, reaching the marketplace [39].

Other success stories for structural biology and SBDD include ligands able to recognize and bind particular sequences of DNA in order to control the transcription of proteins or to prevent the binding of enzymes. The minor groove of DNA is the target for a wide range of anticancer, antiviral, and antiprotozoal agents. Noncovalently binding molecules tend to bind to the minor groove of A/T-rich sequences [40–42], and several are of current clinical use [43]. DNA can also fold and form complex 3D structures that are associated with a particular function. Telomeric DNA sequences can form four-stranded (quadruplex) structures, which may be involved in the structure of telomere ends [44]. SBDD has been successfully applied to this particular DNA folding in order to develop telomerase inhibitors with anticancer activity [45–47].

One of the major benefits of using structural biology in drug discovery has been the development of the SBDD cycle. This multidisciplinary process starts with the resolution of the 3D structure of a ligand bound to a target receptor of interest. 3D visualization and computational tools are then used to analyze the structure and to identify key interactions between ligand and receptor. These interactions can be hydrogen bonds, hydrophobic contacts, water networks, or weaker interactions such as halogen bonds and interactions with aromatic rings [48]. This information is then used to direct structural modifications on the ligand in order to design new molecules with increased potency. Designed molecules are synthesized and tested in vitro. Finally, interesting inhibitors with improved binding affinity and physical–chemical properties are selected for a new run of structure determination. Computational methodologies have played an important role in this drug design cycle, in particular in designing and selecting compounds in silico that bind to the binding site of a protein. A successful in silico structure-based design tool should predict the correct binding mode of the ligand in the protein-binding site, and the binding energy between ligand and protein.

Docking programs are the most widely used in silico techniques that can give answers to the two points highlighted above [49]. The accuracy of docking methods is usually measured by the ability to reproduce the ligand-binding mode observed experimentally. In general, a docking experiment is considered inaccurate when the root mean square deviation between the predicted and experimental binding conformation of the ligand is bigger than 2Å. Currently, state-of-the-art docking programs correctly dock between 70% and 80% of native ligands when they are tested on large sets of protein–ligand complexes, but performance may drop to less than 30% for some docking scenarios [50]. For example, docking accuracy may be significantly reduced for virtual (i.e., designed but not yet synthesized) ligands, as change in the ligand may induce change in the protein conformation, and this is not taken into account in fixed protein-docking protocols [51,52]. Once the ligand has been docked in the binding site, the binding affinity should be predicted in order to rank the quality of the pose with respect to other poses for the compound, and with respect to other molecules. Docking programs use scoring functions to quickly estimate binding energies. Essentially, three types of scoring functions are routinely applied: physical based [53], empirical [54], and knowledge based [55]. All scoring functions make various assumptions and simplifications in the evaluation of the binding energy and do not fully account for a number of physical phenomena that determine molecular recognition. Recently, more rigorous scoring methods that combine molecular mechanics and implicit solvation models, such as MM/PBSA and MM/GBSA, have become available. These methods can be more accurate in ranking docking poses, but require complex calculations that increase computing time [56]. The energetics of displacing binding site waters on ligand binding are thought to be a principal source of binding free energy, and methods to calculate the energetics of this desolvation can also be applied to rank docking poses in congeneric series [57,58].

A major application of docking methods is to dock and rank compounds from different sources (e.g., commercial suppliers, corporate databases, combinatorial libraries, and structure-guided libraries); this approach is known as virtual screening. Virtual-screening methods would be more effective with accurate scoring functions, but to date, and as described in this chapter, only simplistic approximations are available. Despite these difficulties, virtual-screening methods are useful in SBDD. Despite failing to accurately rank active compounds and to distinguish them from inactive ones, the method is useful for discarding inappropriate compounds (which are the majority of screened compounds) so that the top-ranked compounds are enriched with actives. Moreover, it is common practice to visually check a number (300–1000) of high-ranking compounds in order to add to the selection process a level of experience, knowledge, and chemical intuition. Therefore, as long as active compounds are found in the shortlist, their relative ranking becomes less important. Successful examples of virtual screening in the identification of novel hits and the demonstration of significant enrichment have been described in the literature [59,60].

FRAGMENT SCREENING USING X-RAY CRYSTALLOGRAPHY

The first step in fragment-based drug discovery is to develop fragment libraries to be subsequently screened against the target. In general, fragments should have low molecular weight (<300), good solubility or lower lipophilicity (ClogP3), and also the number of hydrogen bond donors and acceptors should be three each. These general principles, known as "the rule of three" [61], allow for the optimization of fragment hits into lead molecules with good physicochemical properties that are compliant with Lipinski's "rule of five" [1]. Different approaches have been used to assemble diverse collections of small molecular fragments. Virtual-screening methods have been applied to create targeted libraries where fragments are selected on the basis of their structural complementarity to the protein. Chemoinformatics tools have been used to generate libraries of fragments that contain functional groups and scaffolds present in known drug molecules [10,62].

In order to screen fragment libraries using high-throughput crystallography, crystals of the target protein are immersed in solutions containing fragments. Protein crystals contain large solvent channels that allow the diffusion of small fragments throughout the crystal. To increase the throughput of the screen, crystals are soaked in cocktails of 2–8-fragment compounds for several hours prior to data collection. Following data collection, automated ligand fitting or refinement software such as AutoSolve™ [63] identifies which if any of the fragments in the cocktail have bound to the protein target. The availability of such software has proved to be a pivotal component of fragment-based screening in a high-throughput manner.

Fragment-based screening has a number of advantages over the conventional screening of drug-like compounds:

1. Only a relatively small number of fragments (between a few hundred and a few thousand) need to be screened because low-complexity molecules have a higher probability of matching the shape and interactions of a receptor when compared with more complex drug-like molecules [64].
2. In order to bind, fragments should form high-quality interactions, whereas the activity in high-throughput screening hits is often due to a large number of lower quality interactions [4]. Therefore, fragments are described as efficient binders and usually possess high ligand efficiency. Here we use Hopkins et al.'s definition of ligand efficiency (LE) [65]:

$$LE = - \Delta G / HAC \approx - RT \ln(IC_{50}) / HAC$$

where ΔG is the free energy of binding of the ligand for a specific protein, HAC (heavy atom count) is the number of atoms that are not hydrogen in the ligand, and the IC_{50} represents the measured potency of the ligand for the protein.

If a drug-like molecule of molecular weight 500 has around 36 heavy atoms, with a target activity of 10 nM, then its ligand efficiency will be about 0.3. A hypothetical fragment with HAC = 11 and an IC_{50} around <2 mM would have an LE = 0.33; one way of viewing this is that the initial fragment potency is sufficient to be optimistic of delivering a 10 nM inhibitor within the molecular weight guidelines of the "rule of five".

3. High lipophilicity and molecular weight have been shown to have a detrimental effect on the permeability, solubility, and toxicity of drug leads [64,66]. Fragments offer low lipophilicity and low-molecular-weight starting points, which can be optimized to high-quality leads with good drug-like properties [67,68]. To ensure that a fragment is grown to a lead with good drug-like properties, the compound's lipophilic ligand efficiency (LLE) is often monitored alongside its LE. A simple measure of LLE that works for drug-sized molecules was proposed by Leeson and Springthorpe [69].

$$LLE = pIC_{50} - \log P$$

To ensure drug-like properties, the LLE should be greater than 5. For fragments, a measure that takes into account the number of heavy atoms in the ligand, LLE_{AT}, works better [70].

CASE HISTORY—PROTEIN KINASE B INHIBITORS FROM FRAGMENT HIT TO CLINICAL CANDIDATE

Introduction

The use of fragment-based approaches in conjunction with high-throughput crystallography provides a powerful drug discovery tool. As a consequence, significant success has been observed by several research groups in developing drug molecules for key therapeutic areas [71,72]. The case history given in this section details the development of orally efficacious inhibitors of protein kinase B (PKB) from fragment hit to clinical candidate. This work was performed as part of a collaboration with scientists from Astex Pharmaceuticals, AstraZeneca, and the Institute for Cancer Research (United Kingdom).

Biology and Rationale

PKB (also known as Akt) is an important biological target for cancer treatment as it plays a pivotal role in the PI3K–PKB–mTOR signaling cascade, as shown in Fig. 4.1 [73]. PKB signals to many cellular pathways involved with cell cycle progression and proliferation, cell survival, protein synthesis, and cell growth. A number of mutations upstream of PKB in this cascade lead to a constitutively active pathway, which leads to proliferation and carcinogenesis. Such mutations may cause activation or amplification of PI3K or PKB expression, or deletion at the genetic level of the tumor suppressor phosphatase and tensin homology (PTEN). As an important node in this cascade, PKB is suitable for targeting with an inhibitor. Inhibitors of this pathway, for example analogs of rapamycin that inhibit mTOR, have shown antitumor efficacy in clinical trials [74]. Furthermore, direct or indirect activation of PKB has been shown to cause resistance to known therapies such as inhibitors of receptor tyrosine kinases [75].

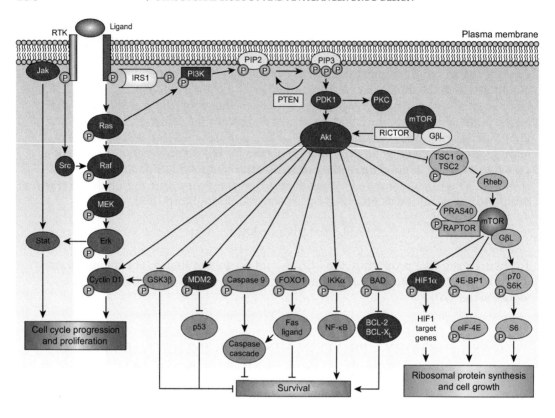

Nature Reviews | Cancer

FIGURE 4.1 The role of PKB in cell signaling. *Source: Reproduced from Yap TA et al., Nature Reviews Cancer 2009.* (This figure is reproduced in color in the color plate section.)

Hit Identification

Whilst the X-ray crystal structure of PKBβ had been published [76], a soakable system suitable for fragment screening was not available. Instead, a PKA–PKB chimera was used, whereby relevant point mutations within the active site of PKA to the appropriate PKB amino acids provided a suitable surrogate to direct PKB crystallography [74].

X-ray crystallography fragment screening of a screening set was undertaken along with hit compounds resulting from a virtual screen of approximately 300,000 low-molecular-weight molecules (<250 Da) using the PKBβ published coordinates. A number of hit compounds were identified binding at the ATP-binding site of the enzyme, known as the hinge region. Compounds **1** and **2** were chosen for further elaboration, as working on more than one series increases the chance of success. Both fragments form two hydrogen bonds to amino acid residues Glu121 and Ala123 (PKA–PKB chimera numbering). Whilst these fragments have relatively low affinity due to their small size, they are very efficient binders (Fig. 4.2).

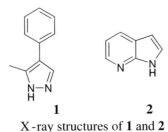

1   **2**

X-ray structures of **1** and **2**

Compound 1   Compound 2

FIGURE 4.2 Fragment hits and binding modes shown by X-ray crystal structures in PKA–PKB chimera. (This figure is reproduced in color in the color plate section.)

A fragment optimization and growing strategy was employed, where binding affinity was increased by growing into other parts of the protein and finding further beneficial interactions through a stepwise process. X-ray crystallography at each stage enabled assessment of the binding mode and further design in the next step.

Example 1: Optimization of Compound 1 Through to Clinical Candidate, AT13148

Compound **1**, with an affinity of 80 µM and a molecular weight of 158, has a high ligand efficiency of 0.47. From analysis of the X-ray crystal structure, growth from the phenyl ring toward an area of negative charge would suggest placement of a positively charged moiety in this region [77]. Therefore, growing with an ethylamine chain to give **3** maintained the high ligand efficiency and furnished a compound with 5.2 µM affinity (Figs 4.3 and 4.4). Interrogation of close structural analogs showed that the methyl substituent on the pyrazole was not required for high ligand efficiency. Then, further growth into a lipophilic pocket of the protein

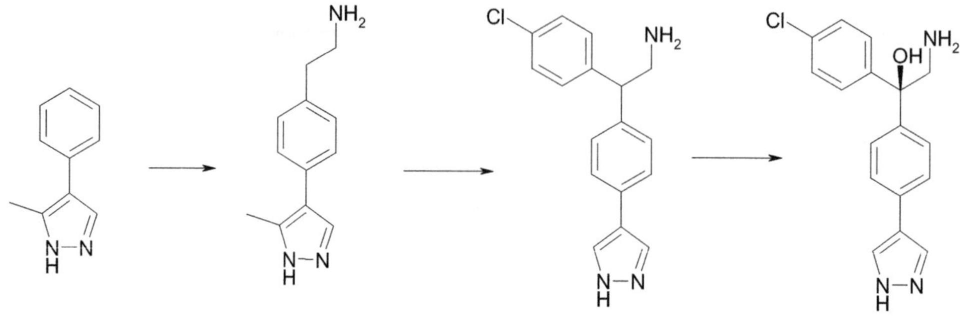

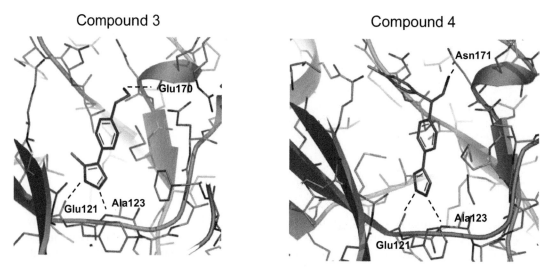

1: 80 μM ±38   **3**: 5.2 μM   **4**: 31 nM ±14   **5, AT13148**
LE 0.47   ±3.3   LE 0.49

FIGURE 4.3   Growth from fragment **1** to clinical candidate AT13148.

Compound 3   Compound 4

FIGURE 4.4   X-ray structures of **3** and **4** bound to PKA–PKB chimera. (This figure is reproduced in color in the color plate section.)

near the glycine-rich loop maintained similar ligand efficiency, thereby improving the affinity to 31 nM for **4**. The chlorophenyl group showed good surface contact with the protein in the X-ray crystal structure (Fig. 4.5). The addition of a hydroxyl group at the benzylic position was required to give a compound with good oral pharmacokinetics, and AT13148 is a clinical candidate in phase I trials.

Preclinical Data for AT13148

AT13148 is an inhibitor of PKB as well as other AGC (cAMP-dependent, cGMP-dependent and protein kinase C) kinases: p70S6 kinase, PKA, ROCK, and SGK [78]. Inhibition

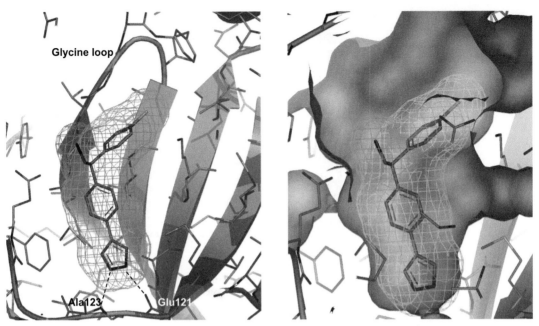

FIGURE 4.5 X-ray structure of **4** rotated by 180° (cf. Fig. 4.4) showing interactions on the left and space filling with surfaces of ligand and protein on the right. (This figure is reproduced in color in the color plate section.)

of multiple AGC kinases may have the advantage of affecting more cellular pathways and providing less opportunity for the cancer to find a resistance mechanism. AT13148 inhibited proliferation of a number of cell lines with deregulation of the PI3K–AKT–mTOR and RAS–RAF pathways, and showed antitumor efficacy in three different tumor xenografts. Figure 4.6(A) shows the concentrations of AT13148 achieved *in vivo* in mice with a HER-2 positive, PIK3CA–mutant BT474 human breast cancer xenograft. Notably, due to the high volume of distribution of the compound, the concentration after a second dose of 40 mg/kg AT13148 is far higher in the tumor than in plasma. Figure 4.6(B) shows the antitumor activity in the same xenograft.

Example 2: Optimization of Compound 2 through to Candidate Compound, AZD5363

The 7-azaindole hit **2** was grown in a similar manner to that in Example 1 to give **6** (Fig. 4.7). The 7-azaindole core was also modified in **6** so as to allow synthetic tractability and rapid exploration of chemical space. Table 4.1 shows the data for PKB and PKA inhibition of compounds in this series along with the cell data obtained. The antiproliferative effect of the compounds was assessed in a sulforhodamine B (SRB) assay in a U87MG glioblastoma cancer cell line, whilst the GSK3β enzyme-linked immunosorbent assay (ELISA) assesses the effect on downstream signaling in a PC3M prostate cancer cell line. Whilst good affinity was attained with **6**, a compound with greater selectivity for PKB compared to other AGC kinases

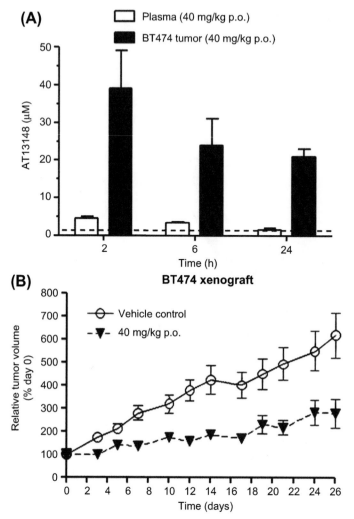

FIGURE 4.6 (A) Concentrations of AT13148 in plasma and tumor with 40 mg/kg oral dose. (B) Reduction in tumor growth in the presence of AT13148.

was desired. This offers an alternative approach to AT13148. Replacement of the phenyl ring with a saturated piperidine ring provided **7** with 15-fold selectivity for PKB over PKA [79]. Compound **7** did not show activity in the cell assays, probably due to poor permeability through the cell membrane. This was improved in **8** by replacing one of the nitrogen atoms in the bicyclic core with a carbon. The reduced polar surface area and higher log P were more suitable for cell penetration.

Further elaboration of this subseries was undertaken due to the selectivity advantage, which was improved further with addition of the chlorobenzyl group in **9**, now accessing the

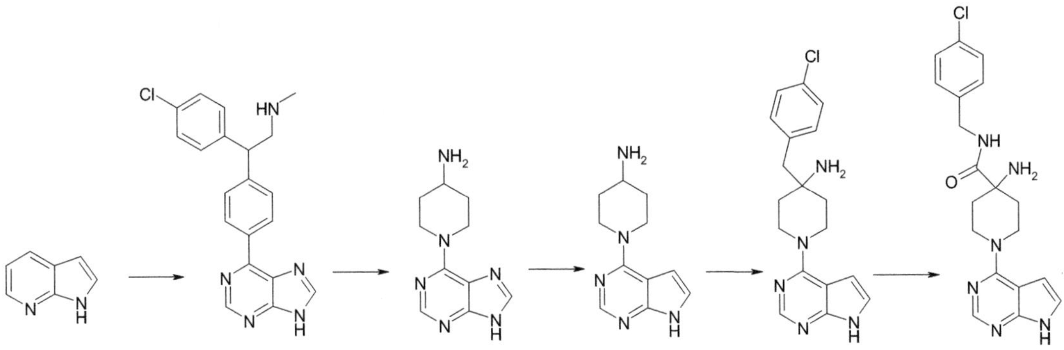

FIGURE 4.7 Fragment growth and modification from 7-azaindole hit **2**.

TABLE 4.1 Activity Data for Compounds in Fig. 4.6

Compound	PKBβ IC$_{50}$ (nM)[1]	PKA IC$_{50}$ (nM)[2]	GSK3β ELISA (PC3M) IC$_{50}$ (μM)[3]	SRB (U87MG) GI$_{50}$ (μM)[4]
6	10 (±3)	15	nd	nd
7	270 (±25)	4100 (±800)	nd	nd
8	180 (±6)	1550 (±120)	15	nd
9	6 (±1.5)	168 (±36)	3.0	5.0
10	2.2 (±1.2)	30	2.3	17

[1] *Inhibition of PKBβ kinase activity in a radiometric filter-binding assay. Mean (±SEM) for n = 3 determinations.*
[2] *Inhibition of PKA kinase activity in a radiometric filter-binding assay. Mean (±SEM) for n = 3 determinations.*
[3] *Cellular ELISA for inhibition of GSK3β phosphorylation in PC3M prostate cancer cells.*
[4] *Cell growth inhibition by sulforhodamine B colorimetric assay; single determination in U87MG glioblastoma cancer cells.*

lipophilic pocket near the glycine-rich loop. Figure 4.8 shows a comparison of binding modes of **9** in PKB and PKA. The amino acid difference thought to be the main cause of the selectivity is Leu173-Met. The charged amine in **9** forms a close interaction with the sulfur of the methionine in the PKB structure, allowing a more favorable conformation of the piperidine ring that results in the chlorophenyl group accessing the lipophilic pocket. This interaction is not possible with leucine, and in PKA the chlorophenyl group adopts a different conformation in a more solvent-exposed position.

Whilst **9** showed good cellular potency, the oral bioavailability of the compound in mouse was poor. This was improved by modifications of the linking atoms between the piperidine and chlorophenyl group, resulting in **10** [80]. The oral bioavailability of **10** was increased to 58%. Further elaboration of this template gave the clinical candidate AZD5363, which is currently in phase I clinical trials.

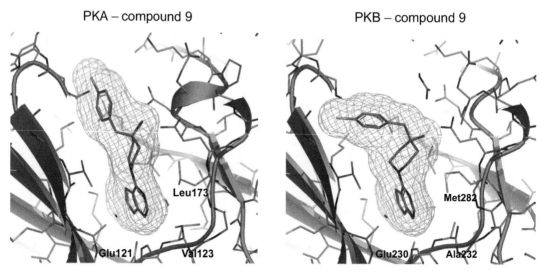

FIGURE 4.8 X-ray structure and comparison of binding modes of **9** in PKA and PKB. Orientation of the ligand in PKB offers better space-filling and surface contact, resulting in higher affinity. (This figure is reproduced in color in the color plate section.)

Preclinical Data for AZD5363

The inhibition of growth of 182 cancer cell lines by AZD5363 was tested, and highly significant activity was seen for cell lines with either an activating mutation at PIKCA or an inactivating mutation or loss of PTEN [75]. The greatest frequency of effect was for cell lines from breast, endometrial, gastric, and hematological and prostate cancers. Resistance to the compound was seen with RAS mutations. Figure 4.9 shows the antitumor effect of AZD5363 monotherapy in a number of cell lines, whereas Fig. 4.10 shows how the compound can sensitize tumors to treatment with other drugs, in this case docetaxel.

CONCLUSIONS

The use of structural biology techniques such as X-ray crystallography and NMR are now widely accepted to be powerful tools in structure-based drug design. Particularly for the case of X-ray crystallography, the continued improvement of equipment, software, and methodologies has resulted in a dramatic improvement in the speed with which structural data can be obtained. Structural biology now has an impact throughout the drug discovery process, from hit identification to late-stage lead optimization. The structure-guided designs of AT13148 and AZD5363 provide a good example of this being put into practice for an oncology target.

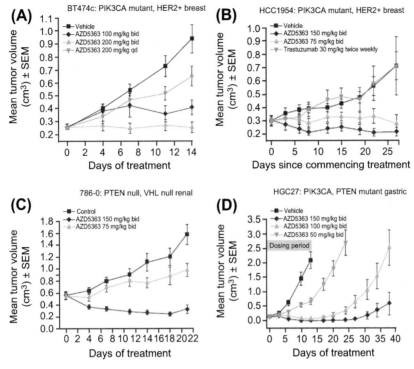

FIGURE 4.9 (A–D) Antitumor effect of AZD5363 in four different human xenograft models. (For color version of this figure, the reader is referred to the online version of this book.)

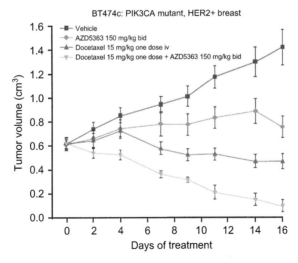

FIGURE 4.10 Effect of combining AZD5363 with a single dose of docetaxel. (For color version of this figure, the reader is referred to the online version of this book.)

References

[1] Lipinski CA, Lombardo F, Dominy BW, Feeney PJ. Experimental and computational approaches to estimate solubility and permeability in drug discovery and development settings. Adv Drug Deliv Rev 2001;46:3–26.

[2] Perola E. An analysis of the binding efficiencies of drugs and their leads in successful drug discovery programs. J Med Chem 2010 Apr 8;53(7):2986–97.

[3] Hann MM. Molecular obesity, potency and other addictions in drug discovery. Med Chem Comm 2011;2(5):349–55.

[4] Carr RA, Congreve M, Murray CW, Rees DC. Fragment-based lead discovery: leads by design. Drug Discov Today 2005;10:987–92.

[5] Lesuisse D, Lange G, Deprez P, Benard D, Schoot B, Delettre G, et al. SAR and X-ray. A new approach combining fragment-based screening and rational drug design: application to the discovery of nanomolar inhibitors of Src SH2. J Med Chem 2002;45:2379–87.

[6] Rees DC, Congreve M, Murray CW, Carr R. Fragment-based lead discovery. Nat Rev Drug Discov 2004;3:660–72.

[7] Murray CW, Verdonk ML, Rees DC. Experiences in fragment-based drug discovery. Trends Pharmacol Sci 2012;33(5):224–32.

[8] Erlanson D. Introduction to fragment-based drug discovery. Fragment-Based Drug Discovery and X-ray Crystallography 2012:1–32.

[9] Erlanson DA, McDowell RS, O'Brien T. Fragment-based drug discovery. J Med Chem 2004;47:3463–82.

[10] Hartshorn MJ, Murray CW, Cleasby A, Frederickson M, Tickle IJ, Jhoti H. Fragment-based lead discovery using X-ray crystallography. J Med Chem 2005;48:403–13.

[11] Wyss D, Wang YS, Eaton H, Strickland C, Voigt J, Zhu Z., et al. Combining NMR and X-ray crystallography in fragment-based drug discovery: discovery of highly potent and selective BACE-1 inhibitors. Fragment-Based Drug Discovery and X-Ray Crystallography 2012:83–114.

[12] Hammarstrom M, Hellgren N, van den Berg S, Berglund H, Härd T. Protein Sci 2002;11:313–21.

[13] Joachimiak A. High-throughput crystallography for structural genomics. Curr Opin Struct Biol 2009;19:573–84.

[14] Islam RS, Tisi D, Levy MS, Lye GJ. Framework for the rapid optimization of soluble protein expression in *Escherichia coli* combining microscale experiments and statistical experimental design. Biotechnol Prog 2007;23(4):785–93.

[15] Blundell TI, Patel S. High-throughput X-ray crystallography for drug discovery. Curr Opin Pharmacol 2004;4:490–6.

[16] Sharff A, Jhoti H. High-throughput crystallization to enhance drug discovery. Curr Opin Chem Biol 2003;7:340–5.

[17] Tickle I, Sharff A, Vinkovic M, Yon J, Jhoti H. High-throughput protein crystallography and drug discovery. Chem Soc Rev 2004;33:558–65.

[18] Caffrey M, Cherezov V. Crystallizing membrane proteins using lipidic mesophases. Nat Protoc 2009;4:706–31.

[19] Trueb P, Sobott BA, Schnyder R, Loeliger T, Schneebeli M, Kobas M, et al. J Synchrotron Radiat 2012;19:347–51.

[20] Wasserman SR, Koss JW, Sojitra ST, Morisco LL, Burley SK. Rapid-access, high-throughput synchrotron crystallography for drug discovery. Trends Pharmacol Sci 2012;33:261–7.

[21] Girard E, Legrand P, Roudenko O, Roussier L, Gourhant P, Gibelin J, et al. Instrumentation for synchrotron-radiation macromolecular crystallography. Acta Crystallogr D Biol Crystallogr 2006;62:12–8.

[22] Neutze R, Moffat K. Time-resolved structural studies at synchrotrons and X-ray free electron lasers: opportunities and challenges. Curr Opin Struct Biol 2012;22:651–9.

[23] Lamzin VS, Perrakis A. Current state of automated crystallographic data analysis. Nat Struct Biol 2000;7(Suppl.):978–81.

[24] Terwilliger TC. Automated structure solution, density modification and model building. Acta Crystallogr D Biol Crystallogr 2002;58:1937–40.

[25] Grant TD, Luft JR, Wolfley JR, Tsuruta H, Martel A, Montelione GT, Snell EH. Small angle X-ray scattering as a complementary tool for high-throughput structural studies. Biopolymers 2011;95:517–30.

[26] Toft KN, Vestergaard B, Nielsen SS, Snakenborg D, Jeppesen MG, Jacobsen JK, et al. High-throughput small angle X-ray scattering from proteins in solution using a microfluidic front-end. Anal Chem 2008;80:3648–54.

[27] Clore GM, Gronenborn AM. Theory and applications of the transferred nuclear overhauser effect to the study of the conformations of small ligands bound to proteins. J Magn Reson 1982;48:402–417.

[28] Dalvit C, Fogliatto G, Stewart A, Veronesi M, Stockman B. WaterLOGSY as a method for primary NMR screening: practical aspects and range of applicability. J Biomol NMR 2001;21:349–59.

[29] Hajduk PJ, Augeri DJ, Mack J, Mendoza R, Yang J, Betz SF, Fesik SW. NMR-based screening of proteins containing ^{13}C-labeled methyl groups. J Am Chem Soc 2000;122:7898–904.

[30] Mayer M, Meyer B. Characterization of ligand binding by saturation transfer difference NMR spectroscopy. Angew Chem Int Ed 1999;38:1784–8.

[31] Parella T, Belloc J. Modern proton-detected 1D ^{1H}–^{15N} NMR experiments. Application to the measurement of ^{1H}, ^{15N} coupling constants at natural abundance. Magn Reson Chem 2002;40:133–8.

[32] Thrippleton MJ, Keeler J. Elimination of zero-quantum interference in two-dimensional NMR spectra. Angew Chem Int Ed 2003;42:3938–41.

[33] Stockman BJ, Dalvit C. NMR screening techniques in drug discovery and drug design. Prog Nucl Magn Reson Spectrosc 2002;41:187–231.

[34] Fejzo J, Lepre C, Xie X. Application of NMR screening in drug discovery. Curr Top Med Chem 2003;3:81–97.

[35] Peng JW, Lepre CA, Fejzo J, Abdul-Manan N, Moore JM. NMR experiments for lead generation in drug discovery. Methods Enzymol 2001;338:202–30.

[36] Matthews DA, Alden RA, Bolin JT, Filman DJ, Freer ST, Hamlin R, et al. Dihydrofolate reductase from *Lactobacillus casei*. X-ray structure of the enzyme methotrexate. NADPH complex. J Biol Chem 1978;253:6946–54.

[37] Kuyper LF, Roth B, Baccanari DP, Ferone R, Beddell CR, Champness JN, et al. Receptor-based design of dihydrofolate reductase inhibitors: comparison of crystallographically determined enzyme binding with enzyme affinity in a series of carboxy-substituted trimethoprim analogues. J Med Chem 1982;25:1120–2.

[38] Tikhe JG, Webber SE, Hostomsky Z, Maegley KA, Ekkers A, Li J, et al. Design, synthesis, and evaluation of 3, 4-dihydro-2H-[1, 4]diazepino[6, 7, 1-hi]indol-1-ones as inhibitors of poly(ADP-ribose) polymerase. J Med Chem 2004;47:5467–81.

[39] Wong S, Witte ON. The BCR-ABL story: bench to bedside and back. Annu Rev Immunol 2004;22:247–306.

[40] Dervan PB, Edelson BS. Recognition of the DNA minor groove by pyrrole-imidazole polyamides. Curr Opin Struct Biol 2003;13:284–99.

[41] Neidle S. DNA minor-groove recognition by small molecules. Nat Prod Rep 2001;18:291–309.

[42] Tidwell RR, Boykin DW. Dicationic DNA minor groove binders as antimicrobial agents. In: Demeunynck M, Bailly C, Wilson WD, editors. DNA and RNA binders: from small molecules to drugs. Weinheim, Germany: Wiley-VCH; 2003. p. 414–60.

[43] Wilson WD, Nguyen B, Tanious FA, Mathis A, Hall JE, Stephens CE, et al. Dications that target the DNA minor groove: compound design and preparation, DNA interactions, cellular distribution and biological activity. Curr Med Chem Anticancer Agents 2005;5:389–408.

[44] Parkinson GN, Lee MP, Neidle S. Crystal structure of parallel quadruplexes from human telomeric DNA. Nature 2002;417:876–80.

[45] Harrison RJ, Cuesta J, Chessari G, Read MA, Basra SK, Reszka AP, et al. Trisubstituted acridine derivatives as potent and selective telomerase inhibitors. J Med Chem 2003;46:4463–76.

[46] Read M, Harrison RJ, Romagnoli B, Tanious FA, Gowan SH, Reszka AP, et al. Structure-based design of selective and potent G quadruplex-mediated telomerase inhibitors. Proc Natl Acad Sci USA 2001;98:4844–9.

[47] Rezler EM, Bearss DJ, Hurley LH. Telomeres and telomerases as drug targets. Curr Opin Pharmacol 2002;2:415–23.

[48] Bissantz C, Kuhn B, Stahl M. A medicinal chemist's guide to molecular interactions. J Med Chem 2010;53:5061–84.

[49] Taylor RD, Jewsbury PJ, Essex JW. A review of protein-small molecule docking methods. J Comput-Aided Mol Des 2002;16:151–66.

[50] Verdonk ML, Giangreco I, Hall RJ, Korb O, Mortenson PN, Murray CW. Docking performance of fragments and druglike compounds. J Med Chem 2011 Aug 11;54(15):5422–31.

[51] Verdonk ML, Mortenson PN, Hall RJ, Hartshorn MJ, Murray CW. Protein–ligand docking against non-native protein conformers. J Chem Inf Model 2008;48(11):2214–25.

[52] Seeliger D, de Groot BL. Conformational transitions upon ligand binding: holo-structure prediction from apo conformations. PLoS Comput Biol 2010;6(1):e1000634. doi:10.1371/journal.pcbi.1000634.

[53] Ewing TJ, Makino S, Skillman AG, Kuntz ID. DOCK 4. 0: search strategies for automated molecular docking of flexible molecule databases. J Comput-Aided Mol Des 2001;15:411–28.

[54] Eldridge MD, Murray CW, Auton TR, Paolini GV, Mee RP. Empirical scoring functions: I. The development of a fast empirical scoring function to estimate the binding affinity of ligands in receptor complexes. J Comput Aided Mol Des 1997;11:425–45.

[55] Mooij WT, Verdonk ML. General and targeted statistical potentials for protein–ligand interactions. Proteins 2005;61:272–87.

[56] Hou T, Wang J, Li Y, Wang W. Assessing the performance of the molecular mechanics/Poisson Boltzmann surface area and molecular mechanics/generalized Born surface area methods. II. The accuracy of ranking poses generated from docking. J Comput Chem 2011 Apr 15;32(5):866–77.

[57] Abel R, Young T, Farid R, Berne BJ, Friesner RA. Role of the active-site solvent in the thermodynamics of factor Xa ligand binding. J Am Chem Soc 2008;130(9):2817–31.

[58] Guimarães CRW, Mathiowetz AM. Addressing limitations with the MM-GB/SA scoring procedure using the WaterMap method and free energy perturbation calculations. J Chem Inf Model 2010;50(4):547–59.

[59] Kitchen DB, Decornez H, Furr JR, Bajorath J. Docking and scoring in virtual screening for drug discovery: methods and applications. Nat Rev Drug Discov 2004;3:935–49.

[60] Leach AR, Shoichet BK, Peishoff CE. Prediction of protein–ligand interactions. Docking and scoring: successes and gaps. J Med Chem 2006;49:5851–5.

[61] Congreve M, Carr R, Murray C, Jhoti H. A 'rule of three' for fragment-based lead discovery? Drug Discov Today 2003;8:876–7.

[62] Lewell XQ, Judd DB, Watson SP, Hann MM. RECAP–retrosynthetic combinatorial analysis procedure: a powerful new technique for identifying privileged molecular fragments with useful applications in combinatorial chemistry. J Chem Inf Comput Sci 1998;38:511–22.

[63] Mooij WT, Hartshorn MJ, Tickle IJ, Sharff AJ, Verdonk ML, Jhoti H. Automated protein–ligand crystallography for structure-based drug design. ChemMedChem 2006;1:827–38.

[64] Hann MM, Leach AR, Harper G. Molecular complexity and its impact on the probability of finding leads for drug discovery. J Chem Inf Comput Sci 2001;41:856–64.

[65] Hopkins AL, Groom CR, Alex A. Ligand efficiency: a useful metric for lead selection. Drug Discov Today 2004;9:430–1.

[66] Walters WP. Going further than Lipinski's rule in drug design. Expert Opin Drug Discov 2012;7(2):99–107.

[67] Leeson PD, St-Gallay SA. The influence of the 'organizational factor' on compound quality in drug discovery. Nat Rev Drug Discov 2011;10(10):749–65.

[68] Murray CW, Verdonk ML, Rees DC. Experiences in fragment-based drug discovery. Trends Pharmacol Sci 2012.

[69] Leeson PD, Springthorpe B. The influence of drug-like concepts on decision-making in medicinal chemistry. Nat Rev Drug Discov 2007;6(11):881–90.

[70] Mortenson PN, Murray CW. Assessing the lipophilicity of fragments and early hits. J Comput-Aided Mol Des 2011;25(7):663–7.

[71] Warner SL, Bashyam S, Vankayalapati H, Bearss DJ, Han H, Mahadevan D, et al. Identification of a lead small-molecule inhibitor of the Aurora kinases using a structure-assisted, fragment-based approach. Mol Cancer Ther 2006;5:1764–73.

[72] Poulsen SA, Bornaghi LF. Fragment-based drug discovery of carbonic anhydrase II inhibitors by dynamic combinatorial chemistry utilizing alkene cross metathesis. Bioorg Med Chem 2006;14:3275–84.

[73] Yap TA, Carden CP, Kaye SB. Beyond chemotherapy: targeted therapies in ovarian cancer. Nat Rev Cancer 2009;9:167–81.

[74] Donald A, McHardy T, Rowlands MG, Hunter LJ, Davies TG, Berdini V, et al. Rapid evolution of 6-phenylpurine inhibitors of protein kinase B through structure-based design. J Med Chem 2007;50:2289–92.

[75] Davies BR, Greenwood H, Dudley P, Crafter C, Yu DH, Zhang J, et al. Preclinical pharmacology of AZD5363, an inhibitor of AKT: pharmacodynamics, antitumour activity, and correlation of monotherapy with genetic background. Mol Cancer Ther 2012;11:873–87.

[76] Yang J, Cron P, Good VM, Thompson V, Hemmings BA, Barford D. Crystal structure of an activated Akt/protein kinase B ternary complex with GSK-3 peptide and AMP-PNP. Nat Struct Biol 2002;9:940–4.

[77] Saxty G, Woodhead SJ, Berdini V, Davies TG, Verdonk ML, Wyatt PG, et al. Identification of inhibitors of protein kinase B using fragment-based lead discovery. J Med Chem 2007;50:2293–2296.

[78] Yap TA, Walton MI, Grimshaw KM, Te Poele RH, Eve PD, Valenti MR, et al. AT13148 is a novel, oral multi-AGC kinase inhibitor with potent pharmacodynamics and antitumour activity. Clin Cancer Res 2012;18:3912–23.

[79] Caldwell JJ, Davies TG, Donald A, McHardy T, Rowlands MG, Aherne GW, et al. Identification of 4-(4-aminopiperidin-1-yl)-7H-pyrrolo[2,3-d]pyrimidines as selective inhibitors of protein kinase B through fragment elaboration. J Med Chem 2008;51:2147–57.

[80] McHardy T, Caldwell JJ, Cheung K, Hunter LJ, Taylor K, Rowlands M, et al. Discovery of 4-amino-1-(7H-pyrrolo[2,3-d]pyrimidin-4-yl)piperidine-4-carbozamides as selective, orally active inhibitors of protein kinase B. J Med Chem 2010;53:2239–2249.

PART II

DRUGS IN THE LABORATORY AND CLINIC

5

Temozolomide: From Cytotoxic to Molecularly Targeted Agent

Malcolm F.G. Stevens

Centre for Biomolecular Sciences, University of Nottingham, Nottingham, UK

INTRODUCTION

It would be easy, but dishonest, to claim that the discovery of temozolomide was a triumph of rational drug design (Figure 5.1). The molecule is a product of an era when "chemistry-driven" drug discovery was the norm and concepts of "molecular target–driven" discovery were two decades away into the future. As with many other drug discoveries of the time, it was a case of "interesting chemistry begetting interesting biology", a concept that today—sadly, but reasonably—raises the hackles of biologists and consequently finds little support from funding bodies. But one aspect hasn't changed: like every drug discovery project that makes it from bench to market, irrespective of starting point, temozolomide has needed its champions operating across the frontiers of chemistry, pharmacology, toxicology, and pharmacy to secure its success. Some of them are shown in a contemporary photograph (Figure 5.2) that is "so 70s".

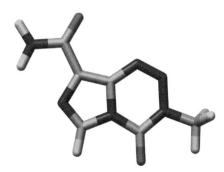

FIGURE 5.1 Structure of temozolomide. (This figure is reproduced in color in the color plate section.) *Source: Thanks to Dr Mark Beardsall for this image.*

Cancer Drug Design and Discovery, Second Edition
http://dx.doi.org/10.1016/B978-0-12-396521-9.00005-X

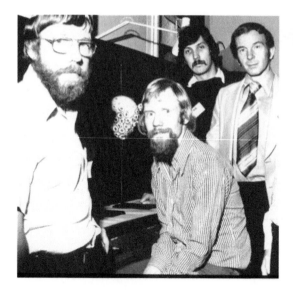

FIGURE 5.2 Some of temozolomide's champions. (From left) Keith Vaughan, Andy Gescher, John Hickman, and Malcolm Stevens in 1976. (For color version of this figure, the reader is referred to the online version of this book.) *Source: Aston University.*

TOWARD IMIDAZOTETRAZINES AND AZOLASTONE (MITOZOLOMIDE)

Chemical inquisitiveness, particularly a focus on the synthesis of nitrogen-rich heterocyclic systems, was at the core of the evolution of the bicyclic imidazotetrazine nucleus of temozolomide, and its lineage can be traced back to PhD days at Nottingham University in the early 1960s. Significant molecules on the track to becoming azolastone and temozolomide are shown in Fig. 5.3.

There were two chemical strands—"triazenes" and "triazines"—with a common starting point that eventually led to the discovery of the antitumor imidazotetrazines. (Note: "triazenes" are acyclic systems with an array of three contiguous nitrogen atoms; "triazines" have the three nitrogen atoms within a six-membered ring system, the other atoms being carbon; and "tetrazines" have four nitrogen atoms in a six-membered ring system.) Over 100 years ago, it was known that 1,2,3-benzotriazinones such as compound **1** underwent ring opening in hot aqueous alkali to generate anthranilic acid [1]. Although the fate of the methyl group was not known at the time, this is precisely the chemistry by which the antitumor imidazotetrazines generate alkylating moieties from triazene intermediates. Compound **1** is devoid of antitumor properties because it cannot ring-open under physiological conditions to afford a monomethyltriazene: had Herr Finger incorporated a powerful electron-withdrawing group *para* to the carbonyl fragment (e.g., CF_3) that would have facilitated ring opening, then the history of cancer chemotherapy might well have dated from the 1880s rather than the 1940s! The aryldimethyltriazene counterparts **2** do have pronounced antitumor properties, and seminal work by Tom Connors and his colleagues on their biochemical pharmacology had revealed that metabolic demethylation to monomethyltriazenes was implicated in their antitumor activity [2]: this discovery had a broad impact on the future development of temozolomide. Significantly, a similar P450-mediated metabolic oxidative demethylation is

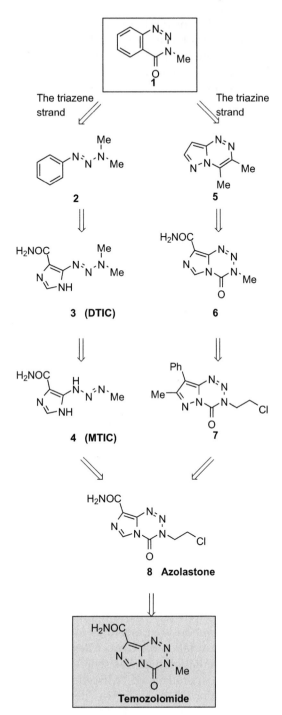

FIGURE 5.3 Molecular milestones from triazenes and triazines to temozolomide. (For color version of this figure, the reader is referred to the online version of this book.)

required to activate the drug dacarbazine (DTIC) **3**, which was marketed as an antimelanoma drug in the 1970s. The first synthesis of α-hydroxylated aryldimethyltriazenes was achieved by Keith Vaughan [3]; a hydroxymethyl metabolite of DTIC had also been identified as a urinary metabolite of DTIC in rats [4] and is the precursor of the monomethyltriazene methylating agent methyl-triazeno-imidazole-carboxamide (MTIC) **4** following loss of a molecule of formaldehyde.

The second discovery strand started with pyrazolotriazines such as **5** and established that the positions of bridgehead nitrogen atoms in these bicyclic heterocycles had a crucial effect in determining their chemical properties, especially their propensity to undergo ring opening under mild conditions [5]. Actually, compound **5** and its N-acyl derivatives had pronounced antitumor actions in vivo against a methylcholanthrene-induced tumor in the rat [6]: the problem was that, at that time, there was no process or funding in academic research to develop a "lead" into a clinical candidate. It wasn't until 1980 in the United Kingdom that Tom Connors and Brian Fox persuaded Cancer Research Campaign to establish a phase I/II committee to select compounds for clinical evaluation. It was good timing for the imidazotetrazines that it transpired.

In the early 1970s, a program of work was initiated at Aston University to explore the chemical and biological properties of bicyclic systems with bridgehead nitrogen atoms exemplified by the imidazotriazinone **6**: these compounds were devoid of antitumor activity [7]. Then, in 1978, a pharmacy postgraduate, Robert Stone (Figure 5.4), was recruited on a May & Baker studentship to work on potentially antiallergic bicyclic compounds, a therapeutic area that the company soon abandoned. At the same time, a German group published a new route to fuse 1,2,3,5-tetrazines from the interaction of diazoazoles and isocyanates [8]. One of the compounds **7** had a critical 2-chloroethyl substituent attached to the tetrazine ring but, sadly for Ege and his colleague, alkyl and aryl groups in the 5-membered azole ring were inimical to antitumor activity. This was another near miss that might well have diverted the temozolomide story in an entirely different direction. But exploiting the Ege reaction Stone, working in collaboration with Eddy Lunt and Chris Newton and their colleagues at May & Baker Ltd, prepared the first example of a bicyclic system from the conjunction of an imidazole ring and a 1,2,3,5-tetrazine ring [9]. The product **8** was given the laboratory name azolastone (subsequently mitozolomide), incorporating the names of the university (Aston) and the student synthesizer (Stone). The early chemical development work and its significance in the emergence of the specific molecular architecture present in the bioactive imidazotetrazines have been reviewed [10,11].

Azolastone was shown by another Aston University PhD student, Neil Gibson, to have remarkable antitumor properties against mouse tumors with high proliferative characteristics, notably mouse leukemias and lymphomas [12]: indeed, it had curative activity against most of the contemporary tumor models of the time—and as a single dose. Presentations of these results were made simultaneously at meetings in the United Kingdom and United States in 1983. At the American Association for Cancer Research (AACR) annual conference, a meager audience heard the presentation that was scheduled in the last session on the last day amongst a medley of others papers labeled "Miscellaneous". It was not a good omen. Undaunted, a parenteral formulation of the drug was developed by pharmacists at Aston led by John Slack and the new agent was fast-tracked to the clinic in 1983 under the direction of Edward Newlands at Charing Cross Hospital, London, and George Blackledge at Queen

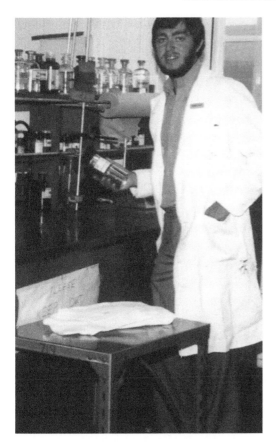

FIGURE 5.4 PhD student Robert Stone in the Pharmacy Department, Aston University, circa 1980. (For color version of this figure, the reader is referred to the online version of this book.)

Elizabeth Hospital, Birmingham, United Kingdom. Beguiled by the remarkable activity of azolastone in the preclinical models of the time, the Aston group were convinced that the elusive "magic bullet" lay within its grasp. A poster was designed—"Azolastone: The Movie"— extolling the classical glory of the new agent (Figure 5.5(A)). Such hubris had to end in tears, of course, and phase I studies on azolastone, which commenced in 1983, revealed that the new molecular miracle provoked profound and irreversible thrombocytopenia in patients [13], particularly so on a repeat-dose schedule [14]. A companion poster from the time spectacularly foreshadowed the demise of azolastone (Figure 5.5(B)), an outcome that might have been predicted from therapeutic index considerations [15]. A competitor teasingly labeled the doomed enterprise "Azo-last-one"!

FROM MITOZOLOMIDE TO TEMOZOLOMIDE

The May & Baker team led by Eddy Lunt and Chris Newton tactically—or sensibly, perhaps, faced with the evidence?—did retire from the fray at this point. Project abandonment is an ever-present threat in industry, but academics will do anything to avoid such drastic

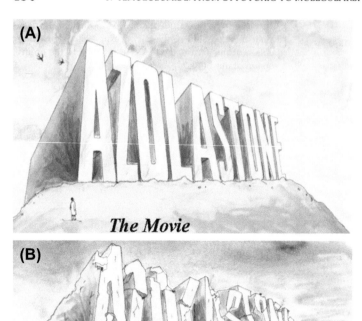

FIGURE 5.5 (A) "Azolastone—The Movie." (B) "Azo-last-one". (For color version of this figure, the reader is referred to the online version of this book.) *Source: Posters designed by Graham Smith, Aston University, ca. 1983.*

action—like their favorite old shirts, something dies within them when they have to be discarded. Luckily, amongst a modest library of analogs (<60) prepared to that date were compounds with different pharmacological properties. The structure–activity relationships are summarized in Fig. 5.6.

The substituent R conveying most potent antitumor properties at N-3 is β-chloroethyl, with methyl much less active: interestingly, replacement of chloroethyl by ethyl, bromoethyl, methoxyethyl, chloropropyl, allyl, and a range of other alkyl substituents gave compounds apparently devoid of useful activity [10]. At C-6, substituent R^1 can be hydrogen or a small straight-chain alkyl group, but not branched alkyl; and at C-8, a rich lode of activity extends through R^2 substituents such as carboxamides, sulfonamides, sulfones and sulfoxides [16]. However, many analogs more potent than mitozolomide with a β-chloroethyl substituent in the tetrazine ring, and particularly sulfur-containing functionalities at C-8, were potentially flawed since the bone marrow toxicities seen in the phase I study of azolastone were linked to the DNA cross-linking properties of this class of molecule [17].

The Aston Pharmacology team, notably Simon Langdon, showed that a minor structural change—replacement of the chloroethyl group of azolastone by methyl, which would

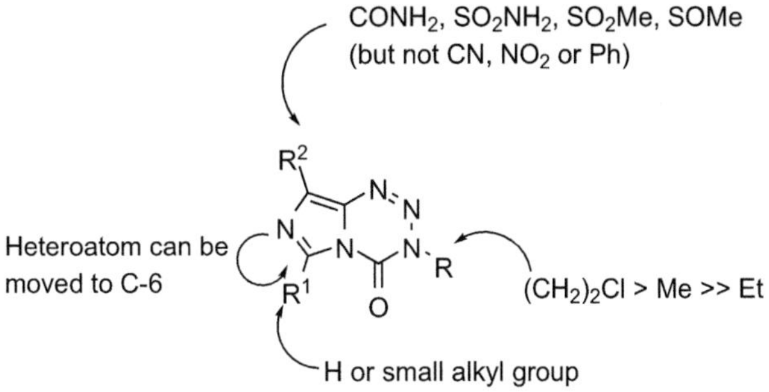

CONH$_2$, SO$_2$NH$_2$, SO$_2$Me, SOMe
(but not CN, NO$_2$ or Ph)

FIGURE 5.6 Structure–activity relationships in imidazotetrazines.

Heteroatom can be moved to C-6

R^2

R^1

R

(CH$_2$)$_2$Cl > Me >> Et

H or small alkyl group

ensure that no DNA cross-linking was possible—conferred significantly changed pharmacological and toxicological properties on the new molecule, and cryptically encoded CCRG 81045, M&B 39831, NSC 362856, but temozolomide to its friends, without compromising its favorable pharmacokinetic features [18]. Actually, scrutinizing the structures of the 3-methylbenzotriazinone 1 and temozolomide, it is apparent that only a small molecular journey has been made in 100 years. But then, the devil is in the details. Unlike mitozolomide, the antitumor activity of temozolomide in the same survival time models previously used was schedule dependent. Temozolomide showed good antitumor activity against mouse hematological (L1210 and P388 leukemia) and solid (M5076 sarcoma, ADJ/PC6A plamacytoma, B16 melanoma, and Lewis lung carcinoma) malignancies on multiple administration schedules. A leukemia L1210 line resistant to cyclophosphamide was still sensitive to temozolomide, whereas L1210 and P388 cell lines resistant to mitozolomide, and an L1210 variant resistant to DTIC 3, were completely cross-resistant with temozolomide, implying common molecular mechanisms with the latter two agents [18].

On the basis of limited information [19], it was regarded that DTIC was poorly demethylated in humans to the active agent MTIC. The chemistry of temozolomide, however, allowed the agent to be ring-opened nonmetabolically to the same methylating species MTIC. Actually, this is only a part of the activation process (see Mode of action of temozolomide section). It was considered that temozolomide might be a suitable clinical alternative to DTIC and provide a test for the hypothesis that DTIC might have been a more effective drug if only it had not suffered from the vagaries of unpredictable metabolism in humans [18]. On this tentative rationale, temozolomide was selected for clinical trial by the Cancer Research Campaign. Subsequent reports that temozolomide demonstrated activity against brain tumor xenografts [20] justified this decision and pointed to a potential use against human brain tumors.

The simple chemical structure and remarkable acid stability of temozolomide suggested that it would be synthetically accessible on a large scale and have appropriate pharmaceutical properties to allow it to be delivered orally. And so it proved.

SYNTHESIS AND CHEMISTRY OF TEMOZOLOMIDE

The original Stone synthesis of temozolomide started with 5-aminoimidazole-4-carboxamide 9, which was converted to the corresponding insoluble diazoimidazole 10, which was further reacted by stirring with methyl isocyanate in a heterogenous system in ethyl

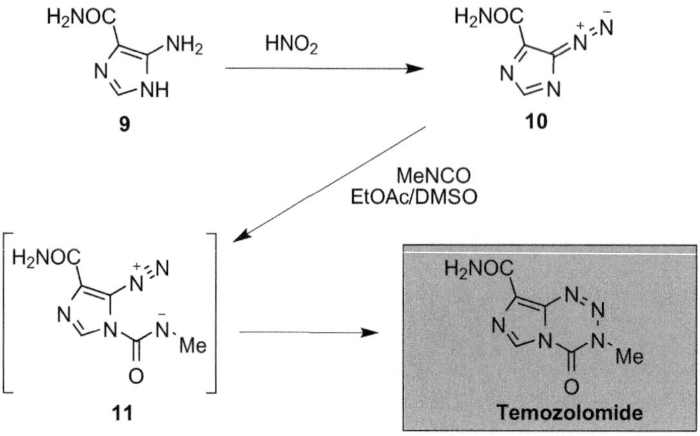

SCHEME 5.1 The Stone synthesis of temozolomide. (For color version of this figure, the reader is referred to the online version of this book.)

acetate at 25 °C for 30 days to afford temozolomide (Scheme 5.1). The second step of the reaction presumably proceeds via an ionic intermediate **11** and is an excellent example of "atom economy", where every atom in the starting materials is incorporated into the product [9].

An atom-economic synthesis, however, should not be confused with an "environmentally friendly" one! The entire project was imperiled by events in Bhopal, India, in December 1984, where a runaway reaction in a tank of methyl isocyanate precipitated a catastrophic toxicological disaster in a densely occupied neighborhood, which still has ramifications on the chemical industry today [21]. Fortunately, a bulk supply of methyl isocyanate had been secured prior to this event because it became impossible to source this pariah molecule on the market afterward. Nor was it considered scientifically or politically prudent to attempt to accelerate the Stone synthesis by confining the reaction in a sealed system, and heating it; or by ultrasonic reduction of solid diazoimidazole **10** to a fine suspension—especially in a laboratory in downtown Birmingham in the United Kingdom! However, the simple trick of using a mixed DMSO–ethyl acetate solvent allowed a kilo of clinical-grade temozolomide to be prepared in 250 g batches in 3 days in near-quantitative yield and to clinical-grade purity.

In the search for safer routes to temozolomide, a range of strategies was adopted (Scheme 5.2). To bypass the requirement for using methyl isocyanate, less volatile isocyanates, such as ethyl isocyanatoacetate and trimethylsilylmethyl isocyanate, were reacted with diazoimidazole carboxamide **10** to give imidazotetrazines **12** [22] and **13** [23], respectively, which could be routinely processed to temozolomide; also, the cyano analog **14** could be hydrolyzed to temozolomide in 10 M-hydrochloric acid at 60 °C, but synthesis of **14** itself was problematic. An alternative approach avoiding the use of methyl isocyanate and potentially unstable diazoimidazoles altogether involved synthesis of 5-amino-1-(N-methylcarbamoyl) imidazole-4-carboxamide **15**. The anion of this imidazole is the putative ionic intermediate **11** in the Stone synthesis (Scheme 5.1). Despite a thorough investigation of cyclization conditions involving variations of the acid, source of nitrosonium ion, solvent, temperature, use of phase transfer catalysts or cyclodextrins, and so on, the optimum process (sodium nitrite in water containing tartaric acid at 0–5 °C) gave only a 45% conversion of **15** to temozolomide—and

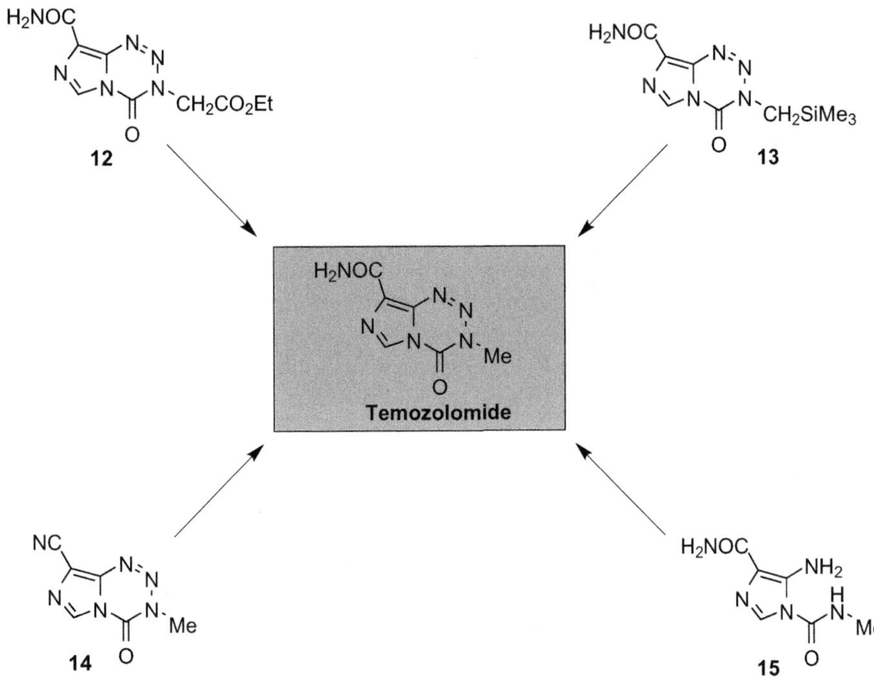

SCHEME 5.2 Alternative syntheses of temozolomide. (For color version of this figure, the reader is referred to the online version of this book.)

this on a good day [24]. In the >25 years since the original discovery of temozolomide, the Stone synthesis hasn't been bettered and is still used for the commercial production of the drug.

EARLY CLINICAL TRIALS ON TEMOZOLOMIDE

In the phase I study, an intravenous (IV) formulation of temozolomide in dimethyl sulfoxide (DMSO) was given as a 1 h infusion at a starting dose of $50 \, mg/m^2$ with a switch to oral administration at $200 \, mg/m^2$, where excellent oral drug bioavailability was confirmed [25]; further dose escalation to $1200 \, mg/m^2$ was continued when leukopenia and thrombocytopenia became dose limiting. The increase in the area under the curve (AUC) was linear with dose, but no responses were seen on this single-dose schedule. Interest was then switched to a five-times-daily schedule in view of the critical schedule dependency noted in preclinical screens. A schedule giving temozolomide at $150 \, mg/m^2$ orally for 5 successive days was well tolerated. In the absence of myelosuppression, subsequent courses were given at $200 \, mg/m^2$ for 5 days on a 4-week cycle. Unusually in a phase I study, responses were observed in melanoma and mycosis fungoides, and two patients with recurrent high-grade gliomas had evidence of clinical activity. Subsequent phase II and later investigations focused on patients with melanoma and particularly high-grade gliomas: these studies have been reviewed [26].

In summary, temozolomide showed confirmed activity against high-grade gliomas either before radiotherapy or on postradiotherapy relapse. Although observed responses were generally of limited duration with modest impact on overall survival, patients benefited from improved cognitive function and mental and physical performance. Further studies also showed that temozolomide could be given on an extended daily schedule [27] and, because of the convenient oral administration of the drug, has become a popular partner in exploratory combination regimens with inter alia radiotherapy, established agents such as BCNU, cisplatin, taxol, biologicals rituximab and pegylated interferon-α-2B, and investigational small molecules such as the tubulin binder epothilone B, thalidomide, 13-cis retinoic acid, the ribonucleotide reductase inhibitors didox and trimidox, the matrix metalloprotease inhibitor marismastat, the angiogenesis inhibitor TNB-470, novel inhibitors of the nuclear enzyme poly(ADP-ribose)polymerase-1 (PARP-1), and especially inhibitors of the repair protein O^6-methylguanine methyltransferase (MGMT, also known as O^6-alkylguanine alkyltransferase or ATase).

MODE OF ACTION OF TEMOZOLOMIDE

Chemical Activation

The chemical mechanism of activation of temozolomide is entirely different from the chemistry utilized in the synthetic pathway [9,28]. The agent is cleaved in a multistep process: activation is initiated by hydrolytic attack at C-4 in a pH-dependent manner ($t_{1/2}$ 1.83 h at 37 °C in phosphate buffer at pH 7.4) to give the unstable monomethyltriazene MTIC **4**, presumably via the tetrahedral adduct **17** and an unstable carbamic acid **18**, which decarboxylates spontaneously. Support for this process comes from the isolation of MTIC from the degradation of temozolomide in aqueous sodium carbonate [9]. MTIC at pH 7.4 has a $t_{1/2}$ of <2 min and cleaves proteolytically to 5-aminoimidazole-4-carboxamide **9** and the highly reactive methanediazonium ion **19**, the active methylating species (Scheme 5.3). In deuteriated phosphate buffer, methyl group transfer to a nucleophile is accompanied by deuterium exchange in the methyl group [29]. The fact that the prodrug temozolomide is stable at acidic pH values and labile above pH 7—exactly the reverse obtained with the ring-opened triazene MTIC—was fortuitous and not a reward for intelligent drug design. A freakish property of temozolomide is that it is actually stable in hot concentrated sulfuric acid. But clearly there is only a small pH window around physiological pH (7.4 ± 0.1) where ring opening of temozolomide is accompanied by fragmentation of MTIC in a methylating mode. The plasma $t_{1/2}$ in patients given IV temozolomide in the phase I study was 1.8 h, (Newlands et.al., 1992) confirming that, unlike DTIC, with temozolomide the chemistry is in control and metabolic processes do not play a significant role in activation of the drug [30].

Exploiting the Stone synthesis, temozolomide has been isotopically labeled with ^{2}H in the carboxamide group, ^{15}N at N-2, ^{11}C and ^{13}C at the methyl group, ^{11}C at C-4, and ^{14}C at C-6. Possibly it is the only pharmaceutical that has been prepared with all $^{11-14}$C isotopes. This has enabled mechanistic questions to be resolved [28], the site of protonation (at N-7) to be determined, and the in vivo fate of every atom in the molecule to be accounted for (Fig. 5.7).

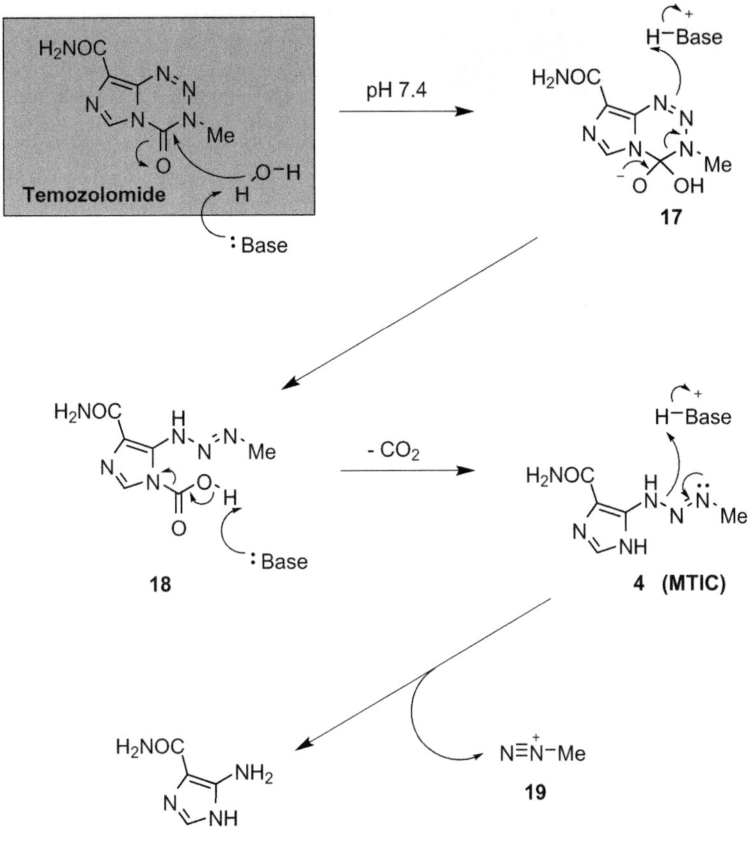

SCHEME 5.3 Chemical activation of temozolomide at pH 7.4. (For color version of this figure, the reader is referred to the online version of this book.)

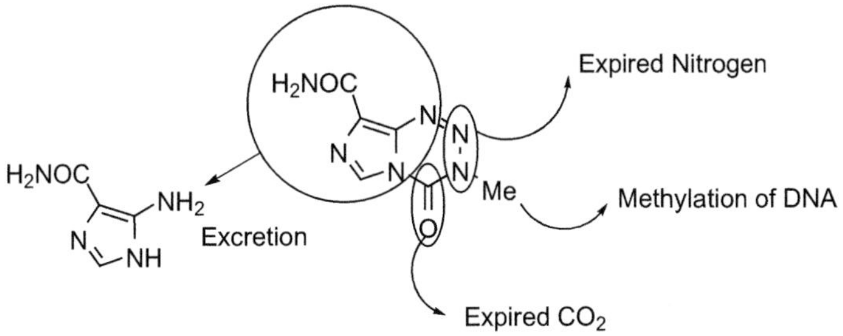

FIGURE 5.7 In vivo fates of C, H, N, and O atoms of temozolomide.

Positron emission tomography (PET) imaging using temozolomide synthesized with a ^{11}C label in the methyl group [31] has confirmed that the drug achieves selective methylation of brain tumors relative to healthy surrounding brain tissue (Figure 5.8). Possibly their slightly different pH environments [32,33] as well as constitutive differential abilities to repair DNA

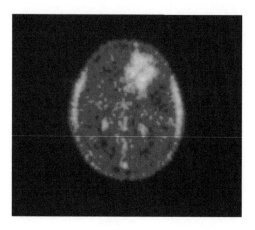

FIGURE 5.8 Positron emission tomography (PET) image of a patient with a glioblastoma tumor treated with temozolomide labeled in the C-4 position with ^{11}C isotope. (This figure is reproduced in color in the color plate section.)

damage account for this phenomenon. In contrast, temozolomide labeled with ^{11}C in the tetrazinone ring carbonyl group is mainly lost as expired carbon dioxide in accordance with the proposed activation chemistry.

Interaction of Temozolomide with DNA and Repair Processes

Temozolomide promiscuously methylates a range of sites in purine residues of DNA, notably at the N^7 position of guanine, the N^3 position of adenine, and the O^6 position of guanine residues [34]. The methanediazonium active species derived from MTIC (or temozolomide), like most short-lived electrophilic reactants, covalently interacts at the most *nucleophilic* micro-environment within DNA—guanine residues in tracts of three or more guanines [35,36]. On this basis, temozolomide was classified as a "cytotoxic agent" (however, see, Epigenetic silencing of the *MGMT* gene section in this chapter). That the primary site of DNA interaction responsible for the drug's cytotoxicity is the O^6-position of guanine residues can be deduced from the observed resistance of tumors that express high levels of MGMT [37–39]. O^6-guanine methylation is a cytotoxic (antitumor) lesion since it provokes mispairing with thymine during DNA replication. Unless repaired by MGMT, mispairing on the daughter strand is recognized by mismatch repair proteins, which trigger futile cycles of thymine excision and reinsertion leading to persistent DNA strand breaks. These lesions eventually engage the DNA damage response mechanisms, leading to cell cycle arrest and apoptosis. Methylations at other sites, such as the N^7 site of guanine and the N^3 site of adenine, are rapidly repaired by base excision repair (BER) processes facilitated by PARP-1 [40].

A simplified overall mechanism of methylation of DNA guanine residues at the O^6 positions by temozolomide, mismatch base pairing, and repair by an active-site cysteine residue of MGMT is shown in Scheme 5.4. MGMT is a member of an exclusive club of proteins that can rotate, or "flip", target nucleotides from an array of stacked bases in DNA for extrahelical processing. A recent crystallographic study reveals how the MGMT protein intrudes Arg128 in its DNA recognition helix into the DNA *minor* groove; bases to be repaired are then flipped out into the *major* groove, with Tyr114 promoting phosphate rotation [41]; the extrahelical base is cushioned in a hydrophobic cleft (Met134 and Val155-Gly160) that provides

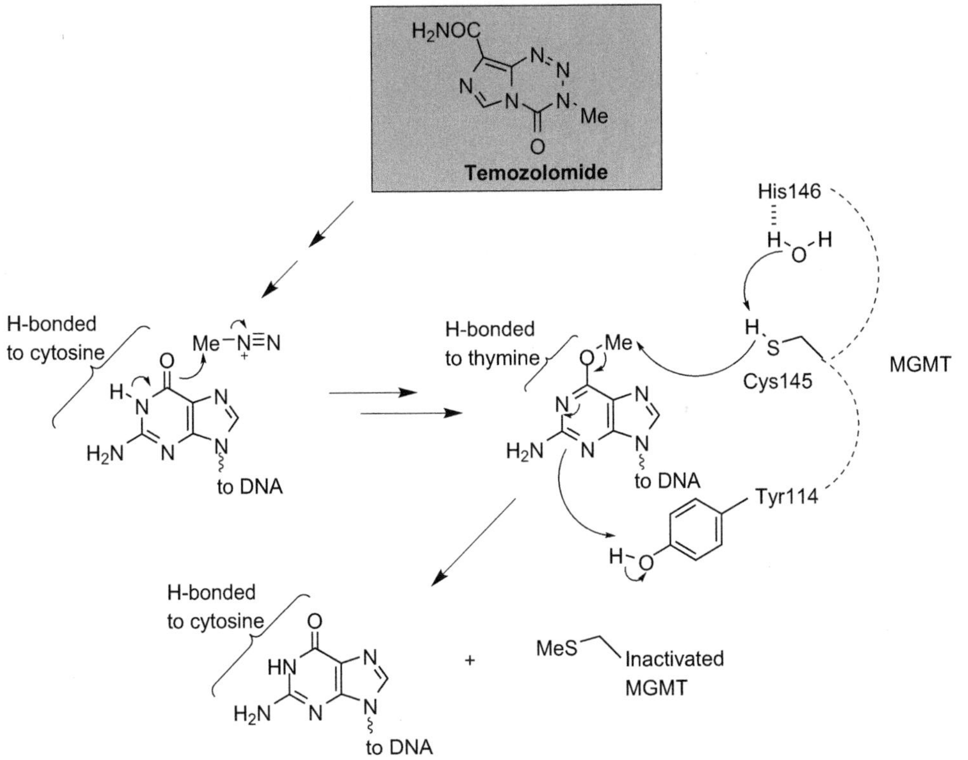

SCHEME 5.4 Mechanism of methylation of a DNA guanine residue at the O^6 position by temozolomide, mismatch base pairing, and repair by an active site cysteine residue of MGMT. (For color version of this figure, the reader is referred to the online version of this book.)

selectivity for 2′-deoxyguanosine nucleotides. A Glu–His–H$_2$O–Cys H-bonded network similar to that found in the Asp-His-Ser catalytic triad of serine proteases aligns a thiolate anion from the activated Cys145 for in-line attack at the methyl group of O^6-methylguanine residues. One molecule of the (suicide) MGMT protein is consumed for each methyl group removed.

Early preclinical studies examining the potential clinical significance(s) of these repair pathways and prospects for their antagonism have been reviewed [26]: these concepts are currently being tested in studies combining temozolomide with novel PARP-1 inhibitors [42] such as AG14447, the phosphate salt of the azepino[5,4,3-cd]indolone **21** [43]; small-molecule pseudo-substrates of MGMT, such as O^6-benzylguanine **22** [44] and the more potent 2-amino-6-[(4-bromo-2-thienyl)methoxy]purine **23** formerly known as Patrin 2 [45]; and the BER inhibitor O-methylhydroxylamine **24** [46] (Fig. 5.9). A depiction of Patrin 2 bound as a noncovalent complex to the active site of MGMT is shown in Figure 5.10.

The key question to be answered in these combination studies is "Do they enhance the clinical spectrum of activity of temozolomide to repair-proficient tumor types without increasing myelosuppression or other toxicities?" However, early studies by the Aston

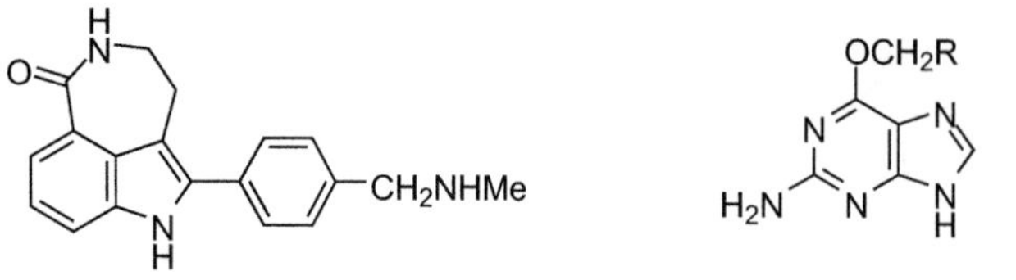

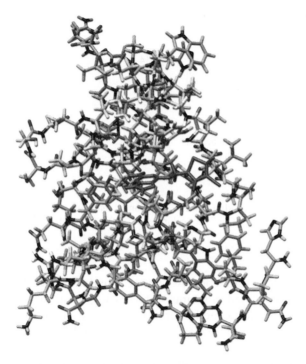

21

22 : R = Ph
23 : R = thien-2-yl

MeONH$_2$

24

FIGURE 5.9 DNA repair inhibitors deployed in combination studies with temozolomide: the PARP-1 inhibitor AG14447 (**21**), MGMT inhibitors O^6-benzylguanine (**22**) and Patrin 2 (**23**), and the BER inhibitor O-methylhydroxylamine (**25**).

FIGURE 5.10 The inhibitor Patrin 2 (in red) in noncovalent association at the active site of MGMT. (This figure is reproduced in color in the color plate section.) *Source: Thanks to Dr Mark Beardsall for this image.*

Group [34,47] showed that DNA methylated at O^6-guanine residues (by temozolomide), but not temozolomide directly, is a potent depletor of MGMT, and it is unlikely that such combinations of temozolomide with **22** or **23**, for example, would be more effective than using temozolomide alone in an extended schedule [27]. Also, it is difficult to envisage how these combination regimes would be brought into clinical practice. The strong commercial position occupied by temozolomide is due, in part, to its suitability for oral administration on an out-patient basis: potential combination partners **21–24** require IV administration and hospitalization.

EPIGENETIC SILENCING OF THE *MGMT* GENE

In a significant development in our understanding of the molecular determinants influencing tumor responses to temozolomide, it is now clear that promoter methylation status (at cytosine C-5 in CpG sequences) of the *MGMT* gene, measured by methylation-specific polymerase chain reaction (PCR), is a powerful predictor of clinical outcome in glioblastoma patients [48,49]. Promoter methylation switches *off* the *MGMT* gene and is associated with longer survival ($P = 0.0051$; log-rank test). At 18 months, survival was 62% (16 of 26) for patients testing positive for a methylated *MGMT* promoter: in the absence of methylation, tumors were repair competent because the *MGMT* gene was switched *on*, and survival was only 8% (1 of 12; $P = 0.002$) [48]. These observations will have a major effect on clinical practice and inform future combination studies with temozolomide.

Intriguingly, experiments coinciding with the discovery phase of temozolomide showed that DNA methylated by temozolomide also inhibits the enzyme cytosine DNA-methyltransferase (DNMT) [50,51]. This enzyme, like MGMT, has an active site cysteine residue and can catalyze the transfer of a methyl group from *S*-adenosylmethionine to the C-5 position of a "flipped-out" cytosine residue within CpG sequences (de novo methylation) [52]. Inhibition of DNMT would lead to DNA *hypo*methylation, and thus activation of genes. Exposure of DNA to methylating agents therefore initiates a cytotoxic event by O^6-guanine methylation, which results in C-G to T-A transitions in DNA, notably in mutagenic "hot spots" in cancer-relevant genes [53]. At the same time, inhibition of the DNMT enzyme could possibly activate the *MGMT* gene to repair the methylation damage. This feedback loop has presumably evolved to protect the genome from the mutagenic consequences of DNA methylation.

NEW ANALOGS OF TEMOZOLOMIDE

The availability of the corresponding 8-carboxylic acids of temozolomide [54] and mitozolomide [55] stimulated efforts to conjugate the imidazotetrazinone pharmacophore via the acid residue to DNA-binding motifs to achieve greater binding selectivity to specific DNA sequences. However, because the chemistry of activation of temozolomide is dominated by cleavage of the tetrazinone ring, and is not perturbed by substituents appended to the imidazole carboxamide fragment, attachments of H-bonding heterocycles, spermidine, peptidic DNA major and minor groove recognition motifs, lexitropsins, and triplex-forming oligonucleotides were not rewarded with evidence of DNA sequence–specific interactions: methylation of multiple guanine sequences in the *major* groove of DNA via the diffusible methanediazonium species was still the inevitable outcome [35,54].

Heterocyclic variants of antitumor imidazotetrazinones with saturated spacer groups such as the bis(imidazotetrazine) **25** had comparable cytotoxicity and alkylation selectivity for DNA guanine sequences as temozolomide and mitozolomide [56], but it is difficult to argue a case that such agents might replace temozolomide. Many of the unusual triazenes and bis(triazenes) synthesized by Vaughan and his colleagues over many years might, in the absence of temozolomide, have made adequate substitutes (for a recent paper, see Ref. [57]).

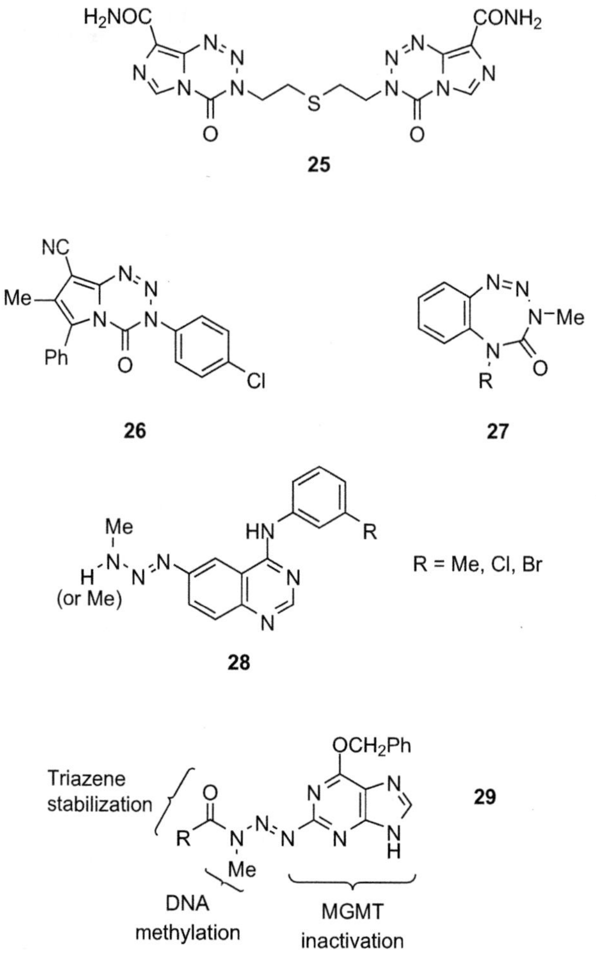

FIGURE 5.11 Compounds 25–29 designed as alternatives to temozolomide.

Other variants of antitumor imidazotetrazines such as the pyrrolo[2,1-*d*]-1,2,3,5-tetrazinone **26** [58] and pyridotetrazepinones **27** [59], although possessing biological activity in their own right, are not convertible to methylating agents and thus are different mechanistically from temozolomide (Fig. 5.11).

"Combitriazenes" are molecular combinations of methyltriazenes and other heterocyclic structures that can fragment to a DNA methylating species (methanediazonium ion) and an agent with a different biological target. Triazenoanilinoquinazolines **28** should undergo proteolysis to liberate a methanediazonium methylating agent (see also Scheme 5.3 for the comparable degradation of MTIC) and an anilinoquinazoline of the general class of adenosine triphosphate (ATP)-antagonistic tyrosine kinase inhibitors [60]. More intriguing is the design of triazenopurines **29** [61], which, following removal of the stabilizing acyl moiety, should fragment to a methanediazonium species and the MGMT inhibitor O[6]-benzylguanine, thus providing, in a molecular combination, the equivalent of the two-drug approach, temozolomide plus O^6-benzylguanine [44].

SUMMARY: TEMOZOLOMIDE, TARGETS, MOLECULAR TARGETS, AND VALIDATED TARGETS

Temozolomide is a prodrug that acts as a molecular delivery device to transport a reactive methylating species to guanine-rich sequences in the major groove of DNA. It is a quintessential "small molecule" of MW 194: every atom in the structure has a role in engineering its favorable chemical, pharmaceutical, and biological profile—ease of synthesis, acid stability, oral bioavailability, freedom from first-pass metabolism, transmission across the blood–brain barrier, and an acceptable toxicological profile unusual for a cytotoxic agent. An esteemed medicinal chemistry journal even allowed the descriptor "cute" in describing its qualities [54]. However, cytotoxic agents emerging from past chemistry-driven programs are now routinely denigrated by the new wave of drug discovery practitioners and analysts wedded to the "validated molecular target"–driven path to anticancer drug discovery (note, however, that despite the Gleevec triumph in chronic myelogenous leukemia, the latter approach has yet to achieve major breakthroughs against metastatic epithelial tumors). Successive clinical disappointments from the new discovery paradigm have been excused because of "sloppy early target validation" [62] or a recognition that the only truly validated target is one proven effective in the crucible of the clinic: anything else is just a "target wannabe" [63].

Temozolomide does, of course, have a *very* precise molecular target—the O^6 position of guanine residues in runs of guanine bases in the major groove of DNA—but, presumably, methylations occur randomly throughout the genome wherever such sequences occur, a hallmark of a cytotoxic agent. However, the propensity of O^6-methylguanine lesions to inflict cellular damage reflected in beneficial antitumor activity is then determined by their persistence, which is controlled by MGMT repair; levels of the MGMT protein, in turn, are controlled by the methylation status of the *MGMT* gene promoter.

There are two apposite definitions of a "validated molecular target" relevant to the rebranding of temozolomide: (1) a target that is perturbed in a patient being treated by a drug selling for >$500 million per annum; and, more seriously, (2) a target that can be measured in a patient population allowing segregation of patients into those suitable for treatment, or those not. Currently temozolomide, marketed as Temodar™ (in the US) and Temodal™ (Europe), fulfills the first criterion with something to spare. The association of the epigenetic inactivation of the *MGMT* gene, readily measurable by PCR, with favorable clinical outcome in temozolomide-treated patients with glioblastoma does, in the opinion of the author, support reclassification of the drug from a cytotoxic to a precision molecularly targeted agent.

Acknowledgments

The author wishes to thank all former colleagues at Aston and Nottingham Universities and at May & Baker Ltd, and a wider college of collaborators worldwide, who have contributed to the discovery and development of temozolomide. The author, and many of these former colleagues, benefit financially from royalties on the sales of temozolomide that accrue to Aston University. Because it has been necessary to restrict the number of cited papers, those quoted, in general, cover work describing the initial and pivotal discoveries only; many very worthy papers have had to be excluded, with apologies.

Finally, the author would like to dedicate this chapter to the memory of three former colleagues who have died over the past few years, but who made exceptional contributions to the broader triazenes and triazines to temozolomide journey—more "champions", in fact. Tom Connors and Edward Newlands both had confidence in the drug when it was still a laboratory curiosity in the 1980s; and Stan McElhinney, operating solo from a small laboratory base in Trinity College, Dublin, synthesized the MGMT inhibitor Patrin 2 (lomeguatrib).

References

[1] Finger H. Beiträge zur Kenntniss des o-Amidobenzamids. J Prakt Chem 1888;37:431–45.
[2] Audette RCS, Connors TA, Mandel HG, Merai K, Ross WCJ. Studies on the mechanism of action of the tumour inhibitory triazenes. Biochem Pharmacol 1973;22:1855–64.
[3] Gescher A, Hickman JA, Simmonds RJ, Stevens MFG, Vaughan K. α-Hydroxylated derivatives of antitumour dimethyltriazenes. Tetrahedron Lett 1978:5041–4.
[4] Kolar GF, Maurer M, Wildschutte M. 5-(3-Hydroxymethyl-3-methyl-1-triazeno)imidazole-4-carboxamide is a metabolite of 5-(3,3-dimethyl-1-triazeno)imidazole-4-carboxamide. Cancer Lett 1980;10:235–41.
[5] Partridge MW, Stevens MFG. Pyrazolo-as-triazines. Part III. Ring fission. J Chem Soc C 1967:1828–30.
[6] Baldwin RW, Partridge MW, Stevens MFG. Pyrazolotriazines: a new class of tumour-inhibitory agents. J Pharm Pharmacol 1966;18S:1S–4S.
[7] Baig GU, Stevens MFG. Triazines and related compounds, Part 22. Synthesis and reactions of imidazo[5,1-c] [1,2,4]triazines. J Chem Soc Perkin Trans I 1981:1424–32.
[8] Ege G, Gilbert K. [7 + 2]- and [11 + 2]-cycloaddition reactions of diazoazoles with isocyanates to azolo[5,1-d] [1,2,3,5]tetrazin-4-ones. Tetrahedron Lett 1979:4253–6.
[9] Stevens MFG, Hickman JA, Stone R, Gibson NW, Baig GU, Lunt E, et al. Antitumor imidazotetrazines. 1. Synthesis and chemistry of 8-carbamoyl-3-(2-chloroethyl)imidazo[5,1-d]-1,2,3,5-tetrazin-4(3H)-one, a novel broad-spectrum antitumor agent. J Med Chem 1984;27:196–201.
[10] Stevens MFG. Second generation azolotetrazinones. In: Harrap KR, Connors TA,, editors. New avenues in developmental cancer chemotherapy. vol. 8 Academic Press; 1987. p. 335–54.
[11] Stevens MFG, Newlands ES. From triazines and triazenes to temozolomide. Eur J Cancer 1993;29A:1045–7.
[12] Hickman JA, Stevens MFG, Gibson NW, Langdon SP, Fizames C, Lavelle F, et al. Experimental antitumor activity against murine tumor model systems of 8-carbamoyl-3-(2-chloroethyl)imidazo[5,1-d]-1,2,3,5-tetrazin-4(3H)-one (mitozolomide), a novel broad-spectrum agent. Cancer Res 1985;45:3008–13.
[13] Newlands ES, Blackledge G, Slack JA, Goddard C, Brindley CJ, Holden L, et al. Phase I clinical trial of mitozolomide (CCRG 81010; M&B 39565; NSC 353451). Cancer Treat Rep 1985;69:801–5.
[14] Schornagel JH, Simonetti G, Dubbelman R, ten Bokkel Huinink WW, McVie JG. Phase I study of mitozolomide on a once daily for 5 days schedule. Cancer Chemother Pharmacol 1990;26:237–8.
[15] Double JA, Bibby MC. Therapeutic index: a vital component in selection of anticancer agents for clinical trial. J Natl Cancer Inst 1989;81:988–94.
[16] Lunt E, Newton CG, Smith C, Stevens GP, Stevens MFG, Straw CG, et al. Antitumor imidazotetrazines. 14. Synthesis and antitumor activity of 6- and 8-substituted imidazo[5,1-d]-1,2,3,5-tetrazinones and 8-substituted pyrazolo[5,1-d]-1,2,3,5-tetrazinones. J Med Chem 1987;30:357–66.
[17] Gibson NW, Hickman JA, Erickson LC. DNA cross-linking and cytotoxicity in normal and transformed human cells treated *in vitro* with 8-carbamoyl-3-(2-chloroethyl)imidazo[5,1-d]-1,2,3,5-tetrazin-4(3H)-one. Cancer Res 1984;44:1772–5.
[18] Stevens MFG, Hickman JA, Langdon SP, Chubb D, Vickers L, Stone R, et al. Antitumor activity and pharmacokinetics in mice of 8-carbamoyl-3-methylimidazo[5,1-d]-1,2,3,5-tetrazin-4(3H)-one (CCRG 81045; M & B 39831), a novel drug with potential as an alternative to dacarbazine. Cancer Res 1987;47:5846–52.
[19] Rutty CJ, Newell DR, Vincent RB, Abel G, Goddard PM, Harland SJ, et al. The species dependent pharmacokinetics of DTIC. Br J Cancer 1983;48:140.
[20] Plowman J, Waud WR, Koutsoukos AD, Rubinstein LV, Moore TD, Grever MR. Pre-clinical antitumor activity of temozolomide in mice: efficacy against human brain tumor xenografts and synergism with 1,3-bis(2-chloroethyl)-1-nitrosourea. Cancer Res 1994;54:3793–9.

[21] Crabb C. Revisiting the Bhopal tragedy. Science 2004;306:1670–1.

[22] Wang Y, Stevens MFG, Thomson WT. Alternative synthesis of the antitumour drug temozolomide avoiding the use of methyl isocyanate. J Chem Soc Chem Commun 1994:1687–8.

[23] Wang Y, Stevens MFG, Thomson WT, Shutts BP. Antitumour imidazotetrazines. Part 33. New syntheses of the antitumour drug temozolomide using 'masked' methyl isocyanates. J Chem Soc Perkin Trans I 1995:2783–7.

[24] Wang Y, Stevens MFG, Chan T-M, DiBenedetto D, Ding Z-X, Gala D, et al. Antitumor imidazotetrazines. 35. New synthetic routes to the antitumor drug temozolomide. J Org Chem 1997;62:7288–94.

[25] Newlands ES, Blackledge GRP, Slack J, Stuart NSA, Stevens MFG. Experimental background and early clinical studies with imidazotetrazine derivatives. In: Giraldi T, Connors TA, Cartei G, editors. Triazenes. New York: Plenum Press; 1990. p. 185–93.

[26] Newlands ES, Stevens MFG, Wedge SR, Wheelhouse RT, Brock C. Temozolomide: a review of its discovery, chemical properties, pre-clinical development and clinical trials. Cancer Treat Rev 1997;23:35–61.

[27] Brock CS, Newlands ES, Wedge SR, Bower M, Evans H, Colquhoun I, et al. Phase I trial of temozolomide using an extended continuous oral schedule. Cancer Res 1998;58:4363–7.

[28] Denny BJ, Wheelhouse RT, Stevens MFG, Tsang LLH, Slack JA. NMR and molecular modelling investigation of the mechanism of activation of the antitumor drug temozolomide and its interaction with DNA. Biochemistry 1994;33:9045–51.

[29] Wheelhouse RT, Stevens MFG. Decomposition of the antitumour drug temozolomide in deuteriated phosphate buffer: methyl group transfer is accompanied by deuterium exchange. J Chem Soc Chem Commun 1993:1177–8.

[30] Tsang LLH, Farmer PB, Gescher A, Slack JA. Characterisation of urinary metabolites of temozolomide in humans and mice and evaluation of their cytotoxicity. Cancer Chemother Pharmacol 1990;27:342–6.

[31] Brown GD, Luthra SK, Brock CS, Stevens MFG, Price PM, Brady F. Antitumor imidazotetrazines. 40. Radiosyntheses of [4-[11]C-*carbonyl*]- and [3-*N*-[11]C-*methyl*]-8-carbamoyl-3-methylimidazo[5,1-*d*]-1,2,3,5-tetrazin-4(3*H*)-one (temozolomide) for positron emission tomography (PET) studies. J Med Chem 2002;45:5448–57.

[32] Rottenberg DA, Ginos JZ, Kearfoot KJ, Junck L, Bigner D. *In vivo* measurement of regional brain tissue pH using positron emission tomography. Ann Neurol 1984;15:S98–102.

[33] Vaupeel P, Kallinowski F, Okunieff P. Blood flow, oxygen and nutrient supply, and metabolic microenvironment of human tumors: a review. Cancer Res 1989;49:6449–65.

[34] Tisdale MJ. Antitumor imidazotetrazines—XV. Role of guanine O^6-alkylation in the mechanism of cytotoxicity of imidazotetrazinones. Biochem Pharmacol 1987;36:457–62.

[35] Clark AS, Deans B, Stevens MFG, Tisdale MJ, Wheelhouse RT, Denny BJ, et al. Antitumor imidazotetrazines. 32. Synthesis of novel imidazotetrazinones and related bicyclic heterocycles to probe the mode of action of the antitumor drug temozolomide. J Med Chem 1995;38:1493–504.

[36] Hartley JA, Mattes WB, Vaughan K, Gibson NW. DNA sequence specificity of guanine N^7 alkylation for a series of structurally related triazenes. Carcinogenesis 1988;9:669–74.

[37] Baer JC, Freeman AA, Newlands E, Watson AJ, Rafferty JA, Margison GP. Depletion of O^6-alkylguanine-DNA alkyltransferase correlates with potentiation of temozolomide and CCNU toxicity in human tumour cells. Br J Cancer 1993;67:1299–302.

[38] Lee SM, Thatcher N, Crowther D, Margison GP. Inactivation of O^6-alkylguanine-DNA alkyltransferase in human peripheral blood mononuclear cells by temozolomide. Br J Cancer 1994;69:452–6.

[39] Wedge SR, Porteous JK, Newlands ES. 3-Aminobenzamide and/or O^6-benzylguanine evaluated as an adjuvant to temozolomide or BCNU treatment in cell lines of variable mismatch repair status and O^6-alkylguanine-DNA alkyltransferase activity. Br J Cancer 1996;74:1030–6.

[40] Plummer ER, Middleton MR, Jones C, Olsen A, Hickson I, McHugh P, et al. Temozolomide pharmacodynamics in patients with metastatic melanoma: DNA damage and activity of repair enzymes O^6-alkylguanine alkyltransferase and poly(ADP-ribose)polymerase-1. Clin Cancer Res 2005;11:3402–9.

[41] Daniels DS, Woo TT, Luu KX, Noll DM, Clarke ND, Pegg AE, et al. DNA binding and nucleotide flipping by the human DNA repair protein AGT. Nat Struct Mol Biol 2004;11:714–20.

[42] Jagtap P, Szabó C. Poly(ADP-ribose) polymerase and the therapeutic effects of its inhibitors. Nat Rev Drug Discov 2005;4:421–40.

[43] Koch SSC, Thorensen LH, Tikhe JG, Maegley KA, Almassy RJ, Li J, et al. Novel tricyclic poly(ADP-ribose) polymerase-1 inhibitors with potent anticancer chemo-potentiating activity: design, synthesis, and X-ray cocrystal structure. J Med Chem 2002;45:4961–74.

[44] Friedman HS, Keir S, Pegg AE, Houghton PJ, Colvin OM, Moschel RC, et al. O^6-Benzylguanine-mediated enhancement of chemotherapy. Mol Cancer Ther 2002;1:943–8.

[45] Ranson M, Middleton MR, Bridgewater J, Lee SM, Dawson M, Jowle D, et al. Lomeguatrib, a potent inhibitor of O^6-alkylguanine-DNA alkyltransferase: phase I safety, pharmacodynamic, and pharmacokinetic trial and evaluation in combination with temozolomide in patients with advanced solid tumours. Clin Cancer Res 2006;12:1577–84.

[46] Liu L, Gerson SL. Targeted modulation of MGMT: clinical implications. Clin Cancer Res 2006;12:328–31.

[47] Bull VL, Tisdale MJ. Antitumour imidazotetrazines—XVI. Macromolecular alkylation by 3-substituted imidazotetrazines. Biochem Pharmacol 1987;36:3215–20.

[48] Hegi ME, Diserens AC, Godard S, Dietrich PY, Regli L, Ostermann S, et al. Clinical trial substantiates the predictive value of O^6-methylguanine-DNA methyltransferase promoter methylation in glioblastoma patients treated with temozolomide. Clin Cancer Res 2004;10:1871–4.

[49] Hegi ME, Diserens AC, Gorlia T, Hamou M, de Tribolet N, Weller M, et al. MGMT gene silencing and benefit from temozolomide in glioblastoma. N Engl J Med 2005;352:997–1003.

[50] Tisdale MJ. Antitumor imidazotetrazines—X. Effect of 8-carbamoyl-3-methylimidazo[5,1-d]-1,2,3,5-tetrazin-4(3H)one (CCRG 81045, M&B 39831, NSC 362856) on DNA methylation during induction of haemoglobin synthesis in human leukaemia cell line K562. Biochem Pharmacol 1986;35:311–6.

[51] Tisdale MJ. Antitumor imidazotetrazines—XVIII. Modification of the level of 5-methylcytosine in DNA by 3-substituted imidazotetrazines. Biochem Pharmacol 1989;38:1097–101.

[52] Winkler FK. DNA totally flipped out by methylase. Structure 1994;2:79–83.

[53] Belinsky SA. Silencing of genes by promoter hypermethylation: key event in rodent and human lung cancer. Carcinogenesis 2005;26:1481–7.

[54] Arrowsmith J, Jennings SA, Clark AS, Stevens MFG. Antitumor imidazotetrazines. 41. Conjugation of the antitumor agents mitozolomide and temozolomide to peptides and lexitropsins bearing DNA major and minor groove-binding structural motifs. J Med Chem 2002;45:5458–70.

[55] Horspool KR, Stevens MFG, Newton CG, Lunt E, Walsh RJA, Pedgrift BL, et al. Antitumor imidazotetrazines. 20. Preparation of the 8-acid of mitozolomide and its utility in the preparation of active antitumor agents. J Med Chem 1990;33:1393–9.

[56] Arrowsmith J, Jennings SA, Langnel DAF, Wheelhouse RT, Stevens MFG. Antitumor imidazotetrazines. Part 39. Synthesis of bis(imidazotetrazine)s with saturated spacer groups. J Chem Soc Perkin Trans I 2000:4432–8.

[57] Glister JF, Vaughan K. A series of 1-[2-aryl-1-diazenyl]-3-({3-[2-aryl-1-diazenyl]perhydrobenzo[d]imidazol-1-yl} methyl)perhydrobenzo[d]imid-azoles. J Heterocyl Chem 2006;43:1–6.

[58] Diana P, Barraja P, Lauria A, Montalbano A, Almerico AM, Dattolo G, et al. Pyrrolo[2,1-d][1,2,3,5]tetrazin-4(3H) ones, a new class of azolotetrazines with potent antitumor activity. Bioorg Med Chem 2003;11:2371–80.

[59] Williams CI, Whitehead MA, Jean-Claude BJ. A semiempirical PM3 treatment of benzotetrazepinone decomposition in acid media. J Org Chem 1997;62:7006–14.

[60] Rachid Z, Brahimi F, Katsoulas A, Teoh N, Jean-Claude BJ. The combi-targeting concept: chemical dissection of the dual targeting properties of a series of combi-triazenes. J Med Chem 2003;46:4313–21.

[61] Wanner MJ, Koch M, Koomen G-J. Synthesis and antitumor activity of methyltriazene prodrugs simultaneously releasing DNA_methylating agents and the antiresistance drug O^6-benzylguanine. J Med Chem 2004;47:6875–83.

[62] Smith C. Hitting the target. Nature 2003;422:341–7; quoting D. Szymkowski, Xencor, Monrovia, California.

[63] Fojo T. Novel_Target.com. Oncologist 2001;6:313–4.

Temozolomide: Patents and the Perils of Invention

Malcolm F.G. Stevens

Centre for Biomolecular Sciences, University of Nottingham, Nottingham, UK

INTRODUCTION

A fortunate inventor involved in the discovery and development of a drug that actually makes it to market usually moves on in their career and loses interest in the drama of what happened often decades earlier. The welcome receipt of a slice, a small percentage, from a royalty stream, shared with former colleagues, reminds him of the successful journey accomplished against all odds. But it doesn't prepare him for an interrogative ordeal where his very integrity as a dedicated and responsible scientist is challenged.

This saga can be considered to start in November 1976, with a draft agreement between Aston University, Birmingham, United Kingdom, and the research director (Dr Kenneth Wooldridge) of May & Baker Ltd, a pharmaceutical company based in Dagenham, Essex, United Kingdom, to fund a postgraduate student under the CASE Scheme (Collaborative Award in Science and Technology) operated by the then UK Science Research Council. The project was originally designed to investigate cyclic compounds with multiple nitrogen atoms that might have antiallergic activity: this disease area was a therapeutic target of May & Baker at that time, but abandoned soon after.

A tenet of this scheme was that the postgraduate student would be based primarily in the Pharmacy Department of the university but spend a 3-month secondment in the company working with industrial colleagues: importantly, under the scheme, the company would be responsible for all intellectual property (IP) issues and the prosecution of patents. Accordingly, Robert Stone was appointed to the May & Baker Studentship and started work in the autumn of 1978. By early 1980, the first syntheses of examples of the new ring system imidazo[5,1-*d*]-1,2,3,5-tetrazine, with intriguing chemical properties, had been achieved by what has become known as the "Stone synthesis" [1]. An entry in a May & Baker laboratory book records that Stone, when working in Dagenham under the supervision of Dr Eddy Lunt, first synthesized the 3-methyl analog (temozolomide) on 29 April 1980. The first paper revealing the synthesis and properties of imidazotetrazines was published in 1984 [1]. The US Food and Drug Administration (FDA) granted a first approval for the treatment of refractory anaplastic astrocytoma in the United States in 1999, and the drug was subsequently marketed by Schering-Plough as a treatment for glioblastoma multiforme in Europe (Temodal™) and in the United States (as Temodar™) (see Chapter 5 for a fuller account of the discovery and development of the drug and photographs of some of the Aston team). Temozolomide has occupied a niche market in cancer chemotherapy, being the only approved drug at the time for this condition, and by 2008 sales of the drug broached the "blockbuster" barrier, exceeding US$1000 million per annum. It was an unlikely, and quite unexpected, outcome; but this success inevitably attracted the interest of predators anxious for their cut of the cash flow, and a challenge to the US patent protecting the temozolomide invention was duly launched in 2007 by Barr Laboratories, Inc., which filed an Abbreviated New Drug Application (ANDA) to launch a generic version of temozolomide on the US market. Cancer Research Technology (CRT, formerly CRCT; the technology transfer arm of the UK charity Cancer Research UK, formerly Cancer Research Campaign), which was the patent assignee, and Schering-Plough, which was the licensee, sued.

So, just when pleasant memories of a rewarding roller-coaster ride had started to fade, this coinventor was wrenched from a state of agreeable and genteel post-Hayflick decline to face an ordeal before a judge in a foreign court, to account for every word and action even three decades earlier, where a wrongly chosen word could jeopardize a successful commercial operation and blight a personal reputation established over half a century. To add insult to injury, a comprehensive archive of laboratory books, references, reports, legal documents, notes, and correspondence, assiduously preserved intact despite many office moves and career changes, were to be used as ammunition by the opposition.

HISTORY OF US PATENT 5,260,291 (1993)

The priority date claiming rights to the temozolomide invention was established by the filing of a UK application on 24 August 1981. The US patent, titled "Tetrazine Derivatives" (Fig. 6.1) and composed by Mr Terry Miller, the patent manager at May & Baker, was filed in 1982.

The patent, at only nine pages, was a masterpiece of economical writing. It exemplified the synthesis of just 13 novel structures (Fig. 6.2) and described their antitumor properties against some of the mouse tumor models of the day—TLX5 lymphoma, leukemia L1210, and B16 melanoma, for example. In wordings that proved to be controversial in court, these compounds were described as "important" and possessing "valuable antineoplastic activity". The compound identified by formula 8-carbamoyl-3-methyl-[3H]-imidazo[5,1-d]-1,2,3, 5-tetrazin-4-one (temozolomide) was highlighted as being "of particular importance," and the 3-(2-chloroethyl) analog (mitozolomide) especially so.

After 1981, patents were granted expeditiously in major national jurisdictions where the patent life was triggered on initial filing. However, in a fact overlooked by the court, patent approval was also completed in Canada (1985), which had a similar policy to that in the United States at the time, in that the patent clock commenced ticking on grant. The progress to granting of the US patent had many elements of a soap opera: the initial application was rejected by the US examiner in 1983 on the grounds of "lack of utility", asserting that

US005260291A

United States Patent [19]

Lunt et al.

[11] **Patent Number:**   **5,260,291**

[45] **Date of Patent:**   **Nov. 9, 1993**

[54] **TETRAZINE DERIVATIVES**

[75] Inventors: **Edward Lunt**, Norfolk; **Malcolm F. G. Stevens**, Birmingham, both of England; **Robert Stone**, Montrose, Australia; **Kenneth R. H. Wooldridge**, Lincolnshire; **Edward S. Newlands**, London, both of England

[73] Assignee: **Cancer Research Campaign Technology Limited**, London, England

[21] Appl. No.: **781,020**

[22] Filed: **Oct. 18, 1991**

Related U.S. Application Data

[63] Continuation-in-part of Ser. No. 607,221, Nov. 1, 1990, abandoned, which is a continuation of Ser. No. 456,614, Dec. 29, 1989, abandoned, which is a continuation of Ser. No. 338,515, Mar. 3, 1989, abandoned, which is a continuation of Ser. No. 135,473, Dec. 21, 1987, abandoned, which is a continuation of Ser. No. 40,716, Apr. 20, 1987, abandoned, which is a continuation of Ser. No. 885,397, Jul. 18, 1986, abandoned, which is a continuation of Ser. No. 798,365, Nov. 18, 1985, abandoned, which is a continuation of Ser. No. 712,462, Mar. 15, 1985, abandoned, which is a continuation of Ser. No. 586,635, Mar. 6, 1984, abandoned, which is a continuation of Ser. No. 410,656, Aug. 23, 1982, abandoned.

[30] **Foreign Application Priority Data**

Aug. 24, 1981 [GB] United Kingdom 8125791

[51] Int. Cl.^{5} **A61K 31/415; C07P 487/04**

[52] U.S. Cl. **514/183; 544/179**

[58] Field of Search 544/179; 514/183

[56] **References Cited**

FOREIGN PATENT DOCUMENTS

571430	8/1988	Australia .
380256	5/1986	Austria .
1001617	12/1984	Bangladesh .
894175	2/1983	Belgium .
1197247	11/1985	Canada .
2932305	2/1981	Fed. Rep. of Germany .
734343	10/1981	Finland .
8214461	1/1985	France .
76863	9/1984	Greece .
186107	8/1984	Hungary .

53408	2/1989	Ireland .
66606	8/1987	Israel .
1152505	1/1987	Italy .
28587	7/1989	Rep. of Korea .
84347	6/1983	Luxembourg .
201668	5/1986	New Zealand .
RP5512	8/1983	Nigeria .
128469	12/1984	Pakistan .
82/6120	8/1982	South Africa .
515176	7/1983	Spain .
8204817.4	6/1987	Sweden .
655114	3/1986	Switzerland .
18691	8/1983	Taiwan . .
1447284	12/1988	U.S.S.R. . .
2104522	6/1985	United Kingdom .

OTHER PUBLICATIONS

Lunt. et. al., J. Med. Chem. vol. 30, pp. 357–366 (1987).

Primary Examiner—Bernard Dentz
Attorney, Agent, or Firm—Klauber & Jackson

[57]   **ABSTRACT**

[3H]-Imidazo[5,1-d]-1,2,3,5-tetrazin-4-one   derivatives of the formula:

wherein R^1 represents hydrogen, or an alkyl, alkenyl or alkynyl group containing up to 6 carbon atoms, each such group being unsubstituted or substituted by from one to three substitutents selected from halogen atoms, alkoxy, alkylthio, alkylsulphinyl and alkylsulphonyl groups containing up to 4 carbon atoms, and optionally substituted phenyl groups, or R^1 represents a cycloalkyl group containing from 3 to 8 carbon atoms, and R^2 represents a carbamoyl group optionally N-substituted by one or two groups selected from alkyl and alkenyl groups containing up to 4 carbon atoms, and cycloalkyl groups containing 3 to 8 carbon atoms, are new therapeutically useful compounds possessing antineoplastic and immunomodulatory activity.

33 Claims, No Drawings

FIGURE 6.1   US Patent 5,260,291.

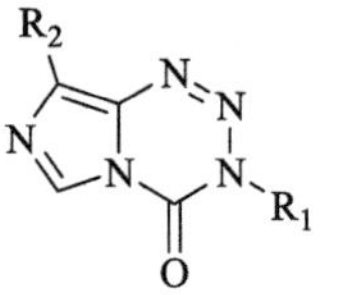

R_1	R_2	
Me	$CONH_2$	(temozolomide)
$(CH_2)_2Cl$	$CONH_2$	(mitozolomide)
$(CH_2)_2Cl$	CONHMe	
$(CH_2)_2Cl$	$CONMe_2$	
$(CH_2)_2Br$	$CONH_2$	
$(CH_2)_2Me$	$CONH_2$	
$(CH_2)_3Cl$	$CONH_2$	
$CH_2CHClCH_2Cl$	$CONH_2$	
$(CH_2)_2OMe$	$CONH_2$	
$CH_2CH=CH_2$	$CONH_2$	
$CH(CH_2)_5$	$CONH_2$	
CH_2Ph	$CONH_2$	
$CH_2C_6H_4OMe$-p	$CONH_2$	

FIGURE 6.2 Novel structures described in US Patent 5,260,291.

the invention should include clinical data in humans and that no such data were included. Mitozolomide entered phase I trials only in 1983. In a perfectly legal tactic, May & Baker abandoned the parent case and filed a continuation; the same examiner reiterated his original rejection. Again, no response was forthcoming, but instead May & Baker abandoned the parent case and filed another continuation. In a corporate complication, May & Baker (through their parent company, Rhône-Poulenc) abandoned the tetrazine project in the mid-1980s, when trials on mitozolomide indicated that only sporadic antitumor activities could be discerned, and then only at unacceptable toxicity levels. This notwithstanding, Miller, concerned that the invention had, in the main, been engendered by ideas from the University of Aston, on his own initiative continued the "ping-pong" duel with the US examiner: in total, over a 10-year period, 10 continuations were filed in response to the lack-of-utility rejoinder.

After the demise of mitozolomide in 1985, clinical attention switched to temozolomide, which entered clinical trial in 1987 under the auspices of the Cancer Research Campaign Phase I Committee. When clear evidence of safety and modest clinical activity, especially against brain tumors and melanoma, emerged, in 1991 May & Baker transferred the tetrazine IP estate to CRCT, which, as assignee, took over responsibility for bringing the vexed and unresolved matter of the US application to a conclusion. As was testified in court by Dr Sue Foden, then CEO of CRCT, to make temozolomide available for cancer patients, it was considered essential to have the manufacturing and marketing clout of a global pharmaceutical company on board, and that a granted US patent would be an essential requirement to secure a deal. In a considerable coup for CRCT and its 2.5 employees at the time, a license agreement was negotiated with Schering-Plough in 1992 following a "road show" to several companies in the United States. A successful substantive response to a new examiner claimed that applicants *did not need* to provide data on clinical efficacy and that animal test data alone *were* sufficient. Such thorough animal data were noted by the examiner in a 1987 paper by the Aston/May & Baker team [2]. On this basis, the examiner mailed a "notice of allowability", and the US patent was duly issued on 9 November 1993, 11 years after the first application. The name of an extra inventor, Dr Edward Newlands, was added to reflect his pivotal role in the preclinical and clinical development of both mitozolomide and temozolomide. In 1999, Schering-Plough filed successfully for a patent term extension, which added 1006 days to the patent's term; the patent was also granted a pediatric exclusivity period and is due to expire in February 2014, some 34 years after the initial synthesis of the drug.

CANCER RESEARCH TECHNOLOGY LTD ET AL. (PLAINTIFFS) VS BARR LABORATORIES INC. ET AL. (DEFENDANTS)

In advance of the trial, fact witnesses may be required to undergo a deposition, which involves answering questions from counsel for the defendants that they deem necessary to establish any facts they consider relevant to the upcoming trial. For inventor Stevens, this event took place in New York in June 2008 and lasted a full day. It was pointed out by plaintiff's counsel that a case "cannot be won on deposition, but can be lost." The core of the questioning by Barr's counsel concerned the provenance of the new compounds, their screening, and, significantly, their structural relationships to dimethyltriazenes (see Chapter 5 for structures), which are well-known in the chemical and biological literature, especially their propensity to undergo metabolic activation to cytotoxic and mutagenic species [3]. A particular focus on the antimelanoma drug dacarbazine (DTIC) carried the implication that Barr was building a case to challenge the patent on the grounds of "obviousness", and that an expert medicinal chemist, given access to all published work in the field, pen, and paper, could have independently designed the same compounds. If only it were that easy! However, nothing in the published work of the Aston team in the 1970s indicated that the imidazotetrazines were in any way conceived as stable variants of MTIC, the ring-opened form of DTIC. Chemical inquisitiveness was the sole motivating factor, and it was only after the postdiscovery phase of the project that the ring-opening relationship with imidazotriazenes was revealed. In another tack, counsel for Barr posited the belief that hydrolytic ring opening of tetrazinones would be "expected". Unfortunately for his argument, the only example he highlighted was that of a monocyclic 1,2,4,5-tetrazinone, not a bicyclic 1,2,3,5-tetrazinone. Chemists will know they are like chalk and cheese.

After this initial skirmish, and to prepare for the real trial and counter the expected attack on "obviousness", this inventor spent many days familiarizing himself with the voluminous literature on dimethyltriazenes from the first publication of their antitumor properties in 1955 [4]. Box files full of reprints on triazenes, some hoarded lovingly for nearly 50 years, provided nostalgic reading; it was like being reunified with faded and dusty old friends. A telling quotation in a paper by Hansch [5] was held in reserve: "Unless one had new biochemical or molecular biological information suggesting that a new triazene might be more effective in some specific way, we would not recommend the synthesis and testing of new congeners." Even more helpful was a comment in a 1986 paper by a competitor group [6] that mitozolomide was "ingeniously designed and synthesized", words that would support the originality claims in US Patent 5,260,291. In any event, Barr dropped the "obviousness" slur and, in the run up to the trial in 2009, charged that the patent was unenforceable due to "prosecution laches"—the deliberate implementation of delaying tactics to extend the life of the patent—and the more personally menacing "inequitable conduct" by inventors and those responsible for prosecuting the patent.

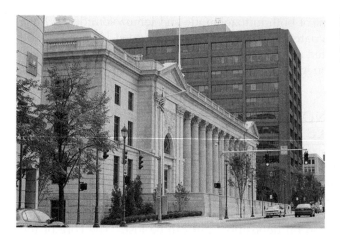

FIGURE 6.3 The courthouse in Wilmington, Delaware. (For color version of this figure, the reader is referred to the online version of this book.)

Other changes had taken place in advance of the trial: May & Baker's parent company Rhône-Poulenc had been reincarnated firstly as Rhône-Poulenc Rorer, then Aventis, and finally Sanofi Aventis; Barr Laboratories had been acquired by Teva Pharmaceuticals; and Schering-Plough had been acquired by Merck and Co. Inc. On the personal front, coinventors Wooldridge and Lunt and patent manager Miller had retired from May & Baker; and, sadly, Newlands was deceased. Stone, who had had no contact with the project since 1981 on completion of his PhD, was originally charged with "inequitable conduct", but this was subsequently dropped. Stevens, whose academic positions had given him the privilege of continuous tenure during the history of the temozolomide story, was confident he had a compelling story to convey to the court as the protagonists assembled in the US District Court for the District of Delaware (Fig. 6.3) on 20 July 2009. For Barr to succeed in its challenge, only one individual had to be successfully charged with "inequitable conduct", but they had to prove that there was an "intent to deceive" the US Patent and Trademark Office (PTO).

As mentioned in this chapter, according to the terms of the CASE Award, May & Baker were to be responsible for all IP issues, including patents. Thus, apart from signing the US application in 1982 and ensuring that the compounds were correctly described and characterized (in some cases, by X-ray structures), Stevens had no further role in its prosecution; he was unaware until patent issuance in 1993 that there had been problems with US examiners. By the mid-1980s, mitozolomide had been abandoned by May & Baker, and there was every expectation that the orphaned temozolomide would suffer the same fate. His career had moved on to other research projects and the responsibility of headship of a large academic department in Aston University at a time of swingeing cuts—known locally as the "decade of the python". He had no role in planning clinical trials or selecting clinicians to run them, on principle never visited wards where patients were treated, and to this day has only ever spoken to one patient treated with temozolomide. At meetings of the CRC Phase I Committee in the 1980s and early 1990s, he had to sign a declaration that on no account could any clinical information be communicated to third parties. Clinical "data"—that is, diagnostic tests, laboratory biochemical investigations, measurements taken at bedside, brain scans, and so on—were deemed to be *utterly* confidential to patients, clinicians, and the hospital concerned. He had no financial interest whatsoever in the success or otherwise of the project until *after* a deal was signed with Schering-Plough in 1992, and then only indirectly through an agreement between CRCT and Aston University.

Of course, none of this cut any ice with Barr's counsel and, ominously, as the trial proceeded, inventor Stevens, the only one of those listed still on active service, found himself in the crosshairs.

Barr's main line of attack was to invoke an applicant's continuing "duty of candor" in its dealings with the PTO and a "duty to disclose" to the PTO any information that may be "material" to the examination of the patent application. (Although this policy may be familiar to non-US laboratory scientists now, it was not in the 1980s.) But ignorance of the scope of these duties, and the severance of the conduit of information from Stevens→Lunt→Miller that had occurred when May & Baker relinquished all further interest in the commercialization of mitozolomide and temozolomide, did not, according to Barr, cancel the obligation on an inventor.

In the patent, all 13 compounds were identified as being "important". Barr asserted that this meant all the compounds had potentially valuable anticancer activity. Not so, claimed Miller: the word indicated that, as the first characterized examples of a novel structural type, they merited being so described. The use of this word was not to be confused with identification of the compounds temozolomide and mitozolomide as having "particular importance", which did teach someone skilled in the art of drug discovery that this was where the seam of useful biological activity lay. Pursuing this line, counsel for Barr then produced several abstracts and publications that described antitumor evaluations of compounds against mouse tumors. Some compounds identified in the patent had T/C values ≤125%; these, by convention, were not considered as showing antitumor outcomes in the test. Several publications used the word "inactive" in such cases, but always in the context of a particular tumor, and not to imply inactivity against *all* tumors. (This point was reinforced by witness Dr Ed Sausville, formerly of the US National Cancer Institute, who explained that it was a normal outcome in drug discovery programs that compounds ineffective against one tumor may well have potent activity against a tumor of different lineage.) A lot of the court's time was spent arguing semantic points around the meaning of a compound being "active" or "inactive" in animal tests and how this information might be of value to the examiner. In exasperation, Miller did make the cutting comment that May & Baker had no intention of developing a drug to treat mouse cancer!

Barr's case was that information from these animal tests—especially negative tests—was "material" and should have been conveyed to the examiner, who might then have made an earlier decision on grant or rejection, thus possibly allowing earlier launch of a generic product in the US market.

Barr also contended that publications on the phase I studies on mitozolomide [7] and temozolomide [8] were "material" in that they revealed clinical information that would have been valuable to the examiner. In court, Stevens explained that he had no inputs into these trials but was listed as a "courtesy author" on the basis that it was reasonable that first clinical publications on a new drug should acknowledge the role of the originator of the product. His injudicious use of the word "disastrous" in deposition to describe the outcome of the phase I study on mitozolomide was claimed by Barr's counsel to indicate that he considered the trial a failure and that such a conclusion was "material" and should have been available to the examiner. However, the word "disastrous" was intended to refer to the extinguishing of the expectation of the inventors and their colleagues that the elusive "magic bullet" lay in their grasp and that immortalization in a Hollywood movie would surely follow. There was even a suggestion that Steve McQueen should be approached for a starring role! This hubristic fantasy had been sustained by the extraordinary, often curative efficacy of mitozolomide against transplanted mouse tumors [9]. (Actually, the mitozolomide phase I trial could have been considered a success as it did just what such trials are designed to accomplish: it defined a maximum tolerated dose and identified the dose-limiting toxicities; and clinicians keenly sought to be involved in phase II trials.) Also, it was explained to the court that this trial was not seeking to identify tumor responses and that the results were preliminary. Although evidence of tumor responses was reported, especially in the temozolomide phase I trial, it is a common experience in oncology trials that seemingly dramatic outcomes at phase I are unlikely to be repeated in formal efficacy trials against specific tumor types.

When questioned in court about his role in the delay of issuance of the US patent, Miller claimed that his being "obdurate" was in response to the similar attitude of the examiner. (In a rare moment of humor appreciated by the court, Miller explained that the unfolding confrontation was an example of "Old Bird's Law" in action. This law, named after a senior colleague at May & Baker, posited thus: "By the time a US patent is granted, the company will have abandoned the project.") How true in this case! Miller also robustly defended his actions on the grounds that he anticipated that the patent would be a significant contribution to cancer research. As subsequent history showed, his dogged persistence was of crucial significance in protecting the commercial standing of temozolomide and securing its availability for many thousands of patients with brain tumors.

Toward the end of the trial, coinventor Stone took the stand and was able to describe his experiences as a postgraduate student at Aston University and working at May & Baker. He especially contrasted the rudimentary equipment and grim laboratories of the Pharmacy Department at Aston in the late 1970s with those of the modern institution in 2008. Much of the investment to finance the transformation was through royalties received by the university from sales of temozolomide. To Stone's disappointment, counsel for Barr declined to cross-examine him: at the very least, a congratulatory comment on his remarkable contribution to a rare event in drug discovery history—a marketed drug, and a blockbuster to boot—would not have gone amiss.

THE VERDICT

Ignoring the fact that CRT (through CRCT) became involved with temozolomide in only 1991 (as discussed in this chapter), the court concluded that it didn't seek to develop the technology prior to the signing of the Schering-Plough license in 1992 (how could it?) and engaged with the PTO only when it had a "profit motive" for doing so. The court also concluded that Stevens withheld information on inactivity data in animal studies, and clinical results in humans that it considered were "highly material". The fact that he and his colleagues had authored some 40 publications on antitumor imidazotetrazines, many in American journals, to the wider scientific community over the period in question was, perversely, taken as evidence from which to infer an "intent to deceive". In pronouncing its verdict in January 2010, the court found CRT's conduct sufficiently egregious to warrant rendering US

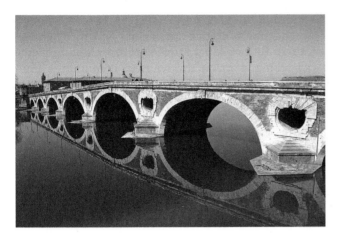

FIGURE 6.4 Bridge over the Garonne in Toulouse, France. (For color version of this figure, the reader is referred to the online version of this book.)

Patent 5,260,291 unenforceable due to "prosecution laches", and found that Stevens committed "inequitable conduct" for disclosure failures with intent to deceive.

The bad news was conveyed to Stevens when he was attending the winter meeting of the European Organisation for the Research and Treatment of Cancer (EORTC) Pharmacology and Molecular Mechanisms (PAMM) group's meeting in Toulouse, France. It was a bitter and humiliating blow, and his blood ran cooler than the icy waters of the river Garonne. But for the steadying support of Secretary Nicola Thomas back in the office, the bridge over the river (Fig. 6.4) might have witnessed a dramatic end to his ordeal.

Had the *CRT* vs *Barr* tussle been a soccer match, then the score at this point would have been Barr-2: CRT-0. But, in a surprise decision in February 2010, the judge granted a temporary restraining order (TRO) preventing Barr (Teva) from launching generic temozolomide on the US market until an appeal before the Federal Circuit Court of Appeals in Washington, DC, had been heard. For the appeal to be successful, it would be necessary for lawyers for CRT to convince two of the three judges to overturn both "prosecution laches" and "inequitable conduct" decisions. Only legal issues could be argued, and no new evidence presented.

THE APPEAL(S)

The US Appeals Court, in its judgment on 9 November 2010, took the view that CRT could not possibly develop and market temozolomide in the United States until Schering-Plough became its licensee, but on securing that liaison speedily moved to secure issuance of its patent. The public interest was secured by the fact that CRT did make the product available for treating cancer patients, and it should not lose that protection because patent issuance was delayed. In the view of the appeals court, Barr had not "invested in temozolomide or any other claimed tetrazine compound between 1982 and 1991, the period of the delay". By a 2:1 majority, they concluded that the district court committed legal error in holding the patent unenforceable for "prosecution laches" and overturned the original decision.

The appeals court also determined that nothing in Stevens's widespread publication of data in the world literature "evidences wrongful intent, but rather the opposite, extreme candor". They also agreed with CRT that the district court erred in finding that Stevens intended to deceive the PTO by not disclosing data on the claimed compounds and thereby relied solely on its finding of materiality to infer intent. Again, by a 2:1 majority they reversed the district court's decision, holding the patent unenforceable for "inequitable conduct".

So the final score was Barr-2: CRT-2, but as the Federal Circuit Appeals Court decision trumped that of the district court, CRT prevailed on what would be, in soccer parlance, the "away-goals-count-double" rule.

There was one final twist: because the decision of the appeals court was not unanimous, Barr sought leave to appeal to the US Supreme Court. This was rejected.

CONCLUSIONS

It could be argued that many drug discoverers would positively welcome the opportunity to sit in the hot seat in a foreign court to defend their actions in respect of a generic challenge to their patented invention. This scenario would happen only if their drug had achieved notable sales. But the charge of "inequitable conduct" does carry an unsavory taste, especially for researchers whose sole motivation is to do their best for patients. Fortunately in the present case, the taint was removed and the threat to a professional reputation nullified, but in other cases mud can stick.

The circumstances surrounding the battle for the US patent protecting temozolomide are unlikely to be repeated since patent terms in the United States are now triggered from filing date. However, there are some lessons that could be learned by researchers lucky (or unlucky?) enough to follow a similar track:

1. Never use the words "active" or "inactive" in any publications or notes reporting biological tests on compounds. Perhaps the terms "prioritized" or "de-prioritized" would be less of a hostage to fortune, but even then a smart counsel might claim some hidden nuance in their meanings.
2. Always keep open the information trail between the laboratory bench and those prosecuting your patent: if in any doubt, disclose the most trivial of data, even if you drive the patent examiner mad.
3. Be wary of agreeing to be a "courtesy author" on a publication where you have not contributed meaningfully to the work. In the 1980s this practice was widespread, but it leaves one open to a challenge in court that, as a listed author, one must somehow have complete knowledge of the totality of the contents of the publication. This is potentially hazardous for laboratory scientists appearing as coauthors on papers reporting clinical results. Some esteemed journals now require every author to make a declaration describing their contribution to the work, and this principle should become standard. "When it comes to apportioning credit, science could learn from the movies" [10].
4. And, finally, be candid and publish because your own career and the careers of your colleagues depend on it. But prepare yourself to be damned.

Acknowledgments

Although this chapter is a personal account of a traumatic milestone in a career, it is also a heartwarming story of how a charity in the United Kingdom prevailed against the odds. The successful outcome of the trans-Atlantic battle for US Patent 5,260,291 could not have been achieved without the testimony of colleagues, some of whose contributions have been highlighted herein. The author would also like to express his thanks and admiration for the legal team of Ropes & Gray LLP led by Jesse Jenner, who spent 2 years mastering a complex brief spanning a third of a century, constructing a compelling case from naïve witnesses, and tutoring them in the do's and don'ts of court etiquette. They were such fun people to be with. But this witness found their instruction "No jokes, please" on the stand somewhat restrictive.

Thanks are also due to legal representatives of CRT, Schering-Plough, and Merck & Co. who attended the trial in a supportive role. And—yes—Barr's counsel and interrogator-in-chief George Lombardi was polite and considerate at all times in his questioning. No hard feelings, George: we both know it was business.

References

[1] Stevens MFG, Hickman JA, Stone R, Gibson NW, Baig GU, Lunt E, et al. Antitumour imidazotetrazines. 1. Synthesis and chemistry of 8-carbamoyl-3-(2-chloroethyl)imidazo[5,1-*d*]-1,2,3,5-tetrazin-4(3*H*)-one, a novel broad-spectrum antitumour agent. J Med Chem 1984;27:196–201.

[2] Lunt E, Newton CJ, Smith C, Stevens GP, Stevens MFG, Straw CG, et al. Antitumor imidazotetrazines. 14. Synthesis and antitumor activity of 6- and 8-substituted imidazo[5,1-*d*]-1,2,3,5-tetrazinones. J Med Chem 1987;30:357–66.

[3] Audette RCS, Connors TA, Mandel HG, Merai K, Ross WC. Studies on the mechanism of action of tumor inhibitory triazenes. Biochem Pharmacol 1973;22:1855–64.

[4] Clark DA, Barclay RK, Stock CC, Rondestvedt CS. Triazenes as inhibitors of mouse sarcoma 180. Proc Soc Exp Biol Med 1955;90:484–9.

[5] Hansch C, Hatheway CJ, Quinn FR, Greenberg N. Antitumour 1-(X-aryl)-3,3-dimethyltriazenes. 2. On the role of correlation analysis in decision making in drug modification. Toxicity quantitative structure-activity relationships of 1-(X-phenyl)-3,3-dialkyltriazenes in mice. J Med Chem 1978;21:574–7.

[6] Cheng CC, Elslager EF, Werbel LM, Leopold III WR. Pyrazole derivatives 5. Synthesis and antineoplastic activity of 3-(2-chloroethyl)-3,4-dihydro-4-oxopyrazolo[5,1-d]-1,2,3,5-tetrazine-8-carboxamide and related compounds. J Med Chem 1986;29:1544–7.

[7] Newlands ES, Blackledge G, Slack JA, Goddard C, Brindley CJ, Holden L, et al. Phase 1 clinical trial of mitozolomide. Cancer Treat Rep 1985;69:801–5.

[8] Newlands ES, Blackledge GRP, Slack JA, Rustin GJ, Smith DB, Stuart NS, et al. Phase 1 clinical trial of temozolomide (CCRG 81045: M&B 39831: NSC 362856). Br J Cancer 1992;65:287–91.

[9] Hickman JA, Stevens MFG, Gibson NW, Langdon SP, Fizames C, Lavelle F, et al. Experimental anti-tumor activity against murine tumor model systems of 8-carbamoyl-3-(2-chloroethyl)imidazo[5,1-*d*]-1,2,3,5-tetrazin-4(3*H*)-one (mitozolomide), a novel broad-spectrum agent. Cancer Res 1985;45:3008–13.

[10] Frische S. It is time for full disclosure of author contributions. Nature 2012;489:475.

7

A New Generation of Cell-Targeted Drugs for Cancer Treatment

Paola B. Arimondo[1,2], Nicolas Guilbaud[1], Christian Bailly[1]

[1]Institut de Recherche Pierre Fabre, Centre de Recherche et Développement, Toulouse, France,
[2]USR 3388 CNRS-Pierre Fabre, CRDPF, Toulouse, France

INTRODUCTION

The beginning of the twenty-first century was marked by a new paradigm in the fight against cancer: the development of targeted therapeutics. Monoclonal antibodies and kinase inhibitors have made a breakthrough in the treatment of tumors, aiming at the control of the action of the therapeutic agent on the chosen target. Today, conventional chemotherapy is frequently associated with (or, in some cases, replaced by) monoclonal antibodies, kinase inhibitors, and cell differentiation or immunomodulatory agents. Great progress has been made, and today about 15 kinase inhibitors and a roughly equal number of monoclonal antibodies are prescribed by clinicians for the treatment of solid tumors and leukemia (Fig. 7.1). One of the first approved monoclonal antibodies was trastuzumab (Herceptin®), a humanized antibody against the HER2 receptor, conceived in the 1990s for the treatment of HER2-positive breast cancers. Other HER2-targeting agents were then developed such as lapatinib (Tykerb®), a chemical agent, and pertuzumab (Perjeta®), another antibody. More recently, metastatic melanoma treatment has experienced a marked revolution with the introduction of ipilimumab (Yervoy®), an antibody, and vemurafenib (Plexxikon®), a small compound directed against the mutated kinase BRAF^{V600E} (see Chapter 18 for a detailed discussion of this topic). Indeed, kinase targeting is very promising: bosutinib (Bosulif®), the dual SRC and ABL kinase inhibitor, has improved the treatment of previously treated Philadelphia chromosome–positive chronic myeloid leukemia patients; and crizotinib (Xalkori®) is changing the management of ALK-positive lung cancers. The multikinase inhibitor regorafenib (Stivarga®) and the vascular endothelial growth factor-directed recombinant fusion protein aflibercept (Zaltrap®) are useful for metastatic colon cancer, while ruxolitinib (Jakafi®) is used for myelofibrosis and axitinib (Inlyta®) is useful in the treatment of renal cell carcinoma. The recent advent of immunoconjugates, with antibodies linked to toxins or radioisotopes, brings a new horizon for

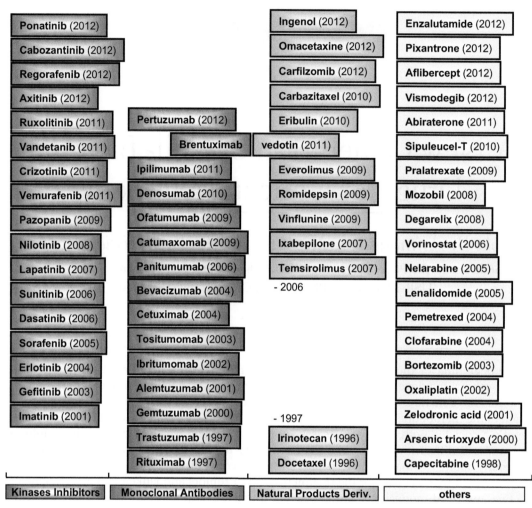

FIGURE 7.1   Four categories of drugs recently approved for the treatment of cancers (year of first US Food and Drug Administration or European Medicines Agency approval). For the sake of clarity, all small molecules are not mentioned. (This figure is reproduced in color in the color plate section.)

antibody-based targeted therapeutics (see Chapter 18). Two examples are the antibody–drug conjugate brentuximab vedotin (Adcetris®), which was approved in 2011 for the treatment of relapsed or refractory Hodgkin's lymphoma, and the immunoconjugate trastuzumab emtansine (T-DM1) for patients with metastatic breast cancer, which is close to registration (Biologics License Application pending). Over the past few years, the number of anticancer agents that has been approved has rapidly increased: more than 60 have been registered in the past 10 years (Fig. 7.1). Among these, natural products and hemisynthetic derivatives are registering a comeback in oncology [1] (see Chapter 17). This is the case, for example, of eribulin (Halaven®) for breast cancer, ingenol mebutate (Picato®) for topical treatment of skin cancer lesions (actinic keratosis), and omacetaxine (homoharringtonine) for chronic myeloid leukemia after

TKI failure. These are examples of new drugs, but there are many others to come in different areas. Take, for example, epigenetics, which has become a promising field for the discovery of new targeted antitumor agents in recent years [2,3]. Four "epigenetic drugs" have been registered since 2004: azacitidine (Vidaza™) and decitabine (Dacogen®) for the treatment of myelodysplastic syndrome and acute myeloid leukemia (AML), and vorinostat (Zolinza®) and romidepsin (Istodax®) for the treatment of cutaneous T-cell lymphoma (CTCL). In 2012, an inhibitor of BRD4 entered clinical trial for the treatment of NUT midline carcinoma [4], and a DOT1L inhibitor for MLL-rearranged leukemia [5]. Interestingly, clinical trials combining DNA methylation inhibitors and histone deacetylase (HDAC) inhibitors gave very positive responses in refractory advanced non-small-cell lung cancers [6]. This domain of cancer chemotherapy is blooming; more epigenetic drugs will no doubt reach the clinic in the near future.

Despite these tremendous progresses with molecularly targeted drugs, conventional cytotoxic agents are still needed [7]. Drugs such as topoisomerase inhibitors, tubulin-targeting drugs, and platinum derivatives, discovered more than 30 years ago, are still widely used, alone (e.g., irinotecan for colon cancer and taxanes in lung cancers) when no other option is available, or frequently in combination with targeted therapeutics (e.g., doxorubicin and cis-platinum). Noteworthy, targeted therapies induce rapid drug resistance, requiring continuous effort in the search for new inhibitors or combination therapies [8]. Therefore, the improvement of conventional cytotoxic agents remains a priority. One of the main drawbacks is the lack of selectivity of these drugs, which may in certain cases cause severe unwanted drug-induced secondary effects (even cancers, in some rare cases). Thus, these nonspecific cytotoxic agents need to be improved, and the targeted therapies have indicated the path: to selectively deliver the cytotoxic agent at the chosen target, the cancer cell. This has led to the use of prodrugs, which combine efficient molecular delivery systems with site-selective drug release, and which represent an emerging class of anticancer agents. An increasing amount of effort is being focused on the optimization of the delivery systems, the cytotoxic agents, and the conjugation playing a role in the release of the molecule at the chosen target. To illustrate the design, conception, and development of this class of drugs and the benefits in safety, tolerability, and thus efficacy that were obtained, we have chosen to describe here two molecules: the prodrug vintafolide and the drug F14512. The advent of targeted therapies, together with genome-wide patient studies, has also introduced the concept of personalized medicine (see Chapter 2 for a detailed discussion of this topic). It is based on the fact that the patients to be treated are chosen because of the presence of the specific target for which the drug is designed. This has required the development of specific biomarkers for each drug. This is the case for vintafolide, which exploits the presence of folate receptors for targeting, and for F14512, which requires active uptake by the polyamide transport system. These two examples, described in this chapter, illustrate the current evolution of cytotoxic therapies in oncology.

VINTAFOLIDE (MK-8109 OR EC145): A NOVEL FOLATE-TARGETED VINCA ALKALOID

Vintafolide is the latest member of a long-established series of *Vinca* alkaloids. As illustrated in Fig. 7.2, starting from vinblastine isolated from the Madagascar periwinkle, vincristine was the first member of this series registered (in 1963) for the treatment of leukemia,

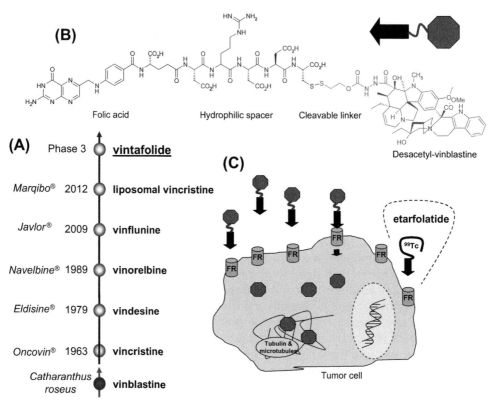

FIGURE 7.2 (A) *Vinca* alkaloids approved for cancer treatments: vinblastine extracted from the Madagascan periwinkle, *Catharanthus roseus*; vincristine (Oncovin®), for leukemia, 1963; vindesine (Eldisine®), for leukemia, 1979; vinorelbine (Navelbine), for NSCLC, 1989, and for breast cancer, 1991; vinflunine (Javlor), for bladder cancer, 2009; liposomal vincristine (Marqibo®), for acute lymphoblastic leukemia, 2012; and vintafolide, currently in phase III for the treatment of ovarian cancer. (B) Structure of vintafolide with its subunits. (C) Illustration of the mode of action of vintafolide: Uptake via the folate receptor (FR) and, after cleavage of the linker, release of the cytotoxic tubulin binder inside the cell to inhibit tubulin polymerization into microtubules and mitotic progression. The technecium (^{99m}Tc)-containing companion imaging agent etarfolatide serves to identify FR-positive tumors by single-photon emission computed tomography. (This figure is reproduced in color in the color plate section.)

followed by vindesine, vinorelbine, and more recently the fluorinated derivative vinflunine (Javlor®), which has been approved in Europe for the treatment of second-line bladder cancer [9]. The first liposomal form of vincristine (Marqibo®) was approved in 2012 to treat adults with Philadelphia chromosome–negative acute lymphoblastic leukemia [10]. The rigid, lipid bilayer of sphingomyelin that encapsulates the drug was designed to allow vincristine to leak out of the liposome slowly, maintaining drug levels for prolonged periods of time. Vintafolide may be the next *Vinca* derivative to be registered, more than 50 years after vincristine, and it represents a novel class of targeted cytotoxic agents as opposed to conventional, non-cell-selective cytotoxic drugs.

Vintafolide exploits the folate receptor (FR) for drug delivery. This concept, introduced in the early 1990s, is based on the high affinity (K_D: 0.1–1 nM) and selectivity of folic acid

(FA, or vitamin B_9) for the FR, which is a glycosylphosphatidylinositol-anchored cell surface glycoprotein. This concept has been successfully exploited to deliver imaging (e.g., the drug surrogate ^{99m}Tc-EC20) [11,12] and therapeutic agents to cells that express FR [13]. Elevated functional FR expression levels have been detected in a variety of cancers, such as ovarian, renal, endometrial, mesothelioma, lung, and breast cancers [14,15]. In a recent study with lung cancers, 72% of adenocarcinomas and 51% of squamous cell carcinomas were found to be strongly positive for the folate receptor, suggesting that folate-linked targeted therapy can potentially be used to treat the majority of lung cancers [16]. Non-small-cell lung cancers (NSCLCs) overexpress folate receptor-alpha (FRα) [17], and the determination of FRα expression would provide prognostic information in patients with lung adenocarcinomas [18]. FRα also plays an important role in the development and progression of other tumors, such as pituitary adenomas [19], but in general FRα status does not influence survival, at least for ovarian cancers [20]. FRα expression is also present in a subset of resected hepatic colorectal cancer metastases [21].

EC145 is a water-soluble *Vinca* alkaloid conjugate incorporating an FA moiety coupled to the microtubule-destabilizing cytotoxic agent desacetyl-vinblastine mono-hydrazine [22]. The FA part acts as a "Trojan horse" for the targeted delivery of the cytotoxic moiety, attached to the carrier via a disulfide-containing peptide-based tether (Fig. 7.2). The molecular spacer controls the proper release of the cytotoxic drug in tumor cells, after delivery. Once the FA–drug conjugate binds the overexpressed FR on epithelial cancer cells (but not in normal tissues), the complex invaginates to form early endosomes inside the tumor cells. The lowering of the pH to <5 via proton pumps located in the endosome membrane causes a conformational change in the FR, enabling release of the FA–drug conjugate. The FR recycles back to the plasma membrane in the late endosome, whereas the FA–drug conjugate remains in the cell to release the cytotoxic moiety, upon reduction of the disulfide bond and self-immolative opening of the acyl hydrazone bond in the acidic milieu of the endosome (Fig. 7.3). The *Vinca* portion escapes endosomal-lysosomal degradation and becomes liberated inside the cell. The Asp–Arg–Asp–Asp–Cys L-peptide moiety (interestingly, the all-D enantiomer is less active) [23], conjugated to the γ-carboxylic acid of folate's glutamyl residue, helps to solubilize the conjugate. The released cytotoxic drug can then diffuse in the cell and play its classical role, disrupting the formation of mitotic spindles and thereby inhibiting cell division and causing cell death, essentially in FR-positive cancer cells, and with little impact on normal tissue unlike the nontargeted drug. In vitro, EC145 was found to bind with high affinity and to produce specific and dose–responsive activity against FR-positive cells. No cell death was observed against FR-negative cells or when FR-positive cells were coincubated with excess FA [24]. In vivo, the activity of EC145 was demonstrated using a variety of FR-positive syngenic and xenograft cancer models, including well-established human nasopharyngeal KB xenografts, even with large tumors (up to 750 mm [3]). Tumor cells within the large malignant mass remain accessible to the FA–drug conjugate, suggesting that the approach may be effective for treating patients with a large inoperable tumor burden. The potent FR-targeted activity and good tolerability of EC145 were confirmed in other in vivo models, including the J6456 lymphoma model [23]. The activity was lost when animals were codosed with an excess of a folate ligand, thus demonstrating the target dependence. Similarly, the unconjugated cytotoxic agent desacetyl-vinblastine was found to be totally inactive when administered at nontoxic doses. Stability of the compound is a concern because premature release of the

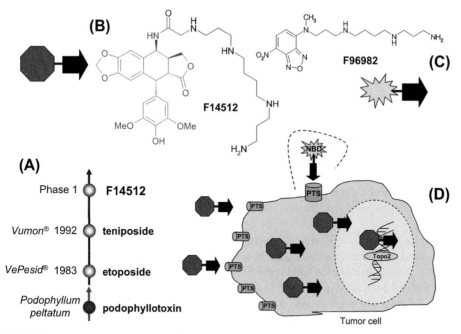

FIGURE 7.3 (A) Podophyllotoxin extracted from *Podophyllum peltatum* is at the origin of the epipodophyllotoxin derivatives etoposide and teniposide, and the new drug candidate F14512. (B) and (C) Structures of F14512 and the probe F96982 containing an NBD fluorescent moiety. (D) Illustration of the cell delivery mechanism and mode of action of F14512: Uptake via the polyamine transport system (PTS) and accumulation into cell nuclei to poison topo-isomerase II–DNA complexes, leading to DNA damage and cell death. The fluorescent probe F96982 is used to analyze the PTS activity in leukemic cells. (This figure is reproduced in color in the color plate section.)

highly cytotoxic payload prior to tumor cell uptake could lead to unwanted nontarget tissue toxicity. But the compound displays rapid blood clearance and concomitantly rapid tumor saturation (a few minutes after intravenous (IV) injection).

The drug entered phase I clinical development in March 2006 for the treatment of patients with refractory or metastatic solid tumors, as an IV bolus injection or a 1 h infusion. The same maximum tolerated dose was determined for the two modes of administration, and for the sake of patient convenience the bolus injection mode was chosen for further clinical studies. Constipation and peripheral neuropathy were the most common and clinically significant tox-icities. During this first-in-humans investigation, the pharmacokinetic profile of EC145 was characterized by rapid distribution and elimination phases of about 6 and 26 min, respectively. The short distribution half-life suggests that the uptake of the conjugate by FR-expressing tissues is very rapid, as anticipated, which is a favorable criterion to limit inactivation reac-tions. The drug is rapidly cleared from the circulation (elimination by both liver and kidney). A systemic clearance of 56.1 L/h with an interindividual variability of 48% in cancer patients was calculated. This phase I study suggested that the toxicity of EC145 is much less than that exhibited during the administration of the free *Vinca* alkaloid. During the phase I trial, one par-tial response to EC145 therapy was observed in a patient with metastatic ovarian cancer [25]. Phase II studies of EC145 were initiated in patients with advanced epithelial ovarian cancer and non-small-cell lung cancer, combined with etarfolatide as a companion imaging agent. Optimal use of vintafolide requires preselection of tumors overexpressing FR. In the clinic, the selection of patients is possible with the use of the radiolabeled conjugate [99mTc]-EC20 as a single-photon emission computed tomography imaging agent for the identification of FR-positive cancers [26], as illustrated in Fig. 7.2. The radiofolate [99mTc]-EC20, also designated FolateScan, is used for both the diagnosis and the staging of FR-positive malignancies and for the localization of inflamed lesions characterized by the accumulation of FR+ macrophages. It can thus be used to image and localize sites of infectious disease [27]. It has been tested for imaging of atherosclerosis in a mice model by selectively targeting FR-positive activated macrophages [28] and for detecting disease activity in patients with rheumatoid arthritis [29]. A randomized phase IIb study (the PRECEDENT trial) in patients with platinum-resistant ovarian cancer—which is an important unmet clinical need—has been completed, and a phase III study (the PROCEED trial) in the same indication is currently accruing patients. The primary endpoint of the trial is progression-free survival as measured by RECIST v. 1.1 (Response Evaluation Criteria in Solid Tumor) criteria in patients with all target tumor lesions positive as assessed by etarfolatide imaging. Overall survival is a secondary endpoint. The trial anticipates recruiting patients at approximately 150 sites in the United States, Canada, Europe, and Asia. Recently, a marketing authorization application has been filed by Merck at the European Medicines Agency for the drug vintafolide and its companion diagnostic imaging agent, etarfolatide, for the targeted treatment of patients with FR-positive platinum-resistant ovarian cancer in combination with pegylated liposomal doxorubicin. Both vinta-folide and etarfolatide have been granted orphan drug status by the European Commission.

In order to try to regulate the biodistribution of EC145 and modulate its gastrointestinal toxicity, a new spacer incorporating a 1-amino-1-deoxy-D-glucitol unit has been designed, without affecting its targeted antitumor activity [30]. The carbohydrate segment spaced in between the FA and *Vinca* moieties confers a shorter elimination half-life, a significant decrease (<70%) in bile clearance, and increased urinary excretion [31]. The new conjugate, EC0489, with an improved therapeutic index, has also been selected as a clinical candidate, with a phase I trial initiated in 2009. But the concept is unchanged. Recently, the very similar compound EC0905, which also incorporates a peptide-based folate spacer with 1-amino-1-deoxy-D-glucitol units, was shown to induce tumor responses of invasive urothelial carcinoma in dogs, suggesting that bladder cancer could be another indication for folate-based drugs [32].

The concept of folate-drug targeting [33] has been exploited with other cytotoxic agents, in particular with mitomycin, but the therapeutic benefit of these FA–mitomycin conjugates was much more modest, and the drugs were apparently not developed clinically [34]. Applied to the microtubule-destabilizing agents tubulysins—secondary metabolites isolated from the myxobacteria *Archangium gephyra* and *Angiococcus disciformis*—it led to a series of FA–tubulysin conjugates and in particular the conjugate of tubulysin B-hydrazide designated EC0305, which displayed antitumor activity superior to EC145 when tested against FR-positive chemo-resistant tumors. Here again, following FR recognition by the FA moiety, tubulysin B is rapidly internalized, entering the cell through FR-mediated endocytosis where the linker is degraded. This conjugate EC0305, which is also well tolerated, was considered for clinical development [35,36]. Other folate-conjugated drugs have been reported, including didemnin B derivatives [37], mitomycin [34,38], epothilone (BMS-753493) [30,39], rapamycin [40], as well as many other polymeric structures (micelles, nanoparticles, dendrimers, etc.) [41]. Other approaches to facilitate the transport of the drug to the target site in tumor cells have been described, such as conjugation to sugars, growth factors, peptides, antibodies, and synthetic polymers. In all cases, the site-specific drug release is achieved by incorporating chemical linkages that are stable under physiological conditions, but cleaved when exposed to specific factors at the delivery site.

A related option consists of targeting the folate receptor with a monoclonal antibody. This is the case of farletuzumab (MORAb-003), a humanized IgG1 antibody targeting FRα that is currently in phase III trial in platinum-sensitive relapsed ovarian cancer [42]. Specifically targeting FRα is essential. Indeed, folic acid and folate-linked drugs bind equally well to both major isoforms of the FR (i.e., FRα, which is primarily expressed on malignant cells, and FRβ, which is upregulated in activated monocytes and macrophages). Drugs targeting only FRα are thus needed. Farletuzumab does not block FRα binding of folates and antifolates, minimally retards folate delivery via FRα-mediated transport, and minimally retards the growth of cells in vitro [43]. This is also a promising anticancer agent. Small molecules, therapeutic drugs, and imaging agents targeting FRα have also been studied [44]. Targeting FRα with small molecules has been investigated as well. The cyclopenta[g]quinazoline-based thymidylate synthase ONX 0801 (formerly BGC 945) is specifically transported into FRα-overexpressing tumors [45,46]. However, this drug does not seem to have been developed further.

F14512: A SPERMINE-CONJUGATED EPIPODOPHYLLOTOXIN

Among various attempts to selectively deliver cytotoxic drugs and improve their efficacy, the polyamine transport system (PTS), which is generally hyperactive in cancer cells, has been considered to be a suitable molecular entry gate for polyamine-based drug delivery [47,48]. Although the importance of polyamine uptake in cancer cells has been extensively documented in the literature, neither the gene(s) nor their molecular structures have yet been identified [49]. Therefore, this approach remains quite empirical, and at present, only indirect methods have been developed and are available to evaluate cytotoxic drug vectorization via the PTS in mammalian cells.

Several examples of polyamine-conjugated anticancer drugs and particularly DNA-interacting agents such as chlorambucil [50], nitroimidazoles [51], enediyenes [52], or camptothecin [53] have contributed to validating the concept of PTS targeting. The enhanced cytotoxicity observed in vitro with these conjugates is largely explained by selective transport via the PTS and the high affinity of polyammonium cations for DNA. However, as a general observation, the increased potency of cytotoxic conjugates has not translated into improved antitumor activity in vivo due to increased side effects in animal models [54].

Whereas the spermine–epipodophyllotoxin conjugate F14512 has been designed by the same strategy [55], recent reviews have emphasized its antitumor potential [55]. The drug features all the required properties of the optimal polyamine drug conjugate: increased cytotoxicity and DNA-binding ability compared to its parent compound, uptake via the PTS, and therefore reduction in toxicity when used in vivo. F14512 can be considered as the most promising anticancer drug in this category, being selected from a large series of compounds derived from a podophyllotoxin core and tethered to natural and unnatural polyamines with a variable spacer. F14512 selection was made from a screening strategy including a topoisomerase II inhibition assay, cytotoxicity studies performed on different PTS-expressing cell lines, and competition experiments with polyamines [56]. Structure–activity relationships displayed a potent specificity for the conjugated tetramine (spermine) compounds, which were more recognized than the triamine (spermidine) ones, while monoamines and diamines showed no selectivity. The importance of the glycyl spacer with an optimal chain length for biological activities of derivatives was also underlined.

Etoposide, discovered in 1961 and launched in 1983 (Fig. 7.3), is still one of the first-line agents in the treatment of NSCLC, testicular tumors, and non-Hodgkin's lymphoma. From a chemical standpoint, F14512 could be simply viewed as another etoposide derivative that contains a spermine in place of the C4 glycosidic moiety. In order to challenge this rather over-simplistic view (or position), an extensive in vitro and in vivo evaluation was performed with the objective to compare and characterize both drugs' pharmacological profiles [57,58]. Etoposide is known as one of the most efficient topoisomerase II inhibitors, endowed with potent anticancer activity. Preliminary results suggested that F14512 can have even more potent (10-fold) topoisomerase II inhibition activity, as observed in a plasmid cleavage assay and potent DNA interaction, on account of its polyamine moiety. While etoposide displays little interaction with DNA in the absence of topoisomerase II, F14512 proved to be a DNA binder capable of protecting DNA from heat denaturation [55]. A subsequent study has confirmed that F14512 functions indeed as a powerful topoisomerase II poison capable of stabilizing topoisomerase II–DNA covalent complexes much more efficiently than etoposide [59]. F14512 produced more single and double DNA strand breaks (DSBs) in vitro than the etoposide derivative TOP-53, which bears a C4 aminoalkyl group that is also involved in the drug–DNA interaction, as is the spermine side chain of F14512. F14512 displayed preferential inhibitory activity toward the α isoform of the enzyme, although it stimulates DNA cleavage mediated by both human topoisomerase IIα and topoisomerase IIβ [59]. A study performed in *Drosophila* models finally confirmed that F14512 induces cleavages at unique sites located in moderately repeated DNA sequences, suggesting that the drug targets a selected and limited subset of genomic sequences [60]. The contribution of DSBs to drug-induced cell death was confirmed with a pair of cell lines harboring respectively normal and deficient DNA repair machinery [55]. In the A549 NSCLC cell line model, F14512 proved to be more than 30-fold more cyto-toxic than etoposide, and triggered less DSBs as demonstrated by cellular phosphor-γH2AX or Comet assays [57]. F14512 is therefore a much more potent topoisomerase II inhibitor than etoposide in vitro, but unexpectedly leads to significantly less DNA breakages *in cellulo*.

The cytotoxic action of F14512 is extremely rapid (within 3 h) but does not lead to a marked accumulation in the S-phase of the cell cycle, in contrast to etoposide. Interestingly, A549 cells treated with F14512 are less prone to undergo apoptosis (neither caspases-dependent nor cas-pases-independent pathways) but preferentially entered into senescence [57]. Drug-induced senescence was characterized qualitatively and quantitatively by increased β-galactosidase activity, both by cytochemical staining and by flow cytometry. Complementary studies indi-cated that senescence arrest induced by F14512 was associated with upregulation of cyclin-dependent kinase inhibitors P16 and cyclin D1, but was also characterized by a marked increase in expression of the protein survivin, a typical inhibitor of apoptosis [61]. It seems obvious that despite close structural similarities and the same mechanism-based cytotoxic activity (topoisomerase II poisoning), differences between F14512 and etoposide in cellular responses, cell cycle arrest, and cell death pathways should reflect distinct pharmacological profiles at the clinical level.

Preclinical evaluation confirmed that F14512 is a far more potent cytotoxic agent than etoposide. In vitro, the polyamine-conjugated drug proved to be superior in 21 out of 29 human solid or hematologic cell lines with a median IC_{50} of 0.18 μM versus 1.4 μM for etoposide [55]. In vivo studies provided evidence of major antitumor activity of F14512 in 13 of 19 models tested [58]. F14512 antitumor effects were demonstrated over a range of 2–5 dose levels, and complete tumor responses were registered in lung LXFL529, sarcoma SXF 1301, and mammary MX1 tumor xenografts. Moreover, F14512 exhibited in vivo activity against the LXFL529/VP tumor subtype, which is partially resistant to etoposide. The 67% tumor response rate obtained with F14512 against the large xenograft panel meets the National Cancer Institute criterion for a new agent and supports its further clinical development [62].

The selective delivery of F14512 in cancer cells via the PTS was validated with two parental or mutated ovarian cell line models (CHO and CHO-MG), respectively expressing high levels of PTS or deficient in PTS. F14512 was found to be 73-fold less cytotoxic against mutated CHO-MG cells as compared to parental ones (IC_{50} values of 8.7 μM and 0.12 μM), while etoposide was equi-cytotoxic against the two cell lines. Competition experiments confirmed that the addition of spermidine to CHO cells resulted in a decrease of sensitivity to F14512. In the same manner, a significant shift in F14512 cytotoxic potency was observed following the addition of 100 μM of spermidine in L1210 murine leukemia cells (PTS+), and resulted in a 2 log increase in the F14512 IC_{50} value. Overall, these data demonstrate that F14512 preferentially uses the PTS to access cells. In A549 NSCLC cells (PTS+), a short contact with F14512 (i.e., a 3 h incubation period) was sufficient to obtain maximal cytotoxic effects, whereas by comparison etoposide needed at least 24 h for maximal effects [57]. The fact that the drug enters cells faster than etoposide underlines the importance of PTS in this gain of efficacy.

The objective of profiling tumor cells according to PTS status has been pursued for several years with fluorescent probes based on the bodipy [63], anthracene [64], or nitrobenzoxadiazole [65] fluorophore scaffolds. The F96982 (N1-methylspermine nitrobenzoxadiazole (NBD)) conjugate was designed and selected from a study assessing 13 probe candidates coupling various linkers to the spermine moiety [66]. F96982 demonstrated optimal stability upon light irradiation, fluorescence yield, and selectivity for PTS-proficient CHO versus PTS-deficient CHO-MG cells. This fluorescent probe (Fig. 7.3) was thus used to validate PTS as a functional biomarker of F14512 sensitivity [67]. Its uptake level was analyzed by fluorescence-activated cell sorting in a panel of hematological cell lines displaying significant differences in term of sensitivity to the drug. As a result, HL-60, BL-41, or CEM cells, for example, gave the highest labeling scores and were found to be among the most sensitive cell lines to F14512, confirming the close correlation between the two parameters. Consistently in the PTS(+) group, F14512 prevented the uptake of the fluorescent probe in a dose-dependent manner. A further study extended these observations ex vivo, the level of fluorescence being higher in cells sampled from solid tumors sensitive to F14512 treatments than those from F14512-refractory tumors [58]. Finally, a radiolabeled ^{99m}Tc-HYNIC spermine probe was successfully injected into mice bearing subcutaneous B16 melanoma, and measurements indicated a tumor-to-muscle scintigraphic ratio of 7.9 ± 2.8 [68]. These results demonstrated that the concept of PTS targeting is valid in vivo and that tumor imaging can be used to identify cancers prone to respond to F14512 treatments or other compounds vectored through the PTS.

F14512 was finally advanced to clinical development based on its high pharmacological activity and acceptable toxicological profile. Particularly, F14512 displayed significant antileukemic activity when examined in vitro in PTS(+) cell lines [67] and in vivo against human AML models. In the disseminated HL-60 model, intermittent administrations of F14512 reduced extensively (and, in a dose-dependent manner, up to 99% of) leukemic cell numbers in mouse bone marrow. It resulted in a significant increase in the life span of F14512-treated HL-60 leukemia-bearing mice, whereas etoposide, tested concurrently, demonstrated a marginal activity only at the highest nontoxic dose. The drug also revealed marked activity against more aggressive AML models directly established from patient samples. These positive results were confirmed and provide a strong rationale for further development of F14512 in oncohematology, either alone or in combination with other antileukemic agents such as cytosine arabinoside (Ara-C). In a first-in-humans multicenter phase I study, 50 patients with refractory or relapsing AML received 1h daily IV infusion for 5 consecutive days every 2 weeks [69]. The main toxicity observed, myelosuppression, was dose dependent and reversible, and the recommended dose was determined as 39 mg/m [2]. Antileukemic activity was observed at different dose levels, with 10% complete responses, 8% complete responses with incomplete recovery, and three patients who experienced hematological improvements. The conclusion of this study was that the clinical outcome of this heavily pretreated population seemed promising, and further clinical development of F14512 is already planned. In conclusion, the concept of selectively targeting cancer cells via PTS still holds great promise, and it is anticipated that the clinical validation of F14512 will continue in the future.

CONCLUSIONS

Despite the fact that they remain widely used, conventional cytotoxic agents are hampered by their lack of specificity, which is often responsible for their undesired side effects. The development of modern targeted therapies has taught us that selectivity based only on the fact that cancerous cells proliferate more than normal cells, and thus are killed more efficiently by cytotoxic agents, is not sufficient, and this is not only because there are also highly proliferating normal cells. It is possible to greatly improve anticancer chemotherapy by directing the drug to the target and, in the case of cytotoxic agents, to tumor cells. This concept is not new, as several prodrugs were conceived in the 1990s to deliver, for example, anthracyclines but it is experiencing today a renaissance thanks to the progress made in antibody technologies, coupling chemistry, and knowledge of the cancer microenvironment. The examples of vintafolide and F14512 reported here illustrate this new challenge in oncology and the benefits that these molecules can bring to patients. Very important is the association of a specific prognostic biomarker that enables the clinician to determine whether the patient will benefit from the targeted agent.

These are just two examples among many new conjugates that have emerged from oncology research to enter clinical development. Efforts are mainly concentrated on finding new ligands that direct and release the cytotoxic agent with high selectivity for tumor cells. We will conclude by citing some further examples, although the list is not exhaustive. The use of positively charged peptides has been largely used. Since findings with penetratin [70], the third helix of the homeodomain of the *Antennapedia* protein, simplified peptides are now exploited such as oligoarginines, and used to overcome efflux-based drug resistance [71]. Due to their synthetic accessibility, peptides that recognize specific proteins or receptors are being used as RGD (arginine–glycine–aspartate) peptides, binding α(v)β(3) integrin [72] or peptide hormones [73]. In the latter case, one of the established key hallmarks of cancerous cells is exploited, the fact that they overexpress receptors transmitting pro-growth signals. The same feature is used in the development of ligands mimicking the high affinity of steroidal estrogens for their receptors [74]. Another class of highly selective ligands is nucleic acids such as aptamers, nucleic acids that, upon folding, bind strongly to particular proteins. Doxorubicin, for example, has been conjugated with success to a DNA aptamer recognizing MUC1 [75].

These are just a few examples. Clearly, cell-targeted drug delivery constitutes a major future direction in the development of the next generation of cytotoxic agents for the management of cancer.

Acknowledgments

We wish to thank colleagues from the Institut de Recherche Pierre Fabre (IRPF, Toulouse, France) for their dedicated work on anticancer agents.

References

[1] Bailly C. Ready for a comeback of natural products in oncology. Biochem Pharmacol 2009;77:1447–57.
[2] Sharma S, Kelly TK, Jones PA. Epigenetics in cancer. Carcinogenesis 2010;31:27–36.
[3] Baylin SB, Jones PA. A decade of exploring the cancer epigenome—biological and translational implications. Nat Rev Cancer 2011;11:726–34.
[4] Schwartz BE, Hofer MD, Lemieux ME, Bauer DE, Cameron MJ, West NH, et al. Differentiation of NUT midline carcinoma by epigenomic reprogramming. Cancer Res 2011;71:2686–96.
[5] Daigle SR, Olhava EJ, Therkelsen CA, Majer CR, Sneeringer CJ, Song J, et al. Selective killing of mixed lineage leukemia cells by a potent small-molecule DOT1L inhibitor. Cancer Cell 2011;20:53–65.
[6] Juergens RA, Wrangle J, Vendetti FP, Murphy SC, Zhao M, Coleman B, et al. Combination epigenetic therapy has efficacy in patients with refractory advanced non-small cell lung cancer. Cancer Discov 2011;1:598–607.
[7] Ismael GF, Rosa DD, Mano MS, Awada A. Novel cytotoxic drugs: old challenges, new solutions. Cancer Treat Rev 2008;34:81–91.
[8] De Palma M, Hanahan D. The biology of personalized cancer medicine: facing individual complexities underlying hallmark capabilities. Mol Oncol 2012;6:111–27.
[9] Schutz FA, Bellmunt J, Rosenberg JE, Choueiri TK. Vinflunine: drug safety evaluation of this novel synthetic vinca alkaloid. Expert Opin Drug Saf 2011;10:645–53.
[10] Heffner Jr L. A new formulation of vincristine for acute lymphoblastic leukemia. Clin Adv Hematol Oncol 2011;9:314–6.
[11] Leamon CP, Parker MA, Vlahov IR, Xu LC, Reddy JA, Vetzel M, et al. Synthesis and biological evaluation of EC20: a new folate-derived, (99m)Tc-based radiopharmaceutical. Bioconjug Chem 2002;13:1200–10.
[12] Reddy JA, Xu LC, Parker N, Vetzel M, Leamon CP. Preclinical evaluation of (99m)Tc-EC20 for imaging folate receptor-positive tumours. J Nucl Med 2004;45:857–66.
[13] Vlahov IR, Leamon CP. Engineering folate-drug conjugates to target cancer: from chemistry to clinic. Bioconjug Chem 2012;23:1357–69.
[14] Parker N, Turk MJ, Westrick E, Lewis JD, Low PS, Leamon CP. Folate receptor expression in carcinomas and normal tissues determined by a quantitative radioligand binding assay. Anal Biochem 2005;338:284–93.
[15] Chen YL, Chang MC, Huang CY, Chiang YC, Lin HW, Chen CA, et al. Serous ovarian carcinoma patients with high alpha-folate receptor had reducing survival and cytotoxic chemo-response. Mol Oncol 2012;6:360–9.
[16] Cagle PT, Zhai QJ, Murphy L, Low PS. Folate receptor in adenocarcinoma and squamous cell carcinoma of the lung: potential target for folate-linked therapeutic agents. Arch Pathol Lab Med 2012.
[17] Nunez MI, Behrens C, Woods DM, Lin H, Suraokar M, Kadara H, et al. High expression of folate receptor alpha in lung cancer correlates with adenocarcinoma histology and EGFR [corrected] mutation. J Thorac Oncol 2012;7:833–40.

[18] O'Shannessy DJ, Yu G, Smale R, Fu YS, Singhal S, Thiel RP, et al. Folate receptor alpha expression in lung cancer: diagnostic and prognostic significance. Oncotarget 2012;3:414–25.

[19] Liu X, Ma S, Yao Y, Li G, Feng M, Deng K, et al. Differential expression of folate receptor alpha in pituitary adenomas and its relationship to tumour behavior. Neurosurgery 2012;70:1274–80. discussion 1280.

[20] Crane LM, Arts HJ, van Oosten M, Low PS, van der Zee AG, van Dam GM, et al. The effect of chemotherapy on expression of folate receptor-alpha in ovarian cancer. Cell Oncol (Dordrecht) 2012;35:9–18.

[21] D'Angelica M, Ammori J, Gonen M, Klimstra DS, Low PS, Murphy L, et al. Folate receptor-alpha expression in resectable hepatic colorectal cancer metastases: patterns and significance. Mod Pathol 2011;24:1221–8.

[22] Vlahov IR, Santhapuram HK, Kleindl PJ, Howard SJ, Stanford KM, Leamon CP. Design and regioselective synthesis of a new generation of targeted chemotherapeutics. Part 1: EC145, a folic acid conjugate of desacetylvinblastine monohydrazide. Bioorg Med Chem Lett 2006;16:5093–6.

[23] Reddy JA, Dorton R, Westrick E, Dawson A, Smith T, Xu LC, et al. Preclinical evaluation of EC145, a folate-vinca alkaloid conjugate. Cancer Res 2007;67:4434–42.

[24] Leamon CP, Reddy JA, Vlahov IR, Westrick E, Parker N, Nicoson JS, et al. Comparative preclinical activity of the folate-targeted *Vinca* alkaloid conjugates EC140 and EC145. Int J Cancer 2007;121:1585–92.

[25] Lorusso PM, Edelman MJ, Bever SL, Forman KM, Pilat M, Quinn MF, et al. Phase I study of folate conjugate EC145 (vintafolide) in patients with refractory solid tumours. J Clin Oncol 2012;30:4011–6.

[26] Low PS, Kularatne SA. Folate-targeted therapeutic and imaging agents for cancer. Curr Opin Chem Biol 2009;13:256–62.

[27] Henne WA, Rothenbuhler R, Ayala-Lopez W, Xia W, Varghese B, Low PS. Imaging sites of infection using a 99mTc-labeled folate conjugate targeted to folate receptor positive macrophages. Mol Pharm 2012;9:1435–40.

[28] Ayala-Lopez W, Xia W, Varghese B, Low PS. Imaging of atherosclerosis in apolipoprotein e knockout mice: targeting of a folate-conjugated radiopharmaceutical to activated macrophages. J Nucl Med 2010;51:768–74.

[29] Matteson EL, Lowe VJ, Prendergast FG, Crowson CS, Moder KG, Morgenstern DE, et al. Assessment of disease activity in rheumatoid arthritis using a novel folate targeted radiopharmaceutical Folatescan. Clin Exp Rheumatol 2009;27:253–9.

[30] Vlahov IR, Vite GD, Kleindl PJ, Wang Y, Santhapuram HK, You F, et al. Regioselective synthesis of folate receptor-targeted agents derived from epothilone analogs and folic acid. Bioorg Med Chem Lett 2010;20:4578–81.

[31] Leamon CP, Reddy JA, Klein PJ, Vlahov IR, Dorton R, Bloomfield A, et al. Reducing undesirable hepatic clearance of a tumour-targeted vinca alkaloid via novel saccharopeptidic modifications. J Pharmacol Exp Ther 2011;336:336–43.

[32] Dhawan D, Ramos-Vara JA, Naughton JF, Cheng L, Low PS, Rothenbuhler R, et al. Targeting folate receptors to treat invasive urinary bladder cancer. Cancer Res 2013;73:875–84.

[33] Low PS, Antony AC. Folate receptor-targeted drugs for cancer and inflammatory diseases. Adv Drug Deliv Rev 2004;56:1055–8.

[34] Reddy JA, Westrick E, Vlahov I, Howard SJ, Santhapuram HK, Leamon CP. Folate receptor specific anti-tumour activity of folate-mitomycin conjugates. Cancer Chemother Pharmacol 2006;58:229–36.

[35] Leamon CP, Reddy JA, Vetzel M, Dorton R, Westrick E, Parker N, et al. Folate targeting enables durable and specific antitumour responses from a therapeutically null tubulysin B analogue. Cancer Res 2008;68:9839–44.

[36] Reddy JA, Dorton R, Dawson A, Vetzel M, Parker N, Nicoson JS, et al. In vivo structural activity and optimization studies of folate-tubulysin conjugates. Mol Pharm 2009;6:1518–25.

[37] Henne WA, Kularatne SA, Ayala-Lopez W, Doorneweerd DD, Stinnette TW, Lu Y, et al. Synthesis and activity of folate conjugated didemnin B for potential treatment of inflammatory diseases. Bioorg Med Chem Lett 2012;22:709–12.

[38] Leamon CP, Reddy JA, Vlahov IR, Westrick E, Dawson A, Dorton R, et al. Preclinical antitumour activity of a novel folate-targeted dual drug conjugate. Mol Pharm 2007;4:659–67.

[39] Gokhale M, Thakur A, Rinaldi F. Degradation of BMS-753493, a novel epothilone folate conjugate anticancer agent. Drug Dev Ind Pharm 2012.

[40] Shillingford JM, Leamon CP, Vlahov IR, Weimbs T. Folate-conjugated rapamycin slows progression of polycystic kidney disease. J Am Soc Nephrol 2012;23:1674–81.

[41] Lu Y, Low PS. Folate targeting of haptens to cancer cell surfaces mediates immunotherapy of syngeneic murine tumours. Cancer Immunol Immunother 2002;51:153–62.

[42] Teng L, Xie J, Teng L, Lee RJ. Clinical translation of folate receptor-targeted therapeutics. Expert Opin Drug Deliv 2012;9:901–8.

[43] Kamen BA, Smith AK. Farletuzumab, an anti-folate receptor alpha antibody, does not block binding of folate or anti-folates to receptor nor does it alter the potency of anti-folates in vitro. Cancer Chemother Pharmacol 2012;70:113–20.

[44] Vaitilingam B, Chelvam V, Kularatne SA, Poh S, Ayala-Lopez W, Low PS. A folate receptor-alpha-specific ligand that targets cancer tissue and not sites of inflammation. J Nucl Med 2012;53:1127–34.

[45] Gibbs DD, Theti DS, Wood N, Green M, Raynaud F, Valenti M, et al. BGC 945, a novel tumour-selective thymidylate synthase inhibitor targeted to alpha-folate receptor-overexpressing tumours. Cancer Res 2005;65:11721–8.

[46] Pillai RG, Forster M, Perumal M, Mitchell F, Leyton J, Aibgirhio FI, et al. Imaging pharmacodynamics of the alpha-folate receptor-targeted thymidylate synthase inhibitor BGC 945. Cancer Res 2008;68:3827–34.

[47] Palmer AJ, Ghani RA, Kaur N, Phanstiel O, Wallace HM. A putrescine-anthracene conjugate: a paradigm for selective drug delivery. Biochem J 2009;424:431–8.

[48] Xie S, Wang J, Zhang Y, Wang C. Antitumour conjugates with polyamine vectors and their molecular mechanisms. Expert Opin Drug Deliv 2010;7:1049–61.

[49] Poulin R, Casero RA, Soulet D. Recent advances in the molecular biology of metazoan polyamine transport. Amino Acids 2012;42:711–23.

[50] Holley JL, Mather A, Wheelhouse RT, Cullis PM, Hartley JA, Bingham JP, et al. Targeting of tumour cells and DNA by a chlorambucil-spermidine conjugate. Cancer Res 1992;52:4190–5.

[51] Holley J, Mather A, Cullis P, Symons MR, Wardman P, Watt RA, et al. Uptake and cytotoxicity of novel nitroimidazole–polyamine conjugates in Ehrlich ascites tumour cells. Biochem Pharmacol 1992;43:763–9.

[52] Suzuki I, Uno S, Tsuchiya Y, Shigenaga A, Nemoto H, Shibuya M. Synthesis and DNA damaging ability of enediyne model compounds possessing photo-triggering devices. Bioorg Med Chem Lett 2004;14:2959–62.

[53] Dallavalle S, Giannini G, Alloatti D, Casati A, Marastoni E, Musso L, et al. Synthesis and cytotoxic activity of polyamine analogues of camptothecin. J Med Chem 2006;49:5177–86.

[54] Verschoyle RD, Carthew P, Holley JL, Cullis P, Cohen GM. The comparative toxicity of chlorambucil and chlorambucil–spermidine conjugate to BALB/c mice. Cancer Lett 1994;85:217–22.

[55] Barret JM, Kruczynski A, Vispe S, Annereau JP, Brel V, Guminski Y, et al. F14512, a potent antitumour agent targeting topoisomerase II vectored into cancer cells via the polyamine transport system. Cancer Res 2008;68:9845–53.

[56] Imbert T, Guminski Y, Cugnasse S, Grousseaud M, Barret J-M, Kruczynski A, et al. Abstract A87: synthesis and structure-activity relationships of a series of epipodophyllotoxin polyamine conjugated derivatives vectorized for active polyamine transporter system in tumour cells, leading to the selection of F14512 for clinical trials. Mol Cancer Ther 2009;8:A87.

[57] Brel V, Annereau JP, Vispe S, Kruczynski A, Bailly C, Guilbaud N. Cytotoxicity and cell death mechanisms induced by the polyamine-vectorized anti-cancer drug F14512 targeting topoisomerase II. Biochem Pharmacol 2011;82:1843–52.

[58] Kruczynski A, Vandenberghe I, Pillon A, Pesnel S, Goetsch L, Barret JM, et al. Preclinical activity of F14512, designed to target tumours expressing an active polyamine transport system. Invest New Drugs 2011;29:9–21.

[59] Gentry AC, Pitts SL, Jablonsky MJ, Bailly C, Graves DE, Osheroff N. Interactions between the etoposide derivative F14512 and human type II topoisomerases: implications for the C4 spermine moiety in promoting enzyme-mediated DNA cleavage. Biochemistry 2011;50:3240–9.

[60] Chelouah S, Monod-Wissler C, Bailly C, Barret JM, Guilbaud N, Vispe S, et al. An integrated *Drosophila* model system reveals unique properties for F14512, a novel polyamine-containing anticancer drug that targets topoisomerase II. PLoS One 2011;6:e23597.

[61] Ballot C, Jendoubi M, Kluza J, Jonneaux A, Laine W, Formstecher P, et al. Regulation by survivin of cancer cell death induced by F14512, a polyamine-containing inhibitor of DNA topoisomerase II. Apoptosis 2012;17:364–76.

[62] Johnson JI, Decker S, Zaharevitz D, Rubinstein LV, Venditti JM, Schepartz S, et al. Relationships between drug activity in NCI preclinical in vitro and in vivo models and early clinical trials. Br J Cancer 2001;84:1424–31.

[63] Soulet D, Gagnon B, Rivest S, Audette M, Poulin R. A fluorescent probe of polyamine transport accumulates into intracellular acidic vesicles via a two-step mechanism. J Biol Chem 2004;279:49355–66.

[64] Phanstiel O t, Kaur N, Delcros JG. Structure-activity investigations of polyamine-anthracene conjugates and their uptake via the polyamine transporter. Amino Acids 2007;33:305–13.

[65] Ware BR, Klein JW, Zero K. Interaction of a fluorescent spermine derivative with a nucleic acid polyion. Langmuir 1988;4:458–63.

[66] Guminski Y, Grousseaud M, Cugnasse S, Brel V, Annereau JP, Vispe S, et al. Synthesis of conjugated spermine derivatives with 7-nitrobenzoxadiazole (NBD), rhodamine and bodipy as new fluorescent probes for the polyamine transport system. Bioorg Med Chem Lett 2009;19:2474–7.

[67] Annereau JP, Brel V, Dumontet C, Guminski Y, Imbert T, Broussas M, et al. A fluorescent biomarker of the polyamine transport system to select patients with AML for F14512 treatment. Leuk Res 2010;34:1383–9.

[68] Pesnel S, Guminski Y, Pillon A, Lerondel S, Imbert T, Guilbaud N, et al. 99mTc-HYNIC-spermine for imaging polyamine transport system-positive tumours: preclinical evaluation. Eur J Nucl Med Mol Imaging 2011;38: 1832–41.

[69] De Botton S, Berthon C, Bulabois CE, Prebet T, Vey N, Chevallier P, et al. F14512 a novel polyamine-vectorized anti-cancer drug targeting topoisomerase II in adult patients with acute myeloid leukemia (AML): results from a phase 1 study. Heamaltologica 2012;97:447.

[70] Dupont E, Prochiantz A, Joliot A. Penetratin story: an overview. Methods Mol Biol 2011;683:21–9.

[71] Wender PA, Galliher WC, Bhat NM, Pillow TH, Bieber MM, Teng NN. Taxol-oligoarginine conjugates overcome drug resistance in-vitro in human ovarian carcinoma. Gynecol Oncol 2012;126:118–23.

[72] Danhier F, Breton AL, Preat V. RGD-based strategies to target alpha(v) beta(3) integrin in cancer therapy and diagnosis. Mol Pharm 2012;9:2961–73.

[73] Mezo G, Manea M. Receptor-mediated tumour targeting based on peptide hormones. Expert Opin Drug Deliv 2010;7:79–96.

[74] Dao KL, Hanson RN. Targeting the estrogen receptor using steroid-therapeutic drug conjugates (hybrids). Bioconjug Chem 2012;23:2139–58.

[75] Hu Y, Duan J, Zhan Q, Wang F, Lu X, Yang XD. Novel MUC1 aptamer selectively delivers cytotoxic agent to cancer cells in vitro. PLoS One 2012;7:e31970.

Inhibition of DNA Repair as a Therapeutic Target

Stephany Veuger, Nicola J. Curtin

Newcastle University, Northern Institute for Cancer Research, Newcastle upon Tyne, UK

INTRODUCTION

Targeting DNA for Cancer Treatment

Cytotoxic radiotherapy and chemotherapy remain the mainstays of treatment despite the introduction of molecularly targeted agents. With the goal of inducing DNA lesions that trigger cell cycle arrest and ultimately cell death, DNA is the main target for a large repertoire of anticancer agents, including ionizing radiation (IR) and most cytotoxic chemotherapeutics. IR induces a plethora of DNA damage of which the double-strand break (DSB) is considered the most cytotoxic. Chemotherapeutic agents include the alkylating agents, which are (or are metabolized into) reactive electrophilic compounds that react with electron-rich moieties in DNA; the antimetabolites that impair the DNA synthesis, either by incorporation of chemically altered nucleotides or by depleting the supply of deoxynucleotides for replication; and the topoisomerase poisons that turn essential enzymes into DNA break inducers.

Several DNA repair pathways have evolved to maintain genomic integrity in the face of endogenous and environmental DNA damage [1,2]. In quiescent normal cells, these repair pathways are adequate to cope with the induced DNA damage before they attempt to replicate the damaged template. However, cancer cells proliferate rapidly, and this partially underlies the success of DNA-damaging anticancer therapy. Antitumor activity results from DNA lesions that persist during DNA replication (S phase of the cell cycle) and obstruct DNA replication forks, causing cell death or potentially lethal mutations, or DNA damage remaining when cells divide (M phase), which leads to chromosomal breakage that is also catastrophic for cell survival. This most likely explains why chemotherapy is tolerable to most normal tissues but highly toxic to cancer cells, and the dose-limiting toxicities are frequently manifest in rapidly dividing normal cells such as the bone marrow and gut epithelium.

Cancer Drug Design and Discovery, Second Edition
http://dx.doi.org/10.1016/B978-0-12-396521-9.00008-5

A second explanation for the efficacy of DNA-damaging anticancer agents in specifically killing cancer cells is the imbalance of DNA damage signaling and repair pathways in cancer cells compared to normal cells. The DNA damage response (DDR) responsible for the signaling and repair of DNA lesions represents a barrier that is inactivated during tumor development [3]. Loss of elements of the DDR, required to create the genomic instability to enable cancer to develop, renders tumors more susceptible to DNA damage.

Roles of DNA Repair in Cancer

Several DNA repair pathways exist to repair specific types of DNA damage. These include pathways repairing one strand of DNA, such as base excision repair (BER), nucleotide excision repair (NER), and mismatch repair (MMR); and those repairing DSBs, such as non-homologous end joining (NHEJ) and homologous recombination repair (HRR). Genomic instability is considered an enabling characteristic of cancer and a prerequisite explaining all the mutations required to develop a malignant tumor [4,5]. Defects in DNA repair are often associated with an increase in mutation rates or gene rearrangements that contribute to genetic instability, which accelerates further genetic changes and progression of cancer development. Redundancy exists within repair pathways, and loss of one pathway may impair but not totally block repair. Therefore, defects in one pathway leading to tumorigenesis may be compensated for by upregulation of a complementary or "back-up" pathway. Cancer cells can become "addicted" to the backup repair pathways to maintain survival.

Genes responsible for DNA damage detection and repair essentially behave as tumor suppressors. Inherited mutations in DNA repair genes are therefore often associated with an increased risk of cancer as a result of increased genomic instability. For example, inherited defects in MMR predispose carriers to hereditary nonpolyposis colon cancer, also known as Lynch syndrome [6]. Furthermore, an inherited defect in HRR, an important DSB repair pathway, predisposes carriers to breast and ovarian cancers [7]. Carriers of these mutations have one functional allele, but tumor development is dependent on somatic inactivation of the second allele rendering tumor cells' repair defective. The success of different treatment regimens may therefore reflect the frequency of a defect in different tumor types.

DNA repair is an important determinant of treatment efficiency. For example, high levels of DNA repair contribute to removal of DNA lesions, resulting in resistance and failed cancer treatments. Defects in DNA mismatch repair confer resistance to a variety of anticancer drugs [8], while HRR-defective tumors are highly sensitive to DNA cross-linkers (bifunctional alkylators) [9]. Thus, it should be possible for patients to be stratified according to the DDR status of their tumor.

Rationale to Inhibit DNA Repair during Cancer Treatment

Targeting DNA is a successful strategy in anticancer therapy; however, as discussed in this chapter, DNA repair can influence therapy outcome. Inhibition of DNA repair therefore represents an excellent strategy for cancer therapy, particularly where repair is amplified in a tumor versus normal tissue or where a tumor is reliant on a pathway for survival. DNA repair inhibitors can reverse repair-mediated resistance and increase the activity of radio- and chemotherapy by increasing the amount or persistence of DNA lesions that lead to cancer cell death. Although upregulated DNA repair pathways can be a mechanism of resistance to anti-cancer agents, the loss of other pathways, creating an imbalance in the DDR, can be exploited through specific inhibition of the remaining or upregulated repair pathway. Thus, the dys-regulated DDR in cancer and differences in repair capabilities between normal and tumor tissue represent both challenges and opportunities for cancer treatment. Here, we describe how inhibitors of enzymes involved in a range of repair pathways may increase the efficacy of anticancer drugs.

O⁶-ALKYLGUANINE DNA ALKYLTRANSFERASE

Development and Mechanism of Action of DNA-Alkylating Agents

DNA-alkylating agents as a class are among the oldest anticancer drugs. They were devel-oped from the chemical warfare agent mustard gas, which was used in the trenches during World War I. Nitrogen mustard, introduced into clinical use in 1942, was the first derivative. This class of anticancer agent still plays an important role in the chemotherapy of several cancers, including leukemia, melanoma, and brain tumors [10]. Their cytotoxic effects are attributable to their ability to alkylate nucleophilic sites (especially nitrogen and oxygen) in DNA. Alkylating agents are generally considered to be cell cycle phase nonspecific, mean-ing that they can kill the cell in all phases of the cell cycle. They are either monofunctional agents, e.g. temozolomide (TMZ) that react with a single DNA base or bifunctional agents e.g. nitrogen mustard analogs, that react with two bases and hence cross-link DNA strands. The most numerous lesions are at the N^7 position of guanine, but the most cytotoxic lesion is alkylation at the O^6 position of guanine. Chemotherapeutically induced alkylation of the O^6 position of guanine results from methylation, following treatment with monofunctional DNA-methylating agents such as TMZ, dacarbazine or procarbazine, and chloroethylation resulting from treatment with chloroethylating nitrogen mustards, N,N'-bis(2-chloroethyl)-N-nitrosourea (BCNU, or carmustine) and N-(2-chloroethyl)-N'-cyclohexyl-N-nitrosourea (CCNU, or lomustine). O^6 methylation of guanine results in mispairing, and cell death is induced by triggering the MMR system into futile cycles of repair and activation of apoptosis. Chloroethylation at the O^6 position of guanine is followed by the reaction of the other alkyl group with an adjacent or opposite base and the formation of an intra- or interstrand cross-link (Fig. 8.1).

Role of O⁶-Alkylguanine DNA Alkyltransferase in Repair and Resistance to Alkylating Agents

The simplest form of repair is the direct reversal of the lesion. O^6-alkylguanine DNA alkyltransferase (AGT) also known as O^6-methylguanine DNA methyltransferase (MGMT), catalyzes the transfer of alkyl substituents (e.g. methyl- and 2-chloroethyl-) from the O^6 position of guanine to an active cysteine (Cys145) acceptor site within the protein (Fig. 8.2). AGT is responsible for the direct demethylation of guanine methylated at the O^6 position. By doing so, AGT impairs the cytotoxic action of both methylating and chloroethylating agents, such as TMZ, and mediates a major resistance pathway to these drugs [11]. The

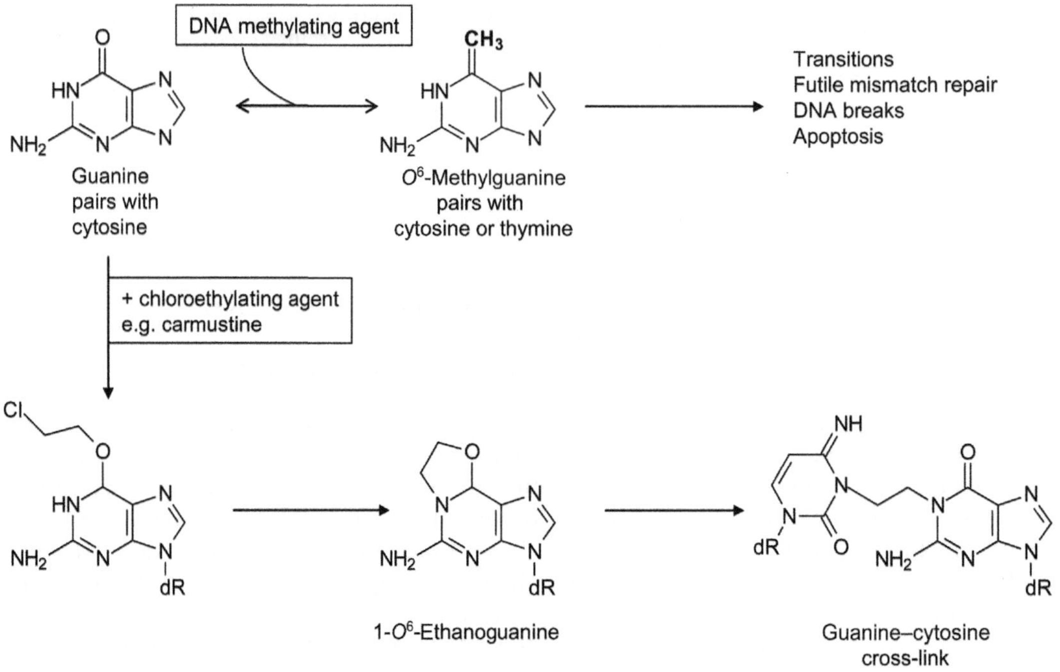

FIGURE 8.1 DNA damage caused by alkylating agents. The cytotoxic effects of both methylating agents (top) and chloroethylating agents (bottom) is largely due to modification at the O^6 position of guanine.

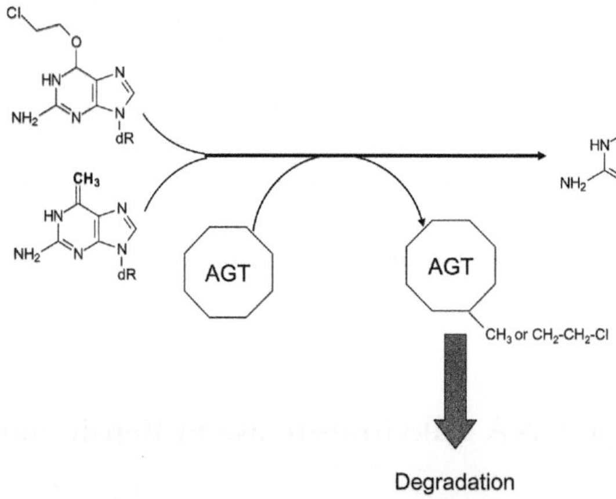

FIGURE 8.2 Repair of O^6-alkylguanine by AGT and its subsequent inactivation and degradation. AGT catalyzes the transfer of the methyl or chloroethyl group attached to the O^6 position of guanine to its active site cysteine, which then targets AGT for degradation.

reaction is stoichiometric and inactivates AGT, which is then ubiquitinated and digested by proteasomes [12]. Importantly, to regenerate AGT activity, synthesis of new molecules is required. Thus, the capacity to repair O^6-alkylguanine lesions is dependent on the abundance of AGT.

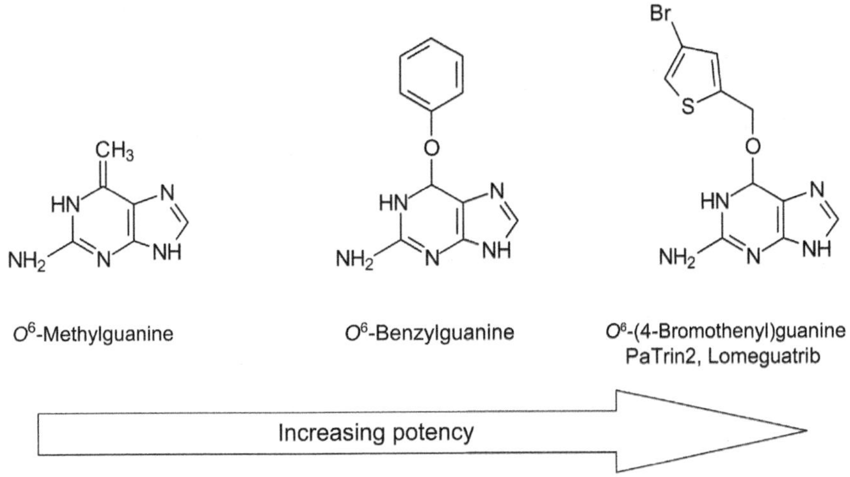

FIGURE 8.3 AGT inactivators.

Tumors have an increased capacity for therapeutic resistance to alkylating agents. AGT levels are generally higher in tumors compared to normal tissues [13], and preclinical studies have demonstrated a strong correlation between AGT activity and resistance to alkylating agents, For example, high-AGT-expressing tumors are fourfold to 10-fold more resistant to TMZ and chloroethylating agents [14,15]. Moreover, clinical studies have shown that reduced AGT protein expression and silencing of the *MGMT* gene (which encodes AGT) by promoter methylation in gliomas are associated with increased sensitivity to TMZ and BCNU [16–18].

Development of AGT Inhibitors: Preclinical Data

On the basis of the correlation of AGT levels with resistance, it was predicted that using a pseudosubstrate to deplete the levels of AGT within the tumor and normal tissues to a similar level would overcome resistance.

The preferred substrate of AGT is O^6-methylguanine in double-stranded DNA (dsDNA), but guanine base derivatives, alkylated at the O^6 position, also deplete AGT. Free O^6-methylguanine was the first AGT inactivator to be developed, but its lack of potency and poor solubility limited its use to "proof-of-principle" studies. O^6-benzylguanine (BG), developed in the 1990s, was around 2000× more potent than O^6-methylguanine with an EC50 of 0.2 μM (Fig. 8.3). BG preexposure completely depleted AGT and substantially increased CCNU cytotoxicity in human colon (HT29) cells in vitro [19]. Sensitization to TMZ was dependent on MMR function, but BCNU sensitization was MMR status independent [20,21]. BG is metabolized to 8-oxo-O^6-BG, which has similar potency and a longer half-life [22]. Advanced preclinical studies demonstrated that BG depleted AGT in tumor and normal tissues in mice bearing human tumor xenografts and increased the antitumor activity of TMZ and BCNU (reviewed in Ref. [23]). However, bone marrow toxicity was also increased. Several other O^6-alkylated guanine analogs have been developed [24], but only O^6-(4-bromothenyl)guanine (PaTrin-2, Lomeguatrib), which is around 10× more potent than O^6-BG and showed promising activity in preclinical studies [25], has undergone clinical evaluation (Fig. 8.3).

Clinical Trials with AGT Inhibitors

The first clinical trial with BG was reported in 1998 [26]. This and subsequent clinical trials showed that BG was nontoxic at doses that depleted AGT activity ($120\,mg/m^2$) in both surrogate normal tissues (lymphocytes) and tumor tissue, including gliomas, confirming its ability to cross the blood–brain barrier. However, it enhanced TMZ- and BCNU-induced myelosuppression, requiring substantial dose reductions of the primary cytotoxic (reviewed in Refs [23,27]). In general, these trials have not shown significant clinical benefit, and despite various administration schedules (e.g., in combination with BCNU-impregnated Gliadel wafers in patients with surgically resected glioma), dose-limiting toxicities were observed and the drug has not progressed beyond phase II trials. PaTrin-2 is also under clinical evaluation; oral administration of $10\,mg/m^2$ inhibited AGT in lymphocytes and tumor biopsies. It was inherently nontoxic and only reduced the MTD (maximum tolerated dose) of TMZ by 25%, and there were some initial responses [28]. However, in subsequent phase II trials with $10\,mg/m^2$ lomeguatrib in combination with TMZ, it failed to show any substantial activity in colon cancer or melanoma patients [29,30]. Confounding effects may have been the high frequency of MMR defects in colon cancer or incomplete MGMT inhibition, as studies show that $120–180\,mg/m^2$ are needed for complete depletion in human tumors [31].

BASE EXCISION REPAIR AND SINGLE-STRAND BREAK REPAIR

The most common endogenous lesions are single base lesions, which arise from processes such as deamination, oxidation, or alkylation of bases, and nicks, which may result from the processing of base lesions or be induced directly from sugar damage (estimated at $10^4–10^5$ lesions/day) [1]. Alkylations result from aberrant methylation by S-adenosyl methionine, and the spontaneous deamination of cytosine to generate uracil in the DNA is a relatively common event. However, the most common lesions are the result of oxidation leading to the formation of 8-oxo-guanine and 5-hydroxycytosine, which mispair with adenine and thymine, respectively [1,32]. The major sources of this damage are reactive oxygen species (ROS) that are largely byproducts of oxidative phosphorylation in mitochondria. In cancer cells, there are high levels of ROS such that the estimated steady-state level of 8-oxo-G lesions is about 10^5 lesions per cell per day in cancer tissues compared to 100-fold lower levels in normal tissues [33].

These lesions are repaired by the BER and single-strand break repair (SSBR) pathways, which are often considered to be synonymous because they involve many of the same components. BER involves the excision of the damaged bases, the generation of a break, and its subsequent repair, whereas SSBR is involved only after the generation of the nick. Therapeutically induced substrates for BER are the methylated DNA bases following treatment with agents such as TMZ. Nicks can also be generated by damage to the deoxyribose backbone by ROS, arising endogenously and therapeutically following irradiation. They can also result from the trapping of topoisomerase I–DNA complexes, for example with topoisomerase I poisons, such as camptothecin derivatives. In practice, the entire pathway is generally referred to as BER. BER is subdivided into short- and long-patch repair corresponding to the removal and replacement of a single nucleotide or 1–13 nucleotides, respectively. The pathway operates throughout the cell cycle. In the first step, the oxidized, deaminated, or alkylated bases are removed by specific glycosylases that bind DNA and flip out the affected base from the minor groove. Endogenous and therapeutically induced alkylation depends on alkyladenine DNA glycosylase (AAG) for this step [34]. The resulting apurinic or apyrimidinic (AP) site is then hydrolyzed by an AP endonuclease, with the major ones being AP endonuclease-1 (APE-1 aka Ref-1 or HAP-1) or AP lyase. The nick in the DNA is then repaired by short- (pre-dominant) or long-patch BER depending on the nature of the 5′ and 3′ ends and, possibly, ATP availability. In short-patch repair, the single nucleotide is replaced by Polβ, and the gap is rejoined by ligase IIIα; in long-patch repair, up to 13 nucleotides are replaced by pol δ/ε and rejoining is completed by ligase I [35–37]. Polynucleotide kinase phosphatase (PNKP) may be necessary to modify the broken ends. PCNA (proliferating cell nuclear antigen), 9-1-1, and Fen-1 are required for the processing of long patches. PARP-1 and XRCC1 facilitate the repair by recruiting repair enzymes and providing the scaffold for short- and long-patch BER.

The BER pathway is an attractive target for the development of inhibitors with the goal of achieving chemo- and radiosensitization. Most studies have focused on the development of inhibitors of PARP-1 or APE-1.

Role of PARP in DNA Repair

Poly(ADP-ribose)polymerase 1 (PARP-1) is the founding, most abundant, and best char-acterized member of a superfamily of 17 PARP enzymes. Only PARP-1 and PARP-2 are direct participants in BER [38]. Both enzymes have DNA damage-recognizing regions at their N-terminus, a central automodification domain, and a highly conserved catalytic domain at the C-terminus (Fig. 8.4).

DNA nicks may be formed by the removal of a damaged base (e.g., N^7-methylguanine) resulting from exposure to DNA-methylating agents, such as TMZ-induced base damage or damaged bases and breaks induced by oxygen radicals after ionizing radiation. PARP-1 and PARP-2 bind to these nicks, which activates their catalytic activity to facilitate repair. Upon activation, PARP-1 (or 2) catalyzes the cleavage of NAD^+, releasing nicotinamide and syn-thesizing long homopolymers of ADP-ribose attached to PARP-1 (or 2) itself (automodifica-tion) or other nuclear proteins (heteromodification), particularly histone H1 and H2B tails. The

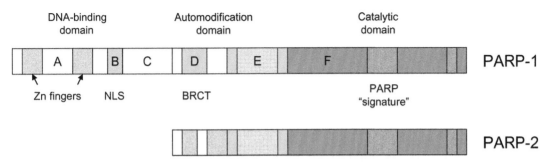

FIGURE 8.4 Structure of PARP-1 and PARP-2. PARP-1 has three functional domains, a DNA-binding domain with two zinc fingers and a nuclear localization signal, an automodification domain containing the BRCT (BRCA1 C terminus) domain, and a catalytic domain containing the highly cross-species conserved "PARP signa-ture". PARP-2 is substantially similar to PARP-1 but with a reduced automodification domain.

synthesis of ADP-ribose polymers in the vicinity of the break is necessary for the recruitment of XRCC1, and the loosening of chromatin to facilitate repair [39] (Fig. 8.5). XRCC1 then recruits and stimulates the other enzymes (DNA polβ and DNA ligase III for short-patch repair, or PNK, DNA Pol δ/ε, PCNA, Fen-1, and ligase I for long-patch repair) with which PARP-1 and -2 also interact [40].

Where investigated, PARP activity is significantly higher in tumor tissue compared with normal tissues, possibly reflecting higher levels of endogenous DNA damage or DNA repair defects that are compensated for by higher PARP activity [41,42]. PARP is a very attractive target for sensitizing tumors to DNA damage that depends on BER or SSBR for its repair.

PARP has also been implicated in DSB repair. DNA double-strand ends provide a powerful stimulus for PARP activation [43], and PARP inhibition has been shown to retard DNA DSB rejoining [44]. PARP-1 may participate in NHEJ and has been shown to exist in a complex with DNA-PKcs and Ku70/80, which are important components of the NHEJ pathway [45,46] and may stimulate DNA-PK activity [47]. Combined use of PARP-1 and DNA-PK inhibitors resulted in synergistic radiosentization [48,49]. Alternatively, PARP is thought to participate in an alternative or backup NHEJ, A-NHEJ (reviewed in Ref. [50]).

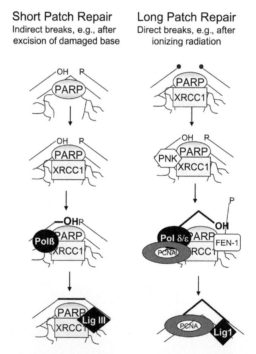

FIGURE 8.5 Base excision repair (BER) and single-strand break repair (SSBR). PARP-1 is involved in both short- and long-patch BER and SSBR. It binds to and is activated by the nick, recruiting the scaffold protein, XRCC1. In the case of simple nicks (e.g., after removal of a damaged base), XRCC1 then recruits DNA polymerase β and ligase II to fill in and religate the gap, respectively. Long-patch BER, in the case of nicks with inappropriate termini, involves the additional recruitment of PNK and PCNA and the synthesis of a short stretch of complementary DNA by DNA polymerase δ/ε, before removal of a short oligo of the damaged strand by Flap endonuclease-1 (FEN-1) and relegation by ligase I.

Development of PARP Inhibitors

The observation that the by-product of NAD$^+$ cleavage by PARP, nicotinamide, is itself a weak PARP inhibitor led to the initial inhibitor development, and most PARP inhibitors today have the nicotinamide pharmacophore incorporated into their structure. The first generation PARP inhibitors were simple analogs of nicotinamide with carbon substituting for the nitrogen at position 3: the 3-substituted benzamides. The prototype PARP inhibitor, 3-aminobenzamide, was first shown to retard the repair of strand breaks and reduce survival following exposure to DNA-methylating agents in 1980 [51]. Although the benzamides helped elucidate the function of PARP, they lacked sufficient potency (requiring millimolar concentrations for cellular activity) or specificity for PARP-1 to allow preclinical evaluation.

Later research led to the development of ever more potent and specific inhibitors, including NU1025 and PD128763, which were as much as 50× more potent than 3AB [52,53]. Using an "analogue by catalogue" approach, Banasik et al. [54] screened commercially available compounds and identified several potent PARP inhibitors, including isoquinolinones and quinazolinones, which have been used as leads for further PARP inhibitor development. These two alternative approaches uncovered structure–activity relationships (SARs) that enabled the identification of features required for potent PARP inhibition: most notably, an electron-rich aromatic or polyaromatic heterocyclic system with a carboxamide group with the carbonyl group in the *anti* conformation to the ring. The reason why these structural features were associated with potency became apparent when the PARP inhibitors PD128763, 4-aminonaphthalimide, and NU1025 were co-crystallized in the NAD$^+$ binding site of PARP-1, revealing important interactions between the carboxamide and critical amino acids, Ser904-OG and Gly863-N in the catalytic domain [55,56]. Using structural biology to direct chemical synthesis resulted in the development of several highly potent inhibitors, in which the carboxamide group was held in the favorable orientation by incorporation into a seven-membered ring [57–60]. AG-014699 (rucaparib) [61] with a K_i of 1.4 nM was the first PARP inhibitor to enter clinical trial for cancer patients [62]. Several other PARP inhibitors have entered clinical investigation such as Veliparib (ABT-888), which also has low nM K_i against both PARP-1 and PARP-2 [63], and olaparib (AZD2281) with nMolar IC$_{50}$ values against PARP-1 and PARP-2 [64] (reviewed in Refs [65–67]) (Fig. 8.6).

Preclinical Radio- and Chemosensitization Studies with PARP Inhibitors

Preclinical studies have revealed that PARP inhibitors potentiate the cytotoxicity and anti-tumor activity of DNA-methylating agents (e.g., TMZ) topoisomerase I poisons, and ionizing radiation, with these observations being confirmed by genetic manipulation of PARP-1 (reviewed in Refs [66–70]). Some studies have also indicated that PARP inhibitors could potentiate cisplatin [71,72], while others do not support these findings, which is perhaps due to cell-specific DNA repair defects.

DNA-Methylating Agents

Monofunctional alkylating agents are the most potent activators of PARP, and PARP plays an important role in the resistance to DNA-methylating agents. Several studies

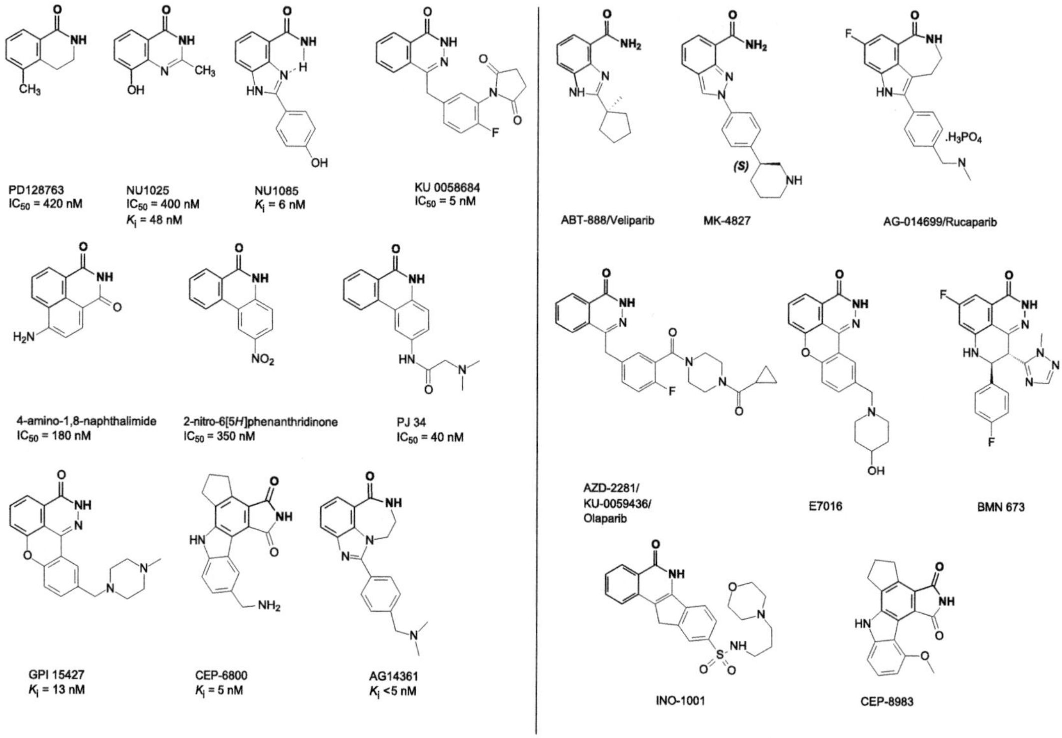

FIGURE 8.6   PARP inhibitors in preclinical and clinical investigation compounds to the left of the vertical line represent preclinical leads; those to the right are compounds under clinical investigation. The nicotinamide pharmacophore is shown in bold.

have investigated TMZ chemosensitization by PARP inhibitors (reviewed in Refs [73,74]). The second-generation inhibitors (e.g., PD128763 and NU1025 (50–100 μM)) increased TMZ-induced DNA strand breakage and caused a four- to sevenfold potentiation of TMZ cytotoxicity at concentrations 50–100× lower than 3AB [75]. Chemosensitization was irrespective of tissue of origin or p53 status [76]. The more potent PARP inhibitors (Fig. 8.6) have also demonstrated marked potentiation of TMZ at submicromolar concentrations. For example, GPI 15427 (1–2 μm) enhanced TMZ growth inhibition in human glioblastoma cells and a panel of colon cancer cell lines [77,78]. Interestingly, ABT-888 preferentially enhanced TMZ cytotoxicity during the S phase, indicating that replication-associated lesions are the most cytotoxic [79].

Several PARP inhibitors have been investigated in xenograft studies. ABT-888 potentiated TMZ-induced tumor growth delay in a variety of subcutaneous, orthotopic, and metastatic xenograft models of some of the most common and difficult-to-treat human cancers [80]. This compound crosses the blood–brain barrier and significantly enhances the antitumor activity of TMZ against intracranial human primary glioblastoma and in models of breast cancer brain metastases [80–82]. AG-014699 (rucaparib) increased TMZ activity against xenograft models of pediatric cancers neuroblastoma and medulloblastoma [83,84]. Complete tumor regressions have been observed in mice bearing U251MG (human glioblastoma) tumors treated with TMZ and CEP-6800 [85], and in SW620 (human colon cancer) xenografts treated with TMZ in combination with AG14361 and AG14447 [57,61]. It was these latter studies that led to the first anticancer clinical trial of a PARP inhibitor (the phosphate salt of AG14447: AG-014699 (rucaparib)) in 2003.

A major mechanism of cellular resistance to TMZ is loss of mismatch repair (MMR), which renders the cell insensitive to the cytotoxicity of O^6-alkyguanine, and MMR deficiency relates to poor response to TMZ in patients with malignant glioma. Various PARP inhibitors (3AB, PD128763, NU1025, AG14361 INO-1001, and ABT-888) were found to enhance TMZ cytotoxicity preferentially in MMR-deficient cells compared to MMR-proficient ones and, in some cases, xenografts, completely overcoming MMR-mediated resistance [21,86–89]. Since only tumors lack MMR, PARP inhibition, in combination with TMZ, represents a potentially selective therapeutic approach.

Topoisomerase I Poisons

Since the initial observations that NU1025 markedly enhanced camptothecin-induced DNA breaks and cytotoxicity and that both NU1025 and NU1085 potentiated topotecan in a panel of human cancer cell lines [76,90], several studies have investigated the therapeutic potential of PARP inhibitors in combination with topoisomerase I poisons. Topoisomerase I is a cellular enzyme that forms a transient complex with DNA catalyzing the cleavage, unwinding, and religation of DNA to reduce torsional stress. The topoisomerase I poisons stabilize the cleavable complex in the broken state. Topoisomerase I poisons, such as the camptothecin derivatives, irinotecan and topotecan, are important components of the arsenal of DNA-damaging agents used in cancer chemotherapy. Cytotoxicity is related to the number of DNA single-strand breaks (SSBs), and the sensitivity to topoisomerase I poisons is therefore directly proportional to topoisomerase I activity.

The mechanisms proposed for the potentiation include de-repression of topoisomerase I activity and inhibition of repair. Although there is some evidence that PARP-1 regulates topoisomerase I activity in response to DNA damage [91], a more likely scenario is that PARP-1 is involved in the repair of topoisomerase I–associated DNA damage. PARP-1 knockout cells and human leukemic cells treated with AG14361 exhibited slower repair of topoisomerase I poison–induced DNA strand breaks and enhanced sensitivity to topoisomerase I–induced cytotoxicity. The mechanism was proposed to be via an effect on BER and SSBR rather than regulation of topoisomerase I activity since BER-defective cells were not sensitized to topoisomerase I poisons by AG14361, and AG14361 did not affect topoisomerase I activity [92]. XRCC1 recruits TDP-1, which removes topoisomerase I from the DNA [93], and PARP-1 may promote this activity by recruiting XRCC1. Poly(ADP-ribosyl)ated PARP-1 and PARP-2, but not the unmodified enzymes, accelerate the removal of camptothecin-stabilized topoisomerase I–DNA cleavable complexes [94].

Several studies have investigated the therapeutic potential of PARP inhibitors in combination with topoisomerase I poisons. Sensitization is generally modest (two- to threefold) compared to the DNA-methylating agents (>fivefold). GPI 15427 increased SN-38 (the active metabolite of irinotecan) cytotoxicity in a panel of colon cancer cell lines [78], and AG14361 potentiated topotecan-induced growth inhibition in human colon and lung cancer cells [57]. AG14447 (the parent compound of AG-014699, rucaparib), caused sensitization of topotecan in human colon cancer cell lines [61]. An indication that PARP inhibitors were acting via inhibition of PARP activity and repair came from the demonstration that in PARP wild-type mouse embryonic fibroblasts (MEFs), but not PARP null MEFs, AG14361 and ABT-888 (veliparib) increased the persistence of topoisomerase I poison–induced DNA breaks and enhanced cytotoxicity [92,95].

In vivo studies have demonstrated that irinotecan-induced tumor growth delay in mice bearing human colon cancer xenografts was enhanced 60% by CEP-6800 (30 mg/kg) [85]. Similarly, AG14361 (5 and 15 mg/kg) and GPI15427 (40 mg/kg) also increased irinotecan-induced tumor growth delay [57,78], confirming the in vitro data. AG014699 (rucaparib) increased tumor growth delay following treatment with topotecan in a neuroblastoma model [84].

Ionizing Radiation

Radiotherapy is a major cancer treatment modality employed in as many as 50% of cancer patients. It causes a variety of DNA damage, which includes base damage and frank DNA breaks that are known targets for PARP-mediated repair. The first PARP inhibitor, 3AB, was shown to increase IR-induced cytotoxicity in mammalian cells [96]. These initial studies have been confirmed by radiosensitization studies using a variety of PARP inhibitors (PARPi) (ANI, NU1025, AZD2281, and E7016) in multiple cell line models with dose enhancement ratios of 1.3–1.7 [90,97–100]. PARP inhibitors have been shown to enhance IR cytotoxicity to cells in both the radiosensitive proliferating state and the radioresistant growth-arrested state. Several PARP inhibitors have been shown to radiosensitize replicating cells [54], possibly by retarding the repair of IR-induced SSBs that convert to DSBs upon collision with replication forks in the S phase [101]. This would be consistent with the observed persistence of IR-induced γH2AX foci (indicative of DNA DSB and collapsed replication forks) following PARPi treatment (AZD2281/olaparib and E7016) [98,99] and increased γH2AX foci and RAD51 foci (indicative of increased homologous recombination at stalled replication forks) [102]. Alternative studies in growth-arrested cells indicate that PARP inhibition inhibits the recovery from potentially lethal IR in colon cancer cells between 50% and 90% [57,61]. These observations have clinical importance as growth-arrested hypoxic radioresistant cells can repopulate the tumor after radiotherapy and are a major contributing factor to failure of radiotherapy treatment [103].

These cell-based data have been confirmed in a variety of xenograft studies. The first studies were using PD128763, which enhanced the therapeutic effect of X-rays up to threefold in mice bearing sarcomas [104]. Later, AG14361 increased the efficacy of fractionated X-rays against human colon cancer xenografts [57], GPI15427 increased the radiosensitivity of head and neck squamous cell carcinoma (HNSCC) xenografts [105], MK-4827 radiosensitized human lung and breast carcinoma xenografts [106], and AZD-2281 (olaparib) radiosensitized small-cell lung cancer xenografts [107]. The PARP inhibitor that has been investigated the most is ABT-888 (veliparib), which significantly increased the antitumor activity of IR in xenograft models of human colon, lung, and prostate cancers [82,108,109]. ABT-888 also significantly potentiated the combination of TMZ and IR in mice bearing intracranial gliomas [81]. Some of the radiosensitization may be due to a vasoactive effect of the PARP inhibitors, which has been demonstrated for AG14361, AG-014699 (rucaparib), and AZD-2281 (olaparib) [107,110,111].

Clinical Trials with PARP Inhibitors

The spectacular responses seen with AG14361 and AG14447 in combination with TMZ in xenograft studies [57,61] led to the first clinical trial of a PARP inhibitor, the phosphate salt of AG14447 (AG-014699, rucaparib), in combination with TMZ in 2003 [62]. In this study, a dose-dependent increase in PARP inhibition in surrogate normal tissues (peripheral blood mononuclear cells, or PBMCs) and tumor biopsies was observed, and a PARP-inhibitory dose (PID) of $12\,mg/m^2$ was not toxic with full-dose TMZ. AG014699 at the PID caused around 90% PARP inhibition in the tumors. Myelosuppression was observed in subsequent phase II studies of the combination in melanoma patients treated with full-dose TMZ ($200\,mg/m^2$) and $12\,mg/m^2$ rucaparib, necessitating TMZ dose reductions [112]. Nevertheless, despite the reduced dose of TMZ, the study reported an increase in the response rate and median time to progression compared to historical reports of TMZ alone. In contrast to these data, olaparib did not improve the response to dacarbazine (DTIC, a closely related drug to TMZ) [113], and dose-limiting myelosuppression was observed with the combination of INO-101 with TMZ [114].

In clinical trials with topoisomerase I poisons, toxicities have also been observed. In a phase I study, the combination of ABT-888 (veliparib) with topotecan resulted in profound myelosuppression. The schedule was revised after further preclinical investigations, and the MTD was established as topotecan $0.6\,mg/m^2/d$ with ABT-888 10 mg twice daily on days 1–5 of a 21-day schedule. In this study, PARP activity was reduced in both tumor cells and PBMCs, and, importantly, increased DNA breaks were detected in circulating tumor cells and PBMCs and some disease stabilization was observed [115]. Dose-limiting diarrhea and neutropenia were observed in a study of veliparib in combination with irinotecan [116], and dose-limiting neutropenia and thrombocytopenia were seen in a phase I study of olaparib and topotecan at low doses, so further dose levels were not explored [117]. A summary of the clinical trials with PARP inhibitors is given in Table 8.1.

Clinical trials with PARP inhibitors in combination with radiotherapy have been initiated, but to date there are no final reports. An interim report, published in abstract form, showed that up to 200 mg ABT-888 (veliparib) twice daily was well tolerated in combination with whole-brain radiotherapy in patients with brain metastases from advanced solid tumors [118]. The appeal of such studies is that the toxicities seen with the chemotherapy combinations may be avoided as the treatment is targeted to the tumour.

Role of APE-1 in BER and SSBR

Another approach to block BER is to inhibit the human AP endonuclease APE-1, also known as Ref-1 or HAP-1. APE-1 is the major mammalian AP endonuclease and acts on abasic or 3′-blocking DNA lesions such as those generated by IR. AP sites block replication and are both cytotoxic and mutagenic. APE-1 recognizes the AP site and cleaves the phosphodiester bond 5′ to the AP site, leaving 5′-deoxyribophosphate and a 3′ hydroxyl terminus, which then becomes the target for the rest of the BER–SSBR pathway. Deletion of APE-1 is embryonically lethal [119], and depletion of APE-1 leads to the accumulation of AP sites, which inhibits proliferation and promotes cell death [120]. DSBs persist under APE-1 deficiency [121]. Moreover, high APE-1 is associated with drug and radiotherapy resistance, it is elevated in several

TABLE 8.1   PARP Inhibitors in Clinical Trial

Name of company and date started	Single agent or combinations	Tumor type	ROUTE or current stage
AG-014699/PF0367338 CO-338 rucaparib Pfizer (now Clovis Oncology) 2003	TMZ combination Various combinations Single agent	Solid tumors Melanoma Solid tumors BRCA mutant breast ovarian	IV Oral Phase II
KU59436/AZD2281 Olaparib AstraZeneca 2005	Single agent Various combinations	Solid tumors BRCA carriers TNBC and HGSOC Solid tumors	Oral Phase II
ABT-888 veliparib Abbott 2006	Single agent Various combinations	Various solid +lymphoblastoid tumours	Oral Phase II
INO-1001 Inotek/Genentek 2003/6	TMZ combinations	Melanoma	IV Phase I (terminated)
MK4827 Merck 2008	Single agent Combinations with TMZ or doxorubicin	Solid and hematological tumors GBM Ovarian	Oral Phase II Phase I
CEP-9722 Cephalon 2009	Single agent Combination with TMZ Gem/cis	Solid tumors Lymphoma	Oral Phase I
GPI21016/E7016 MGIPharma/ Eisai 2010	Combination with TMZ	Melanoma	Oral Phase II
BMN-673 BioMarin 2011	Single agent	Various solid and hematological tumors	Oral Phase I

tumor types, and inactivation of APE-1 confers sensitivity to IR and alkylating agents in the lab setting, making APE-1 an attractive target for the development of inhibitors [122–124].

Development of APE-1 Inhibitors

Several groups have generated small-molecule inhibitors of APE-1. There are two classes of inhibitors: molecules like methoxyamine (MX), which binds to AP sites blocking APE-1 binding and hence function, and those that inhibit the APE-1 endonuclease activity. Like PARP inhibitors, they potentiate DNA-methylating agents such as TMZ, but, unlike PARP inhibitors, they enhance the activity of agents that lead to the misincorporation of fraudulent nucleotides. Such agents include the antifolate inhibitors of thymidylate synthase (e.g., pemetrexed) that deplete the cells of thymidine nucleotides and lead to the misincorporation of uracil.

MX reacts with the aldehyde group in the sugar moiety of the AP site, forming an MX-bound AP site that cannot be repaired by APE-1. In preclinical studies, MX increased TMZ-induced DNA SSBs and DSBs, and potentiated TMZ in a variety of in vitro and in vivo models [125]. Potentiation of TMZ in ovarian cancer cells was shown to be p53 independent, and MX also showed very impressive activity against human colon cancer xenografts [126,127]. MX also enhanced the radiosensitization by iododeoxyuridine (IUdR), which was thought to be due to increased incorporation or persistence of IUdR in the DNA and hence greater radiosensitization [128]. Promising preclinical activity has been documented using MX and pemetrexed combinations, and the mechanism is related to uracil misincorporation and its excision by uracil glycosylase [129]. MX (TRC102) is now undergoing clinical evaluation in several trials in patients with advanced refractory cancers. A phase I trial in combination with pemetrexed has been reported with 14 out of 25 (including four out of five non-small-cell lung cancer (NSCLC)) patients showing a response at tolerable doses, and there is an ongoing study with TMZ [130].

Screening for inhibitors of APE-1 endonuclease activity has been facilitated by HTS (high throughput screening) using a dsDNA substrate that mimics an AP site with a fluorescent label on one strand and a quencher on the other. When the AP site is cut, the strand dissociates and there is an increase in fluorescence. Inhibition of APE-1 therefore results in a reduction of the fluorescence signal [131]. Hits identified by this assay are then subject to more vigorous evaluation. Lucanthone (a topoisomerase II inhibitor) was demonstrated to inhibit APE-1 endonuclease activity and potentiate DNA-methylating agents in breast cancer cells in the laboratory setting [132]. Lucanthone has also been shown to potentiate radiotherapy in patients with brain metastases [133]. APE-1 endonuclease inhibitors identified by in silico modeling and the fluorescence-based assay, including CRT0044876 (7-nitroindole-2-carboxylic acid), increased the persistence of AP sites and cytotoxicity in various in vitro models following alkylating agent treatment [122,131,132,134–136].

MISMATCH REPAIR (MMR)

MMR is a highly conserved pathway to correct replication errors. Those resulting from insertion of the wrong nucleotide are recognized by MSH2 and MSH6, whereas deletions and insertions are recognized by MSH2–MSH3 heterodimers. Downstream processing requires hPMS2 and MLH1–MLH3 heterodimers [137,138]. Importantly, MMR is strand specific, correcting the daughter strand. This is critical for the repair of replication errors inserted opposite the correct template strand under normal circumstances. MMR contributes significantly to genomic stability, and disruption of the MMR pathway increases mutation rates up to 1000-fold [139]. Lynch syndrome, or hereditary nonpolyposis colorectal cancer (HNPCC), which predisposes to gastric, endometrial, and ovarian cancers, is due to MMR defects. MLH1 or MSH2 mutations and silencing of MLH1 by promoter methylation may be responsible for a high proportion of sporadic cancers in these organs [140–146].

MMR is often characterized by microsatellite instability (MSI). Microsatellites are short nucleotide repeats nonrandomly distributed about the genome; polymerase slippage is more common in these repetitive sequences, resulting in the deletions, and sometimes insertions, that are the target of the MMR machinery. Because there are microsatellites in genes involved in other DNA repair pathways, loss of MMR function can result in defects in these repair pathways as well. MMR knockout mice are viable without obvious developmental abnormalities; however, some gene knockouts are sterile. All exhibit the mutator phenotype, and most develop spontaneous tumors, largely lymphomas and gastrointestinal and skin cancers, with the most cancer-prone being Msh2 and Mlh1 null mice (reviewed in Ref. [147]).

The strand specificity of MMR has implications for therapeutically induced DNA damage. Damage on the template strand causes mispairing at replication, but the MMR machinery attempts to repair the newly synthesized strand rather than the damaged one. This results in DNA DSB during the second S phase [148]. Alternatively, cell death may result from signaling by the MMR machinery to ATR–CHK1 and apoptosis [149]. Defects in MMR cause tolerance to DNA-alkylating agents (e.g., TMZ, procarbazine, MNNG N-methyl-N-nitro-N-nitrosoguanidine, and MNU (methylnitrosourea)), platinum agents, and nucleoside analogs: 6TG, mercaptopurine, and 5FU [150]. Whereas studies in colon cancer cell lines indicate that MMR defects are associated with resistance to 5FU, clinical investigations in colon cancer patients with HNPCC or MSI treated with 5FU are somewhat contradictory, no doubt because of the many and varied determinants of sensitivity to 5FU [151–154]. Interestingly, depletion of MSH2 and MSH6 confers sensitivity to Ara-C, fludarabine, and clofarabine, suggesting that these drugs might be useful therapeutically in cancers associated with these defects [155]. Reduced expression of MMR proteins is seen in relapsed glioma after TMZ therapy, and mutations cause TMZ resistance in patients [156,157]. Despite ample preclinical evidence of MMR defects causing resistance to cisplatin, the association with survival of ovarian cancer patients treated with cisplatin is weak, although expression of MMR proteins is reduced after platinum therapy [158].

Since inactivation of MMR confers resistance to many anticancer agents, inhibitors of MMR would not serve to enhance current treatments or circumvent resistance. Rather, the rationale is to attempt to reactivate MMR, particularly through reversal of epigenetic silencing. To this end, it has been shown that methylation of MLH1 can be reversed using the demethylating agent 2′deoxy-5-azacytidine. After promising preclinical data demonstrated chemosensitization of cisplatin, carboplatin, TMZ, and epirubicin [159], clinical trials were initiated in combination with carboplatin and with TMZ, but a phase II trial in combination with carboplatin in gynecological cancer had to be abandoned due to adverse reactions (www.clinical trials. gov, identifier NCT00748527).

DOUBLE-STRAND BREAK REPAIR: NONHOMOLOGOUS END JOINING

DSBs are difficult to repair, and, if left unrepaired, DSBs will trigger cell cycle arrest and/ or cell death [160]. Cells have, out of necessity, developed complex mechanisms to repair DNA DSBs, and such repair constitutes a potential mechanism of therapeutic resistance to therapeutically induced DSBs. Therapeutically induced DSBs result directly from exposure to IR and topoisomerase II poisons, and indirectly from the collision of the replication fork with the single-stranded lesion. Topoisomerase II is an essential enzyme that acts as a dimer to relieve superhelical stress, and the topoisomerase II poisons, which are used to treat nearly one-half of all cancers, lock the complex in the open-gate conformation, creating a persistent protein-associated DSB [161]. IR induces approximately one DSB for every 25 SSBs, but the radiomimetics bleomycin and neocarzinostatin produce a higher frequency of DSBs (10% and 30% of the total breaks, respectively) [162–164].

NHEJ and HRR are the major DSB repair pathways. HRR is a high-fidelity repair pathway using the sister chromatid as a template and can therefore function only during the S and G2 phases of the cell cycle. NHEJ is more error-prone (up to 20 nucleotides can be lost from each end) but is active in all phases of the cell cycle, predominating in G0/G1 [165], and is estimated to repair up to 85% of IR-induced DSBs [166–168].

The Role of DNA-PK in DNA DSB Repair

The core NHEJ proteins are Ku70/80, DNA-PKcs, Artemis XRCC4, ligase IV, and XLF (XRCC4-like factor). DNA-PK, originally identified independently in 1990 by three groups, is a trimeric protein composed of a large catalytic subunit, DNA-PKcs (469 kDa) and the Ku70/80 heterodimer (reviewed in Ref. [169]). The Ku heterodimer binds dsDNA ends, and this promotes the recruitment and activation of the DNA-PK catalytic subunit (DNA-PKcs) to form the DNA-PK holoenzyme necessary to bring about synapsis of the DNA ends (Fig. 8.7). The kinase activity of DNA-PKcs is essential for NHEJ [170]. Although DNA-PKcs can phosphorylate other NHEJ components and H2AX, this does not seem to be essential, and the only conclusively identified physiological target is DNA-PKcs itself allowing dissociation [166,171]. Artemis processes the DNA ends, and the final ligation of the juxtaposed ends is accomplished by the XRCC4–XLF–ligase IV complex [172–174].

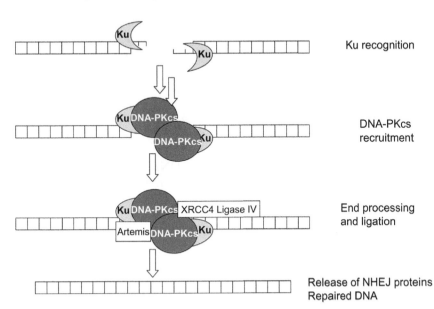

FIGURE 8.7   Model of nonhomologous end joining (NHEJ): the Ku heterodimer binds to the broken DNA ends, recruiting and activating DNA-PKcs to bring about synapsis and to signal the damage to the other NHEJ components. Artemis may be recruited to process the ends, which are then rejoined by XRCC4 and ligase IV, following which the NHEJ complex is released from the repaired DNA.

Cells defective in NHEJ are sensitive to ionizing radiation and topoisomerase II poisons [175,176]. Thus, prevention of the repair of DSBs produced by anticancer agents, including IR, through the inhibition of DNA-PK is an attractive approach to modulating therapy resistance.

Development of DNA-PK Inhibitors

DNA-PK is a serine–threonine protein kinase member of the phosphatidylinositol-3 kinase (PI3K)-related protein kinase (PIKK) family of enzymes. Inhibitors of PI3K, such as wortmanin and LY294002, are noncompetitive and competitive inhibitors of DNA-PK, respectively [177]. Both compounds retard DNA DSB rejoining and enhance the cytotoxicity of IR and the topoisomerase II poison, etoposide, most probably by inhibiting DNA-PKcs, although both can inhibit other members of the PI3K family of enzymes, including ATM (ataxia telangiectasia mutated), at higher concentrations [178–180]. Using LY294002 as a lead, more potent and specific DNA-PK inhibitors have been developed, such as NU7026 (2-(morpholin-4-yl)-benzo[h] chromen-4-one), NU7441 (2-N-morpholino-8-dibenzothiophenyl-chromen-4-one), IC86621, and IC87361 (Fig. 8.8). NU7441 was highly potent and specific with an IC_{50} of only 14 nM and at least 100-fold selectivity for this enzyme compared with other PI3K family kinases [181,182]. CP466722 was identified by library screening [183]. All of the inhibitors substantially slow DSB repair; increase the cytotoxicity and antitumor activity of ionizing radiation, radiomimetics, and topoisomerase II poisons in cells and xenografts in a variety of models; and have been shown to be DNA-PK specific by comparing their sensitization effects in cells with and without DNA-PKcs [48,184–187].

NU7441 showed cellular specificity for DNA-PK, as demonstrated by lack of activity in DNA-PK–deficient V3 cells but profound sensitization of DNA-PKcs–complemented V3-YAC cells to IR and etoposide. NU7441 substantially retarded the repair of IR- and etoposide-induced DNA DSB and increased G2–M accumulation and cytotoxicity induced by IR, etoposide, and doxorubicin in human colon cancer cells [187]. Another structurally different, but less potent, DNA-PK inhibitor, OK-1035, inhibited DNA repair in radioresistant L5178Y cells [188]. SU11752 was identified by library screening as an ATP-competitive DNA-PK inhibitor with comparable potency to wortmanin, but with selectivity for DNA-PK over PI3K and ATM. SU11752 profoundly inhibited DNA DSB repair and sensitized DNA-PK competent M059J cells but not the defective M059K cells to ionizing radiation, but it lacked sufficient potency for in vivo studies [189]. The DNA-PK inhibitor, IC86621, inhibited IR-induced DNA DSB relegation and significantly potentiated IR cytotoxicity in a panel of human colon, ovarian, and prostate cancer cells as well as leukemic and lymphoblastic cells, with the range of enhancements being 1.5- to 4.2-fold. It also enhanced etoposide and bleomycin cytotoxicity in human colon cancer cells [184].

Some DNA-PK inhibitors have been investigated in the tumor xenograft setting. The first was IC86621, which in human colon cancer xenografts increased the IR-induced tumor growth delay and improved survival fourfold [184]. In mice bearing human colon cancer xenografts, NU7441 increased etoposide-induced tumor growth delay twofold [187]. Recently, KU-0060648, a dual inhibitor of DNA-PK and PI3K, has been evaluated for its ability to chemosensitize mice bearing SW620 and MCF-7 xenografts to etoposide. KU-0060648 increased etoposide-induced tumor growth delay by up to 4.5-fold, thus warranting further evaluation of joint DNA-PK and PI3K inhibitors [190].

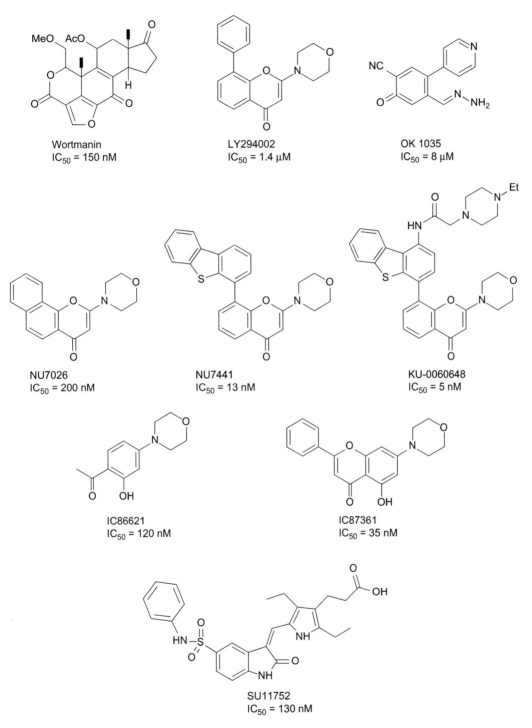

Wortmanin
$IC_{50} = 150$ nM

LY294002
$IC_{50} = 1.4$ μM

OK 1035
$IC_{50} = 8$ μM

NU7026
$IC_{50} = 200$ nM

NU7441
$IC_{50} = 13$ nM

KU-0060648
$IC_{50} = 5$ nM

IC86621
$IC_{50} = 120$ nM

IC87361
$IC_{50} = 35$ nM

SU11752
$IC_{50} = 130$ nM

FIGURE 8.8   DNA-PK inhibitors.

Investigations in clinical samples reveal that both DNA-PKcs levels and activity are higher in poor-prognosis B-cell chronic lymphocytic leukemia (B-CLL) samples derived from patients. The DNA-PK inhibitors NU7026 and NU7441 were shown to enhance sensitivity to fludarabine, chlorambucil, and topoisomerase II poisons, including mitoxantrone. NU7441 sensitized 42 out of 49 patient-derived B-CLL samples to mitoxatrone ex vivo [191].

To date, the only DNA-PK inhibitor to have progressed to clinical trial is CC-115, a dual mTOR and DNA-PK inhibitor, which is undergoing phase I evaluation in multiple myeloma, non-Hodgkin's lymphoma, and various solid tumor types, including Ewing's sarcomas. The study has not been reported yet, but it is anticipated that more studies will appear in the near future with clinical trial data to follow.

DOUBLE-STAND BREAK REPAIR: HOMOLOGOUS RECOMBINATION REPAIR

HRR is a complex pathway of repair, operating only during the S and G2 phases of the cell cycle, and is inextricably linked to the S and G2 checkpoints. This repair pathway deals with stalled or collapsed replication forks and single-ended DSBs that can result from collision of the replication fork with another lesion, as well as frank DNA DSBs. Although this pathway repairs only a minor proportion of DNA DSBs, it may be the most critical as it is high fidelity because it uses the complementary dsDNA on the sister chromatid as a template. HRR is critical for maintaining genomic integrity.

HRR is a multistep pathway in which the MRN complex (MRE11-Rad50-NBS1), facilitated by BRCA1, together with CtIP and EXO resect the ends of the break [192]. The MRN complex recruits ATM to the break and together with DNA-PK phosphorylates histone H2AX, aiding recruitment of 53BP1, RNF168, and BRCA1 [193–195]. The Fanconi anemia (FA) proteins also promote HRR at stalled replication forks via cooperation with BRCA1 (reviewed in Refs [196,197]). ATM stimulates end resection by phosphorylating MRE11, NBS1, CtIP, and EXO [198,199]. The resulting long single-stranded DNA (ssDNA) overhang is rapidly coated with RPA (replication protein A), and the ATRIP–ATR complex is recruited and signals to CHK1 for S and G2 arrest. Stalled replication forks primarily activate ATR rather than ATM [200]. ATR phosphorylates RPA2 and CHK1, which in turn phosphorylates RAD51, both of which are needed for the formation of RAD51 foci [201,202]. BRCA2 delivers RAD51, which displaces the RPA to form the nucleoprotein filament that can invade the complementary duplex DNA [203–205]. Once the invading strand has annealed, it is extended by DNA polymerase and may rejoin the ssDNA on the opposite end of the DSB, to form a noncrossover repair product, or with the other end of the broken DNA to form two Holliday junctions [206]. Resolution of the Holliday junctions is through the actions of various resolvases and helicases (Fig. 8.9) [207–209].

HRR is critical for the maintenance of genomic stability, and the function of the entire repair pathway can be compromised if one or more genes involved in the pathway are mutated. Not surprisingly, many of the genes involved in the pathway are considered to be tumor suppressor genes (e.g., BRCA1 and BRCA2). Germline heterozygote carriers of either defect have a high lifetime risk for breast (up to 85% risk) and ovarian cancer; this carrier status is also associated with prostate, pancreatic, and other gastrointestinal and gynecological cancers, as well as melanoma and hematopoietic cancers [210–212]. The tumors that arise are thought

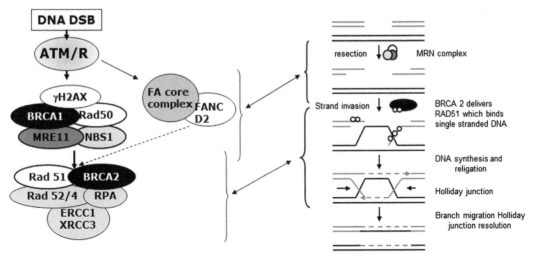

FIGURE 8.9 Pathways for homologous recombination. Homologous recombination involves a complex interaction of DNA damage–sensing signaling and repair proteins, only some of which are shown. Following end resection of the DSB by the MRN complex, facilitated by BRCA1, BRCA2 delivers RAD51 to coat the ssDNA to promote strand invasion of the complementary sister chromatid. Using the complementary DNA as a template resynthesis across the break is followed by religation and branch migration.

to lose the function of the second allele (by mutation, loss of heterozygosity, or epigenetic silencing). In addition, methylation silencing of BRCA1 is associated with breast, ovarian, and NSCLC cancers [213–216]. Homozygous mutation in ATM confers hypersensitivity to ionizing radiation and approximately 100× increased risk of cancer [217,218]. Heterozygous ATM mutations confer a 2× risk of cancer and are linked to breast cancer, pancreatic cancer, leukemia, and lymphoma [219–222]. Epigenetic silencing of ATM is associated with breast, colorectal, HNSCC, and lung cancers [223–227].

Development of HRR Inhibitors

Given the important role that HRR has in dealing with stalled replication forks, many of which occur as a consequence of anticancer agents, HRR represents an excellent therapeutic target for the development of inhibitors. There are few inhibitors of HRR; however, Mirin 1 (6-(4-hydroxyphenyl)-2-thioxo-2,3-dihydro-4(1H)-pyrimidinone), which inhibits MRE11 endonuclease activity, activation of ATM, and phosphorylation of NBS1 and CHK2, G2 checkpoint control, and HRR, has been identified [228]. In addition, cAbl is required for phosphorylation of RAD51 at Tyr315 and DNA damage-induced RAD51 focus formation [229,230]. To this end, the BCR–Abl inhibitor imatinib sensitized not only chronic lymphocytic leukemia (CLL) cells to chlorambucil, but also cell lines derived from solid tumors to MMC and IR [231,232]. The cyclin-dependent kinase CDK1 phosphorylates BRCA1, and loss or inhibition of CDK1 prevents the formation of BRCA1 foci that confer sensitivity to cisplatin [233]. However, the most common way to target HRR is through inhibition of the ATM–CHK2 pathway or ATR–CHK1 pathway that activates cell cycle checkpoints and participates in HRR.

Cell cycle checkpoint signaling is essential to allow time for repair and to prevent DNA damage from becoming fixed or causing cell death following replication and mitosis. The G1 checkpoint is largely activated by ATM signaling to CHK2 and p53 [234]. Damage that has evaded the G1 checkpoint, or that occurs during the S phase, triggers the intra-S phase checkpoint to block further replication, with remaining damage signaled via the G2 checkpoint to prevent cells entering mitosis. These latter checkpoints are triggered by ATR–CHK1 signaling. There is cross-talk between the ATM–CHK2 and ATR–CHK1 pathways, and they share many substrates [235]. ATR plays a role in several DNA repair pathways, particularly HRR, NER, MMR, TLS (trans-lesion synthesis), and BER.

ATM and CHK2

ATM has been investigated as a target for cancer therapy, but there are limited studies with inhibitors due to the lack of availability of potent small-molecule inhibitors Wortmannin and LY294002 were the first compounds used to inhibit ATM but are not specific. Based on the structural similarity of ATM to PI3K, the first selective ATM inhibitor, KU55933, was developed from the PI3K inhibitor LY294002 [236] (Fig. 8.10). KU55933 inhibited the IR-induced phosphorylation of downstream proteins, for example p53, and sensitized cancer cells to IR and topoisomerase I and II inhibitors [237]. Further studies with this compound confirmed its potent radiosensitization in a variety of human cancer models, and its synergistic radio- and chemosensitization in combination with DNA-PK

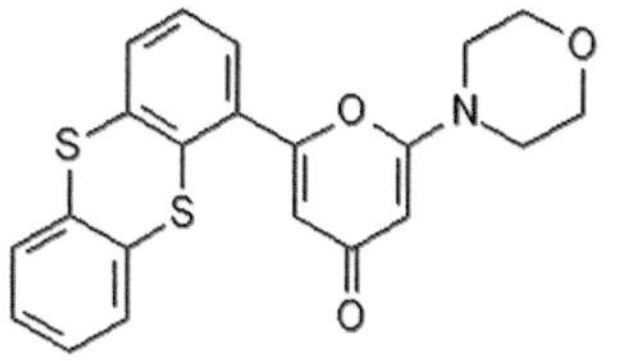

KU55933

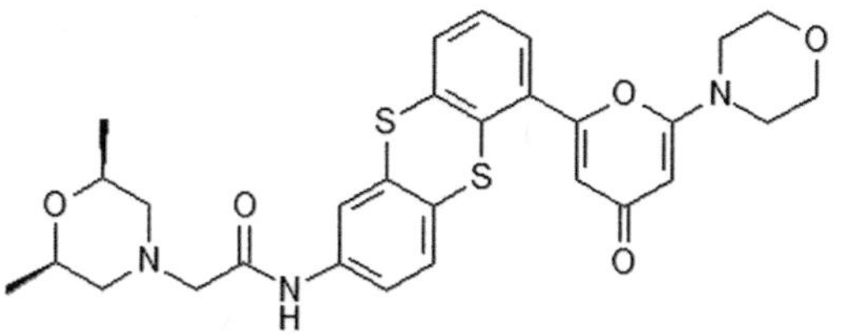

KU-60019

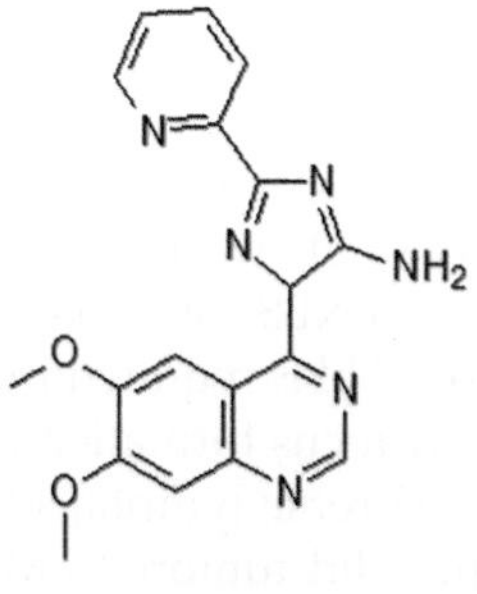

CP466722

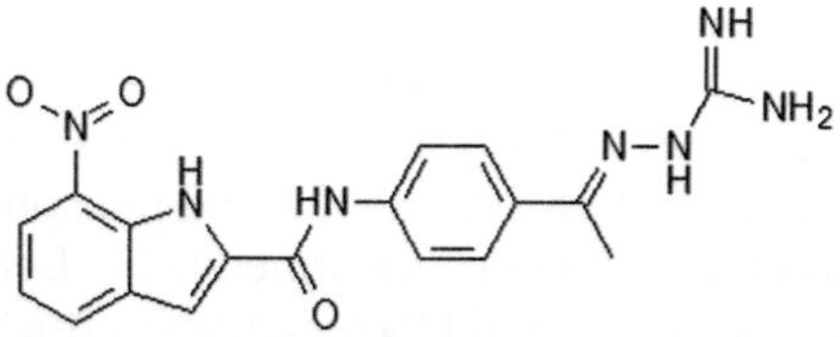

PV1019
CHK2

FIGURE 8.10   ATM and CHK2 inhibitors.

inhibition in prostate cancer cells [238]. Subsequent development of this compound led to the identification of KU-60019 as having increased activity and being a more potent radiosensitizer [239]. Another ATM inhibitor, CP466722, has been identified by library screening. It was necessary to inhibit ATM activity for only 4 h by KU55933 or CP466722 in order to achieve significant radiosensitization [183].

Most CHK2 inhibitors so far developed also inhibit CHK1 and will be considered in the "ATR and CHK1" section; however, CHK2 inhibitors that have nanomolar potency and are selective for CHK2 versus CHK1 have recently been developed [240]. PV1019 is a competitive inhibitor of CHK2 with respect to ATP; it inhibits CHK2 activity in cells and sensitizes human cancer cell lines to topoisomerase I poisons and IR [241]. Other studies have suggested that while CHK2 knockout cells are hypersensitive to oxaliplatin, inhibition of CHK2 protects cells from oxaliplatin [242].

ATR and CHK1

Targeting the S and G2 checkpoints is particularly attractive for cancer therapy because loss of G1 checkpoint control is a common feature of cancer cells, for example, due to defects in the p53 and pRb tumor suppressor genes or an imbalance in cyclins, cyclin-dependent kinases, and their inhibitors. This makes cancer cells more reliant on their S and G2 checkpoints to prevent DNA damage from being translated into cell death [243–245]. Proof-of-principle genetic studies show that dominant negative inhibition of ATR with a kinase-dead ATR mutant, or employing CHK1 small interfering RNA (siRNA) led to abrogation of DNA damage-induced G2 arrest and sensitization of cells to a variety of DNA-damaging chemotherapeutic agents [246–251]. Sensitization was specific to replicating cells, and in some studies inhibition of the ATR–CHK1 pathway selectively sensitized cells that were defective in the G1 checkpoint.

Despite the attractiveness of the target, small-molecule inhibitors of ATR have proved elusive [252]. This may reflect the difficulty of assaying an enzyme that requires a complex of coactivators and regulators, and the progress of ATR research has been hampered by the lack of potent inhibitors. Caffeine, the prototype inhibitor, was weak and nonspecific but provided data that were sufficiently promising for the target to be pursued [253]. Schisandrin B, a natural product, was identified as inhibiting ATR, abrogating the ultraviolet (UV)-induced S and G2/M checkpoint and increasing UV cytotoxicity in human lung cancer cells [254]. In a screen of PI3K inhibitors, PI103 and PI124 were identified as being potent ATR inhibitors with IC_{50} values of 0.9 and 2 μM, respectively [255] (Fig. 8.11). In a HTS assay NVP-BEZ235, which was previously thought to be selective for PI3K and mTOR, was demonstrated to be a potent inhibitor of ATR ($IC_{50} = 100$ nM); and the most potent ATR inhibitor, ETP-46464 ($IC_{50} = 25$ nM), inhibited the restart of stalled replication forks and abrogated S phase arrest after hydroxyurea exposure [256]. VE-821, AZ-20, and NU6027 have recently been identified as being ATR inhibitors [257–260]. All drugs inhibited CHK1 phosphorylation at Ser345 and sensitized cells to a variety of DNA-damaging agents. VE-821 enhanced IR-induced cytotoxicity in a panel of 12 human cancer cell lines, caused a more profound radiosensitization in hypoxic cells. It also increased reoxygenation-induced DNA damage and decreased the survival of cells undergoing reoxygenation [261]. Interestingly, NU6027 inhibited RAD51 focus formation (indicative of HRR suppression) and was more cytotoxic in the presence of a PARP inhibitor or when XRCC1 was defective, suggesting the potential for synthetic lethality. AZ-20 is reported to be an even more potent ATR inhibitor with an IC_{50} of 4.5 nM in

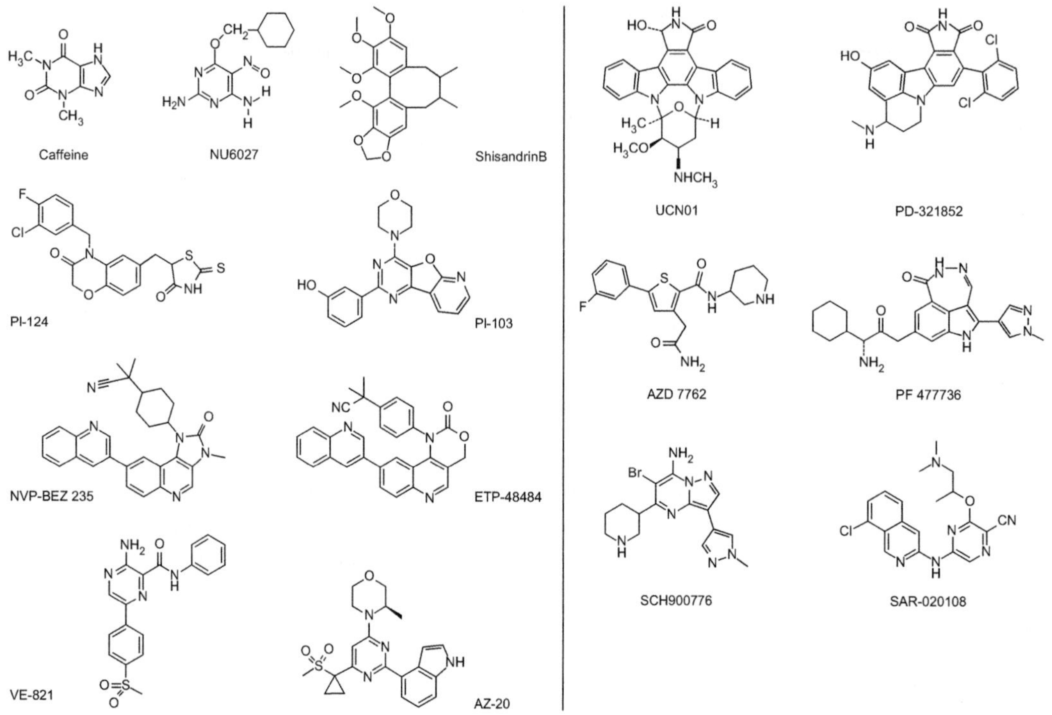

FIGURE 8.11 ATR and CHK1 inhibitors. Compounds to the left of the vertical line are ATR inhibitors; those to the right are CHK1 inhibitors.

biochemical assays and 51 nM in cellular assays. This inhibitor was active as a single agent both in vitro and in vivo, and, at an oral dose of 25 mg/kg bid or 50 mg/kg qd, it inhibited the growth of LoVo xenografts. This is the first report of an ATR inhibitor in an in vivo model, and although only published in abstract form, the full data on this compound are eagerly awaited.

There have been substantial research efforts into the development of CHK1 inhibitors that have culminated in clinical studies. These include the nonspecific staurosporin analog UCN-01 and its derivatives, such as PD321852, the potent dual CHK1 and CHK2 inhibitors AZD7762 and XL9844, and the highly potent selective CHK1 inhibitors PF00477736, CEP-3891, SAR-020106, and SCH900776 (reviewed in Refs [262–265]). When used as a single agent, most of these inhibitors do not affect cell cycle distribution and are not cytotoxic. However, they do prevent cell cycle arrest and increase cytotoxicity after exposure to DNA-damaging agents, including IR and those causing replication stress such as antimetabolites (e.g., gemcitabine), topoisomerase I poisons, and DNA cross-linking agents (e.g., cisplatin), suggesting that the S phase checkpoint is critical. Early studies with UCN-01 demonstrated an abrogation of doxorubicin-induced G2/M arrest and potentiation of cisplatin and camptothecin cytotoxicity in human cancer cell lines [266–268]. The more potent and selective CHK1 inhibitor, SAR-020106 (Sareum) (IC$_{50}$ of 13.3 nM), blocked etoposide-induced cell cycle arrest in HT29 cells [269]; and PF00477736 abrogated gemcitabine- and camptothecin-induced S phase and G2/M arrest, and potentiated the activity of a variety of DNA-damaging agents in several human cancer cell lines [270]. The dual CHK1 and CHK2 inhibitor, AZD7762, inhibited camptothecin-induced G2 arrest and potentiated the cytotoxicity of gemcitabine and topotecan [271,272]. XL-844 blocked gemcitabine-induced S-phase arrest, resulting in premature entry into mitosis [273]. CHK1 inhibitors are also radiosensitizers: AZD7762 markedly increased IR cytotoxicity in a panel of prostate, lung, and colon cancer cell lines [274]; CEP-3891 prevented IR-induced S and G2 arrest in U2OS cells, and increased nuclear fragmentation and cytotoxicity after IR [275].

These in vitro studies translated into positive in vivo xenograft studies, mostly in combination with gemcitabine or IR. For example, PF-00477736 increased the efficacy of gemcitabine against CoLo205 xenografts [270], AZD7762 increased the antitumor activity of gemcitabine and of irinotecan against human cancer xenografts in both mice and rats [272], and XL-844 increased the efficacy of gemcitabine against PANC-1 xenografts [273]. SCH900776 increased gemcitabine-induced DSB accumulation and enhanced the anticancer activity of gemcitabine without exacerbating gemcitabine-induced myelosuppression [276]. Interestingly, SAR-020106 potentiated the antitumor activity of gemcitabine against SW620 xenografts better if administered at the same time than if delayed by 24 h. In vivo radiosensitization data are scarce, but AZD7762 demonstrated radiosensitizing activity in xenograft models of lung cancer with brain metastasis resulting in prolonged survival [269,277].

UCN-01 was the first CHK1 inhibitor to undergo clinical evaluation as a single agent; short infusions were better tolerated than long ones, but after some phase II trials as a single agent and in combination studies, this agent has been discontinued [277,278]. Several of the second-generation inhibitors have been in phase I trials, mostly in combination with gemcitabine, but largely have been reported only in abstract form. Hematological toxicity (neutropenia and thrombocytopenia) was commonly seen with PF00477736 and SCH900776 in combination with gemcitabine and with AZD7762 in combination with gemcitabine and irinotecan (reviewed in Ref. [279]).

EXPLOITING SYNTHETIC LETHALITY FOR CANCER TREATMENTS

Concept of Synthetic Lethality

The term "synthetic lethality" was originally coined by geneticists in the 1940s to describe the process where mutations in two different genes together resulted in cell death but independently did not affect viability [280]. The concept was applied to cancer somewhat later to explain the selective killing of cancer cells with particular molecular defects, by some agents [281]. It is becoming apparent that dysregulation of the DNA damage response (DDR), that contributes to the genomic instability that is an enabling characteristic of cancer, can be exploited by the synthetic lethality approach. Loss of one component of the DDR may be compensated by another backup component in the same (or different) pathway, on which the cancer cell becomes dependent. This has been termed "non-oncogene addiction". Inactivating this compensatory pathway is therefore a means of selectively targeting the tumor (Fig. 8.12). Exploitation of dysregulation of the DDR by the synthetic lethality approach is perhaps the most exciting prospect for the future of cancer treatment [282].

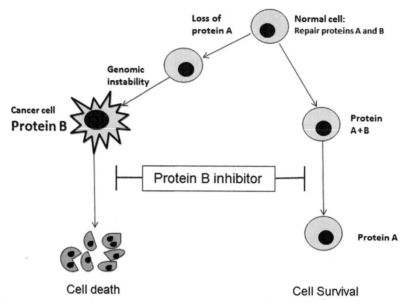

FIGURE 8.12 Synthetic lethality: normal cells contain primary and backup DDR proteins (A and B) to cope with endogenous and induced DNA damage. The genomic instability that enables cancer to develop can be due to loss of one of these pathways (A) leading to hyperdependence on the other (B), which may be amplified. Using an inhibitor of B leads to cell death in the cancer cell but not the normal cell, because this still has protein A to deal with endogenous or induced DNA damage.

Synthetic Lethality between PARP and HRR

PARP inhibition in HRR-defective cells is a clear example of the therapeutic exploitation of "synthetic lethality" to selectively target cancer. The hypothesis that PARP inhibition might be synthetically lethal in HRR-defective cells originally came from the observation that loss or inhibition of PARP resulted in an increase in sister chromatid exchanges [283,284] and an increased dependence on HRR, as indicated by a high level of RAD51 foci [285]. The hyper-recombination phenotype present in PARP-inhibited or -defective cells suggested that HRR has a very important role in PARP-defective cells. The proposed mechanism is that failure to repair the high level of endogenous DNA SSBs by PARP-dependent mechanisms resulted in an accumulation of stalled replication forks requiring HRR for their resolution [285]. These observations were important because, as described in this chapter, defects in aspects of HRR are not uncommon in cancer, with the classic example of BRCA1 and BRCA2 defects and their association with breast and ovarian cancer syndrome [7].

Two seminal papers, published in the same issue of *Nature* in 2005, demonstrated the exquisite sensitivity of HRR-defective cell lines, in particular those homozygous for either the BRCA1 or BRCA2 mutation, to a PARP inhibitor alone [286,287]. These BRCA mutant cells were 100- to 1000-fold more sensitive to PARP inhibitors than the heterozygote or the wild-type cell lines, and regression of tumors derived from the homozygous mutated cells was observed. The relevance to human cancer was further demonstrated by the observation that siRNA-mediated depletion of BRCA2 in MCF7 (wild-type p53) and MDA-MB-231 (mutated p53) breast cancer cell lines also resulted in sensitivity to PARP inhibitor–mediated cytotoxicity [286]. These observations were made in two laboratories using different BRCA1/2-deficient cell lines and PARP inhibitors of different chemical classes, confirming that the sensitivity of the cells to the drugs is mechanism based.

PARP inhibitors may have wider application than just in patients with BRCA1 or BRCA2 mutations. Sporadic breast and ovarian cancers may lose BRCA function through epigenetic silencing or overexpression of other proteins that inhibit their activity, or they may harbor defects in other genes within the HRR pathway [288]. Further studies reveal that inactivation of various other genes involved in HRR also confers sensitivity to PARP inhibitors. For example, ATM-defective cells are also hypersensitive to PARP inhibitor cytotoxicity [289]; and not only are PARP inhibitors synthetically lethal in Chinese hamster ovary (CHO) cells defective in other HRR components (XRCC2 or XRCC3) [286], but also knockdown of other components of the HRR pathway, including RAD51, DSS1, RAD54, RPA1, NBS1, ATR, CHK1, CHK2, FANCD2, FANCA, and FANCC, confers hypersensitivity to PARP inhibitors [290]. Defects in these genes have been associated with a variety of cancers; for example, ATM mutations are commonly observed in leukemias and breast cancers, and both mutation and epigenetic silencing of the FANC genes have been demonstrated in a variety of solid tumors (reviewed in Ref. [291]), suggesting that PARP inhibitors may have a very wide therapeutic application in cancer. Surprisingly, in a siRNA screen, PTEN (phosphatase and tensin homolog) and CDK5 knockdown were also identified as being synthetically lethal with PARP inhibition, CDK5 is involved in checkpoint signaling, and PTEN may regulate RAD51 function [292–294]. PTEN is a tumor suppressor gene that is commonly mutated in cancer and was successfully targeted using the PARP inhibitor olaparib [295]. However, further studies suggest that this may not be universally applicable as PTEN deletion was not associated with defective RAD51 expression or marked hypersensitivity to PARPi in prostate cancer [296].

These studies, largely conducted in mouse and hamster cell lines or using genetic knockdown approaches, have been verified in human cancer cells and xenografts that have evolved to survive despite defective HRR. Significantly, these studies also included a human breast cancer cell line with epigenetic silencing of BRCA1, rather than a mutation, demonstrating the potential in sporadic cancer [297,298]. Interestingly, many HRR genes appear to be suppressed in hypoxic conditions, potentially making hypoxic cells more sensitive to PARP inhibition [299,300]. This "contextual synthetic lethality" has been demonstrated in vivo with increased DSBs and apoptosis and reduced RAD51 foci (indicative of HRR function) seen in hypoxic regions of xenografts in mice treated with a PARP inhibitor [301]. ATM loss in hematological malignancies (e.g., CLL characterized by del 11q and Mantle cell lymphomas with reduced ATM levels) also confers sensitivity to olaparib in in vitro and in vivo xenografts [302,303]. Defects in HRR that arise secondary to MMR defects also confer sensitivity to PARP inhibitors; for example, MRE11 defects due to MSI in colorectal cancer confer sensitivity to the PARP inhibitor, ABT-888, with a significant correlation being observed between MRE11 expression levels and cytotoxicity of ABT-888 at $10 \mu M$ ($R^2=0.915$, $P<0.001$) [304]. Further promising developments suggest that an HRR defect can be created using another targeted agent. CDK1 phosphorylates BRCA1, enabling it to form repair foci, and CDK1 inhibition leads to inactivation of BRCA1. CDK1 inhibition or PARP inhibition alone is nontoxic, but the combination of a CDK1 inhibitor and a PARP inhibitor was cytotoxic in lung cancer cells, xenografts, and spontaneous lung tumors in genetically engineered mice, although it spared normal tissues [305].

However, resistance to PARP inhibitors can develop due to secondary mutations in BRCA1 or BRCA2 that restore their function [306–308]. In addition, it seems that the synthetic lethality of PARP inhibitors in HRR-defective cells is dependent on NHEJ function; HRR function and PARP inhibitor resistance can be restored in BRCA1 mutant cells if 53BP1 and DNA-PKcs (components of NHEJ) are also inactivated [309–311]. This phenomenon of "synthetic viability" reflects studies in FA-defective human cells where the exquisite sensitivity to the DNA cross-linking agent, MMC, can be rescued by inhibition of DNA-PKcs [312]. Deletion of Ku70 and Ligase IV also protects FA cells from interstrand cross-links (ICLs), suggesting that NHEJ and HRR compete for ICL-induced DSBs but that survival is dependent on the error-free HRR [313,314]. Loss of 53BP1 appears to be a relatively common event in BRCA1 mutant and triple-negative breast cancer and in lung cancer, which could compromise the activity of PARP inhibitors in clinical trials against breast cancer [315].

Clinical Application of Synthetic Lethality with PARP Inhibitors

The prospect of nontoxic therapy based on synthetic lethality has real clinical potential, and these experimental observations have provided a boost to PARP research, with nine PARP inhibitors now undergoing clinical evaluation as single agents as well as in combination with conventional cytotoxic therapy (Table 8.1). The first report of a clinical trial of a PARPi as a single agent in patients with BRCA mutations was the pivotal phase I study of the oral PARPi olaparib [316,317]. Olaparib was well tolerated in all patients, toxicities were lower than grade 3 in severity and did not increase in the BRCA mutation carriers. The MTD was 400 mg twice daily. PARP inhibition was confirmed in both surrogate normal tissue and tumor tissue. Importantly, antitumor activity was reported in 12 of the 19 evaluable *BRCA1/2* mutation carriers, including patients with breast, ovarian, and prostate cancer, but no responses were observed in non-*BRCA* mutation carriers. Two parallel phase II studies were undertaken on the basis of this promising phase I data, one in breast and the other in ovarian cancer patients with BRCA1/2 mutations. In each study, cohorts of 27 patients received either 100 or 400 mg olaparib. The common adverse effects were mild, including fatigue, nausea, and vomiting. In the breast study, the overall response rate was 41% (11/27) and progression-free survival (PFS) was 5.7 months with 400 mg, but the response rate (22%) and the PFS (3.8 months) were lower with 100 mg [318]. In the ovarian cancer study, the overall response rate was 33% in the 400 mg group and 12.5% in the 100 mg group, indicating a dose dependency of the response [319].

Several other PARP inhibitors are currently being investigated in patients with germline *BRCA* mutations. In a preliminary report of a phase I trial of MK-4827, in patients with advanced solid tumors enriched for *BRCA*-mutated cancers, the MTD was 300 mg daily with continuous dosing and there was a partial response rate of 20% (12/60) [320]. Interim results of the phase II trial of single-agent rucaparib in patients with *BRCA*-mutated breast and/or ovarian cancer reported a clinical benefit rate of 34% [298].

Clinical studies of PARPi in nongermline *BRCA*-mutated cancers are also underway, in particular high-grade serous ovarian cancers (HGSOCs) and triple-negative breast cancer (TNBC). In a phase II study, the efficacy of continuous olaparib (400 mg twice daily) in HGSOC patients with or without known BRCA mutations and of BRCA-mutated breast cancer or TNBC patients with unknown BRCA status was compared [321]. Encouragingly, in the patients with nongermline BRCA-mutated HGSOC, there was a response rate of 24% compared with 41% in the confirmed BRCA mutation ovarian cancer patients, but curiously, no responses were observed in the two breast cancer arms. This is the *first* study to show single-agent PARP inhibitor activity in nongermline BRCA-mutated cancers, indicating that sporadic HGSOC could be targeted with PARP inhibitors. PARPi are now being investigated as maintenance therapy in HGSOC, and preliminary results showed a significant benefit in PFS (8.4 versus 4.8 months) of olaparib 400 mg twice daily over placebo [322,323].

Other Examples of Synthetic Lethality

There are other examples of synthetic lethality, or synthetic sickness (where a targeted agent specifically sensitizes cancer cells with a specific defect to a cytotoxic agent), emerging. It is possible that such secondary defects in MRE11 (or ATR or PTEN, which also contain microsatellites and are associated with HRR) may contribute to the sensitivity of cells defective in the MMR protein, MSH2, to DNA polβ inhibition [324]. The compensatory roles of BER and HRR that can be exploited by PARP inhibition in HRR-defective cells can also be exploited by inhibition of HRR in BER-defective cells. The ATR inhibitor, NU6027, was more profoundly cytotoxic in cells defective in BER by virtue of mutant XRCC1 or in the presence of a PARP inhibitor [259]. Inhibition of ATM also selectively sensitized DNA polβ mutant cells to irradiation [325]. There seems to be a synthetic interaction between ATM and the FA pathway. FANC defects may be targeted by ATM inactivation; pancreatic cancer cells defective in FANCC or FANCG were hypersensitive to the ATM inhibitor KU55933, and ATM knockdown resulted in synthetic lethality in cells with defects in FANCC, FANCD2, FANCG, and FANCE, which are commonly mutated or lost in cancers [326]. The CHK1 inhibitor Go6976 also reduced cell survival and profoundly increased cisplatin sensitivity in cells with a defective FA pathway [327].

Hyperactive growth factor signaling and oncogenic stress increase DNA breakage that activates ATR/CHK1 [3,328–333]. It is therefore perhaps not surprising to discover that inactivation of ATR or CHK1 is synthetically lethal in oncogene-activated cancer cells. Knocking down ATR to 16% of normal levels was synthetically lethal in ras-transformed cells [334]. Similarly, inhibition of both Chk1 and Chk2 with AZD7762 induced cell death and significantly delayed disease progression of transplanted myc-overexpressing lymphoma cells in vivo [335,336]. Recent studies demonstrate that the ETS (E-twenty six) fusion genes that drive several cancer types, including prostate cancer, Ewing's sarcoma, and acute myeloid leukemia, increase DNA damage and confer hypersensitivity to PARP inhibitors and DNA-PK inhibitors, and the combination of olaparib and TMZ resulted in complete regressions of Ewing's sarcoma xenografts [337,338].

SUMMARY AND CONCLUSIONS

The efficacy of anticancer agents whose main mechanism is to damage DNA can be compromised by DNA repair. Inhibition of DNA repair enzymes has major clinical potential to enhance the persistence of toxic lesions in cancer cells. The disappointing activity of inhibitors of O^6-alkylguanine DNA alkyltransferase in the clinical setting should not be seen as too much of a discouragement to the investigation of other DDR inhibitors as chemo- and radiosensitizers. However, there may need to be careful titration of both the cytotoxic and the inhibitor to avoid toxicity, as clinical combinations with PARP inhibitors have revealed. DNA-PK, ATM, and ATR inhibitors are all showing promising activity in the preclinical setting, and CHK1 inhibitors are undergoing clinical evaluation.

However, the most promising avenue may be the exploitation of DDR defects in cancer by targeting complementary pathways on which the cancers are dependent for survival. This synthetic lethality approach has been successfully demonstrated in both preclinical and clinical settings. It is to be hoped that more examples will be identified in the future.

Acknowledgments

We would like to thank Cancer Research UK and UK Higher Education Funding Council for financial support. Nicola Curtin is also currently in receipt of, or previously received, research funding from pharmaceutical companies involved in the development of the inhibitors described here, namely, Pfizer, BioMarin, AstraZeneca, and Vertex Pharmaceuticals.

Problem Set

1. Give the main reasons for DNA repair being a good drug target for anticancer therapy.

   Answer: Inhibition of DNA repair can increase the tumor-specificity of radio- and chemotherapy. It specifically targets proliferating cells. It may overcome tumor resistance that evolved through upregulation of DNA repair, and it may also function as stand-alone treatments for cancers, exploiting tumor defects that arose during cancer development.

2. There is a clear mechanistic difference between inhibitors of AGT and inhibitors of either PARP or DNA-PK; describe how.

   Answer: AGT is not, strictly speaking, an enzyme as it is consumed as part of the reaction (acceptance of alkyl group from O^6 position of guanine). Inhibitors of AGT bind covalently to AGT to inhibit the function of the protein and target it for degradation. PARP and DNA-PK are enzymes, and their inhibitors are largely competitive with respect to their substrate NAD^+ and ATP, respectively.

3. How can inhibitors of DNA repair function as stand-alone treatments?

   Answer: The inhibitors exploit the fact that tumors carry defects in DNA repair pathways, making other DNA repair pathways essential for cellular survival.

References

[1] Lindahl T. Instability and decay of the primary structure of DNA. Nature 1993;362:709–15.
[2] Lindahl T, Wood RD. Quality control by DNA repair. Science 1999;286:1897–905.
[3] Bartkova J, Horejsi Z, Koed K, Kramer A, Tort F, Zieger K, et al. DNA damage response as a candidate anti-cancer barrier in early human tumorigenesis. Nature 2005;434:864–70.
[4] Hananha D, Weinber RA. Hallmarks of cancer: the next generation. Cell 2011;144:646–74.
[5] Jackson AL, Loeb LA. The contribution of endogenous sources of DNA damage to the multiple mutations in cancer. Mutat Res 2001;477:7–21.
[6] Bronner CE, Baker SM, Morrison PT, Warren G, Smith LG, Lescoe MK, et al. Mutation in the DNA mismatch repair gene homologue hMLH1 is associated with hereditary non-polyposis colon cancer. Nature 1994;368:258–61.

[7] Venkitaraman AR. Cancer susceptibility and the functions of BRCA1 and BRCA2. Cell 2002;108:171–82.

[8] Kaina B, Ziouta A, Ochs K, Coquerelle T. Chromosomal instability, reproductive cell death and apoptosis induced by O^6-methylguanine in Mex–, Mex+ and methylation-tolerant mismatch repair compromised cells: facts and models. Mutat Res 1997;381:227–41.

[9] Tutt A, Bertwistle D, Valentine J, Gabriel A, Swift S, Ross G, et al. Mutation in Brca2 stimulates error-prone homology-directed repair of DNA double-strand breaks occurring between repeated sequences. EMBO J 2001;20:4704–16.

[10] Sabharwal A, Middleton MR. Exploiting the role of O^6-methylguanine-DNA-methyltransferase (MGMT) in cancer therapy. Curr Opin Pharmacol 2006;6:355–63.

[11] Pegg AE. Mammalian O^6-alkylguanine-DNA alkyltransferase: regulation and importance in response to alkylating carcinogenic and therapeutic agents. Cancer Res 1990;50:6119–29.

[12] Ayi TC, Loh KC, Ali RB, Li BF. Intracellular localization of human DNA repair enzyme methylguanine-DNA methyltransferase by antibodies and its importance. Cancer Res 1992;52:6423–30.

[13] Wani G, D'Ambrosio SM. Expression of the O^6-alkylguanine-DNA alkyltransferase gene is elevated in human breast tumor cells. Anticancer Res 1997;17:4311–5.

[14] Schold Jr SC, Brent TP, von Hofe E, Friedman HS, Mitra S, Bigner DD, et al. O^6-alkylguanine-DNA alkyltransferase and sensitivity to procarbazine in human brain-tumor xenografts. J Neurosurg 1989;70:573–7.

[15] Yarosh DB. The role of O^6-methylguanine-DNA methyltransferase in cell survival, mutagenesis and carcinogenesis. Mutat Res 1985;145:1–6.

[16] Esteller M, Garcia-Foncillas J, Andion E, Goodman SN, Hidalgo OF, Vanaclocha V, et al. Inactivation of the DNA-repair gene MGMT and the clinical response of gliomas to alkylating agents. N Engl J Med 2000a;343: 1350–4.

[17] Hegi ME, Diserens AC, Gorlia T, Hamou MF, de Tribolet N, Weller M, et al. MGMT gene silencing and benefit from temozolomide in glioblastoma. N Engl J Med 2005;352:997–1003.

[18] Jaeckle KA, Eyre HJ, Townsend JJ, Schulman S, Knudson HM, Belanich M, et al. Correlation of tumor O^6 methylguanine-DNA methyltransferase levels with survival of malignant astrocytoma patients treated with bis-chloroethylnitrosourea: a Southwest Oncology Group study. J Clin Oncol 1998;16:3310–5.

[19] Dolan ME, Moschel RC, Pegg AE. Depletion of mammalian O^6-alkylguanine-DNA alkyltransferase activity by O^6-benzylguanine provides a means to evaluate the role of this protein in protection against carcinogenic and therapeutic alkylating agents. Proc Natl Acad Sci U S A 1990;87:5368–72.

[20] Liu L, Markowitz S, Gerson SL. Mismatch repair mutations oride alkyltransferase in conferring resistance to temozolomide but not to 1,3-bis(2-chloroethyl)nitrosourea. Cancer Res 1996;56:5375–9.

[21] Wedge SR, Porteous JK, Newlands ES. 3-aminobenzamide and/or O^6-benzylguanine evaluated as an adjuvant to temozolomide or BCNU treatment in cell lines of variable mismatch repair status and O^6-alkylguanine-DNA alkyltransferase activity. Br J Cancer 1996;74:1030–6.

[22] Dolan ME, Roy SK, Fasanmade A, Paras PR, Schilsky RL, Ratain MJ. O^6-benzylguanine in humans: metabolic, pharmacokinetic and pharmacodynamic findings. J Clin Oncol 1998;16:1803–10.

[23] Rabik CA, Njoku MC, Dolan ME. Inactivation of O^6-alkylguanine DNA alkyltransferase as a means to enhance chemotherapy. Cancer Treat Rev 2006;32:261–76.

[24] McElhinney RS, McMurry TB, Margison GP. O^6-alkylguanine-DNA alkyltransferase inactivation in cancer chemotherapy. Mini Rev Med Chem 2003;3:471–85.

[25] Middleton MR, Kelly J, Thatcher N, Donnelly DJ, McElhinney RS, McMurry TB, et al. O(6)-(4-bromothenyl) guanine improves the therapeutic index of temozolomide against A375M melanoma xenografts. Int J Cancer 2000;85:248–52.

[26] Friedman HS, Kokkinakis DM, Pluda J, Friedman AH, Cokgor I, Haglund MM, et al. Phase I trial of O^6-benzylguanine for patients undergoing surgery for malignant glioma. J Clin Oncol 1998;16:3570–5.

[27] Gerson SL. MGMT: its role in cancer aetiology and cancer therapeutics. Nat Rev Cancer 2004;4:296–307.

[28] Ranson M, Middleton MR, Bridgewater J, Lee SM, Dawson M, Jowle D, et al. Lomeguatrib, a potent inhibitor of O^6-alkylguanine-DNA-alkyltransferase: phase I safety, pharmacodynamic, and pharmacokinetic trial and evaluation in combination with temozolomide in patients with advanced solid tumors. Clin Cancer Res 2006;12:1577–84.

[29] Kefford RF, Thomas NP, Corrie PG, Palmer C, Abdi E, Kotasek D, et al. A phase I study of extended dosing with lomeguatrib with temozolomide in patients with advanced melanoma. Br J Cancer 2009;100:1245–9.

[30] Khan OA, Ranson M, Michael M, Olver I, Levitt NC, Mortimer P, et al. A phase II trial of lomeguatrib and temozolomide in metastatic colorectal cancer. Br J Cancer 2008;98:1614–8.

[31] Watson AJ, Sabharwal A, Thorncroft M, McGown G, Kerr R, Bojanic S, et al. Tumor O(6)-methylguanine-DNA methyltransferase inactivation by oral *lomeguatrib*. Clin Cancer Res 2010;16:743–9.

[32] Van Loon B, Markkanen E, Hübscher U. Oxygen as a friend and enemy: how to combat the mutational potential of 8-oxo-guanine. DNA Repair (Amst) 2010;9:604–16.

[33] Wiseman H, Halliwell B. Damage to DNA by reactive oxygen and nitrogen species: role in inflammatory disease and progression to cancer. Biochem J 1996;313:17–29.

[34] O'Connor TR, Laval J. Human cDNA expressing a functional DNA glycosylase excising 3-methyladenine and 7-methylguanine. Biochem Biophys Res Commun 1991;176:1170–7.

[35] Almeida KH, Sobol RW. A unified view of base excision repair: lesion-dependent protein complexes regulated by post-translational modification. DNA Repair (Amst) 2007;6:695–711.

[36] Cox LS, Lane DP, Abbondandolo A, Dogliotti E. Two pathways for base excision repair in mammalian cells. J Biol Chem 1996;271:9573–8.

[37] Petermann E, Ziegler M, Oei SL. ATP-dependent selection between single nucleotide and long patch base excision repair. DNA Repair (Amst) 2003;2:1101–14.

[38] Schreiber V, Dantzer F, Ame JC, de Murcia G. Poly(ADP-ribose): novel functions for an old molecule. Nat Rev Mol Cell Biol 2006;7:517–28.

[39] El-Khamisy SF, Masutani M, Suzuki H, Caldecott KW. A requirement for PARP-1 for the assembly or stability of XRCC1 nuclear foci at sites of oxidative DNA damage. Nucleic Acids Res 2003;31:5526–33.

[40] Caldecott KW. XRCC1 and DNA strand break repair. DNA Repair (Amst) 2003;2:955–69.

[41] Hirai K, Ueda K, Hayaishi O. Aberration of poly(adenosine diphosphate-ribose) metabolism in human colon adenomatous polyps and cancers. Cancer Res 1983;43:3441–6.

[42] Nomura F, Yaguchi M, Togawa A, Miyazaki M, Isobe K, Miyake M, et al. Enhancement of poly-adenosine diphosphate-ribosylation in human hepatocellular carcinoma. J Gastroenterol Hepatol 2000;15:529–35.

[43] Benjamin RC, Gill DM. ADP-ribosylation in mammalian cell ghosts: dependence of poly(ADP-ribose) synthesis on strand breakage in DNA. J Biol Chem 1980;255:10493–501.

[44] Boulton S, Kyle S, Durkacz BW. Interactive effects of inhibitors of poly(ADP-ribose) polymerase and DNA-dependent protein kinase on cellular responses to DNA damage. Carcinogenesis 1999;20:199–203.

[45] Mitchell J, Smith GCM, Curtin NJ. Poly(ADP-ribose) polymerase-1 and DNA-dependent protein kinase have equivalent roles in double strand break repair following ionising radiation. Int J Radiat Oncol Biol Phys 2009;75:1520–7.

[46] Spagnolo L, Barbeau J, Curtin NJ, Morris EP, Pearl LH. Visualisation of a DNA-PK/PARP1 complex. Nucleic Acids Res 2012;40:4168–77.

[47] Ruscetti T, Lehnert BE, Halbrook J, Le Trong H, Hoekstra MF, Chen DJ, et al. Stimulation of the DNA-dependent protein kinase by poly(ADP-ribose) polymerase. J Biol Chem 1998;273:14461–7.

[48] Veuger SJ, Curtin NJ, Richardson CJ, Smith GC, Durkacz BW. Radiosensitization and DNA repair inhibition by the combined use of novel inhibitors of DNA-dependent protein kinase and poly(ADP-ribose) polymerase-1. Cancer Res 2003;63:6008–15.

[49] Veuger SJ, Curtin NJ, Smith GC, Durkacz BW. Effects of novel inhibitors of poly(ADP-ribose) polymerase-1 and the DNA-dependent protein kinase on enzyme activities and DNA repair. Oncogene 2004;23:7322–9.

[50] Iliakis G. Backup pathways of NHEJ in cells of higher eukaryotes: cell cycle dependence. Radiother Oncol 2009;92:310–5.

[51] Durkacz BW, Omidiji O, Gray DA, Shall S. (ADP-ribose)n participates in DNA excision repair. Nature 1980;283:593–6.

[52] Griffin RJ, Pemberton LC, Rhodes D, Bleasdale C, Bowman K, Calvert AH, et al. Novel potent inhibitors of the DNA repair enzyme poly(ADP-ribose)polymerase (PARP). Anticancer Drug Des 1995;10:507–14.

[53] Suto MJ, Turner WR, Arundel-Suto CM, Werbel LM, Sebolt-Leopold JS. Dihydroisoquinolinones: the design and synthesis of a new series of potent inhibitors of poly(ADP-ribose) polymerase. Anticancer Drug Des 1991;6:107–17.

[54] Banasik M, Komura H, Shimoyama M, Ueda K. Specific inhibitors of poly(ADP-ribose) synthetase and mono(ADP-ribosyl)transferase. J Biol Chem 1992;267:1569–75.

[55] Ruf A, de Murcia GM, Schulz G. Inhibitor and NAD+ binding to poly(ADP-ribose) polymerase as derived from crystal structures and homology modeling. Biochemistry 1998;57:3893–900.

[56] Ruf A, Menissier de Murcia J, de Murcia G, Schulz GE. Structure of the catalytic fragment of poly(ADP-ribose) polymerase from chicken. Proc Natl Acad Sci U S A 1996;93:7481–5.

[57] Calabrese CR, Almassy R, Barton S, Batey MA, Calvert AH, Canan-Koch S, et al. Preclinical evaluation of a novel poly(ADP-ribose) polymerase-1 (PARP-1) inhibitor, AG14361, with significant anticancer chemo- and radio-sensitization activity. J Natl Cancer Inst 2004;96:56–67.

[58] Calabrese CR, Batey MA, Thomas HD, Durkacz BD, Wang L-Z, Kyle S, et al. Identification of potent non-toxic poly(ADP-ribose) polymerase-1 (PARP-1) inhibitors: chemopotentiation and pharmacological studies. Clin Cancer Res 2003;9:2711–8.

[59] Canan Koch SS, Thoresen LH, Tikhe JG, Maegley KA, Almassy RJ, Li J, et al. Novel tricyclic poly(ADP-ribose) polymerase-1 inhibitors with potent anticancer chemopotentiating activity: design, synthesis, and X-ray co-crystal structure. J Med Chem 2002;45:4961–74.

[60] Skalitzky DJ, Marakovits JT, Maegley KA, Ekker A, Yu X-H, Hostomsky Z, et al. Tricyclic benzimidazoles as potent PARP-1 inhibitors. J Med Chem 2003;46:210–3.

[61] Thomas HD, Calabrese CR, Batey MA, Canan S, Hostomsky Z, Kyle S, et al. Preclinical selection of a novel poly(ADP-ribose) polymerase inhibitor for clinical trial. Mol Cancer Ther 2007;6:945–56.

[62] Plummer R, Jones C, Middleton M, Wilson R, Evans J, Olsen A, et al. Phase I study of the poly(ADP-ribose) polymerase inhibitor, AG014699, in combination with temozolomide in patients with advanced solid tumors. Clin Cancer Res 2008;14:7917–23.

[63] Penning TD, Zhu GD, Gandhi VB, Gong J, Liu X, Shi Y, et al. Discovery of the poly(ADP-ribose) polymerase (PARP) inhibitor 2-[(R)-2-methylpyrrolidin-2-yl]-1H-benzimidazole-4-carboxamide (ABT-888) for the treatment of cancer. J Med Chem 2009;52:514–23.

[64] Menear KA, Adcock C, Boulter R, Cockcroft XL, Copsey L, Cranston A, et al. 4-[3-(4-cyclopropanecarbonylpiperazine-1-carbonyl)-4-fluorobenzyl]-2H-phthalazin-1-one: a novel bioavailable inhibitor of poly(ADP-ribose) polymerase-1. J Med Chem 2008;51:6581–91.

[65] Ferraris DV. Evolution of poly(ADP-ribose) polymerase-1 (PARP-1) inhibitors: from concept to clinic. J Med Chem 2010;53:4561–84.

[66] Javle M, Curtin NJ. The role of PARP in DNA repair and its therapeutic exploitation. Br J Cancer 2011a;105: 1114–22.

[67] Javle M, Curtin NJ. The potential for poly (ADP-ribose) polymerase inhibitors in cancer therapy. Ther Adv Med Oncol 2011b;3:257–67.

[68] Jagtap P, Szabo C. Poly(ADP-ribose) polymerase and the therapeutic effects of its inhibitors. Nat Rev Drug Discov 2005;4:421–40.

[69] Mangerich A, Burkle A. How to kill tumour cells with inhibitors of poly(ADP-ribose) polymerase. Int J Cancer 2011;128:251–65.

[70] Rouleau M, Patel A, Hendzel MJ, Kaufmann SH, Poirier GG. PARP inhibition: PARP1 and beyond. Nat Rev Cancer 2010;10:293–301.

[71] Boike GM, Petru E, Sevin BU, Averette HE, Chou TC, Penalver M, et al. Chemical enhancement of cisplatin cytotoxicity in a human ovarian and cervical cancer cell line. Gynecol Oncol 1990;38:315–22.

[72] Nguewa PA, Fuertes MA, Cepeda V, Alonso C, Quevedo C, Soto M, et al. Poly(ADP-ribose) polymerase-1 inhibitor 3-aminobenzamide enhances apoptosis induction by platinum complexes in cisplatin-resistant tumour cells. Med Chem 2006;2:47–53.

[73] Curtin NJ. PARP inhibitors for cancer therapy. Expert Rev Mol Med 2005;7:1–20.

[74] Tentori L, Portarena I, Graziani G. Potential clinical applications of poly(ADP-ribose) polymerase (PARP) inhibitors. Pharm Res 2002;45:73–85.

[75] Boulton S, Pemberton LC, Porteous JK, Curtin NJ, Griffin RJ, Golding BT, et al. Potentiation of temozolomide-induced cytotoxicity: a comparative study of the biological effects of poly(ADP-ribose) polymerase inhibitors. Br J Cancer 1995;72:849–56.

[76] Delaney CA, Wang LZ, Kyle S, White AW, Calvert AH, Curtin NJ, et al. Potentiation of temozolomide and topotecan growth inhibition and cytotoxicity by novel poly(adenosine diphosphoribose) polymerase inhibitors in a panel of human tumor cell lines. Clin Cancer Res 2000;6:2860–7.

[77] Tentori L, Leonetti C, Scarsella M, D'Amati G, Vergati M, Portarena I, et al. Systemic administration of GPI 15427, a novel poly(ADP-ribose) polymerase-1 inhibitor, increases the antitumor activity of temozolomide against intracranial melanoma, glioma, lymphoma. Clin Cancer Res 2003;9:5370–9.

[78] Tentori L, Leonetti C, Scarsella M, Muzi A, Mazzon E, Vergati M, et al. Inhibition of poly(ADP-ribose) polymerase prevents irinotecan-induced intestinal damage and enhances irinotecan/temozolomide efficacy against colon carcinoma. FASEB J 2006;20:1709–11.

[79] Liu X, Shi Y, Guan R, Donawho C, Luo Y, Palma J, et al. Potentiation of temozolomide cytotoxicity by poly(ADP)ribose polymerase inhibitor ABT-888 requires a conversion of single-stranded DNA damages to double-stranded DNA breaks. Mol Cancer Res 2008;6:1621–9.

[80] Palma JP, Wang YC, Rodriguez LE, Montgomery D, Ellis PA, Bukofzer G, et al. ABT-888 confers broad in vivo activity in combination with temozolomide in diverse tumors. Clin Cancer Res 2009;15:7277–90.

[81] Clarke MJ, Mulligan EA, Grogan PT, Mladek AC, Carlson BL, Schroeder MA, et al. Effective sensitization of temozolomide by ABT-888 is lost with development of temozolomide resistance in glioblastoma xenograft lines. Mol Cancer Ther 2009;8:407–14.

[82] Donawho CK, Luo Y, Penning TD, Bauch JL, Bouska JJ, Bontcheva-Diaz VD, et al. ABT-888, an orally active poly(ADP-ribose) polymerase inhibitor that potentiates DNA-damaging agents in preclinical tumor models. Clin Cancer Res 2007;13:2728–37.

[83] Daniel RA, Rozanska AL, Mulligan EA, Drew Y, Thomas HD, Castelbuono DJ, et al. Central nervous system penetration and enhancement of temozolomide activity in childhood medulloblastoma models by poly(ADP-ribose) polymerase inhibitor AG014699. Br J Cancer 2010;103:1588–96.

[84] Daniel RA, Rozanska AL, Thomas HD, Mulligan EA, Drew Y, Castelbuono DJ, et al. Inhibition of poly(ADP-ribose) polymerase-1 enhances temozolomide and topotecan activity against childhood neuroblastoma. Clin Cancer Res 2009;15:1241–9.

[85] Miknyoczki SJ, Jones-Bolin S, Pritchard S, Hunter K, Zhao H, Wan W, et al. Chemopotentiation of temozolomide, irinotecan, and cisplatin activity by CEP-6800, a poly(ADP-ribose) polymerase inhibitor. Mol Cancer Ther 2003;2:371–82.

[86] Cheng CL, Johnson SP, Keir ST, Quinn JA, Ali-Osman F, Szabo C, et al. Poly(ADP-ribose) polymerase-1 inhibition reverses temozolomide resistance in a DNA mismatch repair-deficient malignant glioma xenograft. Mol Cancer Ther 2005;4:1364–8.

[87] Curtin NJ, Wang LZ, Yiakouvaki A, Kyle S, Arris CA, Canan-Koch S, et al. Novel poly(ADP-ribose) polymerase-1 inhibitor, AG14361, restores sensitivity to temozolomide in mismatch repair-deficient cells. Clin Cancer Res 2004;10:881–9.

[88] Horton TM, Jenkins G, Pati D, Zhang L, Dolan ME, Ribes-Zamora A, et al. Poly(ADP-ribose) polymerase inhibitor ABT-888 potentiates the cytotoxic activity of temozolomide in leukemia cells: influence of mismatch repair status and O^6-methylguanine-DNA methyltransferase activity. Mol Cancer Ther 2009;8:2232–42.

[89] Tentori L, Turriziani M, Franco D, Serafino A, Levati L, Roy R, et al. Treatment with temozolomide and poly(ADP-ribose) polymerase inhibitors induces early apoptosis and increases base excision repair gene transcripts in leukemic cells resistant to triazene compounds. Leukemia 1999;13:901–9.

[90] Bowman KJ, Newell DR, Calvert AH, Curtin NJ. Differential effects of the poly (ADP-ribose) polymerase (PARP) inhibitor NU1025 on topoisomerase I and II inhibitor cytotoxicity in L1210 cells in vitro. Br J Cancer 2001;84:106–12.

[91] Yung TM, Sato S, Satoh MS. Poly(ADP-ribosyl)ation as a DNA damage-induced post-translational modification regulating poly(ADP-ribose) polymerase-1-topoisomerase I interaction. J Biol Chem 2004;279: 39686–96.

[92] Smith LM, Willmore E, Austin CA, Curtin NJ. The novel poly(ADP-Ribose) polymerase inhibitor, AG14361, sensitizes cells to topoisomerase I poisons by increasing the persistence of DNA strand breaks. Clin Cancer Res 2005;11:8449–57.

[93] Plo I, Liao ZY, Barcelo JM, Kohlhagen G, Caldecott KW, Weinfeld M, et al. Association of XRCC1 and tyrosyl DNA phosphodiesterase (Tdp1) for the repair of topoisomerase I-mediated DNA lesions. DNA Repair (Amst) 2003;2:1087–100.

[94] Malanga M, Althaus FR. Poly(ADP-ribose) reactivates stalled DNA topoisomerase I and induces DNA strand break resealing. J Biol Chem 2004;279:5244–8.

[95] Patel AG, Flatten KS, Schneider PA, Dai NT, McDonald JS, Poirier GG, et al. Enhanced killing of cancer cells by poly(ADP-ribose) polymerase inhibitors and topoisomerase I inhibitors reflects poisoning of both enzymes. J Biol Chem 2012b;287:4198–210.

[96] Ben-Hur E, Chen CC, Elkind MM. Inhibitors of poly(adenosine diphosphoribose) synthetase, examination of metabolic perturbations, and enhancement of radiation response in Chinese hamster cells. Cancer Res 1985;45:2123–7.

[97] Brock WA, Milas L, Bergh S, Lo R, Szabo C, Mason KA. Radiosensitization of human and rodent cell lines by INO-1001, a novel inhibitor of poly(ADP-ribose) polymerase. Cancer Lett 2004;205:155–60.

[98] Dungey FA, Loser DA, Chalmers AJ. Replication-dependent radiosensitization of human glioma cells by inhibition of poly(ADP-ribose) polymerase: mechanisms and therapeutic potential. Int J Radiat Oncol Biol Phys 2008;72:1188–97.

[99] Russo AL, Kwon HC, Burgan WE, Carter D, Beam K, Weizheng X, et al. In vitro and in vivo radiosensitization of glioblastoma cells by the poly (ADP-ribose) polymerase inhibitor E7016. Clin Cancer Res 2009;15(2):607–12.

[100] Schlicker A, Peschke P, Burkle A, Hahn EW, Kim JH. 4-Amino-1,8-naphthalimide: a novel inhibitor of poly(ADP-ribose) polymerase and radiation sensitizer. Int J Radiat Biol 1999;75:91–100.

[101] Saleh-Gohari N, Bryant HE, Schultz N, Parker KM, Cassel TN, Helleday T. Spontaneous homologous recombination is induced by collapsed replication forks that are caused by endogenous DNA single-strand breaks. Mol Cell Biol 2005;25:7158–69.

[102] Harper JV, Anderson JA, O'Neill P. Radiation induced DNA DSBs: contribution from stalled replication forks? DNA Repair (Amst) 2010;9:907–13.

[103] Liu SK, Coackley C, Krause M, Jalali F, Chan N, Bristow RG. A novel poly(ADP-ribose) polymerase inhibitor, ABT-888, radiosensitizes malignant human cell lines under hypoxia. Radiother Oncol 2008;88:258–68.

[104] Leopold WR, Sebolt-Leopold JS. Chemical approaches to improved radiotherapy. In: Valeriote FA, Corbett TH, Baker LH, editors. Cytotoxic anticancer drugs: models and concepts for drug discovery and development. Boston: Kluwer; 1992. p. 179–96.

[105] Khan K, Araki K, Wang D, Li G, Li X, Zhang J, et al. Head and neck cancer radiosensitization by the novel poly(ADP-ribose) polymerase inhibitor GPI-15427. Head Neck 2010;32:381–91.

[106] Wang L, Mason KA, Ang KK, Buchholz T, Valdecanas D, Mathur A, et al. MK-4827, a PARP-1/-2 inhibitor, strongly enhances response of human lung and breast cancer xenografts to radiation. Invest New Drugs 2012;30:2113–220.

[107] Senra JM, Telfer BA, Cherry KE, McCrudden CM, Hirst DG, O'Connor MJ, et al. Inhibition of PARP-1 by olaparib (AZD2281) increases the radiosensitivity of a lung tumor xenograft. Mol Cancer Ther 2011;10:1949–58.

[108] Albert JM, Cao C, Kim KW, Willey CD, Geng L, Xiao D, et al. Inhibition of poly(ADP-ribose) polymerase enhances cell death and improves tumor growth delay in irradiated lung cancer models. Clin Cancer Res 2007;13:3033–42.

[109] Barreto-Andrade JC, Efimova EV, Mauceri HJ, Beckett MA, Sutton HG, Darga TE, et al. Response of human prostate cancer cells and tumors to combining PARP inhibition with ionizing radiation. Mol Cancer Ther 2011;10:1185–93.

[110] Ali M, Telfer BA, McCrudden C, O'Rourke M, Thomas HD, Kamjoo M, et al. Vasoactivity of AG014699, a clinically active small molecule inhibitor of poly(ADP-ribose) polymerase: a contributory factor to chemopotentiation in vivo? Clin Cancer Res 2009;15:6106–12.

[111] Ali M, Kamjoo M, Thomas HD, Kyle S, Pavlovska I, Babur M, et al. The clinically active PARP inhibitor AG014699 ameliorates cardiotoxicity but doesn't enhance the efficacy of doxorubicin despite improving tumour perfusion and radiation response. Molecular Cancer Therapeutics 2011;10:2320–29.

[112] Plummer R, Lorigan P, Evans J, Steven N, Middleton M, Wilson R, et al. First and final report of a phase II study of the poly(ADP-ribose) polymerase (PARP) inhibitor, AG014699, in combination with temozolomide (TMZ) in patients with metastatic malignant melanoma (MM). J Clin Oncol 2006;24(18s):8013.

[113] Khan OA, Gore M, Lorigan P, Stone J, Greystoke A, Burke W, et al. A phase I study of the safety and tolerability of olaparib (AZD2281, KU0059436) and dacarbazine in patients with advanced solid tumours. Br J Cancer 2011;104:750–5.

[114] Bedikian AY, Papadopoulos NE, Kim KB, Hwu WJ, Homsi J, Glass MR, et al. A phase IB trial of intravenous INO-1001 plus oral temozolomide in subjects with unresectable stage-III or IV melanoma. Cancer Invest 2009;27:756–63.

[115] Kummar S, Chen A, Ji J, Zhang Y, Reid JM, Ames M, et al. Phase I study of PARP inhibitor ABT-888 in combination with topotecan in adults with refractory solid tumors and lymphomas. Cancer Res 2011;71:5626–34.

[116] LoRusso P, Ji JJ, Li J, Heilbrun LK, Shapiro G, Sausville EA, et al. Phase I study of the safety, pharmacokinetics (PK), and pharmacodynamics (PD) of the poly(ADP-ribose) polymerase (PARP) inhibitor veliparib (ABT-888; V) in combination with irinotecan (CPT-11; Ir) in patients (pts) with advanced solid tumors. J Clin Oncol 2011;29(Suppl. 15):3000.

[117] Samol J, Ranson M, Scott E, Macpherson E, Carmichael J, Thomas A, et al. Safety and tolerability of the poly(ADP-ribose) polymerase (PARP) inhibitor, olaparib (AZD2281) in combination with topotecan for the treatment of patients with advanced solid tumors: a phase I study. Invest New Drugs 2011;30:1493–500.

[118] Mehta MP, Curran WJ, Wang D, Wang F, Kleinberg L, Brade AM, et al. Phase I safety and pharmacokinetic (PK) study of veliparib in combination with whole brain radiation therapy (WBRT) in patients (pts) with brain metastases. J Clin Oncol 2012;30(Suppl.): abstr. 2013.

[119] Xanthoudakis S, Smeyne RJ, Wallace JD, Curran T. The redox/DNA repair protein Ref-1 is essential for early embryonic development in mice. Proc Natl Acad Sci U S A 1996;93:8919–23.

[120] Fishel ML, He Y, Reed AM, Chin-Sinex H, Hutchins GD, Mendonca MS, et al. Knockdown of the DNA repair and redox signalling protein Ape-1/Ref-1 blocks ovarian cancer cell and tumour growth. DNA Repair (Amst) 2008;7:177–86.

[121] Demple B, Sung JS. Molecular and biological roles of Ape1 protein in mammalian base excision repair. DNA Repair (Amst) 2005;4:1442–9.

[122] Abbotts R, Madhusudan S. Human AP endonuclease 1 (APE1): from mechanistic insights to druggable target in cancer. Cancer Treat Rev 2010;36:425–35.

[123] Fishel ML, Kelley MR. The DNA base excision repair protein Ape1/Ref-1 as a therapeutic and chemopreventive target. Mol Aspects Med 2007;28(3–4):375–95.

[124] Madhusudan S. Human AP endonuclease 1 (APE1): from mechanistic insights to druggable target in cancer. Cancer Treat Rev 2010;36:425–35.

[125] Taverna P, Liu L, Hwang HS, Hanson AJ, Kinsella TJ, Gerson SL. Methoxyamine potentiates DNA single strand breaks and double strand breaks induced by temozolomide in colon cancer cells. Mutat Res 2001;485:269–81.

[126] Fishel ML, He Y, Smith ML, Kelley MR. Manipulation of base excision repair to sensitize ovarian cancer cells to alkylating agent temozolomide. Clin Cancer Res 2007;13:260–7.

[127] Liu L, Nakatsuru Y, Gerson SL. Base excision repair as a therapeutic target in colon cancer. Clin Cancer Res 2002;8:2985–91.

[128] Taverna P, Hwang HS, Schupp JE, Radivoyevitch T, Session NN, Reddy G, et al. Inhibition of base excision repair potentiates iododeoxyuridine-induced cytotoxicity and radiosensitization. Cancer Res 2003;63:838–46.

[129] Bulgar AD, Weeks LD, Miao Y, Yang S, Xu Y, Guo C, et al. Removal of uracil by uracil DNA glycosylase limits pemetrexed cytotoxicity: overriding the limit with methoxyamine to inhibit base excision repair. Cell Death Dis 2012;12(3):e252.

[130] Weiss GJ, Gordon MS, Rosen LS, Savvides P, Ramanathan RK, Mendelson DS, et al. Final results from a phase 1 study of oral TRC102 (methoxyamine HCl), an inhibitor of base-excision repair, to potentiate the activity of pemetrexedin patients with refractory cancer. J Clin Oncol 2010;28(Suppl.):15s; abstr. 2576.

[131] Madhusudan S, Smart F, Shrimpton P, Parsons JL, Gardiner L, Houlbrook S, et al. Isolation of a small molecule inhibitor of DNA base excision repair. Nucleic Acids Res 2005;33:4711–24.

[132] Luo M, Kelley MR. Inhibition of the human apurinic/apyrimidinic endonuclease (APE1) repair activity and sensitization of breast cancer cells to DNA alkylating agents with lucanthone. Anticancer Res 2004;24:2127–34.

[133] Del Rowe JD, Bello J, Mitnick R, Sood B, Filippi C, Moran J, et al. Accelerated regression of brain metastases in patients receiving whole brain radiation and the topoisomerase II inhibitor, lucanthone. Int J Radiat Oncol Biol Phys 1999;43:89–93.

[134] Bapat A, Glass LS, Luo M, Fishel ML, Long EC, Georgiadis MM, et al. Novel small molecule inhibitor of Ape1 endonuclease blocks proliferation and reduces viability of glioblastoma cells. J Pharmacol Exp Ther 2010;334:988–98.

[135] Mohammed MZ, Vyjayanti VN, Laughton CA, Dekker LV, Fischer PM, Wilson 3rd DM, et al. Development and evaluation of human AP endonuclease inhibitors in melanoma and glioma cell lines. Br J Cancer 2011;104: 653–63.

[136] Wilson 3rd DM, Simeonov A. Small molecule inhibitors of DNA repair nuclease activities of APE1. Cell Mol Life Sci 2010;67:3621–31.

[137] Acharya S, Wilson T, Gradia S, Kane MF, Guerrette S, Marsischky GT, et al. hMSH2 forms specific mispair-binding complexes with hMSH3 and hMSH6. Proc Natl Acad Sci U S A 1996;93:13629–34.

[138] Palombo F, Iaccarino I, Nakajima E, Ikejima M, Shimada T, Jiricny J. hMutSbeta, a heterodimer of hMSH2 and hMSH3, binds to insertion/deletion loops in DNA. Curr Biol 1996;6:1181–4.

[139] Modrich P, Lahue R. Mismatch repair in replication fidelity, genetic recombination, and cancer biology. Annu Rev Biochem 1996;65:101–33.

[140] Vasen HF, Watson P, Mecklin JP, Lynch HT. New clinical criteria for hereditary nonpolyposis colorectal cancer (HNPCC, Lynch syndrome) proposed by the international collaborative group on HNPCC. Gastroenterology 1999;116:1453–6.

[141] Backes FJ, Cohn DE. Lynch syndrome. Clin Obstet Gynecol 2011;54:199–214.

[142] Barrow E, Alduaij W, Robinson L, Shenton A, Clancy T, Lalloo F, et al. Colorectal cancer in HNPCC: cumulative lifetime incidence, survival and tumour distribution. A report of 121 families with proven mutations. Clin Genet 2008;74:233–42.

[143] Boland CR, Goel A. Microsatellite instability in colorectal cancer. Gastroenterology 2010;138:2073–87.

[144] Gras E, Catasus L, Arguelles R, Moreno-Bueno G, Palacios J, Gamallo C, et al. Microsatellite instability, MLH-1 promoter hypermethylation, and frameshift mutations at coding mononucleotide repeat microsatellites in ovarian tumors. Cancer 2001;92:2829–36.

[145] Herman JG, Umar A, Polyak K, Graff JR, Ahuja N, Issa JP, et al. Incidence and functional consequences of hMLH1 promoter hypermethylation in colorectal carcinoma. Proc Natl Acad Sci U S A 1998;95:6870–5.

[146] Lynch HT, de la Chapelle A. Genetic susceptibility to non-polyposis colorectal cancer. J Med Genet 1999;36: 801–18.

[147] Hakem R. DNA-damage repair; the good, the bad and the ugly. EMBO J 2008;27:589–605.

[148] Karran P, Bignami M. DNA damage tolerance, mismatch repair and genome instability. Bioessays 1994;16: 833–9.

[149] Yoshioka K, Yoshioka Y, Hsieh P. ATR kinase activation mediated by MutSalpha and MutLalpha in response+ to cytotoxic O^6-methylguanine adducts. Mol Cell 2006;22:501–10.

[150] Irving JA, Hall AG. Mismatch repair defects as a cause of resistance to cytotoxic drugs. Expert Rev Anticancer Ther 2001;1:149–58.

[151] Bracht K, Nicholls AM, Liu Y, Bodmer WF. 5-fluorouracil response in a large panel of colorectal cell lines is associated with mismatch repair deficiency. Br J Cancer 2010;103:340–6.

[152] Jover R, Zapater P, Castells A, Llor X, Andreu M, Cubiella J, et al. Gastrointestinal Oncology Group of the Spanish Gastroenterological Association: the efficacy of adjuvant chemotherapy with 5-fluorouracil in colorectal cancer depends on the mismatch repair status. Eur J Cancer 2009;45:365–73.

[153] Ribic CM, Sargent DJ, Moore MJ, Thibodeau SN, French AJ, Goldberg RM, et al. Tumor microsatellite instability status as a predictor of benefit from fluorouracil-based adjuvant chemotherapy for colon cancer. N Engl J Med 2003;349:247–57.

[154] Sinicrope FA, Foster NR, Thibodeau SN, Marsoni S, Monges G, Labianca R, et al. DNA mismatch repair status and colon cancer recurrence and survival in clinical trials of 5-fluorouracil-based adjuvant therapy. J Natl Cancer Inst 2011;103:863–75.

[155] Fordham SE, Matheson EC, Scott K, Irving JA, Allan JM. DNA mismatch repair status affects cellular response to Ara-C and other anti-leukemic nucleoside analogs. Leukemia 2011;25:1046–9.

[156] Felsberg J, Thon N, Eigenbrod S, Hentschel B, Sabel MC, Westphal M, et al. German Glioma Network Promoter methylation and expression of MGMT and the DNA mismatch repair genes MLH1, MSH2, MSH6 and PMS2 in paired primary and recurrent glioblastomas. Int J Cancer 2011;129:659–70.

[157] Yip S, Miao J, Cahill DP, Iafrate AJ, Aldape K, Nutt CL, et al. MSH6 mutations arise in glioblastomas during temozolomide therapy and mediate temozolomide resistance. Clin Cancer Res 2009;15:4622–9.

[158] Samimi G, Fink D, Varki NM, Husain A, Hoskins WJ, Alberts DS, et al. Analysis of MLH1 and MSH2 expression in ovarian cancer before and after platinum drug-based chemotherapy. Clin Cancer Res 2000;6:1415–21.

[159] Plumb JA, Strathdee G, Sludden J, Kaye SB, Brown R. Reversal of drug resistance in human tumor xenografts by 2'-deoxy-5-azacytidine-induced demethylation of the hMLH1 gene promoter. Cancer Res 2000;60:6039–44.

[160] Ward JF. The yield of DNA double-strand breaks produced intracellularly by ionizing radiation: a review. Int J Radiat Biol 1990;57:1141–50.

[161] McClendon AK, Osheroff N. DNA topoisomerase II, genotoxicity, cancer. Mutat Res 2007;623:83–97.

[162] Nikjoo H, O'Neill P, Wilson WE, Goodhead DT. Computational approach for determining the spectrum of DNA damage induced by ionizing radiation. Radiat Res 2001;156:577–83.

[163] Povirk LF. DNA damage and mutagenesis by radiomimetic DNA-cleaving agents: bleomycin, neocarzinostatin and other enediynes. Mutat Res 1996;355:71–89.

[164] Dedon PC, Jiang ZW, Goldberg IH. Neocarzinostatin-mediated DNA damage in a model AGT-ACT site: mechanistic studies of thiol-sensitive partitioning of C4' DNA damage products. Biochemistry 1992;31:1917–27.

[165] Shrivastav M, De Haro LP, Nickoloff JA. Regulation of DNA double-strand break repair pathway choice. Cell Res 2008;18:134–47.

[166] Mahaney BL, Meek K, Lees-Miller SP. Repair of ionizing radiation-induced DNA double-strand breaks by non-homologous end-joining. Biochem J 2009;417:639–50.

[167] Rothkamm K, Kruger I, Thompson LH, Lobrich M. Pathways of DNA double-strand break repair during the mammalian cell cycle. Mol Cell Biol 2003;23:5706–15.

[168] Shibata A, Conrad S, Birraux J, Geuting V, Barton O, Ismail A, et al. Factors determining DNA double-strand break repair pathway choice in G2 phase. EMBO J 2011;30:1079–92.

[169] Smith GC, Jackson SP. The DNA-dependent protein kinase. Genes Dev 1999;13:916–34.

[170] Kurimasa A, Kumano S, Boubnov NV, Story MD, Tung CS, Peterson SR, et al. Requirement for the kinase activity of human DNA-dependent protein kinase catalytic subunit in DNA strand break rejoining. Mol Cell Biol 1999;19:3877–84.

[171] Merkle D, Douglas P, Moorhead GB, Leonenko Z, Yu Y, Cramb D, et al. The DNA-dependent protein kinase interacts with DNA to form a protein-DNA complex that is disrupted by phosphorylation. Biochemistry 2002;41:12706–14.

[172] Ahnesorg P, Smith P, Jackson SP. XLF interacts with the XRCC4-DNA ligase IV complex to promote DNA nonhomologous end-joining. Cell 2006;124:301–13.

[173] Burma S, Chen BPC, Chen DJ. Role of non-homologous end joining (NHEJ) in maintaining genomic integrity. DNA Repair 2006;5:1042–8.

[174] Lees-Miller SP, Meek K. Repair of DNA double strand breaks by non-homologous end joining. Biochimie 2003;85:1161–73.

[175] Jeggo PA, Caldecott K, Pidsley S, Banks GR. Sensitivity of Chinese hamster ovary mutants defective in DNA double strand break repair to topoisomerase II inhibitors. Cancer Res 1989;49:7057–63.

[176] Tanaka T, Yamagami T, Oka Y, Nomura T, Sugiyama H. The SCID mutation in mice causes defects in the repair system for both double-strand DNA breaks and DNA cross-links. Mutat Res 1993;288:277–80.

[177] Izzard RA, Jackson SP, Smith GC. Competitive and noncompetitive inhibition of the DNA-dependent protein kinase. Cancer Res 1999;59:2581–6.

[178] Boulton S, Kyle S, Durkacz BW. Mechanisms of enhancement of cytotoxicity in etoposide and ionising radiation-treated cells by the protein kinase inhibitor wortmannin. Eur J Cancer 2000;36:535–41.

[179] Price BD, Youmell MB. The phosphatidylinositol 3-kinase inhibitor wortmannin sensitizes murine fibroblasts and human tumor cells to radiation and blocks induction of p53 following DNA damage. Cancer Res 1996;56:246–50.

[180] Rosenzweig KE, Youmell MB, Palayoor ST, Price BD. Radiosensitization of human tumor cells by the phosphatidylinositol 3-kinase inhibitors wortmannin and LY294002 correlates with inhibition of DNA-dependent protein kinase and prolonged G2-M delay. Clin Cancer Res 1997;3:1149–56.

[181] Hardcastle IR, Cockcroft X, Curtin NJ, El-Murr MD, Leahy JJ, Stockley M, et al. Discovery of potent chromen-4-one inhibitors of the DNA-dependent protein kinase (DNA-PK) using a small-molecule library approach. J Med Chem 2005;48:7829–46.

[182] Leahy JJ, Golding BT, Griffin RJ, Hardcastle IR, Richardson C, Rigoreau L, et al. Identification of a highly potent and selective DNA-dependent protein kinase (DNA-PK) inhibitor (NU7441) by screening of chromenone libraries. Bioorg Med Chem Lett 2004;14:6083–7.

[183] Rainey MD, Charlton ME, Stanton RV, Kastan MB. Transient inhibition of ATM kinase is sufficient to enhance cellular sensitivity to ionizing radiation. Cancer Res 2008;68:7466–74.

[184] Kashishian A, Douangpanya H, Clark D, Schlachter ST, Eary CT, Schiro JG, et al. DNA-dependent protein kinase inhibitors as drug candidates for the treatment of cancer. Mol Cancer Ther 2003;2:1257–64.

[185] Shinohara ET, Geng L, Tan J, Chen H, Shir Y, Edwards E, et al. DNA-dependent protein kinase is a molecular target for the development of noncytotoxic radiation-sensitizing drugs. Cancer Res 2005;65:4987–92.

[186] Willmore E, de Caux S, Sunter NJ, Tilby MJ, Jackson GH, Austin CA, et al. A novel DNA-dependent protein kinase inhibitor, NU7026, potentiates the cytotoxicity of topoisomerase II poisons used in the treatment of leukemia. Blood 2004;103:4659–65.

[187] Zhao Y, Thomas HD, Batey MA, Cowell IG, Richardson CJ, Griffin RJ, et al. Preclinical evaluation of a potent novel DNA-dependent protein kinase inhibitor NU7441. Cancer Res 2006;66:5354–62.

[188] Kruszewski M, Wojewodzka M, Iwanenko T, Szumiel I, Okuyama A. Differential inhibitory effect of OK-1035 on DNA repair in L5178Y murine lymphoma sublines with functional or defective repair of double strand breaks. Mutat Res 1998;409:31–6.

[189] Ismail IH, Martensson S, Moshinsky D, Rice A, Tang C, Howlett A, et al. SU11752 inhibits the DNA-dependent protein kinase and DNA double-strand break repair resulting in ionizing radiation sensitization. Oncogene 2004;23:873–82.

[190] Munck JM, Batey MA, Zhao Y, Jenkins H, Richardson CJ, Cano C, et al. Chemosensitization of cancer cells by KU-0060648, a dual inhibitor of DNA-PK and PI-3K. Mol Cancer Ther 2012;11:1789–98.

[191] Elliott SL, Crawford C, Mulligan E, Summerfield G, Newton P, Wallis J, et al. Mitoxantrone in combination with an inhibitor of DNA-dependent protein kinase: a potential therapy for high risk B-cell chronic lymphocytic leukaemia. Br J Haematol 2011;152:61–71.

[192] Zhong Q, Chen CF, Li S, Chen Y, Wang CC, Xiao J, et al. Association of BRCA1 with the hRad50-hMre11-p95 complex and the DNA damage response. Science 1999;285:747–50.

[193] Derheimer FA, Kastan MB. Multiple roles of ATM in monitoring and maintaining DNA integrity. FEBS Lett 2010;584:3675–81.

[194] Paull TT, Lee JH. The Mre11/Rad50/Nbs1 complex and its role as a DNA double-strand break sensor for ATM. Cell Cycle 2005;4:737–40.

[195] Stiff T, O'Driscoll M, Rief N, Iwabuchi K, Lobrich M, Jeggo PA. ATM and DNA-PK function redundantly to phosphorylate H2AX after exposure to ionizing radiation. Cancer Res 2004;64:2390–6.

[196] Kee Y, D'Andrea AD. Expanded roles of the Fanconi anemia pathway in preserving genomic stability. Genes Dev 2010;24:1680–94.

[197] Wang W. Emergence of a DNA-damage response network consisting of Fanconi anaemia and BRCA proteins. Nat Rev Genet 2007;8:735–48.

[198] Bolderson E, Tomimatsu N, Richard DJ, Boucher D, Kumar R, Pandita TK, et al. Phosphorylation of Exo1 modulates homologous recombination repair of DNA double-strand breaks. Nucleic Acids Res 2010;38: 1821–31.

[199] Di Virgilio M, Ying CY, Gautier J. PIKK-dependent phosphorylation of Mre11 induces MRN complex inactivation by disassembly from chromatin. DNA Repair (Amst) 2009;8:1311–20.

[200] Flynn RL, Zou L. A master conductor of cellular responses to DNA replication stress. Trends Biochem Sci 2011;36:133–40.

[201] Shi W, Feng Z, Zhang J, Gonzalez-Suarez I, Vanderwaal RP, Wu X, et al. The role of RPA2 phosphorylation in homologous recombination in response to replication arrest. Carcinogenesis 2010;31:994–1002.

[202] Sorensen CS, Hansen LT, Dziegielewski J, Syljuåsen RG, Lundin C, Bartek J, et al. The cell-cycle checkpoint kinase Chk1 is required for mammalian homologous recombination repair. Nat Cell Biol 2005;7:195–201.

[203] Jensen RB, Carreira A, Kowalczykowski SC. Purified human BRCA2 stimulates RAD51-mediated recombination. Nature 2010;467:678–83.

[204] Liu J, Doty T, Gibson B, Heyer WD. Human BRCA2 protein promotes RAD51 filament formation on RPA-covered single-stranded DNA. Nat Struct Mol Biol 2010;17:1260–2.

[205] Thorslund T, McIlwraith MJ, Compton SA, Lekomtsev S, Petronczki M, Griffith JD, et al. The breast cancer tumor suppressor BRCA2 promotes the specific targeting of RAD51 to single-stranded DNA. Nat Struct Mol Biol 2010;17:1263–5.

[206] Sung P, Klein H. Mechanism of homologous recombination: mediators and helicases take on regulatory functions. Nat Rev Mol Cell Biol 2006;7:739–50.

[207] Bugreev DV, Brosh Jr RM, Mazin AV. RECQ1 possesses DNA branch migration activity. J Biol Chem 2008;283:20231–42.

[208] Gari K, Decaillet C, Stasiak AZ, Stasiak A, Constantinou A. The Fanconi anemia protein FANCM can promote branch migration of Holliday junctions and replication forks. Mol Cell 2008;29:141–8.

[209] Ip SC, Rass U, Blanco MG, Flynn HR, Skehel JM, West SC. Identification of Holliday junction resolvases from humans and yeast. Nature 2008;456:357–61.

[210] Berman DB, Costalas J, Schultz DC, Grana G, Daly M, Godwin AK. A common mutation in BRCA2 that predisposes to a variety of cancers is found in both Jewish Ashkenazi and non-Jewish individuals. Cancer Res 1996;56:3409–14.

[211] Brose MS, Rebbeck TR, Calzone KA, Stopfer JE, Nathanson KL, Weber BL. Cancer risk estimates for BRCA1 mutation carriers identified in a risk evaluation program. J Natl Cancer Inst 2002;94:1365–72.

[212] Vogelstein B, Kinzler KW. Cancer genes and the pathways they control. Nat Med 2004;10:789–99.

[213] Dobrovic A, Simpfendorfer D. Methylation of the BRCA1 gene in sporadic breast cancer. Cancer Res 1997;57:3347–50.

[214] Esteller M, Silva JM, Dominguez G, Bonilla F, Matias-Guiu X, Lerma E, et al. Promoter hypermethylation and BRCA1 inactivation in sporadic breast and ovarian tumors. J Natl Cancer Inst 2000b;92:564–9.

[215] Lahtz C, Pfeifer GP. Epigenetic changes of DNA repair genes in cancer. J Mol Cell Biol 2011;3:51–8.

[216] Lee MN, Tseng RC, Hsu HS, Chen JY, Tzao C, Ho WL. Epigenetic inactivation of the chromosomal stability control genes BRCA1, BRCA2, and XRCC5 in non-small cell lung cancer. Clin Cancer Res 2007;13:832–8.

[217] Taylor AM, Harnden DG, Arlett CF, Harcourt SA, Lehmann AR, Stevens S, et al. Ataxia telangiectasia: a human mutation with abnormal radiation sensitivity. Nature 1975;258:427–9.

[218] Milne RL. Variants in the ATM gene and breast cancer susceptibility. Genome Med 2009;1:12.

[219] Prokopcova J, Kleibl Z, Banwell CM, Pohlreich P. The role of ATM in breast cancer development. Breast Cancer Res Treat 2007;104:121–8.

[220] Roberts NJ, Jiao Y, Yu J, Kopelovich L, Petersen GM, Bondy ML, et al. ATM mutations in patients with hereditary pancreatic cancer. Cancer Discov 2012;2:41–6.

[221] Thompson D, Duedal S, Kirner J. Cancer risks and mortality in heterozygous ATM mutation carriers. J Natl Cancer Inst 2005;97:813–22.

[222] Boultwood J. Ataxia telangiectasia gene mutations in leukaemia and lymphoma. J Clin Pathol 2001;54(7):512–6.

[223] Ai L, Vo QN, Zuo C, Li L, Ling W, Suen JY, et al. Ataxia-telangiectasia-mutated (ATM) gene in head and neck squamous cell carcinoma: promoter hypermethylation with clinical correlation in 100 cases. Cancer Epidemiol Biomarkers Prev 2004;13:150–6.

[224] Bai AH, Tong JH, To KF, Chan MW, Man EP, Lo KW, et al. Promoter hypermethylation of tumor-related genes in the progression of colorectal neoplasia. Int J Cancer 2004;112:846–53.

[225] Flanagan JM, Munoz-Alegre M, Henderson S, Tang T, Sun P, Johnson N, et al. Gene-body hypermethylation of ATM in peripheral blood DNA of bilateral breast cancer patients. Hum Mol Genet 2009;18:1332–42.

[226] Kim WJ, Vo QN, Shrivastav M, Lataxes TA, Brown KD. Aberrant methylation of the ATM promoter correlates with increased radiosensitivity in a human colorectal tumor cell line. Oncogene 2002;21:3864–71.

[227] Pal R, Srivastava N, Chopra R, Gochhait S, Gupta P, Prakash N, et al. Investigation of DNA damage response and apoptotic gene methylation pattern in sporadic breast tumors using high throughput quantitative DNA methylation analysis technology. Mol Cancer 2010;9:303.

[228] Dupré A, Boyer-Chatenet L, Sattler RM, Modi AP, Lee JH, Nicolette ML, et al. A forward chemical genetic screen reveals an inhibitor of the Mre11-Rad50-Nbs1 complex. Nat Chem Biol 2008;4:119–25.

[229] Shimizu H, Popova M, Fleury F, Kobayashi M, Hayashi N, Sakane I, et al. c-ABL tyrosine kinase stabilizes RAD51 chromatin association. Biochem Biophys Res Commun 2009;382:286–91.

[230] Yuan SS, Chang HL, Lee EY. Ionizing radiation-induced Rad51 nuclear focus formation is cell cycle-regulated and defective in both ATM(−/−) and c-Abl(−/−) cells. Mutat Res 2003;525:85–92.

[231] Aloyz R, Grzywacz K, Xu ZY, Loignon M, Alaoui-Jamali MA, Panasci L. Imatinib sensitizes CLL lymphocytes to chlorambucil. Leukemia 2004;18(3):409–14.

[232] Choudhury A, Zhao H, Jalali F, Al Rashid S, Ran J, Supiot S, et al. Targeting homologous recombination using imatinib results in enhanced tumor cell chemosensitivity and radiosensitivity. Mol Cancer Ther 2009;8:203–13.

[233] Johnson N, Cai D, Kennedy RD, Pathania S, Arora M, Li YC, et al. Cdk1 participates in BRCA1-dependent S phase checkpoint control in response to DNA damage. Mol Cell 2009;35:327–39.

[234] Shiloh Y. The ATM-mediated DNA-damage response: taking shape. Trends Biochem Sci 2006;31:402–10.

[235] Smith J, Tho LM, Xu N, Gillespie DA. The ATM-Chk2 and ATR-Chk1 pathways in DNA damage signaling and cancer. Adv Cancer Res 2010;108:73–112.

[236] Hollick JJ, Rigoreau LJM, Cano-Soumillac C, Cockcroft X, Curtin NJ, Frigerio M, et al. Pyranone, thiopyranone, and pyridone inhibitors of phosphatidylinositol 3-kinase related kinases. Structure–activity relationships for DNA-dependent protein kinase inhibition, and identification of the first potent and selective inhibitor of the ataxia telangiectasia mutated kinase. J Med Chem 2007;50:1958–72.

[237] Hickson I, Zhao Y, Richardson CJ, Green SJ, Martin MNB, Orr AI, et al. Identification of a novel and specific inhibitor of the ataxia-telangiectasia mutated kinase ATM. Cancer Res 2004;64:9152–9.

[238] Shaheen FS, Znojek P, Fisher A, Webster M, Plummer R, Gaughan L, et al. Targeting the DNA double strand break repair machinery in prostate cancer. PLoS One 2011;6(5):e20311.

[239] Golding SE, Rosenberg E, Valerie N, Hussaini I, Frigerio M, Cockcroft XF, et al. Improved ATM kinase inhibitor KU-60019 radiosensitizes glioma cells, compromises insulin, AKT and ERK prosurvival signaling, and inhibits migration and invasion. Mol Cancer Ther 2009;8:2894–902.

[240] Lountos GT, Jobson AG, Tropea JE, Self CR, Zhang G, Pommier Y, et al. Structural characterization of inhibitor complexes with checkpoint kinase 2 (Chk2), a drug target for cancer therapy. J Struct Biol 2011;176:292–301.

[241] Jobson AG, Lountos GT, Lorenzi PL, Llamas J, Connelly J, Cerna D, et al. Cellular inhibition of checkpoint kinase 2 (Chk2) and potentiation of camptothecins and radiation by the novel Chk2 inhibitor PV1019 [7-nitro-1H-indole-2-carboxylic acid {4-[1-(guanidinohydrazone)-ethyl]-phenyl}-amide]. J Pharmacol Exp Ther 2009;331:816–26.

[242] Pires IM, Ward TH, Dive C. Oxaliplatin responses in colorectal cancer cells are modulated by CHK2 kinase inhibitors. Br J Pharmacol 2010;159:1326–38.

[243] Massague J. G1 cell cycle control and cancer. Nature 2004;432:298–306.

[244] Sherr CJ. Cancer cell cycles. Science 1996;274:1672–4.

[245] Cimprich KA, Cortez D. ATR: an essential regulator of genome integrity. Nat Rev Mol Cell Biol 2008;9: 616–27.

[246] Caporali S, Falcinelli S, Starace G, Russo MT, Bonmassar E, Jiricny J, et al. DNA damage induced by temozolomide signals to both ATM and ATR: role of mismatch repair system. Mol Pharmacol 2004;66:478–91.

[247] Carrassa L, Broggini M, Erba E, Damia G. Chk1, but not Chk2, is involved in the cellular response to DNA damaging agents: differential activity in cells expressing or not p53. Cell Cycle 2004;3:1177–81.

[248] Cliby WA, Roberts CJ, Cimprich KA, Stringer CM, Lamb JR, Schreiber SL, et al. Overexpression of a kinase-inactive ATR protein causes sensitivity to DNA damaging agents and defects in cell cycle checkpoints. EMBO J 1998;17:159–69.

[249] Harada N, Watanabe Y, Yoshimura Y, Sakumoto H, Makishima F, Tsuchiya M, et al. Identification of a checkpoint modulator with synthetic lethality to p53 mutants. Anticancer Drugs 2011;22:986–94.

[250] Nghiem P, Park PK, Kim Y-S, Vaziri C, Schreiber SL. ATR inhibition selectively sensitizes G_1 checkpoint-deficient cells to lethal premature chromatin condensation. Proc Natl Acad Sci U S A 2001;98:9092–7.

[251] Ward IM, Minn K, Chen J. UV-induced ataxia telangiectasia mutated and RAD3-related (ATR) activation requires replicative stress. J Biol Chem 2004;279:9677–80.

[252] Wagner JM, Kaufmann SH. Prospects for the use of ATR inhibitors to treat cancer. Pharmaceuticals 2010;3:1311–34.

[253] Sarkaria JN, Busby EC, Tibbetts RS, Roos P, Taya Y, Karnitz LM, et al. Inhibition of ATM and ATR kinase activities by the radiosensitizing agent, caffeine. Cancer Res 1999;59:4375–82.

[254] Nishida H, Tatewaki N, Nakajima Y, Magara T, Ko KM, Hamamori Y, et al. Inhibition of ATR protein kinase activity by Schisandrin B in DNA damage response. Nucleic Acids Res 2009;37:5678–89.

[255] Knight ZA, Gonzalez B, Feldman ME, Zunder ER, Goldenberg DD, Williams O, et al. A pharmacological map of the PI3-K family defines a role for p110alpha in insulin signaling. Cell 2006;125:733–47.

[256] Toledo LI, Murga M, Zur R, Soria R, Rodriguez A, Martinez S, et al. A cell-based screen identifies ATR inhibitors with synthetic lethal properties for cancer-associated mutations. Nat Struct Mol Biol 2011;18:721–7.

[257] Charrier JD, Durrant SJ, Golec JM, Kay DP, Knegtel RM, MacCormick S, et al. Discovery of potent and selective inhibitors of ataxia telangiectasia mutated and Rad3 related (ATR) protein kinase as potential anticancer agents. J Med Chem 2011;54:2320–30.

[258] Jacq X, Smith L, Brown E, Hughes A, Odedra R, Heathcote D, et al. *AZ20*, a novel potent and selective inhibitor of ATR kinase with in vivo antitumour activity. Cancer Res 2012;72(8 Suppl. 1); Abstract no. 1823..

[259] Peasland A, Wang L-Z, Rowling E, Kyle S, Chen T, Hopkins A, et al. Identification and evaluation of a potent novel ATR inhibitor, NU6027, in breast and ovarian cancer cell lines. Br J Cancer 2011;105:372–81.

[260] Reaper PM, Griffiths MR, Long JM, Charrier JD, Maccormick S, Charlton PA, et al. Selective killing of ATM- or p53-deficient cancer cells through inhibition of ATR. Nat Chem Biol 2011;7:428–30.

[261] Pires IM, Olcina MM, Anbalagan S, Pollard JR, Reaper PM, Charlton PA, et al. Targeting radiation-resistant hypoxic tumour cells through ATR inhibition. Br J Cancer 2012;107:291–9.

[262] Ashwell S, Zabludoff S. DNA damage detection and repair pathways—recent advances with inhibitors of checkpoint kinases in cancer therapy. Clin Cancer Res 2008;14:4032–7.

[263] Dai Y, Grant S. New insights into checkpoint kinase 1 in the DNA damage response signaling network. Clin Cancer Res 2010;16:376–83.

[264] Garrett MD, Collins I. Anticancer therapy with checkpoint inhibitors: what, where and when? Trends Pharmacol Sci 2011;32:308–16.

[265] Ma CX, Janetka JW, Piwnica-Worms H. Death by releasing the breaks: CHK1 inhibitors as cancer therapeutics. Trends Mol Med 2011;17:88–96.

[266] Furuta T, Hayward RL, Meng LH, Takemura H, Aune GJ, Bonner WM, et al. p21CDKN1A allows the repair of replication-mediated DNA double-strand breaks induced by topoisomerase I and is inactivated by the checkpoint kinase inhibitor 7-hydroxystaurosporine. Oncogene 2006;25:2839–49.

[267] Luo Y, Rockow-Magnone SK, Kroeger PE, Frost L, Chen Z, Han EK, et al. Blocking Chk1 expression induces apoptosis and abrogates the G2 checkpoint mechanism. Neoplasia 2001;3(5):411–9.

[268] Mack PC, Gandara DR, Lau AH, Lara Jr PN, Edelman MJ, Gumerlock PH. Cell cycle-dependent potentiation of cisplatin by UCN-01 in non-small-cell lung carcinoma. Cancer Chemother Pharmacol 2003;51:337–48.

[269] Walton MI, Eve PD, Hayes A, Valenti M, De Haven Brandon A, Box G, et al. The preclinical pharmacology and therapeutic activity of the novel CHK1 inhibitor SAR-020106. Mol Cancer Ther 2010;9:89–100.

[270] Blasina A, Hallin J, Chen E, Arango ME, Kraynov E, Register J, et al. Breaching the DNA damage checkpoint via PF-00477736, a novel small-molecule inhibitor of checkpoint kinase 1. Mol Cancer Ther 2008;7:2394–404.

[271] McNeely S, Conti C, Sheikh T, Patel H, Zabludoff S, Pommier Y, et al. Chk1 inhibition after replicative stress activates a double strand break response mediated by ATM and DNA-dependent protein kinase. Cell Cycle 2010;9:995–1004.

[272] Zabludoff SD, Deng C, Grondine MR, Sheehy AM, Ashwell S, Caleb BL, et al. AZD7762, a novel checkpoint kinase inhibitor, drives checkpoint abrogation and potentiates DNA-targeted therapies. Mol Cancer Ther 2008;7:2955–66.

[273] Matthews DJ, Yakes FM, Chen J, Tadano M, Bornheim L, Clary DO, et al. Pharmacological abrogation of S-phase checkpoint enhances the anti-tumor activity of gemcitabine in vivo. Cell Cycle 2007;6:104–10.

[274] Mitchell JB, Choudhuri R, Fabre K, Sowers AL, Citrin D, Zabludoff SD, et al. In vitro and in vivo radiation sensitization of human tumor cells by a novel checkpoint kinase inhibitor, AZD7762. Clin Cancer Res 2010;16:2076–84.

[275] Syljuasen RG, Sørensen CS, Nylandsted J, Lukas C, Lukas J, Bartek J. Inhibition of Chk1 by CEP-3891 accelerates mitotic nuclear fragmentation in response to ionizing radiation. Cancer Res 2004;64:9035–40.

[276] Guzi TJ, Paruch K, Dwyer MP, Labroli M, Shanahan F, Davis N, et al. Targeting the replication checkpoint using SCH 900776, a potent and functionally selective CHK1 inhibitor identified via high content screening. Mol Cancer Ther 2011;10:591–602.

[277] Yang H, Yoon SJ, Jin J, Choi SH, Seol HJ, Lee JI, et al. Inhibition of checkpoint kinase 1 sensitizes lung cancer brain metastases to radiotherapy. Biochem Biophys Res Commun 2011;406:53–8.

[278] Sausville EA, Arbuck SG, Messmann R, Headlee D, Bauer KS, Lush RM, et al. Phase I trial of 72-hour continuous infusion UCN-01 in patients with refractory neoplasms. J Clin Oncol 2001;19:2319–33.

[279] Chen T, Stephens P, Middleton T, Curtin NJ. Targeting the S and G2 checkpoint. Drug Discov Today 2012;17:194–202.

[280] Dobzhansky T. Genetics of natural populations. Xiii. Recombination and variability in populations of *Drosophila pseudoobscura*. Genetics 1946;31:269–90.

[281] Hartwell LH, Szankasi P, Roberts CJ, Murray AW, Friend SH. Integrating genetic approaches into the discovery of anticancer drugs. Science 1997;278:1064–8.

[282] Kaelin Jr WG. The concept of synthetic lethality in the context of anticancer therapy. Nat Rev Cancer 2005;5:689–98.

[283] Lindahl T, Satoh MS, Poirier GG, Klungland A. Post-translational modification of poly(ADP-ribose) polymerase induced by DNA strand breaks. Trends Biochem Sci 1995;20:405–11.

[284] Oikawa A, Tohda H, Kanai M, Miwa M, Sugimura T. Inhibitors of poly(adenosine diphosphate ribose) polymerase induce sister chromatid exchanges. Biochem Biophys Res Commun 1980;97:1311–6.

[285] Schultz N, Lopez E, Saleh-Gohari N, Helleday T. Poly(ADP-ribose) polymerase (PARP-1) has a controlling role in homologous recombination. Nucleic Acids Res 2003;31:4959–64.

[286] Bryant HE, Schultz N, Thomas HD, Parker KM, Flower D, Lopez E, et al. Specific killing of BRCA2-deficient tumours with inhibitors of poly(ADP-ribose)polymerase. Nature 2005;434:913–7.

[287] Farmer H, McCabe N, Lord CJ, Tutt AN, Johnson DA, Richardson TB, et al. Targeting the DNA repair defect in BRCA mutant cells as a therapeutic strategy. Nature 2005;434:917–21.

[288] Turner N, Tutt A, Ashworth A. Hallmarks of 'BRCAness' in sporadic cancers. Nat Rev Cancer 2004;4:814–9.

[289] Bryant HE, Helleday T. Inhibition of poly(ADP-ribose) polymerase activates ATM which is required for subsequent homologous recombination repair. Nucleic Acids Res 2006;34:1685–91.

[290] McCabe N, Turner NC, Lord CJ, Kluzek K, Bialkowska A, Swift S, et al. Deficiency in the repair of DNA damage by homologous recombination and sensitivity to poly(ADP-ribose) polymerase inhibition. Cancer Res 2006;66:8109–15.

[291] Lord CJ, Garrett MD, Ashworth A. Targeting the double-strand DNA break repair pathway as a therapeutic strategy. Clin Cancer Res 2006;12:4463–8.

[292] Lord CJ, MacDonald S, Swift S, Turner NC, Ashworth A. A high-throughput RNA interference screen for DNA repair determinants of PARP inhibitor sensitivity. DNA Repair (Amst) 2008;7:2010–9.

[293] Shen WH, Balajee AS, Wang J, Wu H, Eng C, Pandolfi PP, et al. Essential role for nuclear PTEN in maintaining chromosomal integrity. Cell 2007;128:157–70.

[294] Turner NC, Lord CJ, Iorns E, Brough R, Swift S, Elliott R, et al. Synthetic lethal siRNA screen identifying genes mediating sensitivity to a PARP inhibitor. EMBO J 2008;27:1368–77.

[295] Mendes-Pereira AM, Martin SA, Brough R, McCarthy A, Taylor JR, Kim JS, et al. Synthetic lethal targeting of PTEN mutant cells with PARP inhibitors. EMBO Mol Med 2009;1:315–22.

[296] Hunt CR, Gupta A, Horikoshi N, Pandita TK. Does PTEN loss impair DNA double-strand break repair by homologous recombination? Clin Cancer Res 2012;18:920–2.

[297] Drew Y, Mulligan EA, Vong W-T, Thomas HD, Kahn S, Kyle S, et al. Therapeutic potential of PARP inhibitor AG014699 in human cancer with mutated or methylated BRCA. J Natl Cancer Inst 2011a;103:334–46.

[298] Drew Y, Ledermann JA, Jones A, Hall G, Jayson GC, Highley M, et al. Phase II trial of the poly(ADP-ribose) polymerase (PARP) inhibitor AG-014699 in BRCA 1 and 2—mutated, advanced ovarian and/or locally advanced or metastatic breast cancer. J Clin Oncol 2011b;29(Suppl.): abstr. 3104.

[299] Bindra RS, Schaffer PJ, Meng A, Woo J, Måseide K, Roth ME, et al. Alterations in DNA repair gene expression under hypoxia: elucidating the mechanisms of hypoxia-induced genetic instability. Ann N Y Acad Sci 2005;1059: 184–95.

[300] Chan N, Koritzinsky M, Zhao H, Bindra R, Glazer PM, Powell S, et al. Chronic hypoxia decreases synthesis of homologous recombination proteins to offset chemoresistance and radioresistance. Cancer Res 2008;68: 605–14.

[301] Chan N, Pires IM, Bencokova Z, Coackley C, Luoto KR, Bhogal N, et al. Contextual synthetic lethality of cancer cell kill based on the tumor microenvironment. Cancer Res 2010;70:8045–54.

[302] Weston VJ, Oldreive CE, Skowronska A, Oscier DG, Pratt G, Dyer MJ, et al. The PARP inhibitor olaparib induces significant killing of ATM-deficient lymphoid tumor cells in vitro and in vivo. Blood 2010;116:4578–87.

[303] Williamson CT, Muzik H, Turhan AG, Zamò A, O'Connor MJ, Bebb DG, et al. ATM deficiency sensitizes mantle cell lymphoma cells to poly(ADP-ribose) polymerase-1 inhibitors. Mol Cancer Ther 2010;9:347–57.

[304] Vilar E, Bartnik CM, Stenzel SL, Raskin L, Ahn J, Moreno V, et al. MRE11 deficiency increases sensitivity to poly(ADP-ribose) polymerase inhibition in microsatellite unstable colorectal cancers. Cancer Res 2011;71: 2632–42.

[305] Johnson N, Li Y-C, Walton ZE, Cheng KA, Li D, Rodig SJ, et al. Compromised CDK1 activity sensitizes BRCA-proficient cancers to PARP inhibition. Nat Med 2011;17:875–83.

[306] Edwards SL, Brough R, Lord CJ, Natrajan R, Vatcheva R, Levine DA, et al. Resistance to therapy caused by intragenic deletion in BRCA2. Nature 2008;451:1111–5.

[307] Sakai W, Swisher EM, Karlan BY, Agarwal MK, Higgins J, Friedman C, et al. Secondary mutations as a mechanism of cisplatin resistance in Brca2-mutated cancers. Nature 2008;451:1116–20.

[308] Swisher EM, Sakai W, Karlan BY, Wurz K, Urban N, Taniguchi T. Secondary Brca1 mutations in Brca1-mutated ovarian carcinomas with platinum resistance. Cancer Res 2008;68:2581–6.

[309] Bouwman P, Aly A, Escandell JM, Pieterse M, Bartkova J, Van Der Gulden H, et al. 53bp1 loss rescues Brca1 deficiency and is associated with triple-negative and Brca-mutated breast cancers. Nat Struct Mol Biol 2010;17:688–95.

[310] Bunting SF, Callen E, Wong N, Chen HT, Polato F, Gunn A, et al. 53bp1 inhibits homologous recombination in Brca1-deficient cells by blocking resection of DNA breaks. Cell 2010;141:243–54.

[311] Patel AG, Sarkaria JN, Kaufmann SH. Nonhomologous end joining drives poly(ADP-ribose) polymerase (PARP) inhibitor lethality in homologous recombination-deficient cells. Proc Natl Acad Sci U S A 2011;108: 3406–11.

[312] Adamo A, Collis SJ, Adelman CA, Silva N, Horejsi Z, Ward JD, et al. Preventing nonhomologous end joining suppresses DNA repair defects of Fanconi anemia. Mol Cell 2010;39:25–35.

[313] Pace P, Mosedale G, Hodskinson MR, Rosado IV, Sivasubramaniam M, Patel KJ. Ku70 corrupts DNA repair in the absence of the Fanconi anemia pathway. Science 2010;329:219–23.

[314] Collins AR. Mutant rodent cell lines sensitive to ultraviolet light, ionizing radiation and cross-linking agents: a comprehensive survey of genetic and biochemical characteristics. Mutat Res 1993;293:99–118.

[315] Bartkova J, Horejsi Z, Sehested M, Nesland JM, Rajpert-De Meyts E, Skakkebaek NE, et al. DNA damage response mediators MDC1 and 53BP1: constitutive activation and aberrant loss in breast and lung cancer, but not in testicular germ cell tumours. Oncogene 2007;26:7414–22.

[316] Fong PC, Boss DS, Yap TA, Tutt A, Wu P, Mergui-Roelvink M, et al. Inhibition of poly(ADP-ribose) polymerase in tumors from BRCA mutation carriers. N Engl J Med 2009a;361:123–34.

[317] Fong PC, Yap TA, Boss DS, Carden CP, Mergui-Roelvink M, Gourley C, et al. Poly(ADP)-ribose polymerase inhibition: frequent durable responses in BRCA carrier ovarian cancer correlating with platinum-free interval. J Clin Oncol 2009;28:2512–9.

[318] Tutt A, Robson M, Garber JE, Domchek SM, Audeh MW, Weitzel JN, et al. Oral poly(ADP-ribose) polymerase inhibitor olaparib in patients with BRCA1 or BRCA2 mutations and advanced breast cancer: a proof-of-concept trial. Lancet 2010;376:235–44.

[319] Audeh MW, Carmichael J, Penson RT, Friedlander M, Powell B, Bell-McGuinn KM, et al. Oral poly(ADP-ribose) polymerase inhibitor olaparib in patients with BRCA1 or BRCA2 mutations and recurrent ovarian cancer: a proof-of-concept trial. Lancet 2010;376:245–51.

[320] Schelman WR, Sandhu SK, Monreno Garcia V, Wilding G, Sun L, Toniatti C, et al. First-in-human trial of a poly(ADP)-ribose polymerase (PARP) inhibitor MK-4827 in advanced cancer patients with antitumor activity in BRCA-deficient tumors and sporadic ovarian cancers (soc). J Clin Oncol 2011;29(Suppl.): abstr. 3102.

[321] Gelmon KA, Tischkowitz M, Mackay H, Swenerton K, Robidoux A, Tonkin K, et al. Olaparib in patients with recurrent high-grade serous or poorly differentiated ovarian carcinoma or triple-negative breast cancer: a phase 2, multicentre, open-label, non-randomised study. Lancet Oncol 2011;12:852–61.

[322] Ledermann JA, Harter P, Gourley C, Friedlander M, Vergote IB, Rustin GJS, et al. Phase II randomized placebo-controlled study of olaparib (AZD2281) in patients with platinum-sensitive relapsed serous ovarian cancer (PSR SOC). J Clin Oncol 2011;29(Suppl. 15):5003.

[323] Oza AM, Cibula D, Oaknin A, Poole CJ, Mathijssen RHJ, Sonke GS, et al. Olaparib plus paclitaxel plus carboplatin (P/C) followed by olaparib maintenance treatment in patients (pts) with platinum-sensitive recurrent serous ovarian cancer (PSR SOC): a randomized, open-label phase II study. J Clin Oncol 2012;30(Suppl.): abstr. 5001.

[324] Martin SA, Martin SA, McCabe N, Mullarkey M, Cummins R, Burgess DJ, et al. DNA polymerases as potential therapeutic targets for cancers deficient in the DNA mismatch repair proteins MSH2 or MLH1. Cancer Cell 2010;17:235–48.

[325] Neijenhuis S, Verwijs-Janssen M, van den Broek LJ, Begg AC, Vens C. Targeted radiosensitization of cells expressing truncated DNA polymerase {beta}. Cancer Res 2010;70:8706–14.

[326] Kennedy RD, Chen CC, Stuckert P, Archila EM, De la Vega MA, Moreau LA, et al. Fanconi anemia pathway-deficient tumor cells are hypersensitive to inhibition of ataxia telangiectasia mutated. J Clin Invest 2007;117:1440–9.

[327] Chen CC, Kennedy RD, Sidi S, Look AT, D'Andrea A. CHK1 inhibition as a strategy for targeting Fanconi anemia (FA) DNA repair pathway deficient tumors. Mol Cancer 2009;16(8):24.

[328] Bartkova J, Rezaei N, Liontos M, Karakaidos P, Kletsas D, Issaeva N, et al. Oncogene-induced senescence is part of the tumorigenesis barrier imposed by DNA damage checkpoints. Nature 2006;444:633–7.

[329] Di Micco R, Fumagalli M, Cicalese A, Piccinin S, Gasparini P, Luise C, et al. Oncogene-induced senescence is a DNA damage response triggered by DNA hyper-replication. Nature 2006;444:638–42.

[330] Dominguez-Sola D, Ying CY, Grandori C, Ruggiero L, Chen B, Li M, et al. Non-transcriptional control of DNA replication by c-Myc. Nature 2007;448:445–51.

[331] Fikaris AJ, Lewis AE, Abulaiti A, Tsygankova OM, Meinkoth JL. Ras triggers ataxia-telangiectasia-mutated and Rad-3-related activation and apoptosis through sustained mitogenic signaling. J Biol Chem 2006;281: 34759–67.

[332] Gorgoulis VG, Vassiliou LV, Karakaidos P, Zacharatos P, Kotsinas A, Liloglou T, et al. Activation of the DNA damage checkpoint and genomic instability in human precancerous lesions. Nature 2005;434:907–13.

[333] Halazonetis TD, Gorgoulis VG, Bartek J. An oncogene-induced DNA damage model for cancer development. Science 2008;319:1352–5.

[334] Gilad O, Nabet BY, Ragland RL, Schloppy DW, Smith KD, Durham AC, et al. Combining ATR suppression with oncogenic Ras synergistically increases genomic instability, causing synthetic lethality or tumorigenesis in a dosage-dependent manner. Cancer Res 2010;70:9693–702.

[335] Hoglund A, Nilsson LM, Muralidharan SV, Hasvold LA, Merta P, Rudelius M, et al. Therapeutic implications for the induced levels of chk1 in myc-expressing cancer cells. Clin Cancer Res 2011;17:7067–79.

[336] Ferrao PT, Bukczynska EP, Johnstone RW, McArthur GA. Efficacy of CHK inhibitors as single agents in MYC-driven lymphoma cells. Oncogene 2012;31:1661–72.

[337] Brenner JC, Ateeq B, Li Y, Yocum AK, Cao Q, Asangani IA, et al. Mechanistic rationale for inhibition of poly(ADP-ribose) polymerase in ETS gene fusion-positive prostate cancer. Cancer Cell 2011;19:664–78.

[338] Brenner JC, Feng FY, Han S, Patel S, Goyal SV, Bou-Maroun LM, et al. PARP-1 inhibition as a targeted strategy to treat Ewing's sarcoma. Cancer Res 2012;72:1608–13.

Recommended Further Reading

Friedberg EC, Walker GC, Siede W, Wood RD, Schultz RA, Ellenberger T. DNA repair and mutagenesis. 2nd ed. Washington DC: ASM Press; 2005.

Useful Websites

http://www.cancerresearchuk.org: For more information on current clinical trials.
http://www.nih.gov/sigs/dna-rep: An interest group for those interested in DNA repair.

Exploiting Cancer Dependence on Molecular Chaperones: HSP90 Inhibitors Past, Present, and Future

Swee Sharp, Keith Jones, Paul Workman

Cancer Research UK Cancer Therapeutics Unit, The Institute of Cancer Research, London, UK

INTRODUCTION

Although considerable progress has been made in a number of malignant diseases, treating cancers with conventional one-size-fits-all cytotoxic drugs has been hugely challenging, especially owing to toxicities and intrinsic or acquired drug resistance. Breakthroughs in our understanding of the genetics and biology of cancer have resulted in the current strategies employed for the discovery of cancer drugs, which involve targeting the molecular pathology driving the progression of individual malignancies, leading to personalized precision medicine [1]. Molecularly targeted drugs that have received approval for use in the clinic include small-molecule kinase inhibitors such as imatinib, gefitinib, erlotinib, lapatinib, vemurafenib, and crizotinib and antibodies exemplified by trastuzumab [2,3].

However, despite significant activity and clinical benefit with molecular therapeutic drugs exploiting a single molecular target, progress has not been as dramatic as might have been expected. Many cancers have multiple oncogenic driver mutations within an individual tumor, and, especially when coupled to the existence of tumor heterogeneity, clonal evolution, and intrinsic and acquired drug resistance involving diverse genetic and epigenetic molecular mechanisms, it has become increasingly apparent that the achievement of maximum clinical efficacy and cure will require a combinatorial targeted approach [1]. Therapeutic inhibition of the heat shock protein 90 (HSP90) molecular chaperone is emerging as an exciting approach to overcome the limitations of single-target therapy and to deliver a combinatorial, multifaceted anticancer effect with the potential to overcome the problems of tumor heterogeneity and drug resistance [4–6]. Indeed, they can be viewed as "network biology drugs". This is because inhibiting HSP90 leads to inactivation and proteasomal degradation of many different oncogenic clients that depend on this molecular chaperone (Fig. 9.1), thereby blocking multiple cancer-causing signaling pathways and delivering a simultaneous combinatorial attack on all of the hallmark traits of malignancy, while also acting on a major stress response mechanism required for cancer cell survival and progression [5,6]. As a result, research on HSP90 inhibitors has evolved over the last 15 years from an initial focus on natural products—used first as preclinical chemical probes to understand chaperone biology and then as clinical pathfinder agents—to the current era of next-generation small-molecule HSP90 drugs that show exciting clinical promise; indeed, from being viewed initially as an unappealing target that attracted little interest from pharmaceutical companies, the situation has changed dramatically so that more than 20 HSP90 inhibitors have entered clinical trials to date and HSP90 is now one of the most aggressively prosecuted targets in the industry, with clear, objective evidence of clinical activity in breast and non-small-cell lung cancer [7,8].

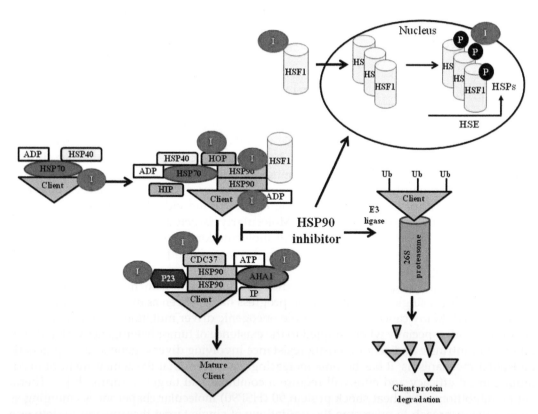

FIGURE 9.1   The HSP90 super-chaperone complex and potential strategies to inhibit its function. The red elipses with the letter I indicate points of interaction for potential inhibitors. (This figure is reproduced in color in the color plate section.)

BIOLOGY OF HSP90

HSP90 is highly conserved and ubiquitously expressed in prokaryotes and eukaryotes. Even under normal homeostatic conditions, HSP90 proteins account for 1–2% of all cellular proteins in most cells [9]. HSP90 performs a range of essential housekeeping functions, especially by assisting in proper folding, activation, and stabilization of proteins in the crowded environment of the cell and by playing a key role in triaging damaged proteins, either for refolding and rescue or for targeting to ubiquitin-mediated proteasomal degradation [10]. When mammalian cells are exposed to physiological stresses such as heat, cytotoxic drugs, UV irradiation, heavy metals, hypoxia, or low pH, the transcription heat shock factor 1 (HSF1) is activated by release from an inhibitory interaction with HSP90, translocates to the nucleus, and binds to heat shock elements within the promoter regions of *HSP* genes, thereby inducing a two- to threefold increase in the expression of HSP90 and other HSPs as part of a concerted effort to maintain protein homeostasis and cell survival [11].

HSPs are traditionally classified into two groups: the high-molecular-weight HSPs (e.g., HSP90, HSP70, and HSP60) and the small HSP family (e.g., HSP27 and αB-crystallin). High-molecular-weight HSPs, like HSP90, are adenosine triphosphate (ATP)-dependent chaperones; indeed, HSP90 operates through a functionally essential ATPase-mediated cycle that is regulated by a range of co-chaperones [12]. In contrast to the high-molecular-weight HSPs, small HSPs are ATP independent [13,14].

There are four highly homologous mammalian isoforms of HSP90: HSP90α, HSP90β, GRP94 (94 kDa glucose-regulated protein), and TRAP1 (tumor necrosis factor receptor-associated protein 1) [9,15]. HSP90α and HSP90β are present in the cytosol, GRP94 mainly resides in the endoplasmic reticulum (ER), while TRAP1 is found in the mitochondria. Most therapeutic attention has focused on the cytosolic isoforms.

HSP90 functions as a homodimer with each monomer consisting of three major domains: an N-terminal ATP-binding domain (25 kDa), a middle domain (35 kDa), and a C-terminal dimerization domain (12 kDa) [16]. The crystal structure of the HSP90 N-terminal domain with ATP and adenosine diphosphate (ADP) [17] provided the first unambiguous evidence for an adenine nucleotide–binding site and led to the elucidation of the now well-accepted mechanism of a chaperone cycle driven by ATP hydrolysis [18]. AHA1 was subsequently identified as a co-chaperone that activates the ATPase activity of HSP90, regulates progress through the chaperone cycle, and thereby controls the efficiency of HSP90 client protein activation [19]. Structural and biochemical studies revealed the molecular basis for recruitment of the kinase-specific co-chaperone CDC37 to HSP90 [20], showed that HSP90-dependent activation of protein kinases is regulated by chaperone-targeted dephosphorylation of the kinase-selective co-chaperone CDC37, yielded the first structural description of a client kinase (CDK4) in complex with HSP90–CDC37 [21], and provided the crystal structure of intact ATP-bound HSP90 [22], confirming the role of the ATPase-coupled conformational cycle.

HSP90 IN CANCER

Consistent with the role of an activated heat shock program in cancer, HSP90 has been reported to be overexpressed in a range of malignancies, including both solid tumors [23–26] and hematological cancers [27–29]. Importantly, high HSP90 expression has been shown to correlate with disease progression in melanoma [30] and to be associated with decreased survival in breast cancer, gastrointestinal stromal tumors (GISTs), and non-small-cell lung cancer (NSCLC) [31–33]. The overexpression of HSP90 helps it to act as a buffer for genetic abnormalities, particularly enabling mutated, overexpressed, and activated oncoprotein clients to perform their malignant functions and avoid proteasomal degradation, while conferring cellular tolerance to the unbalanced signaling produced by these oncoproteins [34]. HSP90 promotes conformational states in client proteins that permit interactions with their specific substrates and ligands [35].

The membership of HSP90's clientele continues to grow and in particular includes numerous oncogenic kinases and transcription factors (see a list at www.picard.ch; the usual criteria are evidence of (1) physical interaction and (2) depletion in cells following pharmacological HSP90 inhibition). Especially important and well-studied oncogenic client proteins include the protein kinases BCR-ABL, ERBB2, ALK, BRAF, CRAF, AKT, and CDK4, together with the androgen receptor (AR) and estrogen receptor (ER). Combinatorial depletion of multiple oncogenic client proteins and simultaneous blockade of many cancer-causing signaling pathways results in biological effects that would be expected to mediate therapeutic benefit by modulating all of the hallmarks of cancer [36], a prediction that is now being realized [4,5]. Moreover, also now being seen is that the potential of HSP90 inhibition to shut down multiple oncogenic signaling pathways simultaneously is particularly useful in situations where feedback loops have been shown to counteract the efficacy of molecularly targeted agents, and also where kinase alleles resistant to pharmacological inhibitors remain dependent on HSP90, as seems generally to be the case [1,7,8,37,39].

Because the oncogenic proteins that are critical for cancer cells are targeted for degradation via the ubiquitin–proteasome pathway following inhibition of the HSP90 chaperone function (Fig. 9.1), this results in cell cycle arrest or cell death [40]. But, of course, it is essential that such effects are preferentially seen in malignant versus healthy cells in order to achieve a therapeutic window and acceptable safety profile. Importantly then, HSP90 inhibition has been shown to result in remarkable selectivity for cancer compared to normal cells. Although the precise explanation is not yet available and is likely to be complex, there appear to be a number of reasons contributing to this selectivity. HSP90 inhibitors have been reported to accumulate in tumor tissue while being rapidly cleared from normal tissue [41]. It is possible that this relates to the overexpression of HSP90 in cancer cells discussed in this chapter, and also to the reported presence of HSP90 in an activated super-chaperone complex in malignant but not healthy cells [42]. Importantly, it has become clear that oncogenic kinases activated by mutation are often much more dependent on HSP90 for stability and function than are their wild-type counterparts. For example, the common V600E and other oncogenic mutant forms of BRAF are much more sensitive to HSP90 inhibition than the wild-type protein [43,44]. Other hypersensitive mutant proteins include v-SRC, BCR-ABL, mutant EGFR, and rearranged ALK. Cancer cells are also more "addicted" than healthy cells to many of HSP90's client proteins, and thus the inactivation and depletion of these oncogenic proteins have more damaging effects on cancer cells versus normal ones [5,45].

The factors responsible for making particular proteins, including oncogenic mutants, dependent on HSP90 have proved elusive as this cannot be explained by the amino acid sequence or known structural features. However, a recent study found that the strength of the interaction of HSP90 with a range of protein kinases was correlated with the thermal instability of the kinase domain, probably reflecting the presence of flexible, unstructured regions of the kinase domain that HSP90 can identify and bind to. Important among such flexible regions is likely to be the "hinge" region of the kinase, a segment of the protein that connects the amino- and carboxy-terminal parts of the kinase domain [46]. These findings suggest not only how the HSP90 acts as a driving force in kinase evolution by stabilizing potentially advantageous but unstable protein forms, but also how the chaperone protects kinases that are activated by mutations in cancer cells and that would otherwise be prone to aggregation or degradation [47].

DISCOVERY AND DEVELOPMENT OF HSP90 INHIBITORS: FROM CHEMICAL PROBES TO DRUGS

Our understanding of the molecular basis of the chaperone function of HSP90, discussed in this chapter, and in particular the use of pharmacological HSP90 ligands to probe mechanisms and explore the consequences of inhibition, has provided the essential validation of HSP90 as a molecular target for cancer therapy [17,48,49] and thereby has led to an explosion in the discovery of HSP90 drugs. Indeed, HSP90 provides a remarkable example of the synergistic interplay between basic research and drug discovery that is enabled by pharmacological inhibitors used as chemical tools and pharmacological pathfinders [50]. As we will review in the chapter, our knowledge of the complex function and regulation of HSP90 provides a number of potential opportunities for pharmacological intervention (Fig. 9.1). However, as we will discuss first, the majority of the activity to date has been focused on chemical tools and drugs that inhibit HSP90 itself, especially via the N-terminal ATP site.

The natural products geldanamycin and radicicol have proved to be especially important in figuring out the structure–function relationship for HSP90 and the druggability of this target. Although the benzoquinone ansamycin antibiotic geldanamycin and the macrolide antibiotic radicicol appear to be unrelated in chemical structure (Fig. 9.2), they both act on the same N-terminal domain, where they bind well into the structurally rather unusual Bergerat fold class of the ATP site that is characteristic of the small GHKL (gyrase, HSP90, histidine kinase, and MutL) family of ATP-binding proteins [51]. The fact that this unusual ATP-binding site of HSP90 shares close three-dimensional similarity to only a relatively small number of proteins such as histidine kinase, topoisomerases, and DNA mismatch repair proteins provides us with the protein structural basis for the design of very potent and highly selective inhibitors that block the ATP-binding and hydrolysis functions of HSP90 that are required for its chaperone activity [18,49,52]. Following this inhibition, ubiquitin ligases are subsequently recruited to the HSP90 chaperone complex, leading to the degradation of client proteins via the proteasome pathway and the subsequent biological and therapeutic effects (Fig. 9.1) [53].

Finding novel compounds as starting points for optimization is a major challenge in all drug discovery research. In the case of HSP90, modification of the natural-product inhibitors was initially productive. Since then, the search for pharmacological HSP90 inhibitors has benefited greatly from the availability of the crystal structure of the N-terminal domain of HSP90, enabling structure-based design. This approach is complemented by the development of biochemical assays that allowed high-throughput screening of large, diverse compound

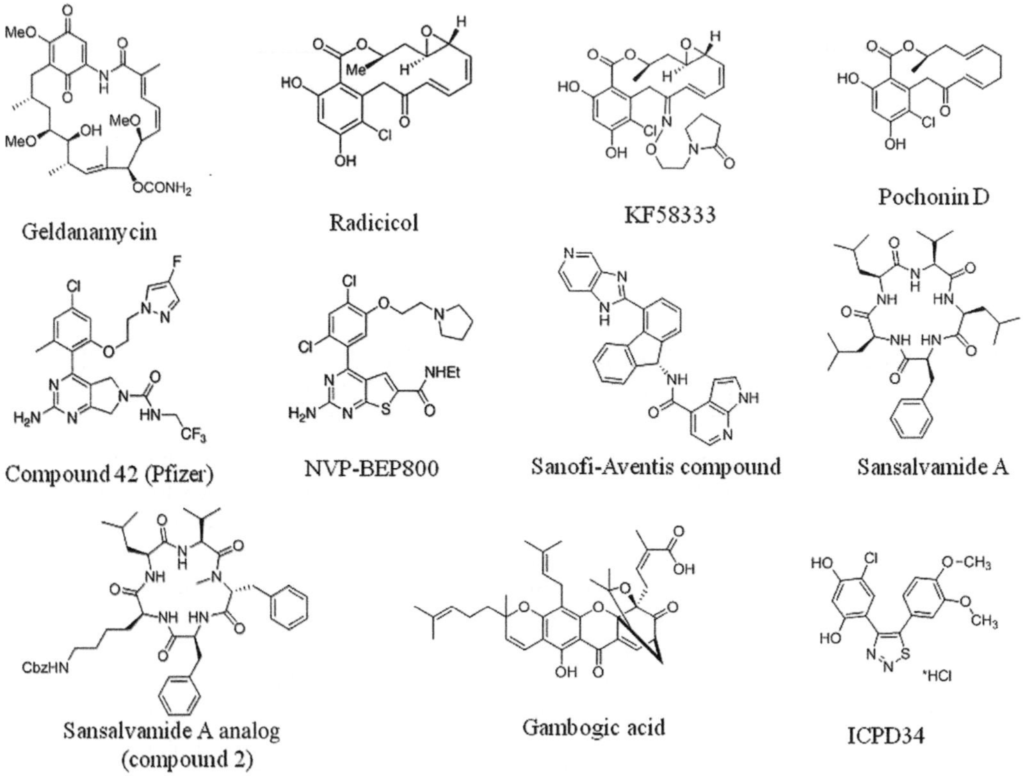

FIGURE 9.2 Chemical structures of selected HSP90 inhibitors studied preclinically.

libraries. Fragment-based approaches have also proved effective, and the optimization of fragment-like hits using structural information from protein X-ray crystallography is now well established as a valuable strategy in the search for new HSP90 inhibitors.

In this chapter, we describe the validation of the HSP90 target with natural compounds, which helps us to understand the complex chaperone biology and define the essential biomarkers, as well as provide the preclinical and clinical pathways to proof-of-concept and therapeutic activity. We then present examples from the plethora of N-terminal ATP-site inhibitors (both natural and synthetic) that have been studied preclinically (Fig. 9.2) or have entered clinical trials (Table 9.1), as well as others acting by different mechanisms.

AGENTS THAT BIND TO THE N-TERMINAL HSP90 ATP-BINDING POCKET

Benzoquinone Ansamycin HSP90 Inhibitors

Geldanamycin was originally thought to act a tyrosine kinase inhibitor [54], until the landmark publication of Whitesell and Neckers in 1994 reported that geldanamycin inhibited the formation of a *v*-Src–HSP90 complex through binding to HSP90 [48]. The subsequent

TABLE 9.1 HSP90 Inhibitors that have Entered Clinical Trials

Structure	Agent	Chemical class	Administration route	Phase	Company
	17-AAG (tanespimycin)	Benzoquinone ansamycin	Intravenous (IV)	II/III	Bristol-Myers Squibb
	17-DMAG (alvespimycin)	Benzoquinone ansamycin	IV	II	Kosan
	IPI-504 (Retaspimycin hydrochloride)	Hydroquinone form of 17-AAG	IV	II	Infinity

Continued

TABLE 9.1 HSP90 Inhibitors that have Entered Clinical Trials *(cont'd)*

Structure	Agent	Chemical class	Administration route	Phase	Company
	IPI-493	Active metabolite of IPI-504 and 17-AAG	Oral	I	Infinity
	NVP-AUY922	Resorcinylic isoxazole	IV	I/II	Novartis
	STA-9090 (ganetespib)	Resorcinol derivative	IV	I/II	Synta/Premiere Oncology
	AT-13387	Resorcinylic benzamide	Oral or IV	I	Astex Therapeutics

Continued

Name	Chemotype	Route	Phase	Company	Structure
KW-2478	Resorcinol	IV	I/II	Kyowa Hakko Kirin	
BIIB021 (CNF-2024)	Purine	Oral	II	Premiere Oncology	
PU-H71	Purine	IV	I	Biogen Idec	
Debio 0932 (CUDC-305)	Imidazopyridine	Oral	I	Debiopharm	

II. DRUGS IN THE LABORATORY AND CLINIC

TABLE 9.1　HSP90 Inhibitors that have Entered Clinical Trials　(cont'd)

Structure	Agent	Chemical class	Administration route	Phase	Company
	MPC-3100	Purine	Oral	I	Myrexis
	SNX-5422 mesylate	2-Amino benzamide	Oral	I	Pfizer
	XL888	2-Amino benzamide	Oral	I	Exelixis
	NVP-HSP990	Pyrido[4,3-d] pyrimidine	Oral	I	Novartis
Structure not disclosed	DS-2248	Not known	Oral	I	Daiichi Sankyo

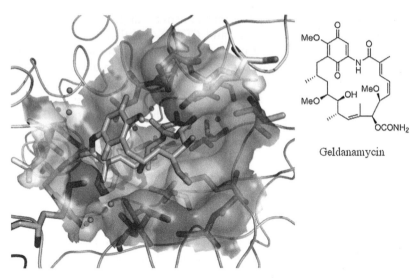

FIGURE 9.3   Geldanamycin bound to the N-terminal domain of human HSP90 (PDB code: 1YET). (This figure is reproduced in color in the color plate section.)

co-crystal structure from the Pearl laboratory in 1997 showed that geldanamycin binds to the ATP-binding site in the N-terminal domain of HSP90 [17,49,55]. The co-crystal structure of geldanamycin and its analogs showed unusual nucleotide mimicry at this site [49,55]. Geldanamycin binds in an orientation in which the macrocyclic ansa ring and the carbamate moiety are directed toward the bottom of the ATP pocket, whereas the benzoquinone ring is oriented toward the top of the pocket (Fig. 9.3). In contrast to the nonbound geldanamycin, the HSP90-bound form is folded over on itself such that the planes of the macrocycle and the benzoquinone are almost parallel. As a critical part of its nucleotide mimicry, geldanamcyin is involved in a series of water-mediated hydrogen-bonding interactions, including interaction of the macrocycle ester carbonyl with a key aspartate residue at the base of the pocket. Additional hydrophobic interactions are also involved. The binding interactions seen with ADP, ATP, and geldanamycin are essentially shared by all other N-terminal ATP-site binders.

Although geldanamycin exhibits compelling in vitro and in vivo antitumor activity, it also showed severe hepatotoxicity in preclinical species (possibly due to the benzoquinone moiety) together with poor solubility [56]. However, semisynthetic geldanamycin analogs in which the 17-methoxy group has been replaced by amine-containing groups gave similar inhibitory effects but with reduced liver toxicity and improved solubility. The two most prominent analogs that have been studied clinically are 17-AAG (17-allylamino-17-demethoxygeldanamycin; tanespimycin) and 17-DMAG (17-demethoxy-17-(2-dimethylamino)-ethylaminogeldanamycin; alvespimycin) (Table 9.1).

17-AAG showed promising anticancer effects in preclinical models in vitro and in vivo [40,57,58] and was the first HSP90 inhibitor to enter clinical trials in 1999. A significant amount of understanding and learning has been obtained from clinical experience with 17-AAG, which was administered intravenously [6–8]. Pharmacokinetic and pharmacodynamic results from the phase I clinical trials of 17-AAG showed that the drug achieved satisfactory exposures at well-tolerated doses and provided proof-of-mechanism for target inhibition, as demonstrated by the depletion of client proteins (CRAF and CDK4), together with the HSF1-dependent induction of HSP72 in peripheral blood mononuclear cells and tumor biopsies (Fig. 9.1) [59]. The pharmacodynamic biomarkers were previously validated in a human tumor xenograft model [60], allowing the Pharmacological Audit Trail (PhAT) to be implemented in the phase I studies of 17-AAG and subsequent HSP90 inhibitors [61,62]. Some early evidence of clinical activity was reported in various malignancies, including melanoma [59,63]. The early signs of therapeutic benefit in melanoma may be due to an increased dependence on HSP90 of mutant or NRAS-activated BRAF and the resulting enhanced sensitivity to depletion by 17-AAG [43,44,64].

The most impressive Response Evaluation Criteria in Solid Tumors (RECIST)-defined responses were seen in a phase II study of 17-AAG combined with trastuzumab in patients with ERBB2-positive, metastatic breast cancer previously progressing on trastuzumab [65]. The investigators reported a response rate of 24%, and overall clinical benefit (including stable disease) was seen in 57% of evaluable patients. This is attributed to the fact that ERBB2, an important driver oncoprotein in this cancer, is a particularly sensitive HSP90 client, together with the achievement, at tolerated doses, of sufficient degradation of this oncogenic client to significantly block tumor growth. In support, preclinical studies have indicated that HSP90 inhibitors may have potential therapeutic activity in cancers harboring amplified or mutant ERBB2 [66,67].

Various combination studies were carried out with 17-AAG in the clinic. In particular, promising results were observed in a phase I/II trial where relapsed or refractory multiple myeloma patients had a durable response following treatment with 17-AAG and the proteasome inhibitor bortezomib [68]. This benefit is attributed to the accumulation of unfolded HSP90 client protein that cannot be degraded in the presence of the proteasome inhibitor, leading to the intolerable proteotoxic stress to which multiple myeloma cells are especially sensitive because of massive immunoglobulin synthesis [68,69].

Studies have shown that degradation of the HSP90 clients CHK1 and WEE1 following HSP90 inhibition resulted in the abrogation of the S and G2/M cell cycle checkpoint controls; hence, combining with DNA-damaging agents may prove beneficial [70,71]. This may explain why a phase I study of 17-AAG and gemcitabine demonstrated some clinical activity [72] leading to a phase II evaluation of this drug combination in ovarian cancer patients.

There is also potential for HSP90 inhibitors such as 17-AAG in leukemia patients where the disease is driven by oncogenic HSP90 client proteins. Preclinical and preliminary data have suggested a benefit for the use of 17-AAG in acute myelogenous leukemia (AML) [73]. The HSP90 client tyrosine kinase FLT3 is frequently mutated and constitutively active in many AML patients and is an oncogenic driver in this disease [74]. Similarly, 17-AAG and other HSP90 inhibitors are being evaluated in chronic myelogenous leukemia and chronic lymphocytic leukemia (CLL) where their HSP90 clients, BCR-ABL and ZAP70 respectively, are particularly sensitive to HSP90 inhibition [75–77].

Despite the promising early clinical results, especially in breast cancer, Bristol-Myers Squibb halted clinical development of 17-AAG, most likely owing to the formulation issues, liver toxicity, and insufficient patent life [78].

Compared to 17-AAG, 17-DMAG (Table 9.1) exhibited potential advantages, especially greater aqueous solubility and ease of formulation, together with reduced metabolic liability and greater oral bioavailability [79–81]. 17-DMAG entered phase I and II clinical trials as an intravenous (IV) agent [82,83]. Indications of clinical activity were reported for 17-DMAG, including a complete response in castration-refractory prostate cancer (CRPC), a partial response in melanoma, and stable disease in chondrosarcoma, CRPC, and renal cancer [82]. The effect seen in CRPC is likely due to the depletion of the AR, which is an HSP90 client protein [84]. Interestingly, given the activity with 17-AAG (as discussed here), clinical antitumor activity (one partial response and seven cases of stable disease) was reported in patients with refractory ERBB2-positive metastatic breast cancer after treatment with 17-DMAG plus trastuzumab [85]. This combination was reported as safe and well tolerated.

The ansamycin HSP90 inhibitors 17-AAG and 17-DMAG have clearly helped pave the way to understanding chaperone inhibition in early clinical trials. However, the difficulties reported with these drugs were clear [7,8]. Although some initial encouraging results emerged from the phase I clinical trials and striking activity was seen in ERBB2-positive breast cancer, a lack of clinical effect was reported for 17-AAG in several phase II studies [86–88]. One of the major limitations for its clinical application is poor solubility [89], masking the true maximum tolerated dose of 17-AAG in patients and making it difficult to achieve the optimal dosing scheduling required to help manage toxicities. This may explain why antitumor responses were not achieved in several phase II trials, including ones involving melanoma, renal cell carcinoma, and CRPC [86,87]. Clinical studies with the more soluble amine-bearing 17-DMAG have been discontinued, apparently due to the overall toxicity profile and other factors [90].

Polymorphic metabolism by cytochrome P450 CYP3A4 [91], efflux by P-glycoprotein [92], and liver toxicity observed in patients [93] have also hampered further clinical development of 17-AAG. The benzoquinone moiety of the ansamycins was long recognized as a potential liability in a pharmaceutical agent, owing to the potential for redox metabolism and resulting hepatotoxicity. Indeed, not only does the benzoquinone in 17-AAG and 17-DMAG introduce the risk of polymorphic quinone metabolism, but in addition loss of expression or the presence of the essentially inactive polymorphic form of the quinone reductase NQO1 (NAD(P)H–quinone oxidoreductase I) gene—an enzyme that catalyzes the reduction of 17-AAG to the hydroquinone, which is a more potent HSP90 inhibitor than the parent quinone—leads to intrinsic resistance to 17-AAG [92,94,95]. Furthermore, loss of NQO1 expression and selection for the inactive polymorphic form have been shown to be the mechanisms of acquired resistance to 17-AAG in preclinical models [96].

One approach to overcome the major solubility limitations of 17-AAG has involved synthesis to the highly soluble hydroquinone hydrochloride IPI-504 (retaspimycin hydrochloride; Table 9.1), which was developed by Infinity Pharmaceuticals [89,97] and has been undergoing phase II trials for patients with advanced NSCLC and traztuzumab-refractory ERBB2-positive breast cancer [98]. Encouraging activity has been reported in NSCLC patients with the ALK gene rearrangements [98]. This responsiveness is likely to be due to the fact that ALK is an HSP90 client. However, trials of IPI-504 in GIST and in patients with CRPC were terminated due to "a higher than anticipated mortality among patients enrolled in the treatment arm" [99,100].

The major metabolite of 17-AAG, the de-allylated analog 17-amino-17-demethoxygeldanamycin (17-AG), has been developed by Infinity Pharmaceuticals and has been evaluated intravenously in phase I clinical trials [55]. Infinity has also developed an oral formulation for 17-AG (IPI-493; Table 9.1).

Resorcinol Class of HSP90 Inhibitors

The 14-membered macrocyclic antibiotic radicicol (Fig. 9.2), like geldanamycin, was originally thought to act as a kinase inhibitor [101,102], but it was later shown to potently inhibit HSP90 function by binding in an L-shaped conformation to its N-terminal ATP pocket [49,103]. The co-crystal structure shows that radicicol makes similar interactions in the ATP pocket to those seen with ADP, ATP, and geldanamycin. Of note is that the resorcinol hydroxyls bind deep in the base of the pocket, with the 3-hydroxyl group binding to the key aspartate mentioned earlier in this article for geldanamycin [49]. Radicicol exhibits potent in vitro antiproliferative activity against a wide variety of human tumor cell lines, but was found to be inactive in in vivo antitumor models [104], apparently due to its reactive electrophilic epoxide moiety. This leads to reaction with a variety of biological nucleophiles, in particular thiols [105]. More stable oxime derivatives such as KF58333 (Fig. 9.2) showed excellent antitumor activity in human tumor xenografts with no apparent liver toxicity; however, problems with eye toxicity have been reported [106]. Pochonin D (Fig. 9.2) is closely related to radicicol and was shown to be a potent HSP90 inhibitor [107]. Similar results have been reported for the synthetic macrolactones and, more recently, for a series of more metabolically stable resorcylic acid macrolactams [108,109]. The macrolactams demonstrated enhanced antitumor activity compared to the equivalent lactones in HCT116 human colon cancer cells. However, none of these radicicol analogs have yet to enter clinical testing.

With the benefit of hindsight, it is clear that the resorcinol motif is an excellent match for the unusual ATP-binding pocket of HSP90, and a number of groups have discovered resorcinol-containing molecules that are potent inhibitors of HSP90. Researchers at The Institute of Cancer Research (ICR) identified a series of the resorcinylic pyrazoles (as exemplified by CCT018159 by high-throughput screening [110,111]. X-ray crystallography with yeast and then human HSP90 demonstrated that these resorcinols bind to N-terminal ATP sites in the same way as radicicol, which helped to define and interpret initial structure–activity relationships in hit-to-lead studies [110]. A subsequent collaboration between the ICR and Vernalis showed improved hydrogen bonding and greater biochemical and cellular potency for resorcinylic pyrazole and isoxazole amides (e.g., VER 49009 and VER50589) as HSP90 inhibitors [112]. Through a structure-based, multiparameter optimization design approach, capitalizing on the crucial network of hydrogen-bonding interactions involving the resorcinol moiety with the key residues in the ATP-binding pocket, as well as a cluster of structurally conserved and highly ordered water molecules (Fig. 9.4), the clinical candidate NVP-AUY922 (Table 9.1) was identified [113,114]. NVP-AUY922 demonstrated extremely high potency against HSP90 ($K_d = 2\,nM$); very high selectivity versus related enzymes, kinases, and various receptors; together with strong efficacy against a broad panel of cancer cells in vitro (with single-digit nanomolar IC_{50}) as well as in a range of subcutaneous and orthotopic human tumor xenograft models covering major cancer types and diverse oncogenic profiles [113]. Significant growth inhibition and/or regressions were seen in vivo, together with therapeutic effects on invasion and metastasis, consistent with the combinatorial action on cancer hallmarks hypothesis proposed for HSP90 inhibitors and discussed in this chapter. As predicted in the design of NVP-AUY922, activity was independent of NQO1 and P-glycoprotein status, and liver toxicity was avoided [113]. Together with the excellent water solubility, these results show significant advantages for NVP-AUY922 over 17-AAG as an IV agent.

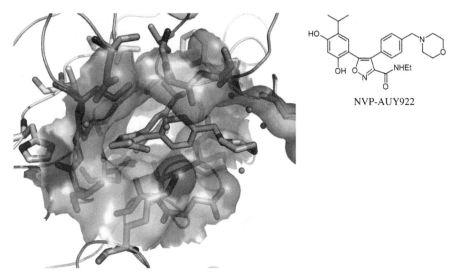

FIGURE 9.4 NVP-AUY922 bound to the N-terminal domain of human HSP90 (PDB code: 2VCI). (This figure is reproduced in color in the color plate section.)

Novartis has taken NVP-AUY922 into clinical testing, and the drug is currently in phase I/II single-agent and combination clinical trials in various malignancies, including NSCLC, ERBB2-positive advanced breast cancer, gastric cancer and refractory GIST (www.clinicaltrials.gov). Phase I studies with IV NVP-AUY922 involving an innovative Bayesian trial design and pharmacokinetic–pharmacodynamic biomarker evaluation have shown a long terminal half-life of 120 h and a dose-dependent increase in exposure in the active range based on mouse models, supporting once-a-week dosing [115]. Inhibition of HSP90 in peripheral blood mononuclear cells and tumor tissue was shown using biomarkers described in this chapter. Dose-dependent metabolic responses were seen by positron emission tomography (PET) scans with labeled fluorodeoxyglucose (FDG-PET). Stable disease was seen in 10 of 171 patients treated. As predicted, liver toxicity was not significant and adverse events included diarrhea, nausea, and fatigue, common with HSP90 inhibitors, together with transient and reversible retinal symptoms that have emerged as mechanism-based class effects.

NVP-AUY922 has been shown to be active in trastuzumab-sensitive as well as both innate and acquired trastuzumab-resistant ERBB2-positive breast cancer cells [116]. Combined with trastuzumab, NVP-AUY922 showed clear synergy in ERBB2-positive BT474 breast cancer cells and in the BT474 tumor xenograft model [117]. Consistent with this, a recent phase II clinical study has shown that NVP-AUY922 in combination with trastuzumab is safe and active in patients with ERBB2-positive metastatic breast cancer who had progressed on trastuzumab-based therapy; the partial response rate was 23%, and the combined partial response and stable disease rate was 74% [118]. The combination was well tolerated, with 5% of patients suffering diarrhea and eye disorders that were reversible with treatment interruption, dose reduction, or discontinuation.

Another significant phase II study assessed NVP-AUY922 in patients with previously treated advanced NSCLC [119]. NVP-AUY922 showed promising clinical activity as a single-agent therapy in EGFR mutant cancers with acquired resistance to EGFR tyrosine kinase inhibitors, ALK-rearranged tumors, and EGFR–KRAS–ALK triple wild-type patients. NVP-AUY922 is currently being evaluated in a range of cancers, with >20 trials listed at ClinicalTrials.gov (www.clinicaltrials.gov).

STA-9090 (ganetespib; Table 9.1), developed by Synta Pharmaceuticals Corporation, is a novel resorcinol containing a triazole moiety; it has been shown to induce degradation of multiple oncogenic HSP90 client proteins and exhibit up to 100-fold greater potency in killing cells and an improved safety profile compared to geldanamycin [120]. Ganetespib has also been shown to be effective as a single agent or combination treatment (e.g., with MEK or PI3K–mTOR inhibitors) in KRAS-driven lung cancer cell lines [121,122]. It is noteworthy that this agent is currently undergoing extensive clinical testing as an IV agent in a broad range of hematological and solid malignancies [123,124]. A recent preclinical study has shown that ganetispib overcame resistance to ALK inhibitors in ALK-rearranged NSCLC, that this agent showed combinatorial activity with ALK inhibitors, and that cancer cells driven by ALK amplification and ROS1 and RET protein kinase gene rearrangements were also sensitive to ganetispib [125]. In addition, a recent publication reported that ganetespib monotherapy demonstrated clinical activity in phase II trials in heavily pretreated patients with advanced NSCLC, particularly in patients with tumors harboring ALK gene rearrangement [126]. Preliminary results of the GALAXY trial (NCT01348126), a randomized phase IIb/III study of ganetespib combined with the taxane docetaxel in advanced NSCLC, have suggested an improvement over docetaxel for second-line therapy [127].

The resorcinylic dihydroxybenzamide AT13387 (Table 9.1), developed by Astex Therapeutics, was discovered through a fragment-based drug discovery approach using nuclear magnetic resonance (NMR) screening and X-ray crystallography [128]. In preclinical studies, this agent is characterized by a long duration of client protein depletion [129]. AT13387 inhibited the proliferation of imatinib-sensitive and -resistant cell lines and tumor xenografts, including those resistant to 17-AAG [130]. A combination of imatinib and AT13387 treatment in the imatinib-resistant GIST430 model significantly enhanced tumor growth inhibition over either of the monotherapies and was well tolerated. A clinical study of AT13887 alone or in combination with the androgen-suppressing drug abiraterone in patients with advanced prostate cancer is ongoing (www.clinicaltrials.gov).

Recent preclinical studies have shown that the resorcinol KW-2478 (developed by Kyowa Hakko Kirin; Table 9.1) could be a promising agent for the treatment of multiple myeloma with various cytogenetic abnormalities [131]. This agent is currently in phase I/II clinical trials as an IV formulation in combination with bortezomib in patients with relapsed and/or refractory multiple myeloma.

The structures of a series of 5-aryl-4-(5-substituted-2-4-dihydroxyphenyl)-1,2,3-thiadiazoles have been determined in complex with the human HSP90α N-terminal domain [132]. These compounds demonstrated antiproliferative activity and induced apoptosis in the HCT116 human colon cancer cell line. Of interest, ICPD 34 (Fig. 9.2) displays a more limited core set of interactions relative to NVP-AUY922 and other developmental resorcinols, and consequently may be less susceptible to resistance derived through mutations in HSP90, which have been reported but only so far in the organisms producing geldanamycin and radicicol [133,134]. However, anticancer activity in cells is modest, indicating a need for further optimization.

Purine and Purine-Like HSP90 Inhibitors

Given that the natural ligand ATP contains an adenine moiety, it is unsurprising that many inhibitors of HSP90 are based on purines or related 6,5-heterocyclic ring systems. Mimicking the unique shape adopted by the natural nucleotide ligand inside the N-terminal pocket of HSP90 by using a structure-based modeling approach, small-molecule purine scaffold inhibitors of HSP90 were designed, as exemplified by PU3 [135,136]. The subsequently determined crystal structure of PU3, complexed with the N-terminal domain of human HSP90β, revealed the true detailed binding mode in which the purine ring of PU3 was confirmed to bind in the same position as the adenine of ATP and ADP as designed, but with an unexpected induced conformational change involving the creation of a channel, produced by the formation of a helix involving flexible residues 104–111 in the phosphate-binding region, which then is able to accommodate the trimethoxy phenyl ring of the purine ligand toward the top of the ATP pocket [137]. Structure–activity relationships were rationalized based on this binding mode, and potent inhibitors designed [137].

Building on this early work, significant improvements of the purine–scaffold HSP90 inhibitors have been achieved, including insensitivity to multidrug resistance, favorable water solubility, oral bioavailability, and metabolic stability [138–141]. This led to the clinical candidates BIIB021 (CNF-2024; administered orally) and PU-H71 (administered IV) from Conforma/Biogen Idec and Memorial Sloan Kettering/Samus Therapeutics, respectively (Table 9.1). BIIB021 is currently being developed by Premiere Oncology and has been reported to be in several phase I clinical trials and two phase II trials in patients with GIST and hormone receptor–positive metastatic breast cancer. A phase II study of BIIB021 in patients with GIST refractory to imatinib and sunitinib showed partial responses as assessed by FDG-PET for five patients [142]. The phase I clinical study for PU-H71 incorporates evaluation of [124]I-labeled PU-H71 to determine intratumoral concentrations (www.clinicaltrials.gov). Recently, Biogen Idec has reported EC144, or 5-(2-amino-4-chloro-7-((4-methoxy-3,5-dimethylpyridin-2-yl) methyl)-7H-pyrrolo[2,3-d]pyrimidin-5-yl)-2-methylpent-4-yn-2-ol, which is a second-generation oral inhibitor of HSP90 and is substantially more potent in vitro and in vivo than BIIB021, with potential for daily or weekly dosing [143].

Although slightly different in structure from the purines, chemically related HSP90 inhibitors with potent oral activity have been developed by Curis/Debiopharm. A phase I clinical trial was initiated by Debiopharm with the orally bioavailable dimethylamino-bearing imidazopyridine, Debio-0932 (formerly CUDC-305; Table 9.1). Of interest, this agent showed extended tumor retention and demonstrated an ability to effectively cross the blood–brain barrier, reaching therapeutic levels and showing efficacy in an intracranial glioblastoma model [144].

The 8-arylthiopurine MPC-3100, developed by Myrexis (Table 9.1; structure not disclosed), is a potent, small-molecule, orally bioavailable HSP90 inhibitor and has shown significant and broad preclinical antitumor activity in tumor xenograft models [145]. A phase I clinical trial was initiated to investigate the safety, tolerability, and pharmacokinetics of MPC-3100 (www.clinicaltrials.gov). In this study, patients have also been evaluated for therapeutic response. The trial is now complete, and results are awaited. In 2012, the pro-drug MPC-0767 was introduced; it is designed to improve upon the poor solubility and bioavailability of MPC-3100 (www.myrexis.com).

Other N-Terminal HSP90 Inhibitors

The orally active 2-aminothieno[2,3-d]pyrimidine development candidate NVP-BEP800 (Fig. 9.2) was discovered in collaborative work between the ICR, Vernalis, and Novartis. Its discovery was based initially on a combination of fragment and in silico screening technologies followed by multiparameter optimization to the candidate [146].

Using an interesting and novel chemical proteomics approach [147], Serenex identified the orally active compound 2-amino benzamide SNX-5422 (Table 9.1). Preclinical studies demonstrated partial tumor regressions in an ERBB2-driven human breast tumor xenograft model, and SNX-5422 was found to be superior to 17-AAG in a mouse model of mutant EGFR NSCLC [148]. Pfizer subsequently acquired this agent (as PF-04929113). Recent phase I results in patients with refractory solid tumor malignancies and lymphomas have shown no objective responses, but long-lasting disease stabilization was observed [149]. However, the development of SNX-5422 was discontinued, likely associated with the ocular toxicity seen in phase I. It is now being developed in the clinic by Esanex.

There has been significant interest among medicinal chemists in the use of macrocyclic compounds as inhibitors of a range of enzymes. As the two original natural-product inhibitors of HSP90, geldanamycin and radicicol, are themselves macrocycles, it was inevitable that synthetic macrocycles would be explored as HSP90 inhibitors. A group at Pfizer has published a series of papers delineating their efforts to develop macrocyclic inhibitors of HSP90. Starting from the structure of the Serenex compound, SNX-5422, they prepared a range of macrocyclic lactams [150]. The basic amine in this original series led to concerns regarding the hERG channel and potential cardiotoxicity issues, but the researchers were subsequently [151] able to eliminate this liability and develop compound 2 (Fig. 9.5) with an IC_{50} value of 92 nM against the ATPase function of HSP90. This potency translated well into cells, with similar activities observed in both biochemical and cellular proliferation assays.

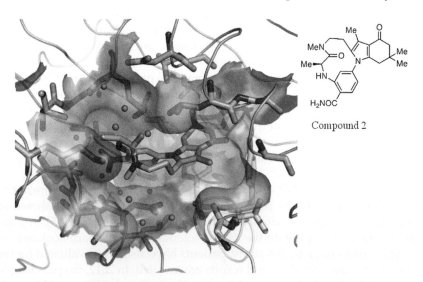

Compound 2

FIGURE 9.5   Pfizer macrocycle 2 bound to the N-terminal domain of human HSP90 (PDB code: 3R91). (This figure is reproduced in color in the color plate section.)

In addition, the Pfizer group was able to obtain an X-ray crystal structure of compound 2 bound to the N-terminal domain of HSP90 (Fig. 9.5). This shows binding in the ATP-site with hydrogen bonds involving the carbonyl group of the tetrahydroindolonone (to Tyr139) and the benzamide (to the canonical Asp93) at the other side of the pocket. In common with many other HSP90 inhibitors, this series showed no kinase inhibitory activity, as expected from the very different ATP-binding conformation found in kinases compared to HSP90. A closely related compound (the N-desmethyl derivative) showed potent activity in proliferation assays across a range of cancer cell lines together with target engagement biomarker changes (HSP70 induction and ERBB2 depletion) in a human breast cancer xenograft, consistent with HSP90 inhibition. This was followed by a report of therapeutic activity using compound 3, which demonstrated good efficacy in a human glioblastoma model when dosed intravenously at 100 mg/kg [152].

Finally, the Pfizer group reported [153] the macrocycle 4 that retains the typical potency of the previously reported compounds but shows enhanced stability in mouse, rat, and human liver microsomes. Macrocycle 4 showed biomarker attenuation in lung cancer and glioblastoma xenograft models and significant tumor growth reduction with weekly IV dosing at 12.5 mg/kg. At 25 mg/kg IV, tumor size reduction was observed.

Recently, a group from Chugai Pharmaceuticals reported on a different class of macrocyclic HSP90 inhibitors based on 2-aminopyrimidines [154]. Compound 5 (Fig. 9.6) was shown to possess a K_d for binding to the N-terminal domain of human HSP90 of 0.52 nM by surface plasma resonance and a 50% growth inhibitory concentration (GI_{50}) of 150 nM against the HCT116 human colorectal cancer cell line. An X-ray structure of this macrocycle bound to the HSP90 N-terminal domain was obtained (Fig. 9.6). In addition, the macrocycle showed very good liver microsomal stability, leading to low clearance and an oral bioavailability of 71% in nude mice. Oral administration once daily at 25 mg/kg led to significant growth inhibition in an HCT116 human colon cancer xenograft model.

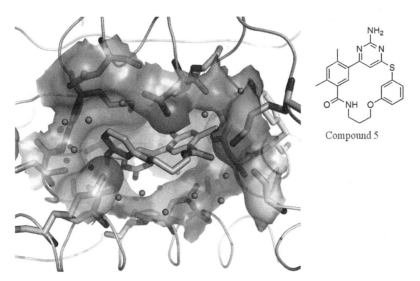

Compound 5

FIGURE 9.6 Chugai macrocycle 5 bound to the N-terminal domain of human HSP90 (PDB code: 3VHC). (This figure is reproduced in color in the color plate section.)

The 2-amino benzamide tropane-derived compound XL888 (Table 9.1) from Exelixis is a potent and selective ATP-competitive inhibitor of HSP90, has a favorable pharmacokinetic profile, and is highly active in multiple human tumor xenograft models [155]. Of interest, XL888 is effective in the vemurafenib-resistant melanoma cell lines that exhibit diverse resistance mechanisms [156]. The preclinical activity profile of XL888 is highly supportive of its clinical development for the treatment of cancers that are driven by proteins regulated by HSP90. XL888 is being evaluated in a phase I trial in patients with solid tumors (www.clinicaltrials.gov).

The pyrido[4,3-d]pyrimidine NVP-HSP990 (Table 9.1) from Novartis is an orally bioavailable, synthetic small-molecule HSP90 inhibitor [157]. NVP-HSP990 exhibits single-digit nanomolar IC_{50} values on three of the Hsp90 isoforms (Hsp90α, Hsp90β, and GRP94) and 320 nM IC_{50} value on TRAP-1, with selectivity against unrelated enzymes, receptors, and kinases [157], including multiple myeloma [158]. Broad-spectrum antitumor activity was seen in multiple tumor cell lines and primary patient samples in vitro and efficacy was seen in various human tumor xenograft models in vivo [157]. HSP990 was progressed toward phase I clinical trials in adult patients with advanced solid tumors.

Merck Serono research has identified hydroxyl-indazole-carboxamides as small-molecule HSP90 inhibitors using a fragment-based approach [159]. The 3-benzylindazole derivatives were shown to bind to the ATP-binding site of HSP90, displayed nanomolar activities in an HSP90-binding assay, inhibited cell proliferation in different human cancer cell lines, and caused the expected upregulation of HSP70 in A2780 ovarian cancer cells.

Pfizer has disclosed a novel class of oral HSP90 inhibitors based on high-throughput screening with subsequent optimization by structure-based design, leading to the identification of an oral development candidate [160]. The 2-amino-4-6-methylphenyl-N-(2,2-difluoropropyl)-5,7-dihydro-6H-pyrrolo[3,4-d]pyrimidine-6-carboxamide (Compound 42; Fig. 9.2) displayed favorable pharmacokinetic–pharmacodynamic relationships and significant efficacy in a melanoma xenograft tumor model. Pfizer has also designed structurally unique macrocycles that have been shown to be potent inhibitors of HSP90 with biomarker activity while being devoid of hERG potency [153]. In vivo efficacy was demonstrated in a glioma xenograft model.

Sanofi-Aventis has reported the discovery of a new class of potent tricyclic HSP90 inhibitors by high-throughput docking using an X-ray structure of the N-terminal domain in a closed conformation of the protein, and shown that they bind to the N-terminal ATP site in a manner not yet previously found for other known HSP90 inhibitors (Fig. 9.7) [161]. X-ray crystallography revealed that these compounds bind into an "induced" hydrophobic pocket 10–15 Å away from the ATP–resorcinol-binding site. Compound 8 was arrived at by structure-based drug design from a tricyclic compound that does not bind at the resorcinol-binding site. Extension of this hit into the resorcinol site gave compound 8, which showed that $K_d = 0.35$ nM in a fluorescence polarization (FP) binding assay, ERBB2 depletion at 30 nM, and GI_{50} values against a panel of tumor cell lines in the range of 20–110 nM. This compound also showed increased survival in a murine leukemia model on twice-daily IV dosing. The researchers hypothesized that more effective inhibitors of HSP90 may be identified by targeting the open conformation of HSP90, to which compound 8 binds, as opposed to the closed form of the protein, which is targeted by 17-AAG.

The conserved water molecules in the ATP-binding site have played an important role in the binding of several inhibitors. A group from Vernalis and Novartis have reported compound 8, a pyrrolopyrimidine carrying a cyano-group with a K_i determined by FP assay of <1 nM [162]. This cyano-group was designed to displace a conserved water molecule, and the compound shows enhanced affinity for HSP90. X-ray crystallography confirmed the design hypothesis (Fig. 9.8).

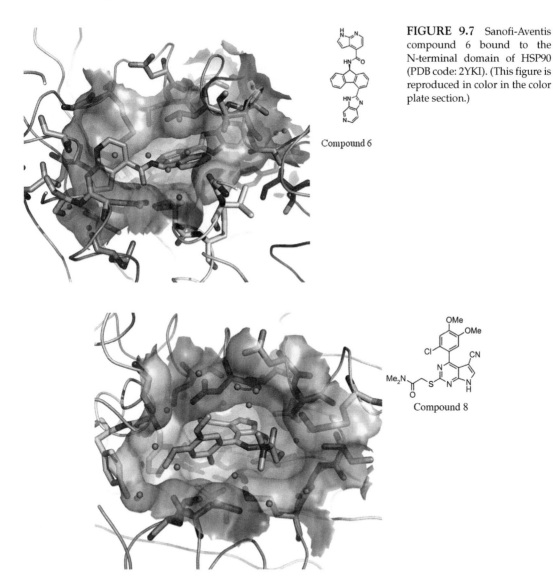

Compound 6

FIGURE 9.7 Sanofi-Aventis compound 6 bound to the N-terminal domain of HSP90 (PDB code: 2YKI). (This figure is reproduced in color in the color plate section.)

Compound 8

FIGURE 9.8 Vernalis–Novartis compound (compound 8) bound to the N-terminal domain of human HSP90 (PDB code: 4FCR). (This figure is reproduced in color in the color plate section.)

AGENTS THAT BIND TO OTHER SITES ON HSP90

Coumarin Antibiotic HSP90 Inhibitors

All of the HSP90 inhibitors that are in clinical trials (Table 9.1) bind to the ATP pocket in the N-terminal of HSP90 (except DS-2248, for which the binding site is unknown, see also later in this chapter). However, studies have shown that other domains of HSP90 can also be targeted. The coumarin antibiotics novobiocin, chlorobiocin, and coumermycin A (Fig. 9.9) target the C-terminal domain of HSP90 and exhibit unique effects on HSP90 conformation, activity and interactions with co-chaperones and clients [163–166]. However, these compounds generally exhibit poor affinity for HSP90, and because of this and the inability to obtain X-ray structures, their further development has been hampered. On the other hand, the novobiocin-derived C-terminal HSP90 inhibitor KU135 (Fig. 9.9) exhibits potent antiproliferative activity against several cell lines and interestingly did not upregulate the expression of HSP70, unlike the N-terminal HSP90 inhibitors (Fig. 9.1) [167,168].

Studies using photoaffinity labeling and protease fingerprinting have demonstrated clear evidence of the binding of novobiocin to the C-terminal domain [169]. Using co-crystal structures of novobiocin bound to the related DNA gyrase, the researchers were able to model the binding of novobiocin and suggested that it interacts at the dimerization interface of HSP90. Various analogs with benzamide side chains (exemplified by compound 83; Fig. 9.9) and possessing low nanomolar antiproliferative activities were synthesized, and these warrant

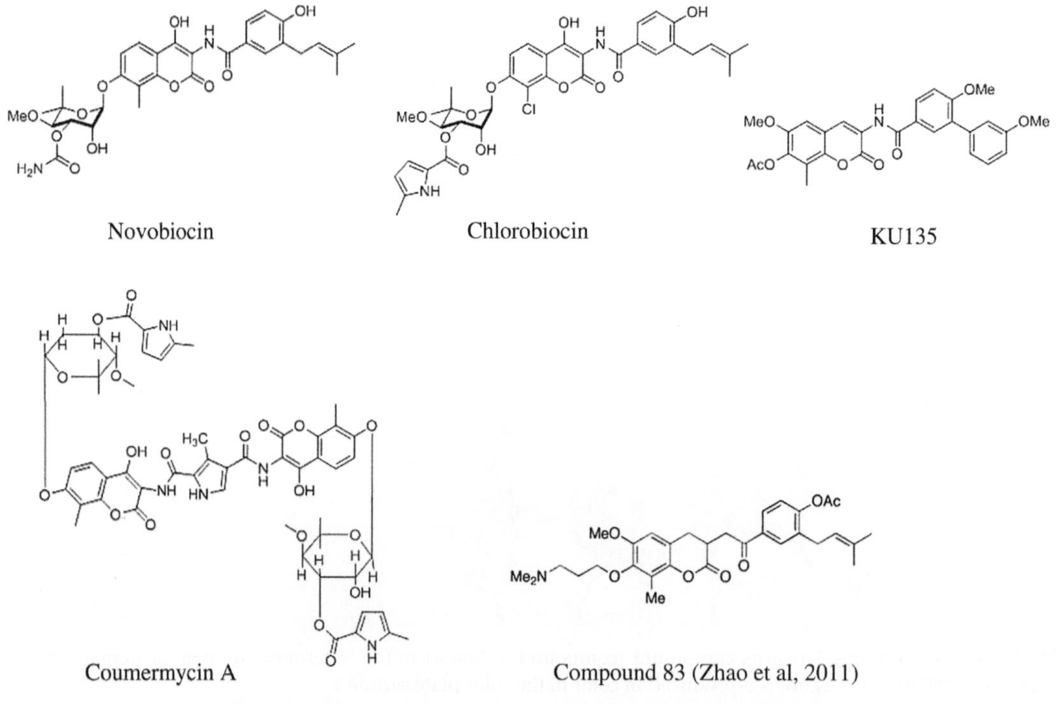

Novobiocin   Chlorobiocin   KU135

Coumermycin A   Compound 83 (Zhao et al, 2011)

FIGURE 9.9 Chemical structures of C-terminal HPS90 inhibitors.

further study [170]. Using the above data, it has been possible to produce analogs of novobiocin that are more potent (compound 13b) but do cause the induction of HSP70 that is more typical of an HSP90 inhibitor [171]. This work enhances the likelihood of developing drugs that act at the C-terminal site as inhibitors of HSP90. If potent drug candidates can be produced that deplete HSP90 clients while avoiding activation of the heat shock response, which protects against apoptosis [172], this could achieve an attractive clinical profile distinct from that of existing N-terminal ATP-site inhibitors.

Other HSP90 Inhibitors

The unspecified oral HSP90 inhibitor from Daiichi Sankyo, DS-2248 (Table 9.1), is currently undergoing phase I evaluation in patients with advanced solid tumors (www.clinicaltrials. gov). The structure of DS-2248 and its binding site to HSP90 are unknown.

The interesting pentapeptide agent Sansalvamide A-amide (San A-amide; Fig. 9.2) and its analogs (particularly compound 2; Fig. 9.2) [173,174] are cytotoxic molecules. Evidence indicates that the San A-amide specifically binds to the N-middle domain of HSP90 in an allosteric manner and disrupts the binding of proteins thought to interact with the HSP90 C-terminal domain, while having no effect on the binding on the client protein ERBB2 to HSP90. Hence, unlike other HSP90 inhibitors, using an in vitro binding assay, the researchers show that these inhibitors appear to inhibit the binding of the C-terminal client proteins IP6K2 and co-chaperones FKBP5 and HOP to HSP90. Interestingly, inhibiting the binding of HOP to HSP90 may affect the ability of HSP70 to dock with HSP90. This interaction is unique, and the Sansalvamide inhibitors may thus be used selectively to inhibit HSP90 client and co-chaperone protein interactions, thereby potentially delivering a distinct biological and clinical effect.

The natural product Gambogic acid (Fig. 9.2) was identified as a novel HSP90 inhibitor by high-throughput screening of natural-product libraries [175]. Gambogic acid inhibited cancer cell proliferation, displayed the molecular signature of HSP90 inhibition, and disrupted the interaction between HSP90, HSP70, and CDC37. Interestingly, this molecule binds to the N-terminal of HSP90 but at a site distinct from the HSP90 ATP-binding pocket. These results may provide a new target for the development of HSP90 inhibitors.

POTENTIAL FUTURE TARGETS

An alternative approach to antagonizing HSP90 is to inhibit other important components of the chaperone and the related stress pathway for the treatment of cancer (Fig. 9.1). Targeting HSP90 co-chaperone proteins, posttranslational modifiers, and elements of HSF1-mediated stress responses has the potential to deliver various biological and clinical profiles distinct from current HSP90 inhibitors. Examples of such approaches are discussed in this section.

Along with depletion of client proteins, HSP90 inhibition is usually accompanied by rapid induction of heat shock proteins such as HSP70 and HSP27 [176]. This is a mechanism-based, HSF1-mediated cytoprotective effect that is observed with all the ATP N-terminal HSP90 inhibitors, resulting in a self-limiting reduction in their effectiveness. Indeed, HSF1 knockout cells have been demonstrated to be more sensitive to HSP90 inhibitors than their wild-type counterparts [177], and dual silencing of HSP72 and HSC70 has been shown not only to inhibit HSP90 indirectly but also to induce tumor-selective apoptosis and sensitize cancer cells to HSP90 inhibitors [178]. Inhibitors of HSP70/HSC70 could exert single-agent activity or be used in combination with HSP90 inhibitors. There is now considerable interest in the discovery of HSF1, HSP70, and HSP27 inhibitors [172,176,179–181].

The co-chaperones CDC37, AHA1 and P23 regulate the function of HSP90 [10] and are highly expressed in cancer cells [182]. Silencing their expression by small interfering RNA (siRNA) has been shown to have direct antitumor effects and also in some cases to increase cancer cell sensitivity to HSP90 inhibitors [183–185]. Thus, targeting these proteins or their interaction with HSP90 may be of therapeutic benefit distinct from that of conventional HSP90 inhibitors. For example, an agent that acted on CDC37, the co-chaperone that directs protein kinases to HSP90, could cause selective kinase depletion while sparing other clients. However, identifying inhibitors that target the primarily hydrophobic protein–protein interaction surfaces has proven to be difficult.

Inhibition of the interactions between HSP90 and its client proteins is of obvious interest, not least because of the potential to achieve selective effects on particular clients or groups of clients. This is, however, very challenging as little is known about the precise molecular basis underlying these interactions. The three-dimensional structure of the HSP90–CDC37–CDK4 complex provided the first view of the interaction between HSP90 and a client protein [22,186]. The peptidomimetic compound shepherdin has been reported to block specifically the interaction between HSP90 and the antiapoptotic client survivin [187]. However, shepherdin can also interact with the ATP pocket of HSP90, hence making the interaction less specific.

HSP90 is subject to a range of posttranslational modifications that can modulate HSP90 function and alter sensitivity to HSP90 inhibitors, including acetylation, phosphorylation, S-nitrosylation, oxidation, and ubiquitination [188,189]. HDAC inhibitors LAQ824 and LBH589 have been shown to induce HSP90 hyperacetylation, leading to inhibition of chaperone functions and subsequent degradation of several client proteins [190]. In a phase I study, LAQ824 was well tolerated at doses that induced accumulation of histone acetylation, with higher doses inducing biomarker changes consistent with HSP90 inhibition [191]. The HSP90 client tyrosine kinase WEE1 has been shown to phosphorylate a conserved tyrosine residue in the N-terminal domain of HSP90, which in turn affects a number of oncogenic kinases (e.g., ERBB2 and CRAF) [188]. Depletion of WEE1 sensitizes prostate and cervical cancer cells to HSP90 inhibition, suggesting that such modulation of posttranslational modifications might be a new strategy to increase the cellular sensitivity of HSP90 inhibitors.

There is significant potential for modulation of chaperone and proteotoxic stress targets to exploit aneuploidy and where there would be selectivity through synthetic lethality. Cancer cells have a limited number of ways to deal with aneuploidy, and these commonly involve the proteasome or the chaperone systems, suggesting the potential for screening for ubiquitin-proteasomal enzymes involved in suppressing the adverse effects of aneuploidy [192]. Interestingly, 17-AAG has been shown to cause lethality in aneuploid but not euploid cells [193].

To date, most of the HSP90 inhibitors are active against HSP90α, HSP90β, and, to some extent, the other two HSP90 isoforms, GRP94 and TRAP1. Using structure-based drug design and measuring the activity of Toll receptors as the functional assay for GRP94 inhibition, compound 2 (Fig. 9.10) was shown to be the most potent inhibitor of GRP94 and to be selective

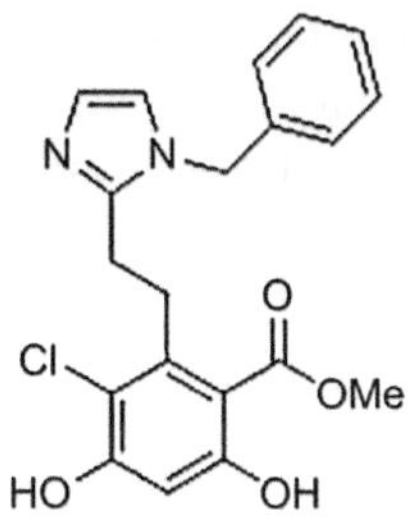

Compound 2

FIGURE 9.10   Chemical structure of a GRP94 inhibitor.

for GRP94 versus HSP90α/β [194]. Compound 2 exhibited no effect on the HSP90α/β client proteins (AKT or CRAF). Interestingly, treatment with compound 2 in cells did not lead to upregulation of BiP (the ER member of the HSP70 family). Hence, there may be value in the development of isoform-selective inhibitors, particularly in understanding which specific isoform or combination of isoforms will be more important for anticancer activity as opposed to toxic side effects.

SUMMARY AND FUTURE DIRECTIONS

As a molecular chaperone, HSP90 was originally seen as an unusual and certainly high-risk cancer drug target, but work over two decades has demonstrated its exciting potential—one that is in tune with emerging concepts of cancer biology, and with inhibitors exploiting or overcoming oncogene and nononcogene addiction, synthetic lethality, cooperative oncogene networks, clonal heterogeneity, and Darwinian selection, together with resistance mechanisms operating at multiple levels.

Early natural-product HSP90 inhibitors were valuable in demonstrating promising preclinical and clinical proof-of-concept activity, particularly the geldanamycin derivative 17-AAG. The natural-product HSP90 inhibitors geldanamycin and radicicol have not only provided extraordinary insights into HSP90 biology but also delivered essential target validation and provided critical evidence of druggability [195]. Early studies using these chemical tools and clinical pathfinders like 17-AAG and 17-DMAG have resulted in the general acceptance in the drug discovery world that HSP90 is a viable therapeutic target in the treatment of cancer. Much of the subsequent drug discovery efforts have focused on the inhibition of HSP90 by small molecules that bind—like geldanamycin and radicicol—to the chaperone's N-terminal nucleotide-binding pocket and are ATP competitive. More than 20 such pharmacological inhibitors of HSP90 have now entered clinical trial with many more progressing through preclinical development.

Although the HSP90 inhibitors were conceived originally as likely to exert broad-spectrum antitumor activity via the blockade of multiple oncogenic client proteins, signaling pathways, and cancer hallmark traits, results from preclinical models and especially from clinical trials have shown particularly strong therapeutic signals in certain disease contexts. In particular, the most convincing activity is seen in patients with cancers that are driven by oncogenic client proteins that are highly dependent on HSP90 for stability and function.

As a key example of this, despite the fact that 17-AAG has been challenging to develop because of drug-related toxicities and liabilities (e.g., hepatotoxicity, poor solubility leading to limitations in formulation and administration, and metabolic instability), this agent has demonstrated impressive activity in trastuzumab-refractory ERBB2-positive breast cancer [65]. Given this positive outcome, it was perhaps surprising that the development of 17-AAG was suspended in 2012 [78]. This is likely because of the aforementioned limitations, as well as commercial considerations owing to limited patent protection and the emergence of next-generation inhibitors with superior pharmaceutical properties. With the inhibitors that are following on, it is noteworthy that the most advanced resorcinol-based compounds, ganetespib and NVP-AUY922, have again shown impressive activity in ERBB2-positive breast cancer and also in NSCLC patients harboring mutant EGFR and rearranged ALK, which are both oncogenic driver client proteins of HSP90.

While it is important to carry out large-scale pivotal studies in the cancers discussed here in which the therapeutic signal seems very strong, broadening the activity profile of HSP90 inhibitors to reveal the full, originally envisaged "network biology drug" potential is also critical. Tumor types that seem to offer particular potential are advanced prostate cancers that remain dependent on the AR, mutant BRAF-driven melanomas and other cancers harboring this oncoprotein, malignancies in addition to breast in which ERBB2 is a key driver (e.g., gastric cancer), mutant KIT-driven GIST, and multiple myeloma, which has unusually high susceptibility to proteotoxic stress.

It has become increasingly clear that to reveal the full potential of HSP90 inhibitors, we need to design clinical trials that evaluate combinations of HSP90 inhibitors with other molecularly targeted agents. While therapeutic inhibition of an oncoprotein leads to silencing of the cognate oncogene-dependent signaling pathway, it also commonly releases negative feedback, resulting in the activation of upstream receptors and parallel compensatory pathways that limit the efficacy of a given therapy [4–6]. The emergence of primary and acquired resistance to a variety of these antitumor agents may be limited by blocking these compensatory pathways, which could result in a synthetic lethality-like effect. Many client proteins of HSP90 are among the key players and effectors of these compensatory mechanisms; hence, the use of HSP90 inhibitors in combination with, in particular, kinase inhibitors and antihormonal agents that also act on the same clients should be beneficial.

The other major reason for combinatorial clinical trials with HSP90 inhibitors is to overcome or prevent resistance through resistant target alleles or bypass pathways [1]. The use of HSP90 inhibitors upfront alongside other targeted agents seems likely to be most effective.

As discussed in this chapter, where the mechanism is disclosed all of the new synthetic small-molecule HSP90 inhibitors in clinical development, from different chemical classes, target the N-terminal ATP site of HSP90. In addition, there is significant potential for discovering novel chemical agents that affect HSP90 function by alternative modes of action (e.g., C-terminal inhibitors or modifiers of posttranslational modification), that affect HSP90 co-chaperone interactions (e.g., CDC37), or that interact elsewhere in the chaperone–stress pathways that are required by cancer cells, for example HSP70 [178] and HSF1 [196]. Laboratory research, including unbiased proteomic screening, continues to uncover specific, cancer-associated HSP90 clients and pathways [8,47,197,198]. This should enhance our understanding of the role of HSP90 in cancer and increase the likelihood of achieving a more personalized HSP90-based treatment for cancer patients.

It is clear that we still have much to learn about HSP90, and results will continue to surprise us. For example, a recent study has shown not only that CDC37 directly antagonizes ATP binding to client kinases, suggesting a role for the HSP90–CDC37 complex in controlling kinase activity, but also, quite unexpectedly, that CDC37 binding to protein kinases is itself antagonized by clinically approved ATP-competitive kinase inhibitors, including vemurafenib, sorafenib, lapatinib, and erlotinib [199]. Furthermore, in cancer cells, such kinase inhibitors deprive their corresponding oncogenic kinases (i.e., BRAF, ERBB2, and EGFR) of access to the HSP90–CDC37 complex, resulting in their degradation. These intriguing results indicate that at least some part of the antitumor effectiveness of inhibitors of HSP90-dependent kinases against cancer cells may result from targeted chaperone deprivation. The new findings provide further support for combining HSP90 and kinase inhibitors, in this case to further enhance chaperone deprivation.

It seems likely that using HSP90 upfront in combination with other targeted therapies will provide the best opportunity to deliver durable therapeutic effects, not least by minimizing the opportunities for drug resistance to develop. However, further work is required to confirm this.

To conclude, the complex and multifaceted HSP90 protein is an attractive molecular target, but there is much yet to understand about its basic biology, and more work needs to be done clinically before an HSP90 inhibitor can achieve regulatory approval for widespread application. Nevertheless, the diversity of chemical classes of HSP90 inhibitors currently in clinical trials along with studies on compounds acting by unknown mechanisms or binding elsewhere than to the ATPase pocket of HSP90 will undoubtedly move the field forward and should increase the likelihood of improved clinical outcomes.

CONFLICT OF INTEREST

All the authors are employees of The Institute of Cancer Research, which has a commercial interest in HSP90 inhibitors and operates a reward-to-inventors scheme. The authors received research funding from Vernalis for the discovery of HSP90 inhibitors, and intellectual property from this program was licensed to Vernalis Ltd and Novartis. Paul Workman has been a consultant to Novartis, is a founder and scientific advisory board member of Chroma Therapeutics, and is a scientific advisory board member of Astex Pharmaceuticals and Nextech Invest.

References

[1] Al-Lazikani B, Banerji U, Workman P. Combinatorial drug therapy for cancer in the post-genomic era. Nat Biotechnol 2012;30:679–92.
[2] Yap TA, Workman P. Exploiting the cancer genome: strategies for the discovery and clinical development of targeted molecular therapeutics. Annu Rev Pharmacol Toxicol 2012;52:549–73.
[3] Collins I, Workman P. New approaches to molecular cancer therapeutics. Nat Chem Biol 2006;2:689–700.
[4] Maloney A, Workman P. HSP90 as a new therapeutic target for cancer therapy: the story unfolds. Expert Opin Biol Ther 2002;2:3–24.
[5] Workman P. Combinatorial attack on multistep oncogenesis by inhibiting the Hsp90 molecular chaperone. Cancer Lett 2004;206:149–57.

[6] Workman P, Burrows F, Neckers L, Rosen N. Drugging the cancer chaperone HSP90: combinatorial therapeutic exploitation of oncogene addiction and tumor stress. Ann N Y Acad Sci 2007;1113:202–16.

[7] Neckers L, Workman P. Hsp90 molecular chaperone inhibitors: are we there yet? Clin Cancer Res 2012;18: 64–76.

[8] Travers J, Sharp S, Workman P. HSP90 inhibition: two-pronged exploitation of cancer dependencies. Drug Discov Today 2012;17:242–52.

[9] Csermely P, Schnaider T, Soti C, Prohaszka Z, Nardai G. The 90-kDa molecular chaperone family: structure, function, and clinical applications. A comprehensive review. Pharmacol Ther 1998;79:129–68.

[10] Pearl LH, Prodromou C, Workman P. The Hsp90 molecular chaperone: an open and shut case for treatment. Biochem J 2008;410:439–53.

[11] Calderwood SK. Heat shock proteins in breast cancer progression—a suitable case for treatment? Int J Hyperthermia 2010;26:681–5.

[12] Mayer MP. Gymnastics of molecular chaperones. Mol Cell 2010;39:321–31.

[13] MacRae TH. Structure and function of small heat shock/alpha-crystallin proteins: established concepts and emerging ideas. Cell Mol Life Sci 2000;57:899–913.

[14] Wang K, Spector A. ATP causes small heat shock proteins to release denatured protein. Eur J Biochem 2001;268:6335–45.

[15] Chen B, Piel WH, Gui L, Bruford E, Monteiro A. The HSP90 family of genes in the human genome: insights into their divergence and evolution. Genomics 2005;86:627–37.

[16] Pearl LH, Prodromou C. Structure and mechanism of the Hsp90 molecular chaperone machinery. Annu Rev Biochem 2006;75:271–94.

[17] Prodromou C, Roe SM, O'Brien R, Ladbury JE, Piper PW, Pearl LH. Identification and structural characterization of the ATP/ADP-binding site in the Hsp90 molecular chaperone. Cell. 1997;90:65–75.

[18] Prodromou C, Panaretou B, Chohan S, Siligardi G, O'Brien R, Ladbury JE, et al. The ATPase cycle of Hsp90 drives a molecular 'clamp' via transient dimerization of the N-terminal domains. EMBO J 2000;19:4383–92.

[19] Panaretou B, Siligardi G, Meyer P, Maloney A, Sullivan JK, Singh S, et al. Activation of the ATPase activity of hsp90 by the stress-regulated cochaperone aha1. Mol Cell. 2002;10:1307–18.

[20] Roe SM, Ali MM, Meyer P, Vaughan CK, Panaretou B, Piper PW, et al. The mechanism of Hsp90 regulation by the protein kinase-specific cochaperone p50 (cdc37). Cell. 2004;116:87–98.

[21] Vaughan CK, Mollapour M, Smith JR, Truman A, Hu B, Good VM, et al. Hsp90-dependent activation of protein kinases is regulated by chaperone-targeted dephosphorylation of Cdc37. Mol Cell 2008;31:886–95.

[22] Ali MM, Roe SM, Vaughan CK, Meyer P, Panaretou B, Piper PW, et al. Crystal structure of an Hsp90-nucleotide-p23/Sba1 closed chaperone complex. Nature 2006;440:1013–7.

[23] Ciocca DR, Clark GM, Tandon AK, Fuqua SA, Welch WJ, McGuire WL. Heat shock protein hsp70 in patients with axillary lymph node-negative breast cancer: prognostic implications. J Natl Cancer Inst 1993;85:570–4.

[24] Kimura E, Enns RE, Alcaraz JE, Arboleda J, Slamon DJ, Howell SB. Correlation of the survival of ovarian cancer patients with mRNA expression of the 60-kD heat-shock protein HSP-60. J Clin Oncol 1993;11:891–8.

[25] Ralhan R, Kaur J. Differential expression of Mr 70,000 heat shock protein in normal, premalignant, and malignant human uterine cervix. Clin Cancer Res 1995;1:1217–22.

[26] Santarosa M, Favaro D, Quaia M, Galligioni E. Expression of heat shock protein 72 in renal cell carcinoma: possible role and prognostic implications in cancer patients. Eur J Cancer 1997;33:873–7.

[27] Yufu Y, Nishimura J, Nawata H. High constitutive expression of heat shock protein 90 alpha in human acute leukemia cells. Leuk Res 1992;16:597–605.

[28] Chant ID, Rose PE, Morris AG. Analysis of heat-shock protein expression in myeloid leukaemia cells by flow cytometry. Br J Haematol 1995;90:163–8.

[29] Mitsiades N, Mitsiades CS, Poulaki V, Chauhan D, Fanourakis G, Gu X, et al. Molecular sequelae of proteasome inhibition in human multiple myeloma cells. Proc Natl Acad Sci U S A 2002;99:14374–9.

[30] McCarthy MM, Pick E, Kluger Y, Gould-Rothberg B, Lazova R, Camp RL, et al. HSP90 as a marker of progression in melanoma. Ann Oncol 2008;19:590–4.

[31] Pick E, Kluger Y, Giltnane JM, Moeder C, Camp RL, Rimm DL, et al. High HSP90 expression is associated with decreased survival in breast cancer. Cancer Res 2007;67:2932–7.

[32] Gallegos Ruiz MI, Floor K, Roepman P, Rodriguez JA, Meijer GA, Mooi WJ, et al. Integration of gene dosage and gene expression in non-small cell lung cancer, identification of HSP90 as potential target. PLoS One 2008;3: e0001722.

[33] Li CF, Huang WW, Wu JM, Yu SC, Hu TH, Uen YH, et al. Heat shock protein 90 overexpression independently predicts inferior disease-free survival with differential expression of the alpha and beta isoforms in gastrointestinal stromal tumors. Clin Cancer Res 2008;14:7822–31.

[34] Whitesell L, Lindquist SL. HSP90 and the chaperoning of cancer. Nat Rev Cancer 2005;5:761–72.

[35] Whitesell L, Bagatell R, Falsey R. The stress response: implications for the clinical development of hsp90 inhibitors. Curr Cancer Drug Targets 2003;3:349–58.

[36] Hanahan D, Weinberg RA. Hallmarks of cancer: the next generation. Cell 2011;144:646–74.

[37] Carracedo A, Ma L, Teruya-Feldstein J, Rojo F, Salmena L, Alimonti A, et al. Inhibition of mTORC1 leads to MAPK pathway activation through a PI3K-dependent feedback loop in human cancer. J Clin Invest 2008;118:3065–74.

[38] O'Reilly KE, Rojo F, She QB, Solit D, Mills GB, Smith D, et al. mTOR inhibition induces upstream receptor tyrosine kinase signaling and activates Akt. Cancer Res 2006;66:1500–8.

[39] Pratilas CA, Taylor BS, Ye Q, Viale A, Sander C, Solit DB, et al. (V600E)BRAF is associated with disabled feedback inhibition of RAF-MEK signaling and elevated transcriptional output of the pathway. Proc Natl Acad Sci U S A 2009;106:4519–24.

[40] Hostein I, Robertson D, DiStefano F, Workman P, Clarke PA. Inhibition of signal transduction by the Hsp90 inhibitor 17-allylamino-17-demethoxygeldanamycin results in cytostasis and apoptosis. Cancer Res 2001;61:4003–9.

[41] Chiosis G, Neckers L. Tumor selectivity of Hsp90 inhibitors: the explanation remains elusive. ACS Chem Biol 2006;1:279–84.

[42] Kamal A, Thao L, Sensintaffar J, Zhang L, Boehm MF, Fritz LC, et al. A high-affinity conformation of Hsp90 confers tumour selectivity on Hsp90 inhibitors. Nature 2003;425:407–10.

[43] da Rocha Dias S, Friedlos F, Light Y, Springer C, Workman P, Marais R. Activated B-RAF is an Hsp90 client protein that is targeted by the anticancer drug 17-allylamino-17-demethoxygeldanamycin. Cancer Res 2005;65:10686–91.

[44] Grbovic OM, Basso AD, Sawai A, Ye Q, Friedlander P, Solit D, et al. V600E B-Raf requires the Hsp90 chaperone for stability and is degraded in response to Hsp90 inhibitors. Proc Natl Acad Sci U S A 2006;103: 57–62.

[45] Weinstein IB, Joe AK. Mechanisms of disease: oncogene addiction—a rationale for molecular targeting in cancer therapy. Nat Clin Pract Oncol 2006;3:448–57.

[46] Taipale M, Krykbaeva I, Koeva M, Kayatekin C, Westover KD, Karras GI, et al. Quantitative analysis of HSP90-client interactions reveals principles of substrate recognition. Cell 2012;150:987–1001.

[47] Samant RS, Workman P. Molecular biology: choose your protein partners. Nature 2012;490:351–2.

[48] Whitesell L, Mimnaugh EG, De Costa B, Myers CE, Neckers LM. Inhibition of heat shock protein HSP90-pp60v-src heteroprotein complex formation by benzoquinone ansamycins: essential role for stress proteins in oncogenic transformation. Proc Natl Acad Sci U S A 1994;91:8324–8.

[49] Roe SM, Prodromou C, O'Brien R, Ladbury JE, Piper PW, Pearl LH. Structural basis for inhibition of the Hsp90 molecular chaperone by the antitumor antibiotics radicicol and geldanamycin. J Med Chem 1999;42: 260–6.

[50] Workman P, Collins I. Probing the probes: fitness factors for small molecule tools. Chem Biol 2010;17:561–77.

[51] Chene P. ATPases as drug targets: learning from their structure. Nat Rev Drug Discov 2002;1:665–73.

[52] Grenert JP, Sullivan WP, Fadden P, Haystead TA, Clark J, Mimnaugh E, et al. The amino-terminal domain of heat shock protein 90 (hsp90) that binds geldanamycin is an ATP/ADP switch domain that regulates hsp90 conformation. J Biol Chem 1997;272:23843–50.

[53] Xu W, Marcu M, Yuan X, Mimnaugh E, Patterson C, Neckers L. Chaperone-dependent E3 ubiquitin ligase CHIP mediates a degradative pathway for c-ErbB2/Neu. Proc Natl Acad Sci U S A 2002;99:12847–52.

[54] Schnur RC, Corman ML, Gallaschun RJ, Cooper BA, Dee MF, Doty JL, et al. Inhibition of the oncogene product p185erbB-2 in vitro and in vivo by geldanamycin and dihydrogeldanamycin derivatives. J Med Chem 1995;38:3806–12.

[55] Porter JR, Ge J, Lee J, Normant E, West K. Ansamycin inhibitors of Hsp90: nature's prototype for anti-chaperone therapy. Curr Top Med Chem 2009;9:1386–418.

[56] Supko JG, Hickman RL, Grever MR, Malspeis L. Preclinical pharmacologic evaluation of geldanamycin as an antitumor agent. Cancer Chemother Pharmacol 1995;36:305–15.

[57] Solit DB, Chiosis G. Development and application of Hsp90 inhibitors. Drug Discov Today 2008;13:38–43.

[58] Munster PN, Basso A, Solit D, Norton L, Rosen N. Modulation of Hsp90 function by ansamycins sensitizes breast cancer cells to chemotherapy-induced apoptosis in an RB- and schedule-dependent manner. See: E. A. Sausville, Combining cytotoxics and 17-allylamino, 17-demethoxygeldanamycin: sequence and tumor biology matters. Clin. Cancer Res 2001;7:2155–8.

[59] Banerji U, O'Donnell A, Scurr M, Pacey S, Stapleton S, Asad Y, et al. Phase I pharmacokinetic and pharmaco-dynamic study of 17-allylamino, 17-demethoxygeldanamycin in patients with advanced malignancies. J Clin Oncol 2005;23:4152–61.

[60] Banerji U, Walton M, Raynaud F, Grimshaw R, Kelland L, Valenti M, et al. Pharmacokinetic–pharmacodynamic relationships for the heat shock protein 90 molecular chaperone inhibitor 17-allylamino, 17-demethoxygeldanamycin in human ovarian cancer xenograft models. Clin Cancer Res 2005;11:7023–32.

[61] Workman P. How much gets there and what does it do? The need for better pharmacokinetic and pharmaco-dynamic endpoints in contemporary drug discovery and development. Curr Pharm Des 2003;9:891–902.

[62] Yap TA, Sandhu SK, Workman P, de Bono JS. Envisioning the future of early anticancer drug development. Nat Rev Cancer 2010;10:514–23.

[63] Pacey S, Gore M, Chao D, Banerji U, Larkin J, Sarker S, et al. A phase II trial of 17-allylamino, 17-demethoxygeldanamycin (17-AAG, tanespimycin) in patients with metastatic melanoma. Invest New Drugs 2012;30:341–9.

[64] Banerji U, Affolter A, Judson I, Marais R, Workman P. BRAF and NRAS mutations in melanoma: potential relationships to clinical response to HSP90 inhibitors. Mol Cancer Ther 2008;7:737–9.

[65] Modi S, Stopeck A, Linden H, Solit D, Chandarlapaty S, Rosen N, et al. HSP90 inhibition is effective in breast cancer: a phase II trial of tanespimycin (17-AAG) plus trastuzumab in patients with HER2-positive metastatic breast cancer progressing on trastuzumab. Clin Cancer Res 2011;17:5132–9.

[66] Rodrigues LM, Chung YL, Al Saffar NM, Sharp SY, Jackson LE, Banerji U, et al. Effects of HSP90 inhibitor 17-allylamino-17-demethoxygeldanamycin (17-AAG) on NEU/HER2 overexpressing mammary tumours in MMTV-NEU-NT mice monitored by magnetic resonance spectroscopy. BMC Res Notes 2012;5:250.

[67] Munster PN, Marchion DC, Basso AD, Rosen N. Degradation of HER2 by ansamycins induces growth arrest and apoptosis in cells with HER2 overexpression via a HER3, phosphatidylinositol 3′-kinase-AKT-dependent pathway. Cancer Res 2002;62:3132–7.

[68] Richardson PG, Chanan-Khan AA, Lonial S, Krishnan AY, Carroll MP, Alsina M, et al. Tanespimycin and bort-ezomib combination treatment in patients with relapsed or relapsed and refractory multiple myeloma: results of a phase 1/2 study. Br J Haematol 2011;153:729–40.

[69] Richardson PG, Mitsiades CS, Laubach JP, Lonial S, Chanan-Khan AA, Anderson KC. Inhibition of heat shock protein 90 (HSP90) as a therapeutic strategy for the treatment of myeloma and other cancers. Br J Haematol 2011;152:367–79.

[70] Tse AN, Sheikh TN, Alan H, Chou TC, Schwartz GK. 90-kDa heat shock protein inhibition abrogates the topoi-somerase I poison-induced G2/M checkpoint in p53-null tumor cells by depleting Chk1 and Wee1. Mol Phar-macol 2009;75:124–33.

[71] Arlander SJ, Felts SJ, Wagner JM, Stensgard B, Toft DO, Karnitz LM. Chaperoning checkpoint kinase 1 (Chk1), an Hsp90 client, with purified chaperones. J Biol Chem 2006;281:2989–98.

[72] Hubbard J, Erlichman C, Toft DO, Qin R, Stensgard BA, Felten S, et al. Phase I study of 17-allylamino-17 deme-thoxygeldanamycin, gemcitabine and/or cisplatin in patients with refractory solid tumors. Invest New Drugs 2011;29:473–80.

[73] Reikvam H, Ersvaer E, Bruserud O. Heat shock protein 90—a potential target in the treatment of human acute myelogenous leukemia. Curr Cancer Drug Targets 2009;9:761–76.

[74] Weisberg E, Barrett R, Liu Q, Stone R, Gray N, Griffin JD. FLT3 inhibition and mechanisms of drug resistance in mutant FLT3-positive AML. Drug Resist Updat 2009;12:81–9.

[75] Peng C, Brain J, Hu Y, Goodrich A, Kong L, Grayzel D, et al. Inhibition of heat shock protein 90 prolongs survival of mice with BCR-ABL-T315I-induced leukemia and suppresses leukemic stem cells. Blood 2007;110:678–85.

[76] O'Hare T, Eide CA, Deininger MW. New Bcr-Abl inhibitors in chronic myeloid leukemia: keeping resistance in check. Expert Opin Investig Drugs 2008;17:865–78.

[77] Castro JE, Prada CE, Loria O, Kamal A, Chen L, Burrows FJ, et al. ZAP-70 is a novel conditional heat shock protein 90 (Hsp90) client: inhibition of Hsp90 leads to ZAP-70 degradation, apoptosis, and impaired signaling in chronic lymphocytic leukemia. Blood 2005;106:2506–12.

[78] Arteaga CL. Why is this effective HSP90 inhibitor not being developed in HER2+ breast cancer? Clin Cancer Res 2011;17:4919–21.

[79] Smith V, Sausville EA, Camalier RF, Fiebig HH, Burger AM. Comparison of 17-dimethylaminoethylamino-17-demethoxy-geldanamycin (17DMAG) and 17-allylamino-17-demethoxygeldanamycin (17AAG) in vitro: effects on Hsp90 and client proteins in melanoma models. Cancer Chemother Pharmacol 2005;56:126–37.

[80] Egorin MJ, Lagattuta TF, Hamburger DR, Covey JM, White KD, Musser SM, et al. Pharmacokinetics, tissue distribution, and metabolism of 17-(dimethylaminoethylamino)-17-demethoxygeldanamycin (NSC 707545) in CD2F1 mice and Fischer 344 rats. Cancer Chemother Pharmacol 2002;49:7–19.

[81] Kaur G, Belotti D, Burger AM, Fisher-Nielson K, Borsotti P, Riccardi E, et al. Antiangiogenic properties of 17-(dimethylaminoethylamino)-17-demethoxygeldanamycin: an orally bioavailable heat shock protein 90 modulator. Clin Cancer Res 2004;10:4813–21.

[82] Pacey S, Wilson RH, Walton M, Eatock MM, Hardcastle A, Zetterlund A, et al. A phase I study of the heat shock protein 90 inhibitor alvespimycin (17-DMAG) given intravenously to patients with advanced solid tumors. Clin Cancer Res 2011;17:1561–70.

[83] Solit DB, Ivy SP, Kopil C, Sikorski R, Morris MJ, Slovin SF, et al. Phase I trial of 17-allylamino-17-demethoxygeldanamycin in patients with advanced cancer. Clin Cancer Res 2007;13:1775–82.

[84] Solit DB, Zheng FF, Drobnjak M, Munster PN, Higgins B, Verbel D, et al. 17-Allylamino-17-demethoxygeldanamycin induces the degradation of androgen receptor and HER-2/neu and inhibits the growth of prostate cancer xenografts. Clin Cancer Res 2002;8:986–93.

[85] Jhaveri K, Miller K, Rosen L, Schneider B, Chap L, Hannah A, et al. A phase I dose-escalation trial of trastuzumab and alvespimycin hydrochloride (KOS-1022; 17 DMAG) in the treatment of advanced solid tumors. Clin Cancer Res 2012;18:5090–8.

[86] Ronnen EA, Kondagunta GV, Ishill N, Sweeney SM, Deluca JK, Schwartz L, et al. A phase II trial of 17-(allylamino)-17-demethoxygeldanamycin in patients with papillary and clear cell renal cell carcinoma. Invest New Drugs 2006;24:543–6.

[87] Solit DB, Osman I, Polsky D, Panageas KS, Daud A, Goydos JS, et al. Phase II trial of 17-allylamino-17-demethoxygeldanamycin in patients with metastatic melanoma. Clin Cancer Res 2008;14:8302–7.

[88] Erlichman C. Tanespimycin: the opportunities and challenges of targeting heat shock protein 90. Expert Opin Investig Drugs 2009;18:861–8.

[89] Ge J, Normant E, Porter JR, Ali JA, Dembski MS, Gao Y, et al. Design, synthesis, and biological evaluation of hydroquinone derivatives of 17-amino-17-demethoxygeldanamycin as potent, water-soluble inhibitors of Hsp90. J Med Chem 2006;49:4606–15.

[90] Taldone T, Gozman A, Maharaj R, Chiosis G. Targeting Hsp90: small-molecule inhibitors and their clinical development. Curr Opin Pharmacol 2008;8:370–4.

[91] Egorin MJ, Zuhowski EG, Rosen DM, Sentz DL, Covey JM, Eiseman JL. Plasma pharmacokinetics and tissue distribution of 17-(allylamino)-17-demethoxygeldanamycin (NSC 330507) in CD2F1 mice1. Cancer Chemother Pharmacol 2001;47:291–302.

[92] Kelland LR, Sharp SY, Rogers PM, Myers TG, Workman P. DT-diaphorase expression and tumor cell sensitivity to 17-allylamino, 17-demethoxygeldanamycin, an inhibitor of heat shock protein 90. J Natl Cancer Inst 1999;91:1940–9.

[93] Pacey S, Banerji U, Judson I, Workman P. Hsp90 inhibitors in the clinic. Handb Exp Pharmacol 2006:331–58.

[94] Guo W, Reigan P, Siegel D, Zirrolli J, Gustafson D, Ross D. Formation of 17-allylamino-demethoxygeldanamycin (17-AAG) hydroquinone by NAD(P)H:quinone oxidoreductase 1: role of 17-AAG hydroquinone in heat shock protein 90 inhibition. Cancer Res 2005;65:10006–15.

[95] Siegel D, Yan C, Ross D. NAD(P)H:quinone oxidoreductase 1 (NQO1) in the sensitivity and resistance to antitumor quinones. Biochem Pharmacol 2012;83:1033–40.

[96] Gaspar N, Sharp SY, Pacey S, Jones C, Walton M, Vassal G, et al. Acquired resistance to 17-allylamino-17-demethoxygeldanamycin (17-AAG, tanespimycin) in glioblastoma cells. Cancer Res 2009;69:1966–75.

[97] Sydor JR, Normant E, Pien CS, Porter JR, Ge J, Grenier L, et al. Development of 17-allylamino-17-demethoxygeldanamycin hydroquinone hydrochloride (IPI-504), an anti-cancer agent directed against Hsp90. Proc Natl Acad Sci U S A 2006;103:17408–13.

[98] Sequist LV, Gettinger S, Senzer NN, Martins RG, Janne PA, Lilenbaum R, et al. Activity of IPI-504, a novel heat-shock protein 90 inhibitor, in patients with molecularly defined non-small-cell lung cancer. J Clin Oncol 2010;28:4953–60.

[99] Janin YL. ATPase inhibitors of heat-shock protein 90, second season. Drug Discov Today 2010;15:342–53.

[100] Oh WK, Galsky MD, Stadler WM, Srinivas S, Chu F, Bubley G, et al. Multicenter phase II trial of the heat shock protein 90 inhibitor, retaspimycin hydrochloride (IPI-504), in patients with castration-resistant prostate cancer. Urology 2011;78:626–30.

[101] Kwon HJ, Yoshida M, Fukui Y, Horinouchi S, Beppu T. Potent and specific inhibition of p60v-src protein kinase both in vivo and in vitro by radicicol. Cancer Res 1992;52:6926–30.

[102] Zhao JF, Nakano H, Sharma S. Suppression of RAS and MOS transformation by radicicol. Oncogene 1995;11:161–73.

[103] Schulte TW, Akinaga S, Soga S, Sullivan W, Stensgard B, Toft D, et al. Antibiotic radicicol binds to the N-terminal domain of Hsp90 and shares important biologic activities with geldanamycin. Cell Stress Chaperones 1998;3:100–8.

[104] Soga S, Neckers LM, Schulte TW, Shiotsu Y, Akasaka K, Narumi H, et al. KF25706, a novel oxime derivative of radicicol, exhibits in vivo antitumor activity via selective depletion of Hsp90 binding signaling molecules. Cancer Res 1999;59:2931–8.

[105] Agatsuma T, Ogawa H, Akasaka K, Asai A, Yamashita Y, Mizukami T, et al. Halohydrin and oxime derivatives of radicicol: synthesis and antitumor activities. Bioorg Med Chem 2002;10:3445–54.

[106] Janin YL. Heat shock protein 90 inhibitors. A text book example of medicinal chemistry? J Med Chem 2005;48:7503–12.

[107] Hellwig V, Mayer-Bartschmid A, Muller H, Greif G, Kleymann G, Zitzmann W, et al. Pochonins A-F, new antiviral and antiparasitic resorcylic acid lactones from *Pochonia chlamydosporia* var. catenulata. J Nat Prod 2003;66:829–37.

[108] Proisy N, Sharp SY, Boxall K, Connelly S, Roe SM, Prodromou C, et al. Inhibition of Hsp90 with synthetic macrolactones: synthesis and structural and biological evaluation of ring and conformational analogs of radicicol. Chem Biol 2006;13:1203–15.

[109] Day JE, Sharp SY, Rowlands MG, Aherne W, Hayes A, Raynaud FI, et al. Targeting the Hsp90 molecular chaperone with novel macrolactams. Synthesis, structural, binding, and cellular studies. ACS Chem Biol 2011;6:1339–47.

[110] Cheung KM, Matthews TP, James K, Rowlands MG, Boxall KJ, Sharp SY, et al. The identification, synthesis, protein crystal structure and in vitro biochemical evaluation of a new 3,4-diarylpyrazole class of Hsp90 inhibitors. Bioorg Med Chem Lett 2005;15:3338–43.

[111] Sharp SY, Boxall K, Rowlands M, Prodromou C, Roe SM, Maloney A, et al. In vitro biological characterization of a novel, synthetic diaryl pyrazole resorcinol class of heat shock protein 90 inhibitors. Cancer Res 2007;67:2206–16.

[112] Sharp SY, Prodromou C, Boxall K, Powers MV, Holmes JL, Box G, et al. Inhibition of the heat shock protein 90 molecular chaperone in vitro and in vivo by novel, synthetic, potent resorcinylic pyrazole/isoxazole amide analogues. Mol Cancer Ther 2007;6:1198–211.

[113] Eccles SA, Massey A, Raynaud FI, Sharp SY, Box G, Valenti M, et al. NVP-AUY922: a novel heat shock protein 90 inhibitor active against xenograft tumor growth, angiogenesis, and metastasis. Cancer Res 2008;68:2850–60.

[114] Brough PA, Aherne W, Barril X, Borgognoni J, Boxall K, Cansfield JE, et al. 4,5-Diarylisoxazole Hsp90 chaperone inhibitors: potential therapeutic agents for the treatment of cancer. J Med Chem 2008;51:196–218.

[115] Sessa C, Shapiro GI, Bhalla KN, Britten C, Jacks KS, Mita M, et al. First-in-human phase I dose-escalation study of the HSP90 inhibitor AUY922 in patients with advanced solid tumors. Clin Can Res. Jun 11, 2013. [Epub ahead of print]

[116] Wainberg ZA, Anghel A, Rogers AM, Desai AJ, Kalous O, Conklin D, et al. Inhibition of HSP90 with AUY922 induces synergy in HER2-amplified trastuzumab-resistant breast and gastric cancer. Mol Cancer Ther 2013;12:509–19.

[117] Jensen MR, Schoepfer J, Radimerski T, Massey A, Guy CT, Brueggen J, et al. NVP-AUY922: a small molecule HSP90 inhibitor with potent antitumor activity in preclinical breast cancer models. Breast Cancer Res 2008;10:R33.

[118] Kong A, Rea D, Ahmed S, Beck JT, López López R, Biganzoli L, et-al. Phase Ib/II study of the HSP90 inhibitor AUY922, in combination with trastuzumab, in patients with HER2+ advanced breast cancer. 2012. ASCO. Abstract No: 530.

[119] Garon EB, Moran T, Barlesi F, Gandhi L, Sequist LV, Kim S-W, et al. Phase II study of the HSP90 inhibitor AUY922 in patients with previously treated, advanced non-small cell lung cancer (NSCLC). 2012. ASCO. Abstract No: 7543.

[120] Ying W, Du Z, Sun L, Foley KP, Proia DA, Blackman RK, et al. Ganetespib, a unique triazolone-containing Hsp90 inhibitor, exhibits potent antitumor activity and a superior safety profile for cancer therapy. Mol Cancer Ther 2012;11:475–84.

[121] Shimamura T, Perera SA, Foley KP, Sang J, Rodig SJ, Inoue T, et al. Ganetespib (STA-9090), a nongeldanamycin HSP90 inhibitor, has potent antitumor activity in in vitro and in vivo models of non-small cell lung cancer. Clin Cancer Res 2012;18:4973–85.

[122] Acquaviva J, Smith DL, Sang J, Friedland JC, He S, Sequeira M, et al. Targeting KRAS-mutant non-small cell lung cancer with the Hsp90 inhibitor ganetespib. Mol Cancer Ther 2012;11:2633–43.

[123] Goldman JW, Raju RN, Gordon GA, El-Hariry I, Teofilivici F, Vukovic VM, et al. A first in human, safety, pharmacokinetics, and clinical activity phase I study of once weekly administration of the Hsp90 inhibitor ganetespib (STA-9090) in patients with solid malignancies. BMC Cancer 2013;13:152.

[124] Choi HK, Lee K. Recent updates on the development of ganetespib as a Hsp90 inhibitor. Arch Pharm Res 2012;35:1855–9.

[125] Sang J, Acquaviva J, Friedland JC, Smith DL, Sequeira M, Zhang C, et al. Targeted inhibition of the molecular chaperone Hsp90 overcomes ALK inhibitor resistance in non-small cell lung cancer. Cancer Discov 2013;3:430–43.

[126] Socinski MA, Goldman J, El-Hariry I, Koczywas M, Vukovic V, Horn L, et al. A multicenter phase II study of ganetespib monotherapy in patients with genotypically-defined advanced non-small cell lung cancer. Clin Cancer Res 2013.

[127] Ramalingam SS, Zaric B, Goss GD, Manegold C Sr., Rosell R, Vukovic V, et-al. Preliminary results from a randomized 2b/3 study of ganetespib and docetaxel combination versus docetaxel in advanced NSCLC (the GALAXY Trial, NCT01348126). 2012. ESMO. Abstract #1248P_PR.

[128] Woodhead AJ, Angove H, Carr MG, Chessari G, Congreve M, Coyle JE, et al. Discovery of (2,4-dihydroxy-5-isopropylphenyl)-[5-(4-methylpiperazin-1-ylmethyl)-1,3-di hydroisoindol-2-yl]methanone (AT13387), a novel inhibitor of the molecular chaperone Hsp90 by fragment based drug design. J Med Chem 2010;53: 5956–69.

[129] Graham B, Curry J, Smyth T, Fazal L, Feltell R, Harada I, et al. The heat shock protein 90 inhibitor, AT13387, displays a long duration of action in vitro and in vivo in non-small cell lung cancer. Cancer Sci 2012; 103:522–7.

[130] Smyth T, Van Looy T, Curry JE, Rodriguez-Lopez AM, Wozniak A, Zhu M, et al. The HSP90 inhibitor, AT13387, is effective against imatinib-sensitive and -resistant gastrointestinal stromal tumor models. Mol Cancer Ther 2012;11:1799–808.

[131] Nakashima T, Ishii T, Tagaya H, Seike T, Nakagawa H, Kanda Y, et al. New molecular and biological mechanism of antitumor activities of KW-2478, a novel nonansamycin heat shock protein 90 inhibitor, in multiple myeloma cells. Clin Cancer Res 2010;16:2792–802.

[132] Sharp SY, Roe SM, Kazlauskas E, Cikotiene I, Workman P, Matulis D, et al. Co-crystallization and in vitro biological characterization of 5-aryl-4-(5-substituted-2-4-dihydroxyphenyl)-1,2,3-thiadiazole hsp90 inhibitors. PLoS One 2012;7:e44642.

[133] Prodromou C, Nuttall JM, Millson SH, Roe SM, Sim TS, Tan D, et al. Structural basis of the radicicol resistance displayed by a fungal hsp90. ACS Chem Biol 2009;4:289–97.

[134] Piper PW, Millson SH. Spotlight on the microbes that produce heat shock protein 90-targeting antibiotics. Open Biol 2012;2:120138.

[135] Chiosis G. Discovery and development of purine-scaffold Hsp90 inhibitors. Curr Top Med Chem 2006;6: 1183–91.

[136] Chiosis G, Timaul MN, Lucas B, Munster PN, Zheng FF, Sepp-Lorenzino L, et al. A small molecule designed to bind to the adenine nucleotide pocket of Hsp90 causes Her2 degradation and the growth arrest and differentiation of breast cancer cells. Chem Biol 2001;8:289–99.

[137] Wright L, Barril X, Dymock B, Sheridan L, Surgenor A, Beswick M, et al. Structure–activity relationships in purine-based inhibitor binding to HSP90 isoforms. Chem Biol 2004;11:775–85.

[138] Biamonte MA, Shi J, Hong K, Hurst DC, Zhang L, Fan J, et al. Orally active purine-based inhibitors of the heat shock protein 90. J Med Chem 2006;49:817–28.

[139] He H, Zatorska D, Kim J, Aguirre J, Llauger L, She Y, et al. Identification of potent water soluble purine-scaffold inhibitors of the heat shock protein 90. J Med Chem 2006;49:381–90.

[140] Zhang L, Fan J, Vu K, Hong K, Le Brazidec JY, Shi J, et al. 7'-substituted benzothiazolothio- and pyridinothiazolothio-purines as potent heat shock protein 90 inhibitors. J Med Chem 2006;49:5352–62.

[141] Rodina A, Vilenchik M, Moulick K, Aguirre J, Kim J, Chiang A, et al. Selective compounds define Hsp90 as a major inhibitor of apoptosis in small-cell lung cancer. Nat Chem Biol 2007;3:498–507.

[142] Dickson MA, Okuno SH, Keohan ML, Maki RG, D'Adamo DR, Akhurst TJ, et al. Phase II study of the HSP90-inhibitor BIIB021 in gastrointestinal stromal tumors. Ann Oncol 2013;24:252–7.

[143] Shi J, Van de Water R, Hong K, Lamer RB, Weichert KW, Sandoval CM, et al. EC144 is a potent inhibitor of the heat shock protein 90. J Med Chem 2012;55:7786–95.

[144] Bao R, Lai CJ, Qu H, Wang D, Yin L, Zifcak B, et al. CUDC-305, a novel synthetic HSP90 inhibitor with unique pharmacologic properties for cancer therapy. Clin Cancer Res 2009;15:4046–57.

[145] Kim SH, Bajji A, Tangallapally R, Markovitz B, Trovato R, Shenderovich M, et al. Discovery of (2S)-1-[4-(2-{6-amino-8-[(6-bromo-1,3-benzodioxol-5-yl)sulfanyl]-9H-purin-9-yl}et hyl)piperidin-1-yl]-2-hydroxypropan-1-one (MPC-3100), a purine-based Hsp90 inhibitor. J Med Chem 2012;55:7480–501.

[146] Brough PA, Barril X, Borgognoni J, Chene P, Davies NG, Davis B, et al. Combining hit identification strategies: fragment-based and in silico approaches to orally active 2-aminothieno[2,3-d]pyrimidine inhibitors of the Hsp90 molecular chaperone. J Med Chem 2009;52:4794–809.

[147] Fadden P, Huang KH, Veal JM, Steed PM, Barabasz AF, Foley B, et al. Application of chemoproteomics to drug discovery: identification of a clinical candidate targeting hsp90. Chem Biol 2010;17:686–94.

[148] Chandarlapaty S, Sawai A, Ye Q, Scott A, Silinski M, Huang K, et al. SNX2112, a synthetic heat shock protein 90 inhibitor, has potent antitumor activity against HER kinase-dependent cancers. Clin Cancer Res 2008;14:240–8.

[149] Rajan A, Kelly RJ, Trepel JB, Kim YS, Alarcon SV, Kummar S, et al. A phase I study of PF-04929113 (SNX-5422), an orally bioavailable heat shock protein 90 inhibitor, in patients with refractory solid tumor malignancies and lymphomas. Clin Cancer Res 2011;17:6831–9.

[150] Zapf CW, Bloom JD, McBean JL, Dushin RG, Nittoli T, Ingalls C, et al. Design and SAR of macrocyclic Hsp90 inhibitors with increased metabolic stability and potent cell-proliferation activity. Bioorg Med Chem Lett 2011;21:2278–82.

[151] Zapf CW, Bloom JD, McBean JL, Dushin RG, Nittoli T, Otteng M, et al. Macrocyclic lactams as potent Hsp90 inhibitors with excellent tumor exposure and extended biomarker activity. Bioorg Med Chem Lett 2011;21: 3411–6.

[152] Zapf CW, Bloom JD, McBean JL, Dushin RG, Golas JM, Liu H, et al. Discovery of a macrocyclic o-aminobenzamide Hsp90 inhibitor with heterocyclic tether that shows extended biomarker activity and in vivo efficacy in a mouse xenograft model. Bioorg Med Chem Lett 2011;21:3627–31.

[153] Zapf CW, Bloom JD, Li Z, Dushin RG, Nittoli T, Otteng M, et al. Discovery of a stable macrocyclic o-aminobenzamide Hsp90 inhibitor which significantly decreases tumor volume in a mouse xenograft model. Bioorg Med Chem Lett 2011;21:4602–7.

[154] Suda A, Koyano H, Hayase T, Hada K, Kawasaki K, Komiyama S, et al. Design and synthesis of novel macrocyclic 2-amino-6-arylpyrimidine Hsp90 inhibitors. Bioorg Med Chem Lett 2012;22:1136–41.

[155] Bussenius J, Blazey CM, Aay N, Anand NK, Arcalas A, Baik T, et al. Discovery of XL888: a novel tropane-derived small molecule inhibitor of HSP90. Bioorg Med Chem Lett 2012;22:5396–404.

[156] Paraiso KH, Haarberg HE, Wood E, Rebecca VW, Chen YA, Xiang Y, et al. The HSP90 inhibitor XL888 overcomes BRAF inhibitor resistance mediated through diverse mechanisms. Clin Cancer Res 2012;18:2502–14.

[157] Menezes DL, Taverna P, Jensen MR, Abrams T, Stuart D, Yu GK, et al. The novel oral Hsp90 inhibitor NVP-HSP990 exhibits potent and broad-spectrum antitumor activities in vitro and in vivo. Mol Cancer Ther 2012;11:730–9.

[158] Khong T, Spencer A. Targeting HSP90 induces apoptosis and inhibits critical survival and proliferation pathways in multiple myeloma. Mol Cancer Ther 2011;10:1909–17.

[159] Buchstaller HP, Eggenweiler HM, Sirrenberg C, Gradler U, Musil D, Hoppe E, et al. Fragment-based discovery of hydroxy-indazole-carboxamides as novel small molecule inhibitors of Hsp90. Bioorg Med Chem Lett 2012;22:4396–403.

[160] Zehnder L, Bennett M, Meng J, Huang B, Ninkovic S, Wang F, et al. Optimization of potent, selective, and orally bioavailable pyrrolodinopyrimidine-containing inhibitors of heat shock protein 90. Identification of development candidate 2-amino-4-{4-chloro-2-[2-(4-fluoro-1H-pyrazol-1-yl)ethoxy]-6-methylphenyl}-N-(2,2-difluoropropyl)-5,7-dihydro-6H-pyrrolo[3,4-d]pyrimidine-6-carboxamide. J Med Chem 2011;54:3368–85.

[161] Vallee F, Carrez C, Pilorge F, Dupuy A, Parent A, Bertin L, et al. Tricyclic series of heat shock protein 90 (Hsp90) inhibitors part I: discovery of tricyclic imidazo[4,5-c]pyridines as potent inhibitors of the Hsp90 molecular chaperone. J Med Chem 2011;54:7206–19.

[162] Davies NG, Browne H, Davis B, Drysdale MJ, Foloppe N, Geoffrey S, et al. Targeting conserved water molecules: design of 4-aryl-5-cyanopyrrolo[2,3-d]pyrimidine Hsp90 inhibitors using fragment-based screening and structure-based optimization. Bioorg Med Chem 2012;20:6770–89.

[163] Yun BG, Huang W, Leach N, Hartson SD, Matts RL. Novobiocin induces a distinct conformation of Hsp90 and alters Hsp90-cochaperone-client interactions. Biochemistry 2004;43:8217–29.

[164] Donnelly A, Blagg BS. Novobiocin and additional inhibitors of the Hsp90 C-terminal nucleotide-binding pocket. Curr Med Chem 2008;15:2702–17.

[165] Allan RK, Mok D, Ward BK, Ratajczak T. Modulation of chaperone function and cochaperone interaction by novobiocin in the C-terminal domain of Hsp90: evidence that coumarin antibiotics disrupt Hsp90 dimerization. J Biol Chem 2006;281:7161–71.

[166] Marcu MG, Neckers LM. The C-terminal half of heat shock protein 90 represents a second site for pharmacologic intervention in chaperone function. Curr Cancer Drug Targets 2003;3:343–7.

[167] Shelton SN, Shawgo ME, Matthews SB, Lu Y, Donnelly AC, Szabla K, et al. KU135, a novel novobiocin-derived C-terminal inhibitor of the 90-kDa heat shock protein, exerts potent antiproliferative effects in human leukemic cells. Mol Pharmacol 2009;76:1314–22.

[168] Samadi AK, Zhang X, Mukerji R, Donnelly AC, Blagg BS, Cohen MS. A novel C-terminal HSP90 inhibitor KU135 induces apoptosis and cell cycle arrest in melanoma cells. Cancer Lett 2011;312:158–67.

[169] Matts RL, Dixit A, Peterson LB, Sun L, Voruganti S, Kalyanaraman P, et al. Elucidation of the Hsp90 C-terminal inhibitor binding site. ACS Chem Biol 2011;6:800–7.

[170] Zhao H, Donnelly AC, Kusuma BR, Brandt GE, Brown D, Rajewski RA, et al. Engineering an antibiotic to fight cancer: optimization of the novobiocin scaffold to produce anti-proliferative agents. J Med Chem 2011;54:3839–53.

[171] Kusuma BR, Zhang L, Sundstrom T, Peterson LB, Dobrowsky RT, Blagg BS. Synthesis and evaluation of novologues as C-terminal Hsp90 inhibitors with cytoprotective activity against sensory neuron glucotoxicity. J Med Chem 2012;55:5797–812.

[172] Powers MV, Jones K, Barillari C, Westwood I, van Montfort RL, Workman P. Targeting HSP70: the second potentially druggable heat shock protein and molecular chaperone? Cell Cycle 2010;9:1542–50.

[173] Kunicki JB, Petersen MN, Alexander LD, Ardi VC, McConnell JR, McAlpine SR. Synthesis and evaluation of biotinylated sansalvamide A analogs and their modulation of Hsp90. Bioorg Med Chem Lett 2011;21:4716–9.

[174] Vasko RC, Rodriguez RA, Cunningham CN, Ardi VC, Agard DA, McAlpine SR. Mechanistic studies of Sansalvamide A-amide: an allosteric modulator of Hsp90. ACS Med Chem Lett 2010;1:4–8.

[175] Davenport J, Manjarrez JR, Peterson L, Krumm B, Blagg BS, Matts RL. Gambogic acid, a natural product inhibitor of Hsp90. J Nat Prod 2011;74:1085–92.

[176] Powers MV, Workman P. Inhibitors of the heat shock response: biology and pharmacology. FEBS Lett 2007;581:3758–69.

[177] Bagatell R, Paine-Murrieta GD, Taylor CW, Pulcini EJ, Akinaga S, Benjamin IJ, et al. Induction of a heat shock factor 1-dependent stress response alters the cytotoxic activity of hsp90-binding agents. Clin Cancer Res 2000;6:3312–8.

[178] Powers MV, Clarke PA, Workman P. Dual targeting of HSC70 and HSP72 inhibits HSP90 function and induces tumor-specific apoptosis. Cancer Cell 2008;14:250–62.

[179] Evans CG, Chang L, Gestwicki JE. Heat shock protein 70 (hsp70) as an emerging drug target. J Med Chem 2010;53:4585–602.

[180] Hadchity E, Aloy MT, Paulin C, Armandy E, Watkin E, Rousson R, et al. Heat shock protein 27 as a new therapeutic target for radiation sensitization of head and neck squamous cell carcinoma. Mol Ther 2009;17:1387–94.

[181] Davenport EL, Zeisig A, Aronson LI, Moore HE, Hockley S, Gonzalez D, et al. Targeting heat shock protein 72 enhances Hsp90 inhibitor-induced apoptosis in myeloma. Leukemia 2010;24:1804–7.

[182] McDowell CL, Bryan Sutton R, Obermann WM. Expression of Hsp90 chaperone [corrected] proteins in human tumor tissue. Int J Biol Macromol 2009;45:310–4.

[183] Smith JR, Clarke PA, de Billy E, Workman P. Silencing the cochaperone CDC37 destabilizes kinase clients and sensitizes cancer cells to HSP90 inhibitors. Oncogene 2009;28:157–69.

[184] Holmes JL, Sharp SY, Hobbs S, Workman P. Silencing of HSP90 cochaperone AHA1 expression decreases client protein activation and increases cellular sensitivity to the HSP90 inhibitor 17-allylamino-17-demethoxygeldanamycin. Cancer Res 2008;68:1188–97.

[185] Forafonov F, Toogun OA, Grad I, Suslova E, Freeman BC, Picard D. p23/Sba1p protects against Hsp90 inhibitors independently of its intrinsic chaperone activity. Mol Cell Biol 2008;28:3446–56.

[186] Vaughan CK, Gohlke U, Sobott F, Good VM, Ali MM, Prodromou C, et al. Structure of an Hsp90-Cdc37-Cdk4 complex. Mol Cell 2006;23:697–707.

[187] Plescia J, Salz W, Xia F, Pennati M, Zaffaroni N, Daidone MG, et al. Rational design of shepherdin, a novel anticancer agent. Cancer Cell 2005;7:457–68.

[188] Mollapour M, Tsutsumi S, Donnelly AC, Beebe K, Tokita MJ, Lee MJ, et al. Swe1Wee1-dependent tyrosine phosphorylation of Hsp90 regulates distinct facets of chaperone function. Mol Cell 2010;37:333–43.

[189] Mollapour M, Neckers L. Post-translational modifications of Hsp90 and their contributions to chaperone regulation. Biochim Biophys Acta 2012;1823:648–55.

[190] Bali P, Pranpat M, Bradner J, Balasis M, Fiskus W, Guo F, et al. Inhibition of histone deacetylase 6 acetylates and disrupts the chaperone function of heat shock protein 90: a novel basis for antileukemia activity of histone deacetylase inhibitors. J Biol Chem 2005;280:26729–34.

[191] de Bono JS, Kristeleit R, Tolcher A, Fong P, Pacey S, Karavasilis V, et al. Phase I pharmacokinetic and pharmacodynamic study of LAQ824, a hydroxamate histone deacetylase inhibitor with a heat shock protein-90 inhibitory profile, in patients with advanced solid tumors. Clin Cancer Res 2008;14:6663–73.

[192] Torres EM, Dephoure N, Panneerselvam A, Tucker CM, Whittaker CA, Gygi SP, et al. Identification of aneuploidy-tolerating mutations. Cell 2010;143:71–83.

[193] Tang YC, Williams BR, Siegel JJ, Amon A. Identification of aneuploidy-selective antiproliferation compounds. Cell 2011;144:499–512.

[194] Duerfeldt AS, Peterson LB, Maynard JC, Ng CL, Eletto D, Ostrovsky O, et al. Development of a Grp94 inhibitor. J Am Chem Soc 2012;134:9796–804.

[195] Patel MN, Halling-Brown MD, Tym JE, Workman P, Al-Lazikani B. Objective assessment of cancer genes for drug discovery. Nat Rev Drug Discov 2013;12:35–50.

[196] Dai C, Whitesell L, Rogers AB, Lindquist S. Heat shock factor 1 is a powerful multifaceted modifier of carcinogenesis. Cell 2007;130:1005–18.

[197] Moulick K, Ahn JH, Zong H, Rodina A, Cerchietti L, Dagama G, et al. Affinity-based proteomics reveal cancer-specific networks coordinated by Hsp90. Nat Chem Biol 2011;7:818–26.

[198] Darby JF, Workman P. Chemical biology: many faces of a cancer-supporting protein. Nature 2011;478:334–5.

[199] Polier S, Samant RS, Clarke PA, Workman P, Prodromou C, Pearl LH. ATP-competitive inhibitors block protein kinase recruitment to the Hsp90-Cdc37 system. Nat Chem Biol 2013;9:307–12.

10

Inhibitors of Tumor Angiogenesis

Adrian L. Harris[1], Daniele Generali[2]

[1]Molecular Oncology Laboratory, Cancer Research UK, Weatherall Institute of Molecular Medicine, John Radcliffe Hospital, Oxford, UK [2]U.O. Multidisciplinare di Patologia Mammaria, U.S. di Terapia Molecolare e Farmacogenomica, Az. Istituti Ospitalieri di Cremona, Cremona, Italy

INTRODUCTION: THE TUMOR ANGIOGENIC PROCESS

The ability of solid tumors to sustain growth beyond a few millimeters (2–3 mm) in size is dependent on their capacity to acquire nutrients and oxygen and to dispose of metabolic waste products and carbon dioxide through the formation of new blood vessels [1,2]. This process, termed angiogenesis, is considered one of the essential hallmarks underlying cancer development and metastasis: tumor cells in areas within the tumor that become depleted of nutrients and oxygen release angiogenic-promoting signals, which drive the angiogenic switch to expand the tumor vascular network [3].

Classically, two distinct types of angiogenesis have been described. The first is sprouting, which involves branching new blood vessels from preexisting blood vessels. The second type is splitting or nonsprouting angiogenesis, which involves the splitting of a lumen of an existing vessel (intussusception). Unlike physiologic angiogenesis, tumor angiogenesis involves endothelial cells that fail to become quiescent [4]. These cells proliferate and grow uncontrollably and have a different phenotype from physiologic vasculature. Morphologically, tumor vasculature is characterized by irregularly shaped vessels, which are dilated, tortuous, and disorganized [5,6].

Recently, other mechanisms of tumor vascularization have been discovered. These include the recruitment of endothelial progenitor cells (EPCs), vessel cooption, vasculogenic mimicry, and lymphangiogenesis. EPCs are circulating cells in the blood that can form new blood vessels. The mobilization and recruitment of EPCs are promoted by several growth factors, chemokines, and cytokines produced during tumor growth [7]. Vessel cooption is a process whereby tumor cells can grow along existing blood vessels without evoking an angiogenic response in such vascular places, such as the brain or lungs [8]. Vasculogenic mimicry is the process of tumor cell plasticity, mainly in aggressive tumors, in which tumor cells dedifferentiate to an endothelial phenotype and make tube-like structures [8]. This mechanism provides an alternate route for tumor vascularization that may be independent of traditional angiogenesis processes. The majority of antiangiogenesis treatments, however, are currently tailored toward the sprouting biology of angiogenesis. Although controversial, angiogenesis may also progress through vascular mimicry in which tumor cells contribute to the formation of vascular channels that resemble endothelial tubes [9,10]. Cancer cells and normal stem cells share many features, such as the expression of similar markers, indicating an undifferentiated state and utilization of similar signaling pathways that may regulate self-renewal in stem cells and cancer cells. Previously, the plasticity (i.e., the ability to differentiate into many cell types) was considered to be more of an attribute of normal stem cells, while the level of tumor malignancy was inversely linked to their level of differentiation. More recently, accumulating evidence suggests that cancer stem cells also possess considerable plasticity. The ability of tumor cells to differentiate into endothelial cells (ECs) and the so-called vasculogenic mimicry (the formation of fluid-conducting channels by tumor cells) has been suggested in various malignancies such as renal, breast, and glioblastoma carcinomas [9,11,12].

Angiogenesis consists of multiple, sequential, and interdependent steps. Briefly, the initial process of angiogenesis involves the stimulation of the endothelial cells lining the luminal surface of the blood vessel by vascular endothelial growth factor (VEGF), resulting in the release of proteases, including matrix metalloproteinases (MMPs), which subsequently leads to degradation of the extracellular matrix (ECM). The second phase of angiogenesis, known as sprouting, is spearheaded by the leading endothelial tip cells that enter the underlying tissue and migrate along the chemotaxic gradient toward the source of the angiogenic stimuli [13]. The exact locations of formed individual vessels are not controlled, and the growing sprouts do not carry blood flow. Thus, this phase of angiogenesis occurs in the absence of any feedback with respect to the effect of the new vessels on hemodynamic and oxygen distribution. Once vessels have formed connections resulting in patent flow pathways, a second phase, pruning, is possible [14], in which responses to hemodynamic and metabolic factors can be used to remove redundant segments, for instance those with low volume flow and high oxygen tension, and to enlarge those that are effectively supplying the tissue, which have higher flow and low distal oxygen levels. For the splitting type of angiogenesis (intussusception) [15], the presence of continuous blood flow allows a faster adaptation of the resulting vascular pattern to tissue demand. In either case, the processes of angiogenesis and pruning, together with the need to distribute capillaries throughout all regions of the tissue, necessarily result in the formation of vascular networks with long and short arterio-venous pathways [16].

However, the structure of tumor vasculature is poorly organized [17]; they are usually irregular, leaky, hemorrhagic, and tortuous. The blood flow is chaotic and poorly oxygenated [18]. Due to these characteristics, the tumor vessels can be selectively targeted. The concept of attacking tumors by shutting their blood supply was first described in the early 1970s [19], and subsequently many studies have demonstrated in preclinical models that targeting tumor angiogenesis will compromise tumor growth.

Numerous agents that are currently in clinical practice and others undergoing clinical development aim to interfere with signals promoting angiogenesis and therefore currently comprise one of the most promising avenues of investigation in the study of tumor biology. Based on the complexity of the tumor angiogenic process, the optimal treatment strategies would target multiple steps of the angiogenic process with widespread applicability, low potential toxicity, and possibly a synergistic effect combined with classical cytotoxic therapy and radiotherapy.

THE COMPLEXITY OF "ANGIO-NETWORK" SIGNALING

The Angiogenic Factors

There are several signaling pathways involved in tumor angiogenesis that represent unbalanced expression of angiogenic factors and inhibitors within the tumor (Table 10.1) [20]. These molecules interplay with the multiple steps of the angiogenic process, interfering with the function of the diverse cell types involved directly or indirectly. The ability of a tumor to induce the formation of a tumor vasculature has been termed the "angiogenic switch" and can occur at different stages of the tumor progression pathway depending on the type of tumor and the environment [21]. Acquisition of the angiogenic phenotype can result from genetic changes or local environmental changes that lead to the activation of endothelial cells. One way for a tumor to activate endothelial cells is through the secretion of proangiogenic growth factors, which then bind to receptors on nearby dormant ECs that line the interior of vessels. Upon EC stimulation, vasodilation and permeability of the vessels increase and the ECs detach from the ECM and grow, as described in this chapter. In the last phase of growth, the vessels mature, a new basal membrane is secreted and differentiated, and the junctions between endothelial cells are recruited and established. The growth factors can also act on more distant cells, recruiting bone marrow–derived precursor endothelial cells and circulating endothelial cells to migrate to the tumor vasculature [22]. Finally, pericytes cover the newly formed vessel. Based on the multiple cytoplasmic processes, distinctive cytoskeletal elements, and envelopment of endothelial cells, pericytes are generally considered to be contractile cells and participate in the regulation of blood flow in the microcirculation [23]. Tumor pericytes appear to play a critical role in regulating vessel maturation, stabilization, quiescence, and function, even where they are less abundant and more loosely attached to vessels compared to healthy tissue [24]. Compared to quiescent pericytes, activated pericytes can change their expression profile, leading to phenotypes that are highly proliferative with the pluripotent ability to differentiate into other pericytes, matrix-forming cells, or adipocytes. They are thought to be at least partially responsible for the irregular, tortuous, and leaky blood vessels found within tumors and involved in resistance to antiangiogenesis drugs [25].

The proangiogenic growth factors responsible for the "angiogenic switch" may be overexpressed due to genetic alterations of oncogenes and tumor suppressors, or in response to the reduced availability of oxygen. Tumors express many of the angiogenic factors, and as the tumor cells proliferate, oxygen becomes depleted and a hypoxic microenvironment occurs within the tumor. Hypoxia-inducible factor (HIF) is degraded in the presence of oxygen, so formation of hypoxic conditions leads to HIF activation and transcription of target genes [26]. The strongest activation of HIF results from hypoxia, but several other factors can contribute to increased expression and activity of HIF, including growth factors such as epidermal growth factor (EGF) [27], and insulin-like growth factor 1 [27], which induce the activation of cell signaling. Oncogenes also induce the activation of growth factors, which stimulate

TABLE 10.1 Pro- and Antiangiogenic Factors

Proangiogenic factors	Antiangiogenic factors
Growth factors and growth factor receptors	*Growth factors and growth factor receptors*
Angiogenin	Angiostatin
Angiotropin	Angiostatin 2
Epidermal growth factor	Endostatin
(Acid and basic) fibroblast growth factor (FGF) and FGFR	Vasostatin
Granulocyte colony-stimulating factor	Chemokines and chemokine receptors
Hepatocyte growth factor	Vascular endothelial growth factor inhibitor
Insulin growth factor (IGF) and IGFR	
Platelet-derived growth factor	
Tumor necrosis factor α	
Vascular endothelial growth factors: VEGF-A, B, C, and D	
Scatter factor	
Neuropilin	
Cox-2	
Genes	*Genes*
c-MYC	p53
K/H-Ras	Rb
c-JUN	
HER-2	
EGFR	
HIF	
NfKb	
Fox	
Cytokines	*Cytokines*
EMAP-II (endothelial monocyte-activating polypeptide)	Interferon α, β, and γ
Inteleukin-1,4,6, and 8	Inteleukin 10 and 12
IP (interferon inducible protein 10)	
Midkine	
MIG (monokine induced by interferon γ)	
Transforming growth factor α and β	
Tumor necrosis factor-α	
Peptide fragments	*Peptide fragments*
Endothelin	Fragment of platelet factor 4
Derivate of prolactine	
Proliferation-related protein	
Endogenous modulators	*Endogenous modulators*
αvβ integrin	Angiopoietin-2
Angiopoietin-1	Angiotensin
Angiostatin II	Angiotensin II
Endothelin	Caveolin I and II
Erythropoietin	Endostatin
Nitric oxide synthase	Isoflavones
Platelet-activating factor	Prolactin
Prostaglandin E2	Thrombospondin-1 and 2
Thrombopoietin	Troponin-1
Adrenomedullin	Retinoic acid
Copper	Arrestin
Eph and Ephrins	Vasohibin
Erythropoietin	$1,25\text{-}(OH)_2$ vitamin D_3
Notch and Dll	Osteopontin cleavage product
Semaphorins, plexins, and roundabouts	
2-Methoxyoestradiol	

TABLE 10.1 Pro- and Antiangiogenic Factors *(cont'd)*

Proangiogenic factors	Antiangiogenic factors
Cell signaling	PTEN
mTOR	
PI3K and AKT	
Ras, MAPK, and ERK	
PKC	
Cell adhesion molecules	
Cadherins (VE-cadherin and N-cadherin)	
Immunoglobulin (Ig) superfamily (JAM-C, ICAM-1, VCAM-1, and PECAM-1)	
Integrins (αVβ3 and αVβ51)	
Selectins (E-selectin)	
Proteases	*Proteases*
Cathepsin	Plasminogen activator inhibitor 1 and 2,
Urokinase type plasminogen activator (uPA) and uPA receptor	TIMPs
MMPs (MMP-2 and MMP-9)	
PEX	
Gelatinase A and B	
METH-1 and 2	
Stromelysin	

HIF expression and activity (e.g., HER2 or mutant Ras), or PI3K and MAPK signaling can contribute to tumor angiogenesis by enhancing the expression of VEGF through increased HIF activity [27–29].

Vascular Endothelial Growth Factor

The VEGF and its receptor tyrosine kinases (vascular endothelial growth factor receptors, or VEGFRs) play a key role in the angiogenesis process [30,31]. While VEGF is actually a family of at least seven members, the term VEGF typically refers to the VEGF-A isoform, one of the most studied members and a major mediator of tumor angiogenesis. VEGF-A is a proangiogenic factor that plays important roles in cell migration, proliferation, and survival. Four major spliced isoforms of VEGF-A are known ($VEGF_{121}$, $VEGF_{165}$, $VEGF_{189}$, and $VEGF_{206}$), with $VEGF_{165}$ being the most predominant form [31]. Other rare ones, as well as inhibitory variants, are present; these isoforms, the most common of which is $VEGF_{165}b$, form a substantial portion of total VEGF in many tissues, including normal colon tissue. $VEGF_{165}b$ binds bevacizumab with the same affinity as $VEGF_{165}$, and the overexpression of $VEGF_{165}b$ in human colon carcinomas grown in mice conferred resistance to bevacizumab treatment [32]. Studies on these isoforms, which may be useful in clinical routine, showed that a low $VEGF_{165}b$:$VEGF_{total}$ ratio may be a predictive marker for bevacizumab in metastatic colorectal cancer, and individuals with high relative levels may not benefit [32]. The VEGF and VEGF family of receptors is fundamental for endothelial cell growth and the angiogenic process [33]. For this reason, the majority of angiogenesis inhibitors that have been investigated in clinical trials have targeted VEGF or VEGF receptors.

$VEGF$-A_{165} is commonly overexpressed by a wide variety of human tumors, and overexpression has been correlated with progression, invasion and metastasis, microvessel density, and poorer survival and prognosis in patients [34,35]. When VEGF is secreted from tumor cells, it interacts with cell surface receptors, including VEGFR-1 and -2, located on vascular endothelial cells and bone marrow–derived cells. VEGFR-2 is believed to mediate the majority of the angiogenic effects of VEGF-A, while the role of VEGFR-1 is complex and not fully understood [31]. A soluble form of VEGFR-1 can act as a decoy receptor, preventing VEGF-A by acting on VEGFR-2 and activating signaling pathways. However, there is also evidence that indicates that VEGFR-1 plays an important role in developmental angiogenesis [31]. A third receptor, VEGFR-3, is involved in lymphangiogenesis and does not bind VEGF-A [31].

Platelet-Derived Growth Factors

The family of platelet-derived growth factors (PDGFs) and receptors (PDGFRs) is involved in vessel maturation and the recruitment of pericytes [36]. There are two forms of the PDGF tyrosine kinase receptors, PDGFR-α and -β [37]. Endothelial cells express PDGF and generally act in a paracrine manner, recruiting PDGFR-expressing cells, particularly pericytes and smooth muscle cells, to the developing vessels [38]. Overexpression of PDGFR has been associated with poor prognosis in ovarian cancer [39], indicating a likely role for the PDGF pathway in human cancers.

Fibroblast Growth Factors

The mammalian fibroblast growth factor (FGF) family is composed of 21 different proteins, which are classified into six different groups based on their sequence similarities [37]. The FGF ligands are involved in promoting the proliferation, migration, and differentiation of vascular endothelial cells [40]. Fibroblast Growth Factors Receptors (FGFRs) are often overexpressed in tumors, and mutations of the FGFR genes have been found in human cancers, making it particularly significant that FGFR activation in endothelial cell culture and animal models leads to angiogenesis [37]. Overexpression of various FGF ligands in different types of tumors has been documented [37]. FGF-2, in particular, has been shown to possess potent angiogenic activity and is also commonly overexpressed in tumors [41].

Epidermal Growth Factors

The EGF family consists of 11 known members, which bind to one of four epidermal growth factor receptors (EGFRs). All of the receptors, except HER3, contain an intracellular tyrosine kinase domain [42,43]. HER2 does not have any known ligands that bind with high affinity, despite it being a potent oncoprotein [42,43]. Activation of EGFR has been linked to angiogenesis in xenograft models in addition to metastasis, cell proliferation, survival, migration, transformation, adhesion, and differentiation [43]. The family is expressed on and functions in endothelial cells. However, in tumors, activation of the EGFR pathway upregulates the production of proangiogenic factors such as VEGF, and it can be viewed as more of an indirect regulator of angiogenesis, making the role of the EGF–EGFR system less important to angiogenesis than more direct regulators, such as the VEGF and PDGF systems [42,43].

Hepatocyte Growth Factor

Hepatocyte growth factor (HGF) is a heparin-binding glycoprotein and binds to the tyrosine kinase receptor, c-Met. HGF–Met signaling is implicated in the proliferation, migration, and differentiation of various types of cells, including endothelium. It is involved in angiogenesis processes in vitro and in vivo [44]. Furthermore, a proteolytic fragment of HGF (NK4) has antiangiogenic activity, blocking both HGF and VEGF–bFGF effects. NK4 gene therapy inhibited tumor invasion, metastasis, and angiogenesis in experimental models [45]. These results support the concept that targeting tumor invasion, metastasis, and angiogenesis with NK4 could have a considerable therapeutic potential for cancer patients. This factor and its receptor cMet are induced by hypoxia and may comprise a main mechanism for induced resistance (discussed further in this chapter). In the matter of angiogenesis, the HGF along with its receptor (c-Met) are promising targets [46]. HGF increases expression of angiogenic mediators, including VEGF and its receptor, in endothelial cells [47]. The c-Met receptor and VEGF receptor (VEGFR) have also been found to cooperate to promote tumor survival, and c-Met has additional roles in tumor angiogenesis, as an independent angiogenic factor and one that may interact with the angiogenic proliferation and survival signals promoted through VEGF and other angiogenic proteins. Hypoxia increases hypoxia-inducible factor 1a (HIF-1a), which subsequently increases HGF expression in tumor and surrounding normal interstitial cells with an increase in Met expression in endothelial and tumor cells. HGF–c-Met signaling increases VEGF levels in tumors and VEGFR-2 in endothelial cells [48].

Because HGF–c-Met signaling is activated in angiogenesis and tumor growth, several strategies have been explored for inhibiting the pathway [49]. Thus, when combined clinically, the inhibition of VEGF and HGF–c-Met signaling should have a greater effect on the induction of endothelial cell apoptosis and the decrease of vascular tubulogenesis as shown in vitro, as well as a reduction in the formation of capillaries or a decrease of the microvessel density within tumors in vivo [27]. Thus, targeting inhibition of HGF/c-Met is both a means of enhanced VEGF and VEGFR axis-mediated inhibition of angiogenesis at the time of initial therapy and a response to the expected hypoxia within tumors induced by antiangiogenic therapy. Targeting both axes should have clinical benefits. At the moment, dual cMET–VEGF blockers are being tested in clinical trials [50,51]. Cabozantinib, a potent inhibitor of both MET and VEGFR-2, showed in its early clinical experience promising signs of antitumor activity at doses not associated with toxicity. Most notably, results of 17 patients with medullary thyroid cancer treated with cabozantinib indicated a >50% response rate and a 100% disease control rate [51].

Angiopoietins and Tie Receptors

The angiopoietin ligands and Tie receptor tyrosine kinases (RTKs) play a regulatory role in vascular homeostasis [52]. The angiopoietin (Ang) family of ligands (Ang-1, 2, and 3/4) binds to the RTK Tie-2. No ligand has been identified as yet for the Tie-1 receptor [52–54]. Ang-1 behaves as an agonist, activating the Tie-2 receptor, while Ang-2 acts as an antagonist for Tie-2 [54]. In the presence of VEGF-A, Ang-2 will promote angiogenesis, and in the absence of VEGF-A, Ang-2 will cause vessel regression [54]. Overexpression of Ang-2 has been found to correlate with increased angiogenesis, malignancy, and aggressive tumor growth in some cancers, and in other tumor types overexpression led to decreased tumor growth and metastasis and vessel regression [52–54]. While the angiopoietins and Tie receptors appear to play an important role during tumor angiogenesis, the specific mechanisms are controversial. A further understanding of the specific roles of the members of the Ang–Tie system may enable targeting of this system for antiangiogenic and anticancer purposes.

New drugs targeting Ang–Tie are in ongoing clinical development. AMG-386 is a peptide–Fc fusion protein that targets both Ang 1 and 2 to the Tie-2 receptor [55]. In a phase I trial of AMG 386, one patient with advanced refractory ovarian cancer achieved a partial response (PR) and durable CA-125 response [56]. A phase II randomized trial has been evaluated with weekly paclitaxel 80 mg (3 weeks on and 1 week off) plus weekly AMG 386 10 mg/kg, AMG 386 3 mg/kg, or placebo in 161 patients with recurrent epithelial ovarian cancer, primary peritoneal cancer, or fallopian tube cancer, with progression-free survival (PFS) as the primary endpoint [57]. Median PFS with AMG 386 10 mg/kg and 3 mg/kg was 7.2 months and 5.7 months, respectively, versus 4.6 months with placebo (HR for AMG 386 arms combined, 0.76; 95% CI, 0.52–1.12; $P = 0.165$), with evidence of a significant dose–response effect ($P = 0.037$). AMG 780 in a phase I trial enrolling solid tumors or PF04856884 in metastatic renal cancer and metastatic colon cancer is undergoing ongoing study (www.clinicaltrials.gov).

Delta and Jagged Ligands and Notch Signaling

The family of Notch receptors (Notch 1–4) and their transmembrane ligands Delta-like (Dll1, 3, 4) and Jagged (Jagged1, 2) play important roles in cells undergoing differentiation, acting primarily to determine and regulate cell fate, as well as playing a part in developmental and tumor angiogenesis. Activation of Notch signaling is dependent upon cell-to-cell interactions and occurs when the extracellular domain of the cell surface receptor interacts with a ligand found on a nearby cell [58]. Delta-like 4 (Dll4) and Jagged1 have particularly been implicated in tumor angiogenesis, with strong expression of Dll4 seen in the endothelium of tumor blood vessels and much weaker expression in nearby normal blood vessels [59,60]. The expression of Dll4 appears to be regulated directly by VEGF in the setting of tumor angiogenesis, and increased levels of VEGF lead to increased expression of Dll4 [60]; however, Dll4 plays a role as an angiogenesis modulator regulating excessive VEGF-induced vessel branching, allowing vessel formation to occur at a productive and efficient rate [61]. Overexpression of Jagged1, a Notch ligand, is dependent on MAPK signaling and has been associated with angiogenic endothelial cells in vitro [62]. Jagged1 is thought to promote angiogenesis, as overexpression in head and neck squamous cell carcinoma cells leads to increased vascularization and tumor growth [62]. Inhibition of specific components of the Notch signaling pathway, such as Dll4 or Jagged1, or more broad inhibition of Notch signaling may prove to be effective for inhibiting functional angiogenesis and neovascularization in tumors, and some of the preclinical studies appear promising. However, further studies are needed to better understand the role that Notch signaling and its individual components play in tumor angiogenesis, as therapeutic antibodies to Dll4 are in phase I trials exploited for clinical use [63].

A recent study assessed the maximum tolerated dose, safety, pharmacokinetics, pharmacodynamics, and antitumor activity of RO4929097, a gamma secretase inhibitor of Notch signaling in patients with advanced solid malignancies [64]. Tumor responses included one partial response in a patient with colorectal adenocarcinoma with neuroendocrine features, one mixed response (stable disease) in a patient with sarcoma, and one nearly complete 2-[18-F] fluoro-2-deoxy-ᴅ-glucose (FDG)–positron emission tomography (PET) response in a patient with melanoma. Transient grade 3 hypophosphatemia and grade 3 pruritus were observed, suggesting that RO4929097 was well tolerated, but further studies are warranted on the basis of its favorable safety profile and its preliminary evidence of clinical antitumor activity [64]. Similar results were obtained with another compound, MK-0752, targeting Dll4-Notch signaling; however, MK-0752 toxicity was schedule dependent. Weekly dosing was generally well tolerated and resulted in strong modulation of a Notch gene signature. Clinical benefit was observed, and rational combination trials are currently ongoing to maximize clinical benefit with this novel agent [65]. New ongoing trials are reported at www.clinicaltrials.gov.

Hypoxia-Inducible Factor

HIF is a transcription factor involved in cellular adaptation to hypoxia. HIF transcriptional activity is regulated by the presence of oxygen and becomes active in low-oxygen conditions (hypoxia). As reviewed by Harris [66], because HIF regulates genes that enable cell survival in a hypoxic environment, including those involved in glycolysis, angiogenesis, and expression of growth factors, it plays an important role in the biology and regulation of tumor growth [66]. The central role of HIF in the activation of angiogenic-related genes makes it a promising target for the treatment of solid tumors, particularly since HIF-1α is reported to be overexpressed in the majority of solid tumors [67] and positively correlates with angiogenesis, aggressiveness, metastasis, and resistance to radiation or chemotherapy and negatively correlates with progression, survival, and outcome [68]. To date, some agents have been tested in clinical trials, but unfortunately with no particularly relevant clinical activity, and no specific anti-HIF drugs have been approved. However, agents on clinical trial or on the market inhibit the HIF pathway through indirect mechanisms such as affecting HIF-α mRNA expression, protein translation, and protein degradation (see the review by Jones and Harris [69]).

Receptor Tyrosine Kinase Signaling

RTKs are transmembrane proteins that mediate the transmission of extracellular signals (such as growth factors) to the intracellular environment, therefore controlling important cellular functions and initiating processes like angiogenesis. Structurally, the RTKs generally consist of an extracellular ligand-binding domain, a single transmembrane domain, a catalytic cytoplasmic tyrosine kinase region, and regulatory sequences. RTKs are activated by the binding of a growth factor ligand to the extracellular domain, leading to receptor dimerization and subsequent autophosphorylation of the receptor complex by the intracellular kinase domain, utilizing adenosine triphosphate (ATP) [70]. The phosphorylated receptor then interacts with a variety of cytoplasmic signaling molecules, leading to signal transduction and eventually angiogenesis, among other processes involved in cell survival, proliferation, migration, and differentiation of endothelial cells [70]. RTKs that become deregulated can contribute to the transformation of a cell. The dysregulation can occur through several different mechanisms, including (1) amplification and/or overexpression of RTKs, (2) gain of function mutations or deletions that result in constitutively active kinase activity, (3) genomic rearrangements that produce constitutively active kinase fusion proteins, and (4) constant stimulation of RTKs from high levels of proangiogenic growth factors, all of which lead to increased downstream signaling [70].

Complex signaling networks uses multiple factors to determine the biological outcome of the receptor activation. While the pathways are often depicted as linear pathways for simplicity, they are actually a network of pathways with various cross-talk and overlapping functions, as well as distinct functions. Some of the known signaling cascades include the Raf kinase–MEK–MAPK and PI3K–AKT–mTOR pathways [71,72]. Thus, most drugs in this class will have an effect on angiogenesis as well as on tumor cells. Recently, the use of these inhibitors has revealed their surprising ability to enhance the effect of local radiation therapy without increasing toxicity. The mechanism is partly related to a decrease in oxygen consumption, hence increased oxygen levels, with concomitant durable changes in the vasculature [73]. This leads to increased perfusion and maintained oxygen delivery, but in contrast to the vascular normalization reported on VEGF inhibitor therapy, this has a much more durable effect [74].

Endothelial Metabolism

The switch to a glycolytic metabolism is a rapid adaptation of tumor cells to hypoxia during their growth. Although this metabolic conversion may primarily represent a rescue pathway to meet the bioenergetic and biosynthetic demands of proliferating tumor cells, it also creates a gradient of lactate that mirrors the gradient of oxygen in tumors. More than just metabolic waste, the lactate anion is known to participate in cancer aggressiveness, in part through activation of the hypoxia-inducible factor 1 (HIF-1) pathway in tumor and endothelial cells [75]. Endothelial cells derive most of their energy anaerobically through glycolysis [76]; lactate, a by-product of glycolysis, stimulates angiogenesis by inactivating prolyl hydroxylases [77], thereby activating HIF and thus VEGF expression [78]. Therefore, they already have the metabolism to survive in acute highly hypoxic conditions, and to generate sufficient energy to continue sprouting [79]. Endothelial cells can consume oxygen when forming either sprouts [80] or vascular networks [81], if it is available. However, metabolic adaptation and utilization of lactate mean that endothelial cells are well suited to growing in the harsh environmental conditions of severe hypoxia.

Several regulators of metabolism modulate angiogenesis, including peroxisome proliferator-activated receptors (PPARs), PGC-1α, and AMP-dependent kinase (AMPK). PPARs are transcription factors that regulate nutrient utilization and energy homeostasis. The isoform PPARβ, which is a regulator of lipid oxidation [82], stimulates microvessel maturation [83]. Its activators upregulate the expression of VEGF, resulting in enhanced endothelial cell proliferation, microvessel sprouting, and tube formation [84].

The transcriptional coactivator PGC-1α augments energy production in tissues by stimulating mitochondrial biogenesis and cellular respiration [85]. It also stimulates angiogenesis by inducing VEGF expression through interacting with estrogen-related receptor alpha (ERR-α), thereby preparing the tissue for oxidative metabolism [86]. AMPK is activated upon energy deprivation and promotes nutrient uptake and oxidation, but also attenuates energy-consuming processes [87]. Pharmacological activation of AMPK upregulates VEGF levels, resulting in improved revascularization of ischemic limbs [88]. These findings support the concept that regulators of oxidative metabolism ensure sufficient O_2 and nutrient supply through boosting vessel growth. Angiogenesis also stimulates the growth of adipose tissue, and adipogenic factors have been increasingly recognized as modulators of angiogenesis. The adipokine leptin, which regulates food intake, stimulates angiogenesis and endothelial cell fenestration, in part by inducing VEGF expression [89], and it promotes angiogenesis together with VEGF [90].

Tumor-Associated Stroma

Stromal contribution to the development and progression of a wide variety of tumors has been supported by extensive clinical evidence and the use of experimental mouse models of cancer pathogenesis. The stroma in human carcinomas consists of ECM and various types of noncarcinoma cells, mainly leukocytes, endothelial cells, fibroblasts, myofibroblasts, and bone marrow–derived progenitors. Each cell type can potentially communicate with others, or with tumor cells, through secretion of growth factors, chemokines, proteases, and ECM components [91]. Cumulatively, these cellular interactions influence the composition and order of the tumor microenvironment to support tumor progression: the tumor-associated stroma actively supports tumor growth by stimulating neoangiogenesis, as well as proliferation and invasion of apposed carcinoma cells [92].

The tumor-associated stroma, or tumor microenvironment, can grossly be categorized into two types of cells: (1) cells that are present in the normal tissue parenchyma before tumor development, and (2) cells that are recruited to the tumor-associated stroma from distal sites (e.g., the circulation or the bone marrow). The first type is largely composed of fibroblasts and endothelial cells, whereas the second type of cells is largely composed of immune or inflammatory cells, including T- and B-cells, macrophages, neutrophils, mast cells, and other bone marrow–derived cells.

Inflammation and the Immune System

Briefly, inflammatory pathways, meant to defend the organism against infection and injury, as a by-product can promote an environment that favors tumor growth and metastasis. Inflammation has therefore been mentioned as the seventh hallmark of cancer [93,94]. Macrophages are among the first cells to infiltrate infected or damaged tissue. Tumor-associated macrophages (TAMs), which constitute a significant part of the tumor-infiltrating immune cells, have been linked to the growth, angiogenesis, and metastasis of a variety of cancers, most likely through polarization of TAM to the M2 (alternative) phenotype [95]. Intratumoral TAM count has been correlated with depth of invasion, lymph node metastasis, and staging of cancer, suggesting that intratumoral macrophages cause cancer cells to have a more aggressive behavior associated with a worse prognosis as seen in several type of cancers (intestinal type gastric cancer, pancreatic cancer, and thyroid cancer) [96–99]. However, the peritumoral TAMs can prevent tumor development; patients with high peritumoral TAM numbers have better prognosis and a higher survival rate [100].

The induction of angiogenesis is mediated by not only TAM but also myeloid-derived suppressor cells (MDSC), which produce proinflammatory cytokines, endothelial growth factors (VEGF and bFGF), and protease (MMP9) implicated in neoangiogenesis. MDSCs inhibit effector T-cell function and thus prevent the formation and execution of an effective antitumor immune response [101]. Recently reported studies have shown that MDSCs also function to promote tumor-dependent angiogenesis as well as tumor metastasis, and to provide tumor resistance to antiangiogenic drugs (see the review by Ko et al. [101]).

Bone marrow–derived endothelial progenitor cells (EPCs) contribute to angiogenesis-mediated pathological neovascularization, and recent studies have begun to recognize the biological significance of this contribution [103]. EPCs are reportedly important for the repair and remodeling of the vasculature (they home to sites of damage and promote vascular integrity) and are implicated in tumor angiogenesis [104]. EPCs have also been shown to give rise to up to 16% of the neovasculature in spontaneous tumors growing in transgenic mice, and they also contribute to human tumor vessels [105]. It is important to mention that many conflicting reports exist as to whether these EPCs arise from the bone marrow hematopoietic compartment or are nonhematopoietic in origin, and these differences could be attributed to the wide variances in the assays used to identify the cells and in the time points at which the data are collected [106]. However, in tumor angiogenesis, the tumor-derived paracrine signals activate the bone marrow compartment, resulting in the mobilization and recruitment of subsets of bone marrow–derived cells to the tumor bed. In response to tumor cytokines, including VEGF, the VEGFR-2$^+$ EPCs mobilize into the peripheral circulation and move to the tumor bed, where they incorporate into sprouting of new intratumoral vessels [107].

The "Angio-Network"

These factors could potentially initiate several signaling cascades, such as phosphatidylinositol 3-kinase (PI3K)–AKT–mammalian target of rapamycin (mTOR) and protein kinase C (PKC)–Raf-mitogen-activated protein kinase kinase (MEK)–mitogen-activated protein kinase (MAPK), to facilitate increased vascular permeability as well as increased endothelial cell proliferation, migration, and survival [108]. Similar to VEGF-mediated signaling, binding of the fibroblast growth factors (FGFs) to their RTK FGF receptors 1–4 on the surface of endothelial cells activates the Ras–Raf–MAPK and PI3K–AKT–mTOR pathways, suggesting the possibility of considerable cross-talk between VEGF–VEGFR and FGF–FGFR signaling. PDGFs regulate vessel maturation as well as the recruitment of pericytes and smooth muscle cells to the vasculature, and their activity is mediated by two RTKs, PDGFR-α and PDGFR-β [37]. Importantly, signaling through the PDGFRs activates a broad range of intracellular pathways, including MAPK, PI3K–AKT, and Ras–Raf–MEK, resulting in pericyte precursor cell proliferation and migration [109]. However, tumor cells also promote erythropoietin (EPO) production in perivascular cells via PDGF–PDGFR signaling to stimulate erythropoiesis and tumor oxygenation [110], indicating that PDGF inhibition could in fact worsen tumor hypoxia. Further evidence suggests that the angiopoietin (Ang)–Tie-2 pathway is critical for tumor angiogenesis [111,112]. In the presence of VEGF, Ang-2 facilitates sprouting angiogenesis by interrupting Ang-1-mediated vessel normalization and stabilization, causing impaired pericyte coverage, vessel destabilization, and increased vascular permeability [113]. Ang-2 binding to Tie-2 triggers PI3K–AKT–NF-kB (nuclear factor kappa-light-chain-enhancer of activated B cells) and Ras–Raf–MEK activity, promoting endothelial cell survival as well as proliferation or migration, respectively associated with a possible interplay between various signaling pathways such as mTOR and MAPK. This means that several endothelial growth factors can function in parallel to stimulate angiogenesis via the same pathways, which is demonstrated by the VEGF–VEGFR-2 and HGF–MET pathways, both converging on the

AKT–mTOR and Ras–MAPK signaling axes in endothelial cells [114]. This suggests that combined inhibition of VEGFR-2 and MET is necessary to efficiently block angiogenesis, and that targeting downstream targets such as mTOR and MAPK can block the response to several proangiogenic receptors simultaneously.

Ligands and RTKs involved in neovascularization are present on many different cell compartments within a malignant tumor, introducing another level of complexity to angiogenesis regulation. Cancer-associated fibroblasts are the major source of the MET ligand HGF, emphasizing the important proangiogenic role of nonmalignant cell populations within the tumor microenvironment. Apart from endothelial cells, MET is also present on tumor cells, and MET-induced signaling facilitates endothelial cell growth by inducing VEGF expression and impairing thrombospondin-1 (TSP-1) expression in tumor cells [48]. This VEGF–TSP-1 imbalance mediated by MET suggests that the HGF–MET pathway may contribute to the angiogenic switch within the tumor microenvironment. This suggests that the angiogenic switch is not mediated by the acquisition of mutations alone, but is regulated by the interplay between malignant and nonmalignant cell populations in the tumor microenvironment. The extensive interplay between various signaling pathways and cell compartments in the tumor can be seen as an "angio-network" (Fig. 10.1). Accordingly, the analysis of a single pathway is too simplistic, and more comprehensive assays where all the key players are analyzed simultaneously are needed in order to assess how the angiogenesis process should be targeted.

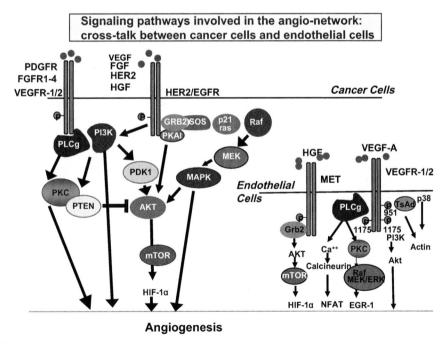

Angiogenesis

FIGURE 10.1 The angio-network: cross-talk between cancer cells and endothelial cells. ERK, extracellular signal-regulated kinase; MAPK, mitogen-activated protein kinase; PI3K, phosphatidylinositol 3′ kinase; PKB, protein kinase B. (This figure is reproduced in color in the color plate section.)

This is a feasible approach today, as from tumor biopsies we can assess which and how receptor kinases are deregulated [115].

ANTIANGIOGENIC STRATEGIES

There are two main classes of approved drugs in this area: monoclonal antibodies, such as bevacizumab, and oral small-molecule tyrosine kinase inhibitors (TKIs), for example sunitinib (Sutent®), sorafenib (Nexavar®), pazopanib (Votrient), and axitinib (Inlyta®). Whereas bevacizumab binds circulating and local VEGF and hence neutralizes its biologic activity, the TKIs inhibit the intracellular catalytic function of VEGF receptors expressed by vascular endothelial cells, particularly VEGFR-2, the major signaling receptor for VEGF-mediated (tumor) angiogenesis. The TKIs are not totally specific for VEGF receptors; invariably, they also antagonize the function of other kinase domain RTKs similar in structure to VEGF receptors (e.g., PDGFRs, c-kit, Flt-3, and Raf, which is also targeted in the case of sorafenib or pazopanib). Most TKIs are taken orally, continuously, on a daily basis or with regular break periods (e.g., sunitinib), whereas bevacizumab is administered intravenously every 2 or 3 weeks depending on the dose used [46]. It is worthwhile mentioning that chemotherapy could also have antiangiogenic activity, particularly metronomic therapy (e.g., cyclophosphamide, methotrexate, or capecitabine) [116,117].

Antiangiogenic Activity of Conventional Therapies

Recent studies have suggested that several classes of chemotherapeutic drugs have antiangiogenic activity in vitro or in vivo, including several agents that are routinely used in the clinic [118], such as cyclophosphamide, paclitaxel, doxorubicin, and thalidomide [119]. Paclitaxel, a microtubule inhibitor that is an active agent in the treatment of many different cancers, was shown to possess antiangiogenic properties independent of its antiproliferative action in in vivo models [120]. The weekly regimen as used routinely with paclitaxel could be viewed as "metronomic-like" (discussed further in this chapter) and thus may be a factor in the results that were obtained compared to regimens such as once-every-3-week docetaxel plus bevacizumab (i.e., the AVADO trial) [121].

Thalidomide has been shown to be a useful drug in cancer therapy. As a first-in-class immunomodulatory orally bioavailable drug, it was found to have significant single-agent activity in relapsed refractory multiple myeloma. The antiangiogenic effect seems to be mediated via inhibition of VEGF and bFGF [122]. Thalidomide and the new compound lenalidomide are currently used in treatment of multiple myeloma (MM). Because of the large production of VEGF and bFGF by the bone marrow (BM) [122], angiogenesis is an attractive target for the treatment of MM [123–125]. Recent investigations into the antiangiogenic activity of lenalidomide, based on its structural characteristics and reduced toxicity compared to thalidomide, are currently ongoing. Lenalidomide impacts angiogenesis in vivo and in vitro and selectively blocks migration of the BM endothelial cells (ECs) of patients with active MM [126,127]. It downregulates key angiogenic genes and VEGF–VEGFR-2-mediated downstream signaling pathways involved in MM-EC migration and the NF-κB pathway [127]. Proteomics analysis shows that lenalidomide-treated MM-ECs specifically modulate the expression levels of angiogenesis-related molecules governing MM-EC migration, cell shape and cytoskeletal remodeling, energy metabolism, and protein clearance [126]. Altogether, these data imply the intrinsic complexity of the signaling pathways modulated by lenalidomide at the cellular and molecular levels. Data also suggest that lenalidomide, by targeting angiogenesis, may exert an indirect anti-MM effect [128].

Among the various approaches to inhibiting angiogenesis, metronomic therapy is now broadly used in cancer treatment. The "metronomic therapy" approach refers to the frequent, even daily, administration of chemotherapy at doses below the maximum tolerated dose, for long periods of time, with no prolonged drug-free breaks [129]. Administering chemotherapy in this investigational fashion is thought to cause antitumor effects by a variety of mechanisms that include inhibition of angiogenesis [119], stimulation of the immune system, targeting HIF-1 expression, as well as possibly direct tumor cell targeting [130].

The phase II trials based on this approach involved a daily oral metronomic methotrexate plus cyclophosphamide [131], or this chemotherapy drug combined with a targeted agent such as trastuzumab [132], a selective estrogen receptor antagonist (e.g., fulvestrant or letrozole) [133,134], or an EGFR antagonist such as erlotinib or bevacizumab [135]. However, in order to validate the clinical data obtained so far, there are three other randomized phase III trials, in either the adjuvant or metastatic setting, currently underway evaluating oral metronomic chemotherapy regimens alone or in combination with a targeted agent such as bevacizumab. There are also a number of phase II clinical trials currently underway evaluating the combination of a small-molecule antiangiogenic TKIs plus metronomic chemotherapy, including for the treatment of breast cancer (www.clinicaltrials.gov).

COX-2 inhibitors suppress growth factor–induced angiogenesis in endothelial cells, suggesting that endothelial-derived COX-2 is essential in directly regulating angiogenesis [136]. Emerging data suggest that celecoxib may cause a time-dependent reduction in circulating angiogenic markers. A phase II study of lung cancer patients receiving celecoxib (400 mg orally twice a day) concurrently with paclitaxel and carboplatin plus radiation therapy found that serum and plasma levels of VEGF declined at 2, 5, and 7 months following treatment [137]. Treatment with celecoxib 400 mg twice daily was sufficient to normalize the increased levels of PGE2 found in non-small-cell lung cancer (NSCLC) after treatment with paclitaxel and carboplatin. Another COX-2 inhibitor, rofecoxib, has been shown to inhibit angiogenesis in a number of in vivo systems [138]. In view of these properties, the combination of antiangiogenic chemotherapy with a COX-2 inhibitor warrants clinical evaluation [139].

Apart from their specific activity on bone resorption by suppressing osteoclast activity, pamidronate and zoledronic acid, both potent bisphosphonates, also may have direct antitumor activity arising from inhibition of tumor cell adhesion, invasion, and viability, and antiproliferative and proapoptotic effects, possibly due to the presence of the nitrogen atom [140]. The bisphosphonates may have antiangiogenic effects [140]. In clinical trials with zoledronate, there was a significant reduction of VEGF and PDGF serum levels induced by a single administration in a "window of opportunity" trial [141].

Antiangiogenic Drugs

Bevacizumab

Bevacizumab has been studied in a number of solid tumors and has been approved by the US Food and Drug Administration (FDA) for the treatment of advanced colorectal cancer,

NSCLC, advanced renal cell cancer (RCC), and recurrent glioblastoma multiforme. Bevacizumab is a humanized monoclonal antibody that binds to VEGF-A, preventing it from binding to its cognate receptors and activating signaling cascades that lead to angiogenesis. Initial proof of the concept that targeting VEGF-A could inhibit the growth of tumors (despite its having no effect on the growth rate of the tumor cells in vitro) was demonstrated in a mouse model in 1993 using a monoclonal antibody against VEGF-A-121, which led to the clinical development of bevacizumab.

Colon Cancer

In colorectal cancer, bevacizumab, in combination with irinotecan, 5-fluorouracil (5-FU), and leucovorin (IFL), as first-line therapy for metastatic colorectal cancer showed an improvement of PFS and overall survival (OS) to 10.6 months compared to the control arm. Bevacizumab is also approved for second-line therapy in combination with 5-FU, leucovorin, and oxaliplatin (FOLFOX4) [142]. Even as second-line therapy, the response rate, PFS, and OS rates were improved with the addition of bevacizumab, highlighting its benefits in metastatic colorectal cancer. In the adjuvant setting of colorectal cancer, bevacizumab was tested in association with FOLFOX6, and at 3 years of median follow-up, no advantage in disease-free survival or OS has been observed [143]. The lack of efficacy of bevacizumab in this adjuvant trial raises the possibility that micrometastatic disease has not yet established the aberrant vasculature targeted by bevacizumab.

Lung and Breast Cancers

In lung cancer, the addition of bevacizumab to paclitaxel and carboplatin improved the response rate, PFS, and OS compared with carboplatin and paclitaxel alone [144].

In breast cancer, the first combination trial in advanced breast cancer was based on capecitabine alone or capecitabine in combination with bevacizumab. Unfortunately, despite the significant overall response rate (ORR) in favor of the combination, the primary endpoint of improved PFS was not achieved [145]. The higher response rate suggested a potential benefit with bevacizumab, and any improvements in survival may have been masked by the fact that the patients enrolled had been heavily pretreated. The E2100 trial, based on newly metastatic HER2-negative cancers to receive either paclitaxel or paclitaxel in combination with bevacizumab, had a significantly higher response rate and improvement in PFS but not OS, and led to the accelerated approval of bevacizumab in this setting [145].

The subsequent clinical trials of bevacizumab in metastatic breast cancer have failed to support the encouraging data from E2100. Two additional FDA reviews by the Oncology Drug Advisory Committee ultimately led to the removal of the breast cancer indication for bevacizumab. The AVADO trial was a three-arm trial comparing docetaxel as a single agent with docetaxel and bevacizumab at two dose levels: 7.5 and 15 mg/kg. A 1-month improvement was observed in PFS favoring the bevacizumab arms, but no difference was observed in OS. The median OS in the control arm was 31.9 months compared with 30.8 months with low-dose bevacizumab and 30.2 months with high-dose bevacizumab. Patients receiving bevacizumab experienced more treatment disruptions [146].

The RIBBON-1 trial randomized patients to receive or not receive bevacizumab. The data were analyzed in two distinct chemotherapy groups: "anthracycline-based" or "taxane-based" chemotherapy with or without bevacizumab. A significant improvement in both response rate and PFS was reported when bevacizumab was added to each chemotherapy regimen. However, OS was not improved [147].

Bevacizumab was studied in the second-line setting in RIBBON-2. Women with HER2-negative disease that progressed after first-line therapy were randomly assigned to receive chemotherapy according to the choice of the treating oncologist with or without bevacizumab. With subsequent disease progression, bevacizumab could be added to the third-line regimen. PFS favored the bevacizumab-treated patients, but, again, no improvement in OS was observed [148].

In the neoadjuvant setting, the GeparQuinto trial showed that pathological complete response rates (pCRs) were higher for those assigned to bevacizumab: 18.4% versus 14.9% for those receiving chemotherapy alone ($P=0.04$) [149]. The same results were obtained by the National Surgical Adjuvant Breast and Bowel Project (NSABP) B40 trial, showing that a significant increase in pCR rate was observed for those women assigned to bevacizumab (34.5% versus 28.2%; $P=0.02$). Consistently higher response rates with bevacizumab added to chemotherapy are reported in all stages of breast cancer. However, clinically meaningful endpoints of improved OS in advanced disease have not been seen. Despite a clear signal of increased efficacy, we have yet to identify a population of women who clearly benefit from bevacizumab.

Renal Cancer

In RCC, the AVOREN study demonstrated an improvement in PFS with bevacizumab therapy combined with interferon compared to interferon alone, but not an improvement in OS [150]. In an open-label study, bevacizumab was again associated with a significant benefit in PFS and a nonsignificant improvement in OS [151].

Glioblastoma

In glioblastoma, VEGF is highly expressed [152], and for this reason a phase II trial of bevacizumab in combination with irinotecan was conducted in 35 patients with recurrent glioblastoma multiforme, resulting in a 6-month PFS rate of 46% and an OS rate of 77% [153]. A randomized trial was performed in 167 patients comparing the combination of bevacizumab and irinotecan to bevacizumab alone. The objective tumor response was observed in 28.2% of patients treated with bevacizumab and 37.8% of those treated with combination therapy. Based on these data, bevacizumab has been approved for use as a single agent in patients with recurrent glioblastoma multiforme.

The VEGF-Trap

The VEGF-Trap, known as Aflibercept, is a soluble fusion protein of some of the human extracellular domains of VEGFR-1 and VEGFR-2 and the Fc portion of human immunoglobulin (Ig) G. Aflibercept binds to both VEGF-A and PlGF with a high affinity and essentially renders the VEGF-A and PlGF ligands unable to bind and activate cell receptors [154]. Aflibercept inhibited tumor growth in xenograft models and blocked all tumor-associated angiogenesis. Aflibercept in phase II trials on ovarian cancer produced stable disease in 41% of patients [55]. In contrast, in metastatic breast cancer it demonstrated a response rate of 5%, and the PFS rate at 6 months was only 10% [154].

VEGF Receptor Tyrosine Kinase Inhibitors

The RTK inhibitors are particularly useful in treating cancer because of their dual block of oncoprotein signal transduction and downstream angiogenic processes. They also often target more than one type of receptor and affect both ECs and cancer cells because the receptors are expressed on both types of cell [155].

Sunitinib (SU11248)

This is an orally available compound that inhibits VEGFR, PDGFR, Flt-3,c-kit, and Rearrenged during transfection (RET) kinases [156]. In a phase III trial in patients with metastatic RCC, sunitinib provided a statistically significant improvement in both the median PFS and the ORR compared to interferon. Also, in gastrointestinal stromal tumors (GISTs) it diminished disease progression [157]. Unfortunately, it failed to improve the ORR and PFS in metastatic breast cancer when compared to bevacizumab [158].

Sorafenib (BAY 43-9006)

This is an oral inhibitor of the intracellular Raf kinase (B-Raf and C-Raf), but it also targets the VEGFR (VEGFR-2 and VEGFR-3), PDGFR, and c-kit kinases [159]. In a phase III trial of advanced RCC, sorafenib was found to increase the median PFS compared to placebo. In metastatic breast cancer data from a trial named SOLTI-0721 based on a sorafenib and capecitabine combination, it showed an advantage in PFS but was unfortunately accompanied by significantly increased toxicity. As a result, the phase III trial evaluating this regimen (termed RESILENCE) [160] will involve a lower dose of sorafenib [161].

Imatinib

This drug inhibits cytoplasmic and nuclear protein PDGFR and c-kit tyrosine kinases [162]. Imatinib has been reported to demonstrate antiangiogenesis activity in vitro, through inhibition of PDGFR [163].

A great number of other antiangiogenic TKIs are currently under investigation. Pazopanib targets VEGFR-1, 2, and 3; PDGFR-α and -β; and c-Kit kinases [164]. In a phase III study, pazopanib demonstrated significant improvement in PFS and tumor response rate compared with a placebo in treatment-naïve and cytokine-pretreated patients with advanced or metastatic RCC [165]. Vandetanib inhibits VEGFR-2, EGFR, and RET receptor kinases. This agent showed promising results against advanced NSCLC in a phase II study [166] and was proved to be effective in a phase III trial in combination with docetaxel [167]. However, its benefit was modest, and the application for FDA approval in NSCLC was withdrawn. However, there is a growing awareness of the efficacy of blocking both VEGFR-2 and EGFR signaling [168], because EGFR signaling might activate the VEGFR-2 pathway. In the Biomarker-integrated Approaches of Targeted Therapy for Lung Cancer Elimination (BATTLE) trial, which selected a treatment modality depending on the character of the cancer biomarkers, lung cancer with expression of VEGFR-2 responded well to vandetanib, which inhibited both VEGFR-2 and EGFR [169]. Vandetanib also showed benefits against medullary thyroid cancer and has been approved by the FDA for the treatment of this type of cancer. Axitinib acts against VEGFR-1, 2, and 3 [170]. Positive phase III trial results for axitinib in patients with previously treated metastatic RCC have been recently reported, with axitinib significantly prolonging PFS compared with sorafenib.

Monoclonal Antibodies to EGFR

Cetuximab and panitumumab are indirect RTKs that bind to the inactive form of EGFR on the extracellular domain [171]. They prevent the ligand from being able to bind to the receptor and therefore any downstream signaling activation. They are approved by the FDA for use in patients with EGFR-expressing metastatic colorectal cancer and unresectable head and neck cancer. With regard to their antiangiogenic activity, studies have shown that EGF and EGFR inhibitors cause a reduction in the synthesis of proangiogenic cytokines, rather than direct inhibition of angiogenesis [172].

PI3K Signaling Inhibition

PI3K signaling contributes to many cell processes, including angiogenesis, cell proliferation, survival, and motility, and is initiated by RTK activation [72]. Upregulation of the PI3K pathway can increase angiogenesis through multiple pathways, including increasing the levels of HIF-1α under normoxic conditions [27,173]. Initial evidence that PI3K and AKT were involved in the regulation of angiogenesis in vivo was obtained when constitutively active PI3K and AKT were shown to induce angiogenesis and increase levels of VEGF [27]. Inhibitors of the PI3K pathway have been found to decrease tumor angiogenesis and demonstrate HIF inhibition, including rapamycin analogs such as temsirolimus (CCI-779) and everolimus (RAD001) [29,174,175]. The block of angiogenesis is believed to be due at least partially to the inhibition of HIF-1α caused by the inhibition of mTOR [29,174,175].

Clinical trials of temsirolimus and everolimus as single agents have demonstrated improved survival in patients with advanced RCC, metastatic breast cancer, and neuroendocrine cancer, leading to FDA approval for these indications.

The MAPK signaling pathway is another pathway that can lead to increased angiogenesis and increased levels of HIF-1α, making it a logical target for antiangiogenesis strategies. One approach has been to inhibit *Ras* and Rho, which are activators of the MAPK pathway. During *Ras* activation, a farnesyl group is transferred onto a cysteine residue in the C-terminal end of *Ras*, enabling *Ras* to interact with intracellular membranes via the farnesyl group [71]. *Ras* is also involved in stabilizing HIF-1α, and targeting *Ras* has been shown to destabilize HIF-1α and decrease HIF transcriptional activity [28]. Tipifarnib has been the most studied farnesyltransferase inhibitor to date, with antiangiogenic, antiproliferative, and proapoptotic activity demonstrated in preclinical studies [176,177]. However, clinical trials of tipifarnib in multiple cancers have failed to demonstrate significant anticancer activity.

Chaperones and Redox Control

The chaperone heat shock protein 90 (HSP90) possesses a wide range of functions including oncoproteins and/or angiogenic-related proteins as HIF-1α and AKT. By inhibiting HSP90 from binding to HIF-1α, the protein RACK1 is able to bind HIF-1α, recruiting a ubiquitin ligase complex, inducing ubiquitination, and leading to proteasomal degradation [178]. Clinical trials of several HSP90 inhibitors are currently ongoing for anticancer use (see Chapter 9), and the effects on HIF-1α and angiogenesis are of interest [179].

The thioredoxins (Trx) are redox proteins that function to reduce oxidized cysteines in proteins through a nicotinamide adenine dinucleotide phosphate (NADPH)-dependent reaction. One member, thioredoxin-1 (Trx-1), is overexpressed in many human tumors and has been associated with decreased patient survival [180]. Trx-1 participates in the regulation of transcription factors, including HIF-1α [181]. Overexpression of Trx-1 has been shown to increase levels of HIF-1α protein and VEGF expression in vitro, and increase angiogenesis in vivo, making it an attractive target for HIF and angiogenesis inhibition [182]. PX-12 is the first Trx-1 inhibitor to enter a phase I trial of 38 patients with various types of solid tumors. It demonstrates some preliminary antitumor activity [183], and further development is ongoing (www.clinicaltrials.gov).

Endogenous Antiangiogenic Proteins

Also, since tumor angiogenesis is the net result of the balance between pro- and antiangiogenic endogenous proteins, the focus should be directed not only at inhibiting activators such as VEGF, PDGF, and FGF, but also at activating natural inhibitors such as TSP-1 and collagen-derived degradation products such as endostatin and tumstatin [184]. These endogenous antiangiogenic compounds are categorized as "direct" angiogenesis inhibitors. Instead of "indirect" angiogenesis inhibition of ligands and receptors, these direct-acting agents induce endothelial cell apoptosis via simultaneous inhibition of several signaling pathways. Thus, it has been suggested that "direct" angiogenesis inhibitors would be less prone to resistance [72]. However, the use of such endogenous angiogenesis inhibitors still needs to be refined, in particular with respect to the stability and solubility of the drugs if administered to humans [184].

Concepts in Antiangiogenic Therapy: Normalization of Tumor Vasculature

In most cases, antiangiogenic therapy is combined with other types of treatments against cancer such as radiation and chemotherapy. This combination is believed to give better results compared to only one type of treatment. However, the chemotherapy needs to be delivered directly to the target (tumor) via blood flow. At the same time, the patient is treated with agents to inhibit tumor vasculature growth by decreasing oxygen and nutrient uptake. Apparently, there is an inconsistency in the way this patient is treated. How can we achieve a maximal delivery of the chemotherapeutic when we try to shut down the vessels through which the chemotherapeutic needs to be delivered? To try to answer this question, a new concept in antiangiogenic therapy came into view in a study by Jain [74], which proposed the hypothesis that trying to normalize the tumor vasculature will positively help different anticancer treatments. Normalization of the tortuous and leaky tumor blood vessels would improve blood flow in the tumor. In addition, the microenvironment generated by a heterogeneous blood flow is characterized by hypoxia, interstitial hypertension, and acidosis. Hypoxia in itself is responsible for the fact that tumor cells become resistant to radiation and some cytotoxic drugs [66]. Moreover, it induces genetic instability and selects for more malignant cells with increased metastatic potential [185]. Abnormal vasculature and the abnormal microenvironment are the two major issues that impair, to a large extent, drug delivery and efficacy in cancer therapy. If we are able to develop normal vasculature, we may be able improve the delivery system to get to the tumor cells, and in this way we may also achieve a sufficient concentration of drugs delivered and taken up by the tumor. VEGF seems to be a very promising target for the tumor vasculature normalization hypothesis. In embryos, overexpression of VEGF or deletion of a single allele results in embryonic lethality [185]. In adults, ectopic overexpression of VEGF results in very abnormal vasculature [186]. These findings point out that for the normal development of tumor vasculature, VEGF spatial expression levels and their temporal control are extremely important.

In a study by Jain, blockade of VEGF signaling showed a reversal effect on tumor vasculature characteristics, showing furthermore a normalization of these vessels [185]. The normalized vasculature was characterized by less dilated and winding vessels, with a more normal basement membrane and a larger pericyte-covered area. Jain et al. showed that besides morphological changes, blocking VEGF signaling showed functional alterations as well. The interstitial fluid pressure decreased, the tumor oxygenation increased, and an improvement in drug penetration was demonstrated [185]. Recently, an improvement in immune response was found, based on the immunosuppressive effects of VEGF being reversed, in a similar fashion [187].

In a clinical study, treatment of rectal carcinoma patients with bevacizumab combined with chemotherapy and radiation showed very interesting results [188]. After a single-dose treatment with bevacizumab, in a time period of 2 weeks the global blood flow of tumors measured by computed tomography (CT) was decreased by 30–50% in six consecutive patients. Moreover, tumor microvascular density, vascular volume, and interstitial fluid pressure were reduced as well. This suggests that the remaining vessels nourishing the tumor were competent in delivering the radioactive agents to the tumor parenchyma.

These findings were different when bevacizumab was not included in the study: in the patients treated only with chemotherapy and radiation, the uptake of radioactive tracers was much lower. Thus, we can hypothesize that the use of bevacizumab potentially helps in the normalization of the tumor vasculature and improvement of the drug delivery system [188]. A window-of-opportunity study, in which bevacizumab was administered as a short-term first-line treatment to 43 primary breast cancer patients, showed a considerable heterogeneity in the patients' responses to bevacizumab therapy, divided into three intrinsic patterns of early response to bevacizumab [189]. In conclusion, all these data from preclinical and clinical studies show the relevance of VEGF in normalization of tumor vasculature. Blocking VEGF activity and its downstream signaling can be a starting point to initiate and carry out different projects on the normalization hypothesis. However, some recent clinical evidence has actually shown that bevacizumab treatment can reduce, rather than increase, intratumoral low-molecular-weight drug chemotherapy (e.g., docetaxel) delivery [190]. Clearly, further clinical studies of this kind are required to verify or refute this result and the theory itself.

While highly specific inhibition can be advantageous in targeting only the specific signaling transduction cascade, it can also mean modest outcomes in the clinical setting, especially when complicated processes such as angiogenesis, known to have signaling redundancy, are involved. Therefore, other strategies for anti-VEGF treatment potentially include using TKIs, soluble receptors, antisense oligonucleotides, and RNA interference. Of these, the TKIs are the most extensively studied. Whereas antibodies recognize specific epitopes in their target protein, the TKIs are less specific because they typically inhibit the function of other factors as well. For example, sunitinib and sorafenib were the first two TKI-targeting VEGFRs to be widely explored in a variety of solid tumor types. Both drugs have shown clinical efficacy as single therapy agents, possibly due to their ability to inhibit multiple proangiogenic signaling pathways.

At present, normalizing the disorganized tumor vasculature, rather than disrupting or blocking it, has emerged as a new but controversial option for anticancer therapy. Preclinical and clinical data have shown that tumor vascular normalization using monoclonal antibodies, proteins, peptides, small molecules, and pericytes resulted in decreased tumor size and reduced metastasis. Accumulated data have shown that a variety of vasculogenic and angiogenic tumor cells and genes play important roles in tumor neovascularization, growth, and metastasis. Therefore, multiple targeting of vasculogenic tumor cells and genes may improve the efficacy of tumor vascular normalization (see the review by Shang et al. [191]).

RESISTANCE: THE ANTIANGIOGENIC THERAPY LOOP

Antiangiogenic therapy was originally thought of as a therapy "resistant to drug resistance" [192]. It was assumed that drugs directed at the nonmalignant part of the cancer, such as the endothelial cells, would target the "vulnerable part" of cancer since these cells have a stable genome and lack the evading mechanisms inherent in cancer cells. Although a controversial hypothesis, angiogenesis may also progress through vascular mimicry in which tumor cells contribute to the formation of vascular channels that resemble endothelial tubes [9,10]. This phenomenon, if relevant, would facilitate acquired resistance to angiogenesis inhibitors similar to resistance to therapy designed to target the malignant cell population.

Unlike chemotherapy, most or perhaps even all types of cancer were hypothesized to be vulnerable to antiangiogenic drug therapy. However, it is well known that there are cancers such as renal and hepatocellular cancer that are intrinsically resistant or less responsive to every class of chemotherapy independent of their cell proliferation rate. The same variability in response seems to apply to antiangiogenic drugs targeting the VEGF pathway. There are cancers, such as renal or colorectal, where the use of antivascular therapy has improved the survival rate, but others such as pancreatic cancer seem to be refractory [1,193]. Again, the marked difference in ovarian cancer, as opposed to breast cancer, is unexplained. At present, phase III data are available in ovarian cancer only for the VEGF-targeted monoclonal antibody bevacizumab, and that has demonstrated a progression-free survival benefit when used in combination with first-line paclitaxel and carboplatin and continued as maintenance therapy [194].

Various mechanisms are thought to underlie the resistance to the VEGF blockade observed in some patients with cancer; they include, for example, induction or upregulation of compensatory and alternative pathways mediating angiogenesis once one particular pathway has been therapeutically blocked [195]. The extent of each mechanism responsible is highly variable from one cancer to another and differs depending on the type of anti-VEGF used. Understanding the molecular bases of these cancer type–dependent resistance mechanisms against the VEGF blockade offers opportunities to improve antiangiogenic treatment.

Hypoxia Induced by Antiangiogenic Therapy

VEGF inhibition induced vessel regression, leading to hypoxia in tumor tissues; this circumstance favors the induction of a high rate of tumor cell death. However, some cells are hypoxia tolerant; these are likely to be so-called cancer stem cells, survive in poorly oxygenated niches, and elicit tumor adaptation to antiangiogenesis. Some reports suggest that the resultant selection of tumor cells renders tumors even more invasive and metastatic [196]. In this setting, new research using preclinical models further suggests that antiangiogenic agents actually increase the invasive and metastatic properties of breast cancer cells. Conly et al. have demonstrated that by generating intratumoral hypoxia in human breast cancer xenografts, the antiangiogenic agents sunitinib and bevacizumab increase the population of cancer stem cells. In vitro studies revealed that hypoxia-driven stem and progenitor cell enrichment is primarily mediated by HIF-1α. They showed that the cancer stem cell regulatory pathway is activated in breast cancer cells under hypoxic conditions in vitro and in sunitinib-treated mouse xenografts, demonstrating that hypoxia-driven cancer stem cell stimulation limits the effectiveness of antiangiogenic agents [197] and suggesting that to improve patient outcome, these agents might have to be combined with cancer stem cell–targeting drugs [72]. However, contradictory results from other preclinical and clinical studies indicate that the concept of cancer aggravation by VEGF blockade is still unproven. Randomized, placebo-controlled phase III studies in 4205 cancer patients did not support a decreased time to disease progression, increased mortality, or altered disease progression pattern after cessation of bevacizumab therapy [198]. Infiltrative growth is, however, facilitated by fibroblasts activated by the tumor cells to secrete serineproteinases and MMPs to enable endothelial and tumor cell invasion. In line with this, novel strategies are warranted where tumor cell migration or glycolysis is targeted when such resistance mechanisms develop.

Additional targeting of HIF-1α, or the carbonic anhydrase (CA9) induced by HIF and protecting against acid pH, has shown synergistic effects in xenograft experiments. Disrupting the pH homeostasis by targeting carbonic anhydrases in hypoxic tumor cells has been proposed as a tumor-selective approach. Drug development efforts have identified a range of compounds with varying selectivity for CAIX. Treatment of mice with CAIX-positive mammary tumors with sulfonamides resulted in significant inhibition of tumor growth and metastasis formation in both spontaneous and experimental models of metastasis. Therefore, it represents an important clinical avenue for window-of-opportunity studies to select appropriate combinations for randomized trials. To date, indisulam (chloro-indolyl sulfonamide) is in phase II clinical trials treating various tumor types such as renal clear cell carcinoma and metastatic breast cancer [69].

Cytokine and Growth Factor Upregulation by Therapy

A number of preclinical studies have shown that interfering with the VEGF pathway using antibodies can result in the upregulation of higher levels of the proangiogenic molecule known as basic fibroblast growth factor (bFGF) [199]. Depending on the antiangiogenic drug and the tumor model, a number of other growth factors have been implicated, mostly in preclinical models, including interleukin-8, stromal derived factor-1, and various inflammatory cytokines, among a number of others [200,201]. The induction or upregulation of such growth factors may be the consequence of the original antiangiogenic treatment causing an increase in tumor hypoxia and hence also upregulating the transcription factor hypoxia-inducible factor-1 (HIF-1), which in turn can act as a master switch to upregulate several compensatory proangiogenic growth factors [202,203]. Consequently, targeting HIF-1 or HIF-1-regulated specific molecular mediators of angiogenesis (such as bFGF or interleukin-8) represents a possible strategy to prolong the tumor inhibition caused by an antiangiogenic drug treatment [202].

For small-molecule TKIs, mechanisms include downregulation of VEGF receptors in endothelial cells, selection of hypoxia-resistant cells, lysosomal intracellular degradation of TKIs, and suboptimal pharmacokinetics (e.g., reduced blood levels of drug) [204]. Anti-VEGFR-2 therapy failed both in preclinical tumor models and in human gliomas due to upregulation of FGF, PDGF, as well as several other signaling molecules [205]. However, alternative signaling can be prevented, as exemplified by resistance to anti-VEGFR-2 therapy, which is avoided if an antibody to another member of the VEGF family, PlGF, is added [206].

Tumor Characteristics and Mutations

A major resistance mechanism is derived from the inherent plasticity of malignant cells themselves. The tumor microenvironment is characterized by hypoxia, which the cancer cells have adapted to and survive in [20]. Hypoxia also promotes a more aggressive genotype, selecting for cancer cells harboring TP53-inactivating mutations [207]. There is increasing evidence that antiangiogenic therapy can lead to metabolic changes from oxidative respiration to glycolysis [208] where ATP for DNA synthesis and cell growth is provided by the pentose phosphate shunt. Thus, the requirement for oxygen and neovascularization is reduced. Anti-apoptotic mechanisms are also induced by hypoxia, as is autophagy [209,210].

Since many signaling pathways converge on the same downstream signaling molecules, another way of avoiding resistance due to signaling cross-talk is to target downstream hubs, such as mTOR and MAPK, if the signaling converges downstream of the receptors [20]. Apart from acquired resistance to angiogenesis inhibitors, upfront resistance due to the inherent characteristics of a particular malignant tumor can also occur (e.g., p53 mutations) [72]. A malignant tumor can simply lack dependency on a particular angiogenic signaling pathway, in which case a single-target angiogenesis inhibitor will fail [195]. This is very evident in RCC, where most patients respond, but close to 20% progress directly on bevacizumab [211].

The Microenvironment

Furthermore, tumor cells and other components of the tumor microenvironment, such as myeloid cells and stromal cells, produce a multitude of proangiogenic growth factors, exposing endothelial cells to the essential growth factors needed [20]. Inhibition of a single cytokine is therefore in many cases not enough to block the angiogenesis process. Furthermore, proangiogenic growth factors can be secreted by various cell populations within a malignant tumor. This is exemplified by VEGF, which is secreted by malignant cells, endothelial cells, and fibroblasts within the tumor, indicating that several cell compartments need to be targeted simultaneously to stop VEGF production. Accordingly, if VEGFR-2 is blocked on the endothelium, VEGF can still be produced by tumor cells and cancer-associated fibroblasts to stimulate angiogenesis via VEGFR-1 and VEGFR-3 [212]. Furthermore, components of tissue microenvironments are recognized to profoundly influence cellular phenotypes, including susceptibilities to toxic insults. Thus, the tumor microenvironment can promote drug resistance in a passive way by preventing penetration of drugs into the tumor, or in an active way by secreting protective cytokines or changing gene transcription within the tumor cells to override the cytotoxic effects of anticancer agents [213]. Also, damage responses in benign cells comprising the tumor microenvironment may directly contribute to enhancing tumor growth kinetics [214].

Tumor Endothelial Marker Biology

Tumor-associated endothelial cells differ from endothelial cells outside of the tumor, as shown by their differential survival properties and gene expression profiles [69,215]. This provides the endothelial cells with alternative growth factor receptors and downstream signaling pathways if one receptor is blocked, pointing again to the necessity of drug combinations or "cocktails" to counteract angiogenesis [72]. This can occur even if endothelial cells harbor a stable and normal genome, and an emerging body of data is focusing on such cellular plasticity as a reason for drug resistance [72,216].

A major controversy in the field of angiogenesis inhibition is whether endothelial cells harbor mutations that will contribute to drug resistance. At present, data in support of such a phenomenon are limited [72]. Therefore, endothelial genetic alterations are probably not the basis for drug resistance, and they should retain a partial sensitivity to anti-VEGF therapy. This is supported by a recent clinical study showing that bevacizumab had a significant therapeutic effect when added to chemotherapy in second-line treatment, beyond progression on bevacizumab in the first-line setting [217]. This could imply that drug resistance develops against the chemotherapeutic agent(s) that bevacizumab is combined with, and that a therapeutic benefit from anti-VEGF treatment can still be derived if another type of chemotherapy is added in the second-line setting.

Another proposed and intriguing mechanism relates to vascular phenotype regarding the presence of subtypes of tumor-associated blood vessels that are refractory to VEGF deprivation. Dvorak's group has described the extensive heterogeneity of the tumor vasculature: there are six major types of tumor-associated blood vessels, which can be broadly classified into "early" versus "late" vessels. Late vessels appear to be insensitive to VEGF inhibition [218], in contrast to the "early" vessels. However, such "resistant" vessels may be sensitive to antiangiogenic attack using other types of antiangiogenic drugs or vascular-targeting therapeutic strategies. Thus, determining the heterogeneity and composition of blood vessels in human breast cancer may shed light on helping to explain the limited benefits thus far that VEGF pathway–targeting drugs have when treating this type of cancer, especially since long-established spontaneous human tumors may have a preponderance of "late" vessels in contrast to rapidly growing, recently transplanted tumors in mice [218].

The Epithelial-to-Mesenchymal Transition

Alternatively, if the neovascularization process is halted, cancer cells can grow along pre-existing blood vessels to obtain adequate oxygen and nutrient supply, so-called vascular cooption [219]. Another avoidance mechanism has been observed in malignant brain and pancreatic tumors where angiogenesis inhibition switches the cancer from solid tumor growth into diffuse infiltrative growth to obviate the need for neovascularization [208]. This invasive phenotype seems related to the epithelial-to-mesenchymal transition (EMT) [220]. A crucial mechanism by which carcinoma cells enhance their invasive capacity is the dissolution of intercellular adhesions and the acquisition of a more motile mesenchymal phenotype as part of an EMT. Although many transcription factors can trigger it, the full molecular reprogramming occurring during an EMT is mainly orchestrated by three major groups of transcription factors: the ZEB, Snail, and Twist families. Upregulated expression of these EMT-activating transcription factors promotes tumor invasiveness in cell lines and xenograft mice models, and has been associated with poor clinical prognosis in human cancers. Evidence accumulated in the last few years indicates that EMT-related factors also regulate an expanding set of cancer cell capabilities beyond tumor invasion. Thus, EMT-related factors have been shown to cooperate in oncogenic transformation, regulate cancer cell stemness, override safeguard programs against cancer like apoptosis and senescence, determine resistance to chemotherapy, and promote tumor angiogenesis [221].

Pericytes

Pericytes are adventitial cells located within the basement membrane of capillary and postcapillary venules. Because of their multiple cytoplasmic processes, distinctive cytoskeletal elements, and envelopment of endothelial cells, pericytes are generally considered to be cells that stabilize the vessel wall, controlling endothelial cell proliferation and thereby the growth of new capillaries. Several molecules are involved in the control and modulation of the interactions occurring between pericytes and endothelial cells, such as PDGF-B, TGF-b, VEGF, and angiopoietins [222].

During the initial phase of angiogenesis, activated pericytes in parent vessels increase their proliferation and move into the perivascular spaces [223]. Although initially endothelial cell sprouts may form without pericyte involvement, pericytes are among the first cells to invade newly vascularized tissues and locate at the growing front of the endothelial sprouts by determining the location of sprout formation and by guiding newly formed vessels [224]. Alternatively, pericytes can invade tissues in the absence of endothelial cells and can form tubes enabling the subsequent penetration of endothelial cells [225]. Overall, these data suggest the existence of a mutual interplay between endothelial cells and pericytes in the direction of the angiogenic process, assigning to the pericytes a putative morphogenetic role.

Antiangiogenic treatment directed against endothelial cells using VEGF inhibitors induces the regression of tumor vessels and decreases tumor size [5], leading to vessel normalization, characterized by increased pericyte coverage, tumor perfusion, and chemotherapeutic sensitivity [185]. Moreover, removal of VEGF inhibition causes tumor regrowth due to the fact that pericytes provide a scaffold for the rapid regrowth of tumor vessels. Pericytes have been indicated as putative targets in the pharmacological therapy of tumors by using the synergistic effect of antiendothelial and antipericytic molecules. Removal of pericyte coverage leads to exposed tumor vessels, which may explain the enhanced effect of combining inhibitors that target both tumor vessels and pericytes. Finding drugs that allow manipulation of pericyte–endothelial cell interactions will provide physicians with a potent tool capable of controlling and blocking vascular proliferation and permeability. The future use of molecules interfering with the endothelial cell–pericyte unit will be also of interest in tissue engineering as well as the development of multitissue organs [226].

CLINICAL AND BIOLOGICAL MARKERS FOR ANTIANGIOGENIC STRATEGIES

Improved therapeutic strategies need to be developed. One is to obtain upfront tumor biopsies in order to determine which proangiogenic pathways are upregulated, followed by a tailor-made treatment to the individual patient [227]. Also, targeting signaling molecules far upstream in the pathways, such as ligands or RTKs, probably increases the possibility of escape mechanisms due to cross-talk between pathways and alternative signaling further downstream. Therefore, drugs that target central, downstream hubs, such as mTOR and MAPK, might theoretically be less prone to trigger escape mechanisms.

The potential for mTOR inhibition to prevent resistance to signaling inhibitors in breast cancer cells is elegantly demonstrated in the recent BOLERO-2 trial where the rapalog everolimus was added to the aromatase inhibitor exemestane. However, the targeting of such central signaling molecules is clearly associated with toxicity issues, probably due to interference with the many pathways necessary for normal tissue homeostasis [228].

Clinically, it is well known that some patients have a much more favorable response to antiangiogenic therapy than others with the same malignancy. The search for predictive biomarkers in order to identify the patients who will benefit from treatment beforehand has therefore been extensive. A large number of potential biomarkers have been studied, but so far none has been successfully identified and more research is needed [229]. An obvious approach is to assess whether tumors that are heavily vascularized are more sensitive to angiogenesis inhibitors than those that are not [102]. Evaluation of angiogenesis could be used as a prognostic marker to evaluate the aggressiveness of tumor and as a potential predictive marker of antiangiogenic treatment response. There is a growing need for rapid and effective biomarkers to establish dosage and to monitor clinical response. However, no marker of angiogenic activity of a tumor is available in predicting response to antiangiogenic agents.

Clinical Pathology of Angiogenesis

Microvascular density (MVD) indexes have been developed to evaluate and quantify angiogenesis on tissue samples with labeling of activated and proliferating endothelial cells to facilitate identification of small vessels. Immunohistochemical (IHC) studies for CD34, CD31, and Factor VIII are currently used. MVD indexes can be determined with various methods using average, center, and highest microvessel counts (see the review by Fox and Harris [230]). MVD is well known as an independent prognostic indicator in a variety of human cancers [231], but it does not reveal the degree of the angiogenic activity in a tumor and cannot be considered a surrogate marker for efficacy of antiangiogenic agents [232]. Apart from its prognostic value in some studies, the MVD of malignant tumors has no value in predicting who will respond to antiangiogenic therapy [233]. Moreover, histopathologic techniques have several limitations: they need to be standardized, require tissue sampling, and do not explore the entire tumor volume, which can lead to errors due to the heterogeneity of malignant tumors.

Plasma Markers

VEGF expression, evaluated by IHC, plasma, or urine levels, is of potential value for prognosis and also for predicting the effectiveness of radiotherapy, chemotherapy, and hormone therapy in tumors [234]. A decrease in circulating VEGF levels is not usually observed in trials evaluating antiangiogenic agents, but it has been reported [235].

More recently, preliminary evidence of a positive correlation between clinical benefit and efficacy and VEGF levels has been reported using a new VEGF ELISA assay, which detects the short circulating form of VEGF (the isoforms 111 and 121) [236]. Using this new analysis, recent findings support a potential role for plasma VEGF as a predictive marker for the therapeutic benefit of adding bevacizumab to chemotherapy in metastatic breast cancer and advanced NSCLC [237]. Positive correlations were also detected in the AVADO trial involving bevacizumab and docetaxel [236].

The VEGFR Receptor and Single-Nucleotide Polymorphisms

Being the main targets of antiangiogenic therapy, VEGF and VEGFRs have been extensively studied as biomarkers. For VEGF, there have been a large number of studies with varying results, but measuring this growth factor is fraught with a multitude of potential pitfalls. A particular problem is the low stability of VEGF, whereas soluble VEGFR-1 seems to be more robust and could be a better biomarker for the angiogenesis inhibitor response [238]. Moreover, additional biomarkers involving the single-nucleotide polymorphisms (SNPs) in angiogenesis-related genes are under investigation. Distinct VEGF (VEGF-2578AA and VEGF-1154AA) single-nucleotide genetic polymorphisms in a retrospective analysis of the E2100 trial have been shown to predict improved outcome in terms of prolonged OS, but not PFS, and less grade 3 or 4 hypertension in metastatic breast cancer patients receiving bevacizumab and paclitaxel [239]. VEGF SNPs (VEGF-2578 and VEGF-1154) have also been identified to be potentially predictive in assessing outcome in metastatic colorectal patients treated with irinotecan-based chemotherapy plus bevacizumab [240]. A recent study has shown that an SNP in VEGFR-1 was also found to predict poor response to bevacizumab in two clinical trials where the anti-VEGF antibody was combined with chemotherapy [241]. In another single-arm study of patients with recurrent ovarian cancer, multivariate analyses showed that polymorphisms in *VEGF-936*, which is reported to affect regulation of VEGF concentrations and the 3′ untranslated region of neuropilin-1 (a VEGF coreceptor), predicted PFS [242].

EPC Assays

Willet et al. have shown that bevacizumab leads to a reduction in circulating endothelial cells, which could be a potential new biomarker [188]. VEGF-driven tumor angiogenesis is believed to depend partly on the mobilization of endothelial precursors from bone marrow, which integrate into growing tumors and form a functional vascular bed [1]. Raised concentrations of circulating endothelial cells are thought to reflect active angiogenesis and, therefore, might serve as biomarkers of bevacizumab efficacy [1]. Findings from small-scale studies support this theory [243]. However, the results are very difficult to compare for baseline or changing concentrations of circulating endothelial cells in bevacizumab-treated patients, and better assays are needed for further studies on the role of circulating endothelial cells in defining the response to bevacizumab.

Imaging

A precise assessment of the biological activity of antiangiogenic therapies in vivo is important. Functional imaging techniques may provide more specific data than morphological approaches (tumor volume, reduction, tumor size, etc.). Noninvasive techniques have the potential to measure functional parameters and offer surrogate markers for therapy, regardless of tumor type or location. Such techniques include dynamic contrast-enhanced magnetic resonance imaging (DCE-MRI), CT scan, or fluorodeoxyglucose-18 PET [244,245]. By using this type of approach, it is possible to obtain several parameters such as tissue blood flow, tissue blood volume, tissue interstitial volume, mean transit time, and capillary permeability expressed as the product of permeability and the surface of capillary wall [246].

DCE-MRI is a noninvasive molecular and functional imaging technique that is performed after injection of a contrast agent. MR sequences can be designed to be sensitive to the vascular phase of contrast medium delivery, and from these images, data on tissue perfusion and blood volume can be extracted. To date, there are no definite criteria based on DCE-MRI. However, changes in its parameters were reported to correlate with the effect of some targeted agents, including sorafenib, bevacizumab, trastuzumab, and cetuximab [189,247,248]. Patients with inflammatory or locally advanced breast cancer showed a statistically significant decrease in the DCE-MRI pharmacokinetic parameter K_{trans} after one cycle of bevacizumab [247,248]. Mehta et al. are now conducting a study to assess the early therapeutic response to bevacizumab in primary breast cancer using DCE-MRI and gene expression profiles. The study has identified three intrinsic patterns of early response to bevacizumab: (1) significant reduction in permeability and blood flow over the extent of the tumor, (2) the development of a large central necrotic core, and (3) little or no change in the tumor vasculature. Their primary results imply that the second response group may ultimately correspond to the subset of patients who receive the greatest benefit from bevacizumab [189].

DCE-MRI measurements correlate with MVD as measured by IHC surrogates of tumor angiogenesis. DCE-MRI can monitor the effectiveness of a variety of treatments, including chemotherapy, hormonal manipulation, radiotherapy, and novel therapeutic approaches such as antiangiogenic drugs [249]. Furthermore, observations that MRI kinetic measurements can detect the suppression of vascular permeability after the administration of anti-VEGF antibodies and inhibitors of VEGF signaling support the important role played by VEGF in determining MRI enhancement (see the review by Atri [250]), but these observations need to be correlated with outcome in randomized trials.

CT is the most commonly used imaging technique in oncology since it is widely available, fast, and convenient. CT can provide high anatomical resolution, and, by using Hounsfield units (HUs), it gives information about tissue density. Recently, some new CT response criteria along with RECIST have been developed in targeted therapy with regard to antiangiogenic drugs. Chun et al. have devised novel tumor response criteria based on morphologic changes observed on CT scans in patients with colorectal cancer harboring liver metastases that were treated with bevacizumab-containing regimens [251]. The new morphologic criteria assigned each metastatic lesion into one of three different groups. A group 3 metastasis was characterized by heterogeneous attenuation and a thick, poorly defined tumor–liver interface. A group 1 metastasis was characterized by homogeneous low attenuation with a thin, sharply defined tumor–liver interface. A group 2 metastasis had morphology that could not be rated as 3 or 1. When present, a peripheral rim of hyperattenuating contrast enhancement was designated a group 3 characteristic, and resolution of this enhancement was classified as group 1. Morphologic response criteria were defined as optimal if the metastasis changed from a group 3 or 2 to a 1, incomplete if the group changed from 3 to 2, and none if the group had not changed or if it increased. They found that among patients treated with bevacizumab, CT-based morphologic criteria had a statistically significant association with both pathologic response and overall survival, compared to RECIST criteria, which did not correlate with survival and showed a trend in relation to pCR.

The new dynamic CT is a molecular and functional imaging technique that is able to provide information about blood flow, blood volume, capillary permeability, and microvessel density. Several studies have proven that CT perfusion (CTP) is a valuable technique for evaluating antivascular drugs such as bevacizumab. According to a study of neoadjuvant bevacizumab treatment in rectal cancer, CTP at day 12 post bevacizumab alone showed significant decreases in blood flow and permeability of the surface area product compared with before treatment. It was also demonstrated that blood flow and blood volume of the lesions were significantly reduced after 2 days of bevacizumab infusion in patients with metastatic carcinoid tumors [252–254].

PET is a common radionuclide imaging technique. FDG is the most commonly used radiopharmaceutical for PET. FDG uptake on PET, expressed as standardized uptake values (SUVs), reflects the metabolic activity of cells. There are no generally accepted criteria for a metabolic response in tumor therapy. The European Organization for Research and Treatment of Cancer (EORTC) PET response criteria and the PET Response Criteria in Solid Tumors (PERCIST) are both based on the magnitude of the change in SUV relative to baseline [255].

However, PET–CT seems to be an early predictor of the response to antiangiogenic therapies such as sorafenib or bevacizumab [236,256]. Goshen et al. investigated the value of FDG–PET in the response evaluation of colorectal cancer patients with liver metastasis treated with bevacizumab and irinotecan. They concluded that FDG–PET correlated better than CT with pathology, and was more indicative of pathological changes [257]. These data suggest that functional imaging obtained by PET could help to assess whether the drug inhibits the target, as demonstrated by the reduction of tumor perfusion; select an adequate dosage for phase II studies, in relation to the identification of the doses able to reduce tumor perfusion; identify the best schedule of administration for phase II studies; and, finally, distinguish responsive versus unresponsive patients to antiangiogenesis drugs. However, an improvement in the use of PET–CT is needed in clinical studies to assess the tumor flow and metabolism as biologic endpoints of response to antiangiogenic agents [258,259].

Hypertension

Although controversial, the onset of hypertension during bevacizumab treatment has been associated with improved outcome in patients with advanced lung cancer, metastatic colorectal cancer, renal cancer, and melanoma. In particular, increased diastolic blood pressure appears to define who will respond to angiogenesis inhibitors [260]. It has been suggested that the development of hypertension and proteinuria during bevacizumab treatment could reflect decreased nitric oxide synthesis due to a more effective blockade of VEGF signaling, translating into improved patient outcome [261,262]. These initial findings were tested in several retrospective subset analyses, as in the E2100 trial related to metastatic breast cancer patients where the presence of grade 3 or 4 hypertension was significantly associated with increased duration of OS, compared with patients who had no hypertension, or in a phase III trial in NSCLC where the same results were obtained [263]. Hypertension was also predictive of bevacizumab efficacy in a retrospective subset analysis of a CALGB90206 trial on metastatic RCC [151]. However, a retrospective analysis of six trials on different tumor subtypes showed that the onset of hypertension after starting was predictive of OS and PFS in only one study. Based on this, it might be possible that bevacizumab-induced hypertension is related to a particular type of cancer or treatment.

In clinical practice, it would of importance to establish the cutoff values for the rise of blood pressure, and to time the onset in patients receiving bevacizumab. Certain factors might be predictive of bevacizumab-induced hypertension and could help in selecting which patients will have benefits from bevacizumab-based treatment. Regular monitoring of hypertension in patients receiving bevacizumab is important, especially early in the course of treatment. Research is required to further understand the mechanistic links between the hypertensive and antiangiogenic effects of bevacizumab before hypertension can be advocated to guide treatment. In this direction, some polymorphisms in VEGFA (VEGF-634 CC and VEGF-1498 TT) have also been associated with bevacizumab-induced hypertension, but did not predict an OS benefit from bevacizumab in breast carcinoma [239]. However, given the modest effect of antiangiogenic therapy in most cases, good biomarkers are clearly needed. The potential clinical utility of these biomarkers needs to be prospectively validated in larger cohorts.

CONCLUSIONS

Angiogenesis plays a critical role in the local growth and metastasis of many different solid tumors, and thus has been identified as a hallmark of cancer. Over recent years, great progress has been made in developing molecules with antiangiogenic activity. However, the efficiency of the angiogenesis inhibitors clinically used has so far not resulted in drugs that completely and permanently interrupt neovascularization; and although clinical benefits were obtained in the treatment of various cancers such as renal cancer or colon cancer, concern by oncologists arose at the evidence of clinical observations of resistance to antiangiogenic therapy and subsequent tumor regrowth during or after treatment. Antiangiogenic agents such as bevacizumab and TKIs have been approved for the treatment of several solid cancers in combination with chemotherapy, or as single agents based on phase III clinical trials. Thus, if targeting VEGF signaling seems to be crucial as it has caused a survival benefit in particular types of cancer, we should consider VEGF or VEGFR inhibitors integrated with the standard oncological treatments. However, the PFS improvement is still only a few months, and is not frequently associated with an increase in OS; these data highlight the importance of the resistance phenomenon that could reflect a tumor's ability to acquire resistance or to activate preexisting or intrinsic resistance. In this scenario, a full understanding of tumor biology is crucial in the proper selection of the adequate drug and/or the adequate patients. An in-depth study of new markers able to identify tumors that are responsive or resistant to antiangiogenic inhibitors or tumor vascular imaging-related techniques is fundamental to daily clinical practice. Critical comparisons of early imaging changes after even 1 week of antiangiogenic therapy, objective response criteria, and analysis of these changes in randomized trials to test their predictive value are essential to put antiangiogenic therapy forward as a personalized medicine. These approaches of angiogenesis will serve an important role in predicting a particular patient's clinical course, guiding which patients may benefit most from antiangiogenic therapies and developing biomarkers to monitor patients' responses to these therapies.

As the tumor angiogenesis process is complex and, as with all biological systems, cells adapt when antiangiogenic therapy is given, it will be important to reanalyze tumor biology after treatment failure in order to assess which alternative signaling pathways have been upregulated and thus which therapy the clinicians should administer. In the future, tailored treatments based on dynamic assessment of response should result in individualized patient therapy and improved progression-free and survival outcomes, as well as being more cost-effective and, importantly, reducing unnecessary toxicity in patients.

Acknowledgments

ALH is funded by Cancer Research UK, the Breast Cancer Research Fund, Oxford Cancer Imaging Centre, the NIHR Oxford Biomedical Research Centre, and the Kennington Cancer Fund.

References

[1] Kerbel RS. Tumour angiogenesis. N Engl J Med 2008;358:2039–49.
[2] Carmeliet P. Cardiovascular biology. Creating unique blood vessels. Nature 2001;412:868–9.
[3] Hanahan D, Weinberg RA. The hallmarks of cancer. Cell 2000;100:57–70.
[4] Hanahan D, Folkman J. Patterns and emerging mechanisms of the angiogenic switch during tumourigenesis. Cell 1996;86:353–64.
[5] Baluk P, Hashizume H, McDonald DM. Cellular abnormalities of blood vessels as targets in cancer. Curr Opin Genet Dev 2005;15:102–11.
[6] Nagy JA, Chang SH, Shih SC, Dvorak AM, Dvorak HF. Heterogeneity of the tumour vasculature. Semin Thromb Hemost 2010;36:321–31.
[7] Ahn GO, Brown JM. Role of endothelial progenitors and other bone marrow-derived cells in the development of the tumour vasculature. Angiogenesis 2009;12:159–64.
[8] Dome B, Hendrix MJ, Paku S, Tovari J, Timar J. Alternative vascularization mechanisms in cancer: pathology and therapeutic implications. Am J Pathol 2007;170:1–5.
[9] Hendrix MJ, Seftor EA, Hess AR, Seftor RE. Vasculogenic mimicry and tumour-cell plasticity: lessons from melanoma. Nat Rev Cancer 2003;3:411–21.
[10] Kirschmann DA, Seftor EA, Hardy KM, Seftor RE, Hendrix MJ. Molecular pathways: vasculogenic mimicry in tumour cells: diagnostic and therapeutic implications. Clin Cancer Res 2012;18:2726–32.
[11] Bussolati B, Grange C, Sapino A, Camussi G. Endothelial cell differentiation of human breast tumour stem/progenitor cells. J Cell Mol Med 2009;13:309–19.

[12] El Hallani S, Boisselier B, Peglion F, Rousseau A, Colin C, Idbaih A, et al. A new alternative mechanism in glioblastoma vascularization: tubular vasculogenic mimicry. Brain 2010;133:973–82.

[13] Gerhardt H. VEGF and endothelial guidance in angiogenic sprouting. Organogenesis 2008;4:241–6.

[14] Carmeliet P. Angiogenesis in life, disease and medicine. Nature 2005;438:932–6.

[15] Djonov V, Baum O, Burri PH. Vascular remodeling by intussusceptive angiogenesis. Cell Tissue Res 2003;314:107–17.

[16] Pries AR, Secomb TW. Origins of heterogeneity in tissue perfusion and metabolism. Cardiovasc Res 2009;81:328–35.

[17] McDonald DM, Baluk P. Significance of blood vessel leakiness in cancer. Cancer Res 2002;62:5381–5.

[18] Munn LL. Aberrant vascular architecture in tumours and its importance in drug-based therapies. Drug Discov Today 2003;8:396–403.

[19] Folkman J. Tumour angiogenesis: therapeutic implications. N Engl J Med 1971;285:1182–6.

[20] Weis SM, Cheresh DA. Tumour angiogenesis: molecular pathways and therapeutic targets. Nat Med 2011;17:1359–70.

[21] Bergers G, Benjamin LE. Tumourigenesis and the angiogenic switch. Nat Rev Cancer 2003;3:401–10.

[22] Carmeliet P. Angiogenesis in health and disease. Nat Med 2003;9:653–60.

[23] Shepro D, Morel NM. Pericyte physiology. FASEB J 1993;7:1031–8.

[24] Hellstrom M, Gerhardt H, Kalen M, Li X, Eriksson U, Wolburg H, et al. Lack of pericytes leads to endothelial hyperplasia and abnormal vascular morphogenesis. J Cell Biol 2001;153:543–53.

[25] Abramsson A, Lindblom P, Betsholtz C. Endothelial and nonendothelial sources of PDGF-B regulate pericyte recruitment and influence vascular pattern formation in tumours. J Clin Invest 2003;112:1142–51.

[26] Pugh CW, Ratcliffe PJ. Regulation of angiogenesis by hypoxia: role of the HIF system. Nat Med 2003;9:677–84.

[27] Jiang BH, Jiang G, Zheng JZ, Lu Z, Hunter T, Vogt PK. Phosphatidylinositol 3-kinase signalling controls levels of hypoxia-inducible factor 1. Cell Growth Differ 2001;12:363–9.

[28] Blancher C, Moore JW, Robertson N, Harris AL. Effects of ras and von Hippel-Lindau (VHL) gene mutations on hypoxia-inducible factor (HIF)-1alpha, HIF-2alpha, and vascular endothelial growth factor expression and their regulation by the phosphatidylinositol 3'-kinase/Akt signalling pathway. Cancer Res 2001;61:7349–55.

[29] Land SC, Tee AR. Hypoxia-inducible factor 1alpha is regulated by the mammalian target of rapamycin (mTOR) via an mTOR signalling motif. J Biol Chem 2007;282:20534–43.

[30] Grothey A, Galanis E. Targeting angiogenesis: progress with anti-VEGF treatment with large molecules. Nat Rev Clin Oncol 2009;6:507–18.

[31] Ferrara N, Gerber HP, LeCouter J. The biology of VEGF and its receptors. Nat Med 2003;9:669–76.

[32] Varey AH, Rennel ES, Qiu Y, Bevan HS, Perrin RM, Raffy S, et al. VEGF 165 b, an antiangiogenic VEGF-A isoform, binds and inhibits bevacizumab treatment in experimental colorectal carcinoma: balance of pro- and antiangiogenic VEGF-A isoforms has implications for therapy. Br J Cancer 2008;98:1366–79.

[33] Ferrara N. Role of vascular endothelial growth factor in physiologic and pathologic angiogenesis: Therapeutic implications. Semin Oncol 2002;29:10–4.

[34] Ishigami SI, Arii S, Furutani M, Niwano M, Harada T, Mizumoto M, et al. Predictive value of vascular endothelial growth factor (VEGF) in metastasis and prognosis of human colorectal cancer. Br J Cancer 1998;78:1379–84.

[35] Inoue K, Ozeki Y, Suganuma T, Sugiura Y, Tanaka S. Vascular endothelial growth factor expression in primary esophageal squamous cell carcinoma. Association with angiogenesis and tumour progression. Cancer 1997;79:206–13.

[36] Lindahl P, Johansson BR, Leveen P, Betsholtz C. Pericyte loss and microaneurysm formation in PDGF-B-deficient mice. Science 1997;277:242–5.

[37] Cao Y, Cao R, Hedlund EM. Regulation of tumour angiogenesis and metastasis by FGF and PDGF signalling pathways. J Mol Med (Berl) 2008;86:785–9.

[38] Andrae J, Gallini R, Betsholtz C. Role of platelet-derived growth factors in physiology and medicine. Genes Dev 2008;22:1276–312.

[39] Dabrow MB, Francesco MR, McBrearty FX, Caradonna S. The effects of platelet-derived growth factor and receptor on normal and neoplastic human ovarian surface epithelium. Gynecol Oncol 1998;71:29–37.

[40] Abraham JA, Mergia A, Whang JL, Tumolo A, Friedman J, Hjerrild KA, et al. Nucleotide sequence of a bovine clone encoding the angiogenic protein, basic fibroblast growth factor. Science 1986;233:545–8.

[41] Lindner V, Majack RA, Reidy MA. Basic fibroblast growth factor stimulates endothelial regrowth and proliferation in denuded arteries. J Clin Invest 1990;85:2004–8.

[42] Gullick WJ. The epidermal growth factor system of ligands and receptors in cancer. Eur J Cancer 2009;45 (Suppl. 1):205–10.

[43] Yarden Y, Sliwkowski MX. Untangling the ErbB signalling network. Nat Rev Mol Cell Biol 2001;2:127–37.

[44] Gao CF, Vande Woude GF. HGF/SF-Met signalling in tumour progression. Cell Res 2005;15:49–51.

[45] Maemondo M, Narumi K, Saijo Y, Usui K, Tahara M, Tazawa R, et al. Targeting angiogenesis and HGF function using an adenoviral vector expressing the HGF antagonist NK4 for cancer therapy. Mol Ther 2002;5:177–85.

[46] Ferrara N, Kerbel RS. Angiogenesis as a therapeutic target. Nature 2005;438:967–74.

[47] Gerritsen ME, Tomlinson JE, Zlot C, Ziman M, Hwang S. Using gene expression profiling to identify the molecular basis of the synergistic actions of hepatocyte growth factor and vascular endothelial growth factor in human endothelial cells. Br J Pharmacol 2003;140:595–610.

[48] Zhang YW, Su Y, Volpert OV, Vande Woude GF. Hepatocyte growth factor/scatter factor mediates angiogenesis through positive VEGF and negative thrombospondin 1 regulation. Proc Natl Acad Sci U S A 2003;100: 12718–23.

[49] Comoglio PM, Giordano S, Trusolino L. Drug development of MET inhibitors: Targeting oncogene addiction and expedience. Nat Rev Drug Discov 2008;7:504–16.

[50] Smith DC, Smith MR, Sweeney C, Elfiky AA, Logothetis C, Corn PG, et al. Cabozantinib in patients with advanced prostate cancer: results of a phase II randomised discontinuation trial. J Clin Oncol 2012.

[51] Nagilla M, Brown RL, Cohen EE. Cabozantinib for the treatment of advanced medullary thyroid cancer. Adv Ther 2012;29:925–34.

[52] Augustin HG, Koh GY, Thurston G, Alitalo K. Control of vascular morphogenesis and homeostasis through the angiopoietin-Tie system. Nat Rev Mol Cell Biol 2009;10:165–77.

[53] Shim WS, Ho IA, Wong PE. Angiopoietin: a TIE(d) balance in tumour angiogenesis. Mol Cancer Res 2007;5: 655–65.

[54] Thomas M, Augustin HG. The role of the angiopoietins in vascular morphogenesis. Angiogenesis 2009;12: 125–37.

[55] Coxon A, Bready J, Min H, Kaufman S, Leal J, Yu D, et al. Context-dependent role of angiopoietin-1 inhibition in the suppression of angiogenesis and tumour growth: implications for AMG 386, an angiopoietin-1/2-neutralizing peptibody. Mol Cancer Ther 2010;9:2641–51.

[56] Herbst RS, Hong D, Chap L, Kurzrock R, Jackson E, Silverman JM, et al. Safety, pharmacokinetics, and antitumour activity of AMG 386, a selective angiopoietin inhibitor, in adult patients with advanced solid tumours. J Clin Oncol 2009;27:3557–65.

[57] Karlan BY, Oza AM, Richardson GE, Provencher DM, Hansen VL, Buck M, et al. Randomised, double-blind, placebo-controlled phase II study of AMG 386 combined with weekly paclitaxel in patients with recurrent ovarian cancer. J Clin Oncol 2012;30:362–71.

[58] Thurston G, Noguera-Troise I, Yancopoulos GD. The Delta paradox: DLL4 blockade leads to more tumour vessels but less tumour growth. Nat Rev Cancer 2007;7:327–31.

[59] Noguera-Troise I, Daly C, Papadopoulos NJ, Coetzee S, Boland P, Gale NW, et al. Blockade of Dll4 inhibits tumour growth by promoting non-productive angiogenesis. Nature 2006;444:1032–7.

[60] Patel NS, Li JL, Generali D, Poulsom R, Cranston DW, Harris AL. Up-regulation of delta-like 4 ligand in human tumour vasculature and the role of basal expression in endothelial cell function. Cancer Res 2005;65:8690–7.

[61] Hellstrom M, Phng LK, Hofmann JJ, Wallgard E, Coultas L, Lindblom P, et al. Dll4 signalling through Notch1 regulates formation of tip cells during angiogenesis. Nature 2007;445:776–80.

[62] Zeng Q, Li S, Chepeha DB, Giordano TJ, Li J, Zhang H, et al. Crosstalk between tumour and endothelial cells promotes tumour angiogenesis by MAPK activation of Notch signalling. Cancer Cell 2005;8:13–23.

[63] Ridgway J, Zhang G, Wu Y, Stawicki S, Liang WC, Chantery Y, et al. Inhibition of Dll4 signalling inhibits tumour growth by deregulating angiogenesis. Nature 2006;444:1083–7.

[64] Tolcher AW, Messersmith WA, Mikulski SM, Papadopoulos KP, Kwak EL, Gibbon DG, et al. Phase I study of RO4929097, a gamma secretase inhibitor of Notch signalling, in patients with refractory metastatic or locally advanced solid tumours. J Clin Oncol 2012;30:2348–53.

[65] Krop I, Demuth T, Guthrie T, Wen PY, Mason WP, Chinnaiyan P, et al. Phase I pharmacologic and pharmacodynamic study of the gamma secretase (Notch) inhibitor MK-0752 in adult patients with advanced solid tumours. J Clin Oncol 2012;30:2307–13.

[66] Harris AL. Hypoxia—a key regulatory factor in tumour growth. Nat Rev Cancer 2002;2:38–47.

[67] Talks KL, Turley H, Gatter KC, Maxwell PH, Pugh CW, Ratcliffe PJ, et al. The expression and distribution of the hypoxia-inducible factors HIF-1alpha and HIF-2alpha in normal human tissues, cancers, and tumour-associated macrophages. Am J Pathol 2000;157:411–21.

[68] Mabjeesh NJ, Amir S. Hypoxia-inducible factor (HIF) in human tumourigenesis. Histol Histopathol 2007;22:559–72.

[69] Jones DT, Harris AL. Small-molecule inhibitors of the HIF pathway and synthetic lethal interactions. Expert Opin Ther Targets 2012.

[70] Madhusudan S, Ganesan TS. Tyrosine kinase inhibitors in cancer therapy. Clin Biochem 2004;37:618–35.

[71] Downward J. Targeting RAS signalling pathways in cancer therapy. Nat Rev Cancer 2003;3:11–22.

[72] Engelman JA. Targeting PI3K signalling in cancer: opportunities, challenges and limitations. Nat Rev Cancer 2009;9:550–62.

[73] Fokas E, McKenna WG, Muschel RJ. The impact of tumour microenvironment on cancer treatment and its modulation by direct and indirect antivascular strategies. Cancer Metastasis Rev 2012;31:823–42.

[74] Jain RK. Normalizing tumour vasculature with anti-angiogenic therapy: a new paradigm for combination therapy. Nat Med 2001;7:987–9.

[75] De Saedeleer CJ, Copetti T, Porporato PE, Verrax J, Feron O, Sonveaux P. Lactate activates HIF-1 in oxidative but not in Warburg-phenotype human tumour cells. PLoS One 2012;7:e46571.

[76] Quintero M, Colombo SL, Godfrey A, Moncada S. Mitochondria as signalling organelles in the vascular endothelium. Proc Natl Acad Sci U S A 2006;103:5379–84.

[77] Lu C, Bonome T, Li Y, Kamat AA, Han LY, Schmandt R, et al. Gene alterations identified by expression profiling in tumour-associated endothelial cells from invasive ovarian carcinoma. Cancer Res 2007;67:1757–68.

[78] Hunt TK, Aslam R, Hussain Z, Beckert S. Lactate, with oxygen, incites angiogenesis. Adv Exp Med Biol 2008;614:73–80.

[79] DeBerardinis RJ, Lum JJ, Hatzivassiliou G, Thompson CB. The biology of cancer: metabolic reprogramming fuels cell growth and proliferation. Cell Metab 2008;7:11–20.

[80] Helmlinger G, Endo M, Ferrara N, Hlatky L, Jain RK. Formation of endothelial cell networks. Nature 2000;405:139–41.

[81] Hansen-Algenstaedt N, Stoll BR, Padera TP, Dolmans DE, Hicklin DJ, Fukumura D, et al. Tumour oxygenation in hormone-dependent tumours during vascular endothelial growth factor receptor-2 blockade, hormone ablation, and chemotherapy. Cancer Res 2000;60:4556–60.

[82] Evans RM, Barish GD, Wang YX. PPARs and the complex journey to obesity. Nat Med 2004;10:355–61.

[83] Muller-Brusselbach S, Komhoff M, Rieck M, Meissner W, Kaddatz K, Adamkiewicz J, et al. Deregulation of tumour angiogenesis and blockade of tumour growth in PPARbeta-deficient mice. EMBO J 2007;26:3686–98.

[84] Piqueras L, Reynolds AR, Hodivala-Dilke KM, Alfranca A, Redondo JM, Hatae T, et al. Activation of PPARbeta/delta induces endothelial cell proliferation and angiogenesis. Arterioscler Thromb Vasc Biol 2007;27:63–9.

[85] Finck BN, Kelly DP. PGC-1 coactivators: inducible regulators of energy metabolism in health and disease. J Clin Invest 2006;116:615–22.

[86] Arany Z, Foo SY, Ma Y, Ruas JL, Bommi-Reddy A, Girnun G, et al. HIF-independent regulation of VEGF and angiogenesis by the transcriptional coactivator PGC-1alpha. Nature 2008;451:1008–12.

[87] Long YC, Zierath JR. AMP-activated protein kinase signalling in metabolic regulation. J Clin Invest 2006;116:1776–83.

[88] Ouchi N, Shibata R, Walsh K. AMP-activated protein kinase signalling stimulates VEGF expression and angiogenesis in skeletal muscle. Circ Res 2005;96:838–46.

[89] Suganami E, Takagi H, Ohashi H, Suzuma K, Suzuma I, Oh H, et al. Leptin stimulates ischemia-induced retinal neovascularization: possible role of vascular endothelial growth factor expressed in retinal endothelial cells. Diabetes 2004;53:2443–8.

[90] Cao R, Brakenhielm E, Wahlestedt C, Thyberg J, Cao Y. Leptin induces vascular permeability and synergistically stimulates angiogenesis with FGF-2 and VEGF. Proc Natl Acad Sci U S A 2001;98:6390–5.

[91] Bhowmick NA, Moses HL. Tumour–stroma interactions. Curr Opin Genet Dev 2005;15:97–101.

[92] Albini A, Sporn MB. The tumour microenvironment as a target for chemoprevention. Nat Rev Cancer 2007;7:139–47.

[93] Mantovani A, Sica A. Macrophages, innate immunity and cancer: balance, tolerance, and diversity. Curr Opin Immunol 2010;22:231–7.

[94] Mantovani A, Allavena P, Sica A, Balkwill F. Cancer-related inflammation. Nature 2008;454:436–44.

[95] Pollard JW. Tumour-educated macrophages promote tumour progression and metastasis. Nat Rev Cancer 2004;4:71–8.

[96] Kawahara A, Hattori S, Akiba J, Nakashima K, Taira T, Watari K, et al. Infiltration of thymidine phosphorylase-positive macrophages is closely associated with tumour angiogenesis and survival in intestinal type gastric cancer. Oncol Rep 2010;24:405–15.

[97] Lee CH, Espinosa I, Vrijaldenhoven S, Subramanian S, Montgomery KD, Zhu S, et al. Prognostic significance of macrophage infiltration in leiomyosarcomas. Clin Cancer Res 2008;14:1423–30.

[98] Ryder M, Ghossein RA, Ricarte-Filho JC, Knauf JA, Fagin JA. Increased density of tumour-associated macrophages is associated with decreased survival in advanced thyroid cancer. Endocr Relat Cancer 2008;15:1069–74.

[99] Kang JC, Chen JS, Lee CH, Chang JJ, Shieh YS. Intratumoural macrophage counts correlate with tumour progression in colorectal cancer. J Surg Oncol 2010;102:242–8.

[100] Funada Y, Noguchi T, Kikuchi R, Takeno S, Uchida Y, Gabbert HE. Prognostic significance of CD8+ T cell and macrophage peritumoural infiltration in colorectal cancer. Oncol Rep 2003;10:309–13.

[101] Ko JS, Bukowski RM, Fincke JH. Myeloid-derived suppressor cells: a novel therapeutic target. Curr Oncol Rep 2009;11:87–93.

[102] Tartour E, Pere H, Maillere B, Terme M, Merillon N, Taieb J, et al. Angiogenesis and immunity: a bidirectional link potentially relevant for the monitoring of antiangiogenic therapy and the development of novel therapeutic combination with immunotherapy. Cancer Metastasis Rev 2011;30:83–95.

[103] Mund JA, Case J. The role of circulating endothelial progenitor cells in tumour angiogenesis. Curr Stem Cell Res Ther 2011;6:115–21.

[104] Asahara T, Murohara T, Sullivan A, Silver M, van der Zee R, Li T, et al. Isolation of putative progenitor endothelial cells for angiogenesis. Science 1997;275:964–7.

[105] Peters BA, Diaz LA, Polyak K, Meszler L, Romans K, Guinan EC, et al. Contribution of bone marrow-derived endothelial cells to human tumour vasculature. Nat Med 2005;11:261–2.

[106] Li Calzi S, Neu MB, Shaw LC, Kielczewski JL, Moldovan NI, Grant MB. EPCs and pathological angiogenesis: when good cells go bad. Microvasc Res 2010;79:207–16.

[107] Kopp HG, Ramos CA, Rafii S. Contribution of endothelial progenitors and proangiogenic hematopoietic cells to vascularization of tumour and ischemic tissue. Curr Opin Hematol 2006;13:175–81.

[108] Norden AD, Drappatz J, Wen PY. Antiangiogenic therapies for high-grade glioma. Nat Rev Neurol 2009;5:610–20.

[109] Ribatti D, Nico B, Crivellato E. The role of pericytes in angiogenesis. Int J Dev Biol 2011;55:261–8.

[110] Xue Y, Lim S, Yang Y, Wang Z, Jensen LD, Hedlund EM, et al. PDGF-BB modulates hematopoiesis and tumour angiogenesis by inducing erythropoietin production in stromal cells. Nat Med 2012;18:100–10.

[111] Oliner J, Min H, Leal J, Yu D, Rao S, You E, et al. Suppression of angiogenesis and tumour growth by selective inhibition of angiopoietin-2. Cancer Cell 2004;6:507–16.

[112] Mazzieri R, Pucci F, Moi D, Zonari E, Ranghetti A, Berti A, et al. Targeting the ANG2/TIE2 axis inhibits tumour growth and metastasis by impairing angiogenesis and disabling rebounds of proangiogenic myeloid cells. Cancer Cell 2011;19:512–26.

[113] Cascone T, Heymach JV. Targeting the angiopoietin/Tie2 pathway: cutting tumour vessels with a double-edged sword? J Clin Oncol 2012;30:441–4.

[114] Gherardi E, Birchmeier W, Birchmeier C, Vande Woude G. Targeting MET in cancer: rationale and progress. Nat Rev Cancer 2012;12:89–103.

[115] Saelen MG, Flatmark K, Folkvord S, de Wijn R, Rasmussen H, Fodstad O, et al. Tumour kinase activity in locally advanced rectal cancer: angiogenic signalling and early systemic dissemination. Angiogenesis 2011;14:481–9.

[116] Penel N, Adenis A, Bocci G. Cyclophosphamide-based metronomic chemotherapy: after 10 years of experience, where do we stand and where are we going? Crit Rev Oncol Hematol 2012;82:40–50.

[117] Kerbel RS. Reappraising antiangiogenic therapy for breast cancer. Breast 2011;20(Suppl. 3):S56–60.

[118] Miller KD, Sweeney CJ, Sledge Jr GW. Redefining the target: chemotherapeutics as antiangiogenics. J Clin Oncol 2001;19:1195–206.

[119] Browder T, Butterfield CE, Kraling BM, Shi B, Marshall B, O'Reilly MS, et al. Antiangiogenic scheduling of chemotherapy improves efficacy against experimental drug-resistant cancer. Cancer Res 2000;60:1878–86.

[120] Klauber N, Parangi S, Flynn E, Hamel E, D'Amato RJ. Inhibition of angiogenesis and breast cancer in mice by the microtubule inhibitors 2-methoxyestradiol and taxol. Cancer Res 1997;57:81–6.

[121] Pivot X, Schneeweiss A, Verma S, Thomssen C, Passos-Coelho JL, Benedetti G, et al. Efficacy and safety of bevacizumab in combination with docetaxel for the first-line treatment of elderly patients with locally recurrent or metastatic breast cancer: results from AVADO. Eur J Cancer 2011;47:2387–95.

[122] Singhal S, Mehta J, Desikan R, Ayers D, Roberson P, Eddlemon P, et al. Antitumour activity of thalidomide in refractory multiple myeloma. N Engl J Med 1999;341:1565–71.

[123] Vacca A, Scavelli C, Montefusco V, Di Pietro G, Neri A, Mattioli M, et al. Thalidomide downregulates angiogenic genes in bone marrow endothelial cells of patients with active multiple myeloma. J Clin Oncol 2005;23:5334–46.

[124] Vacca A, Ribatti D, Presta M, Minischetti M, Iurlaro M, Ria R, et al. Bone marrow neovascularization, plasma cell angiogenic potential, and matrix metalloproteinase-2 secretion parallel progression of human multiple myeloma. Blood 1999;93:3064–73.

[125] Ria R, Vacca A, Russo F, Cirulli T, Massaia M, Tosi P, et al. A VEGF-dependent autocrine loop mediates proliferation and capillarogenesis in bone marrow endothelial cells of patients with multiple myeloma. Thromb Haemost 2004;92:1438–45.

[126] Dredge K, Marriott JB, Macdonald CD, Man HW, Chen R, Muller GW, et al. Novel thalidomide analogues display anti-angiogenic activity independently of immunomodulatory effects. Br J Cancer 2002;87:1166–72.

[127] Dredge K, Horsfall R, Robinson SP, Zhang LH, Lu L, Tang Y, et al. Orally administered lenalidomide (CC-5013) is anti-angiogenic in vivo and inhibits endothelial cell migration and Akt phosphorylation in vitro. Microvasc Res 2005;69:56–63.

[128] De Luisi A, Ferrucci A, Coluccia AM, Ria R, Moschetta M, de Luca E, et al. Lenalidomide restrains motility and overangiogenic potential of bone marrow endothelial cells in patients with active multiple myeloma. Clin Cancer Res 2011;17:1935–46.

[129] Kerbel RS, Kamen BA. The anti-angiogenic basis of metronomic chemotherapy. Nat Rev Cancer 2004;4:423–36.

[130] Pasquier E, Kavallaris M, Andre N. Metronomic chemotherapy: new rationale for new directions. Nat Rev Clin Oncol 2010;7:455–65.

[131] Colleoni M, Rocca A, Sandri MT, Zorzino L, Masci G, Nole F, et al. Low-dose oral methotrexate and cyclophosphamide in metastatic breast cancer: antitumour activity and correlation with vascular endothelial growth factor levels. Ann Oncol 2002;13:73–80.

[132] Orlando L, Cardillo A, Ghisini R, Rocca A, Balduzzi A, Torrisi R, et al. Trastuzumab in combination with metronomic cyclophosphamide and methotrexate in patients with HER-2 positive metastatic breast cancer. BMC Cancer 2006;6:225.

[133] Aurilio G, Munzone E, Botteri E, Sciandivasci A, Adamoli L, Minchella I, et al. Oral metronomic cyclophosphamide and methotrexate plus fulvestrant in advanced breast cancer patients: a mono-institutional case-cohort report. Breast J 2012;18:470–4.

[134] Bottini A, Generali D, Brizzi MP, Fox SB, Bersiga A, Bonardi S, et al. Randomised Phase II trial of letrozole and letrozole plus low-dose metronomic oral cyclophosphamide as primary systemic treatment in elderly breast cancer patients. J Clin Oncol 2006;24:3623–8.

[135] Montagna E, Cancello G, Bagnardi V, Pastrello D, Dellapasqua S, Perri G, et al. Metronomic chemotherapy combined with bevacizumab and erlotinib in patients with metastatic HER2-negative breast cancer: clinical and biological activity. Clin Breast Cancer 2012;12:207–14.

[136] Jones MK, Wang H, Peskar BM, Levin E, Itani RM, Sarfeh IJ, et al. Inhibition of angiogenesis by nonsteroidal anti-inflammatory drugs: insight into mechanisms and implications for cancer growth and ulcer healing. Nat Med 1999;5:1418–23.

[137] Altorki NK, Keresztes RS, Port JL, Libby DM, Korst RJ, Flieder DB, et al. Celecoxib, a selective cyclo-oxygenase-2 inhibitor, enhances the response to preoperative paclitaxel and carboplatin in early-stage non-small-cell lung cancer. J Clin Oncol 2003;21:2645–50.

[138] Gately S, Li WW. Multiple roles of COX-2 in tumour angiogenesis: a target for antiangiogenic therapy. Semin Oncol 2004;31:2–11.

[139] Gasparini G, Longo R, Sarmiento R, Morabito A. Inhibitors of cyclo-oxygenase 2: a new class of anticancer agents? Lancet Oncol 2003;4:605–15.

[140] Wood J, Bonjean K, Ruetz S, Bellahcene A, Devy L, Foidart JM, et al. Novel antiangiogenic effects of the bisphosphonate compound zoledronic acid. J Pharmacol Exp Ther 2002;302:1055–61.

[141] Santini D, Vincenzi B, Dicuonzo G, Avvisati G, Massacesi C, Battistoni F, et al. Zoledronic acid induces significant and long-lasting modifications of circulating angiogenic factors in cancer patients. Clin Cancer Res 2003;9:2893–7.

[142] Giantonio BJ, Catalano PJ, Meropol NJ, O'Dwyer PJ, Mitchell EP, Alberts SR, et al. Bevacizumab in combination with oxaliplatin, fluorouracil, and leucovorin (FOLFOX4) for previously treated metastatic colorectal cancer: results from the Eastern Cooperative Oncology Group Study E3200. J Clin Oncol 2007;25:1539–44.

[143] Allegra CJ, Yothers G, O'Connell MJ, Sharif S, Petrelli NJ, Colangelo LH, et al. Phase III trial assessing bevacizumab in stages II and III carcinoma of the colon: results of NSABP protocol C-08. J Clin Oncol 2011;29:11–6.

[144] Sandler A, Gray R, Perry MC, Brahmer J, Schiller JH, Dowlati A, et al. Paclitaxel-carboplatin alone or with bevacizumab for non-small-cell lung cancer. N Engl J Med 2006;355:2542–50.

[145] Miller K, Wang M, Gralow J, Dickler M, Cobleigh M, Perez EA, et al. Paclitaxel plus bevacizumab versus paclitaxel alone for metastatic breast cancer. N Engl J Med 2007;357:2666–76.

[146] Miles DW, Chan A, Dirix LY, Cortes J, Pivot X, Tomczak P, et al. Phase III study of bevacizumab plus docetaxel compared with placebo plus docetaxel for the first-line treatment of human epidermal growth factor receptor 2-negative metastatic breast cancer. J Clin Oncol 2010;28:3239–47.

[147] Robert NJ, Dieras V, Glaspy J, Brufsky AM, Bondarenko I, Lipatov ON, et al. RIBBON-1: randomised, double-blind, placebo-controlled, phase III trial of chemotherapy with or without bevacizumab for first-line treatment of human epidermal growth factor receptor 2-negative, locally recurrent or metastatic breast cancer. J Clin Oncol 2011;29:1252–60.

[148] Brufsky AM, Hurvitz S, Perez E, Swamy R, Valero V, O'Neill V, et al. RIBBON-2: a randomised, double-blind, placebo-controlled, phase III trial evaluating the efficacy and safety of bevacizumab in combination with chemotherapy for second-line treatment of human epidermal growth factor receptor 2-negative metastatic breast cancer. J Clin Oncol 2011;29:4286–93.

[149] von Minckwitz G, Eidtmann H, Rezai M, Fasching PA, Tesch H, Eggemann H, et al. Neoadjuvant chemotherapy and bevacizumab for HER2-negative breast cancer. N Engl J Med 2012;366:299–309.

[150] Escudier B, Bellmunt J, Negrier S, Bajetta E, Melichar B, Bracarda S, et al. Phase III trial of bevacizumab plus interferon alfa-2a in patients with metastatic renal cell carcinoma (AVOREN): final analysis of overall survival. J Clin Oncol 2010;28:2144–50.

[151] Rini BI, Halabi S, Rosenberg JE, Stadler WM, Vaena DA, Archer L, et al. Phase III trial of bevacizumab plus interferon alfa versus interferon alfa monotherapy in patients with metastatic renal cell carcinoma: final results of CALGB 90206. J Clin Oncol 2010;28:2137–43.

[152] Godard S, Getz G, Delorenzi M, Farmer P, Kobayashi H, Desbaillets I, et al. Classification of human astrocytic gliomas on the basis of gene expression: a correlated group of genes with angiogenic activity emerges as a strong predictor of subtypes. Cancer Res 2003;63:6613–25.

[153] Vredenburgh JJ, Desjardins A, Herndon 2nd JE, Marcello J, Reardon DA, Quinn JA, et al. Bevacizumab plus irinotecan in recurrent glioblastoma multiforme. J Clin Oncol 2007;25:4722–9.

[154] Holash J, Davis S, Papadopoulos N, Croll SD, Ho L, Russell M, et al. VEGF-Trap: a VEGF blocker with potent antitumour effects. Proc Natl Acad Sci U S A 2002;99:11393–8.

[155] Young RJ, Reed MW. Anti-angiogenic therapy: concept to clinic. Microcirculation 2012;19:115–25.

[156] Gan HK, Seruga B, Knox JJ. Sunitinib in solid tumours. Expert Opin Investig Drugs 2009;18:821–34.

[157] Demetri GD, van Oosterom AT, Garrett CR, Blackstein ME, Shah MH, Verweij J, et al. Efficacy and safety of sunitinib in patients with advanced gastrointestinal stromal tumour after failure of imatinib: a randomised controlled trial. Lancet 2006;368:1329–38.

[158] Yang L, Shi L, Fu Q, Xiong H, Zhang M, Yu S. Efficacy and safety of sorafenib in advanced renal cell carcinoma patients: results from a long-term study. Oncol Lett 2012;3:935–9.

[159] Wilhelm SM, Adnane L, Newell P, Villanueva A, Llovet JM, Lynch M. Preclinical overview of sorafenib, a multikinase inhibitor that targets both Raf and VEGF and PDGF receptor tyrosine kinase signalling. Mol Cancer Ther 2008;7:3129–40.

[160] Rugo HS. Inhibiting angiogenesis in breast cancer: the beginning of the end or the end of the beginning? J Clin Oncol 2012;30:898–901.

[161] Baselga J, Segalla JG, Roche H, Del Giglio A, Pinczowski H, Ciruelos EM, et al. Sorafenib in combination with capecitabine: an oral regimen for patients with HER2-negative locally advanced or metastatic breast cancer. J Clin Oncol 2012;30:1484–91.

[162] Steeghs N, Nortier JW, Gelderblom H. Small molecule tyrosine kinase inhibitors in the treatment of solid tumours: an update of recent developments. Ann Surg Oncol 2007;14:942–53.

[163] Kim R, Emi M, Arihiro K, Tanabe K, Uchida Y, Toge T. Chemosensitization by STI571 targeting the platelet-derived growth factor/platelet-derived growth factor receptor-signalling pathway in the tumour progression and angiogenesis of gastric carcinoma. Cancer 2005;103:1800–9.

[164] Sonpavde G, Hutson TE. Pazopanib: a novel multitargeted tyrosine kinase inhibitor. Curr Oncol Rep 2007;9:115–9.

[165] Sternberg CN, Davis ID, Mardiak J, Szczylik C, Lee E, Wagstaff J, et al. Pazopanib in locally advanced or metastatic renal cell carcinoma: results of a randomised phase III trial. J Clin Oncol 2010;28:1061–8.

[166] Kiura K, Nakagawa K, Shinkai T, Eguchi K, Ohe Y, Yamamoto N, et al. A randomised, double-blind, phase IIa dose-finding study of vandetanib (ZD6474) in Japanese patients with non-small cell lung cancer. J Thorac Oncol 2008;3:386–93.

[167] Herbst RS, Sun Y, Eberhardt WE, Germonpre P, Saijo N, Zhou C, et al. Vandetanib plus docetaxel versus docetaxel as second-line treatment for patients with advanced non-small-cell lung cancer (ZODIAC): a double-blind, randomised, phase 3 trial. Lancet Oncol 2010;11:619–26.

[168] Herbst RS, Ansari R, Bustin F, Flynn P, Hart L, Otterson GA, et al. Efficacy of bevacizumab plus erlotinib versus erlotinib alone in advanced non-small-cell lung cancer after failure of standard first-line chemotherapy (BeTa): a double-blind, placebo-controlled, phase 3 trial. Lancet 2011;377:1846–54.

[169] Tsao AS, Liu S, Lee JJ, Alden C, Blumenschein G, Herbst R, et al. Clinical outcomes and biomarker profiles of elderly pretreated NSCLC patients from the BATTLE trial. J Thorac Oncol 2012;7:1645–52.

[170] Hu-Lowe DD, Zou HY, Grazzini ML, Hallin ME, Wickman GR, Amundson K, et al. Nonclinical antiangiogenesis and antitumour activities of axitinib (AG-013736), an oral, potent, and selective inhibitor of vascular endothelial growth factor receptor tyrosine kinases 1, 2, 3. Clin Cancer Res 2008;14:7272–83.

[171] Mauriz JL, Gonzalez-Gallego J. Antiangiogenic drugs: current knowledge and new approaches to cancer therapy. J Pharm Sci 2008;97:4129–54.

[172] Perrotte P, Matsumoto T, Inoue K, Kuniyasu H, Eve BY, Hicklin DJ, et al. Anti-epidermal growth factor receptor antibody C225 inhibits angiogenesis in human transitional cell carcinoma growing orthotopically in nude mice. Clin Cancer Res 1999;5:257–65.

[173] Laughner E, Taghavi P, Chiles K, Mahon PC, Semenza GL. HER2 (neu) signalling increases the rate of hypoxia-inducible factor 1alpha (HIF-1alpha) synthesis: novel mechanism for HIF-1-mediated vascular endothelial growth factor expression. Mol Cell Biol 2001;21:3995–4004.

[174] Hudson CC, Liu M, Chiang GG, Otterness DM, Loomis DC, Kaper F, et al. Regulation of hypoxia-inducible factor 1alpha expression and function by the mammalian target of rapamycin. Mol Cell Biol 2002;22:7004–14.

[175] Guba M, von Breitenbuch P, Steinbauer M, Koehl G, Flegel S, Hornung M, et al. Rapamycin inhibits primary and metastatic tumour growth by antiangiogenesis: involvement of vascular endothelial growth factor. Nat Med 2002;8:128–35.

[176] Delmas C, End D, Rochaix P, Favre G, Toulas C, Cohen-Jonathan E. The farnesyltransferase inhibitor R115777 reduces hypoxia and matrix metalloproteinase 2 expression in human glioma xenograft. Clin Cancer Res 2003;9:6062–8.

[177] End DW, Smets G, Todd AV, Applegate TL, Fuery CJ, Angibaud P, et al. Characterization of the antitumour effects of the selective farnesyl protein transferase inhibitor R115777 in vivo and in vitro. Cancer Res 2001;61:131–7.

[178] Liu YV, Baek JH, Zhang H, Diez R, Cole RN, Semenza GL. RACK1 competes with HSP90 for binding to HIF-1alpha and is required for O(2)-independent and HSP90 inhibitor-induced degradation of HIF-1alpha. Molecular Cell 2007;25:207–17.

[179] Taldone T, Gozman A, Maharaj R, Chiosis G. Targeting Hsp90: small-molecule inhibitors and their clinical development. Curr Opin Pharmacol 2008;8:370–4.

[180] Powis G, Montfort WR. Properties and biological activities of thioredoxins. Annu Rev Pharmacol Toxicol 2001;41:261–95.

[181] Huang LE, Arany Z, Livingston DM, Bunn HF. Activation of hypoxia-inducible transcription factor depends primarily upon redox-sensitive stabilization of its alpha subunit. J Biol Chem 1996;271:32253–9.

[182] Welsh SJ, Bellamy WT, Briehl MM, Powis G. The redox protein thioredoxin-1 (Trx-1) increases hypoxia-inducible factor 1alpha protein expression: Trx-1 overexpression results in increased vascular endothelial growth factor production and enhanced tumour angiogenesis. Cancer Res 2002;62:5089–95.

[183] Ramanathan RK, Kirkpatrick DL, Belani CP, Friedland D, Green SB, Chow HH, et al. A phase I pharmacokinetic and pharmacodynamic study of PX-12, a novel inhibitor of thioredoxin-1, in patients with advanced solid tumours. Clin Cancer Res 2007;13:2109–14.

[184] Sund M, Xie L, Kalluri R. The contribution of vascular basement membranes and extracellular matrix to the mechanics of tumour angiogenesis. APMIS 2004;112:450–62.

[185] Jain RK. Normalization of tumour vasculature: an emerging concept in antiangiogenic therapy. Science 2005;307:58–62.

[186] Nagy JA, Vasile E, Feng D, Sundberg C, Brown LF, Detmar MJ, et al. Vascular permeability factor/vascular endothelial growth factor induces lymphangiogenesis as well as angiogenesis. J Exp Med 2002;196:1497–506.

[187] Huang Y, Yuan J, Righi E, Kamoun WS, Ancukiewicz M, Nezivar J, et al. Vascular normalizing doses of anti-angiogenic treatment reprogram the immunosuppressive tumour microenvironment and enhance immuno-therapy. Proc Natl Acad Sci U S A 2012;109:17561–6.

[188] Willett CG, Boucher Y, di Tomaso E, Duda DG, Munn LL, Tong RT, et al. Direct evidence that the VEGF-specific antibody bevacizumab has antivascular effects in human rectal cancer. Nat Med 2004;10:145–7.

[189] Mehta S, Hughes NP, Buffa FM, Li SP, Adams RF, Adwani A, et al. Assessing early therapeutic response to bevacizumab in primary breast cancer using magnetic resonance imaging and gene expression profiles. J Natl Cancer Inst Monogr 2011:71–4.

[190] Van der Veldt AA, Lubberink M, Bahce I, Walraven M, de Boer MP, Greuter HN, et al. Rapid decrease in delivery of chemotherapy to tumours after anti-VEGF therapy: implications for scheduling of anti-angiogenic drugs. Cancer Cell 2012;21:82–91.

[191] Shang B, Cao Z, Zhou Q. Progress in tumour vascular normalization for anticancer therapy: challenges and perspectives. Front Med 2012;6:67–78.

[192] Kerbel RS. A cancer therapy resistant to resistance. Nature 1997;390:335–6.

[193] Hurwitz H, Fehrenbacher L, Novotny W, Cartwright T, Hainsworth J, Heim W, et al. Bevacizumab plus irinotecan, fluorouracil, and leucovorin for metastatic colorectal cancer. N Engl J Med 2004;350:2335–42.

[194] Kroep JR, Nortier JW. The role of bevacizumab in advanced epithelial ovarian cancer. Curr Pharm Des 2012;18:3775–83.

[195] Bergers G, Hanahan D. Modes of resistance to anti-angiogenic therapy. Nat Rev Cancer 2008;8:592–603.

[196] Lu X, Kang Y. Hypoxia and hypoxia-inducible factors: master regulators of metastasis. Clin Cancer Res 2010;16:5928–35.

[197] Conley SJ, Gheordunescu E, Kakarala P, Newman B, Korkaya H, Heath AN, et al. Antiangiogenic agents increase breast cancer stem cells via the generation of tumour hypoxia. Proc Natl Acad Sci U S A 2012;109:2784–9.

[198] Smith IE, Pierga JY, Biganzoli L, Cortes-Funes H, Thomssen C, Pivot X, et al. First-line bevacizumab plus taxane-based chemotherapy for locally recurrent or metastatic breast cancer: safety and efficacy in an open-label study in 2,251 patients. Ann Oncol 2011;22:595–602.

[199] Casanovas O, Hicklin DJ, Bergers G, Hanahan D. Drug resistance by evasion of antiangiogenic targeting of VEGF signalling in late-stage pancreatic islet tumours. Cancer Cell 2005;8:299–309.

[200] Shojaei F, Lee JH, Simmons BH, Wong A, Esparza CO, Plumlee PA, et al. HGF/c-Met acts as an alternative angiogenic pathway in sunitinib-resistant tumours. Cancer Res 2010;70:10090–100.

[201] Huang D, Ding Y, Zhou M, Rini BI, Petillo D, Qian CN, et al. Interleukin-8 mediates resistance to antiangio-genic agent sunitinib in renal cell carcinoma. Cancer Res 2010;70:1063–71.

[202] Rapisarda A, Melillo G. Overcoming disappointing results with antiangiogenic therapy by targeting hypoxia. Nat Rev Clin Oncol 2012;9:378–90.

[203] Semenza GL. Targeting HIF-1 for cancer therapy. Nat Rev Cancer 2003;3:721–32.

[204] Gotink KJ, Broxterman HJ, Labots M, de Haas RR, Dekker H, Honeywell RJ, et al. Lysosomal sequestration of sunitinib: a novel mechanism of drug resistance. Clin Cancer Res 2011;17:7337–46.

[205] Batchelor TT, Sorensen AG, di Tomaso E, Zhang WT, Duda DG, Cohen KS, et al. AZD2171, a pan-VEGF receptor tyrosine kinase inhibitor, normalizes tumour vasculature and alleviates edema in glioblastoma patients. Cancer Cell 2007;11:83–95.

[206] Fischer C, Jonckx B, Mazzone M, Zacchigna S, Loges S, Pattarini L, et al. Anti-PlGF inhibits growth of VEGF(R)-inhibitor-resistant tumours without affecting healthy vessels. Cell 2007;131:463–75.

[207] Yu JL, Rak JW, Coomber BL, Hicklin DJ, Kerbel RS. Effect of p53 status on tumour response to antiangiogenic therapy. Science 2002;295:1526–8.

[208] Keunen O, Johansson M, Oudin A, Sanzey M, Rahim SA, Fack F, et al. Anti-VEGF treatment reduces blood supply and increases tumour cell invasion in glioblastoma. Proc Natl Acad Sci U S A 2011;108:3749–54.

[209] Pike LR, Singleton DC, Buffa F, Abramczyk O, Phadwal K, Li JL, et al. Transcriptional up-regulation of ULK1 by ATF4 contributes to cancer cell survival. Biochem J 2013;449:389–400.

[210] Mazure NM, Pouyssegur J. Atypical BH3-domains of BNIP3 and BNIP3L lead to autophagy in hypoxia. Autophagy 2009;5:868–9.

[211] Escudier B, Pluzanska A, Koralewski P, Ravaud A, Bracarda S, Szczylik C, et al. Bevacizumab plus interferon alfa-2a for treatment of metastatic renal cell carcinoma: a randomised, double-blind phase III trial. Lancet 2007;370:2103–11.

[212] Nyberg P, Salo T, Kalluri R. Tumour microenvironment and angiogenesis. Front Biosci 2008;13:6537–53.

[213] Meads MB, Hazlehurst LA, Dalton WS. The bone marrow microenvironment as a tumour sanctuary and contributor to drug resistance. Clin Cancer Res 2008;14:2519–26.

[214] Sun Y, Campisi J, Higano C, Beer TM, Porter P, Coleman I, et al. Treatment-induced damage to the tumour microenvironment promotes prostate cancer therapy resistance through WNT16B. Nat Med 2012;18:1359–68.

[215] Horimoto Y, Polanska UM, Takahashi Y, Orimo A. Emerging roles of the tumour-associated stroma in promoting tumour metastasis. Cell Adh Migr 2012;6:193–202.

[216] Fernando NT, Koch M, Rothrock C, Gollogly LK, D'Amore PA, Ryeom S, et al. Tumour escape from endogenous, extracellular matrix-associated angiogenesis inhibitors by up-regulation of multiple proangiogenic factors. Clin Cancer Res 2008;14:1529–39.

[217] Bennouna J, Sastre J, Arnold D, Osterlund P, Greil R, Van Cutsem E, et al. Continuation of bevacizumab after first progression in metastatic colorectal cancer (ML18147): a randomised phase 3 trial. Lancet Oncol 2012.

[218] Sitohy B, Nagy JA, Jaminet SC, Dvorak HF. Tumour-surrogate blood vessel subtypes exhibit differential susceptibility to anti-VEGF therapy. Cancer Res 2011;71:7021–8.

[219] Rubenstein JL, Kim J, Ozawa T, Zhang M, Westphal M, Deen DF, et al. Anti-VEGF antibody treatment of glioblastoma prolongs survival but results in increased vascular cooption. Neoplasia 2000;2:306–14.

[220] Foroni C, Broggini M, Generali D, Damia G. Epithelial–mesenchymal transition and breast cancer: role, molecular mechanisms and clinical impact. Cancer Treat Rev 2012;38:689–97.

[221] Sanchez-Tillo E, Liu Y, de Barrios O, Siles L, Fanlo L, Cuatrecasas M, et al. EMT-activating transcription factors in cancer: beyond EMT and tumour invasiveness. Cell Mol Life Sci 2012;69:3429–56.

[222] Hughes CC. Endothelial-stromal interactions in angiogenesis. Curr Opin Hematol 2008;15:204–9.

[223] Diaz-Flores L, Gutierrez R, Varela H. Behavior of postcapillary venule pericytes during postnatal angiogenesis. J Morphol 1992;213:33–45.

[224] Nehls V, Drenckhahn D. The versatility of microvascular pericytes: from mesenchyme to smooth muscle? Histochemistry 1993;99:1–2.

[225] Ozerdem U, Stallcup WB. Early contribution of pericytes to angiogenic sprouting and tube formation. Angiogenesis 2003;6:241–9.

[226] Mancuso MR, Davis R, Norberg SM, O'Brien S, Sennino B, Nakahara T, et al. Rapid vascular regrowth in tumours after reversal of VEGF inhibition. J Clin Invest 2006;116:2610–21.

[227] Stommel JM, Kimmelman AC, Ying H, Nabioullin R, Ponugoti AH, Wiedemeyer R, et al. Coactivation of receptor tyrosine kinases affects the response of tumour cells to targeted therapies. Science 2007;318:287–90.

[228] Baselga J, Campone M, Piccart M, Burris 3rd HA, Rugo HS, Sahmoud T, et al. Everolimus in postmenopausal hormone-receptor-positive advanced breast cancer. N Engl J Med 2012;366:520–9.

[229] Pircher A, Hilbe W, Heidegger I, Drevs J, Tichelli A, Medinger M. Biomarkers in tumour angiogenesis and anti-angiogenic therapy. Int J Mol Sci 2011;12:7077–99.

[230] Fox SB, Harris AL. Histological quantitation of tumour angiogenesis. APMIS 2004;112:413–30.

[231] Gasparini G. The rationale and future potential of angiogenesis inhibitors in neoplasia. Drugs 1999;58:17–38.

[232] Hlatky L, Hahnfeldt P, Folkman J. Clinical application of antiangiogenic therapy: microvessel density, what it does and doesn't tell us. J Natl Cancer Inst 2002;94:883–93.

[233] Vermeulen PB, Gasparini G, Fox SB, Colpaert C, Marson LP, Gion M, et al. Second international consensus on the methodology and criteria of evaluation of angiogenesis quantification in solid human tumours. Eur J Cancer 2002;38:1564–79.

[234] Toi M, Matsumoto T, Bando H. Vascular endothelial growth factor: its prognostic, predictive, and therapeutic implications. Lancet Oncol 2001;2:667–73.

[235] Gordon MS, Margolin K, Talpaz M, Sledge Jr GW, Holmgren E, Benjamin R, et al. Phase I safety and pharmacokinetic study of recombinant human anti-vascular endothelial growth factor in patients with advanced cancer. J Clin Oncol 2001;19:843–50.

[236] Jayson GC, Hicklin DJ, Ellis LM. Antiangiogenic therapy—evolving view based on clinical trial results. Nat Rev Clin Oncol 2012;9:297–303.

[237] An SJ, Huang YS, Chen ZH, Su J, Yang Y, Chen JG, et al. Posttreatment plasma VEGF levels may be associated with the overall survival of patients with advanced non-small cell lung cancer treated with bevacizumab plus chemotherapy. Med Oncol 2012;29:627–32.

[238] Duda DG, Willett CG, Ancukiewicz M, di Tomaso E, Shah M, Czito BG, et al. Plasma soluble VEGFR-1 is a potential dual biomarker of response and toxicity for bevacizumab with chemoradiation in locally advanced rectal cancer. Oncologist 2010;15:577–83.

[239] Schneider BP, Wang M, Radovich M, Sledge GW, Badve S, Thor A, et al. Association of vascular endothelial growth factor and vascular endothelial growth factor receptor-2 genetic polymorphisms with outcome in a trial of paclitaxel compared with paclitaxel plus bevacizumab in advanced breast cancer: ECOG 2100. J Clin Oncol 2008;26:4672–8.

[240] Koutras AK, Antonacopoulou AG, Eleftheraki AG, Dimitrakopoulos FI, Koumarianou A, Varthalitis I, et al. Vascular endothelial growth factor polymorphisms and clinical outcome in colorectal cancer patients treated with irinotecan-based chemotherapy and bevacizumab. Pharmacogenomics J 2012;12:468–75.

[241] Lambrechts D, Claes B, Delmar P, Reumers J, Mazzone M, Yesilyurt BT, et al. VEGF pathway genetic variants as biomarkers of treatment outcome with bevacizumab: an analysis of data from the AViTA and AVOREN randomised trials. Lancet Oncol 2012;13:724–33.

[242] Schultheis AM, Lurje G, Rhodes KE, Zhang W, Yang D, Garcia AA, et al. Polymorphisms and clinical outcome in recurrent ovarian cancer treated with cyclophosphamide and bevacizumab. Clin Cancer Res 2008;14:7554–63.

[243] Ronzoni M, Manzoni M, Mariucci S, Loupakis F, Brugnatelli S, Bencardino K, et al. Circulating endothelial cells and endothelial progenitors as predictive markers of clinical response to bevacizumab-based first-line treatment in advanced colorectal cancer patients. Ann Oncol 2010;21:2382–9.

[244] Collins JM. Imaging and other biomarkers in early clinical studies: one step at a time or re-engineering drug development? J Clin Oncol 2005;23:5417–9.

[245] Miller JC, Pien HH, Sahani D, Sorensen AG, Thrall JH. Imaging angiogenesis: applications and potential for drug development. J Natl Cancer Inst 2005;97:172–87.

[246] Anderson H, Price P, Blomley M, Leach MO, Workman P; Cancer Research Campaign PK/PD Technologies Advisory Committee. Measuring changes in human tumour vasculature in response to therapy using functional imaging techniques. Br J Cancer 2001;85(8):1085–93.

[247] Wedam SB, Low JA, Yang SX, Chow CK, Choyke P, Danforth D, et al. Antiangiogenic and antitumour effects of bevacizumab in patients with inflammatory and locally advanced breast cancer. J Clin Oncol 2006;24:769–77.

[248] Thukral A, Thomasson DM, Chow CK, Eulate R, Wedam SB, Gupta SN, et al. Inflammatory breast cancer: dynamic contrast-enhanced MR in patients receiving bevacizumab—initial experience. Radiology 2007;244:727–35.

[249] Padhani AR, Husband JE. Dynamic contrast-enhanced MRI studies in oncology with an emphasis on quantification, validation and human studies. Clin Radiol 2001;56:607–20.

[250] Atri M. New technologies and directed agents for applications of cancer imaging. J Clin Oncol 2006;24:3299–308.

[251] Chun YS, Vauthey JN, Boonsirikamchai P, Maru DM, Kopetz S, Palavecino M, et al. Association of computed tomography morphologic criteria with pathologic response and survival in patients treated with bevacizumab for colorectal liver metastases. JAMA 2009;302:2338–44.

[252] Koukourakis MI, Mavanis I, Kouklakis G, Pitiakoudis M, Minopoulos G, Manolas C, et al. Early antivascular effects of bevacizumab anti-VEGF monoclonal antibody on colorectal carcinomas assessed with functional CT imaging. Am J Clin Oncol 2007;30:315–8.

[253] Yao JC, Phan A, Hoff PM, Chen HX, Charnsangavej C, Yeung SC, et al. Targeting vascular endothelial growth factor in advanced carcinoid tumour: a random assignment phase II study of depot octreotide with bevacizumab and pegylated interferon alpha-2b. J Clin Oncol 2008;26:1316–23.

[254] Jiang T, Kambadakone A, Kulkarni NM, Zhu AX, Sahani DV. Monitoring response to antiangiogenic treatment and predicting outcomes in advanced hepatocellular carcinoma using image biomarkers, CT perfusion, tumour density, and tumour size (RECIST). Invest Radiol 2012;47:11–7.

[255] Young H, Baum R, Cremerius U, Herholz K, Hoekstra O, Lammertsma AA, et al. Measurement of clinical and subclinical tumour response using [18F]-fluorodeoxyglucose and positron emission tomography: review and 1999 EORTC recommendations. European Organization for Research and Treatment of Cancer (EORTC) PET Study Group. Eur J Cancer 1999;35:1773–82.

[256] Colavolpe C, Chinot O, Metellus P, Mancini J, Barrie M, Bequet-Boucard C, et al. FDG-PET predicts survival in recurrent high-grade gliomas treated with bevacizumab and irinotecan. Neuro-oncol 2012;14:649–57.

[257] Goshen E, Davidson T, Zwas ST, Aderka D. PET/CT in the evaluation of response to treatment of liver metastases from colorectal cancer with bevacizumab and irinotecan. Technol Cancer Res Treat 2006;5:37–43.

[258] Herbst RS, Mullani NA, Davis DW, Hess KR, McConkey DJ, Charnsangavej C, et al. Development of biologic markers of response and assessment of antiangiogenic activity in a clinical trial of human recombinant endostatin. J Clin Oncol 2002;20:3804–14.

[259] Liu G, Rugo HS, Wilding G, McShane TM, Evelhoch JL, Ng C, et al. Dynamic contrast-enhanced magnetic resonance imaging as a pharmacodynamic measure of response after acute dosing of AG-013736, an oral angiogenesis inhibitor, in patients with advanced solid tumours: results from a phase I study. J Clin Oncol 2005;23:5464–73.

[260] Rini BI, Cohen DP, Lu DR, Chen I, Hariharan S, Gore ME, et al. Hypertension as a biomarker of efficacy in patients with metastatic renal cell carcinoma treated with sunitinib. J Natl Cancer Inst 2011;103:763–73.

[261] van Heeckeren WJ, Ortiz J, Cooney MM, Remick SC. Hypertension, proteinuria, and antagonism of vascular endothelial growth factor signalling: clinical toxicity, therapeutic target, or novel biomarker? J Clin Oncol 2007;25:2993–5.

[262] Shim JH, Chen HM, Rich JR, Goddard-Borger ED, Withers SG. Directed evolution of a beta-glycosidase from *Agrobacterium* sp. to enhance its glycosynthase activity toward C3-modified donor sugars. Protein Eng Des Sel 2012;25:465–72.

[263] Dahlberg SE, Sandler AB, Brahmer JR, Schiller JH, Johnson DH. Clinical course of advanced non-small-cell lung cancer patients experiencing hypertension during treatment with bevacizumab in combination with carboplatin and paclitaxel on ECOG 4599. J Clin Oncol 2010;28:949–54.

The Renaissance of CYP17 Inhibitors for the Treatment of Prostate Cancer

Qingzhong Hu[1], Rolf W. Hartmann[1,2]

[1]Pharmaceutical & Medicinal Chemistry, Saarland University, Saarbrücken, Germany
[2]Helmholtz Institute for Pharmaceutical Research Saarland (HIPS), Saarbrücken, Germany

PROSTATE CANCER: EPIDEMIOLOGY, DIAGNOSIS, AND CURRENT THERAPIES

Prostate cancer (PCa) has the second highest incidence among cancers, accounting for 14% of newly diagnosed cancer cases worldwide in 2008, and more than a quarter of a million people died of it in the same year [1]. PCa has an even higher morbidity when looking at only industrialized countries, where it ranked first, followed by cancers in the lung and bronchus [1,2]. In 2012, 241,740 new cases were estimated in the United States, which accounts for 29% of all incident cancer cases. At the same time, 28,170 PCa patients are expected to die, representing 9% of the total of all cancer-related deaths.

The difference in incidences between industrialized and developing countries is caused to some degree by the extensive employment of prostate-specific antigen (PSA) screening in economically developed regions. PSA is a "chymotrypsin-like" serine protease [3] that is specifically produced by the prostate and therefore is exploited as a biomarker in the treatment of PCa [4]. When patients show more than $4\,ng/mL$ of PSA concentration in plasma, they are suspected of having PCa. This test frequently triggers false alarms [5] because elevated PSA levels can also be induced by prostatitis or benign prostatic hyperplasia. In spite of the criticism on this, PSA screening is acknowledged to be successful in reducing prostate cancer mortality [6]. The other screening method—digital rectal examination (DRE)—involves the inspection of the prostate gland regarding size, shape, and texture with a finger through the rectum. Although only the rear part of the prostate is detectable by DRE, it is still reliable because most PCas originate there. Observations of irregular shapes, lumps, and increased stiffness indicate potential PCa cases. Unfortunately, most cancers identified via DRE are in advanced stages with a poor prognosis. All suspected PCa cases identified via PSA tests or DRE are subsequently scrutinized with ultrasound or magnetic resonance imaging and ultimately confirmed by prostate biopsy to distinguish types, stages, and grades under the microscope.

Prostatic adenocarcinoma is the most frequently diagnosed PCa, which presents shrinkage or even disappearance of stroma and gland lumen compared to normal prostate. Irregular tumorous glands and prominent large nucleoli are also characteristic for prostatic adenocarcinoma. According to these histological observations, PCa patients are classified according to the Gleason grading system. The grades have been exploited as prognostic factors to predict the time to progression. PCa can also be staged based on the degree of metastasis. The primary localized PCa is divided into stage I or II regarding its size and visibility, whereas cancer spreading outside of the prostate to nearby tissues, the seminal vesicles for instance, is defined as stage III. Cases with metastasis to local lymph nodes and/or distant organs are categorized as stage IV. PCa metastasizes to the rectum, bladder, liver, and lungs; bones are the most favorable sites because of the abundant transferrin in bone tissue promoting cancer cells to proliferate [7].

Currently, several therapies are available. The treatment is chosen based on not only the grades and stages of the tumor but also the patients' situation such as age, health, and life expectancy [8].

Active surveillance implies no treatment but only monitoring PSA levels. It usually applies to patients with a life expectancy of less than 10 years, if the tumor is not aggressive, until the quality of life is reduced, for instance by pain or dysfunction in urination. For these patients, it is very likely that the cause of their death will not be PCa; therefore, it is not necessary to suffer the possible side effects of the treatment.

Local therapy consists of a set of nonpharmaceutical approaches to treating PCa, including prostatectomy, radiation therapy, and cryotherapy. However, these are suitable only for early-stage patients. *Prostatectomy* is the excision of the prostate and seminal vesicles and is currently the first-line therapy for PCa patients in stages I or II if they are younger than 70 and otherwise healthy. Because it is difficult to remove sufficient tissue to prevent recurrence, prostatectomy is not recommended for advanced diseases, although sometimes application in combination with hormone therapy is attempted. As an alternative, *radiation therapy* can be performed in two different ways depending on the location of the radiation source: external-beam radiation therapy (outside the body) and brachytherapy (implanted into the tumor tissue). Normally, brachytherapy is advantageous as maximum curative effects are achieved and at the same time the damage to the nearby normal tissues is minimal. *Cryotherapy*, on the other hand, is a minimally invasive surgery that is effective for recrudescent and radio-resistant PCa in the early stages by freezing the prostate gland and sometimes seminal vesicles with liquid nitrogen. It is of lower risk, elicits less discomfort compared to other local therapies, and can be exploited as a secondary treatment when other primary therapies fail.

Although local PCa in early stages can be cured with these treatments and the five-year survival can even approach 100% [9], advanced diseases, especially cases with metastasis, ineluctably result in death if not effectively controlled. These patients are commonly treated with *hormone therapy*; while chemotherapy is usually reserved as the last option due to severe side effects. *Chemotherapy* involves the employment of cytotoxic agents that destroy cancer cells in various ways, such as destruction of the cell membrane integrity resulting in necrosis, induction of apoptosis, and arrest of mitosis to block proliferation and differentiation. From docetaxel, approved in 2004 as the first cytotoxic agent for the treatment of PCa, to the latest cytotoxic agent for PCa, cabazitaxel (launched in 2010), the taxanes have been demonstrated to improve median survival time when applied in combination with prednisone [10]. However, cytotoxic agents affect all cells undergoing rapid mitosis; normal cells are therefore simultaneously damaged, especially cells in the bone marrow, digestive tract, and hair follicles, leading to common side effects such as myelosuppression, mucositis, and alopecia.

Radiopharmaceuticals targeting bone metastasis such as Strontium-89, Samarium-153, and Rhenium-186 were employed only for pain palliation until Radium-223 demonstrated an improvement of overall survival of 19 weeks [11]. Alpharadin (Radium-223 chloride) is an α-emitter with a short track length (<100 μm, about 2–10 cell diameters). Since it is also a calcium mimic, it can be maximally uptaken by bones (40–60% of applied dose), while the rest is rapidly excreted. These features render alpharadin to cause less damage to normal tissue, especially bone marrow, compared to other radiopharmaceuticals and traditional radiation therapy. Alpharadin is now on fast track to be granted approval by the US Food and Drug Administration (FDA) and is expected to be launched in 2013.

Cancer *immunotherapy* consists of several approaches stimulating the patients' immune system to kill cancer cells after the intervention of vaccines. Sipuleucel-T was the first vaccine, approved by FDA in 2010. This personalized treatment demonstrated an improvement in median survival of 4.1 months [12].

ANDROGENS AND HORMONE THERAPY

Hormone therapy as the first choice for patients with advanced PCa is based on the finding that the growth of up to 80% of PCa depends on androgen stimulation [13,14]. Therefore, segregation of androgens from tumor cells will effectively prevent these cells from further proliferation.

Androgen Secretion and Androgen Receptor Binding

The production of androgens is regulated by the hypothalamic–pituitary–gonadal–adrenal axes (Fig. 11.1). The hypothalamus as a vital modulator controls many basic functions of the body, such as blood pressure, immune response, and body temperature. It secretes several hormones directly targeting the pituitary via the hypophyseal portal system, for example the gonadotropin-releasing hormone (GnRH, also known as hypothalamic luteinizing hormone–releasing hormone (LHRH)) and the corticotropin-releasing hormone (CRH). GnRH and CRH stimulate the release of gonadotropins (Gn, including follicle-stimulating hormone (FSH) and luteinizing hormone (LH)) and the adrenocortico-tropic hormone (ACTH) from the anterior pituitary, respectively. Consequently, after binding to the corresponding receptors, Gn and ACTH trigger the production of androgens in testes and adrenals that is catalyzed by 17α-hydroxylase-17,20-lyase (CYP17) and other steroidogenic enzymes. An estimated 90% of androgens are produced in the testes, and less than 10% in the adrenals. Moreover, the adrenals secrete only testosterone, whereas in testes the testosterone generated in situ can be converted into dihydrotestosterone (DHT, the strongest androgen)—a process that is catalyzed by 5α-reductase (5α-R). Circulating testosterone is predominantly bound to the sex hormone–binding globulin and albumin, while only approximately 2% is available as free unbound

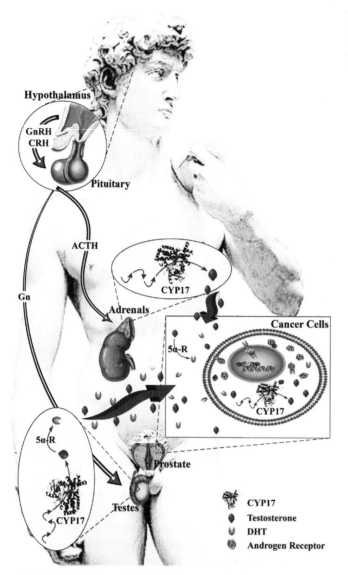

FIGURE 11.1 The regulation of androgen biosynthesis and the binding of androgen to androgen receptors in prostate cancer cells.

hormone. When the plasma concentration of testosterone is sufficient, it downregulates the production of GnRH and CRH via a negative feedback mechanism. Due to the presence of 5α-R in the prostate, DHT can also be formed in this gland from testosterone. Besides, de novo androgen biosynthesis in PCa cells from adrenal steroids or even cholesterol has recently been demonstrated [15], and this is a major reason why PCa becomes castration resistant [16].

These androgens subsequently bind to the androgen receptor (AR), which is overexpressed in PCa cells, resulting in cancer cell proliferation. The AR is a member of the steroid and nuclear receptor superfamily, and is similar in its structure and function manner [17] to other steroid receptors such as estrogen receptors, mineralocorticoid receptors, and progesterone receptors. AR floats in the cytoplasm, acting as an intracellular transcription factor. Unbound ARs are associated with heat shock proteins. After the binding of androgens, a series of sequential conformational changes is triggered to disassociate, dimers are formed, and phosphorylation happens. It is notable that phosphorylation or dephosphorylation of ARs has been deemed essential for agonism or antagonism [18]. These ARs subsequently translocate into the nucleus and bind to the androgen response element located in the promoter or enhancer region of the target gene. Recruitment of other transcriptional coregulators (e.g., steroid receptor coactivator 3) stimulates the transcriptional machinery and initiates the expression of AR-regulated genes, leading to mitogenic effects in prostate cancer cells. The recruitment of different coregulators (coactivator or corepressor) has been proven to be another switch of agonistic or antagonistic activity [19]. Besides the genomic effects, AR has also been observed to directly interact with cytosolic proteins from various signaling pathways in the prostate [20,21]. These nongenomic actions rapidly activate kinase signaling cascades or modulate the intracellular calcium levels, and therefore possibly contribute to the survival and proliferation of PCa cells [22].

Targets Relating to Androgen Stimulation

Two approaches are possible to separate PCa cells from the androgen stimulation: blockade of the AR by AR antagonists, which have been applied in the clinic for many years, and interruption of androgen biosyntheses (androgen deprivation therapy (ADT)). As for the latter, several nodes in the androgen secretion system are crucial (Fig. 11.1); however, not all of them are suitable targets. Reducing androgen secretion via interference with the hypothalamus–pituitary–testes axis is feasible. Castration can directly eradicate androgen production from testes, while application of GnRH analogs leads to the same effects by decreasing the Gn secretion via either desensitizing the gonadotrope cells (GnRH agonists) or antagonizing GnRH receptors in the pituitary (GnRH antagonists). On the contrary, the hypothalamus–pituitary–adrenals axis should be left alone because ACTH also controls the biosynthesis of glucocorticoids and mineralocorticoids besides that of androgens. Interference with the production and function of CRH or ACTH will lead to severe side effects. Moreover, enzymes in androgen biosynthesis are also promising targets. CYP17 is the pivotal enzyme responsible for the conversion of progestogens into androgens. Its inhibition can reduce the plasma testosterone level to less than 1 ng/dL [23]. On the contrary, despite the fact that 5α-R inhibitors [24] reduce intracellular prostatic DHT concentration and are therefore employed in the treatment of benign prostatic hyperplasia, they do not show effects in PCa patients because testosterone as the precursor of DHT can stimulate cancer cells to proliferate as well.

Treatments Using Hormone Therapy

Estrogen and Progestin

Applications of estrogens or progestins [25] as early attempts to suppress androgen production were soon abandoned because of gynecomastia and elevated cholesterol levels that lead to a higher risk of cardiovascular diseases.

Orchiectomy

Castration is a reasonable treatment due to the fact that more than 90% of the androgens are produced in the testes. It is a simple operation and inexpensive compared to other long-term therapies. However, not everyone is willing to take permanent impotency as a consequence.

GnRH Analogs (Agonists and Antagonists)

Application of GnRH analogs is also known as "chemical castration". Both agonists and antagonists can suppress Gn secretion and thus block the production of testicular androgens. As for agonists, initial application leads to a surge of FSH and LH secretion after their binding to GnRH receptors in gonadotrope cells in the pituitary. This surge causes a large amount of testosterone and DHT to be produced in the testes, and thus leads to a tumor growth spurt (termed "tumor flare"). Nevertheless, after around 10 days, these gonadotrope cells are no longer sensitive to endogenous GnRH or GnRH agonists, leading to a major reduction in Gn concentration and consequently to the decline of androgen levels comparable to that after castration. This suppression of androgen production lasts as long as GnRH agonists are consecutively administered [26]. On the other hand, GnRH antagonists competitively bind to the GnRH receptor and consequently block Gn release directly. Although GnRH analogs, such as leuprolide, goserelin, and buserelin (Fig. 11.2), annihilate the androgen production in testes, they have no effect on adrenals. Despite the fact that the plasma testosterone concentration is reduced to less than 50 ng/dL, the androgens inside the prostate, which either originate from adrenals or are synthesized de novo in the tumor, are still in concentrations high enough to promote cancer cell growth [27,28]. Moreover, side effects such as testicular atrophy and loss

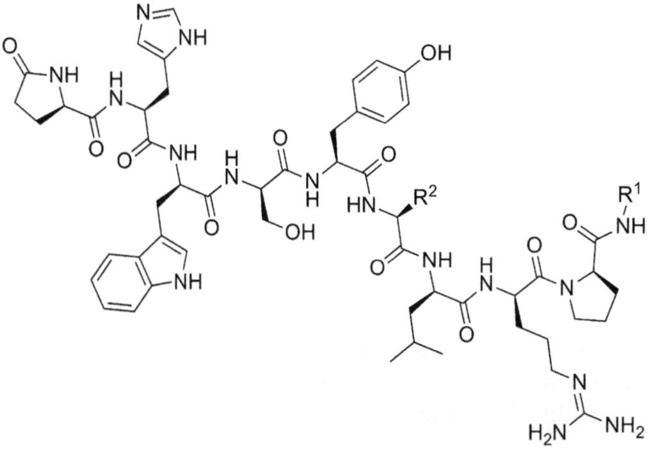

FIGURE 11.2 GnRH analogs in clinical use.

Compd	R¹	R²
Leuprolide	Et	*i*-Pr
Goserelin	ureido	*t*-BuO
Buserelin	Et	*t*-BuO
Histrelin	Et	1-benzyl-1*H*-imidazol-4-yl
Nafarelin	2-amino-2-oxoethyl	naphthalen-2-ylmethyl
Deslorelin	Et	1*H*-indol-3-yl

of bone mineral density are also observed as the consequences of the application of GnRH analogs.

AR Antagonists (Antiandrogens)

Since GnRH analogs show no blockade of adrenal androgen production, they are combined with AR antagonists (Fig. 11.3). This is the current standard therapy, the so-called combined androgen blockade (CAB), which has been demonstrated to be more effective than AR antagonists alone. Since steroidal AR antagonists are less potent than nonsteroidal ones and additionally suppress the production of some adrenal steroids, nonsteroidal AR antagonists are mainly employed. CAB is successful in delaying the progression of the disease and improving overall survival [29]. However, some cases progress to castration-resistant prostate cancer (CRPC). Several reasons could be responsible for this progression, such as intratumoral androgen biosynthesis and ligand-independent activation of AR. Moreover, early AR antagonists like bicalutamide exhibit mixed agonistic and antagonistic activities, and this partial agonism can be boosted by overexpression of AR and some other transcriptional factors, such as the forkhead box transcription factor A (FoxA1), consequently leading to resistance. Furthermore, the long-term application of antiandrogens induces AR mutations, such as T877A and W741C, which reduce the receptor's capability to recognize AR antagonists [30,31] and glucocorticoids [32] as agonists. Fortunately, CRPC has recently been demonstrated to be still hormone dependent by the brilliant performance of the CYP17 inhibitor abiraterone [23]. This finding has also been confirmed by the second-generation AR antagonist enzalutamide (MDV3100). It has higher AR affinity compared to previous AR antagonists, reduces AR translocation into the nucleus, and impairs DNA binding and coactivator recruitment [33]. It shows no agonism, even in the presence of highly overexpressed AR and FoxA1 [34]. Furthermore, greater than 50% reduction in the serum PSA level has been reported in over half of the PCa patients under enzalutamide treatment [35]. More importantly, improvement

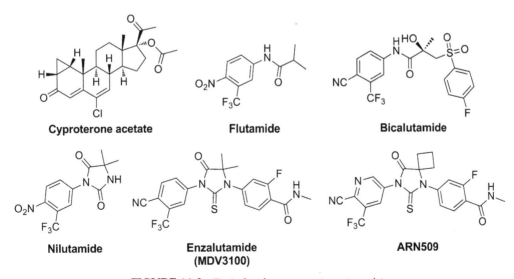

FIGURE 11.3 Typical androgen receptor antagonists.

of overall survival by 4.8 months has been achieved [36]. Enzalutamide has been launched in 2012, while a rather similar analog, ARN-509, is presently in a late clinical-trial phase [37].

INHIBITION OF CYP17 AS A PROMISING TREATMENT FOR PROSTATE CANCER

The Central Role of CYP17 in Androgen Biosynthesis

The biosynthesis of androgens (Fig. 11.4) starts with cholesterol, which is produced during the metabolism of fatty acids. After the side chain of cholesterol is cleaved by CYP11A1 (cholesterol side-chain cleavage enzyme, P450scc), pregnenolone is generated. This is actually the rate-limiting step in the biosynthesis route of steroidal hormones. Pregnenolone is subsequently converted into progesterone after further dehydrogenation catalyzed by 3β-hydroxysteroid dehydrogenase/Δ4-5 isomerase (3β-HSD). These two precursors are then hydroxylated at the 17α position followed by cleavage of the C17-20 bond. Both steps are catalyzed by CYP17, yielding dehydroepiandrosterone (DHEA) and androstenedione, which are subsequently converted to testosterone and finally DHT.

CYP17 is the hinge of steroid biosynthesis; its presence and activity determine which hormones are produced. In adrenal zonaglomerulosa lacking CYP17 expression, steroidogenesis goes directly to the mineralocorticoid aldosterone (Fig. 11.4). On the contrary, in the zona fasciculata and zona reticularis, the presence of CYP17 facilitates the production of other steroids. This enzyme switches the direction of steroid biosynthesis due to its catalytic bifunctionality, namely, 17α-hydroxylase and C17,20-lyase activities. In the zona fasciculata, 17α-hydroxylation predominates, leading to the formation of 17α-hydroxypregnenolone and 17α-hydroxyprogesterone, which are then converted to glucocorticoids by 11β-hydroxylase (CYP11B1); whereas in the zona reticularis and in the gonads, the presence of both activities leads to the production of DHEA and androstenedione [38]. Although the reasons for this interesting phenomenon and the mechanism of one enzyme having two activities are still unclear, several regulators of 17,20-lyase activity have been identified, such as the abundance of osidoreductase [39] and cytochrome b5 [40] as well as the phosphorylation of serine and threonine residues [41].

Androgens can be produced not only in testes and adrenals, but also inside PCa cells, and their biosynthesis is also dependent on CYP17. Therefore, inhibition of CYP17 can totally block androgen production and thus prevent further stimulation of PCa cells.

It is notable that other cytochrome P450 (CYP) enzymes are also very important for steroidogenesis. CYP11A1 starts the whole route; CYP11B1 is responsible for the production of glucocorticoids such as cortisol, and aldosterone synthase (CYP11B2) is the key enzyme of the mineralocorticoid (e.g., aldosterone) biosynthesis (Fig. 11.4); while steroid 21-hydroxylase (CYP21) is involved in both. The interference with these enzymes will lead to severe side effects and toxicity; selectivity over these steroidogenic CYPs is therefore a crucial safety factor for CYP17 inhibitors.

CYP17: Biochemistry and Crystal Structure

CYP17 is a cysteinato-heme enzyme belonging to the cytochrome P450 superfamily. It contains a heme group, which is covalently linked to the protein through the sulfur atom of a

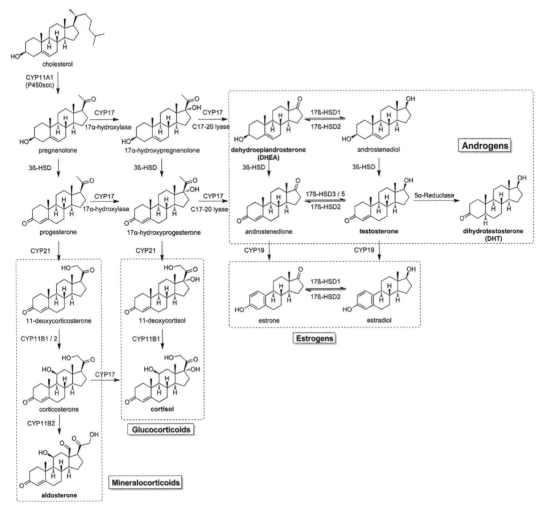

FIGURE 11.4 CYP17 in the biosynthesis route of androgens.

proximal cysteine. The heme is the reactive center to activate molecule oxygen and to oxidize the substrate. CYP17 comprises 508 amino acids with an approximate molecular weight of 57 kDa; it is coded by gene *CYP17*, which is located in chromosome 10 q24.3.

CYP17 adopts the common oxidation mechanism proposed for CYP enzymes (Fig. 11.5) that involves the sequential two-electron reduction, spin state alternation of the iron, and two protonations [42]. In the resting state, water coordinates to the iron (A) until the substrate binds in the active site of the enzyme. After displacement of the water molecule, the state of the heme iron changes from low spin to high spin, which facilitates the transfer of an electron from NAD(P)H via an electron transfer system, reducing the ferric ion to a ferrous ion (C). This intermediate species is then bound by oxygen at the distal axial coordination position of the heme iron, leading to an oxy-P450 complex (D). Interestingly, it can also coordinate with CO, showing a maximum absorption at a wavelength of approximately 450 nM, which is the

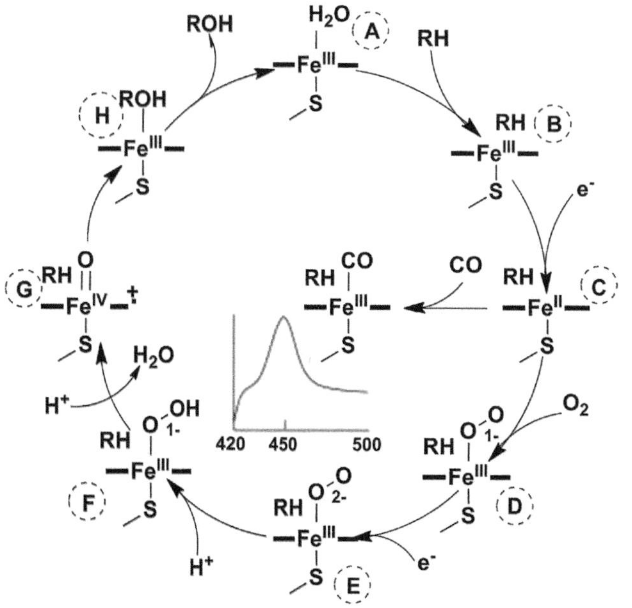

FIGURE 11.5 Catalytic mechanism of cytochrome P450.

origin of the name P450. The oxy-P450 complex as the last relatively stable intermediate is subsequently reduced by a second electron to a peroxo-ferric intermediate (E), which is then rapidly protonated twice by local transfer from water or surrounding amino acid side chains, releasing one water molecule and forming a highly reactive iron(IV)-oxo species (G). After the subsequent oxygenation of the substrate (H) and the release of the product, the heme returns to its resting state.

CYP17 binds to the endoplasmic reticulum, and the consequent difficulties of crystallization have meant that its crystal structure was not determined until 2012. CYP17 presents a similar folding configuration and topology to other CYP enzymes with highly conserved helices A–L. The I- and L-helices bind the heme; while residues in the B-, F- and I-helices are involved in the recognition, binding of the substrates, and release of the products. The most significant feature distinguishing CYP17 from other CYP enzymes like CYP19 is that the steroidal substrates lean on the I-helix, orienting to helices F and G instead of positioning against the K–L loop [43] (Fig. 11.6).

STEROIDAL CYP17 INHIBITORS

CYP17 inhibitors have been designed predominately by a ligand-based approach. This was due to the long-term absence of a crystal structure, which was solved very recently [43], and it can be expected that the first compound derived from structure-based approaches will be published soon. So far, the natural substrates (pregnenolone and progesterone; Fig. 11.7) were therefore used as the best templates to work on, leading to a large number of steroidal CYP17 inhibitors. Three different inhibitory mechanisms have been exploited

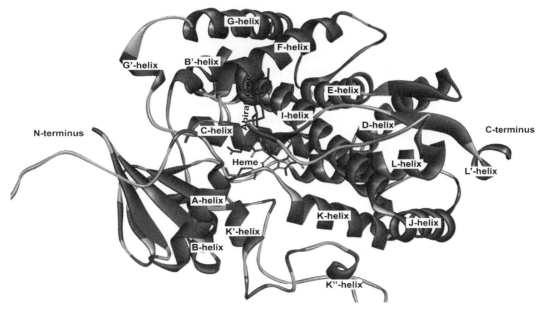

FIGURE 11.6 Crystal structure of CYP17 bound with abiraterone (PDB ID: 3RUK).

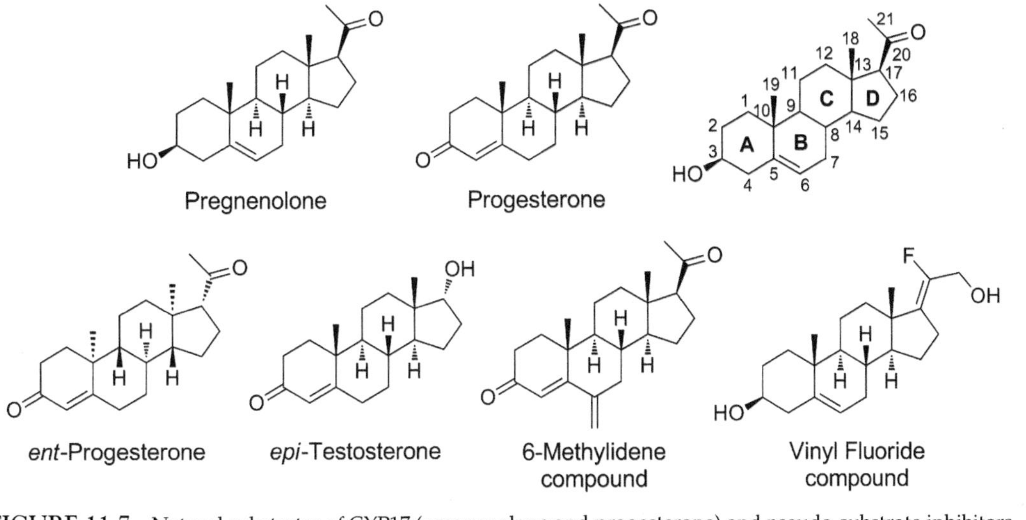

Pregnenolone

Progesterone

ent-Progesterone

epi-Testosterone

6-Methylidene compound

Vinyl Fluoride compound

FIGURE 11.7 Natural substrates of CYP17 (pregnenolone and progesterone) and pseudo-substrate inhibitors.

in the development of steroidal inhibitors: competition using pseudo-substrates, covalent binding attack after activation by the enzyme (mechanism inactivators), and coordination to the heme iron. Interestingly, only the last mechanism has been applied to nonsteroidal CYP17 inhibitors.

Pseudo-substrates

Endogenous steroidal hormones exhibit conservative stereo-configuration (e.g., 10β, 13β, and 17β), which is important for the recognition and the interaction with their targets. Artificial stereoisomers (Fig. 11.7) *ent*-progesterone [44] and *epi*-testosterone [45] cannot be metabolized by CYP17 after their binding and thus achieve competitive inhibition with weak potency. Moreover, 6-methylidene substituted progesterone has been reported as a dual inhibitor of CYP17 and 5α-R with similar potency. It also prevents androgen uptake by the prostate and thus leads to prostatic regression [46]. Furthermore, vinyl fluoride has been introduced at the 17 position of the pregnenolone scaffold to mimic the enol state of the acetyl group, resulting in high inhibition against cynomolgus monkey testicular CYP17 [47].

Mechanism Inactivators

The interesting finding that cyclopropyl amino or ether groups irreversibly bind to the P450 enzymes was reported in the 1980s [48] and was soon applied in the design of CYP17 inhibitors [49]. It was shown that the cyclopropyl amino or ether compounds were activated by the enzymatic one-electron oxidation of nitrogen or oxygen atoms, leading to the cleavage of the cyclopropyl ring and subsequently the formation of reactive radicals. These radicals covalently bind to the CYP enzyme while still binding in the active site, and therefore inactivate the enzyme [50]. Since CYP17 oxidizes the 17 position of the steroidal scaffold, cyclopropyl amino or ether moieties were introduced at the corresponding position (Fig. 11.8). Further modifications were also performed, such as furnishing substituents, rearranging the double bonds, replacing C with N at the 4 position, and inserting methylidene in the steroidal scaffold [51–53]. These efforts led to some potent CYP17 inhibitors acting in a time-dependent manner [51]. Although these compounds arrested the growth of androgen-dependent human prostatic tumors in mice, they were less effective than castration [52].

Ligands Coordinating to the Heme Iron

In CYP enzymes, an iron atom is chelated by the quadridentate protoporphyrin while the evolutionary conserved cysteine as the proximal ligand of this iron attaches the whole heme to the enzyme. The sixth coordination position, however, is reserved because the heme iron is the reaction center to activate the molecule oxygen and subsequently insert one of the

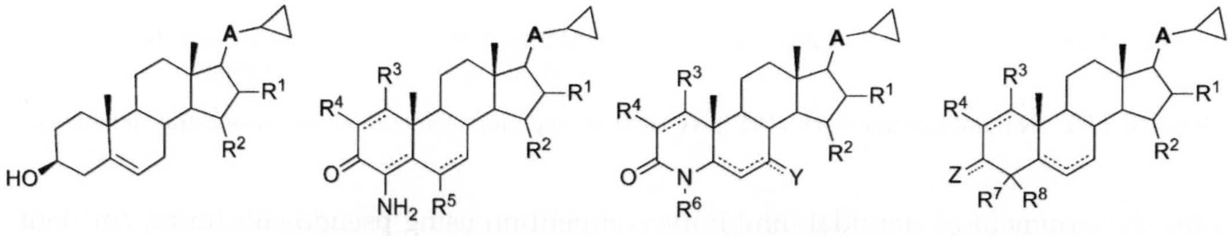

A = NH, O;   Y = O, alkyl, hydroxyl, alkyloxy, halo;   Z = O, OH, alkanoyloxy; R^1, R^6 = H, alkyl;
R^2 = halo, phenylsulfinyl, alkyl; R^3, R^4 = halo, alkyl; R^7, R^8 = H, halo, alkyl

FIGURE 11.8   General structures of mechanism-based inactivators.

oxygen atoms into the substrate, leading to product formation. Therefore, occupation of the heme iron with coordinating ligands will block the binding of endogenous substrate and dislodge it from the active site, resulting in a competitive reversible inhibition of the enzyme. Heterocycles containing sp^2 hybrid N were demonstrated to be the most effective coordinating groups. Besides, other moieties such as oxime [54–57], aziridine [54,58], diaziridine and diazirine [59], azetidine [59], thiirane [59], oxirane [59], N-methylformamide [55,60], amino [58], hydroxyl [54], thiophene [61], and furan [61] were also inserted into pregnenolone or progesterone scaffolds (Fig. 11.9). Nearly all analogs showed only weak to moderate activity except the oxime compounds, whose inhibitory potency can be very high toward human CYP17 (IC_{50} values up to 10 nM). These compounds also reduce serum testosterone and DHT levels without hypothalamic LH being affected [54]. Moreover, hydroxamates as bidentate donors to metal ions were speculated to be able to remove the heme iron from the porphyrin complex and thus inactivate the enzyme in a noncompetitive manner. However, only weak inhibition was observed [62]. Furthermore, it has also been revealed that the Δ16-17 double bond can significantly increase inhibitory potency [54,56], while the stereo-configuration of the 20 position is also crucial [55].

The coordination of the sp^2 hybrid N to the heme iron was initially demonstrated between some antifungal agents and CYP enzymes, characterized by the red shift in ultraviolet absorption [63], and subsequently between CYP19 inhibitors and their target enzyme [64]. The finding was soon successfully exploited in designing inhibitors of CYP19 [65–70], CYP11B1 [71–73], and CYP11B2 [74–83]. Many CYP17 inhibitors have also been designed with different sp^2 hybrid nitrogen-containing heterocycles substituted at the 17 position of modified pregnenolone or progesterone scaffolds in which a Δ16-17 double bond was commonly inserted. In contrast to many other potent steroidal CYP17 inhibitors, abiraterone was approved by the FDA in 2011 and gleterone is in phase II clinical trial now.

Abiraterone (Zytiga®: Abiraterone Acetate)

Abiraterone as the first-in-class of CYP17 inhibitors was launched as its acetate prodrug form with the brand name of Zytiga®. Abiraterone is based on the pregnenolone scaffold with an additional Δ16-17 double bond. 3-Pyridyl was employed as the coordinating group replacing the acetyl group of prognenolone at the 17 position (Fig. 11.10). Although the logP

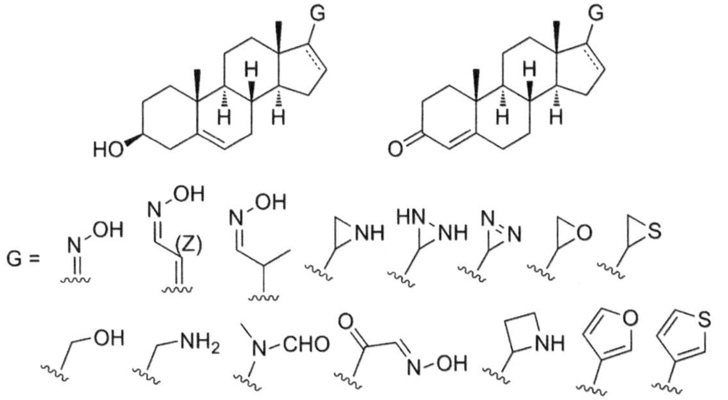

FIGURE 11.9 Steroidal inhibitors of CYP17 with coordinating groups other than heterocycles containing sp^2 hybrid N.

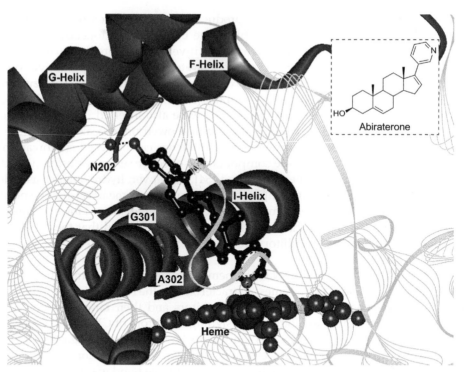

FIGURE 11.10   Abiraterone and its binding in CYP17 active site.

value of abiraterone acetate is 5.19, which actually breaks Lipinski's rule of 5, it is orally applied [84]. Abiraterone strongly inhibits both 17α-hydroxylase (IC$_{50}$ = 4nM) and C17-20 lyase (IC$_{50}$ = 2.9nM) activities of CYP17 in a human testicular microsome assay [85]. The Δ16-17 double bond was demonstrated to be responsible for its irreversible inhibition and promoted the inhibitory potency by around 12-fold compared to the 17β-pyridyl analog without a double bond [86]. Abiraterone does not interfere with CYP19 and 5α-R (IC$_{50}$s > 50μM), but showed moderate inhibition of CYP11B1 (IC$_{50}$ = 1610nM) and CYP11B2 (IC$_{50}$ = 1750nM) [87]. It is also a potent inhibitor of hepatic CYP1A2, CYP2D6, and CYP2C8, as well as a moderate inhibitor of CYP2B6, CYP2C9, CYP2C19, CYP3A4, and CYP3A5 [84,88]. Accordingly, it is not surprising that abiraterone elevated both the maximal concentration (C_{max}) and the area under the curve (AUC) of dextromethorphan, a known CYP2D6 substrate, by around threefold in a drug–drug interaction trial [84]. Abiraterone itself is a substrate of CYP3A4, which oxidizes aromatic N, leading to an inability to coordinate to the heme iron. Moreover, abiraterone inhibits 3β-hydroxysteroid dehydrogenase, which is responsible for the conversion of DHEA and androstenediol to androstenedione and testosterone, respectively (Fig. 11.4), with an IC$_{50}$ value below 1μM [89]. This inhibition may also contribute to its antitumor effect. Furthermore, recent studies revealed that abiraterone interferes with AR as well. Abiraterone decreased up to approximately 80% of the steady-state AR levels in LNCaP cells at a concentration of 15μM after a three-day application [90]. This was achieved by interfering with the cap-dependent translational machinery to reduce AR synthesis because abiraterone does not affect the degradation of AR. Moreover, abiraterone showed low binding affinity for the AR but moderate blockade of AR-mediated transactivation [90]. Its ability to inhibit AR translocation to the nucleus has also been demonstrated [89,90].

The co-crystal structure of CYP17 and abiraterone illustrates its binding to the active site. Abiraterone coordinates to the heme iron with its pyridyl N in a nearly perpendicular manner (Fig. 11.10), while the steroidal scaffold presents an angle of 60° to the heme plane leaning to the I-helix, more precisely: the hydrophobic surface formed by Gly301 and Ala302. Moreover, the OH group at the 3β position interacts with Asn202 via a hydrogen bond. All these interactions endow abiraterone with high affinity for the CYP17 enzyme [43].

Abiraterone exhibits potent inhibition of rat CYP17 with an IC_{50} value of 220 nM [88]. Although no information about its inhibition of mouse CYP17 is available, abiraterone has been shown to significantly reduce plasma testosterone concentration (<0.1 nM) as well as the weights of prostate, seminal vesicles, kidneys, and testes in mice; however, this is at the expense of an elevation of plasma LH by three- to fourfold [91].

Around 60 clinical trials on abiraterone had been registered by November 2012 according to www.clinicaltrial.gov. Fourteen of them have been completed, while eight and 38 clinical trials are still ongoing or are recruiting to start soon, respectively. The success of the completed clinical trials ensured the approval of abiraterone.

It has been revealed that until the dose of abiraterone acetate was increased to 500 mg, no constant effects on plasma testosterone levels were observed. On the other hand, application of 500 mg abiraterone acetate per day to advanced PCa patients who were castrated or maintaining GnRH analogs was successful in reducing testosterone concentrations to undetectable levels (<0.14 nM/L) or less than 25% of baseline levels [92]. Similarly, the same dose led to a 50% reduction of baseline testosterone levels in noncastrated patients, although the targeted levels of <0.7 nM/L were not reached. However, this suppression was overcome after 6–9 days because of an increase (up to threefold) of LH as the consequence of negative feedback [92]. This provides a reason for using GnRH analogs in combination. In contrast, 1000 mg per day of abiraterone acetate reduces testosterone to undetectable levels within 8 days [23]. Due to the plateau of observed pharmacodynamic effects [23], the dose of 1000 mg/day was selected for further clinical trials and as the final prescribing dose. The single dosing of abiraterone exhibited protracted suppression of androgen production [92], consistent with its irreversible inhibition behavior.

After oral application of the acetate prodrug, abiraterone can be detected only in doses over 200 mg [92]. Abiraterone acetate plasma levels were below detectable levels (<0.2 ng/mL) even at 1000 mg doses [84,93], indicating rapid conversion from acetate prodrug to free abiraterone. As for the standard 1000 mg per day dosing, the median time to reach the maximum plasma concentration (t_{max}) was 2 h with C_{max} of 226 ± 178 ng/mL and AUC of 1173 ± 690 ng h/mL [84]. The latter two parameters increased proportionally according to the elevation of the dose from 250 to 1000 mg [84]. However, discrepancies in findings were reported [23,92,93] from early phase I clinical trials, probably due to the limited number of patients. The exposure of abiraterone was also significantly promoted by food ingestion: C_{max} and AUC values were 17 and 10 times higher, respectively, with a high-fat diet [84]. Abiraterone can be oxidized at the aromatic nitrogen atom by hepatic CYP3A4 to form the N-oxide analog. This leads to deactivation due to the loss of coordinating ability to the heme iron. The N-oxide analog and parent abiraterone can also be transformed by sulfotransferase SULT2A1 to inactive metabolite N-oxide abiraterone sulfate and abiraterone sulfate, respectively. These two major circulating metabolites each accounted for 43% of the total metabolites [84]. Furthermore, the mean terminal half-life ($t_{1/2}$) of abiraterone in plasma is around 12h, which makes an oral application once a day possible. Approximately 88% of abiraterone acetate was excreted by feces with only about 5% by urine. Since abiraterone acetate hydrolyzes to free abiraterone in blood very rapidly, the fact that approximately 55% of the compound in feces was original abiraterone acetate [84] might indicate poor gastrointestinal absorption. As for the sources of free abiraterone in feces, which accounted for around 22% [84], both excretion via bile and hydrolysis from acetate prodrug assisted by bacteria are possible.

After abiraterone acetate was administrated to castrated (either by orchiectomy or with GnRH analogs applied) CRPC patients, not only were the plasma concentrations of testosterone suppressed to undetectable levels (<1ng/dL), but also other hormones were influenced. DHEA was downregulated by threefold to a median concentration of 79.2ng/dL, dehydroepiandrostenedione sulfate (DHEA-S) was undetectable in plasma (<15µg/dL), and androstenedione was suppressed by 16-fold to less than 2ng/dL [23,93]. The production of downstream estradiol was blocked as well, leading to concentrations of <80pg/dL [93]. Unfortunately, no information on the alteration of pregnenolone, progesterone, 17α-hydroxypregnenolone, and 17α-hydroxyprogesterone has been published. Moreover, the plasma concentrations of 11-deoxycorticosterone (DOC) and corticosterone increased by 10- and 40-fold to 69 and 6514ng/dL, respectively. These elevations of mineralocorticoids were explained as being the consequence of the fivefold increase of ACTH secretion, which is probably due to negative feedback of downregulated cortisol levels (twofold) [23]. The reduction of aldosterone concentrations by 1.5-fold was speculated to be caused by the negative feedback from the renin–angiotensin–aldosterone system that was activated by the high levels of DOC and corticosterone [23]. However, another possibility was not considered: the decrease of aldosterone could be a result of the inhibition of CYP11B2 by abiraterone, which is the pivotal enzyme in aldosterone production (IC$_{50 \text{ CYP11B2}}$ = 1750nM). Similar inhibition of CYP11B1 (responsible for the biosynthesis of cortisol) by abiraterone (IC$_{50 \text{ CYP11B1}}$ = 1610nM) could also account for the reduction of cortisol levels, which are in contrast to the fourfold elevated concentrations of precursor 11-deoxycortisol [23]. Furthermore, the concentrations of FSH and LH remained in the normal range in these orchiectomized CRPC patients [23,92].

As the major biomarker in the treatment of PCa, PSA levels were significantly reduced in most of the patients who were treated with abiraterone. However, the probability and extent of the PSA decline largely depended on the situation and treatment history of patients, such as the baseline concentrations of testosterone and PSA, metastases, and the history of ketoconazaole and docetaxel treatment. In ketoconazole-naïve patients, the median percentage to achieve PSA decline by 50% or more was 68% (ranges found: 57% [23], 64% [93], 67% [94], and 79% [95]) for the docetaxel chemotherapy-naïve cohort, which was much higher than the 45% [96] for postdocetaxel patients. Analogical results were observed in a postketoconazole cohort: 47% of chemotherapy-naïve patients [93] exhibited a PSA decline of more than 50%, whereas only 26% of postdocetaxel patients [96] achieved this. Similarly, ketoconazole-naïve patients showed a higher probability of a decrease in PSA of over 50% than postketoconazole ones in both chemotherapy-naïve and postdocetaxel cohorts (64% vs 47% and 45% vs 26%, respectively) [93,96]. The same trend was observed for the median PSA progression time, namely, 169 days for postdocetaxel patients [96,97], which was apparently shorter than that for docetaxel-naïve patients

(234 days [93] and 225 days [94]). Moreover, around half of the patients showed a reduction in the number of circulating tumor cells to fewer than five per 7.5 mL blood [94,95,97]. Partial responses defined according to Response Evaluation Criteria in Solid Tumors (RECIST) were also identified in 18–37% of patients [94,96,97]. Furthermore, an interesting phenomenon called "bone scan flare" was observed in up to 48% of patients [95]. The bone scan results of these patients were interpreted as "disease progression" characterized by the increase in the number or intensity of lesions despite the fact that the PSA level was reduced by 50% or more. These patients eventually showed improvement or stability in the bone scan after another 3 months of treatment. Although this bone scan flare has been reported before in the treatment of PCa, the high incidence of 48% in the abiraterone clinical trial is surprising.

The improvement of these clinical parameters is associated with an increase of overall survival. In the multicenter, double-blind, placebo-controlled phase III study (COU-AA-301), 1195 postdocetaxel patients with metastatic CRPC were recruited. Of these patients, 797 were administered abiraterone acetate 1000 mg per day, in combination with prednisone 5 mg twice daily; the rest were given placebos and prednisone. The median overall survival for the abiraterone group was 15.8 months, which is clearly longer than that of the placebo arm (11.2 months) [98,99]. Of the patients in the abiraterone group, 29.5% showed reductions of PSA levels by 50% or more, and the median PSA progression time was 8.5 months [98,99]. Moreover, in another phase III clinical trial (COU-AA-302) for docetaxel-naïve CRPC patients, the Independent Data Monitoring Committee decided to unblind the study and cross all patients from placebo to abiraterone acetate at the interim analysis [100].

Abiraterone was well tolerated, and no dose-limiting toxicity was observed even when the dose was increased to 2000 mg per day [23,92]. However, large clinical trials revealed some side effects. Hypokalemia, hypertension, and edema are symptoms that result from the above-mentioned elevated levels of mineralocorticoids. They were managed with eplerenone or glucocorticoids such as prednisone and dexamethasone. Moreover, elevations of aspartate aminotransferase, alanine aminotransferase, and total bilirubin, indicating liver dysfunction, were also observed. The incidence of cardiac disorders, such as arrhythmia and cardiac failure, was higher in the abiraterone arm compared to the placebo group. Although only few patients reached grade 3 or 4, further monitoring is needed after the drug has been launched to market, because cardiovascular mortality has been proven to be higher in PCa patients under androgen deprivation [101]. Other common adverse reactions, such as fatigue, muscle discomfort, hot flushes, diarrhea, urinary tract infection, and coughs, were mild [84,98–100].

The combined application of glucocorticoids, such as prednisone and dexamethasone, not only relieved the secondary mineralocorticoid excess by suppressing ACTH secretion, but also partially reversed the resistance to abiraterone. As a mechanism for the latter effect, a reduction was proposed of steroids upstream to testosterone that were speculated to be able to activate AR [98–100].

By now, several clinical trials examining the performance of abiraterone in combination with other agents are ongoing or about to be started, for example with cabazitaxel (a chemotherapeutic), enzalutamide (an AR antagonist), veliparib (a poly ADP ribose polymerase (PARP) inhibitor), sipuleucel-T (a PCa vaccine), and ipilimumab (a monoclonal antibody). Besides, the application of abiraterone for other indications is also being evaluated, such as in adult women with the 21-hydroxylase deficiency and postmenopausal women with advanced or metastatic breast cancer.

Gleterone (TOK-001, VN/124-1)

Despite the minor difference between abiraterone (3-pyridyl) and gleterone (Fig. 11.11, 1-benzimidazolyl, whose 1-N connects to steroidal scaffold directly), the latter is reported to be 2.7-fold more potent in an assay using CYP17 expressed from *Escherichia coli* [102]. Gleterone exhibits a similar binding mode for CYP17 as abiraterone, with the exception that it occupies an additional hydrophobic pocket demarcated by Val366, Ala367, Ile371, and Val483 with its benzene moiety [43]. Gleterone downregulates both wild-type (WT) and mutated AR in LNCaP cells to a similar level as abiraterone, in a dose-dependent reversible manner [90,103]. However, in LAPC-4 cells its performance was worse than abiraterone [88]. It is debatable whether gleterone can promote AR degradation [90,103], but the impairment of the cap-dependent translational machinery to decrease AR protein expression was demonstrated [90]. Gleterone has much higher affinity toward AR than abiraterone in both WT and mutated (W741C and W741C) enzymes. It showed comparable blockade of the AR transactivation to the antiandrogen bicalutamide in WT AR and sustained the ability toward the above-mentioned mutated AR. No agonist or partial-agonist activity of gleterone was observed for these three types of AR. Bicalutamide, by contrast, was recognized as an agonist for mutated AR [90]. It is notable that gleterone also reduced the androgen-stimulated nuclear translocation of AR. Moreover, induction of the endoplasmic reticulum stress response by gleterone was disputed in different studies [90,104]. All these effects contributed to the antiproliferative effects in vitro [90,103] and the antitumor activity in mouse LAPC-4 xenografts [103,105]. Furthermore, gleterone has a dose-independent pharmacokinetic profile in mice after subcutaneous application, with a half-life of 44min [102].

The recently released phase I clinical trial data for gleterone [106] indicates that this multimechanism CYP17 inhibitor is well tolerated even at a high dose of 2600mg per day with only minor side effects, such as fatigue, nausea, and diarrhea. Eleven out of 49 patients exhibited reductions of PSA levels by 50% or more. Tumor regression was also identified with computed tomography (CT) scans for some patients. Gleterone will be further evaluated in a phase II clinical trial for long-term safety and efficacy in CRPC patients who are hormone therapy naïve. This drug candidate has been granted fast-track designation by the FDA and will hopefully be approved in the near future.

Other Heterocycles

Besides 3-pyridyl in abiraterone and 1-benzimidazolyl in gleterone, further heterocycles have been exploited as coordinating groups leading to various activity profiles in vitro and in vivo (Fig. 11.12), such as imidazolyl [107–110], 1,2,3-triazolyl [107–109], 1,2,4-triazolyl [109], tetrazolyl [107,108], pyrazolyl [107,108,110], oxazolyl [110,111], isoxazolyl [110],

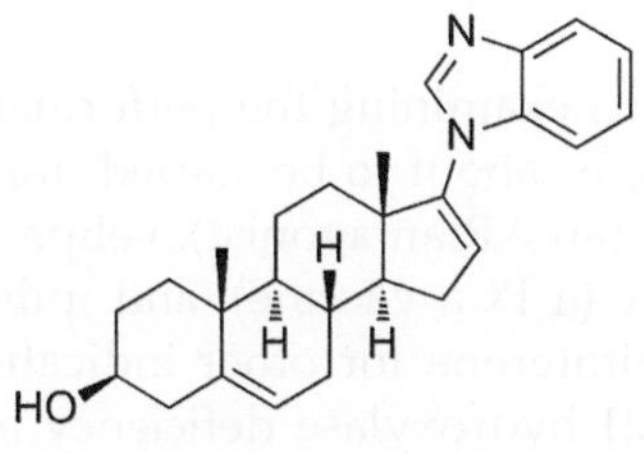

FIGURE 11.11   Structure of gleterone (TOK-001).

thiazolyl [61,111], pyrazinyl [102], pyrimidinyl [102,112], benzotriazolyl [102], and indazolyl [113]. It is notable that almost all compounds have a Δ16-17 double bond in their steroidal scaffolds. Moreover, the inhibitors based on a progesterone scaffold were normally weaker toward CYP17 than the corresponding pregnenolone analogs. However, they also inhibited 5α-R [107,109], which is responsible for the conversion of testosterone to DHT. This dual inhibition of two key enzymes in the androgen biosynthesis route might be advantageous for the treatment of PCa. Several compounds emerge from the others with superior in vitro activity and selectivity as well as the ability to reduce testosterone levels in vivo. SA40 is a structural analog of abiraterone with 3-pyrimidyl instead of 3-pyridyl as the coordinating group (Fig. 11.1). It showed threefold more potent inhibition of CYP17 than abiraterone in an irreversible and noncompetitive manner when tested in a human testicular microsome assay [112]. No inhibition of CYP11B2 and only a weak effect on CYP19 were observed. SA40 strongly reduced the plasma testosterone concentration as well as prostate and seminal vesicle weights when administrated intraperitoneally to rats as the 3-acetyl ester prodrug [114]. However, as does abiraterone, it also increases adrenal and pituitary weights [114]. VN/85-1 and VN/87-1 (Fig. 11.12) are analogs of gleterone with

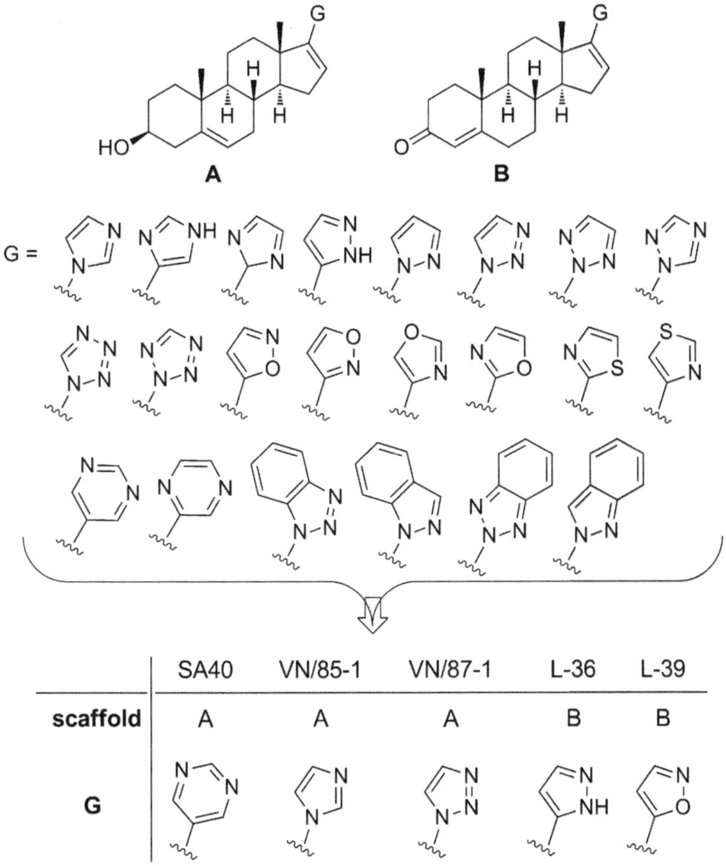

FIGURE 11.12 Steroidal CYP17 inhibitors with various *sp²* hybrid nitrogen-containing heterocycles as coordinating groups. The five most potent examples in vitro and in vivo are SA40, VN/85-1, VN/87-1, L-36, and L-39.

1-imidazolyl and 1-triazolyl replacing 1-benzimidazolyl, respectively. In a human testicular microsome assay, both compounds were potent, noncompetitive inhibitors of CYP17 with K_i values of about 1 nM and also showed some antiandrogen activity [109]. They not only reduced the concentrations of testosterone and DHT in serum, testes, and prostate, but also diminished prostate and seminal vesicle weights in rats [109]. Additionally, these two compounds also inhibited the proliferation of WT LNCaP tumor cells in vitro and in mice [115]. However, they showed high clearance from the circulation and thus short half-lives of around 1 h after oral, subcutaneous, or intravenous applications in mice [116,117]. Moreover, as dual inhibitors of CYP17 and 5α-R, L-36, and L-39 (Fig. 12.12), they significantly reduced testosterone and DHT levels in serum and testicular and prostatic tissue, as well as prostate weights in rats [118]. L-39 exhibited similar effects in reducing tumor growth as castration and decreased serum PSA levels by more than 80% in a human prostate cancer (PC-82) xenograft model in mice [119]. However, rapid clearance and low bioavailability were also observed [116,119].

Modifications of the Steroidal Scaffold

Besides the introduction of the Δ16-17 double bond, further modifications have been performed to the steroidal scaffold (Fig. 11.13), such as the insertion of N, O, or S into the A or B ring at the 2, 4, or 6 position; variations at the 3-Oxo group; and the expansion or reduction of the A or B ring [120,121].

NONSTEROIDAL CYP17 INHIBITORS

Although the steroidal CYP17 inhibitor abiraterone has been launched into the clinic and gleterone is in late clinical development, there are potential drawbacks attributed to their steroidal scaffold, such as poor absorption and consequent low bioavailability, first-pass effects, and affinity for steroid receptors. Nonsteroidal CYP17 inhibitors are therefore discussed as being favorable alternatives. Among numerous potent nonsteroidal CYP17 inhibitors identified, ketoconazole, orteronel, TD464, and CFG920 were or are being evaluated in clinical trials. Some of them are expected to be superior to the current drugs in use.

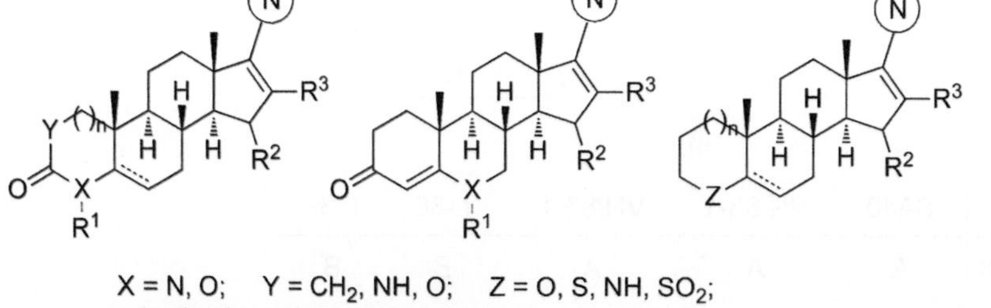

X = N, O;   Y = CH$_2$, NH, O;   Z = O, S, NH, SO$_2$;
R^1, R^2, R^3 = H, alkyl, aryl, halogen

(N) = pyridyl, benzimidazolyl, pyrimidyl, imidazolyl

FIGURE 11.13   Modifications on the steroidal scaffolds.

Ketoconazole

The application of CYP17 inhibitors for the treatment of PCa started with the off-label use of ketoconazole (Fig. 11.14). Ketoconazole is an antimycotic agent exhibiting unselective inhibition toward CYP17, CYP11B1, CYP11B2, CYP11A1, and some hepatic CYP enzymes like CYP3A4. This poor selectivity profile led to severe side effects and grade 3 or 4 toxicities, such as adrenal insufficiency, neuropathy, and hepatotoxicity [122]. Although reduced doses of 200 or 300 mg three times per day were attempted instead of the standard 400 mg dose, side effects and toxicity were reduced but not avoided [123,124]. Nevertheless, ketoconazole is still widely employed in combination with hydrocortisone replacement therapy. In several phase II studies of ketoconazole, 31–62% of chemotherapy-naïve patients exhibited a decline in PSA levels of 50% or more, and the median PSA progression time was up to 7.7 months [123–127]. It has been shown that PCa patients with progression under flutamide withdrawal still retained responses to ketoconazole [125], and the combination of ketoconazole with anti-androgens was more effective than antiandrogen alone, although no difference in overall survival was observed [122]. However, the combination of ketoconazole with doxorubicin or alendronate was not superior to ketoconazole treatment [126,127].

Orteronel (TAK700)

Takeda Chemical Industries Ltd. has developed a series of imidazol-4-yl methanols and dihydropyrroloimidazol-7-ols (Fig. 11.15), which contained a bulky aromatic moiety attached to the methylene such as naphthyl and biphenyl. These compounds showed potent inhibition ($IC_{50} < 50$ nM) against human and rat CYP17 C17-20 lyase in assays using recombinant human CYP17 expressed in *E. coli* and rat testicular microsomes, respectively [128–131]. Besides its contribution of lowering logP, the hydroxyl group was demonstrated to be crucial for improving selectivity over CYP11B1 and hepatic CYP enzymes as well as for avoiding an increase of liver weight in rats [128]. The *S*-enantiomers were always more potent than the corresponding *R*-enantiomers [128–130]. The efforts in optimizing these compounds led to orteronel (TAK700, Fig. 11.15) with a dihydropyrroloimidazole as the heme-coordinating group. Orteronel showed a fivefold more potent inhibition toward C17-20 lyase than 17α-hydroxylase, with IC_{50} values of 140 and 760 nM, respectively; whereas abiraterone was more potent but less selective in the same assays, with IC_{50} values of 27 and 30 nM toward C17-20 lyase and 17α-hydroxylase, respectively [131]. However, orteronel was not selective regarding the cynomolgus monkey enzymes (27 nM for lyase vs 38 nM for hydroxylase), which was probably the reason for the observed reduction of aldosterone and cortisol levels in adrenal cells [131]. Multiple dosing of orteronel (15 mg/kg) to castrated cynomolgus monkeys reduced the plasma concentrations of DHEA and cortisol

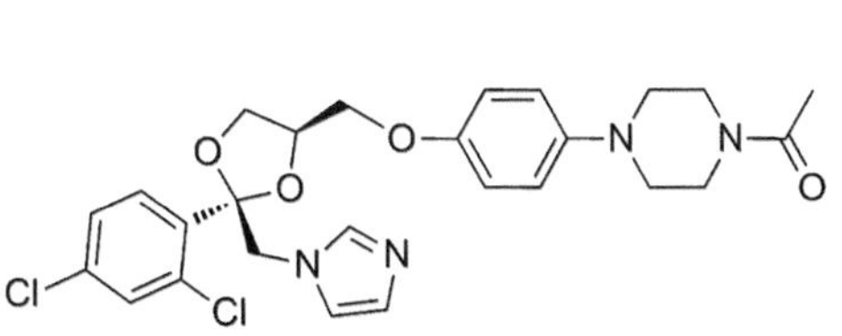

FIGURE 11.14 Structure of ketoconazole.

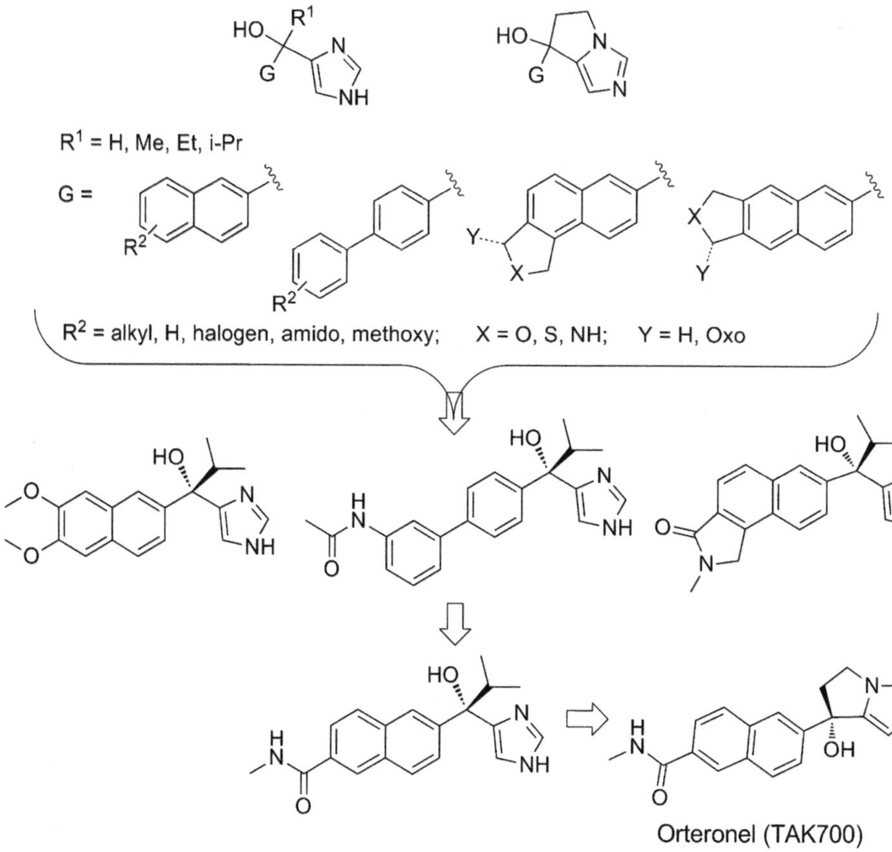

FIGURE 11.15   Structures of orteronel (TAK700) and analogs.

by 93% and 83%, respectively. The plasma testosterone levels were decreased to 0.2–0.3 ng/ mL [131]. Intact cynomolgus monkeys exhibited a similar suppression of the DHEA and cortisol concentrations, but circadian rhythms were observed. Moreover, after the oral application of orteronel (1 mg/kg) to cynomolgus monkeys, the maximal plasma concentration (0.147 μg/ mL) was reached after 1.7 h, and a $t_{1/2}$ of 3.8 h and an AUC of 0.727 μg h/mL were observed [131]. Since orteronel was also selective over CYP11B1 ($IC_{50} > 1000$ nM) and a series of hepatic CYP enzymes, such as CYP1A2, CYP2A6, CYP2B6, CYP2C8, CYP2C9, CYP2D6, CYP2E1, and CYP3A4 [132] with $IC_{50} > 3$ μM, it was further evaluated in clinical trials.

It was shown that after dose escalation to more than 300 mg twice daily, all patients exhibited a reduction in PSA levels [133–135]. Although no dose-limiting toxicity was observed, nearly all patients experienced more than one treatment-emergent adverse event, and around 20% patients discontinued therapy. The most common and severe side effects were fatigue and hypokalemia, respectively. Although orteronel has been claimed to have better selectivity over 17α-hydroxylase and CYP11B1 than abiraterone, elevation of ACTH by 171% and decline of cortisol by 21% were observed. After balancing efficacy and toxicity, 300–400 mg twice daily were recommended for the subsequent evaluations. After administration of 300 mg twice daily, the concentrations of testosterone and DHEA-S were significantly reduced to <1 ng/dL and 9 μg/dL, respectively [136]. From 60% to 70% of patients showed a PSA decline of 50% or more, and the median PSA progression time was 14.8 months [136]. The mean circulating tumor cell count also decreased, from 16.6 per 7.5 mL blood to 3.9 [135]. Although prednisone has been shown to not result in any improvement in antitumor effects, it was still employed in combination with orteronol in the subsequent phase III clinical trials [137], probably for the suppression of ACTH and mineralocorticoid levels.

VT-464

From 2011 to 2012, Viamet Pharmaceuticals Inc. published four patents with broad claims covering almost all derivatives of 1- or 4-triazoles, 2-tetrazoles, and 4-pyrimidines except published compounds [138–141]. However, a close look at these patents revealed that the synthesized examples were focused on the methylene naphthalenes or (iso)quinolines substituted by the above-mentioned heterocycles (Fig. 11.16). The naphthalene or (iso)quinoline core can be furnished with various substituents, such as alkoxyl and aryl. Alkyl, especially *iso*-propyl, can be introduced onto the methylene bridge with or without an additional hydroxy group. The most potent example showed an IC_{50} value of 30 nM toward CYP17 in an assay using rat testicular microsomes. In January 2012, Viamet Pharmaceuticals Inc. announced the start of a phase I/II clinical trial with the CYP17 inhibitor VT-464 for the treatment of chemotherapy-naïve patients with CRPC. VT-464 has been claimed to be a potent, orally available CYP17 lyase inhibitor. Unfortunately, no structure information was released. Nevertheless, it can be assumed that the structure is similar to the examples presented in Fig. 11.16. VT-464 has been

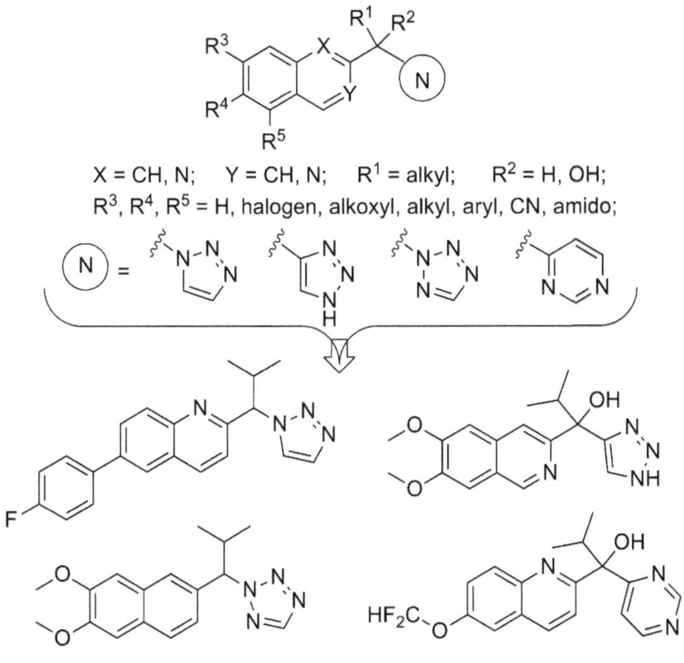

FIGURE 11.16 Structures of CYP17 inhibitors from Viamet Pharmaceuticals, Inc.

X = CH, N;   Y = CH, N;   R¹ = alkyl;   R² = H, OH;
R³, R⁴, R⁵ = H, halogen, alkoxyl, alkyl, aryl, CN, amido;

reported to exhibit a 10-fold selective inhibition of human C17-20 lyase over 17α-hydroxylase with IC_{50} values of 69 and 670 nM, respectively [142], while abiraterone showed IC_{50} values of 15 and 2.5 nM in the same assay. Although VT-464 is less potent, it is 58-fold more selective toward C17-20 lyase than abiraterone. Since 17α-hydroxylase is at the node branching mineralocorticoids and other downstream steroidal hormones, such as glucocorticoids and androgens (Fig. 11.4), the inhibition of the hydroxylase should lead to an increase in mineralocorticoids and a reduction of cortisol, as observed in the clinical trials of abiraterone. In contrast, selective inhibition of C17-20 lyase should have little effect on progestagens, glucocorticoids, and mineralocorticoids. This hypothesis was demonstrated by comparison between abiraterone and VT-464 in chemically castrated male rhesus monkeys [143,144]. Abiraterone led to elevated concentrations of progesterone, pregnenolone, corticosterone, and DOC by factors of 21, 7, 2.8, and 7, respectively, whereas VT-464 resulted in slightly decreased levels of progesterone, pregnenolone, and corticosterone by factors of 2, 3.8, and 2.8, respectively, as well as similar DOC levels [143]. On the other hand, abiraterone reduced cortisol levels by 11-fold in contrast to VT-464, which led to nearly unchanged cortisol concentrations [144]. It is apparent that since VT-464 has almost no influence on the upstream steroid hormones, prednisone is no longer necessary. Furthermore, VT-464 suppressed the plasma testosterone concentration by 90% in monkeys after a subcutaneous administration of 12.5 mg/kg [142,144] and dose-dependent inhibition of tumor growth in an LNCaP mouse xenograft model [145]. VT-464 is now in a phase I/II, open-label, multiple-dose study without prednisone to evaluate its safety, tolerability, pharmacokinetics, and pharmacodynamics in chemotherapy-naïve CRPC patients.

Heterocycle Methylene Substituted Carbazoles, Fluorenes, and Dibenzofurans

A series of carbazoles, fluorenes, and dibenzofurans, substituted by an sp^2 hybrid N-containing heterocycle via a methylene bridge, were synthesized as CYP17 inhibitors with YM116 (Fig. 11.17) as a representative example [146–150]. YM116 exhibited potent inhibition of C17-20 lyase with an IC_{50} value of 4.2 nM using human testicular microsomes, and was claimed to be 50-fold more specific over 17α-hydroxylase [148]. YM116 suppressed the production

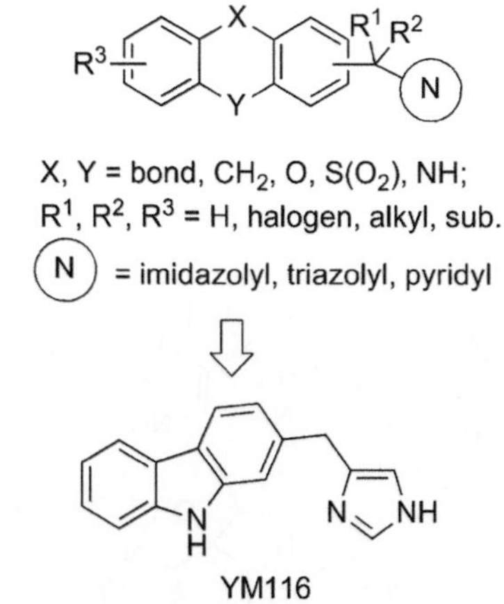

X, Y = bond, CH₂, O, S(O₂), NH;
R¹, R², R³ = H, halogen, alkyl, sub. Ph;
Ⓝ = imidazolyl, triazolyl, pyridyl

YM116

FIGURE 11.17 Heterocycle methylene substituted carbazoles, fluorenes, and dibenzofurans with YM116 as a representative.

of DHEA, androstenedione, and cortisol in NCI-H295 cells with IC_{50} values of 2.1, 3.6, and 50.4 nM, respectively. Moreover, YM116 significantly reduced DHEA-S levels with an ED_{50} value of 11 mg/kg and slightly decreased serum aldosterone concentration in guinea pigs, whereas plasma cortisol levels were not reduced even at a dose of 100 mg/kg [149].

Imidazolyl or Pyridyl Methylene Substituted Biphenyls

In mimicking the steroidal scaffold of natural substrates, a series of sp^2 hybrid N-containing heterocycle methylene substituted biphenyls (Fig. 11.18) have been designed, synthesized, and evaluated as CYP17 inhibitors [87,88,150–160]. These compounds showed potent inhibitions of human CYP17, with some of them being more potent than abiraterone in an assay using recombinant human enzyme expressed in *E. coli*. It has been shown that the hydrogen bond–forming groups on the A ring significantly elevated inhibitory potency, and it has been speculated that this was due to interactions with R109, K231, and H235 [151,153]. Substituents on the methylene bridge were crucial as well, with an ethyl group strongly promoting CYP17 inhibition [150]. Isopropylidene, on the other hand, not only further increased inhibition but also strongly improved selectivity over CYP11B1, CYP11B2, CYP19, and a series of hepatic CYP enzymes such as CYP3A4 [87]. Although exchanging the phenyl moiety with other heterocycles [88] and fusing the alkyl substituents to the biphenyl core [160] showed only a little improvement, the replacement of the imidazolyl by a 4-pyridyl as the coordinating group strongly increased inhibitory potency [152]. Some fluorine analogs (Fig. 12.18) were more effective than abiraterone and

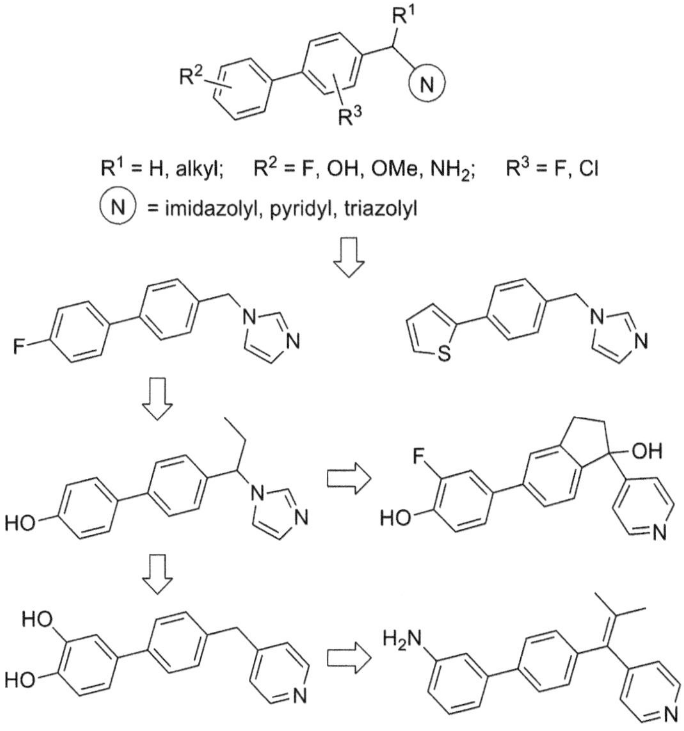

FIGURE 11.18 General structure of imidazolyl, pyridyl, or triazolyl methylene substituted biphenyls and representative compounds.

R^1 = H, alkyl; R^2 = F, OH, OMe, NH_2; R^3 = F, Cl

(N) = imidazolyl, pyridyl, triazolyl

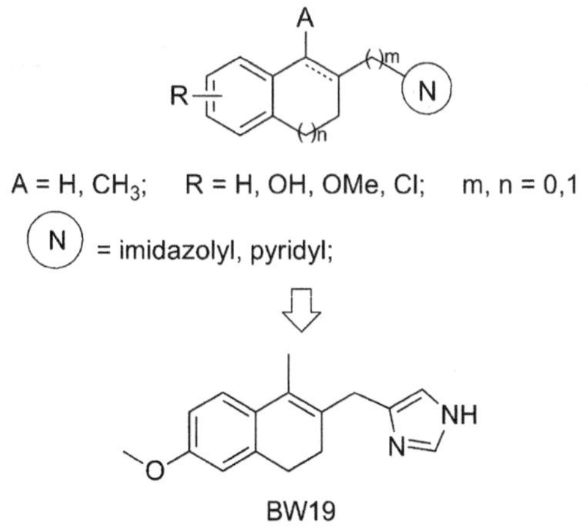

A = H, CH$_3$;   R = H, OH, OMe, Cl;   m, n = 0,1

(N) = imidazolyl, pyridyl;

BW19

FIGURE 11.19   General structure of semisaturated naphthalenes and representative compound BW19.

suppressed the plasma testosterone concentration in rats by more than 80% after oral administration of 50mg/kg. Importantly, the suppression lasted more than 24h, in contrast to the increase of testosterone levels above control observed after 24h when abiraterone was applied. This inability of long-term suppression is probably due to the poor pharmacokinetic properties of abiraterone in rats since its $t_{1/2}$ was 1.6h and the AUC was 11488nM/h, significantly less than the tested F substituted biphenyl compound ($t_{1/2} = 12.8$h and AUC$\geq$80488nM/h) [151].

Semisaturated Naphthalenes

BW19 (Fig. 11.19) is a representative of the semisaturated naphthalene type of CYP17 inhibitors [114,161–165]. Its potency is similar to that of abiraterone in assays using human testicular microsomes or recombinant CYP17 expressed in *E. coli*, with a similar IC$_{50}$ value of 110nM [114]. Notably, this compound also inhibits CYP19 (IC$_{50} = 1.2\mu$M), but shows no inhibition of CYP11B2. After an intraperitoneal administration to rats at a dose of 0.1mmol/kg for 14 days, BW19 not only significantly reduced the plasma testosterone concentration to castration level, being twofold more effective than abiraterone, but also decreased prostate and seminal vesicle weights [114].

Branched Bis-Aryl Substituted Heterocycles

Bayer, Novartis, and Bristol-Myers Squibb have developed various bis-aryl substituted heterocycles as CYP17 inhibitors [166–177]. Most of these compounds strongly inhibit CYP17 with IC$_{50}$ values less than 100nM. Although they were claimed to be C17-20 lyase inhibitors, no data on selectivity over 17α-hydroxylase have been published. (Fig. 11.20)

Others

More examples of CYP17 inhibitors are presented in Fig. 11.21. Although CB7645 as an adamantine carboxylate strongly inhibited human CYP17 and was resistant to esterase hydrolysis [178], it exhibited little activity in mice and had a poor pharmacokinetic profile [179].

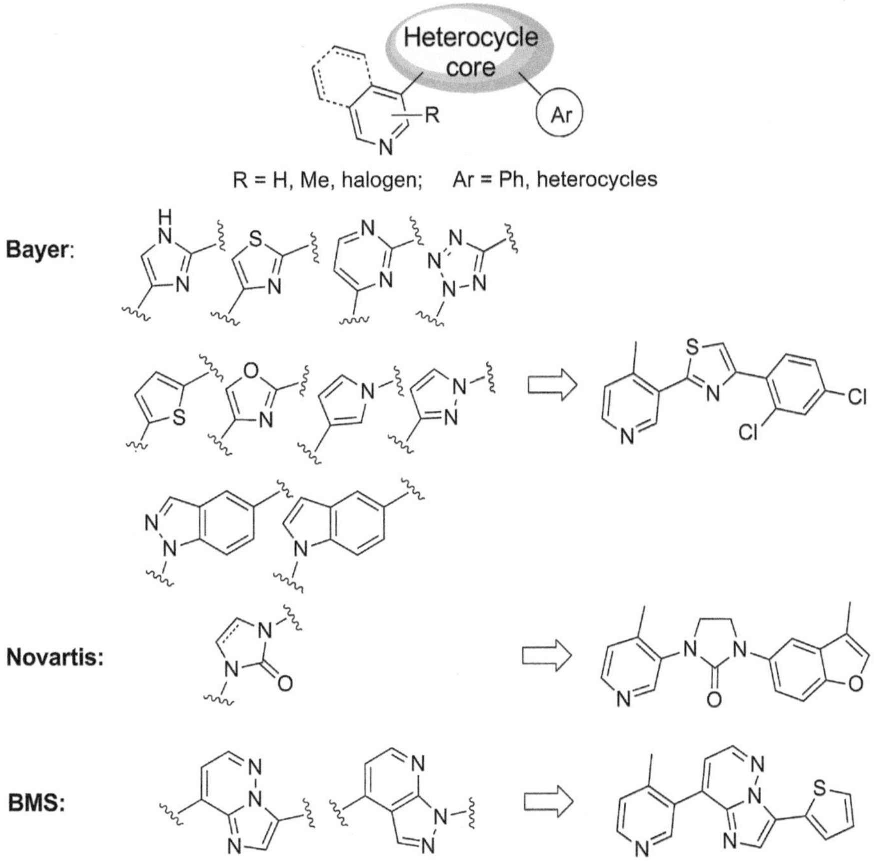

FIGURE 11.20 General structure of branched bis-aryl substituted heterocycles and representative compounds.

Furthermore, Bristol-Myers Squibb and Novartis published several types of CYP17 inhibitors in 2012 characterized by a sulfonamide moiety [180] and cores of an aryl annelated with a piperidin-2-one, respectively [181]. Recently, Novartis announced a phase I/II, multicenter, open-label, dose-finding study of CFG920 for patients with metastatic CRPC. No structure information on CFG920 is available.

CYP17 INHIBITORS IN THE POST-ABIRATERONE ERA

Despite the improvements in overall survival, some drawbacks for abiraterone have to be mentioned, such as a secondary mineralocorticoid excess leading to hypokalemia and edema, poor pharmacokinetic properties requiring high doses, eventual binding to steroid receptors, as well as modest selectivity over CYP11B1 and CYP11B2. Safer CYP17 inhibitors with better profiles are therefore necessary.

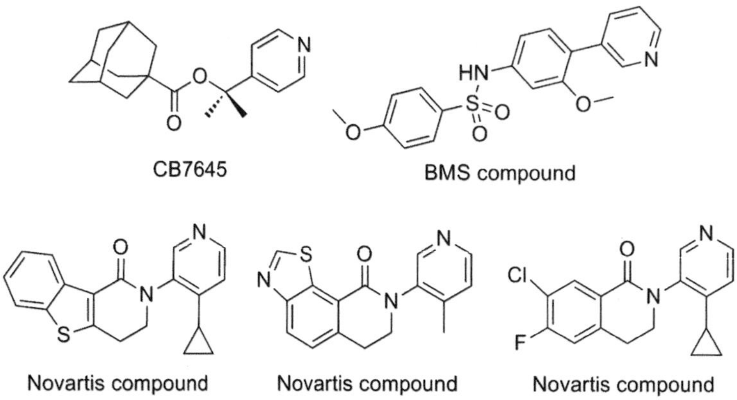

FIGURE 11.21 Miscellaneous types of CYP17 inhibitors.

CB7645

BMS compound

Novartis compound   Novartis compound   Novartis compound

Selective C17-20 Lyase Inhibitors

As discussed in this chapter, CYP17 is actually one enzyme with two activities, namely, 17α-hydroxylase and C17-20 lyase. The inhibition of 17α-hydroxylase can lead to the accumulation of progestagens and, accordingly, elevation of mineralocorticoids. Glucocorticoids, on the contrary, will be downregulated. This hypothesis, which has been recently demonstrated by the in vivo study of VT464 in monkeys [143], provides answers to the origin of secondary mineralocorticoid excess caused by abiraterone. Therefore, selective inhibitors of C17-20 lyase would lead to safer treatment. Although some compounds have been previously claimed to be C17-20 lyase inhibitors, selectivity data over 17α-hydroxylase were mostly absent. Novel, rapid, and easy-to-handle assays are therefore urgently needed [182].

Dual Inhibitors of CYP17 C17-20 Lyase and CYP11B1

Many possible reasons for castration resistance of PCa have been identified, such as intratumoral androgen biosynthesis, overexpression of AR, and AR mutations. Some types of mutated ARs can be activated by glucocorticoids, especially cortisol [32], and thus further stimulate cancer cell proliferation. Therefore, cortisol production needs to be controlled together with androgen production in patients expressing these types of mutated ARs. Since CYP11B1 is the pivotal enzyme in cortisol biosynthesis, its inhibition would effectively reduce cortisol levels. Although the production of cortisol ought to be blocked, the upstream enzyme 17α-hydroxylase needs to be left unaffected to avoid elevation of mineralocorticoids. Since multitargeting agents exhibit advantages over drugs in combination such as compliance and less risk of drug–drug interactions, dual inhibitors of CYP17 C17-20 lyase and CYP11B1 have been proposed [152]. In the clinic, determination of the AR status should be performed before a treatment decision is finally made.

Dual CYP17 C17-20 Lyase and CYP11B2 Inhibitors

The deficiency of androgens leads to an elevation of aldosterone via accumulation of progesterone, reduction of estrogens, and increased serum low- and high-density lipoproteins [153]. Excessive aldosterone, which is a proinflammatory factor, can lead to deleterious effects on the kidneys, vessels, brain, and heart. Although the risk of cardiovascular diseases as a result of CYP17 inhibition has not yet been emphasized, an increased mortality caused by

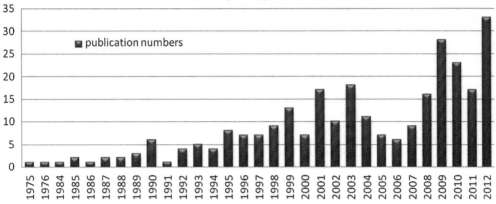

FIGURE 11.22 Publications regarding CYP17 inhibitors from 1975 to 2012.

cardiovascular complications has been reported to be associated with ADT [101]. Therefore, dual inhibitors of CYP17 C17-20 lyase and CYP11B2 could be a promising option for the treatment of PCa in reducing cardiovascular complications [183]. Selectivity over 17α-hydroxylase prevents reduction of cortisol levels while the remaining corticosterone can act as a mineralocorticoid to avoid side effects caused by aldosterone suppression.

RENAISSANCE: SUMMARY AND CONCLUSIONS

According to Scifinder records, there have been 279 publications on CYP17 inhibitors since 1975 (Fig. 11.22). It can be seen that the number of publications increased every year after various pseudo-substrates had been identified as CYP17 inhibitors, and ketoconazole was used off-label until 2003. Then a decline in publication numbers followed, probably due to the fact that some researchers and companies left the field. Nevertheless, before long, as the clinical success of abiraterone has been published, the research area started to flourish again with more than 30 publications in 2012. From only ketoconazole being used off-label as a CYP17 inhibitor to nowadays one drug (abiraterone) on the market and another four drug candidates in clinical trials, the development of CYP17 inhibitors has not only resulted in a novel treatment option but also demonstrated that androgens still play a crucial role in this disease even after its progression to castration resistance. Although abiraterone still shows some drawbacks, the solution of these problems by identification of more selective and/or multitargeting agents [184] could provide safer treatments and thus increase the quality of life and survival time of patients.

References

[1] Jemal A, Bray F, Center MM, Ferlay J, Ward E, Forman D. Global cancer statistics. CA Cancer J Clin 2011;61:69–90.
[2] Siegel R, Naishadham D, Jemal A. Cancer statistics, 2012. CA Cancer J Clin 2012;62:10–29.
[3] LeBeau AM, Singh P, Isaacs JT, Denmeade SR. Prostate-specific antigen is a "chymotrypsin-like" serine protease with unique P1 substrate specificity. Biochemistry 2009;48:3490–6.
[4] Makarov DV, Carter HB. The discovery of prostate specific antigen as a biomarker for the early detection of adenocarcinoma of the prostate. J Urol 2006;176:2383–5.

[5] Welch HG, Albertsen PC. Prostate cancer diagnosis and treatment after the introduction of prostate-specific antigen screening: 1986–2005. J Natl Cancer Inst 2009;101:1325–9.

[6] van Leeuwen PJ, Connolly D, Gavin A, Roobol MJ, Black A, Bangma CH, et al. Prostate cancer mortality in screen and clinically detected prostate cancer: estimating the screening benefit. Eur J Cancer 2010;46:377–83.

[7] Weinzimer SA, Gibson TB, Collett-Solberg PF, Khare A, Liu B, Cohen P. Transferrin is an insulin-like growth factor-binding protein-3 binding protein. J Clin Endocrinol Metab 2001;86:1806–13.

[8a] Meng MV. Prostate cancer. In: McPhee SJ, Papadakis MA, editors. Current medical diagnosis & treatment 2011. 50th ed. McGraw-Hill Companies, Inc; 2011.

[8b] Yin L, Hu Q, Hartmann RW. Recent progress in pharmaceutical therapies for castration-resistant prostate cancer. Int J Mol Sci 2013; in press.

[9] Siegel R, DeSantis C, Virgo K, Stein K, Mariotto A, Smith T, et al. Cancer treatment and survivorship statistics, 2012. CA Cancer J Clin 2012;62:220–41.

[10] Tannock IF, de Wit R, Berry WR, Horti J, Pluzanska A, Chi KN, et al. Docetaxel plus prednisone or mitoxantrone plus prednisone for advanced prostate cancer. N Engl J Med 2004;351:1502–12.

[11] Nilsson S, Franzén L, Parker C, Tyrrell C, Blom R, Tennvall J, et al. Bone-targeted radium-223 in symptomatic, hormonerefractory prostate cancer: a randomised, multicentre, placebo-controlled phase II study. Lancet Oncol 2007;8:587–9.

[12] Kantoff PW, Higano CS, Shore ND, Berger ER, Small EJ, Penson DF, et al. for the IMPACT Study Investigators Sipuleucel-T immunotherapy for castration-resistant prostate cancer. N Engl J Med 2010;363:411–22.

[13] Geller J. Basis for hormonal management of advanced prostate cancer. Cancer 1993;71:1039–45.

[14] Imamoto T, Suzuki H, Yano M, Kawamura K, Kamiya N, Araki K, et al. The role of testosterone in the pathogenesis of prostate cancer. Int J Urol 2008;15:472–80.

[15] Cai C, Chen S, Ng P, Bubley GJ, Nelson PS, Mostaghel EA, et al. Intratumoral de novo steroid synthesis activates androgen receptor in castration-resistant prostate cancer and is upregulated by treatment with CYP17A1 inhibitors. Cancer Res 2011;71:6503–13.

[16] Montgomery RB, Mostaghel EA, Vessella R, Hess DL, Kalhorn TF, Higano CS, et al. Maintenance of intratumoral androgens in metastatic prostate cancer: a mechanism for castration-resistant tumor growth. Cancer Res 2008;68:4447–54.

[17] Gao W, Bohl CE, Dalton JT. Chemistry and structural biology of androgen receptor. Chem Rev 2005;105:3352–70.

[18] Wang LG, Liu XM, Kreis W, Budman DR. Phosphorylation/dephosphorylation of androgen receptor as a determinant of androgen agonistic or antagonistic activity. Biochem Biophys Res Commun 1999;259:21–8.

[19] Masiello D, Cheng S, Bubley GJ, Lu ML, Balk SP. Bicalutamide functions as an androgen receptor antagonist by assembly of a transcriptionally inactive receptor. J Biol Chem 2002;277:26321–6.

[20] Zagar Y, Chaumaz G, Lieberherr M. Signaling cross-talk from Gbeta4 subunit to Elk-1 in the rapid action of androgens. J Bio Chem 2004;279:2403–13.

[21] Kampa M, Papakonstanti EA, Hatzoglou A, Stathopoulos EN, Stournaras C, Castanas E. The human prostate cancer cell line LNCaP bears functional membrane testosterone receptors, which increase PSA secretion and modify actin cytoskeleton. FASEB J 2002;16:1429–31.

[22] Migliaccio A, Castoria G, Di Domenico M, de Falco A, Bilancio A, Lombardi M, et al. Steroid-induced androgen receptor-oestradiol receptor beta-Src complex triggers prostate cancer cell proliferation. EMBO J 2000;19:5406–17.

[23] Attard G, Reid AHM, Yap TA, Raynaud F, Dowsett M, Settatree S, et al. Phase I clinical trial of a selective inhibitor of CYP17, abiraterone acetate, confirms that castration-resistant prostate cancer commonly remains hormone driven. J Clin Oncol 2008;26:4563–71.

[24] Picard F, Schulz T, Hartmann RW. 5-Phenyl substituted 1-methyl-2-pyridones and 4′-substituted biphenyl-4-carboxylic acids: synthesis and evaluation as inhibitors of steroid-5α-reductase type 1 and 2. Bioorg Med Chem 2002;10:437–48.

[25] Huggins C, Hodges CV. Studies in prostatic cancer. I. The effect of castration, estrogens and androgen injections on serum phosphatases in metastatic carcinoma of the prostate. Cancer Res 1941;1:293–7.

[26] Huhtaniemi I, Nikula H, Parvinen M, Rannikko S. Histological and functional changes of the testis tissue during GnRH agonist treatment of prostatic cancer. Am J Clin Oncol 1988;11:S11–5.

[27] Titus MA, Schell MJ, Lih FB, Tomer KB, Mohler JL. Testosterone and dihydrotestosterone tissue levels in recurrent prostate cancer. Clin Cancer Res 2005;11:4653–7.

[28] Stanbrough M, Bubley GJ, Ross K, Golub TR, Rubin MA, Penning TM, et al. Increased expression of genes converting adrenal androgens to testosterone in androgen-independent prostate cancer. Cancer Res 2006;66:2815–25.

[29] Crawford ED, Eisenberger MA, McLeod DG, Spaulding JT, Benson R, Dorr FA, et al. A controlled trial of leuprolide with and without flutamide in prostatic carcinoma. N Engl J Med 1989;321:419–24.

[30] Suzuki H, Akakura K, Komiya A, Aida S, Akimoto S, Shimazaki J. Codon 877 mutation in the androgen receptor gene in advanced prostate cancer: relation to antiandrogen withdrawal syndrome. Prostate 1996;29:153–8.

[31] Hara T, Miyazaki J, Araki H, Yamaoka M, Kanzaki N, Kusaka M, et al. Novel mutations of androgen receptor: a possible mechanism of bicalutamide withdrawal syndrome. Cancer Res 2003;63:149–53.

[32] Zhao XY, Malloy PJ, Krishnan AV, Swami S, Navone NM, Peehl DM, et al. Glucocorticoids can promote androgen-independent growth of prostate cancer cells through a mutated androgen receptor. Nat Med 2000;6:703–6.

[33] Tran C, Ouk S, Clegg NJ, Chen Y, Watson PA, Arora V, et al. Development of a second-generation antiandrogen for treatment of advanced prostate cancer. Science 2009;324:787–90.

[34] Belikov S, Öberg C, Jääskeläinen T, Rahkama V, Palvimo JJ, Wrange Ö. FoxA1 corrupts the antiandrogenic effect of bicalutamide but only weakly attenuates the effect of MDV3100 (Enzalutamide™). Mol Cell Endocrinol 2013;365:95–107.

[35] Scher HI, Beer TM, Higano CS, Anand A, Taplin ME, Efstathiou E, et al. Antitumour activity of MDV3100 in castration-resistant prostate cancer: a phase 1–2 study. Lancet 2010;375:1437–46.

[36] Scher HI, Fizazi K, Saad F, Taplin ME, Sternberg CN, Miller K, et al. Increased survival with enzalutamide in prostate cancer after chemotherapy. N Engl J Med 2012;367:1187–97.

[37] Clegg NJ, Wongvipat J, Joseph JD, Tran C, Ouk S, Dilhas A, et al. ARN-509: a novel antiandrogen for prostate cancer treatment. Cancer Res 2012;72:1494–503.

[38] Miller WL, Auchus RJ, Geller DH. The regulation of 17,20 lyase activity. Steroids 1997;62:133–42.

[39] Yanagibashi K, Hall PF. Role of electron transport in the regulation of the lyase activity of C-21 side-chain cleavage P450 from porcine adrenal and testicular microsomes. J Biol Chem 1986;261:8429–33.

[40] Kominami S, Ogawa N, Morimune R, Huang DY, Takemori S. The role of cytochrome b5 in adrenal microsomal steroidogenesis. J Steroid Biochem Mol Biol 1992;42:57–64.

[41] Zhang LH, Rodriguez H, Ohno S, Miller WL. Serine phosphorylation of human P450c17 increases 17,20-lyase activity: implications for adrenarche and the polycystic ovary syndrome. Proc Natl Acad Sci U S A 1995;92:10619–23.

[42] Denisov LG, Makris TM, Sligar SG, Schlichting I. Structure and chemistry of cytochrome P450. Chem Rev 2005;105:2253–77.

[43] DeVore NM, Scott EE. Structures of cytochrome P450 17A1 with prostate cancer drugs abiraterone and TOK-001. Nature 2012;482:116–20.

[44] Auchus RJ, Kumar AS, Boswell CA, Gupta MK, Bruce K, Rath NP, et al. The enantiomer of progesterone (ent-progesterone) is a competitive inhibitor of human cytochromes P450c17 and P450c21. Arch Biochem Biophys 2003;409:134–44.

[45] Bičíková M, Hampl R, Hill M, Stárka L. Inhibition of steroid 17 alpha-hydroxylase and C17,20-lyase in the human testis by epitestosterone. J Steroid Biochem Mol Biol 1993;46:515–8.

[46] Neubauer BL, Best KL, Blohm TR, Gates C, Goode RL, Hirsch KS, et al. Ly207320 (6-methylene-4-pregnene-3,20-dione) inhibits testosterone biosynthesis, androgen uptake, 5 alpha-reductase, and produces prostatic regression in male rats. Prostate 1993;23:181–99.

[47] Burkhart JP, Weintraub PM, Gates CA, Resvick RJ, Vaz RJ, Friedrich D, et al. Novel steroidal vinyl fluorides as inhibitors of steroid C17(20) lyase. Bioorg Med Chem 2002;10:929–34.

[48] Guengerich FP, Willard RJ, Shea JP, Richards LR, Macdonald TL. Mechanism-based inactivation of cytochrome P-450 by heteroatom-substituted cyclopropanes and formation of ring-opened products. J Am Chem Soc 1984;106:6446–7.

[49] Angelastro MR, Laughlin ME, Schatzman GL, Bey P, Blohm TR. 17β-(cyclopropylamino)-androst-5-en-3β-ol, a selective mechanism-based inhibitor of cytochrome P450 17α (steroid 17α-hydroxylase/C_{17-20}lyase). Biochem Biophys Res Commun 1989;162:1571–7.

[50] Hanzlik RP, Tullman RH. Suicidal inactivation of cytochrome P-450 by cyclopropylamines: evidence for cation-radical intermediates. J Am Chem Soc 1982;104:2048–50.

[51] Angelastro MR, Marquart AL, Weintraub PM, Gates CA, Laughlin ME, Blohm TR, et al. Time-dependent inactivation of steroid $C_{17(20)}$ lyase by 17β-cyclopropyl ether-substituted steroids. Bioorg Med Chem Lett 1996;6:97–100.

[52] Weintraub PM, Gates CA, Angelastro MR, Johnston JO, Curran TT. 4-Amino-17β-(cyclopropyloxy)androst-4-en-3-one, 4-amino-17β-(cyclopropylamino)androst-4-en-3-one and related compounds as C17–20 lyase and 5α-reductase inhibitors WO9428010. 1994.

[53] Pribish JR, Gates CA, Weintraub PM. 17-Beta-cyclopropyl- (amino/oxy) 4-aza steroids as active inhibitors of testosterone 5-alpha-reductase and C17-20 lyase WO9730069. 1997.

[54] Ling YZ, Li JS, Kato K, Liu Y, Wang X, Klus GT, et al. Synthesis and in vitro activity of some epimeric 20α-hydroxy, 20-oxime and aziridine pregnene derivatives as inhibitors of human 17α-hydroxylase/C17,20-lyase and 5α-reductase. Bioorg Med Chem 1998;6:1683–93.

[55] Li JS, Li Y, Son C, Brodie AMH. Synthesis and evaluation of pregnane derivatives as inhibitors of human testicular 17α-hydroxylase/c17,20-lyase. J Med Chem 1996;39:4335–9.

[56] Hartmann RW, Hector M, Haidar S, Ehmer PB, Reichert W, Jose J. Synthesis and evaluation of novel steroidal oxime inhibitors of P450 17 (17α-hydroxylase/C17-20-lyase) and 5α-reductase types 1 and 2. J Med Chem 2000;43:4266–77.

[57] Li JS, Li Y, Son C, Brodie AMH. Inhibition of androgen synthesis by 22-hydroximino-23,24-bisnor-4-cholen-3-one. Prostate 1995;26:140–50.

[58] Njar VCO, Hector M, Hartmann RW. 20-Amino and 20, 21-aziridinyl pregnene steroids: development of potent inhibitors of 17α-hydroxylase/C17,20-lyase (P450 17). Bioorg Med Chem 1996;4:1447–53.

[59] Hartmann RW, Hector M, Wachall BG, Paluszczak A, Palzer M, Huch V, et al. Synthesis and evaluation of 17-aliphatic heterocycle- substituted steroidal inhibitors of 17α-hydroxylase/C17-20-lyase (P450 17). J Med Chem 2000;43:4437–45.

[60] Haidar S, Hartmann RW. C16 and C17 substituted derivatives of pregnenolone and progesterone as inhibitors of 17α-hydroxylase-C17,20-lyase: synthesis and biological evaluation. Arch Pharm Pharm Med Chem 2002;11:526–34.

[61] Burkhart JP, Gates CA, Laughlin ME, Resvick RJ, Peet NP. Inhibition of steroid C17(20)-lyase with C17-heteroaryl steroids. Bioorg Med Chem 1996;4:1411–20.

[62] Haidar S, Klein CDP, Hartmann RW. Synthesis and evaluation of steroidal hydroxamic acids as inhibitors of P450 17 (17α-hydroxylase/C17-20-lyase). Arch Pharm Pharm Med Chem 2001;334:138–40.

[63] Yoshida Y, Aoyama Y. Interaction of azole antifungal agents with cytochrome P-450 purified from *Saccharomyces cerevisiae* microsomes. Biochem Pharmacol 1987;36:229–35.

[64] Hartmann RW, Bayer H, Grün G. Aromatase inhibitors: syntheses and structure-activity studies of novel pyridyl-substituted indanones, indans, and tetralins. J Med Chem 1994;37:1275–81.

[65] Abadi AH, Abou-Seri SM, Hu Q, Negri M, Hartmann RW. Synthesis and biological evaluation of imidazolyl-methylacridones as cytochrome P-450 enzymes inhibitors. MedChemComm 2012;3:663–6.

[66] Yin L, Hu Q. Drug discovery for breast cancer and coinstantaneous cardiovascular disease: what is the future? Future Med Chem 2013;5:359–62.

[67] Leze MP, Paluszczak A, Hartmann RW, Le Borgne M. Synthesis of 6- or 4-functionalized indoles via a reductive cyclization approach and evaluation as aromatase inhibitors. Bioorg Med Chem Lett 2008;18:4713–5.

[68] Gobbi S, Hu Q, Negri M, Zimmer C, Belluti F, Rampa A, et al. Modulation of cytochromes P450 with xanthone-based molecules: from aromatase to aldosterone synthase and steroid 11β-hydroxylase inhibition. J Med Chem 2013;56:1723–9.

[69] Gobbi S, Cavalli A, Rampa A, Belluti F, Piazzi L, Paluszcak A, et al. Lead optimization providing a series of flavone derivatives as potent nonsteroidal inhibitors of the cytochrome P450 aromatase enzyme. J Med Chem 2006;49:4777–80.

[70] Cavalli A, Bisi A, Bertucci C, Rosini C, Paluszcak A, Gobbi S, et al. Enantioselective nonsteroidal aromatase inhibitors identified through a multidisciplinary medicinal chemistry approach. J Med Chem 2005;48:7282–9.

[71] Yin L, Lucas S, Maurer F, Kazmaier U, Hu Q, Hartmann RW. Novel imidazol-1-ylmethyl substituted 1,2,5,6-tetrahydro-pyrrolo[3,2,1-ij]-quinolin-4-ones as potent and selective CYP11B1 inhibitors for the treatment of Cushing's syndrome. J Med Chem 2012;55:6629–33.

[72] Emmerich J, Hu Q, Hanke N, Hartmann RW. Cushing's syndrome: development of highly potent and selective CYP11B1 inhibitors of the (pyridylmethyl)pyridine type. J Med Chem Lett 2013; in press.

[73] Hille UE, Zimmer C, Haupenthal J, Hartmann RW. Optimization of the first selective steroid-11β-hydroxylase (CYP11B1) inhibitors for the treatment of cortisol dependent diseases. ACS Med Chem Lett 2011;2:559–64.

[74] Lucas S, Heim R, Ries C, Schewe KE, Birk B, Hartmann RW. In vivo active aldosterone synthase inhibitors with improved selectivity: lead optimization providing a series of pyridine substituted 3,4-dihydro-1H-quinolin-2-one derivatives. J Med Chem 2008;51:8077–87.

[75] Lucas S, Heim R, Negri M, Antes I, Ries C, Schewe KE, et al. Novel aldosterone synthase inhibitors with extended carbocyclic skeleton by a combined ligand-based and structure-based drug design approach. J Med Chem 2008;51:6138–49.

[76] Heim R, Lucas S, Grombein CM, Ries C, Schewe KE, Negri M, et al. Overcoming undesirable CYP1A2 inhibition of pyridylnaphthalene-type aldosterone synthase inhibitors: influence of heteroaryl derivatization on potency and selectivity. J Med Chem 2008;51:5064–74.

[77] Hu Q, Yin L, Hartmann RW. Novel heterocycle substituted 4,5-dihydro-[1,2,4]triazolo[4,3-a]quinolines as potent and selective aldosterone synthase inhibitors for the treatment of aldosterone-related cardiovascular diseases. J Med Chem 2013; in press.

[78] Voets M, Antes I, Scherer C, Müller-Vieira U, Biemel K, Barassin C, et al. Heteroaryl-substituted naphthalenes and structurally modified derivatives: selective inhibitors of CYP11B2 for the treatment of congestive heart failure and myocardial fibrosis. J Med Chem 2005;48:6632–42.

[79] Yin L, Hu Q, Hartmann RW. Novel pyridyl or isoquinolinyl substituted indolines and indoles as potent and selective aldosterone synthase inhibitors. J Med Chem 2013; in press.

[80] Lucas S, Negri M, Heim R, Zimmer C, Hartmann RW. Fine-tuning the selectivity of aldosterone synthase inhibitors: insights from studies from studies of heteroaryl substituted 1,2,5,6-tetrahydropyrrolo[3,2,1-ij]quinoline-4-one derivatives. J Med Chem 2011;54:2307–19.

[81] Yin L, Hu Q, Hartmann RW. 3-Pyridinyl substituted aliphatic cycles as CYP11B2 inhibitors: aromaticity abolishment of the core significantly increased selectivity over CYP1A2. PLoS ONE 2012;7(11):e4804810.1371/journal.pone.0048048.

[82] Hu Q, Yin L, Hartmann RW. Selective dual inhibitors of CYP19 and CYP11B2: targeting cardiovascular diseases hiding in the shadow of breast cancer. J Med Chem 2012;55:7080–9.

[83] Yin L, Hu Q, Hartmann RW. Tetrahydropyrroloquinolinone type dual inhibitors of aromatase/aldosterone synthase as a novel strategy for breast cancer patients with elevated cardiovascular risks. J Med Chem 2013;56:460–70

[84] Zytiga prescribing information, http://www.zytigahcp.com/pdf/full_prescribing_info.pdf; 2012 [accessed 08.11.12].

[85] Potter GA, Banie SE, Jarman M, Rowlands MG. Novel steroidal inhibitors of human cytochrome P450 17, (l7α-hydroxylase- Cl7,20-lyase): potential agents for the treatment of prostatic cancer. J Med Chem 1995;38:2463–71.

[86] Jarman M, Barrie SE, Llera JM. The 16,17-double bond is needed for irreversible inhibition of human cytochrome P450 17α by abiraterone (17-(3-pyridyl)androsta-5,16-dien-3β-ol) and related steroidal inhibitors. J Med Chem 1998;41:5375–81.

[87] Hu Q, Yin L, Jagusch C, Hille UE, Hartmann RW. Isopropylidene substitution increases activity and selectivity of biphenyl methylene 4-pyridine type CYP17 inhibitors. J Med Chem 2010;53:5049–53.

[88] Jagusch C, Negri M, Hille UE, Hu Q, Bartels M, Jahn-Hoffmann K, et al. Synthesis, biological evaluation and molecular modeling studies of methyleneimidazole substituted biaryls as inhibitors of human 17α-hydroxylase-17,20-lyase (CYP17)—part I: heterocyclic modifications of the core structure. Bioorg Med Chem 2008;16: 1992–2010.

[89] Li R, Evaul K, Sharma KK, Chang KH, Yoshimoto J, Liu JY, et al. Abiraterone inhibits 3β-hydroxysteroid dehydrogenase: a rationale for increasing drug exposure in castration-resistant prostate cancer. Clin Cancer Res 2012;18:3571–9.

[90] Soifer HS, Souleimanian N, Wu S, Voskresenskiy AM, Collak FK, Cinar B, et al. Direct regulation of androgen receptor activity by potent CYP17 inhibitors in prostate cancer cells. J Bio Chem 2012;287:3777–87.

[91] Barrie SE, Potter GA, Goddard PM, Haynes BP, Dowsett M, Jarman M. Pharmacology of novel steroidal inhibitors of cytochrome P450 17 (17α-hydroxylase/C17-20 lyase). J Steroid Biochem Mol Biol 1994; 50:267–73.

[92] O'Donnell A, Judson I, Dowsett M, Raynaud F, Dearnaley D, Mason M, et al. Hormonal impact of the 17α-hydroxylase/C(17,20)-lyase inhibitor abiraterone acetate (CB7630) in patients with prostate cancer. Br J Cancer 2004;90:2317–25.

[93] Ryan CJ, Smith MR, Fong L, Rosenberg JE, Kantoff P, Raynaud F, et al. Phase I clinical trial of the CYP17 inhibitor abiraterone acetate demonstrating clinical activity in patients with castration-resistant prostate cancer who received prior ketoconazole therapy. J Clin Oncol 2010;28:1481–8.

[94] Attard G, Reid AHM, A'Hern R, Parker C, Oommen NB, Folkerd E, et al. Selective inhibition of CYP17 with abiraterone acetate is highly active in the treatment of castration-resistant prostate cancer. J Clin Oncol 2009;27:3742–8.

[95] Ryan CJ, Shah S, Efstathiou E, Smith MR, Taplin ME, Bubley GJ, et al. Phase II study of abiraterone acetate in chemotherapy-naïve metastatic castration-resistant prostate cancer displaying bone flare discordant with serologic response. Clin Cancer Res 2011;17:4854–61.

[96] Danila DC, Morris MJ, de Bono JS, Ryan CS, Denmeade SR, Smith MR, et al. Phase II multicenter study of abiraterone acetate plus prednisone therapy in patients with docetaxel-treated castration-resistant prostate cancer. J Clin Oncol 2010;28:1496–501.

[97] Reid AHM, Attard G, Danila DC, Oommen NB, Olmos D, Fong PC, et al. Significant and sustained antitumor activity in postdocetaxel, castration-resistant prostate cancer with the CYP17 inhibitor abiraterone acetate. J Clin Oncol 2010;28:1489–95.

[98] de Bono JS, Logothetis CJ, Molina A, Fizazi K, North S, Chu L, et al. Abiraterone and increased survival in metastatic prostate cancer. N Engl J Med 2011;364:1995–2005.

[99] Fizazi K, Scher HI, Molina A, Logothetis CJ, Chi KN, Jones RJ, et al. Abiraterone acetate for treatment of metastatic castration-resistant prostate cancer: final overall survival analysis of the COU-AA-301 randomised, double-blind, placebo-controlled phase 3 study. Lancet Oncol 2012;13:983–92.

[100] Ryan CJ, Smith MR, De Bono JS, Molina A, Logothetis C, De Souza PL, et al. Interim analysis (IA) results of COU-AA-302, a randomized, phase III study of abiraterone acetate (AA) in chemotherapy-naive patients (pts) with metastatic castration-resistant prostate cancer (mCRPC). Proc Am Soc Clin Oncol 2012;30(Suppl.); abstr. LBA4518.

[101] Efstathiou JA, Bae K, Shipley WU, Hanks GE, Pilepich MV, Sandler HM, et al. Cardiovascular mortality after androgen deprivation therapy for locally advanced prostate cancer: RTOG 85-31. J Clin Oncol 2008;27:92–9.

[102] Handratta VD, Vasaitis TS, Njar VCO, Gediya LK, Kataria R, Chopra P, et al. Novel C-17-heteroaryl steroidal CYP17 inhibitors/antiandrogens: synthesis, in vitro biological activity, pharmacokinetics, and antitumor activity in the LAPC4 human prostate cancer xenograft model. J Med Chem 2005;48:2972–84.

[103] Vasaitis T, Belosay A, Schayowitz A, Khandelwal A, Chopra P, Gediya KZ, et al. Androgen receptor inactivation contributes to antitumor efficacy of 17α-hydroxylase/17,20-lyase inhibitor 3β-hydroxy-17-(1H-benzimidazole-1-yl)-androsta-5,16-diene in prostate cancer. Mol Cancer Ther 2008;7:2348–57.

[104] Bruno R, Gover T, Burger A, Brodie AMH, Njar VCO. 17α-Hydroxylase/17,20 lyase inhibitor VN/124-1 inhibits growth of androgen independent prostate cancer cells via induction of the endoplasmic reticulum stress response. Mol Cancer Ther 2008;7:2828–36.

[105] Bruno RD, Vasaitis TS, Gediya LK, Purushottamachar P, Godbole AM, Ates-Alagoz Z, et al. Synthesis and biological evaluations of putative metabolically stable analogs of VN/124-1 (TOK-001): head to head antitumor efficacy evaluation of VN/124-1 (TOK-001) and abiraterone in LAPC-4 human prostate cancer xenograft model. Steroids 2011;76:1268–79.

[106] Early clinical data show galeterone safe, effective against prostate cancer, http://www.aacr.org/home/public–media/aacr-press-releases.aspx?d=2769; [accessed 03.11.12].

[107] Njar VCO, Kato K, Nnane IP, Grigoryev DN, Long BJ, Brodie AMH. Novel 17-azolyl steroids, potent inhibitors of human cytochrome 17α-hydroxylase-C17,20-lyase (P450 17α): potential agents for the treatment of prostate cancer. J Med Chem 1998;41:902–12.

[108] Njar VCO, Klus GT, Brodie AMH. Nucleophilic vinylic 'addition-elimination' substitution reaction of 3β-acetoxy-17-chloro-16- formylandrosta-5,16-diene: a novel and general route to 17-substituted steroids. Part 1—synthesis of novel 17-azolyl-Δ16-steroids; inhibitors of 17α-hydroxylase/17,20-lyase (17α-lyase). Bioorg Med Chem Lett 1996;6:2777–82.

[109] Nnane IP, Njar VCO, Liu Y, Lu Q, Brodie AMH. Effects of novel 17-azolyl compounds on androgen synthesis in vitro and in vivo. J Steroid Biochem Mol Biol 1999;71:145–52.

[110] Ling YZ, Li JS, Liu Y, Kato K, Klus GT, Brodie AMH. 17-Imidazolyl, pyrazolyl, and isoxazolyl androstene derivatives: novel steroidal inhibitors of human cytochrome C17,20-lyase (P450 17α). J Med Chem 1997;40:3297–304.

[111] Zhu N, Ling Y, Lei X, Handratta V, Brodie AMH. Novel P450 17α inhibitors: 17-(2′-oxazolyl)- and 17-(2′-thiazolyl)-androstene derivatives. Steroids 2003;68:603–11.

[112] Haidar S, Ehmer PB, Hartmann RW. Novel steroidal pyrimidyl inhibitors of P450 17 (17α-hydroxylase/C17,20-lyase). Arch Pharm Pharm Med Chem 2001;334:373–4.

[113] Moreira VA, Vasaitis TS, Njar VCO, Salvador JAR. Synthesis and evaluation of novel 17-indazole androstene derivatives designed as CYP17 inhibitors. Steroids 2007;72:939–48.

[114] Haidar S, Ehmer PB, Barassin S, Batzl-Hartmann C, Hartmann RW. Effects of novel 17α-hydroxylase/C17, 20-lyase (P450 17, CYP 17) inhibitors on androgen biosynthesis in vitro and in vivo. J Steroid Biochem Mol Biol 2003;84:555–62.

[115] Grigoryev DN, Long BJ, Nnane IP, Njar VCO, Liu Y, Brodie AMH. Effects of new 17α-hydroxylase/C17, 20-lyase inhibitors on LNCaP prostate cancer cell growth in vitro and in vivo. Br J Cancer 1999;81:622–30.

[116] Nnane IP, Njar VCO, Brodie AMH. Pharmacokinetics of novel inhibitors of androgen synthesis after intravenous administration in mice. Cancer Chemother Pharmacol 2003;51:519–24.

[117] Nnane IP, Njar VCO, Brodie AMH. Pharmacokinetic profile of 3β-hydroxy-17-(1H-1,2,3-triazol-1-yl) androsta-5,16-diene (VN/87-1), a potent androgen synthesis inhibitor, in mice. J Steroid Biochem Mol Biol 2001;78:241–6.

[118] Nnane IP, Kalo K, Liu Y, Lu Q, Wang X, Ling YZ, et al. Effects of some novel inhibitors of C17,20-lyase and 5α-reductase in vitro and in vivo and their potential role in the treatment of prostate cancer. Cancer Res 1998;58:3826–32.

[119] Nnane IP, Long BJ, Ling YZ, Grigoryev DN, Brodie AMH. Anti-tumour effects and pharmacokinetic profile of 17-(5'-isoxazolyl)androsta-4,16-dien-3-one (L-39) in mice: an inhibitor of androgen synthesis. Br J Cancer 2000;83:74–82.

[120] Chu D, Myers PL, Wang B. Decahydro-1H-indenoquinolinone and decahydro-3H-cyclopentaphenanthridinone CYP17 inhibitors US20100105700. 2010.

[121] Chu D, Wang B, Tao Y. Novel CYP17 inhibitors. WO2011088160. 2011.

[122] Small EJ, Halabi S, Dawson NA, Stadler WM, Rini BI, Picus J, et al. Antiandrogen withdrawal alone or in combination with ketoconazole in androgen-independent prostate cancer patients: a phase III trial (CALGB 9583). J Clin Oncol 2004;22:1025–33.

[123] Harris KA, Weinberg V, Bok RA, Kakefuda M, Small EJ. Low dose ketoconazole with replacement doses of hydrocortisone in patients with progressive androgen independent prostate cancer. J Urol 2002;168:542–5.

[124] Wilkinson S, Chodak G. An evaluation of intermediate-dose ketoconazole in hormone refractory prostate cancer. Eur Urol 2004;45:581–4.

[125] Small EJ, Baron AD, Fippin L, Apodaca D. Ketoconazole retains activity in advanced prostate cancer patients with progression despite flutamide withdrawal. J Urol 1997;157:1204–7.

[126] Figg WD, Liu Y, Arlen P, Gulley J, Steinberg SM, Liewehr DJ, et al. A randomized, phase II trial of ketoconazole plus alendronate versus ketoconazole alone in patients with androgen independent prostate cancer and bone metastases. J Urol 2005;173:790–6.

[127] Millikan R, Baez L, Banerjee T, Wade J, Edwards K, Winn R, et al. Randomized phase 2 trial of ketoconazole and ketoconazole/doxorubicin in androgen independent prostate cancer. Urol Oncol 2001;6:111–5.

[128] Matsunaga N, Kaku T, Ojida A, Tanaka T, Hara T, Yamaoka M, et al. C17,20-lyase inhibitors. Part 2: design, synthesis and structure–activity relationships of (2-naphthylmethyl)-1H-imidazoles as novel C17,20-lyase inhibitors. Bioorg Med Chem 2004;12:4313–36.

[129] Kaku T, Tsujimoto S, Matsunaga N, Tanaka T, Hara T, Yamaoka M, et al. 17,20-Lyase inhibitors. Part 3: design, synthesis, and structure–activity relationships of biphenylylmethylimidazole derivatives as novel 17,20-lyase inhibitors. Bioorg Med Chem 2011;19:2428–42.

[130] Kaku T, Matsunaga N, Ojida A, Tanaka T, Hara T, Yamaoka M, et al. 17,20-Lyase inhibitors. Part 4: design, synthesis and structure–activity relationships of naphthylmethylimidazole derivatives as novel 17,20-lyase inhibitors. Bioorg Med Chem 2011;19:1751–70.

[131] Yamaoka M, Hara T, Hitaka T, Kaku T, Takeuchi T, Takahashi J, et al. Orteronel (TAK-700), a novel non-steroidal 17,20-lyase inhibitor: effects on steroid synthesis in human and monkey adrenal cells and serum steroid levels in cynomolgus monkeys. J Steroid Biochem Mol Biol 2012;129:115–28.

[132] Kaku T, Hitaka T, Ojida A, Matsunaga N, Adachi M, Tanaka T, et al. Discovery of orteronel (TAK-700), a naphthylmethylimidazole derivative, as a highly selective 17,20-lyase inhibitor with potential utility in the treatment of prostate cancer. Bioorg Med Chem 2011;19:6383–99.

[133] Dreicer R, Agus DB, MacVicar GR, MacLean D, Zhang T, Stadler WM. Safety, pharmacokinetics, and efficacy of TAK-700 in metastatic castration-resistant prostrate cancer: a phase I/II, open-label study. J Clin Oncol 2010;28(Suppl. 15); abstr. 3084.

[134] Dreicer R, Agus DB, MacVicar GR, MacLean D, Zhang T, Stadler WM. Safety, pharmacokinetics, and efficacy of TAK-700 in castration-resistant, metastatic prostate cancer: a phase I/II, open-label study. Genitourinary Cancers Symposium 2010. abstr. 103.

[135] Agus DB, Stadler WM, Shevrin DH, Hart L, MacVicar GR, Hamid O, et al. Safety, efficacy, and pharmaco-dynamics of the investigational agent orteronel (TAK-700) in metastatic castration-resistant prostate cancer (mCRPC): updated data from a phase I/II study. J Clin Oncol 2012;30(Suppl. 5); abstr. 98.

[136] George DJ, Corn PG, Michaelson MD, Hammers HJ, Alumkal JJ, Ryan CJ, et al. Safety and activity of the inves-tigational agent orteronel (ortl) without prednisone in men with nonmetastatic castration-resistant prostate cancer (nmCRPC) and rising prostate-specific antigen (PSA): updated results of a phase II study. J Clin Oncol 2012;30(Suppl); abstr. 4549.

[137] Dreicer R, Agus DB, Bellmunt J, De Bono JS, Petrylak DP, Tejura B, et al. A phase III, randomized, double-blind, multicenter trial comparing the investigational agent orteronel (TAK-700) plus prednisone (P) with placebo plus P in patients with metastatic castration-resistant prostate cancer (mCRPC) that has progressed during or following docetaxel-based therapy. J Clin Oncol 2012;30(Suppl. 15); abstr. TPS4693.

[138] Hoekstra WJ, Schotzinger RJ, Rafferty SW. Metalloenzyme inhibitor compounds. WO2012082746. 2012.

[139] Hoekstra WJ, Schotzinger RJ, Rafferty SW. Metalloenzyme inhibitor compounds. WO2012064943. 2012.

[140] Hoekstra WJ, Schotzinger RJ, Rafferty SW. Metalloenzyme inhibitor compounds. WO2012058529. 2012.

[141] Hoekstra WJ, Schotzinger RJ, Rafferty SW. Metalloenzyme inhibitor compounds. WO2011082245. 2011.

[142] Eisner JR, Abbott DH, Bird IM, Rafferty SW, Moore WR, Schotzinger RJ. VT-464: a novel, selective inhibitor of P450c17(CYP17)-17,20 lyase for castration-refractory prostate cancer (CRPC). J Clin Oncol 2012;30(Suppl. 5); abstr. 198.

[143] Eisner JR, Abbott DH, Bird IM, Rafferty SW, Moore WR, Schotzinger RJ. Assessment of steroid hormones upstream of P450c17 (CYP17) in chemically castrate male rhesus monkeys following treatment with the CYP17 inhibitors VT-464 and abiraterone acetate (AA). Endocr Rev 2012;33; (03_MeetingAbstracts), SAT-266.

[144] Abbott DH, Eisner JR, Rafferty SW, Moore WR, Schotzinger RJ. Plasma steroid concentrations in male rhesus monkeys following treatment with the P450c17 (CYP17) inhibitors VT-464 and abiraterone acetate: a compari-son to human 17,20-lyase (lyase) and combined lyase/17α-hydroxylase (hydroxylase) deficiencies. Endocr Rev 2012;33; (03_MeetingAbstracts), SAT-256.

[145] Pisle ST, Pressler HM, Troutman SM, Eisner JR, Rafferty SW, Schotzinger RJ, et al. Activity of VT-464, a selective CYP17 lyase inhibitor, in the LNCaP prostate cancer xenograft model. J Clin Oncol 2012;30(Suppl. 5); abstr. 64.

[146] Minoru O, Toru Y, Eiji K, Yoshiaki S, Tsukasa I, Masafumi K. Azole derivative and pharmaceutical composition thereof. WO9509157. 1995.

[147] Cherry PC, Cocker JD, Searle AD. Carbazole derivatives with 17,20-lyase inhibiting activity. WO9427989. 1994.

[148] Ideyama Y, Kudoh M, Tanimoto K, Susaki Y, Nanya T, Nakahara T, et al. YM116, 2-(1H-imidazol-4-ylmethyl)-9H-carbazole, decreases adrenal androgen synthesis by inhibiting C17,20-lyase activity in NCI-H295 human adrenocortical carcinoma cells. Jpn J Pharmacol 1999;79:213–20.

[149] Ideyama Y, Kudoh M, Tanimoto K, Susaki Y, Nanya T, Nakahara T, et al. Novel nonsteroidal inhibitor of cytochrome P450 17α (17α-hydroxylase/C17,20-lyase), YM116, decreased prostatic weights by reducing serum concentrations of testosterone and adrenal androgens in rats. Prostate 1998;37:10–8.

[150] Hu Q, Negri M, Jahn-Hoffmann K, Zhuang Y, Olgen S, Bartels M, et al. Synthesis, biological evaluation, and molecular modeling studies of methylene imidazole substituted biaryls as inhibitors of human 17α-hydroxylase-17,20-lyase (CYP17)—part II: core rigidification and influence of substituents at the methylene bridge. Bioorg Med Chem 2008;16:7715–27.

[151] Hu Q, Negri M, Olgen S, Hartmann RW. The role of fluorine substitution in biphenyl methylene imidazole type CYP17 inhibitors for the treatment of prostate carcinoma. ChemMedChem 2010;5:899–910.

[152] Hu Q, Jagusch C, Hille UE, Haupenthal J, Hartmann RW. Replacement of imidazolyl by pyridyl in biphe-nyl methylenes results in selective CYP17 and dual CYP17/CYP11B1 inhibitors for the treatment of prostate cancer. J Med Chem 2010;53:5749–58.

[153] Hille UE, Hu Q, Vock C, Negri M, Bartels M, Mueller-Vieira U, et al. Novel CYP17 inhibitors: synthesis, biologi-cal evaluation, structure-activity relationships and modeling of methoxy- and hydroxy-substituted methyle-neimidazolyl biphenyls. Eur J Med Chem 2009;44:2765–75.

[154] Pinto-Bazurco Mendieta MAE, Negri M, Hu Q, Hille UE, Jagusch C, Jahn-Hoffmann K, et al. CYP17 inhibitors. Annulations of additional rings in methylene imidazole substituted biphenyls: synthesis, biological evaluation and molecular modeling. Arch Pharm (Weinheim, Ger) 2008;341:597–609.

[155] Hille UE, Hu Q, Pinto-Bazurco Mendieta MAE, Bartels M, Vock CA, Lauterbach T, et al. Steroidogenic cyto-chrome P450 (CYP) enzymes as drug targets: combining substructures of known CYP inhibitors leads to com-pounds with different inhibitory profile. C R Chim 2009;12:1117–26.

[156] Wachall BG, Hector M, Zhuang Y, Hartmann RW. Imidazole substituted biphenyls: a new class of highly potent and in vivo active inhibitors of P450 17 as potential therapeutics for treatment of prostate cancer. Bioorg Med Chem 1999;7:1913–24.

[157] Zhuang Y, Wachall BG, Hartmann RW. Novel imidazolyl and triazolyl substituted biphenyl compounds: synthesis and evaluation as nonsteroidal inhibitors of human 17α-hydroxylase-C17, 20-lyase (P450 17). Bioorg Med Chem 2000;8:1245–52.

[158] Leroux F, Hutschenreuter TU, Charriere C, Scopelliti R, Hartmann RW. N-(4-biphenylmethyl)imidazoles as potential therapeutics for the treatment of prostate cancer: metabolic robustness due to fluorine substitution? Helv Chim Acta 2003;86:2671–86.

[159] Pinto-Bazurco Mendieta MAE, Negri M, Jagusch C, Hille UE, Müller-Vieira U, Schmidt D, et al. Synthesis, biological evaluation and molecular modelling studies of novel ACD- and ABD-ring steroidomimetics as inhibitors of CYP17. Bioorg Med Chem Lett 2008;18:267–73.

[160] Pinto-Bazurco Mendieta MAE, Negri M, Jagusch C, Müller-Vieira U, Lauterbach T, Hartmann RW. Synthesis, biological evaluation, and molecular modeling of abiraterone analogues: novel CYP17 inhibitors for the treatment of prostate cancer. J Med Chem 2008;51:5009–18.

[161] Hutschenreuter TU, Ehmer PE, Hartmann RW. Synthesis of hydroxy derivatives of highly potent non-steroidal CYP 17 inhibitors as potential metabolites and evaluation of their activity by a non cellular assay using recombinant human enzyme. J Enzyme Inhib Med Chem 2004;19:17–32.

[162] Wächter GA, Hartmann RW, Sergejew T, Grün GL, Ledergerber D. Tetrahydronaphthalenes: influence of heterocyclic substituents on inhibition of steroidogenic enzymes P450 arom and P450 17. J Med Chem 1996;39:834–41.

[163] Zhuang Y, Hartmann RW. Synthesis of novel oximes of 2-aryl-6-methoxy-3,4-dihydronaphthalene and their evaluation as inhibitors of 17α-hydroxylase-C$_{17,20}$-lyase (P450 17). Arch Pharm (Weinheim, Ger) 1998;331: 36–40.

[164] Zhuang Y, Hartmann RW. Synthesis and evaluation of azole-substituted 2-aryl-6-methoxy-3,4-dihydronaphthalenes and -naphthalenes as inhibitors of 17α-hydroxylase-C$_{17,20}$-lyase (P450 17). Arch Pharm (Weinheim, Ger) 1999;332:25–30.

[165] Hartmann RW, Palusczak A, Lacan F, Ricci G, Ruzziconi R. CYP 17 and CYP 19 inhibitors: evaluation of fluorine effects on the inhibiting activity of regioselectively fluorinated 1-(naphthalen-2-ylmethyl)imidazoles. J Enzyme Inhib Med Chem 2004;19:145–55.

[166] Bierer D, McClure A, Fu W, Achebe F, Ladouceur GH, Burke MJ, et al. 3-Pyridyl or 4-isoquinolinyl thiazoles as C17,20 lyase inhibitors. WO03027085. 2003.

[167] Ladouceur GH, Burke MJ, Wong WC, Bierer, D. Substituted 3-pyridyl indoles and indazoles as C17,20 lyase inhibitors. WO03027094. 2003.

[168] Scott WJ, Johnson J, Fu W, Bierer D. Substituted 3-pyridyl tetrazoles as steroid C17,20 lyase inhibitors. WO03027095. 2003.

[169] Hart B, Sibley R, Dumas J, Bierer D, Zhang C. Substituted 3-pyridyl imidazoles as C17,20 lyase inhibitors. WO03027096. 2003.

[170] Scott WJ, Fu W, Monahan MK, Bierer D. Substituted 3-pyridyl pyrimidines as C17,20 lyase inhibitors. WO03027100. 2003.

[171] Scott WJ, Johnson J, McClure A, Fu W, Zhang C, Bierer, D. Substituted 3-pyridyl pyrroles and 3-pyridyl pyrazoles as C17,20 lyase inhibitors. WO03027101. 2003

[172] Achebe F, McClure A, Bierer D. Substituted 3-pyridyl thiophenes as C17,20 lyase inhibitors. WO03027105. 2003.

[173] Hart B, Bierer D, Zhang C. Substituted 3-pyridyl oxazole as C17,20 lyase inhibitors. WO03027107. 2003.

[174] Bock MG, Gaul C, Gummadi VR, Sengupta, S. 1, 3-Disubstituted imidazolidin-2-one derivatives as inhibitors of CYP17. WO2020149755. 2010.

[175] Velapapthi U, Liu P, Balog JA. Imidazopyridazinyl compounds and their uses for cancer. WO2011137155. 2011.

[176] Velapapthi U, Frennesson DB, Saulnier MG, Austin JF, Huang A, Balog JA. Azaindazole compounds. WO2012009510. 2012.

[177] Austin JF, Frennesson DB, Saulnier MG. Substituted azaindazole compounds. WO20120064815. 2012.

[178] Rowlands MG, Barrie SE, Chan F, Houghton J, Jarman M, McCague R. Esters of 3-pyridylacetic acid that combine potent inhibition of 17α-hydroxylase/C17,20-lyase (cytochrome P450 17α) with resistance to esterase hydrolysis. J Med Chem 1995;38:4191–7.

[179] Barrie SE, Haynes BP, Potter GA, Chan FC, Goddard PM, Dowsett M. Biochemistry and pharmacokinetics of potent non-steroidal cytochrome P450 17α inhibitors. J Steroid Biochem Mol Biol 1997;60:347–51.

[180] Austin JF, Sharma LS, Balog JA, Huang A, Velaparthi U, Darne CP, et al. Sulfonamide compounds useful as CYP17 inhibitors. WO2012015723. 2012.

[181] Bock MG, Gaul C, Gummadi VR, Moebitz H, Sengupta S. 17α-Hydroxylase/C17,20-lyase inhibitors. WO2012035078. 2012.

[182] Krug SJ, Hu Q, Hartmann RW. Hits identified in library screening demonstrate selective CYP17A1 lyase inhibition. J Steroid Biochem Mol Biol 2013;134:75–9.

[183] Hu Q, Pinto-Bazurco Mendieta MAE, Hartmann RW. Highly potent and selective non-steroidal dual inhibitors of CYP17/CYP11B2 for the treatment of prostate cancer in reducing cardiovascular complications. J Med Chem in press.

[184] Yin L, Hu Q. CYP17 inhibitors: from promiscuous abiraterone to selective C17-20 lyase inhibitors and multi-targeting agents. Nat Rev Urol 2013; in press.

12

Apoptosis in Cancer: Mechanisms, Deregulation, and Therapeutic Targeting

Zahid H. Siddik

Department of Experimental Therapeutics, The University of Texas,
MD Anderson Cancer Center, Houston, TX, USA

INTRODUCTION

Apoptosis is a genetic program of cell death that is inherent to mammalian and plant cells, and it empowers cells to activate the program and commit suicide when self-destruction signals are generated. In mammals, this process is vital for eliminating cells in a range of physiological processes, including normal embryonic development, homeostatic regulation of tissue mass in adults, and immune system functions. Apoptosis is also critical for cellular response to stress, but in this case, the threshold for the stressful stimuli to induce death in normal cells can be high, so that only extreme conditions, such as irreparable genomic damage, will activate programmed cell death. The reason for the limited sensitivity is easy to comprehend: Throughout evolution, eukaryotic cells have been exposed to harsh environments, and have progressively adapted and acquired the ability to become more resilient. This resiliency is encrypted into the genome and passed on through cytokinesis to the next generation, ensuring that daughter cells have an identical copy of the genetic material to cope with environmental stress. Therefore, when mammalian cells are stressed by genetic damage or other causes, such as oxidative stress and hypoxia, the normal response of the cells is to mitigate the stress and survive, and only if the stress is excessive will cells then activate the apoptotic program.

It is noteworthy that apoptosis is a frequent occurrence in an adult human body, destroying some 50–70 million defective cells every day [1]. On rare occasions, however, genetic damage may escape surveillance mechanisms and induce the development of cancer, which may or may not retain the apoptotic program. If tumor cells retain the program and if this is also associated with an acquired reduced stress threshold for activating apoptosis, as in many cancers, then a narrow therapeutic window is afforded for the specific antitumor modality to induce responses and even cures. In contrast, defects in the apoptotic program, either *ab initio* or attained during the course of therapy, can lead to poor therapeutic outcomes. Since apoptosis is an indispensable component of cancer therapy, much effort has been devoted by the cancer research community to restore in resistant cells, and even enhance in sensitive cells, facile activation of this cell death process. To understand the specific rationale for each of the various approaches that are presently in preclinical and clinical development for targeting apoptosis, it becomes important to discuss the apoptotic mechanism and how defects in this cell death program can render tumor cells resistant to therapy.

MECHANISMS OF APOPTOSIS

Apoptosis is morphologically similar across various cell types and species, and manifests as a series of cellular changes that include chromatin condensation, nuclear fragmentation, cell shrinkage, blebbing, and phagocytosis [2,3]. The process is highly regulated to avoid an inflammatory response and is complex, involving a large number of proteins. However, apoptosis can essentially be divided into two major pathways, extrinsic and intrinsic. These two pathways are activated in an independent manner but are linked, and they have some common cysteinyl aspartate proteinases (caspases) that are intimately involved in affecting the morphological features of apoptosis. However, a distinguishing feature is that the extrinsic pathway is mediated through caspase-8, whereas the intrinsic pathway involves caspase-9 (Fig. 12.1). There are some

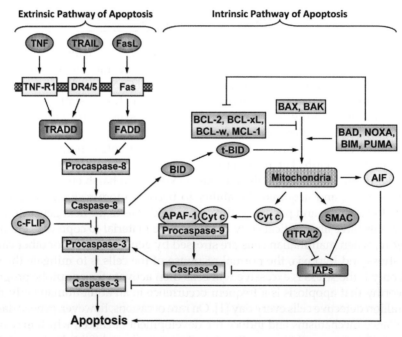

FIGURE 12.1 Extrinsic and intrinsic pathways of apoptosis. The two pathways are independent but connected through BID, and they share caspase-3 as the common effector protease. (This figure is reproduced in color in the color plate section.)

14 members in the caspase family that are usually present in cells in inactive procaspase forms, and they become activated only through a series of cleavage reactions when stress signals are received by the cell death machinery. Although apoptosis is largely dependent on caspases, it can also occur in a caspase-independent manner [4].

Extrinsic Death Receptor (DR) Apoptotic Pathway

As the name suggests, the extrinsic pathway is activated by extracellular apoptotic signals, which are transduced into cells when specific death-inducing ligands bind to transmembrane death receptors on the cell surface. The most common interactions are between tumor necrosis factor (TNF), TNF-related apoptosis-inducing ligands (TRAILs), or FasL ligands and, respectively, their cognitive receptors TNF-R1 (TNF receptor type 1), DR4 (TRAIL-R1) and DR5 (TRAIL-R2), or Fas (also known as Apo-1 or CD95) (Fig. 12.1). This binding induces oligomerization of the receptor and allows the intracellular extension of the receptor to recruit the corresponding TNF or TRAIL receptor-associated death domain (TRADD) or Fas-associated death domain (FADD) adapter protein that then permits the binding of procaspase-8 to form the death-inducing signaling complex (DISC). Formation of DISC allows autoactivation of procaspase-8 to the initiator caspase-8, which then activates the downstream effector caspases caspase-3, 6, and 7, which ultimately target cellular structures to effect cell death [5]. Of these, caspase-3 is most often implicated in the cell death process following exposure to therapeutic agents.

Intrinsic Mitochondrial Apoptotic Pathway

In contrast to the extrinsic pathway, the intrinsic pathway of apoptosis is initiated by stress stimuli generated within the cell and involves the critical change in the mitochondrial outer membrane potential in order to increase its permeability and release proapoptotic biochemicals and proteins. In cancer therapy, a typical example of the onset of proapoptotic stress stimuli comes from DNA damage induced by cytotoxic agents, such as adriamycin, methotrexate, and cisplatin. In such situations, the DNA damage is recognized by specialized damage recognition proteins, which then transduce stress signals through a series of protein–protein interactions that eventually result in mitochondrial release of cytochrome c, together with second mitochondria-derived activator of apoptosis (SMAC), also known as DIABLO (the direct inhibitor of apoptosis protein (IAP)-binding protein with low pI), and the serine protease HTRA2 (Omi). The functions of these proteins are coordinated to activate or enhance potency of the effector caspase. First, the cytosolic release of cytochrome c promotes its binding to the adapter protein APAF-1 and recruitment of procaspase-9 to form the "apoptosome" structure, and the resultant formation of active caspase-9 converts procaspase-3, 6, and 7 to the corresponding active form [5]. The SMAC/DIABLO and HTRA2 proteins potentiate the apoptotic process by inhibiting or inactivating IAPs, such as XIAP, and alleviating the latter's inhibitory effects on caspases [6]. Depending on the cytotoxic agent, the mitochondria may also release the apoptosis-inducing factor (AIF), which translocates to the nucleus and induce apoptosis in a caspase-independent manner [7].

The independence of the intrinsic pathway from the extrinsic pathway has been demonstrated in a series of gene knockout studies. Thus, knockout of FADD or caspase-8 inhibits apoptosis by death receptor stimulation, but not by cytotoxic drugs, and, conversely, knock-out of caspase-9 or APAF-1 renders cells insensitive to cytotoxic drugs, but not to agents activating the death receptor pathway [8–11]. However, the two pathways are linked through BID, a member of the BCL-2 family, but in a unidirectional manner [12,13]. That is, activated caspase-8 in the extrinsic pathway can cleave BID, and the cleaved product t-BID then trans-locates to the mitochondria to modulate the process for the cytoplasmic release of cytochrome c and activate the intrinsic apoptotic pathway. This pathway is also critically regulated by other members of the BCL-2 family, although reports indicate that BCL-2 proteins can also impact the extrinsic pathway [14].

Regulation of the Intrinsic Pathway of Apoptosis by the BCL-2 Family

Members of the BCL-2 family modulate the mitochondrial outer membrane potential, and their presence in the regulatory oligomeric complex is a determinant of whether or not the mitochondrial release of cytochrome c, SMAC/DIABLO, and HTRA2 will occur. The original member BCL-2 was identified in non-Hodgkin lymphoma, but is present in many cell types and functions as a negative regulator of apoptosis. Other proteins with BCL-2-like features and homology were subsequently identified so that the BCL-2 family now comprises some 20–25 members, which are subdivided into two groups [15,16]. One group is composed of members that, like BID (BCL-2-interacting domain death agonist), are proapoptotic and include BAX (BCL-2-associated x protein), BAK (BCL-2 antagonist killer 1), BAD (BCL-2 antagonist of cell death), BIM (BCL-2-interacting mediator of cell death), NOXA, and PUMA (p53-upregulated modulator of apoptosis) (Fig. 12.1). In contrast, the second group has antiapoptotic members that function like BCL-2; it includes BCL-xL (BCL-2-related long isoform), BCL-w (also called BCL-2-like protein 2, or BCL-2-L2), and MCL-1 (myeloid cell leukemia 1). This antiapoptotic group has four BCL-2 homology domains (BH1, BH2, BH3, and BH4), whereas the proapop-totic forms can either have all four domains and function as "effectors" (BAX and BAK), or have only the BH3 domain that functions as "direct activators", "sensitizers" or "derepres-sors" (e.g., BAD, BID, BIM, NOXA, and PUMA). The relative cellular expression of antiapop-totic, effector, and direct activator, sensitizer, or derepressor proteins will dictate the final mitochondrial pore-forming capability of the oligomeric regulatory complex, which in turn will determine the permeability of the mitochondrial outer membrane and whether the cell undergoes apoptosis or resists the stress signal and survives [15,17]. For instance, BIM and BID interact with and oligomerize BAX and BAK for a proapoptotic effect, whereas the pres-ence of an antiapoptotic member, such as BCL-2, in the oligomer will inhibit apoptosis. On the other hand, the BH3 domain protein can also negatively interact with the antiapoptotic member, thereby promoting BAX and BAK oligomerization and potentiating apoptosis.

Induction of Apoptosis by the Tumor Suppressor p53

The greater drug sensitivity of tumor cells compared to normal cells may depend on a specific gene signature profile that lowers the threshold for stress signals to induce apop-tosis in tumor cells following exposure to antitumor agents. In this context, a specific gene that commands greater attention is the tumor suppressor *TP53*, which is generally hailed as the "guardian of the genome". In its wild-type conformation, the p53 protein product is

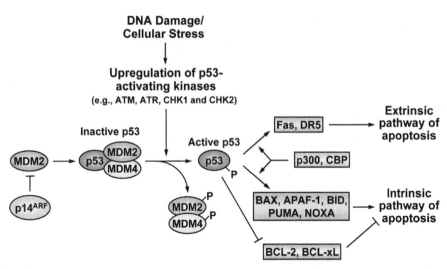

FIGURE 12.2 Induction of apoptosis by the tumor suppressor p53. Binding to MDM2 and MDM4 inactivates p53, but posttranslational phosphorylation releases p53 to transactivate downstream target genes and induce apoptosis via the extrinsic and intrinsic pathways. (This figure is reproduced in color in the color plate section.)

critical for antitumor drug response and for imparting drug sensitivity to tumor cells [18]. It accomplishes this function by transcriptionally activating downstream target genes that are intimately involved in DNA damage response, including cell cycle arrest and apoptosis [19]. Although p53-induced apoptosis usually requires transcriptional activation, it can also occur in a transcription-independent manner (discussed further in this chapter). In either situation, the activity of p53 is tightly regulated: under basal conditions, p53 activity is kept in check by the interaction with the proteins mouse double minute 2 homolog (MDM2) and the structurally related MDM4, which promote proteosomal degradation and attenuate proapoptotic functions of the tumor suppressor [20]. Therefore, to activate apoptotic response with antitumor agents, p53 must first be released from the MDM2/4–p53 complex (Fig. 12.2). This is accomplished by upregulation of upstream kinases, such as ATM (ataxia telangiectasia mutated), ATR (ataxia telangiectasia and Rad3-related), CHK1, and CHK2, which posttranslationally modify p53 at several sites. However, phosphorylation at Ser15, Thr18, and Ser20 are the most critical to release and stabilize p53 from the complex; allow recruitment of transcription co-activators, such as p300 and CREB (cyclic adenosine monophosphate response element-binding protein)-binding protein (CBP); and activate its apoptotic function [21]. Posttranslational modifications at distinct sites of MDM2 (e.g., Tyr394) and MDM4 (e.g., Tyr99) also occur in parallel to enhance dissociation of the complex and release p53 [20].

Apoptosis signaling induced by p53 can be transduced along both the extrinsic and intrinsic pathways (Fig. 12.2). In the extrinsic pathway, the most significant transcriptional targets of p53 are the *Fas* and the *DR5* genes [22,23]. The intrinsic pathway, on the other hand, has several proapoptotic genes that are targeted by p53, including *BAX*, *NOXA*, *APAF-1* (apoptotic protease-activating factor 1), *PUMA*, and *BID* [23]. In each case, the apoptotic response to antitumor agents is slow since p53 itself must first be stabilized and activated, then it must translocate to the nucleus to transcriptionally increase the levels of mRNA of target genes that subsequently translate into higher levels of the corresponding proteins to activate the respective cell death pathway. In contrast, the transcription-independent mechanism of apoptosis is relatively fast since the mechanism is simply dependent on translocation of p53 to the mitochondria and its negative interaction with antiapoptotic BCL-xL and BCL-2 proteins to indirectly enhance proapoptotic oligomerization of BAK and BAX [24,25]. In a similar manner, p53 binds directly to BAK to facilitate BAK oligomerization by disrupting the negative antiapoptotic interaction between BAK and MCL-1 [26]. Downregulation of antiapoptotic BCL-2 by p53 through transcriptional repression can also tip the balance in favor of apoptosis [27].

DEFECTS IN APOPTOSIS AND ANTITUMOR DRUG RESISTANCE

Most anticancer agents that act through DNA damage or stress-inducing signaling mechanisms require an intact apoptotic pathway for facile antitumor response [28]. Thus, defects in any part of the pathway will render tumor cells resistant to the antitumor agent. Moreover, because the pathway is shared by many antitumor agents, tumor cells demonstrating resistance to one agent will be cross-resistant to structurally diverse, unrelated drugs. Defects in apoptosis can arise through a variety of mechanisms, which in general include (1) failure to detect DNA damage, (2) functional failure in the proapoptotic protein or receptor, (3) upregulation of survival pathways, and (4) decrease in levels of the proapoptotic protein. Some of the specific mechanisms involved are shown in Fig. 12.3. Although a thorough treatise on each of these mechanisms is beyond the scope of this chapter, a brief examination is warranted to better understand, in general terms, which mechanisms can be most effectively targeted to induce apoptosis.

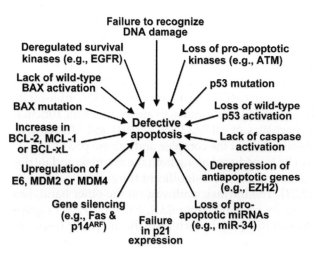

FIGURE 12.3 Mechanisms inhibiting apoptosis and inducing resistance to antitumor agents. Tumor cells may express several resistance mechanisms at the same time, and this essentially inhibits antitumor response. The number of mechanisms involved in inhibiting apoptosis is extensive, and only a selection is shown.

Failure to Detect DNA Damage

The ability to respond to cellular insult from a therapeutic modality first requires recognition of the damage that then induces stress signals to affect a favorable apoptotic response. The most common source of stress with antitumor modalities is DNA damage, but the specific proteins that recognize this damage depend on the type of lesion induced, such as single- or double-strand DNA breaks. DNA damage is recognized by the PI3K-like kinase ATM, ATR, or DNA-dependent protein kinase (DNA-PK), which then initiates a cascade of phosphorylation steps to transmit the DNA damage signal to the apoptotic machinery [29]. Failure in DNA damage recognition impedes apoptosis. Defect in the ATM pathway, for instance, has been reported in the form of low ATM expression or mutation, and this impacts negatively on the response of B-cell chronic lymphocytic leukemia (CLL) patients to the therapy [30–33]. Poor apoptosis and response can also occur if the downstream protein substrate of ATM becomes deregulated instead, and this is exemplified by downregulation of CHK2 in non-small-cell lung cancer (NSCLC) [34,35].

Another form of DNA damage is through the formation of DNA adducts induced by antitumor agents. Such adducts are typical of platinum-based antitumor agents, and the best example of this is cisplatin. This agent binds to N7 sites of both adenine and guanine to form DNA interstrand and intrastrand adducts, which induce local unwinding and kinking of the DNA [36]. These physical distortions by cisplatin are recognized by some 20 different specialized DNA damage recognition proteins to transduce DNA damage signals and affect apoptosis. One such protein is hMSH2, which is a member of the mismatch repair group of proteins and recognizes intrastrand GpG adducts. Absence of hMSH2 has indeed been observed in cisplatin-resistant tumor cells, and this directly attenuates apoptosis [36].

Functional Failure in the Proapoptotic Protein or Receptor

Proteins involved in the apoptotic pathway may fail for several reasons: they may mutate, their expression downregulated by gene deletion or silencing, or they do not become activated in their wild-type state to transduce the cell death signal. The tumor suppressor CHK2 is an example that, as indicated in the previous section, is an important substrate for phosphorylation in ATM-mediated apoptotic signaling, but either is silenced, as in NSCLC [34], or becomes redundant due to ATM defects upstream, as in CLL [30]. Several isoforms of the microRNA miR-34 also play an effective role in promoting apoptosis, but in 60–100% of renal, breast, urothelial, colorectal, pancreatic, and ovarian cancers, miR-34 expression is reduced due to gene silencing from promoter hypermethylation [37]. Downregulation of BAX expression can also occur and leads to therapy failure, but this is ascribed to mutation in the *BAX* gene that has been observed in ~50% of gastric and colorectal cancer patients [38–40]. In addition, failure of therapy to activate wild-type BAX has been reported as a mechanism for the poor outcome in Hodgkin disease [41].

Perhaps the most important example of a proapoptotic gene gone awry in cancer is *p53*, and its mutation in about half of all human cancers is one of the most frequently occurring genetic abnormalities that inhibits apoptosis, reduces antitumor drug response, and reduces survival rates in patients [42–44]. The clearest example of this is in pediatric patients, where choroid plexus carcinoma is universally curable with a chemoradiation regimen if wild-type p53 is expressed, but ~80% patients die within 6 months of diagnosis if tumors harbor mutant p53 [45]. Similar, but not as dramatic, observations have been made in advanced breast cancer, which responds positively in the presence of wild-type p53 to the 5-fluorouracil (5-FU)–epirubicin–cyclophosphamide regimen in 45–64% of patients, and this contrasts strikingly with the absence of any response when mutant p53 is present in the tumor [46,47]. It is also useful to consider CLL in this context: in this disease, the 5-year survival rate was reduced threefold when mutant p53 was expressed (20% vs 59%) [48]. In chronic myelogenous leukemia (CML), the availability of the targeted BCR–ABL inhibitor imatinib (STI-571, or Gleevec) has revolutionized its treatment, but the treatment fails when mutant p53 is present [49]. Likewise, gefitinib, a targeted inhibitor of epidermal growth factor receptor (EGFR) tyrosine kinase that is effective in NSCLC, loses antitumor activity when tumor cells express mutant p53 [50]. In some cancers, mutant p53 may express a gain-of-function phenotype, and such tumor cells express supra-resistance to a variety of apoptosis-inducing agents [35]. Interestingly, such a high level of resistance is not confined to the mutant p53 category; evidence indicates that some wild-type p53 cancers not only are resistant to therapy but also may express a gain-of-resistance phenotype [35]. This is observed in a number of tumor tissue types, including NSCLC and ovarian, mesothelioma, renal cell, and bladder cancers. In such cancers, the wild-type p53 is prevented from becoming activated by the antitumor agent. Several mechanisms have been reported for this, including increased p53 degradation from upregulated MDM2 and MDM4 in ~10–70% of several cancer types [51,52] and loss of posttranslational modification by downregulation of upstream kinases, such as ATM in CLL [53], CHK2 in NSCLC [34], and HIPK2 (homeodomain-interacting protein kinase 2) in colorectal cancers [54]. Much of the resistance to therapeutic agents in wild-type p53 cancers is due to loss of its transactivation function that impacts the expression of genes directly involved in apoptosis, such as BAX, Fas, p21, and miR-34 [55–58]. Indeed, defective expression of BAX and miR-34 has been correlated to poor clinical response in several cancers [37–40,59]. Another p53 target that is important in apoptosis and that negatively impacts clinical antitumor response in NSCLC and ovarian cancer when it becomes deregulated is p21 [60,61]. This cyclin-dependent kinase (CDK) inhibitor is also classified as a tumor suppressor, but its apoptotic effect is mediated through an indirect role—specifically, through p21-dependent repression of survivin, stathmin, telomerase, and other antiapoptotic proteins, which effectively lowers the apoptotic threshold [62–65].

Loss of apoptosis and onset of therapeutic resistance can also arise through attenuation of death receptor stimulation in the extrinsic apoptotic pathway. In this regard, reduced expression of Fas has been reported in leukemia, neuroblastoma, and other cancers that are associated with resistance to several antitumor agents, including doxorubicin, methotrexate, and cytarabine [66,67]. More recently, overexpression of the antiapoptotic protein c-FLIP has been demonstrated to antagonize TRAIL, prevent activation of the caspase-8/3 cascade (Fig. 12.1), and thereby inhibit the antitumor activity of 5-FU, cisplatin, and gemcitabine in pancreatic cancer [68]. The mechanism for this increase in c-FLIP and resistance to TRAIL was investigated in NSCLC cells and ascribed to stabilization of the antiapoptotic protein as a direct effect of upregulated AKT (also known as protein kinase B) expression and activity [69].

Upregulation of Survival Pathways

Over the past several decades, a number of survival pathways have been identified that, when upregulated, interfere with facile apoptotic signaling induced by antitumor agents. Some of the survival pathways involve upregulation of specific kinases, such as EGFR, HER2/neu, BCR/ABL, PI3K, and AKT, that can positively increase the function of antiapoptotic proteins, as exemplified above with c-FLIP. Deregulated constitutive activity of these kinases can also modulate function of the proapoptotic protein, as has been demonstrated by the phosphorylation of p21 at Thr^{145} and/or Ser^{146} sites, which then leads to sequestration of p21 in the cytoplasm, resulting in the loss of nuclear proapoptotic facilitative functions of this CDK inhibitor [70–72]. For instance, p21-dependent repression of antiapoptotic genes (*EZH2*, *survivin*, *telomerase*, etc.) is lost by nuclear exclusion [63,64,73]. However, the negative impact of phosphorylated p21 is not entirely due to its nuclear exclusion. Indeed, phosphorylated p21 sequestered in the cytoplasm also downregulates apoptosis by binding to procaspase-3 and preventing conversion to active caspase-3 [74]. The significance of this cytoplasmic sequestration of p21 becomes apparent from its reported correlation with resistance in testicular, breast, and ovarian cancers to antitumor agents, such as cisplatin [75–77]. The kinase AKT can also directly inactivate proapoptotic BAD [78,79] and indirectly downregulate the proapoptotic BIM, FasL, and IGF-BP1 proteins by phosphorylating and inactivating the transcriptional capacity of the forkhead target FKHRL1 [80,81].

BCL-2, MDM2, and IAP proteins are perhaps the three best known inhibitors of apoptosis, and their upregulation in cancers is well documented. The antiapoptotic BCL-2 is overexpressed in many cancers, and increase in its levels inhibits apoptosis by directly interfering with the oligomerization of proapoptotic BAD and BAK to release cytochrome c [15,17]. Similarly, an increase in MDM2 levels also attenuates apoptosis, but by downregulating p53 (discussed further in this chapter). A greater propensity for survival in tumor cells from increased levels of IAP proteins is ascribed to loss of their negative regulation by SMAC/DIABLO and HTRA2 proteins that then prevent caspase activation (see above). Overexpression of IAPs occurs frequently and is associated with poor therapeutic outcomes in several cancers, including NSCLC and pancreatic cancer [82–84]. IAPs are essentially a family of eight proteins in human cells and include the well-known XIAP, c-IAP1, c-IAP2, survivin, and ML-IAP, which impact caspase activity by either direct caspase binding or indirect high-affinity binding to SMAC/DIABLO. All IAPs have one (survivin and ML-IAP) or three (XIAP, c-IAP1, and c-IAP2) copies of the baculoviral IAP repeat (BIR) domain, which is important for negative protein–protein interactions that inhibit apoptosis, and many have a RING domain at the carboxy terminus that appears to be important for their E3 ubiquitin ligase activity and proteosomal degradation [82]. These IAPs have different targets for inhibiting apoptosis. Overexpressed XIAP, for instance, binds directly to caspase-3, caspase-7, and caspase-9, whereas c-IAP1, c-IAP2, and ML-IAP inhibit SMAC/SIABLO to prevent it from inactivating XIAP. These effects of IAPs can also be upregulated by other survival factors, such as the nuclear transcription factor NF-κB, which can exert a strong antiapoptotic influence when activated upon immediate proteosomal degradation of the inhibitor IκB by other deregulated pro-survival pathways, such as the PI3K–AKT pathway [85]. Activated NF-κB can also upregulate other antiapoptotic proteins, such as c-FLIP and the BCL-2 homologs BCL-xL and BFL-1/A1 [86,87].

An unusual role of p53 is in nuclear export of the BRCA1 protein in order to enhance the potency of DNA damage response. BRCA1 is normally involved in DNA repair, and its nuclear export potentiates apoptosis by not only increasing the persistence of DNA damage but also facilitating cell death processes in the cytosol [88,89]. However, dysfunctional p53 loses this ability to export BRCA1 in breast cancer and reduces antitumor response. Upregulation of survival pathways that mediate overexpression of BRCA1 in MCF-7 cells and result in cisplatin resistance has also been reported, and this may well be due to the inability of wild-type p53 to affect sufficient nuclear reduction of the repair protein to relieve its inhibitory effects on apoptosis [90].

Decrease in Levels of the Proapoptotic Protein

Apoptosis is dependent on a large number of proteins, and it is readily appreciated that reduced expression of a rate-limiting protein will inhibit the apoptotic process. This premise is consistent with decrease in levels of wild-type p53 through gene deletion or increased proteosomal degradation. The latter case is exemplified in cervical cancers, where infection by the human papillomavirus type 16 (HPV-16) results in frequent expression of the E6 oncogene product, which promotes p53 degradation via the ubiquitin pathway and prevents apoptotic response to therapeutic agents, such as camptothecin and cisplatin [91,92]. As discussed in this chapter, reduction in wild-type p53 levels from increased degradation is also affected by overexpression of MDM2 or MDM4, and this causes the consequential reduction in proapoptotic proteins (e.g., p21 and BAX) that are normally transactivated by p53. This overexpression of MDM2 is usually mediated through gene amplification, transcriptional upregulation, or increased translation [93,94], but failure to sequester it in the nucleolus following loss of the tumor suppressor p14^{ARF} has also been reported [95,96]. Like p53, frequent reduction in p14^{ARF} levels, as observed in neuroblastoma and colon cancer, can be attributable to homozygous gene deletion, but gene silencing can also contribute to its deregulation [97,98]. Indeed, epigenetic mechanisms are responsible for reductions in a cadre of other apoptotic proteins, typically through promoter hypermethylation, as has been shown with p21 in 40% of acute lymphocytic leukemia (ALL) patients, and this was associated with a lower patient survival rate compared to cases where the p21 promoter was hypomethylated and fully functional (6–8% vs ~60%) [99].

In apoptosis, the ultimate goal of the various signaling pathways is to activate caspases, which can execute the process of cell death. Therefore, reduction in caspase activity will inhibit apoptosis and impact response to therapy. There is, indeed, strong evidence to demonstrate that reduction in levels of the apoptosome adapter protein APAF-1 and/or caspase-3, 8, and 9 induces drug resistance in head and neck, ovarian, cervical, and breast cancers and in neuroblastoma [100–104]. In colorectal cancer, caspase-9 expression was similarly downregulated over twofold in 68% of cases, and this was associated with a poor clinical outcome [105].

THERAPEUTIC TARGETING OF APOPTOSIS

Under basal conditions, tumor cells are constantly fine-tuning homeostatic controls so that pro-survival signals always have an edge or even substantially exceed pro-death signals in order that the tumor cells survive. When the imbalance is slight, cytotoxic or targeted therapy can disrupt this homeostasis so that proapoptotic signals become dominant and induce cell death. However, a greater imbalance of signals toward survival will render tumor cells resistant to therapy, and, therefore, more specific and potent strategies have to be devised for targeting apoptosis. This may be accomplished by approaches that directly stimulate the apoptotic pathway, raise intracellular stress further to activate apoptosis, target antiapoptotic proteins for downregulation, or increase or activate intracellular proapoptotic proteins.

Directly Stimulating the Apoptotic Pathway

The extrinsic apoptotic pathway has attracted much attention for the development of apoptosis-targeted therapy, primarily since death receptors on the cell membrane are directly and easily accessible targets for apoptotic agonists that do not require entry into the tumor cell. Moreover, the pathway can bypass signaling defects upstream, such as those attributed to mutations in p53. Dulanermin (AMG-951), a recombinant human rhTRAIL composed of extracellular domain amino acids 114–281 of the wild-type ligand, is a prototype agonist that has shown much promise. This agonist was selectively active against tumor cells, has demonstrated effectiveness in murine xenograft models, and is a subject of clinical trials [106]. Preliminary phase I studies in non-Hodgkin lymphoma have demonstrated the therapy to be well tolerated and to have some clinical benefits, and this has encouraged its further development toward phase II trials [107]. Targeting Fas receptor with APO010 (a synthetic hexameric FasL ligand) and Fasaret (a recombinant adenoviral construct encoding FasL) is also being tested in clinical trials against solid tumors [108,109]. In a similar approach, agonistic antibodies have been developed to directly target DR4 and DR5 death receptors, and these include apomab, mapatumumab, lexatumumab, TRA-8/CS-1008, AMG-655, and LBY135, which are in various stages of clinical development [107,110,111].

The therapeutic potential of targeting death receptors is likely to be enhanced in combination with other antitumor agents, particularly since both the intrinsic and extrinsic pathways will be activated. This has been demonstrated with TRAIL in cisplatin-resistant cells, where the combination with cisplatin was highly effective, requiring upregulation of caspase-8 by the platinum drug as a dependent variable [112]. Similarly, pancreatic cancer, melanoma, and renal cancer cells resistant to TRAIL were sensitized to this ligand when combined with targeted reduction in XIAP, survivin, and BCL-2 levels [113–115]. Resistance to TRAIL can also arise if death ligand activation is inhibited in some systems by upregulation of NF-κB, but combination of TRAIL with NF-κB inhibition has demonstrated some success against colorectal cancer and melanoma tumor cells [116,117]. Combining agonists with cytotoxic drugs, targeting agents, and/or biologics in several cancers has, therefore, generated much clinical interest, and trials of combinations are ongoing [107]. Preliminary results are encouraging, as gleaned from a phase 1b NSCLC trial in 24 patients, where the combination of dulanermin with paclitaxel, carboplatin, and bevacizumab not only was well tolerated but also demonstrated good antitumor activity, which was defined by one complete and 13 partial responses [118].

Elevating Intracellular Stress

Tumor cells generate increased levels of reactive oxygen species (ROS, such as superoxide, hydrogen peroxide, hydroxyl radicals, and nitric oxide), which can interact with intracellular macromolecules (lipids, proteins, and DNA) and elevate stress signaling [119]. The precise mechanism for increased ROS is unclear, but survival signals from upregulated *c-MYC, RAS, SRC,* and other oncogenes are implicated. Moreover, such oncogenic stimulation promotes tumor cell proliferation, which increases demand for ATP from the inefficient glycolytic pathway in mitochondria and affects greater leakage of injury-causing electrons as a consequence [120]. The sustained stress would normally be intolerable, but cells survive using adaptive mechanisms, primarily by upregulating redox-buffering systems, which include glutathione (GSH), thioredoxin, superoxide dismutase (SOD), peroxidase, and catalase. This has the net effect of increasing ROS tolerance in tumor cells. However, such adaptive mechanisms have limited capacities, and this understanding has defined the use of specific therapeutic agents that further increase oxidative stress to exceed the cellular threshold above normally tolerated levels and induce apoptosis. Moreover, since tumor cells expressing high endogenous ROS will be more susceptible to such a therapeutic strategy than normal cells, this will also improve the therapeutic index.

The concept of increasing ROS within already-stressed tumor cells as a cell death strategy was initially tested with rotenone, which disrupts mitochondrial respiratory chain and promotes the leakage of electrons to further increase ROS and induce apoptosis [121,122]. ROS can also be generated by US Food and Drug Administration (FDA)-approved antitumor agents, and these offer an immediate opportunity for translation in the clinic. Indeed, the potential has been tested in tumor cells with such agents as arsenic trioxide, bleomycin, doxorubicin, bortezomib, and cisplatin, which in oxidatively stressed tumor cells were highly potent at inducing apoptosis [121,123–128]. Elesclomol (STA-4783), on the other hand, is an ROS-generating agent that entered clinical trials in combination with paclitaxel, but failed because of unmanageable side effects of the combination [119]. However, other ROS-inducing agents in clinical trials, motexafin gadolinium and β-lapachone, show promise and may progress further. Resveratrol, a naturally occurring compound found in red grapes and blueberries, is also drawing increasing attention; it promotes nitric oxide production to elevate oxidative stress and induce apoptosis in a p53-dependent manner [129]. In some of the studies noted here, the mechanism of cell death was also investigated in parallel and attributed to classical changes associated with the intrinsic and extrinsic pathways of apoptosis, such as an increase in BAX; FasL; DR4; cytosolic cytochrome c; activation of caspase-3, 8, and 9; and DNA fragmentation that could be prevented by the antioxidant N-acetylcysteine [124,125,127–129]. The intermediate mechanisms included activation of the p38 and JNK MAPK pathways [122,123], but information in this respect is limited.

Increased levels of ROS can also be generated by disrupting cellular buffering systems, and this is well illustrated following the inhibition of SOD by 2-methoxyestradiol, which has a striking apoptotic effect in leukemia and ovarian tumor cells, where a high endogenous basal level of ROS was a prerequisite for facile cell death [130,131]. In an analogous manner, inhibition of catalase with 3-amino-1,2,4-triazol enhanced the apoptotic activity of ROS-inducing arsenic trioxide [128]. Some naturally occurring compounds also have demonstrated the capacity to interfere with the cellular buffering system and increase ROS levels, which may explain their chemoprevention activity. One promising compound is β-phenylisothiocyanate (PEITC), which is derived from cruciferous vegetables and is highly effective against tumor cells resistant to several clinical antitumor agents, including cisplatin, fludarabine, and Gleevec [132]. The high potency of PEITC is ascribed to its ability to covalently interact with GSH and rapidly reduce levels of this thiol, which then loses its capacity to buffer oxidative stress and permits increases in ROS levels. Also, reduction in GSH will further promote apoptosis by attenuating thiolation reactions, which are important in the functioning of some pro-survival proteins, such as NF-κB and MCL-1; in inhibiting DNA repair; and in reducing the antiapoptotic effectiveness of BCL-2 [36,133–135]. These effects of PEITC, together with its selectivity for tumor cells, make this agent an ideal candidate for continued development, which has reached the phase I level in the clinic. Other agents impacting the buffering system include imexon (which depletes GSH), buthionine sulfoximine (which inhibits GSH synthesis), and tetrathiomolybdate (which inhibits SOD-1), which have also entered clinical trials either as single agents or in combination with established antitumor drugs, such as arsenic trioxide, melphalan, docetaxel, and gemcitabine; their development is ongoing [119].

Downregulating Antiapoptotic Proteins

Reducing the levels or effects of antiapoptotic proteins will lower the stress threshold for activating the apoptosis program, and this was briefly discussed in this chapter in relation to sensitizing tumor cells to TRAIL following the targeted reduction of BCL-2, XIAP, or survivin [113–115]. Various approaches have been used to downregulate such proteins in a targeted manner, and they range from RNA interference to small-molecule antagonists and inhibitors. Some of the approaches and agents emerging from these investigations are shown in Fig. 12.4.

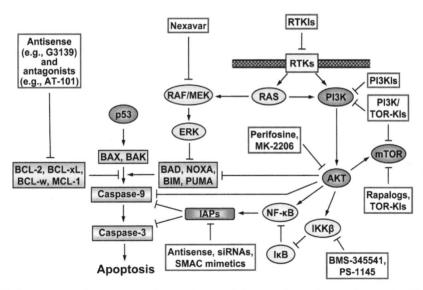

FIGURE 12.4 Activating the intrinsic pathway of apoptosis by targeting antiapoptotic proteins. The antitumor agents, shown in the red box, induce apoptosis by downregulating antiapoptotic BCL-2 family members or inhibitor of apoptosis proteins (IAPs), or via inhibition of receptor tyrosine kinases (RTKs) and the PI3K–AKT–mTOR, IKKβ–IκB–NF-κB, or RAS–RAF–MEK–ERK pathway. (This figure is reproduced in color in the color plate section.)

Targeting the BCL-2 Family

Measures to subdue BCL-2 include the 18-mer antisense oblimersen (G3139; Genasense), which reduces BCL-2 levels and induces cell death in vitro and in vivo, but demonstrates greater activity in combination with existing clinically active agents, including antimetabolites, alkylating agents, monoclonal antibodies, and γ-irradiation [85]. Based on these preclinical antitumor characteristics, oblimersen entered clinical trials, but it demonstrated limited activity in melanoma and CLL when administered in combination with dacarbazine or a fludarabine–cyclophosphamide doublet [85]. Similarly, a recent phase I study, in combination with gemcitabine against solid refractory cancers, reported minimal activity, although a 75% reduction in BCL-2 levels was achieved [136]. It is possible that a greater reduction in BCL-2 levels is required at the clinical level for activity to become meaningful, but this has not been explored. Another antisense ASO-15999 has been used in combination with cisplatin against mesothelioma cells to target BCL-xL, the levels of which are substantially upregulated in this disease. The combination was effective in reducing BCL-xL levels and inducing apoptosis in tissue culture cells and in orthotopic xenografts [137,138], but no follow-up clinical studies have yet been reported with this antisense.

An alternative approach to target BCL-2 and related family members relies on novel inhibitors or antagonists, including AT-101 (the R-(−)-enantiomer of gossypol acetic acid), obatoclax (GX15-070), and navitoclax (ABT-263), that interfere with protein–protein interactions between proapoptotic and antiapoptotic members of the BCL-2 family [17,107]. More specifically, these agents are predicted to antagonize this interaction by fitting into the hydrophobic pocket of the BH3-binding groove of BCL-2 and also of antiapoptotic family members BCL-xL, MCL-1, and BCL-w (Fig. 12.4). AT-101, a biphenolic molecule isolated from cottonseeds, induces apoptosis via activation of caspase-9, 7, and 3 in preclinical studies [139]. However, recent results from clinical trials of AT-101 alone in chemotherapy-sensitive small-cell lung cancer (SCLC) or second-line in NSCLC in combination with docetaxel appear disappointing, and did not show any antitumor benefit with this gossypol derivative [140,141]. On the other hand, a preliminary clinical report of AT-101 in combination with cisplatin and etoposide indicates some promise, with partial responses noted in three out of 12 SCLC patients [142]. Therefore, the clinical utility of AT-101 may depend on the appropriate combination with the cytotoxic agent and/or the tumor type. Obatolclax, another pan-BCL-2 antagonist, also overcomes apoptotic resistance from overexpression of antiapoptotic members. In particular, obatoclax potently inhibits the interaction between BAK and MCL-1 without altering MCL-1 levels and restores sensitivity of melanoma, B-cell lymphoma, and ALL cells to the proteosome inhibitor bortezomib (Velcade) or glucocorticoid [143–145]. The clinical trials with obatoclax continue, but early indications from phase I studies are that it has minimal or no activity in heavily pretreated patients with advanced Hodgkin lymphoma or CLL cancer [146,147]. Navitoclax also binds the BH3-only antiapoptotic BCl-2 members, but with an affinity substantially greater than those of previously described antagonists [148,149]. It has demonstrated good apoptotic activity in cell lines and xenografts, with SCLC tumor models showing substantial sensitivity to the agent, including regression of large established tumors [150–152]. The clinical activity of navitoclax has been investigated, and thrombocytopenia from BCL-xL inhibition was consistently shown to be dose limiting [153–156]. The antitumor activity of navitoclax as a single agent against several tumor types, on the other hand, was not consistent. In SCLC and other nonhematologic cancers, navitoclax was minimally effective, as indicated by 2–3% partial response and 23–25% stable disease [155,156]. This was contrary to expectations from preclinical investigations, where SCLC xenograft studies predicted high tumor sensitivity of this disease to the drug. In contrast, this antagonist was highly active against refractory CLL and other lymphoid malignancies, inducing 22–35% partial response, with 24–27% stable disease [153,154]. These responses correlated with reduced MCL-1 expression and proapoptotic-favorable high BIM:MCL-1 or BIM:BCL-2 ratios.

Targeting IAP Family

IAPs prevent apoptosis by downregulating caspase activities, and several approaches to inhibit IAPs have been developed to explore their potential in the clinical management of cancers (Fig. 12.4). Of the IAPs, XIAP and survivin are perhaps the most potent at inhibiting apoptosis. Both antisense oligonucleotides and small interfering RNAs (siRNAs) to target these IAPs have been developed to test their feasibility as modulators of apoptosis. Indeed, these agents have demonstrated significant reductions in IAP levels (up to 85%) that led to the expected enhancement in antitumor effects of radiotherapy and cytotoxics (e.g., taxol, etoposide, vinorelbine, and doxorubicin) in lung tumor models grown in tissue culture or in mice as xenografts [157,158]. In these studies, PARP (poly ADP ribose polymerase) degradation and DNA condensation and fragmentation were observed, indicating that the antitumor effects were directly attributable to apoptosis. Such beneficial antitumor effects of siRNAs and antisense molecules against IAPs have also been observed in other models, particularly hepatoma, melanoma, and head and neck and pancreatic cancers [159–162]. These studies encouraged further preclinical development of the approach that resulted in the second-generation antisense molecule AEG-35156 (GEM-640) entering clinical trials [82]. In preclinical studies, this antisense also reduced XIAP by over 80% at both the transcript and protein levels, and although it displayed single-agent antitumor activity, its combination with taxanes was the most effective, even curative, against several xenograft models, including ovarian, colon, lung, and prostate cancers [163,164]. Clinically, the antisense was well tolerated, confirmed the ability to reduce XIAP levels, and produced antitumor responses in nonrandomized phase I trials with AML (acute myeloid leukemia) patients, but the results from a randomized phase II trial in AML were not encouraging [82], which was consistent with outcomes in other trials [165]. The IAP survivin has also been targeted by the antisense approach, and phase I clinical studies of LY-2181308 have reported that the agent is well tolerated, but the reductions in tumor survivin levels were only 20%, and although apoptotic signaling was restored, it was insufficient to affect antitumor benefits [166,167]. Nevertheless, LY-2181308 has entered phase II trials to more thoroughly evaluate its therapeutic potential [107].

The seminal interest in targeting IAPs has resulted in alternative approaches that rely on molecules to directly interact with and neutralize these inhibitors of apoptosis. SMAC/DIABLO mimetics have been developed to investigate their potential to bind and antagonize XIAP, ML-IAP, and c-IAP1/2 and permit activation of caspases. Indeed, SMAC/DIABLO peptides derived from its N-terminus bind IAPs at the BIR domain with high affinity and have validated that such an approach can sensitize tumor models to apoptotic stimuli, such as that demonstrated with TRAIL in a malignant glioma xenograft model [168,169]. Unfortunately, the physico-chemical and pharmacologic properties of peptidomimetics (i.e., their poor in vivo stability and cell permeability) are not conducive to optimal therapeutic application, and this has shifted attention to the development of nonpeptide small-molecule

SMAC/DIABLO mimetics using high-throughput screens for initial hits [82]. These mimetics are either single monomeric small molecules (e.g., AT-406, GDC-0917, LCL-161, CS-3, ML-101, and LBW-242) or dimeric molecules (e.g., SM-164, TL-32711, BV-6, HGS-1029, and AEG-40730) formed from two identical monomers connected with a chemical linker. Both types are presently in development for their demonstrated ability to promote apoptosis alone or in combination, although the dimeric forms have higher potencies. Nevertheless, members from each class (AT-406, GDC-0917, LCL-161, HGS-1029, and TL-32711) have entered clinical trials recently [14,82], and this suggests that properties of SMAC/DIABLO mimetics other than potency must also be important determinants for advancing the compound to the clinic. In this regard, AT-406 demonstrates higher uptake in tumors than in normal tissue; binds avidly to XIAP, c-IAP1, and c-IAP2 with Ki of 2–66,nM; antagonizes XIAP BIR3 protein; degrades cellular c-IAP1; displays excellent apoptotic activity in a variety of sensitive and resistant human cell lines and xenografts; potentiates activity in a combination setting; and demonstrates good oral bioavailability in primates and nonprimate animals [170,171], all of which contribute to making the monomeric AT-406 a good oral candidate for clinical trials. The other two monomeric chemical mimetics, GDC-0917 and LCL-161, are also orally bioavailable. In contrast, the dimeric HGS-1029 and TL-32711 (birinapant) are not suited to oral administration; indeed, recent preliminary reports indicate that phase I studies have adopted a 15–30min intravenous (IV) infusion as standard procedure for drug administration [172–175]. Whether the easier oral route of administration will favor monomeric compounds for further development will depend on their clinical activity relative to dimeric mimetics, but the limited data on activity from phase I trials of the mimetics do not permit this assessment at the present time and must await further studies. However, it should be noted that like the monomeric AT-406, the dimeric TL32711 also appears to have a high potential for clinical success based on its good preclinical profile that includes a >70% reduction in c-IAP1 levels, reversal of caspase-3 and caspase-7 inhibition by XIAP, high tumor drug uptake and slow elimination in xenografts, and high activity in various established and primary human tumor xenografts as a single agent [174].

Alternative Targets for Downregulation

A number of indirect targets have also been explored to lower the cellular stress threshold in order to activate apoptosis. NF-κB can upregulate a number of antiapoptotic genes, including BCL-xL and XIAP, which can have potent pro-survival effects [87]. Therefore, this transcription factor represents a viable target in cancer therapy, and its inhibition by nitrosylcobalamin or sorafenib has indeed confirmed antitumor effects against melanoma and colon cancer cells when combined with TRAIL [116,117]. Targeted inhibition of NF-κB can be affected by increasing the levels of the endogenous inhibitor IκB, and this molecular understanding has resulted in the rational development of PS-1145, which is a selective inhibitor of IKKβ that normally suppresses expression of its downstream target IκB. Inhibition of IKKβ, therefore, allows IκB to increase (Fig. 12.4). In preclinical studies with prostate and imatinib-resistant CML cancer cells, which express constitutively active NF-κB, PS-1145 effectively inhibited the transcription factor, suppressed IAP1/2, and induced caspase-3/7–dependent apoptosis [176,177]. Similar studies with another IKKβ-selective inhibitor, BMS-345541, in a melanoma model that expressed constitutive IKKβ activity validated the target by directly linking the in vitro and in vivo antitumor activity to a reduction in NF-κB activity and resultant mitochondrial release of AIF [178]. Both of these IKKβ inhibitors have remained at the experimental level, and the future clinical development of these or other such inhibitors is uncertain. However, clinical downregulation of NF-κB activity is already possible with the drug bortezomib, which increases IκB levels by inhibiting its proteosomal degradation [87], but since other pathways are also impacted in parallel, the contribution of the anti–NF-κB effect in the antitumor activity of the proteosomal inhibitor is not clear.

Another potential target for therapeutic benefits is the PI3K–AKT pathway, which is upregulated in many cancers from multiple mechanisms, and which has profound anti-apoptotic effects by chronically impacting the function of downstream targets [179–182]. The upregulated downstream phosphorylation can be activating, as with the pro-survival IKKβ–NF-κB pathway and the mammalian target of rapamycin (mTOR), or inactivating, as with the proapoptotic BAD and c-FLIP. Therefore, substantial effort has been devoted to the identification of small molecules that inhibit pro-survival downstream targets or the PI3K–AKT pathway itself (Fig. 12.4). The inhibition of IKKβ–NF-κB has been discussed in this chapter, and the search for inhibitors of mTOR has led to the discovery of the now clinically approved Sirolimus (rapamycin) and analogs Everolimus (RAD-001) and Temsirolimus (CCI-779) [85]. These "rapalogs" irreversibly sequester mTOR, prevent formation of mTOR complex 1 (mTORC1), and inhibit signaling to downstream pro-survival effectors. Although these inhibitors in combination regimens have demonstrated good activity against several cancers, including those that are refractory to standard therapies, they have limitations, including feedback activation of oncogenic pathways and failure to inhibit protein synthesis, that have spurred the presently ongoing preclinical and/or clinical development of mTOR kinase inhibitors (TOR-KIs) (e.g., OSI-027, AZD-8055, and INK-128) as the next generation of more potent drugs selectively targeting mTOR activity rather than irreversible sequestration of mTOR [183]. One pathway activated by feedback mechanisms involves PI3K, which has generated a parallel track for the development of the new generation of PI3K–TOR-KIs (e.g., BEZ-235, BGT-226, XL-765, GSK-2126458, and PF-04691502). These second-generation bimodal drugs do inhibit both mTOR and PI3K, promote apoptosis, and are presently in clinical development [183].

The development of PI3K–TOR-KIs has not deterred the ongoing clinical development of the first-generation PI3K–AKT inhibitors, as it is understood that potent inhibition of this pathway alone can nullify multiple mechanisms involved in inhibiting apoptosis. The discovery of the original PI3K inhibitor (PI3KI), the fungal product wortmannin, was the catalyst for the concerted search and eventual identification of more effective first-generation inhibitors (e.g., GSK-1059615, XL-147, PX-866, BKM-120, and GS-1101/CAL-101) [184]. Although these inhibitors also limit the serine–threonine kinase activity of downstream AKT, inhibitors targeting AKT directly have also been developed to provide additional options for attenuating PI3K–AKT signaling. Several lead inhibitors have been described, with the lipid-based perifosine and the small-molecule MK-2206 undergoing clinical development [185]. At the preclinical level, these AKT inhibitors have demonstrated antitumor benefits and shown synergy in combinations with irradiation, established cytotoxics, and targeted therapeutics. However, in the clinic, the persistent declines in phospho-AKT have resulted in only limited partial responses, with the less significant disease stabilization being more frequently observed [185,186]. Therefore, further interest in AKT inhibitors is likely to depend on evidence of greater clinical activity in forthcoming studies.

Deregulation of the PI3K–AKT pathway can also occur from defects upstream in EGFR (ErbB-1) and the closely related HER-2 (ErbB-2); these receptor tyrosine kinases (RTKs) are overexpressed or carry activating mutations in many cancers and, thereby, inhibit apoptosis and induce resistance to therapy [179,181]. Over the past two decades, concerted research efforts eventually resulted in a number of clinically approved targeting agents: panitumumab (Vectibix), cetuximab (Erbitux), gefitinib (Iressa), and erlotinib (Tarceva) for EGFR, and trastuzumab (Herceptin) for HER-2. These RTK inhibitors (RTKIs) have the capacity to upregulate BAX activation and p21 and p27 expression, which are central to their antitumor apoptotic effects [187–190]. Many of these RTKIs mediate apoptosis via the intrinsic pathway, with the apoptotic signals going through BIM [191]. For instance, erlotinib and another agent, sorafenib (Nexavar), an inhibitor of the downstream RAF–MEK–ERK pathway, are heavily dependent on BIM upregulation—with associated increases in BAX, BAK, and BAD and concomitant decreases in MCL-1, XIAP, and survivin protein levels—for their intrinsic apoptotic activity [192,193]. Moreover, pretreatment BIM RNA expression is also highly predictive for apoptotic effects with EGFR, HER2, and PI3K inhibitors, but not the traditional chemotherapeutic agents taxol (paclitaxel), gemcitabine, and cisplatin [194]. Thus, high BIM levels, whether preexisting, or upregulated by RTKIs, or both, appear to be a strong determinant of apoptosis for these targeted therapeutic agents.

Intracellular Increase in Proapoptotic Protein Expression or Activation

The tumor suppressor p53 has an important role in apoptosis, and it accomplishes this by transactivating downstream proapoptotic genes and transrepressing antiapoptotic genes. Therefore, directly activating p53 and overexpressing or activating its downstream proapoptotic targets represent two potentially effective options for inducing apoptosis.

Modulating Proapoptotic Targets Downstream of p53

Gene therapy using the DNA vector technology is the most direct way to overexpress proapoptotic genes to kill cancer cells, but this would also be toxic to normal cells. For selective expression, therefore, the vector must be administered directly into the tumor and/or be driven by a tumor-specific and inducible promoter element. In this regard, an inducible adenoviral vector expressing the BAX gene has indeed demonstrated effectiveness at activating apoptosis in several cancer cell lines, including cervical tumor and glioma models [195,196]. The concept has advanced to the treatment of patients, but the clinical trials underway selectively target the extrinsic apoptosis pathway through overexpression of TNF-α, FasL, or TRAIL with such adenoviral vectors [109,165]. However, it is well acknowledged that most cancer patients die from the metastatic disease, and the difficulty of making gene therapy effective in the tumor-inaccessible metastatic setting is a limiting factor in implementing this technology over a wider tumor spectrum. Also, activation of apoptosis from ectopic increase in these ligands is dependent on endogenous expression of the corresponding death receptor being normal, which is not always the case. For instance, basal expression of Fas can be reduced by gene silencing in several cancers, as exemplified by prostate and bladder cancers [197], and Fas downregulation not only limits the benefits of *FasL* gene therapy but also induces resistance to therapeutic agents even when endogenous FasL expression is normal. However, Fas expression can be restored by use of a hypomethylating agent, such as Azacitidine or Decitabine, or use of the histone deacetylase inhibitor Vorinostat that is able to open the chromatin structure and reactivate the silenced gene [109].

Unmistakably, caspases are critical terminal components of the apoptotic pathway, but they are prone to downregulation in cancers through gene silencing as a result of DNA hypermethylation [198], FLIP overexpression [68], or increase in IAPs [82–84]. Caspase-8 is one example that is frequently impacted, and its upregulation to reestablish facile apoptosis can be affected by desilencing the gene with Decitabine [198], activating the gene through HDAC (histone deacetylase) inhibition with Vorinostat [109], downregulating FLIP with siRNA [199], or inhibiting IAP with siRNA or antisense [14]. Caspases may also fail to become activated by defects further upstream in the DNA damage pathway, and, therefore, there is much interest in the design of small molecules that will directly activate procaspases to induce apoptosis [200]. The specific focus has been on procaspase-3, since it immediately generates an active effector caspase, and also because procaspase-3 is generally present in abundance in cancer cells as compared to normal cells [201]. This was evident from reports demonstrating high tumor cell levels of procaspase-3 that were expressed in a variety of cancer types but particularly in breast, melanoma, lung, and renal tumor models in the National Cancer Institute (NCI)-60 tumor cell line panel [202]. In the search for a small molecule that cleaves procaspase-3 to the active form, 20,000 small molecules were screened in one reported study, which identified four hits, but only the procaspase-activating compound PAC-1 was selected for its high potency (EC_{50} of $0.2\,\mu M$) to form the caspase-3 product and its ability to rapidly activate apoptosis [201]. PAC-1 as a single agent demonstrated apoptosis in a number of cell lines, and the antitumor effects were inversely correlated with target levels; that is, it was most potent in tumor cells expressing the highest levels of procaspase-3 (e.g., IC_{50} of $0.35\,\mu M$ vs NCI-H226 lung tumor cells) and least potent against cells lacking procaspase-3 (e.g., IC_{50} of $>75\,\mu M$ vs MCF-7 breast tumor cells). Another advantage demonstrated by PAC-1 was its selectivity against primary colon cancer versus normal colon tissue cultures from 23 patients [201]. Recent reports suggest that more potent versions of PAC-1 are under preclinical development [203].

Directly Activating p53

Wild-type p53 is the most effective and potent activator of a tightly controlled apoptotic process: it can coordinately transactivate several proapoptotic genes, such as *BAX*, *APAF-1*, *NOXA*, *Fas*, *PUMA*, and *DR5*, and transrepress antiapoptotic genes, such as *BCL-2* and *survivin*. Loss of wild-type p53 function, therefore, typically leads to an absence of apoptotic stimulus, which induces chemoresistance in tumor cells to a variety of unrelated antitumor agents, including ionizing radiation, etoposide, paclitaxel, vinblastine, and cisplatin [204]. Dysfunction of p53 occurs frequently through both mutational and nonmutational mechanisms; therefore, activating apoptosis by restoring wild-type p53 function represents a logical strategy to promote or enhance antitumor benefits. Moreover, there is strong evidence to support the notion that once p53 is activated, it will induce apoptotic cell death, even though tumor cells may express pro-survival genes [205]. Thus, efforts to activate p53 have been extensive, and a number of options have emerged. One approach has been adenoviral-based p53 gene therapy. Indeed, Gendicine has been approved for clinical use in China, but in the United States and Europe, a similar product (Aldexin) demonstrated some benefit but failed to reach approval endpoints, partly due to issues of p53 gene delivery to metastatic sites [206]. This has served to intensify interest in small molecules to restore the activity of both mutant and wild-type p53.

TARGETING MUTANT P53

Mutation in p53 is one of the most frequently observed genetic alterations in cancer, and with about 1500 missense mutations identified in human tumors so far, the ability of p53 mutants to attenuate or inhibit apoptosis is a persistent barrier to clinical antitumor response. Most mutations are located in the DNA-binding domain, which induces a change in p53 conformation that reduces its thermodynamic stability; this hinders p53 from binding to its consensus sites in genomic DNA, transactivating proapoptotic genes, and transrepressing pro-survival genes. Also, p53 interacts with >100 proteins to regulate its multiple functions, including transcriptional-independent apoptosis, and its mutation results in a loss-of-function phenotype, which is seen in part as loss of these protein–protein interactions that hinder coordinated signal transduction pathways from converging on the apoptotic machinery to induce cell death [35]. The six frequently mutated sites in p53 of human tumor cells are at amino acid positions 175, 245, 248, 249, 273, and 282. Mutations in these "hot spot" positions are particularly formidable since the mutants formed, such as R175H-p53, R248W-p53, R249S-p53, and R273H-p53, may not only lose normal p53 functions but also acquire additional antiapoptotic functions not normally associated with wild-type p53. For instance, mutants R248W-p53 and R273H-p53, but not wild-type p53, interact with the Mre11 protein and inhibit the formation of the Mre11–Rad50–NBS1 (MRN) complex that is important for ATM activation following DNA double-strand breaks [207]. More importantly, some of these so-called gain-of-function mutants induce in tumor cells greater resistance to therapeutic agents than loss-of-function mutants, not only through restriction in their transactivation of proapoptotic genes, such as *FAS*, *BAX*, and *Puma*, but also through an acquired ability to upregulate pro-survival genes, such as *BAG-1*, *EGFR*, and *NFKB2* [35]. However, both loss-of-function and gain-of-function p53 mutants debilitate effective cancer therapy and, therefore, have been targeted in small-molecule drug discovery programs to restore p53-dependent apoptosis [208], as depicted in Fig. 12.5.

Efforts to discover small molecules to interact with mutant p53 were rationally prompted by an earlier study demonstrating that a synthetic peptide based on the C-terminus of p53 restored normal p53 functions in several p53 mutants and induced apoptosis in cancer cells, but not nonmalignant human cell lines [209]. *In silico* screens of NCI's database have been conducted in an effort to identify small molecules with a similar effect, and three hits of interest belonging to the thiosemicarbazone family were reported recently [210]. These compounds were preferentially effective against cell lines

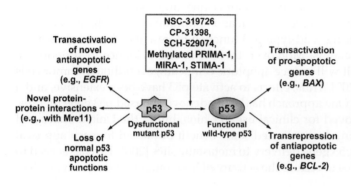

FIGURE 12.5 Rescuing mutant p53. Mutation in p53 can cause loss of normal p53 functions, but may also enable mutant p53 to acquire novel functions. Small-molecule modifiers, as exemplified in the red box, interact with mutant p53, alter the conformational structure, and restore wild-type p53 apoptotic functions. (This figure is reproduced in color in the color plate section.)

harboring mutations at hotspot sites 175, 248, and 273. The lead thiosemicarbazone compound NSC-319726 induced the gain-of-function R175H-p53 mutant to function as wild-type p53 in cell cultures and xenografts, as evidenced by expression of target genes *p21* and *PUMA* and induction of apoptosis.

Cell-based high-throughput assays using chemical libraries have also resulted in several hits that interact with mutant p53. The small molecule CP-31398 is an example and one of the earliest to be identified from a library of over 300,000 chemicals. This styrylquinazoline drug restored p53 function in several mutant p53 human cell lines and induced p21, cell cycle arrest, and apoptosis [211,212]. However, the cell death was caspase independent, was insensitive to BCL-xL, and did not require phosphorylation of p53 at serines 15 and 20, which has raised uncertainty regarding whether the exact mode of action of CP-31398 is through restoration of wild-type p53 function [211,212]. In another screen of a chemical library, a DNA-binding assay was used that focused on the DNA-binding domain where most p53 mutations become inactivating, and this resulted in the identification of the quinazoline-based SCH-529074. This modifier restores p53 stability and function in hotspot mutants R175H-p53, R273H-p53, and R249S-p53 by binding to the intended core domain in tumor cells, inhibiting ubiquitination of p53 by MDM2, transactivating p21 and BAX, inducing apoptosis, and inhibiting growth of tumor cells in vitro and of murine tumor xenografts [213]. Evidence was provided that the specific position for binding of SCH-529074 in the DNA-binding domain is at or near amino acid 268 of p53. Studies with both CP-31398 and SCH-529074 continue at the preclinical level [213,214].

The interest in rescuing mutant p53 and restoring wild-type p53 function has been further stimulated by the recent introduction of the small molecule PRIMA-1/Met (APR-246) into phase I studies against hematological and prostate cancers; the drug was well tolerated, induced p53 target genes, demonstrated apoptosis, and showed early signs of clinical activity [215]. This agent is a methylated analog of PRIMA-1 (p53 reactivation and induction of massive apoptosis 1) that was identified in a cell-based screening assay [216]. PRIMA-1 and the methylated analog converted gain-of-function mutant R175H-p53 or R273H-p53 to wild-type conformation, induced p21 and NOXA in mutant p53 cells, activated apoptotic pathways, demonstrated antitumor activity against mutant p53 cell lines, and inhibited the growth of human tumor xenografts [216–219]. Further studies have demonstrated that PRIMA-1 and the analog have a unique mechanism that requires biological activation and subsequent covalent interaction with cysteines in the core domain to stabilize mutant p53 and induce wild-type functions [220]. Covalent interactions also play a role in the ability of structurally distinct small molecules MIRA-1 and STIMA-1 to rescue mutant R175H-p53 or R273H-p53 in preclinical investigations [221,222].

TARGETING WILD-TYPE P53

Although wild-type p53 is a strong inducer of apoptosis, it can often fail not only from mutation but also from dysfunction of pathways regulating p53 activity. Thus, tumors harboring wild-type p53 can lose apoptotic activity and become resistant to a variety of therapeutic agents, including cisplatin, paclitaxel, and 5-FU. Of the several options available for reversing negative regulation of wild-type p53 activity and restoring p53-dependent apoptosis, the two with significant interest and/or potential involve the MDM2/MDM4 axis and posttranslational modification (Fig. 12.6).

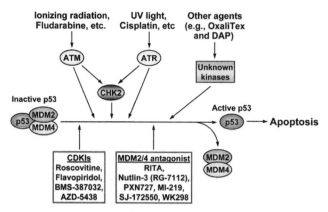

FIGURE 12.6 Activating wild-type p53 by disrupting its binding to MDM2/MDM4. Wild-type p53 is kept inactive by its interaction with MDM2/MDM4 proteins. The CDK inhibitors (CDKIs) and MDM2/4 antagonists, shown in their respective red boxes, interfere with p53 binding and thereby release and activate wild-type p53 to induce apoptosis. Also, p53 may be activated by agents activating independent DNA damage pathways. Thus, inactive wild-type p53, by virtue of loss of a posttranslational modifying kinase (e.g., ATM), can be reactivated by another agent inducing an alternative kinase (e.g., ATR). (This figure is reproduced in color in the color plate section.)

The apoptotic activity of wild-type p53 in cells is normally kept in check by its binding to MDM2/MDM4, which can be overexpressed in some tumors to exacerbate this negative interaction. This has stimulated the search for small molecules that can attenuate or antagonize MDM2/4–p53 interactions and increase p53 activity. CDK inhibitors (CDKIs) provide an option to suppress MDM2 levels at the transcription level and increase p53 levels by reducing the negative interaction between MDM2 and p53. The CDKIs roscovitine and flavopiridol accomplish repression of MDM2 by concerted inhibition of CDK7, CDK8, and CDK9, which are normally responsible for activating RNA polymerase II to complete transcription [223,224]. Improved CDKIs are designed to also target CDK1, CDK2, and CDK4 for greater efficacy, and some, such as BMS-387032 and AZD-5438, have entered clinical trials [223]. The other option explored to upregulate p53 activity is to more directly inhibit the binding between p53 with MDM2/4. A number of molecules have been identified as a result, and these target binding sites on p53, MDM2, or MDM4 to disrupt the MDM2/4–p53 complex. RITA (reactivation of p53 and induction of tumor cell apoptosis), for instance, was identified from a cell-based screen of a chemical library [225]. It is a thiophene agent that binds to p53, prevents its interaction with MDM2 in vitro and in vivo, and induces potent apoptotic activity in tumor cell lines harboring wild-type p53. Similar effects have also been observed with the cis-imidazoline compound Nutlin-3 (RG-7112), which emerged from structural knowledge of the p53–MDM2 interaction [226]. This compound binds MDM2 in the p53-binding pocket to facilitate stabilization and activation of wild-type p53 in tumor cells. It is presently undergoing clinical trials in patients with leukemia as well as solid tumors [227]. Another antagonist in clinical trials that targets MDM2 and disrupts binding to p53 is the tryptamine derivative JNJ-26854165, which has a different mode of action: it induces apoptosis in a transcription-independent manner and suppresses induction of p21 [228]. The agent induces apoptosis in a p53-independent manner also, and this suggests a complex underlying mechanism for its activity. Two other small molecules targeting MDM2 are the spiro-oxindole MI-219 and the isoquinolinone PXN727 (PXN822), which are in preclinical development [206,229]. MI-219 is of particular interest for its high potency and its 10,000-fold selectivity for MDM2 over MDM4. In contrast, the imidazo-indole derivative WK298 binds to both MDM2 and MDM4, whereas the small molecule SJ-172550 appears to interact more selectively with MDM4 [230,231]. These MDM4 antagonists are also currently in development at the preclinical level.

Defects in activation of wild-type p53 can also arise from deregulation in its posttranslational modifications, which are required for its stabilization and activation. Several types of p53 modifications can become deregulated to inhibit apoptosis, but the failure to phosphorylate p53 is probably the most important. Also, defective phosphorylation of MDM2 and/or MDM4 will also impact p53 function by preventing the robust release of wild-type p53 from the MDM2/4–p53 complex. However, the drug development options are presently conceptual and can be discussed only in relation to wild-type p53 phosphorylation where some supportive evidence is available. For instance, ATM and CHK2 are known to be downregulated in CLL [32,53,232] and NSCLC [34], respectively, and this can attenuate phosphorylation at the Ser15, Thr18, and Ser20 sites, which are necessary for p53 to be released from the complex, become stabilized, and be activated. Replacing deficient kinases by gene therapy for p53-dependent sensitization of tumor cells to therapeutic agents is possible, and this is amply demonstrated in preclinical studies (e.g., ectopic ATM expression [233]), but such a strategy may not always be possible in a clinical metastatic setting. Where silenced by promoter hypermethylation, as with CHK2, the kinase may be amenable to re-expression through the application of demethylating agents or HDAC inhibitors, but this is not always easy [34,35]. Thus, other approaches need to be considered.

One concept that is in its infancy for restoring p53 regulation through posttranslational phosphorylation is the potential induction of alternative DNA damage–signaling pathways. This is analogous to differential regulation of p53 in ataxia telangiectasia (AT) cells, where ATM is mutated. Thus, p53 regulation through ATM-dependent DNA damage signaling is defective in these cells so that ionizing radiation, for instance, cannot activate p53, but other DNA-damaging agents, such as UV light and cisplatin, can use the intact ATR-dependent pathway to restore p53 function [234,235] (Fig. 12.6). Such a strategy may have utility in the treatment of 20–40% of CLL patients, where mutated ATM prevents response to fludarabine and other agents due to the failure of wild-type p53 to become stabilized and activated [32,53,232], but the success of such a strategy may be possible only with a carefully developed DNA-damaging agent specific for CLL. This thesis is amply supported by preclinical investigations in ovarian tumor cells with the clinically active cisplatin, which is dependent on ATR, CHK1, and CHK2 to phosphorylate, stabilize, and activate wild-type p53 for its antitumor activity [35,36]. Paradoxically, cisplatin is not active against all tumor cells that harbor wild-type p53, and in resistant cells this failure is ascribed to a lack of p53 stabilization and/or activation [35,236]. The resistant cells, however, are highly sensitive to ionizing radiation, which stabilizes and activates p53 through independent DNA damage pathways [237]. Similar sensitivity of cisplatin-resistant tumor cells is also observed with designer platinum analogs, such as *1R,2R*-diaminocyclohexane(*trans*-diacetato)(dichloro)platinum(IV) (DAP) and the texaphyrin–oxaliplatin conjugate oxaliTex, which activate p53, but independently of ATR, ATM, CHK1, or CHK2 [236,238,239] (Fig. 12.6). Such studies must continue to develop alternative options that are becoming increasingly important in this era of personalized medicine.

CONCLUSION

Apoptosis is an important physiological process in normal cells, but it is equally important in tumor cells for significant therapeutic response and even cures as a desirable endpoint. Loss of apoptosis in tumors invariably results in treatment failure. However, therapeutic options that enhance apoptosis in sensitive tumor cells and restore or activate apoptosis in resistant cells are becoming available, and their success will potentially advance the cause for increasing cure rates in the clinic. Some of the strategies for activating apoptosis have been discussed, but others, such as synthetic lethality, are in various stages of development, and their impact will be felt in the coming years. A concerted effort by the cancer research community is an absolute imperative to ensure that successful strategies to target apoptosis emerge and change the standard of treatment at the clinical level, particularly against refractory cancers.

Acknowledgments

Research support from US Public Health Service grants CA127263 and CA160687 to ZHS and Support Grant CA16672 to MD Anderson Cancer Center awarded by the National Cancer Institute, and in part from the Megan McBride Franz Endowed Research Fund, are gratefully acknowledged.

References

[1] Karam JA, Hsieh J-T. Anti-cancer strategy of transitional cell carcinoma of bladder based on induction of different types of programmed cell deaths. In: Chen GG, Lai PBS, editors. Apoptosis in carcinogenesis and chemotherapy: apoptosis in cancer. Netherlands: Springer; 2009. p. 25–50.

[2] Saraste A, Pulkki K. Morphologic and biochemical hallmarks of apoptosis. Cardiovasc Res 2000;45:528–37.

[3] Hacker G. The morphology of apoptosis. Cell Tissue Res 2000;301:5–17.

[4] Galluzzi L, Maiuri MC, Vitale I, Zischka H, Castedo M, Zitvogel L, et al. Cell death modalities: classification and pathophysiological implications. Cell Death Differ 2007;14:1237–43.

[5] Slee EA, Adrain C, Martin SJ. Serial killers: ordering caspase activation events in apoptosis. Cell Death Differ 1999;6:1067–74.

[6] Verhagen AM, Ekert PG, Pakusch M, Silke J, Connolly LM, Reid GE, et al. Identification of DIABLO, a mammalian protein that promotes apoptosis by binding to and antagonizing IAP proteins. Cell 2000;102:43–53.

[7] Joza N, Pospisilik JA, Hangen E, Hanada T, Modjtahedi N, Penninger JM, et al. AIF: not just an apoptosis-inducing factor. Ann NY Acad Sci 2009;1171:2–11.

[8] Yeh WC, Pompa JL, McCurrach ME, Shu HB, Elia AJ, Shahinian A, et al. FADD: essential for embryo development and signaling from some, but not all, inducers of apoptosis. Science 1998;279:1954–8.

[9] Varfolomeev EE, Schuchmann M, Luria V, Chiannilkulchai N, Beckmann JS, Mett IL, et al. Targeted disruption of the mouse caspase 8 gene ablates cell death induction by the TNF receptors, Fas/Apo1, and DR3 and is lethal prenatally. Immunity 1998;9:267–76.

[10] Hakem R, Hakem A, Duncan GS, Henderson JT, Woo M, Soengas MS, et al. Differential requirement for caspase 9 in apoptotic pathways in vivo. Cell 1998;94:339–52.

[11] Yoshida H, Kong YY, Yoshida R, Elia AJ, Hakem A, Hakem R, et al. Apaf1 is required for mitochondrial pathways of apoptosis and brain development. Cell 1998;94:739–50.

[12] Fulda S, Debatin KM. Extrinsic versus intrinsic apoptosis pathways in anticancer chemotherapy. Oncogene 2006;25:4798–811.

[13] Zhao Y, Li R, Xia W, Neuzil J, Lu Y, Zhang H, et al. Bid integrates intrinsic and extrinsic signaling in apoptosis induced by alpha-tocopheryl succinate in human gastric carcinoma cells. Cancer Lett 2010;288:42–9.

[14] Wong RS. Apoptosis in cancer: from pathogenesis to treatment. J Exp Clin Cancer Res 2011;30:87.

[15] Chipuk JE, Moldoveanu T, Llambi F, Parsons MJ, Green DR. The BCL-2 family reunion. Mol Cell 2010;37:299–310.

[16] Boumela I, Assou S, Aouacheria A, Haouzi D, Dechaud H, De Vos J, et al. Involvement of BCL2 family members in the regulation of human oocyte and early embryo survival and death: gene expression and beyond. Reproduction 2011;141:549–61.

[17] Lessene G, Czabotar PE, Colman PM. BCL-2 family antagonists for cancer therapy. Nat Rev Drug Discov 2008;7:989–1000.

[18] O'Connor PM, Jackman J, Bae I, Myers TG, Fan S, Mutoh M, et al. Characterization of the p53 tumor suppressor pathway in cell lines of the National Cancer Institute anticancer drug screen and correlations with the growth-inhibitory potency of 123 anticancer agents. Cancer Res 1997;57:4285–300.

[19] Zilfou JT, Lowe SW. Tumor suppressive functions of p53. Cold Spring Harb Perspect Biol 2009;1:a001883.

[20] Perry ME. The regulation of the p53-mediated stress response by MDM2 and MDM4. Cold Spring Harb Perspect Biol 2010;2:a000968.

[21] Meek DW, Anderson CW. Posttranslational modification of p53: cooperative integrators of function. Cold Spring Harb Perspect Biol 2009;1:a000950.

[22] Muller M, Wilder S, Bannasch D, Israeli D, Lehlbach K, Li-Weber M, et al. p53 activates the CD95 (APO-1/Fas) gene in response to DNA damage by anticancer drugs. J Exp Med 1998;188:2033–45.

[23] Haupt S, Berger M, Goldberg Z, Haupt Y. Apoptosis—the p53 network. J Cell Sci 2003;116:4077–85.

[24] Erster S, Mihara M, Kim RH, Petrenko O, Moll UM. In vivo mitochondrial p53 translocation triggers a rapid first wave of cell death in response to DNA damage that can precede p53 target gene activation. Mol Cell Biol 2004;24:6728–41.

[25] Galluzzi L, Morselli E, Kepp O, Tajeddine N, Kroemer G. Targeting p53 to mitochondria for cancer therapy. Cell Cycle 2008;7:1949–55.

[26] Leu JI, Dumont P, Hafey M, Murphy ME, George DL. Mitochondrial p53 activates Bak and causes disruption of a Bak-Mcl1 complex. Nat Cell Biol 2004;6:443–50.

[27] el Deiry WS. The role of p53 in chemosensitivity and radiosensitivity. Oncogene 2003;22:7486–95.

[28] Brown JM, Attardi LD. The role of apoptosis in cancer development and treatment response. Nat Rev Cancer 2005;5:231–7.

[29] Rich T, Allen RL, Wyllie AH. Defying death after DNA damage. Nature 2000;407:777–83.

[30] Stankovic T, Weber P, Stewart G, Bedenham T, Murray J, Byrd PJ, et al. Inactivation of ataxia telangiectasia mutated gene in B-cell chronic lymphocytic leukaemia. Lancet 1999;353:26–9.

[31] Starostik P, Manshouri T, O'Brien S, Freireich E, Kantarjian H, Haidar M, et al. Deficiency of the ATM protein expression defines an aggressive subgroup of B-cell chronic lymphocytic leukemia. Cancer Res 1998;58:4552–7.

[32] Kojima K, Konopleva M, McQueen T, O'Brien S, Plunkett W, Andreeff M. Mdm2 inhibitor Nutlin-3a induces p53-mediated apoptosis by transcription-dependent and transcription-independent mechanisms and may overcome Atm-mediated resistance to fludarabine in chronic lymphocytic leukemia. Blood 2006;108:993–1000.

[33] Ripolles L, Ortega M, Ortuno F, Gonzalez A, Losada J, Ojanguren J, et al. Genetic abnormalities and clinical outcome in chronic lymphocytic leukemia. Cancer Genet Cytogenet 2006;171:57–64.

[34] Zhang P, Wang J, Gao W, Yuan BZ, Rogers J, Reed E. CHK2 kinase expression is down-regulated due to promoter methylation in non-small cell lung cancer. Mol Cancer 2004;3:14.

[35] Martinez-Rivera M, Siddik ZH. Resistance and gain-of-resistance phenotypes in cancers harboring wild-type p53. Biochem Pharmacol 2012;83:1049–62.

[36] Siddik ZH. Cisplatin: mode of cytotoxic action and molecular basis of resistance. Oncogene 2003;22:7265–79.

[37] Vogt M, Munding J, Gruner M, Liffers ST, Verdoodt B, Hauk J, et al. Frequent concomitant inactivation of miR-34a and miR-34b/c by CpG methylation in colorectal, pancreatic, mammary, ovarian, urothelial, and renal cell carcinomas and soft tissue sarcomas. Virchows Arch 2011;458:313–22.

[38] Sturm I, Kohne CH, Wolff G, Petrowsky H, Hillebrand T, Hauptmann S, et al. Analysis of the p53/BAX pathway in colorectal cancer: low BAX is a negative prognostic factor in patients with resected liver metastases. J Clin Oncol 1999;17:1364–74.

[39] Krajewski S, Blomqvist C, Franssila K, Krajewska M, Wasenius VM, Niskanen E, et al. Reduced expression of proapoptotic gene BAX is associated with poor response rates to combination chemotherapy and shorter survival in women with metastatic breast adenocarcinoma. Cancer Res 1995;55:4471–8.

[40] Friess H, Lu Z, Graber HU, Zimmermann A, Adler G, Korc M, et al. Bax, but not bcl-2, influences the prognosis of human pancreatic cancer. Gut 1998;43:414–21.

[41] Kashkar H, Kronke M, Jurgensmeier JM. Defective Bax activation in Hodgkin B-cell lines confers resistance to staurosporine-induced apoptosis. Cell Death Differ 2002;9:750–7.

[42] Mandinova A, Lee SW. The p53 pathway as a target in cancer therapeutics: obstacles and promise. Sci Transl Med 2011;3; 64rv1.

[43] Goldstein I, Marcel V, Olivier M, Oren M, Rotter V, Hainaut P. Understanding wild-type and mutant p53 activities in human cancer: new landmarks on the way to targeted therapies. Cancer Gene Ther 2011;18:2–11.

[44] Robles AI, Harris CC. Clinical outcomes and correlates of TP53 mutations and cancer. Cold Spring Harb Perspect Biol 2010;2:a001016.

[45] Tabori U, Shlien A, Baskin B, Levitt S, Ray P, Alon N, et al. TP53 alterations determine clinical subgroups and survival of patients with choroid plexus tumors. J Clin Oncol 2010;28:1995–2001.

[46] Schmidt M, Bachhuber A, Victor A, Steiner E, Mahlke M, Lehr HA, et al. p53 expression and resistance against paclitaxel in patients with metastatic breast cancer. J Cancer Res Clin Oncol 2003;129:295–302.

[47] Kandioler-Eckersberger D, Ludwig C, Rudas M, Kappel S, Janschek E, Wenzel C, et al. TP53 mutation and p53 overexpression for prediction of response to neoadjuvant treatment in breast cancer patients. Clin Cancer Res 2000;6:50–6.

[48] Gonzalez D, Martinez P, Wade R, Hockley S, Oscier D, Matutes E, et al. Mutational status of the TP53 gene as a predictor of response and survival in patients with chronic lymphocytic leukemia: results from the LRF CLL4 trial. J Clin Oncol 2011;29:2223–9.

[49] Wendel HG, de Stanchina E, Cepero E, Ray S, Emig M, Fridman JS, et al. Loss of p53 impedes the antileukemic response to BCR-ABL inhibition. Proc Natl Acad Sci USA 2006;103:7444–9.

[50] Rho JK, Choi YJ, Ryoo BY, Na II, Yang SH, Kim CH, et al. p53 enhances gefitinib-induced growth inhibition and apoptosis by regulation of Fas in non-small cell lung cancer. Cancer Res 2007;67:1163–9.

[51] Toledo F, Wahl GM. Regulating the p53 pathway: in vitro hypotheses, in vivo veritas. Nat Rev Cancer 2006;6:909–23.

[52] Lavin MF, Gueven N. The complexity of p53 stabilization and activation. Cell Death Differ 2006;13:941–50.

[53] Pettitt AR, Sherrington PD, Stewart G, Cawley JC, Taylor AM, Stankovic T. p53 dysfunction in B-cell chronic lymphocytic leukemia: inactivation of ATM as an alternative to TP53 mutation. Blood 2001;98:814–22.

[54] Puca R, Nardinocchi L, Gal H, Rechavi G, Amariglio N, Domany E, et al. Reversible dysfunction of wild-type p53 following homeodomain-interacting protein kinase-2 knockdown. Cancer Res 2008;68:3707–14.

[55] Bargonetti J, Manfredi JJ. Multiple roles of the tumor suppressor p53. Curr Opin Oncol 2002;14:86–91.

[56] Hermeking H. The miR-34 family in cancer and apoptosis. Cell Death Differ 2010;17:193–9.

[57] Wade M, Rodewald LW, Espinosa JM, Wahl GM. BH3 activation blocks Hdmx suppression of apoptosis and cooperates with Nutlin to induce cell death. Cell Cycle 2008;7:1973–82.

[58] Lin K, Adamson J, Johnson GG, Carter A, Oates M, Wade R, et al. Functional analysis of the ATM-p53-p21 pathway in the LRF CLL4 trial: blockade at the level of p21 is associated with short response duration. Clin Cancer Res 2012;18:4191–200.

[59] Sturm I, Papadopoulos S, Hillebrand T, Benter T, Luck HJ, Wolff G, et al. Impaired BAX protein expression in breast cancer: mutational analysis of the BAX and the p53 gene. Int J Cancer 2000;87:517–21.

[60] Shoji T, Tanaka F, Takata T, Yanagihara K, Otake Y, Hanaoka N, et al. Clinical significance of p21 expression in non-small-cell lung cancer. J Clin Oncol 2002;20:3865–71.

[61] Rose SL, Goodheart MJ, DeYoung BR, Smith BJ, Buller RE. p21 expression predicts outcome in p53-null ovarian carcinoma. Clin Cancer Res 2003;9:1028–32.

[62] Nawrocki ST, Carew JS, Douglas L, Cleveland JL, Humphreys R, Houghton JA. Histone deacetylase inhibitors enhance lexatumumab-induced apoptosis via a p21Cip1-dependent decrease in survivin levels. Cancer Res 2007;67:6987–94.

[63] Lohr K, Moritz C, Contente A, Dobbelstein M. p21/CDKN1A mediates negative regulation of transcription by p53. J Biol Chem 2003;278:32507–16.

[64] Shats I, Milyavsky M, Tang X, Stambolsky P, Erez N, Brosh R, et al. p53-dependent down-regulation of telomerase is mediated by p21waf1. J Biol Chem 2004;279:50976–85.

[65] Wu Q, Kirschmeier P, Hockenberry T, Yang TY, Brassard DL, Wang L, et al. Transcriptional regulation during p21WAF1/CIP1-induced apoptosis in human ovarian cancer cells. J Biol Chem 2002;277:36329–37.

[66] Friesen C, Fulda S, Debatin KM. Deficient activation of the CD95 (APO-1/Fas) system in drug-resistant cells. Leukemia 1997;11:1833–41.

[67] Fulda S, Los M, Friesen C, Debatin KM. Chemosensitivity of solid tumor cells in vitro is related to activation of the CD95 system. Int J Cancer 1998;76:105–14.

[68] Haag C, Stadel D, Zhou S, Bachem MG, Moller P, Debatin KM, et al. Identification of c-FLIP(L) and c-FLIP(S) as critical regulators of death receptor-induced apoptosis in pancreatic cancer cells. Gut 2011;60:225–37.

[69] Wang X, Chen W, Zeng W, Bai L, Tesfaigzi Y, Belinsky SA, et al. Akt-mediated eminent expression of c-FLIP and Mcl-1 confers acquired resistance to TRAIL-induced cytotoxicity to lung cancer cells. Mol Cancer Ther 2008;7:1156–63.

[70] Keeshan K, Cotter TG, McKenna SL. Bcr-Abl upregulates cytosolic p21WAF-1/CIP-1 by a phosphoinositide-3-kinase (PI3K)-independent pathway. Br J Haematol 2003;123:34–44.

[71] Li Y, Dowbenko D, Lasky LA. AKT/PKB phosphorylation of p21Cip/WAF1 enhances protein stability of p21Cip/WAF1 and promotes cell survival. J Biol Chem 2002;277:11352–61.

[72] Zhou BP, Liao Y, Xia W, Spohn B, Lee MH, Hung MC. Cytoplasmic localization of p21Cip1/WAF1 by Akt-induced phosphorylation in HER-2/neu-overexpressing cells. Nat Cell Biol 2001;3:245–52.

[73] Tang X, Milyavsky M, Shats I, Erez N, Goldfinger N, Rotter V. Activated p53 suppresses the histone methyltransferase EZH2 gene. Oncogene 2004;23:5759–69.

[74] Suzuki A, Tsutomi Y, Miura M, Akahane K. Caspase 3 inactivation to suppress Fas-mediated apoptosis: identification of binding domain with p21 and ILP and inactivation machinery by p21. Oncogene 1999;18:1239–44.

[75] Koster R, di Pietro A, Timmer-Bosscha H, Gibcus JH, van den BA, Suurmeijer AJ, et al. Cytoplasmic p21 expression levels determine cisplatin resistance in human testicular cancer. J Clin Invest 2010;120:3594–605.

[76] Xia X, Ma Q, Li X, Ji T, Chen P, Xu H, et al. Cytoplasmic p21 is a potential predictor for cisplatin sensitivity in ovarian cancer. BMC Cancer 2011;11:399.

[77] Xia W, Chen JS, Zhou X, Sun PR, Lee DF, Liao Y, et al. Phosphorylation/cytoplasmic localization of p21Cip1/WAF1 is associated with HER2/neu overexpression and provides a novel combination predictor for poor prognosis in breast cancer patients. Clin Cancer Res 2004;10:3815–24.

[78] Hayakawa J, Ohmichi M, Kurachi H, Kanda Y, Hisamoto K, Nishio Y, et al. Inhibition of BAD phosphorylation either at serine 112 via extracellular signal-regulated protein kinase cascade or at serine 136 via Akt cascade sensitizes human ovarian cancer cells to cisplatin. Cancer Res 2000;60:5988–94.

[79] Mabuchi S, Ohmichi M, Kimura A, Hisamoto K, Hayakawa J, Nishio Y, et al. Inhibition of phosphorylation of BAD and Raf-1 by Akt sensitizes human ovarian cancer cells to paclitaxel. J Biol Chem 2002;277:33490–500.

[80] Brunet A, Bonni A, Zigmond MJ, Lin MZ, Juo P, Hu LS, et al. Akt promotes cell survival by phosphorylating and inhibiting a Forkhead transcription factor. Cell 1999;96:857–68.

[81] Dijkers PF, Medema RH, Lammers JW, Koenderman L, Coffer PJ. Expression of the pro-apoptotic Bcl-2 family member Bim is regulated by the forkhead transcription factor FKHR-L1. Curr Biol 2000;10:1201–4.

[82] Fulda S, Vucic D. Targeting IAP proteins for therapeutic intervention in cancer. Nat Rev Drug Discov 2012;11:109–24.

[83] Krepela E, Dankova P, Moravcikova E, Krepelova A, Prochazka J, Cermak J, et al. Increased expression of inhibitor of apoptosis proteins, survivin and XIAP, in non-small cell lung carcinoma. Int J Oncol 2009;35:1449–62.

[84] Lopes RB, Gangeswaran R, McNeish IA, Wang Y, Lemoine NR. Expression of the IAP protein family is dysregulated in pancreatic cancer cells and is important for resistance to chemotherapy. Int J Cancer 2007;120:2344–52.

[85] Ghobrial IM, Witzig TE, Adjei AA. Targeting apoptosis pathways in cancer therapy. CA Cancer J Clin 2005;55:178–94.

[86] Zong WX, Edelstein LC, Chen C, Bash J, Gelinas C. The prosurvival Bcl-2 homolog Bfl-1/A1 is a direct transcriptional target of NF-kappaB that blocks TNFalpha-induced apoptosis. Genes Dev 1999;13:382–7.

[87] Eberle J, Kurbanov BM, Hossini AM, Trefzer U, Fecker LF. Overcoming apoptosis deficiency of melanoma—hope for new therapeutic approaches. Drug Resist Updat 2007;10:218–34.

[88] Wang H, Yang ES, Jiang J, Nowsheen S, Xia F. DNA damage-induced cytotoxicity is dissociated from BRCA1's DNA repair function but is dependent on its cytosolic accumulation. Cancer Res 2010;70:6258–67.

[89] Jiang J, Yang ES, Jiang G, Nowsheen S, Wang H, Wang T, et al. p53-dependent BRCA1 nuclear export controls cellular susceptibility to DNA damage. Cancer Res 2011;71:5546–57.

[90] Husain A, He G, Venkatraman ES, Spriggs DR. BRCA1 up-regulation is associated with repair-mediated resistance to cis-diamminedichloroplatinum(II). Cancer Res 1998;58:1120–3.

[91] Talis AL, Huibregtse JM, Howley PM. The role of E6AP in the regulation of p53 protein levels in human papillomavirus (HPV)-positive and HPV-negative cells. J Biol Chem 1998;273:6439–45.

[92] Padilla LA, Leung BS, Carson LF. Evidence of an association between human papillomavirus and impaired chemotherapy-induced apoptosis in cervical cancer cells. Gynecol Oncol 2002;85:59–66.

[93] Momand J, Jung D, Wilczynski S, Niland J. The MDM2 gene amplification database. Nucleic Acids Res 1998;26:3453–9.

[94] Freedman DA, Wu L, Levine AJ. Functions of the MDM2 oncoprotein. Cell Mol Life Sci 1999;55:96–107.

[95] Lain S. Protecting p53 from degradation. Biochem Soc Trans 2003;31:482–5.

[96] Bell HS, Ryan KM. Targeting the p53 family for cancer therapy: 'big brother' joins the fight. Cell Cycle 2007;6:1995–2000.

[97] Carr-Wilkinson J, O'Toole K, Wood KM, Challen CC, Baker AG, Board JR, et al. High frequency of p53/MDM2/p14ARF pathway abnormalities in relapsed neuroblastoma. Clin Cancer Res 2010;16:1108–18.

[98] Shen L, Kondo Y, Hamilton SR, Rashid A, Issa JP. P14 methylation in human colon cancer is associated with microsatellite instability and wild-type p53. Gastroenterology 2003;124:626–33.

[99] Roman-Gomez J, Castillejo JA, Jimenez A, Gonzalez MG, Moreno F, Rodriguez MC, et al. 5' CpG island hypermethylation is associated with transcriptional silencing of the p21(CIP1/WAF1/SDI1) gene and confers poor prognosis in acute lymphoblastic leukemia. Blood 2002;99:2291–6.

[100] Kim PK, Mahidhara R, Seol DW. The role of caspase-8 in resistance to cancer chemotherapy. Drug Resist Updat 2001;4:293–6.

[101] Ding Z, Yang X, Pater A, Tang SC. Resistance to apoptosis is correlated with the reduced caspase-3 activation and enhanced expression of antiapoptotic proteins in human cervical multidrug-resistant cells. Biochem Biophys Res Commun 2000;270:415–20.

[102] Mueller T, Voigt W, Simon H, Fruehauf A, Bulankin A, Grothey A, et al. Failure of activation of caspase-9 induces a higher threshold for apoptosis and cisplatin resistance in testicular cancer. Cancer Res 2003;63:513–21.

[103] Kojima H, Endo K, Moriyama H, Tanaka Y, Alnemri ES, Slapak CA, et al. Abrogation of mitochondrial cytochrome c release and caspase-3 activation in acquired multidrug resistance. J Biol Chem 1998;273:16647–50.

[104] Kuwahara D, Tsutsumi K, Oyake D, Ohta T, Nishikawa H, Koizuka I. Inhibition of caspase-9 activity and Apaf-1 expression in cisplatin-resistant head and neck squamous cell carcinoma cells. Auris Nasus Larynx 2003;30(Suppl.):S85–8.

[105] Shen XG, Wang C, Li Y, Wang L, Zhou B, Xu B, et al. Downregulation of caspase-9 is a frequent event in patients with stage II colorectal cancer and correlates with poor clinical outcome. Colorectal Dis 2010;12:1213–8.

[106] Bellail AC, Qi L, Mulligan P, Chhabra V, Hao C. TRAIL agonists on clinical trials for cancer therapy: the promises and the challenges. Rev Recent Clin Trials 2009;4:34–41.

[107] Storey S. Targeting apoptosis: selected anticancer strategies. Nat Rev Drug Discov 2008;7:971–2.

[108] Call JA, Eckhardt SG, Camidge DR. Targeted manipulation of apoptosis in cancer treatment. Lancet Oncol 2008;9:1002–11.

[109] Villa-Morales M, Fernandez-Piqueras J. Targeting the Fas/FasL signaling pathway in cancer therapy. Expert Opin Ther Targets 2012;16:85–101.

[110] Ashkenazi A. Targeting the extrinsic apoptosis pathway in cancer. Cytokine Growth Factor Rev 2008;19:325–31.

[111] Ashkenazi A. Directing cancer cells to self-destruct with pro-apoptotic receptor agonists. Nat Rev Drug Discov 2008;7:1001–12.

[112] Duiker EW, Meijer A, van der Bilt AR, Meersma GJ, Kooi N, van der Zee AG, et al. Drug-induced caspase 8 upregulation sensitises cisplatin-resistant ovarian carcinoma cells to rhTRAIL-induced apoptosis. Br J Cancer 2011;104:1278–87.

[113] Mohr A, Albarenque SM, Deedigan L, Yu R, Reidy M, Fulda S, et al. Targeting of XIAP combined with systemic mesenchymal stem cell-mediated delivery of sTRAIL ligand inhibits metastatic growth of pancreatic carcinoma cells. Stem Cells 2010;28:2109–20.

[114] Chawla-Sarkar M, Bae SI, Reu FJ, Jacobs BS, Lindner DJ, Borden EC. Downregulation of Bcl-2, FLIP or IAPs (XIAP and survivin) by siRNAs sensitizes resistant melanoma cells to Apo2L/TRAIL-induced apoptosis. Cell Death Differ 2004;11:915–23.

[115] Stadel D, Mohr A, Ref C, MacFarlane M, Zhou S, Humphreys R, et al. TRAIL-induced apoptosis is preferentially mediated via TRAIL receptor 1 in pancreatic carcinoma cells and profoundly enhanced by XIAP inhibitors. Clin Cancer Res 2010;16:5734–49.

[116] Ricci MS, Kim SH, Ogi K, Plastaras JP, Ling J, Wang W, et al. Reduction of TRAIL-induced Mcl-1 and cIAP2 by c-Myc or sorafenib sensitizes resistant human cancer cells to TRAIL-induced death. Cancer Cell 2007;12:66–80.

[117] Chawla-Sarkar M, Bauer JA, Lupica JA, Morrison BH, Tang Z, Oates RK, et al. Suppression of NF-κB survival signaling by nitrosylcobalamin sensitizes neoplasms to the anti-tumor effects of Apo2L/TRAIL. J Biol Chem 2003;278:39461–9.

[118] Soria JC, Smit E, Khayat D, Besse B, Yang X, Hsu CP, et al. Phase 1b study of dulanermin (recombinant human Apo2L/TRAIL) in combination with paclitaxel, carboplatin, and bevacizumab in patients with advanced non-squamous non-small-cell lung cancer. J Clin Oncol 2010;28:1527–33.

[119] Trachootham D, Alexandre J, Huang P. Targeting cancer cells by ROS-mediated mechanisms: a radical therapeutic approach? Nat Rev Drug Discov 2009;8:579–91.

[120] Pelicano H, Carney D, Huang P. ROS stress in cancer cells and therapeutic implications. Drug Resist Updat 2004;7:97–110.

[121] Pelicano H, Feng L, Zhou Y, Carew JS, Hileman EO, Plunkett W, et al. Inhibition of mitochondrial respiration: a novel strategy to enhance drug-induced apoptosis in human leukemia cells by a reactive oxygen species-mediated mechanism. J Biol Chem 2003;278:37832–9.

[122] Newhouse K, Hsuan SL, Chang SH, Cai B, Wang Y, Xia Z. Rotenone-induced apoptosis is mediated by p38 and JNK MAP kinases in human dopaminergic SH-SY5Y cells. Toxicol Sci 2004;79:137–46.

[123] Benhar M, Dalyot I, Engelberg D, Levitzki A. Enhanced ROS production in oncogenically transformed cells potentiates c-Jun N-terminal kinase and p38 mitogen-activated protein kinase activation and sensitization to genotoxic stress. Mol Cell Biol 2001;21:6913–26.

[124] Tsang WP, Chau SP, Kong SK, Fung KP, Kwok TT. Reactive oxygen species mediate doxorubicin induced p53-independent apoptosis. Life Sci 2003;73:2047–58.

[125] Hug H, Strand S, Grambihler A, Galle J, Hack V, Stremmel W, et al. Reactive oxygen intermediates are involved in the induction of CD95 ligand mRNA expression by cytostatic drugs in hepatoma cells. J Biol Chem 1997;272:28191–3.

[126] Miyajima A, Nakashima J, Yoshioka K, Tachibana M, Tazaki H, Murai M. Role of reactive oxygen species in cis-dichlorodiammineplatinum-induced cytotoxicity on bladder cancer cells. Br J Cancer 1997;76:206–10.

[127] Ling YH, Liebes L, Zou Y, Perez-Soler R. Reactive oxygen species generation and mitochondrial dysfunction in the apoptotic response to Bortezomib, a novel proteasome inhibitor, in human H460 non-small cell lung cancer cells. J Biol Chem 2003;278:33714–23.

[128] Jing Y, Dai J, Chalmers-Redman RM, Tatton WG, Waxman S. Arsenic trioxide selectively induces acute promyelocytic leukemia cell apoptosis via a hydrogen peroxide-dependent pathway. Blood 1999;94:2102–11.

[129] Kim MY, Trudel LJ, Wogan GN. Apoptosis induced by capsaicin and resveratrol in colon carcinoma cells requires nitric oxide production and caspase activation. Anticancer Res 2009;29:3733–40.

[130] Hileman EO, Liu J, Albitar M, Keating MJ, Huang P. Intrinsic oxidative stress in cancer cells: a biochemical basis for therapeutic selectivity. Cancer Chemother Pharmacol 2004;53:209–19.

[131] Zhou Y, Hileman EO, Plunkett W, Keating MJ, Huang P. Free radical stress in chronic lymphocytic leukemia cells and its role in cellular sensitivity to ROS-generating anticancer agents. Blood 2003;101:4098–104.

[132] Chen G, Wang F, Trachootham D, Huang P. Preferential killing of cancer cells with mitochondrial dysfunction by natural compounds. Mitochondrion 2010;10:614–25.

[133] Trachootham D, Zhou Y, Zhang H, Demizu Y, Chen Z, Pelicano H, et al. Selective killing of oncogenically transformed cells through a ROS-mediated mechanism by beta-phenylethyl isothiocyanate. Cancer Cell 2006;10:241–52.

[134] Trachootham D, Zhang H, Zhang W, Feng L, Du M, Zhou Y, et al. Effective elimination of fludarabine-resistant CLL cells by PEITC through a redox-mediated mechanism. Blood 2008;112:1912–22.

[135] Kelland LR. New platinum antitumor complexes. Crit Rev Oncol Hematol 1993;15:191–219.

[136] Galatin PS, Advani RH, Fisher GA, Francisco B, Julian T, Losa R, et al. Phase I trial of oblimersen (Genasense(R)) and gemcitabine in refractory and advanced malignancies. Invest New Drugs 2011;29:971–7.

[137] Ozvaran MK, Cao XX, Miller SD, Monia BA, Hong WK, Smythe WR. Antisense oligonucleotides directed at the bcl-xl gene product augment chemotherapy response in mesothelioma. Mol Cancer Ther 2004; 3:545–50.

[138] Littlejohn JE, Cao X, Miller SD, Ozvaran MK, Jupiter D, Zhang L, et al. Bcl-xL antisense oligonucleotide and cisplatin combination therapy extends survival in SCID mice with established mesothelioma xenografts. Int J Cancer 2008;123:202–8.

II. DRUGS IN THE LABORATORY AND CLINIC

[139] Moretti L, Li B, Kim KW, Chen H, Lu B. AT-101, a pan-Bcl-2 inhibitor, leads to radiosensitization of non-small cell lung cancer. J Thorac Oncol 2010;5:680–7.

[140] Baggstrom MQ, Qi Y, Koczywas M, Argiris A, Johnson EA, Millward MJ, et al. A phase II study of AT-101 (Gossypol) in chemotherapy-sensitive recurrent extensive-stage small cell lung cancer. J Thorac Oncol 2011;6:1757–60.

[141] Ready N, Karaseva NA, Orlov SV, Luft AV, Popovych O, Holmlund JT, et al. Double-blind, placebo-controlled, randomized phase 2 study of the proapoptotic agent AT-101 plus docetaxel, in second-line non-small cell lung cancer. J Thorac Oncol 2011;6:781–5.

[142] Leal TA, Schelman WR, Traynor AM, Kolesar J, Marnocha RM, Eickhoff JC, et al. A phase I study of r-(–)-gossypol (AT-101, NSC 726190) in combination with cisplatin (P) and etoposide (E) in patients with advanced solid tumors and extensive-stage small cell lung cancer (ES-SCLC). J Clin Oncol 2010;28(Suppl.); Abstract e13030.

[143] Nguyen M, Marcellus RC, Roulston A, Watson M, Serfass L, Murthy Sr M, et al. Small molecule obatoclax (GX15-070) antagonizes MCL-1 and overcomes MCL-1-mediated resistance to apoptosis. Proc Natl Acad Sci USA 2007;104:19512–7.

[144] Heidari N, Hicks MA, Harada H. GX15–070 (obatoclax) overcomes glucocorticoid resistance in acute lympho-blastic leukemia through induction of apoptosis and autophagy. Cell Death Dis 2010;1:e76.

[145] Dasmahapatra G, Lembersky D, Son MP, Patel H, Peterson D, Attkisson E, et al. Obatoclax interacts synergisti-cally with the irreversible proteasome inhibitor carfilzomib in GC- and ABC-DLBCL cells in vitro and in vivo. Mol Cancer Ther 2012;11:1122–32.

[146] O'Brien SM, Claxton DF, Crump M, Faderl S, Kipps T, Keating MJ, et al. Phase I study of obatoclax mesylate (GX15-070), a small molecule pan-Bcl-2 family antagonist, in patients with advanced chronic lymphocytic leukemia. Blood 2009;113:299–305.

[147] Oki Y, Copeland A, Hagemeister F, Fayad LE, Fanale M, Romaguera J, et al. Experience with obatoclax mesyl-ate (GX15-070), a small molecule pan-Bcl-2 family antagonist in patients with relapsed or refractory classical Hodgkin lymphoma. Blood 2012;119:2171–2.

[148] Degterev A, Lugovskoy A, Cardone M, Mulley B, Wagner G, Mitchison T, et al. Identification of small-molecule inhibitors of interaction between the BH3 domain and Bcl-xL. Nat Cell Biol 2001;3:173–82.

[149] Oltersdorf T, Elmore SW, Shoemaker AR, Armstrong RC, Augeri DJ, Belli BA, et al. An inhibitor of Bcl-2 family proteins induces regression of solid tumours. Nature 2005;435:677–81.

[150] Shoemaker AR, Mitten MJ, Adickes J, Ackler S, Refici M, Ferguson D, et al. Activity of the Bcl-2 family inhibitor ABT-263 in a panel of small cell lung cancer xenograft models. Clin Cancer Res 2008;14:3268–77.

[151] Tse C, Shoemaker AR, Adickes J, Anderson MG, Chen J, Jin S, et al. ABT-263: a potent and orally bioavailable Bcl-2 family inhibitor. Cancer Res 2008;68:3421–8.

[152] Hann CL, Daniel VC, Sugar EA, Dobromilskaya I, Murphy SC, Cope L, et al. Therapeutic efficacy of ABT-737, a selective inhibitor of BCL-2, in small cell lung cancer. Cancer Res 2008;68:2321–8.

[153] Roberts AW, Seymour JF, Brown JR, Wierda WG, Kipps TJ, Khaw SL, et al. Substantial susceptibility of chronic lymphocytic leukemia to BCL2 inhibition: results of a phase I study of navitoclax in patients with relapsed or refractory disease. J Clin Oncol 2012;30:488–96.

[154] Wilson WH, O'Connor OA, Czuczman MS, LaCasce AS, Gerecitano JF, Leonard JP, et al. Navitoclax, a targeted high-affinity inhibitor of BCL-2, in lymphoid malignancies: a phase 1 dose-escalation study of safety, pharma-cokinetics, pharmacodynamics, and antitumour activity. Lancet Oncol 2010;11:1149–59.

[155] Rudin CM, Hann CL, Garon EB, Ribeiro dO, Bonomi PD, Camidge DR, et al. Phase II study of single-agent navitoclax (ABT-263) and biomarker correlates in patients with relapsed small cell lung cancer. Clin Cancer Res 2012;18:3163–9.

[156] Gandhi L, Camidge DR, Ribeiro dO, Bonomi P, Gandara D, Khaira D, et al. Phase I study of navitoclax (ABT-263), a novel Bcl-2 family inhibitor, in patients with small-cell lung cancer and other solid tumors. J Clin Oncol 2011;29:909–16.

[157] Hu Y, Cherton-Horvat G, Dragowska V, Baird S, Korneluk RG, Durkin JP, et al. Antisense oligonucleotides tar-geting XIAP induce apoptosis and enhance chemotherapeutic activity against human lung cancer cells in vitro and in vivo. Clin Cancer Res 2003;9:2826–36.

[158] Cao C, Mu Y, Hallahan DE, Lu B. XIAP and survivin as therapeutic targets for radiation sensitization in pre-clinical models of lung cancer. Oncogene 2004;23:7047–52.

[159] Grossman D, McNiff JM, Li F, Altieri DC. Expression and targeting of the apoptosis inhibitor, survivin, in human melanoma. J Invest Dermatol 1999;113:1076–81.

[160] Sharma H, Sen S, Lo ML, Mariggio A, Singh N. Antisense-mediated downregulation of anti-apoptotic proteins induces apoptosis and sensitizes head and neck squamous cell carcinoma cells to chemotherapy. Cancer Biol Ther 2005;4:720–7.

[161] Kami K, Doi R, Koizumi M, Toyoda E, Mori T, Ito D, et al. Downregulation of survivin by siRNA diminishes radioresistance of pancreatic cancer cells. Surgery 2005;138:299–305.

[162] Yamaguchi Y, Shiraki K, Fuke H, Inoue T, Miyashita K, Yamanaka Y, et al. Targeting of X-linked inhibitor of apoptosis protein or survivin by short interfering RNAs sensitize hepatoma cells to TNF-related apoptosis-inducing ligand- and chemotherapeutic agent-induced cell death. Oncol Rep 2005;14:1311–6.

[163] LaCasse EC, Cherton-Horvat GG, Hewitt KE, Jerome LJ, Morris SJ, Kandimalla ER, et al. Preclinical characterization of AEG35156/GEM 640, a second-generation antisense oligonucleotide targeting X-linked inhibitor of apoptosis. Clin Cancer Res 2006;12:5231–41.

[164] Shaw TJ, LaCasse EC, Durkin JP, Vanderhyden BC. Downregulation of XIAP expression in ovarian cancer cells induces cell death in vitro and in vivo. Int J Cancer 2008;122:1430–4.

[165] Jia LT, Chen SY, Yang AG. Cancer gene therapy targeting cellular apoptosis machinery. Cancer Treat Rev 2012;38:868–76.

[166] Talbot DC, Ranson M, Davies J, Lahn M, Callies S, Andre V, et al. Tumor survivin is downregulated by the antisense oligonucleotide LY2181308: a proof-of-concept, first-in-human dose study. Clin Cancer Res 2010;16:6150–8.

[167] Tanioka M, Nokihara H, Yamamoto N, Yamada Y, Yamada K, Goto Y, et al. Phase I study of LY2181308, an antisense oligonucleotide against survivin, in patients with advanced solid tumors. Cancer Chemother Pharmacol 2011;68:505–11.

[168] Vucic D, Deshayes K, Ackerly H, Pisabarro MT, Kadkhodayan S, Fairbrother WJ, et al. SMAC negatively regulates the anti-apoptotic activity of melanoma inhibitor of apoptosis (ML-IAP). J Biol Chem 2002;277:12275–9.

[169] Fulda S, Wick W, Weller M, Debatin KM. Smac agonists sensitize for Apo2L/T. Nat Med 2002;8:808–15.

[170] Brunckhorst MK, Lerner D, Wang S, Yu Q. AT-406, an orally active antagonist of multiple inhibitor of apoptosis proteins, inhibits progression of human ovarian cancer. Cancer Biol Ther 2012;13:804–11.

[171] Cai Q, Sun H, Peng Y, Lu J, Nikolovska-Coleska Z, McEachern D, et al. A potent and orally active antagonist (SM-406/AT-406) of multiple inhibitor of apoptosis proteins (IAPs) in clinical development for cancer treatment. J Med Chem 2011;54:2714–26.

[172] Eckhardt SG, Gallant G, Sikic BI, Camidge DR, Burris III HA, Wakelee HA, et al. Phase I study evaluating the safety, tolerability, and pharmacokinetics (PK) of HGS1029, a small-molecule inhibitor of apoptosis protein (IAP), in patients (pts) with advanced solid tumors. ; Abstract J Clin Oncol 2010;28(Suppl.):2580.

[173] Sikic BI, Eckhardt SG, Gallant G, Burris HA, Camidge DR, Colevas AD, et al. Safety, pharmacokinetics (PK), and pharmacodynamics (PD) of HGS1029, an inhibitor of apoptosis protein (IAP) inhibitor, in patients (Pts) with advanced solid tumors: results of a phase I study. ; Abstract J Clin Oncol 2011;29(Suppl.):3008.

[174] Graham MA, Mitsuuchi Y, Burns J, Chunduru S, Benetatos C, McKinlay M, et al. Phase I PK/PD analysis of the Smac-mimetic TL32711 demonstrates potent and sustained cIAP1 suppression in patient PBMCs and tumor biopsies. ; Abstract Mol Cancer Ther 2011;10(11 Suppl.):A25.

[175] Fetterly GJ, Liu B, Senzer NN, Amaravadi RK, Schilder RJ, Martin LP, et al. Clinical pharmacokinetics of the Smac-mimetic birinapant (TL32711) as a single agent and in combination with multiple chemotherapy regimens. ; Abstract J Clin Oncol 2012;30(Suppl.):3029.

[176] Yemelyanov A, Gasparian A, Lindholm P, Dang L, Pierce JW, Kisseljov F, et al. Effects of IKK inhibitor PS1145 on NF-κB function, proliferation, apoptosis and invasion activity in prostate carcinoma cells. Oncogene 2006;25:387–98.

[177] Cilloni D, Messa F, Arruga F, Defilippi I, Morotti A, Messa E, et al. The NF-κB pathway blockade by the IKK inhibitor PS1145 can overcome imatinib resistance. Leukemia 2006;20:61–7.

[178] Yang J, Amiri KI, Burke JR, Schmid JA, Richmond A. BMS-345541 targets inhibitor of kappaB kinase and induces apoptosis in melanoma: involvement of nuclear factor kappaB and mitochondria pathways. Clin Cancer Res 2006;12:950–60.

[179] Navolanic PM, Steelman LS, McCubrey JA. EGFR family signaling and its association with breast cancer development and resistance to chemotherapy (review). Int J Oncol 2003;22:237–52.

[180] Berns K, Horlings HM, Hennessy BT, Madiredjo M, Hijmans EM, Beelen K, et al. A functional genetic approach identifies the PI3K pathway as a major determinant of trastuzumab resistance in breast cancer. Cancer Cell 2007;12:395–402.

[181] Knuefermann C, Lu Y, Liu B, Jin W, Liang K, Wu L, et al. HER2/PI-3K/Akt activation leads to a multidrug resistance in human breast adenocarcinoma cells. Oncogene 2003;22:3205–12.

[182] West KA, Castillo SS, Dennis PA. Activation of the PI3K/Akt pathway and chemotherapeutic resistance. Drug Resist Updat 2002;5:234–48.

[183] Wander SA, Hennessy BT, Slingerland JM. Next-generation mTOR inhibitors in clinical oncology: how pathway complexity informs therapeutic strategy. J Clin Invest 2011;121:1231–41.

[184] Brana I, Siu LL. Clinical development of phosphatidylinositol 3-kinase inhibitors for cancer treatment. BMC Med 2012;10:161.

[185] Pal SK, Reckamp K, Yu H, Figlin RA. Akt inhibitors in clinical development for the treatment of cancer. Expert Opin Investig Drugs 2010;19:1355–66.

[186] Yap TA, Yan L, Patnaik A, Fearen I, Olmos D, Papadopoulos K, et al. First-in-man clinical trial of the oral pan-AKT inhibitor MK-2206 in patients with advanced solid tumors. J Clin Oncol 2011;29:4688–95.

[187] Le XF, Pruefer F, Bast Jr RC. HER2-targeting antibodies modulate the cyclin-dependent kinase inhibitor p27Kip1 via multiple signaling pathways. Cell Cycle 2005;4:87–95.

[188] Ariyama H, Qin B, Baba E, Tanaka R, Mitsugi K, Harada M, et al. Gefitinib, a selective EGFR tyrosine kinase inhibitor, induces apoptosis through activation of Bax in human gallbladder adenocarcinoma cells. J Cell Biochem 2006;97:724–34.

[189] Mohsin SK, Weiss HL, Gutierrez MC, Chamness GC, Schiff R, Digiovanna MP, et al. Neoadjuvant trastuzumab induces apoptosis in primary breast cancers. J Clin Oncol 2005;23:2460–8.

[190] Zhao YF, Wang CR, Wu YM, Ma SL, Ji Y, Lu YJ. P21 (waf1/cip1) is required for non-small cell lung cancer sensitive to Gefitinib treatment. Biomed Pharmacother 2011;65:151–6.

[191] Green DR. Fas Bim boom!. Immunity 2008;28:141–3.

[192] Zhang W, Konopleva M, Ruvolo VR, McQueen T, Evans RL, Bornmann WG, et al. Sorafenib induces apoptosis of AML cells via Bim-mediated activation of the intrinsic apoptotic pathway. Leukemia 2008;22:808–18.

[193] Deng J, Shimamura T, Perera S, Carlson NE, Cai D, Shapiro GI, et al. Proapoptotic BH3-only BCL-2 family protein BIM connects death signaling from epidermal growth factor receptor inhibition to the mitochondrion. Cancer Res 2007;67:11867–75.

[194] Faber AC, Corcoran RB, Ebi H, Sequist LV, Waltman BA, Chung E, et al. BIM expression in treatment-naive cancers predicts responsiveness to kinase inhibitors. Cancer Discov 2011;1:352–65.

[195] Huh WK, Gomez-Navarro J, Arafat WO, Xiang J, Mahasreshti PJ, Alvarez RD, et al. Bax-induced apoptosis as a novel gene therapy approach for carcinoma of the cervix. Gynecol Oncol 2001;83:370–7.

[196] Huang J, Gao J, Lv X, Li G, Hao D, Yao X, et al. Target gene therapy of glioma: overexpression of BAX gene under the control of both tissue-specific promoter and hypoxia-inducible element. Acta Biochim Biophys Sin (Shanghai) 2010;42:274–80.

[197] Santourlidis S, Warskulat U, Florl AR, Maas S, Pulte T, Fischer J, et al. Hypermethylation of the tumor necrosis factor receptor superfamily 6 (APT1, Fas, CD95/Apo-1) gene promoter at rel/nuclear factor kappaB sites in prostatic carcinoma. Mol Carcinog 2001;32:36–43.

[198] Fulda S, Kufer MU, Meyer E, van Valen F, Dockhorn-Dworniczak B, Debatin KM. Sensitization for death receptor- or drug-induced apoptosis by re-expression of caspase-8 through demethylation or gene transfer. Oncogene 2001;20:5865–77.

[199] Watanabe K, Okamoto K, Yonehara S. Sensitization of osteosarcoma cells to death receptor-mediated apoptosis by HDAC inhibitors through downregulation of cellular FLIP. Cell Death Differ 2005;12:10–8.

[200] MacKenzie SH, Schipper JL, Clark AC. The potential for caspases in drug discovery. Curr Opin Drug Discov Devel 2010;13:568–76.

[201] Putt KS, Chen GW, Pearson JM, Sandhorst JS, Hoagland MS, Kwon JT, et al. Small-molecule activation of pro-caspase-3 to caspase-3 as a personalized anticancer strategy. Nat Chem Biol 2006;2:543–50.

[202] Svingen PA, Loegering D, Rodriquez J, Meng XW, Mesner Jr PW, Holbeck S, et al. Components of the cell death machine and drug sensitivity of the National Cancer Institute Cell Line Panel. Clin Cancer Res 2004;10:6807–20.

[203] Peterson QP, Hsu DC, Goode DR, Novotny CJ, Totten RK, Hergenrother PJ. Procaspase-3 activation as an anticancer strategy: structure-activity relationship of procaspase-activating compound 1 (PAC-1) and its cellular co-localization with caspase-3. J Med Chem 2009;52:5721–31.

[204] Wosikowski K, Regis JT, Robey RW, Alvarez M, Buters JT, Gudas JM, et al. Normal p53 status and function despite the development of drug resistance in human breast cancer cells. Cell Growth Differ 1995;6:1395–403.

[205] Kastan MB. Wild-type p53: tumors can't stand it. Cell 2007;128:837–40.

[206] Cheok CF, Verma CS, Baselga J, Lane DP. Translating p53 into the clinic. Nat Rev Clin Oncol 2011;8:25–37.

[207] Song H, Hollstein M, Xu Y. p53 gain-of-function cancer mutants induce genetic instability by inactivating ATM. Nat Cell Biol 2007;9:573–80.

[208] Maslon MM, Hupp TR. Drug discovery and mutant p53. Trends Cell Biol 2010;20:542–55.

[209] Kim AL, Raffo AJ, Brandt-Rauf PW, Pincus MR, Monaco R, Abarzua P, et al. Conformational and molecular basis for induction of apoptosis by a p53 C-terminal peptide in human cancer cells. J Biol Chem 1999;274:34924–31.

[210] Yu X, Vazquez A, Levine AJ, Carpizo DR. Allele-specific p53 mutant reactivation. Cancer Cell 2012;21:614–25.

[211] Wischhusen J, Naumann U, Ohgaki H, Rastinejad F, Weller M. CP-31398, a novel p53-stabilizing agent, induces p53-dependent and p53-independent glioma cell death. Oncogene 2003;22:8233–45.

[212] Wang W, Takimoto R, Rastinejad F, el Deiry WS. Stabilization of p53 by CP-31398 inhibits ubiquitination without altering phosphorylation at serine 15 or 20 or MDM2 binding. Mol Cell Biol 2003;23:2171–81.

[213] Demma M, Maxwell E, Ramos R, Liang L, Li C, Hesk D, et al. SCH529074, a small molecule activator of mutant p53, which binds p53 DNA binding domain (DBD), restores growth-suppressive function to mutant p53 and interrupts HDM2-mediated ubiquitination of wild type p53. J Biol Chem 2010;285:10198–212.

[214] Kapetanovic IM, Muzzio M, McCormick DL, Thompson TN, Johnson WD, Horn TL, et al. Pharmacokinetics and tissue and tumor exposure of CP-31398, a p53-stabilizing agent, in rats. Cancer Chemother Pharmacol 2012;69:1301–6.

[215] Lehmann S, Bykov VJ, Ali D, Andren O, Cherif H, Tidefelt U, et al. Targeting p53 in vivo: a first-in-human study with p53-targeting compound APR-246 in refractory hematologic malignancies and prostate cancer. J Clin Oncol 2012;30:3633–9.

[216] Bykov VJ, Issaeva N, Shilov A, Hultcrantz M, Pugacheva E, Chumakov P, et al. Restoration of the tumor suppressor function to mutant p53 by a low-molecular-weight compound. Nat Med 2002;8:282–8.

[217] Bao W, Chen M, Zhao X, Kumar R, Spinnler C, Thullberg M, et al. PRIMA-1Met/APR-246 induces wild-type p53-dependent suppression of malignant melanoma tumor growth in 3D culture and in vivo. Cell Cycle 2011;10:301–7.

[218] Lambert JM, Moshfegh A, Hainaut P, Wiman KG, Bykov VJ. Mutant p53 reactivation by PRIMA-1MET induces multiple signaling pathways converging on apoptosis. Oncogene 2010;29:1329–38.

[219] Zache N, Lambert JM, Wiman KG, Bykov VJ. PRIMA-1MET inhibits growth of mouse tumors carrying mutant p53. Cell Oncol 2008;30:411–8.

[220] Lambert JM, Gorzov P, Veprintsev DB, Soderqvist M, Segerback D, Bergman J, et al. PRIMA-1 reactivates mutant p53 by covalent binding to the core domain. Cancer Cell 2009;15:376–88.

[221] Bykov VJ, Issaeva N, Zache N, Shilov A, Hultcrantz M, Bergman J, et al. Reactivation of mutant p53 and induction of apoptosis in human tumor cells by maleimide analogs. J Biol Chem 2005;280:30384–91.

[222] Zache N, Lambert JM, Rokaeus N, Shen J, Hainaut P, Bergman J, et al. Mutant p53 targeting by the low molecular weight compound STIMA-1. Mol Oncol 2008;2:70–80.

[223] Wesierska-Gadek J, Schmid G. Dual action of the inhibitors of cyclin-dependent kinases: targeting of the cell-cycle progression and activation of wild-type p53 protein. Expert Opin Investig Drugs 2006;15:23–38.

[224] Dey A, Tergaonkar V, Lane DP. Double-edged swords as cancer therapeutics: simultaneously targeting p53 and NF-κB pathways. Nat Rev Drug Discov 2008;7:1031–40.

[225] Issaeva N, Bozko P, Enge M, Protopopova M, Verhoef LG, Masucci M, et al. Small molecule RITA binds to p53, blocks p.53-HDM-2 interaction and activates p53 function in tumors. Nat Med 2004;10:1321–8.

[226] Vassilev LT, Vu BT, Graves B, Carvajal D, Podlaski F, Filipovic Z, et al. In vivo activation of the p53 pathway by small-molecule antagonists of MDM2. Science 2004;303:844–8.

[227] Beryozkina A, Nichols GL, Reckner M, Vassilev LT, Rueger R, Jukofsky L, et al. Pharmacokinetics (PK) and pharmacodynamics (PD) of RG7112, an oral murine double minute 2 (MDM2) antagonist, in patients with leukemias and solid tumors. ; Abstract J Clin Oncol 2011;29(Suppl.):3039.

[228] Kojima K, Burks JK, Arts J, Andreeff M. The novel tryptamine derivative JNJ-26854165 induces wild-type p53- and E2F1-mediated apoptosis in acute myeloid and lymphoid leukemias. Mol Cancer Ther 2010;9:2545–57.

[229] Shangary S, Qin D, McEachern D, Liu M, Miller RS, Qiu S, et al. Temporal activation of p53 by a specific MDM2 inhibitor is selectively toxic to tumors and leads to complete tumor growth inhibition. Proc Natl Acad Sci USA 2008;105:3933–8.

[230] Popowicz GM, Czarna A, Wolf S, Wang K, Wang W, Domling A, et al. Structures of low molecular weight inhibitors bound to MDMX and MDM2 reveal new approaches for p53-MDMX/MDM2 antagonist drug discovery. Cell Cycle 2010;9:1104–11.

[231] Reed D, Shen Y, Shelat AA, Arnold LA, Ferreira AM, Zhu F, et al. Identification and characterization of the first small molecule inhibitor of MDMX. J Biol Chem 2010;285:10786–96.

[232] Johnson GG, Sherrington PD, Carter A, Lin K, Liloglou T, Field JK, et al. A novel type of p53 pathway dysfunction in chronic lymphocytic leukemia resulting from two interacting single nucleotide polymorphisms within the p21 gene. Cancer Res 2009;69:5210–7.

[233] Fan Z, Chakravarty P, Alfieri A, Pandita TK, Vikram B, Guha C. Adenovirus-mediated antisense ATM gene transfer sensitizes prostate cancer cells to radiation. Cancer Gene Ther 2000;7:1307–14.

[234] Zhang N, Song Q, Lu H, Lavin MF. Induction of p53 and increased sensitivity to cisplatin in ataxia-telangiectasia cells. Oncogene 1996;13:655–9.

[235] Harris SL, Levine AJ. The p53 pathway: positive and negative feedback loops. Oncogene 2005;24:2899–908.

[236] Mujoo K, Watanabe M, Nakamura J, Khokhar AR, Siddik ZH. Status of p53 phosphorylation and function in sensitive and resistant human cancer models exposed to platinum-based DNA damaging agents. J Cancer Res Clin Oncol 2003;129:709–18.

[237] Siddik ZH, Mims B, Lozano G, Thai G. Independent pathways of p53 induction by cisplatin and X-rays in a cisplatin-resistant ovarian tumor cell line. Cancer Res 1998;58:698–703.

[238] He G, Kuang J, Khokhar AR, Siddik ZH. The impact of S- and G2-checkpoint response on the fidelity of G1-arrest by cisplatin and its comparison to a non-cross-resistant platinum(IV) analog. Gynecol Oncol 2011;122:402–9.

[239] Arambula JF, Sessler JL, Siddik ZH. A texaphyrin-oxaliplatin conjugate that overcomes both pharmacologic and molecular mechanisms of cisplatin resistance in cancer cells. Med Chem Commun 2012;3:1275–81.

Targeting the MDM2–p53 Protein–Protein Interaction: Design, Discovery, and Development of Novel Anticancer Agents

Ian R. Hardcastle

Newcastle Cancer Centre, Northern Institute for Cancer Research,
Newcastle University, Newcastle upon Tyne, UK

INTRODUCTION

Cancer drug discovery activities in the postgenomic era have sought to identify small molecules able to modulate molecular targets identified as being intimately linked to the "hallmark" characteristics of cancer. Enzymes, such as kinases, frequently linked to angiogenesis, growth, or survival pathways, have been regarded as highly "druggable" and have been investigated with notable success (see Chapters 1, 10, 12 and 18). New agents have been discovered and improved clinical outcomes delivered in many cases. Initially, other potential targets identified were viewed as less tractable, in particular protein–protein interactions and protein–DNA interactions, and were not deemed attractive by many.

The tractability of protein–protein interactions as molecular targets for small-molecule drugs has been examined. Many protein–protein binding sites cover large surface areas (>600 Å^2); they may be relatively flat and featureless, lacking obvious small-molecule binding sites, and have high binding energies as a result of the sum of many weak attractive interactions. However, analysis of binding energies by alanine scanning has revealed the presence of "hotspots" (i.e., residues that contribute a large fraction of the binding energy) [1,2]. Hotspot residues are frequently found in clusters near the center of the interface, often forming hydrophobic clefts. These observations raise the possibility that small molecules, able to bind with sufficient affinity to hotspot clusters, would be able to antagonize a given protein–protein interaction [3].

Cancer Drug Design and Discovery, Second Edition
http://dx.doi.org/10.1016/B978-0-12-396521-9.00013-9

A number of clinically used cancer drugs act at protein–protein interfaces, either stabilizing or inhibiting the interaction (Table 13.1). The majority are complex natural products with the ability to present precise molecular recognition over a significant area of the protein-binding site. The Bcl family inhibitors (e.g., Navitoclax) were the first rationally designed small-molecule inhibitors of protein–protein interactions to enter clinical studies. Despite the large molecular weight of this family of agents, they demonstrate excellent proof-of-concept for protein–protein interaction inhibitors.

p53 AND CANCER

The transformation-related protein 53 (*TP53*) gene encodes a 53 KDa protein—p53—which, along with p63 and p73, is a descendant of a family of transcription factors that has an ancient evolutionary heritage [4]. The p53 protein acts principally as a tumor suppressor, but has additional roles in other physiological processes, including autophagy, cell adhesion, cell metabolism, fertility, and stem cell aging and development (Fig. 13.1) [5]. p53 functions as a molecular signaling node and is activated by a number of posttranslational modifications, including phosphorylation, acetylation, and methylation. The best understood pathways result from cellular stress, resulting in direct phosphorylation of p53 at a number of serine or threonine residues throughout the protein. In the absence of stress, p53 is maintained at low levels, with a short half-life of <20 min. Cellular insults resulting from DNA damage caused by ionizing radiation, ultraviolet (UV) light, or cytotoxic chemotherapeutics can be signaled to p53 via a number of kinase enzymes, including ATM, ATR, CDK2, CHK1/CHK2, CK1, DNA-PK, ERK2, JNK, MAPKAPK2, and p38 kinase [6]. Phosphorylation of latent p53 results in a conformational switch in the tetrameric protein and a rapid increase in the levels of the transcriptionally active protein. p53 is then able to activate ≥150 genes to transcription that are responsible for committing the cell to apoptosis, cell cycle arrest, DNA repair, senescence, or altered metabolism. Alternatively, activation of oncogenic signaling pathways leading to activation of p19^{ARF} results in p53 activation by inactivation of MDM2 [4]. The response to p53 activation depends on the tissue and cell type [7]. The response of different tissues of mice to γ-irradiation in vivo is heterogeneous [8]. In some tissues, p53 activation results in the accumulation of p53 and the activation of proapoptotic genes (e.g., *Bax*, *Fas*, *Puma*, and *Noxa*), whereas in other tissues, p53 accumulation is observed without apoptosis or p53 induction is not seen. Differences in response have also been observed to be dependent on the duration and intensity of irradiation [9]. The complexity of p53 activation appears to be the result of the numerous activation pathways and additional posttranslational modifications possible on p53, allowing the recruitment of different transcriptional promoters and different cellular responses.

p53 inactivation by mutation occurs in around 50% of human cancers [10]. Inactivation is caused principally by point mutation, usually affecting the DNA-binding domain. These mutations fall into two groups, one that affects the DNA contacts and another that alters the conformation of the scaffold required for DNA binding [11]. p53 mutants have been demonstrated to inhibit transcription as dominant negatives by a variety of mechanisms, including oligomerization with wild-type protein [12,13].

TABLE 13.1 Drugs that Modulate Protein–Protein Interactions

Drug	Structure	Target
Vincristine		α,β-Tubulin
Taxol		α,β-Tubulin
Rapamycin		mTOR (Tor1 and Tor 2)
Navitoclax		Bcl-2 and Bcl-XL

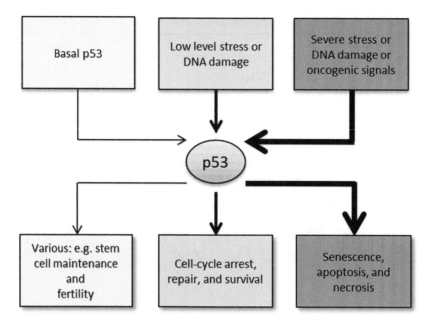

FIGURE 13.1   p53 activation and response.

MDM2, MDMX, and p53 Control

The murine double-minute 2 (*Mdm2*) gene was identified from amplified regions of double-minute (DM) chromosomes from NIH-3T3 DM mice [14]. Subsequently, MDM2 was shown to be a p53-associated protein in human sarcomas, and to be oncogenic [15,16]. The paralog MDMX (or MDM4) was identified as a p53-interacting protein from a mouse c-DNA library and subsequently in humans [17,18].

The essential nature of p53 regulation by MDM2 and MDMX has been demonstrated by knockout mouse models. *Mdm2−/−* knockout mice are embryonically lethal around the time of implantation. Lethality is rescued in the double knockout for *Mdm2* and *Trp53* [19,20]. Similarly, *Mdmx*-null mice died at 7.5–8.5 days gestation, owing to loss of cell proliferation, but the loss of *p53* completely rescued the embryos and the mice developed normally [21,22]. *Mdmx−/−* lethality has been rescued by the overexpression of MDM2, indicating some overlap in developmental roles for the proteins [23]. These data indicate that MDM2 and MDMX are able to act independently, providing essential p53 control mechanisms that are nonredundant.

MDM2 inhibits the activity of p53 directly, by binding to and occluding the p53 transactivation domain, and by promoting the destruction of the complex, through its E3-ubiquitin ligase activity [24,25]. In addition, MDM2 is a transcriptional target of p53, so the two proteins are linked in an autoregulatory feedback loop, ensuring that p53 activation is transient.

Similar to MDM2, MDMX is able to bind to the transactivation domain and inactivate p53, but it lacks E3–ubiquitin ligase activity. MDM2 and MDMX are able to form heterodimers with enhanced E3-ligase activity, possibly regulating MDM2 activity [26]. MDMX is not transcriptionally activated by p53 [27].

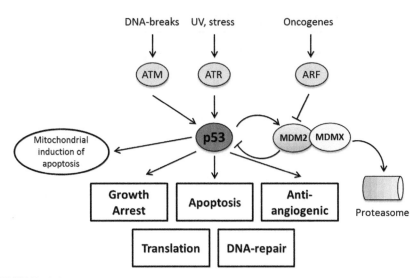

FIGURE 13.2 Mechanistic model for p53, MDM2, and MDMX response to cellular stressors.

The tumor suppressor protein p19[ARF], an alternate reading frame product of *CDKN2A*, is a negative regulator of MDM2 [28,29]. Oncogenic growth signals induce the transcription of p19[ARF] and result in the destruction of MDM2. p53 is stabilized through the inhibition of ubiquitination by MDM2 and p53 export from the nucleus, and proteasomal destruction is blocked [30].

A model for p53 activation can now be proposed. Initially, cellular levels of MDM2 and p53 are maintained at low concentration by MDM2-mediated proteasomal degradation and MDMX blocking p53 transcription. In response to cellular stress or genotoxic insult, p53 is phosphorylated and liberated from the MDM2–MDMX complex; it is then able to directly activate apoptosis at microsomes and initiate transcription in the nucleus. Alternatively, p53 can be activated by oncogenic signaling via p19[ARF] and inactivation of MDM2. Transcriptional activation of p53 results in an accumulation of p53, providing positive feedback and amplification of the signal. Transcription of MDM2 results in inactivation of p53, and a negative feedback loop ensures that the p53 response does not remain unchecked (Fig. 13.2).

Gene amplification of *MDM2*, giving rise to overexpression of the MDM2 protein, has been observed in tumor samples taken from common sporadic cancers. Overall, around 10% of tumors had *MDM2* amplification, with the highest incidence found in hepatocellular carcinoma (44%), lung cancer (15%), sarcomas and osteosarcomas (28%), and Hodgkin's disease (67%). The amplification *MDMX* has been reported in a smaller selection of tumors with variable incidence, for example brain or nervous system tumors (5–12%), breast tumors (5–40%), and sarcomas (17%). Interestingly, overexpression (three- to fivefold) of MDMX in the absence of gene amplification appears to be more common, as observed in breast (19%), uterine (15%), testicular (27%), stomach or small intestine (42%), colorectal (19%), laryngeal (23%), and lung (18%) cancers as well as melanoma (65%) [26,31,32]. Gene amplification of *MDM2* or *MDMX* and p53 mutations appear to be mutually exclusive, suggesting that a single mechanism for disabling the p53 tumor suppressor function is necessary and sufficient for carcinogenesis.

TARGETING THE MDM2–p53 INTERACTION

The therapeutic hypothesis for MDM2–p53 inhibition proposes that a potent inhibitor of the protein–protein interaction will liberate p53 from the repressive control of MDM2, and then subsequently activate p53-mediated cell death in the tumor. In tumors, selectivity is envisioned to result from p53 sensing preexisting DNA damage or oncogenic activation signals that had previously been blocked by the action of MDM2 at normal or overexpressed levels. In normal cells, p53 activation is anticipated to result in activation of nonapoptotic pathways. The addition of DNA-damaging agents or ionizing radiation is expected to be synergistic with MDM2–p53 inhibition.

Preliminary experiments using antisense oligodeoxyribonucleotides provided evidence consistent with the therapeutic hypothesis. SJSA and JAR cell lines (MDM2 amplified, p53 wild-type) treated with MDM2-specific phosphorothioate oligos showed decreased expression of MDM2 protein levels, upregulated p21, and induction of apoptosis, and a p53-responsive luciferase gene reporter was activated. The oligos were also synergistic with the topoisomerase-1 poison camptothecin [33]. Similarly, a 2'-O-methoxyethyl-modified hemimer targeted to MDM2 mRNA completely inhibited MDM2 expression in SJSA-1 cells and induced p53 and p21 expression, but in this case did not induce apoptosis in the absence of the DNA-damaging agents carboplatin and mitomycin-C [34].

MDM2 Structural Biology

The first X-ray crystal structures of human and *Xenopus laevis* MDM2 with a p53 peptide bond were reported in 1996 [35]. The structure shows that MDM2 forms a hydrophobic cleft into which the 15-mer p53 peptide binds as an amphipathic α-helix (Protein Data Bank identification number (PDB ID): 1YCR; Fig. 13.3). The key p53 residues filling the cleft are Phe[19], Trp[23], and Leu[26], which make van der Waals interactions with good shape complementarity. Two intermolecular hydrogen bonds are present: between the Phe[19] backbone amide of p53 and the side chain of Gln[72] of MDM2, and between the indole NH of Trp[23] of p53 and the Leu[54] backbone carbonyl within the MDM2 hydrophobic cleft.

X-ray structures of the apo-MDM2 structure are not available; however, a high-resolution nuclear magnetic resonance (NMR) structure has been solved, showing that the protein adopts multiple conformations (PDB ID: 1Z1M; Fig. 13.4) [36]. A portion of the N-terminal region of MDM2 (residues 16–24) acts as a "lid" and closes over the p53-binding site [37]. The lid region easily displaced by p53 and the MDM2 binding cleft widens to allow binding, forming a more stable complex [38]. The MDM2 lid region is thought to play an important role in the regulation of the MDM2–p53 interaction by placing phosphorylatable residues of both proteins in close proximity.

A number of groups have investigated the molecular dynamics of MDM2 between the apo- and p53-bound state [39,40]. The results show the mobility of the N-terminal "lid" portion of MDM2, which exists in two main conformations: "open", which is found predominantly in the p53-bound state; and "closed", which is found for the apo state. The apo-closed state is stabilized by a network of interactions with the lid, produced by two salt-bridge interactions between Glu[23] and either Arg[97] or Arg[105], and Glu[25] and Lys[51].

(A)

(B)

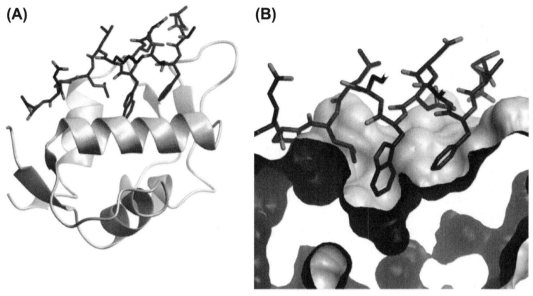

FIGURE 13.3 X-ray structure of MDM2 and p53 peptide (PDB ID: 1YCR). (A): Ribbon view; and (B): surface showing the binding interaction. (This figure is reproduced in color in the color plate section.)

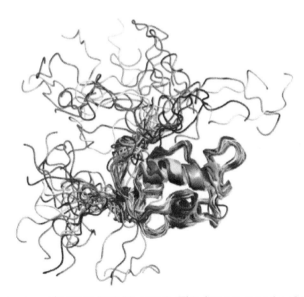

FIGURE 13.4 NMR structure of MDM2 (PDB ID: 1Z1M). (This figure is reproduced in color in the color plate section.)

MDM2–p53 INHIBITORS

Peptide Inhibitors

The initial observation of inhibition of the MDM2–p53 interaction arose from immunoprecipitation experiments. One antibody from a panel was unable to co-immunoprecipitate the MDM2–p53 complex from cell extracts, suggesting that the antibody recognized the same region on p53 to which MDM2 binds [41]. A complete library of 15-mer peptides corresponding to the p53 protein was immobilized on enzyme-linked immunosorbent assay (ELISA) plates and screened with MDM2 protein, revealing the consensus binding site on MDM2 to be –QETFSDLWKL–. The consensus sequence was confirmed from phage display libraries screened against an immobilized MDM2 protein or an anti-p53 antibody [42]. The IP3 peptide (**1**) (Table 13.2) showed greater than 20-fold increased affinity for MDM2 over the wild-type p53 sequence. Expression of an IP3–GST fusion peptide in the SA-1 cell line (MDM2 amplified, p53wt) produced specific effects on p53 activity, the cell cycle, and cell survival [43].

Optimization of the IP3 peptide was achieved through the introduction of α,α-disubstituted amino acids at residues free from strong interactions with the MDM2 protein, the best being α-aminobutyric acid (Aib) for Asp21 and cyclopropanecarboxylic acid (Ac$_3$c) for Gly25. The introduction of steric constraint and stabilization of the α-helix was confirmed by NMR experiments. The reduced entropic penalties for binding to MDM2 gave a fourfold improved inhibitory activity for 8-mer peptide **3** compared with 8-mer peptide **2**. Guided by the NMR model, affinity was improved a further sevenfold by replacement of the tyrosine residue with a phosphonomethylphenylalanine residue (Pmp; peptide **4**), enabling the formation of a salt-bridge interaction with the ε-amino group of Lys94 of MDM2. Analysis of the MDM2 X-ray structure suggested that Trp23 indole rings do not completely fill the hydrophobic cleft and that small lipophilic groups at the 6-position would fill the space. As predicted, 6-substitution with fluorine, methyl, or chlorine gave a 20- to 63-fold improvement in binding affinity, as exemplified by the 6-chloro substituted AP peptide **5** (IC$_{50}$ = 5 nM) [44]. The importance of this residue for binding affinity is confirmed by the low activity of the control peptide **6**, which includes an alanine substitution for Trp23. The X-ray structure of the AP peptide bound to MDM2 has been solved (PDB ID: 2GV2; Fig. 13.5), showing the 6-chloro group occupying

TABLE 13.2　Peptide Inhibitors of the MDM2–p53 Interaction

	Peptide	Sequence	IC$_{50}$ (nM)
	p53wt	Ac-Gln16-Glu-Thr-Phe-Ser-Asp21-Leu-Trp-Lys-Leu-Leu-Pro27-NH$_2$	8673 ± 164
1	IP3	Ac-Met-Pro-Arg-Phe19-Met-Asp-Tyr-Trp-Glu-Gly-Leu26-Asn-NH$_2$	313 ± 10
2	8 mer	Ac-Phe19-Met-Asp-Tyr-Trp-Glu-Gly-Leu26-NH$_2$	8949 ± 85
3		Ac-Phe19-Met-Aib-Tyr-Trp-Glu-Ac$_3$c-Leu26-NH$_2$	2210 ± 346
4		Ac-Phe19-Met-Aib-Pmp-Trp-Glu-Ac$_3$c-Leu26-NH$_2$	314 ± 88
5	AP	Ac-Phe19-Met-Aib-Pmp-6-Cl-Trp-Glu-Ac$_3$c-Leu26-NH$_2$	5 ± 1
6		Ac-Phe19-Met-Aib-Pmp-Ala -Glu-Ac$_3$c-Leu26-NH$_2$	>2000
7		Biotin-Ser-Gly-Antennapedia43–58-Cys-*Linker*-Phe19-Met-Aib-Pmp-6-Cl-Trp-Glu-Ac$_3$c-Leu26-NH$_2$	9 ± 1

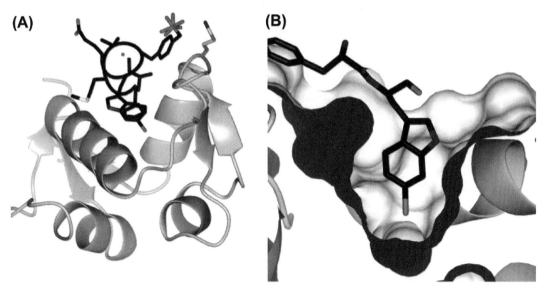

FIGURE 13.5 X-ray structure of MDM2 and AP peptide (PDB ID: 2GV2). (A): End on ribbon view; and (B): surface showing Trp[23] binding pocket. (This figure is reproduced in color in the color plate section.)

space below the Trp[23] site, and making additional van der Waals contacts with Phe[86] and Ile99 as predicted. The Pmp residue, however, does not make the predicted salt-bridge and is observed projecting into solvent. Despite its poor cellular penetration, the AP peptide (at 100 µM) has been shown to induce accumulation of p53, p21, and MDM2 in HCT116 cells (p53wt, MDM2wt), but not in the p53 mutant SKBR-3 line. In addition, the AP peptide induced apoptosis in OSA-CL cells (p53wt, MDM2 amplified) in a dose-dependent way [45]. The cellular permeability of the AP peptide **5** was addressed by linking it to the Antennapedia third helix via a maleimido bridge, giving compound **7**, which retained affinity for MDM2 [46].

Peptide-Mimetic Inhibitors

A number of approaches have been employed to address the predicted poor pharmaceutical properties of peptide MDM2–p53 inhibitors. These have included stabilization of the peptide by hydrocarbon "staples" and incorporation into mini-proteins, or the use of inherently more stable backbones with the ability to array the key groups in an optimal conformation.

The stapled peptide approach relies on the ability of a hydrocarbon link between distant residues in a peptide chain to lock its helical structure and provide improved cellular penetration and metabolic stability [47]. The 15-residue α-helical loop of p53 that interacts with MDM2 provided the basis for a library of eight stapled peptides linked between residues i and $i + 7$. Linking between Phe[19] and Leu[26] gave a potent inhibitor (**8**) (Table 13.3) with good α-helicity (62%) but poor cellular penetration [48]. Improved cellular permeability was achieved by the substitution of charged aspartic and glutamic acid residues with asparagines and glutamines, without compromising the activity (**9**). In addition, residues involved in p53 nuclear export or ubiquitination were mutated, with a 50-fold loss of binding affinity for MDM2 but improved cellular uptake and activity (**10**). The optimized compound **10** showed dose-dependent inhibition of SJSA-1 cell viability ($EC_{50} = 8.8$ µM) and induction of apoptosis

TABLE 13.3   Hydrocarbon Stapled Peptide Inhibitors of the MDM2–p53 Interaction [48]

	Peptide	Sequence	K_d (nM)	α-helicity
	p53wt	Ac-Leu-Ser-Gln16-Glu-Thr-Phe-Ser-Asp21-Leu-Trp-Lys-Leu-Leu-Pro27-Glu-Asn-NH2	410 ± 19	11%
8	SAH-p53–4	Ac-Leu-Ser-Gln16-Glu-Thr-Phe19-*-Asp-Leu-Trp-Lys-Leu-Leu26-*-Glu-Asn-NH2	0.92 ± 0.11	59%
9	SAH-p53–5	Ac-Leu-Ser-Gln16-Glu-Thr-Phe19-*-*Asn*-Leu-Trp-Lys-Leu-Leu26-*-*Gln*-Asn-NH2	0.80 ± 0.05	20%
10	SAH-p53–8	Ac-*Gln*-Ser-Gln16-Glu-Thr-Phe19-*-*Asn*-Leu-Trp-*Arg*-Leu-Leu26-*-*Gln*-Asn-NH2	55 ± 11	85%

*= Hydrocarbon linker residue.

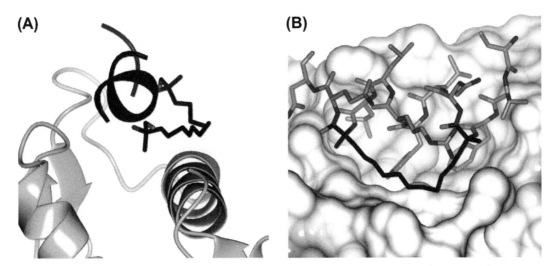

(A)   **(B)**

FIGURE 13.6   X-ray structure of MDM2 and stapled peptide **10** (PDB ID: 3V3B). (A): End on ribbon view; and (B): surface showing interaction of hydrocarbon staple. (This figure is reproduced in color in the color plate section.)

measured by activation of caspase-3 (EC_{50} = 5.8 µM). The X-ray crystal structure of **10** bound to MDM2 (PDB ID: 3V3B; Fig. 13.6) shows that the peptide makes a short α-helix from residues 19–27, with the key binding residues Phe19, Trp23, and Leu26 occupying similar space to the native structure [49]. Minor changes are observed in MDM2, notably the movement of the Met62 side chain to accommodate the hydrocarbon staple that overlays the Met50–Lys64 helix that forms the rim of the binding pocket. Importantly, stapled peptide **10** is also a potent inhibitor of the MDMX–p53 interaction in cell-free and cellular assays (K_d = 2.3 ± 0.2 nM), and is cytotoxic to cells overexpressing MDM2, MDMX, or both proteins through a p53-mediated mechanism.

An alternative approach to stapling used a heterocyclic linker to staple a 3_{10} helical peptide targeted to MDM2 and MDMX (Table 13.3; the peptide dual-inhibitor (pDI) peptide) [50]. A range of stapled peptides (**11–13**) (Table 13.4), synthesized by the photoinduced

TABLE 13.4 Stapled Peptide Inhibitors of the MDM2–p53 and MDMX–p53 Interaction [51]

	Peptide	Sequence	IC$_{50}$ (nM) MDM2	IC$_{50}$ (nM) MDMX
	pDI	Ac-Leu-Thr-Phe-Glu-His-Tyr-Trp-Ala-Gln-Leu-Leu-Thr-Ser-NH$_2$	44	550
11		Ac-Leu-Thr-Phe-α-His-Tyr-Trp-β-Gln-Leu-Leu-Thr-Ser-NH$_2$	61	540
12		Ac-Leu-Thr-Phe-α-His-Tyr-Trp-Ala-Gln-Leu-Leu-β-Ser-NH$_2$	6.2	340
13		Ac-Leu-Thr-Phe-α-Arg-Tyr-Trp-Ala-Arg-Leu-Leu-β-Ser-NH$_2$	39	550

α = alkene modified lysine; β = tetrazole-modified lysine.

cycloaddition of alkene- and tetrazole-modified lysine residues, showed similar activity to the parent peptide [51]. Substitution with arginine at two nonessential residues increased the positive charge on the compound and improved cellular uptake for **13** without compromising binding affinity; however, activation of a p53 reporter in U2OS cells was modest.

Other approaches to improving the metabolic stability of peptide-derived inhibitors rely on the use of alternative backbones, capable of recapitulating the side chain interactions of p53 with the MDM2-binding site. Examples of MDM2–p53 inhibitors based on a range of scaffolds have been reported, including D-peptides, β-peptides, di-proline β-hairpins, and peptoids.

Peptides synthesized from D-amino acids show improved resistance to metabolic degradation. The retroinverso peptide **14** has the reverse sequence of amino acids to the p53 peptide and is synthesized from D-amino acids. These D-peptides usually form left-handed helices; however, the modest activity of **14** (IC$_{50}$ = 14 μM) suggests that it may also be able to form right-handed turns [52]. The use of mirror-image phage display and native chemical ligation gave the D-peptide ligands ^{D}PMI-α (**15**), ^{D}PMI-β (**16**), and ^{D}PMI-γ (**17**), with good binding affinity for MDM2 (Table 13.5) and resistance to proteolysis [53,54]. Co-crystallization of **15** and with MDM2 yielded X-ray structures (PDB ID: 3LNJ; Fig. 13.7). In both structures, the peptide adopts a left-handed helix with the triplet of residues ^{D}Trp^3–^{D}Leu^7–^{D}Leu^{77} or ^{D}Trp^3–^{D}Phe^7–^{D}Leu^{11} occupying the p53-binding cleft. Structure-based optimization of **16** by the introduction of ^{D}6-F-Trp^3 and ^{D}4-CF$_3$-Phe^7 (^{D}PMI-γ; [18]) resulted in a 400-fold improvement in potency [55]. The D-peptides are not active in cell lines, presumably due to poor uptake, so arginine–glycine–aspartic acid (RGD)-liposomal encapsulation was used to demonstrate dose-dependent growth inhibition in U87 human glioma cells (p53wt) and induction of p53-dependent proteins. Significant tumor growth delay was seen in vivo in U87 xenografts treated intravenously (IV) with 7 mg/kg of liposomal **15**.

β-Peptides have an additional backbone carbon atom that confers resistance to proteolysis and metabolism. A β^3-decapeptide, which formed a stable 14-helix in aqueous solution, was used as the scaffold for the p53 residues Phe^{19}, Trp^{23}, and Leu^{26} arrayed on sequential turns of the helix, giving a modest MDM2 inhibitory potency [56]. Computational de novo design and screening methods yielded β^3-decapeptides with improved potency for MDM2 (K_d < 30 nM) through the inclusion of 6-chlorotryptophan or 3-trifluoromethyl- or 3,4-dichlorophenylalanine residues at the 6-position [57].

TABLE 13.5   D-Peptide Inhibitors of MDM2–p53

		D-**Amino acid sequence**	K_d **(nM)**[1]
14		Ac-Asn-Gln-Pro-Leu-Leu-Lys-Trp-Leu-Asp-Ser-Phe-Thr-Glu-Gln-Ser-NH$_2$	1400[2]
15	DPMIα	Thr-Asn-Trp-Tyr-Ala-Gln- Leu-Glu-Lys-Leu-Leu-Arg-NH$_2$	219 ± 11
16	DPMIβ	Thr-Ala-Trp-Tyr-Ala-Gln-Phe-Glu-Lys-Leu-Leu-Arg-NH$_2$	34.5 ± 0.6
17	DPMIγ	LHis-Asp-Trp-Trp-Pro-Leu-Ala-Phe-Ala-Lys-Leu-Leu-Arg-NH$_2$	53 ± 6
18	DPMIδ	Thr-Ala-**6-F-Trp**-Tyr-Ala-Gln-**4-CF₃-Phe**-Glu-Lys-Leu-Leu-Arg-NH$_2$	0.22 ± 0.21

[1] *By competition SPR.*
[2] *IC$_{50}$ by ELISA.*

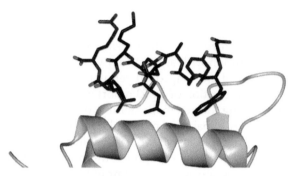

FIGURE 13.7   X-ray structure of MDM2 and DPMI-α (**15**) (PDB ID: 3LNJ). (This figure is reproduced in color in the color plate section.)

The D-Pro–L-Pro dipeptide template forms a β-hairpin motif, which has been used as an α-helix mimetic scaffold to orientate the critical p53 residues correctly for binding to MDM2. The Asp^2, 6-Cl-Trp^3 analog (**19**) (IC$_{50}$ = 140 nM)—identified from a β-hairpin library—co-crystallized with MDM2 (PDB ID: 2AXI), showing interactions between the hydrophobic side chains of Phe^1, 6-Cl-Trp^3, and Leu^4, buried in the p53-binding site [58,59].

19

Oligomeric *N*-substituted glycines or peptoids are resistant to proteolysis, and the introduction of chiral side chains can be used to sterically tune the helical conformation. Peptoids (e.g., **20**) designed to correctly orientate the important p53 side chain groups and including achiral polar functional groups, such as phosphonate, sulfonamide, and p-nitrophenyl, to improve water solubility and form additional interactions with MDM2, showed modest inhibition of the MDM2–p53 interaction (**20**; IC$_{50}$ = 9.9 μM) [60].

20

A number of oligomeric structures have been designed to mimic one face of short α-helical structures important in protein–protein interactions, including MDM2–p53. Terphenyl **21** aligns the isobutyl–2-naphthylmethylene–isobutyl sequence in the correct orientation for binding to MDM2 (K_i = 0.182 μM). NMR studies showed binding to the p53-binding site of MDM2 with the 2-naphthylmethylene occupying the Trp^{23} binding pocket [61]. Oligoamides have similar ability to form α-helix mimetic structures with better physicochemical properties than terphenyls. A library of 8000 oligobenzamides was screened against MDM2, from which a few compounds with modest potency were identified (e.g., **22**; IC$_{50}$ = 8 μM) [62]. A similar small series of *ortho*-O-alkyl oligobenzamides designed to mimic the p53–helix showed similar potency (e.g., **23**; IC$_{50}$ = 1.0 μM) [63]. The N-alkyl oligobenzamide series from the same research group showed similar binding to MDM2 (e.g., **24**; IC$_{50}$ = 2.8) [64]. The pyrrolopyrimidine scaffold was designed as an α-helix mimetic to replace the oligobenzamide H-bonded structure [65]. Screening of a 900-member library identified **25** and **26** as inhibitors of MDM2–p53 (K_i = 0.62 and 0.84 μM, respectively) that also showed similar inhibition of MDMX–p53. A small series of α-1,4-linked tri-2-deoxygalactose trisaccharides (e.g., **26**), designed to mimic the p53 peptide, showed only weak inhibitory activity, suggesting that this scaffold was not well optimized [66].

21   **22**   **23**   **24**

Small-Molecule Inhibitors

The possibility of inhibiting the MDM2–p53 interaction with small, drug-like molecules has attracted a significant amount of attention from the drug discovery community. The protein–protein target has been the subject of high-throughput screening (HTS) campaigns, virtual screening, pharmacophore screening, and structure-based design approaches that have yielded a number of chemotypes with excellent potency and potential for development.

cis-*Imidazolines or Nutlins*

A series of cis-imidazolines (**28–30**) (Table 13.6) were identified by HTS of a diverse library of compounds, and named "Nutlins" after their place of origin in Nutley, New Jersey [67]. Each of these compounds has submicromolar activity in a competitive surface plasmon resonance (SPR) assay as racemates. The enantiomers of Nutlin-3 (**30**) were separated by chiral high-performance liquid chromatography, and one enantiomer, Nutlin-3a (**30a**), showed potent activity (IC$_{50}$ = 90 nM), whereas Nutlin-3b (**30b**) was 150-fold less potent and provided a useful control compound. The co-crystal structure of Nutlin-2 (**29**) with MDM2 shows that the inhibitor makes mostly hydrophobic interactions with the protein, occupying the p53-binding site on MDM2 (PDB ID: 1RV1; Fig. 13.8). One bromophenyl ring fills the Trp pocket, and the other occupies the Leu^{26} site. The Phe^{19} site is partially filled by the ethyl ether side chain. The piperidine side chain overlays the surface of MDM2 and presumably aids the aqueous solubility of the compound. In addition, the binding mode for Nutlin-1 (**28**) has been determined by NMR (PDB ID: 1TTV) and is in good agreement with the X-ray structure of **29** [68].

TABLE 13.6 *cis*-Imidazoline Inhibitors

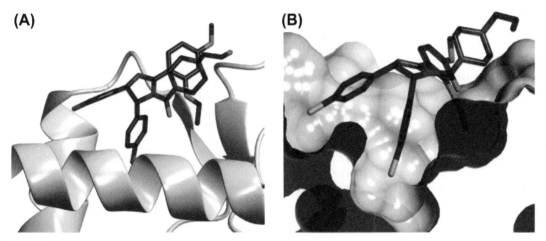

Compound	Name	X	R^1	R^2	IC$_{50}$ (μM)[1]
28	Nutlin-1	Cl	COCH$_3$	CH$_3$	0.26
29	Nutlin-2	Br	CH$_2$CH$_2$OH	H	0.14
30a	Nutlin-3a	Cl	H	CH$_3$	0.09
30b	Nutlin-3b	Cl	H	CH$_3$	13.6

[1] *Measured by competition SPR.*

FIGURE 13.8 X-ray structure of MDM2 and Nutlin-2 (**29**) (PDB ID: 1RV1). (A): Ribbon view; and (B): surface showing binding interaction. (This figure is reproduced in color in the color plate section.)

Nutlin-1 (**28**) was investigated in cell lines with defined MDM2 and p53 status, and, as expected, it showed a dose-dependent increase in p53, MDM2, and p21 in HCT116, RKO, and SJSA-1 cells (p53wt) but not in the SW480 and MDA-MB-453 lines (p53−/−). Cell cycle analysis using bromodeoxyuridine in HCT116, RKO, and SJSA-1 cells showed G$_1$ and G$_2$/M blocks, but not in the p53 mutant lines examined. Similarly, growth inhibition in p53 wild-type cells was greater (IC$_{50}$s = 1.4–1.8 μM) compared with p53 mutant lines (IC$_{50}$s = 13–21 μM) either by an MTT (3-(4,5-dimethylthiazol-2-yl)-2,5-diphenyltetrazolium bromide) assay or by clonogenic survival. Apoptosis was observed in SJSA-1 cells by TUNEL (terminal deoxynu-cleotidyl transferase dUTP nick end labeling) staining. A genotoxic mechanism for Nutlin-1 (**28**) was excluded by measurement of p53 Ser15 phosphorylation, a marker for DNA damage.

The cellular activity of Nutlin-3a (**30a**) has been investigated in a panel of cell lines, includ-ing engineered lines, using a variety of methods [69]. Nutlin-3a (**30a**) was growth inhibitory in mouse embryonic fibroblasts from animals with normal p53, and mdm2 was inactive in cells derived from the p53−/− mdm2−/− double-knockout mice. The global pattern of gene expression in p53wt and p53−/− cells following treatment with **30a** and **30b** was evaluated using Affymetric GeneChip, which showed that 143 of 40,000 genes were affected by the active enantiomer **30a** in p53wt HCT116 cells, but no effect was seen for the control com-pound **30b**, or for either compound in the p53-null line. In a panel of p53wt cell lines, the active enantiomer **30a** showed dose-dependent induction of p21, cell cycle arrest, and induc-tion of apoptosis.

Racemic Nutlin-3 (**30**; 200 mg/kg, twice daily [BD], 20 days) showed in vivo efficacy in an SJSA-1 osteosarcoma xenograft, giving 90% inhibition of tumor growth, with no significant toxicity or weight loss [67]. Similarly, the active Nutlin-3a enantiomer (**30a**) showed substan-tial activity in a 3-week antitumor efficacy study with SJSA xenografts (**30a**; 200 mg/kg, BD, 21 days), giving eight partial and one full tumor regression, without significant weight loss or toxicity. Antitumor activity was also seen in MHM, LnCaP, and 22Rv1 xenografts. The *mdm2* amplified tumors (MHM and SJSA-1) showed similar sensitivity to the inhibitor. These results confirmed Nutlin-3a (**30a**) as a potent and selective MDM2–p53 inhibitor that meets the tool compound criteria [70], and so it has been used in many subsequent studies exploring the role of MDM2 and p53 in different settings.

Further developments to the imidazoline class of inhibitors have been described in the patent literature [71,72]. The modifications introduced have addressed the need for improved potency and drug-like properties (e.g., compounds **31–35**). The two chlorophenyl groups are unchanged, with variation introduced at the 2-aryl substituent and the urea side chain. Recently, the structure of a clinical candidate from the Nutlin series, RG7112 (**36**), was reported [73,74]. It differs from the parent (**30a**) by the addition of two methyl groups to the imidazo-line ring, the addition of a 6-*t*-butyl group to the 2-phenyl substituent, and the addition of a 3-methylsulfonylpropyl side chain to the piperazine. The clinical development of RG7112 will be discussed further in this chapter.

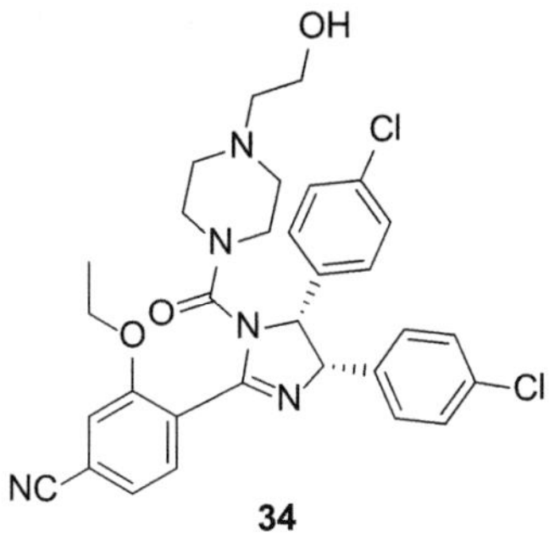

34

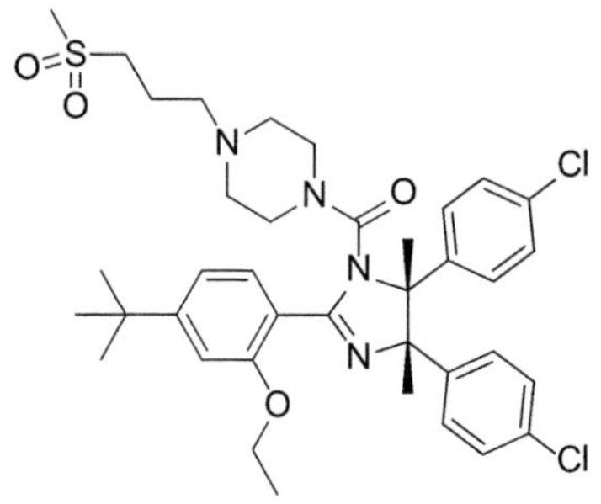

36: RG-7112

1,4-Benzodiazepine-2,5-diones

A 1,4-benzodiazepine-2,5-dione library provided the initial hits from a fluorescence thermal denaturation affinity HTS of over 338,000 diverse library compounds for MDM2 binding [75,76]. The ability of hit compounds, such as **37**, to inhibit the binding of a p53 peptide to MDM2 was confirmed by a fluorescence polarization (FP) assay. Structure-activity studies for the active (*S,S*) diastereomer showed that a 4-chlorobenzyl group was optimal (**39**) (Table 13.7). The X-ray structure of **39** bound to MDM2 (PBD ID: 1T4E; Fig. 13.9) shows the inhibitor occupying the hydrophobic binding cleft, making largely van der Waals interactions with the protein. In common with the Nutlin-2 structure, the halophenyl groups occupy the Trp[23] and Leu[26] pockets on MDM2, while the heterocyclic scaffold lies flat against the protein surface and the Phe[19] binding site. Poor pharmacokinetics and lack of oral bioavailability were observed for **39**, so further optimization sought to address these limitations [77].

TABLE 13.7   1,4-Benzodiazepine-2,5-diones

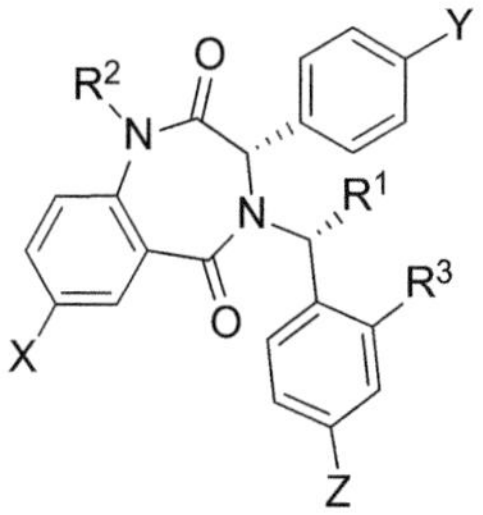

Compound	X	Y	Z	R^1	R^2	R^3	IC_{50} (μM)[1]
37	I	CF_3	H	CO_2CH_3	H	H	2.2
39	I	Cl	Cl	CO_2H	H	H	0.22
40	I	Cl	Cl	CO_2H	$(CH_2)_4CO_2H$	H	0.51
41	CCH	Cl	Cl	CH_3	$(CH_2)_4CO_2H$	H	0.71
42	I	Cl	Cl	CH_3	$(CH_2)_3N(C_2H_4)_2NCH_3$	NH_2	0.55

[1] *Measured by competition FP.*

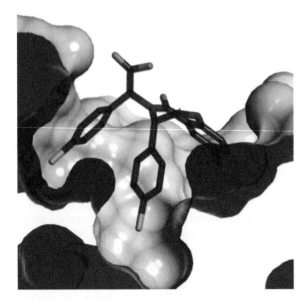

FIGURE 13.9 X-ray structure of MDM2 and **39** (PDB ID: 1T4E). (This figure is reproduced in color in the color plate section.)

Introduction of a pentanoic acid group at N^1 of the benzodiazepinedione ring (**40**) (Table 13.7) improved solubility without significant loss of potency. The 7-ethynyl compound **41** and 2-anilino-4-chlorobenzyl derivative **43**, bearing basic water-solubilizing groups, gave the best combination of cell-free inhibition of MDM2–p53 binding in the FP assay and cellular activity as measured by the induction of the p53-inducible gene PIG3 [78]. In a panel of cell lines, selective growth inhibition in p53wt cells was demonstrated for **39** and **41**, although the potencies observed were low ($GI_{50} = 10$–58 μM) [79]. In common with Nutlin-3a (**30a**), phosphorylation of Ser15 on p53 or H2AX phosphorylation was not observed for **41**, showing that the compound does not cause DNA damage. Hep2G hepatocellular carcinoma cells treated with **41** showed a rapid induction of p21 and MDM2, followed by a slower induction of PIG3 mRNA levels by real-time polymerase chain reaction (RT-PCR), and PUMAα, p21, p53, and MDM2 protein levels by Western blotting.

Further structural modifications resulting in **43** gave improved cellular activity. In A375 melanoma cells, **43** was synergistic with doxorubicin, 5-fluorouracil, and irinotecan, probably due to stabilization of p53. However, combination with cisplatin resulted in antagonism. A pharmacodynamic assay measuring the induction of p21 mRNA by RT-PCR in mice treated with **43** (25 and 50 mg/kg, intraperitoneal, BD) showed a 30-fold induction at 25 mg/kg, similar to that seen with the doxorubicin-positive control, and >150-fold at the 50 mg/kg dose. No apparent toxicity was seen at the 25 mg/kg dose, but weight loss was noted at 50 mg/kg.

Based on the in vitro results, the antitumor efficacy of **43** alone and in combination with doxorubicin was assessed in an A375 xenograft model. Treatment with **43** alone (100 mg/kg, by mouth or orally [PO], BD × 10) produced a modest effect on tumor growth, whereas the lower dose of doxorubicin alone (1.5 mg/kg, IV, every day [QD] × 5) was not significantly inhibitory. The combination of **43** and doxorubicin (100 and 1.5 mg/kg) produced a similar inhibitory effect to the higher dose of doxorubicin (3 mg/kg, IV, QD × 5). The combination

TABLE 13.8 Spirooxindoles

Compound	X	Y	Z	R^1	R^2	IC_{50} (nM)[1]	K_i (nM)[1]
43	Cl	H	H	CH_3	CH_3	86	
44	Cl	H	H	$-(CH_2)_2N(C_2H_4)_2O$	H	13	
45	Cl	F	H	$-(CH_2)_2N(C_2H_4)_2O$	H		1.7 ± 0.5
46	Br	H	H	$-(CH_2)_2N(C_2H_4)O$	H	18	
47	Cl	F	H	$-(CH_2)_2N(C_2H_4)_2NCH_3$	H		1.5 ± 0.4
48	Cl	F	H	$-(CH_2)_2CH(C_2H_4)_2NCH_3$	H		2.0 ± 0.5
49	Cl	F	H	$-(CH_2)_2CH(S)OHCH_2OH$	H		0.6 ± 0.1
50	Cl	H	F	$-(CH_2)_2CH(S)OHCH_2OH$	H		13.3 ± 1.8
51	Cl	F	F	$-(CH_2)_2CH(S)OHCH_2OH$	H		9.6 ± 3.9

[1] Measured by competition FP.

was significantly less toxic than doxorubicin alone. Despite promising results, activity on this compound series has not continued.

Spirooxindoles

The spirooxindole series of MDM2–p53 inhibitors was discovered initially using substructure searching to identify natural products containing an oxindole ring, intended to mimic the Trp[23] of p53 [80]. Two alkaloids (i.e., spirotryprostatin A and alstonisine) contained the spiro(oxindole-3,3′-pyrrolidine) core that was used as a scaffold to design possible inhibitors, by docking into the MDM2 structure. Spirooxindole (43) (Table 13.8) displayed potent activity in an FP assay. Docking studies suggested that the chlorooxindole ring occupies the Trp[23] pocket, the 3-chlorophenyl group projects into the Phe[19] pocket, and the t-butyl group fills the Leu[26] pocket. Further compounds based on the same scaffold and designed to mimic the additional interactions of Leu[22] from p53 gave rise to the oxindole (44), which showed improved potency. The docked structure of 44 showed that the morpholine ring carbons and the linker mimic the Leu[22] interaction and the morpholine oxygen in proximity to the amine group of Lys94 in MDM2. The introduction of a fluorine atom at the 2-phenyl position gave a threefold improvement in activity (45) (in MI-63) [81]. Spirooxindole 45 showed p53-dependent growth inhibition and dose-dependent induction of p53 transcription products, by Western blotting, in the LNCaP prostate cancer cell line but not in the PC3-deleted p53 line. Selectivity against other α-helix binding proteins was demonstrated, and 45 has >10,000 fold selectivity for MDM2 over Bcl2 or Bcl-xL proteins. The bromo analog **46** was investigated in a panel of colon cancer cell lines and showed significant upregulation of p53-dependent genes, with similar potency to Nutlin-3 (**30**) [82]. The paired isogenic cell lines, HCT116 (p53wt and p53−/−) and RKO (p53wt and p53shRNA), were used to demonstrate that growth inhibition was p53 dependent with 11- and 20-fold ratios. Similarly, apoptosis was shown to be p53 dependent. HCT116 cells engineered to lack p21 were resistant to the induction of cell cycle arrest by **46**.

The potency and oral activity of the spirooxindole series were optimized further [83]. The parent compound **45** displayed poor oral bioavailability and pharmacokinetics in rats ($T_{1/2}$ = 1.3 h; F = 10%). Substitution of the morpholine side chain with N-methylpiperazine (**47**) or N-methylpiperidine (**48**) gave improved potency and modest improvements in pharmacokinetics ($T_{1/2}$ = 3.8 and 7.1 h, and F = 31% and 14%, respectively). Replacement of the basic side chain with a neutral 1,3-diol (**49**) gave improved potency and pharmacokinetics ($T_{1/2}$ = 3.9 h; F = 21%). Interestingly, switching the fluorine to the 5-position on the oxindole ring system (**50**) (MI-219) resulted in a significant loss of potency in the cell-free assay, but only a modest reduction of the cellular activity along with improved oral bioavailability ($T_{1/2}$ = 1.4 h; F = 65%). Introduction of two fluorine substituents (**51**) gave a similar potency [84]. Oxindoles **49** and **50** showed potent dose-dependent activation of p53-dependent genes in SJSA-1 cells, but not in the p53-deleted Saos-2 line. The fluorinated inhibitors **50** and **51** were investigated with a panel of lymphoma cell lines with defined p53 status. In the p53 wild-type follicular small cleaved-cell lymphoma (FSCCL) line, **50** and **51** showed good growth-inhibitory activity, induction of apoptosis, and cell cycle arrest.

Compound **49** gave a significant growth delay in vivo in an SJSA-1 xenograft model, similar to that achieved with irinotecan and without significant toxicity. Combination of **48** with irinotecan was more effective than single-agent treatment. Oxindole (MI-219 [**50**]) was investigated further in normal and tumor cell lines [85]. In primary human normal cells, the inhibitor activates the p53 pathway, but failed to induce PUMA and thus initiate apoptosis. Cell cycle arrest was observed in both normal and tumor cells exposed to **50** by a p53- and p21-dependent mechanism. The antitumor activity of **50** was demonstrated in SJSA-1 and LNCaP xenograft mouse models at nontoxic doses. The difluoro compound **51** showed significant activity in the FSCCL systemic severe combined immunodeficiency mouse model at nontoxic doses [84].

A clinical candidate from the spirooxindole series has been disclosed (SAR-405838); however, to date, results from the phase I trials have not been reported.

Isoindolinones

The isoindolinone series of inhibitors originated from the optimization of weak inhibitors, in the first instance through in silico library screening and synthesis of test examples yielding isoindolinones **52** and **53** (IC$_{50}$s = 5.3 and 16 μM, respectively) that showed modest cellular activity [86,87]. In the absence of an X-ray structure for an isoindolinone bound to MDM2, the binding interactions of a selection of isoindolinones with MDM2 were investigated in solution by NMR [88,89]. The results highlighted a number of experimentally plausible binding modes for the inhibitors, with either the 4-chlorophenyl residue or the isoindolinone ring system occupying the Trp^{23} binding pocket for the (R)-enantiomers of **52** or **53**. Structure–activity studies showed that optimization of the ether side chain could be achieved by the introduction of a cyclopropyl group, and that a 4-nitrobenzyl substituent gave a significant

TABLE 13.9 Isoindolinones

Compound	X	Y	IC$_{50}$ (nM)[1]
54	NO$_2$	H	170
55	NO$_2$	Cl	44
56	Br	Cl	137
57	CN	Cl	136

[1] Measured by ELISA.

improvement in potency (**54**) (Table 13.9). Introduction of a chloro substituent at the 4-position of the isoindolinone ring system gave improved potency (**55**) and allowed the replacement of the undesirable 4-nitro substituent with the more pharmaceutically acceptable bromo or cyano groups (**56** and **57**). Isoindolinone **55** showed improved cellular activity over earlier compounds, inducing transcription of p53-dependent genes at comparable levels to Nutlin-3a (**30a**), and was growth inhibitory in p53 wild-type HCT116 cells (GI$_{50}$ = 3.7 μM) and three-fold less growth inhibitory in the paired p53−/− HCT116 line.

52   **53**

Isoquinolin-1-ones

The isoquinolin-1-one series (e.g., **59**) originated from a scaffold-hopping approach based on published potent MDM2–p53 inhibitors and a three-dimensional shape fitting to the p53-binding site of MDM2, extracted from the X-ray structure of MDM2 with Nutlin-2 bound [90]. Selected analogs were synthesized and screened using a combination of NMR spectroscopy, isothermal colorimetry, and SPR methods. Hit compound **60** showed promising activity (K_D^{ITC} = 2 μm) but was devoid of cellular activity in PA-1 ovarian teratocarcinoma cells. Introduction of a hydrophilic amide side chain retained MDM2–p53 inhibitory activity (**61**;

$K_D^{ITC} = 4\ \mu m$) and gave some p53-dependent cellular activity. Further introduction of a 6-chloroindole substituent and an *N*-methyl piperidinyl group to the side chain (**62**; $K_D^{ITC} = 2.5\ \mu m$) improved cellular activity in the PA-1 line ($GI_{50} = 6.3\ \mu M$) with twofold selectivity over the E6 p53-degraded paired cell line. Isoquinolin-1-one (**60**) induced apoptosis in AP-1 cells (at 20 and 40 μM) and showed some induction of p53-dependent genes, by RT-PCR and Western blotting.

59; X = F; Y = OCH3; R = H
60; X = Cl; Y = Cl; R = H
61; X = Cl; Y = Cl; R = NHCH₂CH₂OCH₃

62

Chromenotriazolopyrimidines

The chromenotriazolopyrimidine ([*rac*]-**63**) (Table 13.10) was identified from a HTS of 1.4 million library compounds using a homogeneous time-resolved fluorescence assay (HTRF), and the *syn*-(6R,7S) configuration was identified as the active stereoisomer [91]. The authors note that the stereoisomers of **63** equilibrated in solution favoring the more stable but less active isomer. Introduction of a methyl group at N11 (**64**) provided stability without affecting the MDM2–p53 inhibitory potency. Structure–activity studies showed that the di-chloro and 7-(4-bromophenyl)-6-(4-chlorophenyl) analogs (**65** and **66**) were equipotent with the hit compound. Substitution at the *para*-position of the 6-phenyl ring with a cyano or methyl group (**67** and **68**) was tolerated, but introduction of an ethyl residue (**69**) abolished activity. The X-ray structure of **63** bound to MDM2 (PDB ID: 3JZK; Fig. 13.10) shows the 7-(4-bromophenyl) group occupying the Leu[26] binding site, the Trp[23] pocket filled by the 6-(4-bromophenyl) group, and the chromenotriazolopyrimidine spanning the surface of the protein from the phenyl D-ring in the Phe[19] binding site to the triazole ring close to Val93 of MDM2.

Further optimization of the potency and pharmacokinetic properties was achieved by variation of the group at N11 [92]. The introduction of a polar or acidic group improved potency (e.g., **70** and **71**), whereas basic groups did not improve potency. The acids **70** and **71** were moderately orally bioavailable (*F* = 14% and 54%, respectively) and showed improved solubility over the parent.

Imidazoles

A structure-based approach was used by the Novartis Group, resulting in the design of potent nonpeptidic inhibitors of MDM2–p53 based on an imidazole scaffold [93]. The design approach sought to retain the chloroaryl group present in the 6-chlorotryptophan of the AP peptide and other published inhibitors, in addition to filling the Phe[19] and Leu[26] pockets. The placement of an aromatic ring in contact with the side chain of Val93 on MDM2 readily gave access to the three pockets. Substructure searching of the in-house compound collection

TABLE 13.10   Chromenotriazolopyrimidines

Compound	X	Y	R	IC$_{50}$ (µM)[1]
63	Br	Br	H	1.2
64	Br	Br	CH$_3$	1.2
65	Cl	Cl	CH$_3$	1.2
66	Br	Cl	CH$_3$	0.89
67	Br	CN	CH$_3$	2.1
68	Br	CH$_3$	CH$_3$	4.6
69	Br	CH$_2$CH$_3$	CH$_3$	>100
70	Br	Br	CH$_2$CO$_2$H	0.48
71	Br	Br	(CH$_2$)$_4$CO$_2$H	0.35

[1] *Measured by HTRF.*

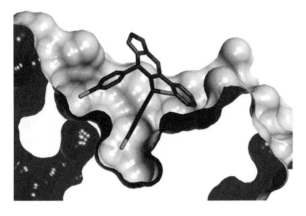

FIGURE 13.10   X-ray structure of MDM2 and **63** (PDB ID: 3JZK) surface showing binding interaction. (This figure is reproduced in color in the color plate section.)

provided imidazole **72**, which showed promising activity in a time-resolved fluorescence resonance energy transfer (TR-FRET) assay (IC$_{50}$ = 3.8 µM). Modeling of compound **72** in the MDM2 structure suggested that replacement of the 4-chloroaryl ring with a 6-chloroindole could allow the formation of a hydrogen bond to MDM2, as seen in the peptide X-ray structures. In addition, removal of the methylene spacer to the 4-substituent was predicted to improve activity by fitting the Phe[19] pocket more favorably. Inhibitors **73** and **74** (IC$_{50}$s = 0.9

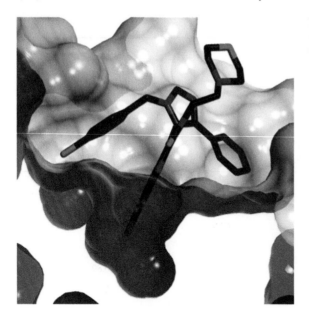

FIGURE 13.11 X-ray structure of MDM2 and **74** (PDB ID: 4DIJ). (This figure is reproduced in color in the color plate section.)

and 0.2 µM, respectively) demonstrated the benefits of these changes and showed that the Leu[26] pocket could be filled with aromatic or aliphatic substituents. The physicochemical properties of the series were improved by the addition of a morpholino side chain via a carboxamide at the indole 2-position (**75**; IC_{50} = 0.03 µM), which unexpectedly improved potency. The X-ray structure of **75** bound to MDM2 (PDB ID: 4DIJ; Fig. 13.11) confirms the anticipated binding mode and shows additional interactions contributing to the inhibitory activity, that is, a stacking interaction between His96 and the 1-chlorobenzyl group, and the amide carbonyl forming a network of water-mediated H-bonds to MDM2 residues.

Interestingly, this compound series shows some inhibitory activity for MDMX (e.g., **75**; MDMX IC_{50} = 19 µM). The X-ray structure of a related inhibitor (**76**) (MDM2 IC_{50} = 0.19 µM and MDMX IC_{50} = 20 µM) bound to MDMX (PDB ID: 4LBJ; Fig. 13.12) shows a comparable binding interaction with the protein, which has a similar hotspot binding region to p53 [94]. Substantial induced fit movements are seen in the structure (e.g., the 6-chloroindole occupies the Trp[23] pocket, requiring the repositioning of the side chains of surrounding residues). The N,N-dimethylpropylamine group occludes the Phe[19] binding pocket by overlying the hydrophobic α-helical rim of the binding pocket. Overall, the energetically unfavorable movements in the MDMX protein result in a lower binding affinity, compared with MDM2.

72   **73**   **74**

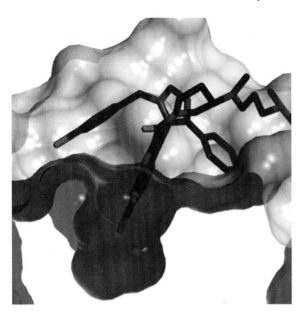

FIGURE 13.12 X-ray structure of MDMX and **76** (PDB ID: 4LBJ). (This figure is reproduced in color in the color plate section.)

75; R =

76; R =

Piperidinones

Analysis of the binding modes of published MDM2 inhibitors provided the design concept for novel scaffolds, including the 1,3,5,6-tetrasubstituted piperidinone (**77**; IC_{50} = 2.4 µM) [95]. Interestingly, a switch from the *cis*-diaryl configuration to the *trans*-diaryl and inversion at the C3 center gave a 50-fold improvement in activity for the active enantiomer (**78**) (Table 13.11). The predicted binding mode for **78** places the 5-(3-chlorophenyl) group into the Leu[26] pocket, the 6-(4-chlorophenyl) group into the Trp[23] pocket, and the cyclopropyl-methyl group overlaying the Phe[19] binding site. The 2-carboxylate was proposed to form an electrostatic interaction with the imidazole side chain of His96, an interaction not seen in other MDM2 inhibitor structures.

TABLE 13.11   Piperidinones

Compound	R^1	R^B	R^2	R^3	IC$_{50}$ (nM)[1]	IC$_{50}$ (nM)[2]
78	A	–	COOH	H	34	372
79	A	–	T	H	14	190
80	B	CO_2Et	COOH	H	7.6	86
81	B	CO_2tBu	COOH	H	4.2	43
82	B	CO_2tBu	T	H	1.8	20
83	B	CO_2tBu	COOH	CH_3	2.2	20
84	B	CO_2tBu	T	CH_3	0.9	9.0
85	B	Et	COOH	CH_3	2.8	36
86	B	CH_2OH	COOH	CH_3	1.7	6.8
87	B	(S)–$CH(CH_3)OH$	COOH	CH_3	1.1	4.2
88	B	CH_2OH	COOH	H	6.2[3]	–

[1] Measured by HTRF.
[2] Measured by HTRF in 15% human serum.
[3] K_D measured by SPR with full-length MDM2.

Optimization of the structure started with variation of the N-alkyl group. The cyclopropyl-methyl group found in **78** was the best unsubstituted alkyl substituent. Similarly, variation of the C3 substituent returned the (3R)-methylenecarboxylic acid (**78**) and the (3R)-methylenetetrazole (**79**) as the favored substituents. Introduction of an alkyl ester group at the α-methylene of the N-propyl substituent, designed to direct the group into the optimal configuration, resulted in a greater than threefold improvement in activity for the ethyl ester **80** and eightfold improvement for the t-butyl ester **81**. Further improvement in potency was gained for the tetrazole derivative **82**.

The high-resolution X-ray structure of **81** bound to MDM2 (PDB ID: 4ERE) confirmed the proposed binding mode, showing the two aryl groups in a *gauche* conformation when bound. Computational experiments on the core structure suggested that the bound conformation was not the most energetically favorable and so the compound would suffer a penalty for binding. The addition of a C3-methyl substituent was predicted to stabilize the binding conformation via the introduction of a steric clash between the methyl group and the C5-chlorophenyl group in the *anti* configuration. The prediction was borne out by the twofold gain in activity

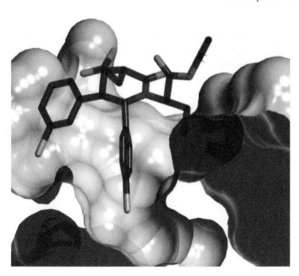

FIGURE 13.13 X-ray structure of MDM2 and **87** (PDB ID: 4ERF). (This figure is reproduced in color in the color plate section.)

for compounds **83** and **84**, and by ^{1}H NMR measurements of vicinal coupling constants at two different temperatures. In vitro profiling of **83** and **84** showed that the tetrazole analog carried a greater liability for human pregnane X receptor (hPXR) activation and CYP3A4 inhibition.

Further optimization of the *N*-substituent showed a threefold loss of potency on replacement of the *t*-butyl ester with an ethyl group (**85**). Potency was regained by the replacement of the terminal methyl group with a hydroxyl group (**86**) or the introduction of an (*S*)-secondary alcohol (**87**); for both examples, the potency in the presence of 15% human serum was improved over that for **84**, indicating lower protein binding.

The X-ray structure of **87** bound to MDM2 (PDB ID: 4ERF; Fig. 13.13) shows the compound bound in a similar orientation to **81**. The C6 4-chlorophenyl group fills the Trp[23] pocket, and the C5 3-chlorophenyl group occupies the Leu[23] pocket, forming a favorable π-stacking interaction with the imidazole of His96 that also forms an electrostatic interaction with the carboxylic acid at C3. The Phe[19] pocket is occupied by the ethyl group of the *N*-substituent, directed by the steric constraint of the α-substituent, and the hydroxyl group is exposed to solvent. Further NMR and X-ray structural studies using an extended MDM2 construct (amino acids 6–125) that includes N-terminal residues usually absent in MDM2–ligand complexes have given greater information about the interaction of the N-terminal "lid" domain of MDM2 with the ligand [96]. Both the deposited NMR structures of **78** (PDB ID: 2LZJ) and the X-ray structure of **88** (PDB ID: 4HBM, Fig. 13.14) show the same global structure with significant ordering of the N-terminal domain into a short α-helical segment, a β-turn, and a short β-strand close to the ligand. Additional interactions are seen between the side chains of Val14 and Thr16 and the C5 3-chlorophenyl group, in addition to the side chain hydroxyl of Thr16 forming an additional H-bond to the imidazole nitrogen of His96. Interestingly, in the crystal structure, the β-strand from one MDM2 molecule forms an antiparallel β-sheet with another MDM2 molecule, giving rise to a dimeric protein–ligand complex.

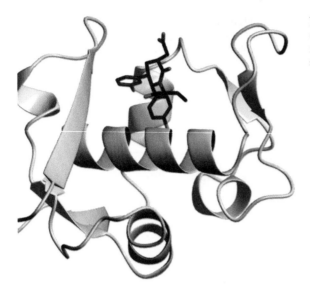

FIGURE 13.14 X-ray structure of MDM2 (amino acids 6–125) and **88** (PDB ID: 4HBM). (This figure is reproduced in color in the color plate section.)

77

Compounds **83** and **87** showed potent growth inhibition in SJSA-1 cells ($GI_{50}s$ = 0.19 and 0.07 μM, respectively), and HCT116 p53wt cells ($GI_{50}s$ = 0.85 and 0.20 μM, respectively). Both compounds showed >100-fold p53-dependent selectivity when compared with the HCT116 p53−/− cell line. As expected, inhibitors **83** and **87** gave prominent dose-dependent induction of p21 mRNA in HCT116 cells. Both compounds **83** and **87** have been examined in SJSA-1 tumor xenograft models. In a pharmacodynamic study, **83** showed dose-dependent induction of p21 mRNA, with a 15-fold induction at the 300 mg/kg dose. In a 14-day study, **83** showed antitumor efficacy (ED_{50} = 118 mg/kg) with 91% growth inhibition at 200 mg/kg. Compound **87** showed an improved pharmacokinetic profile over **83** with lower hPXR activation, CYP3A4 inhibition, and clearance in human hepatocytes. In SJSA-1 xenografts, **87** showed improved p21 induction over time compared with **81**, and improved efficacy (ED_{50} = 78 mg/kg) and tumor regression at 200 mg/kg QD, without significant observed toxicity. A BD dosing schedule was adopted to address the high clearance and short half-life of **87**, in mice, and either 75 or 100 mg/kg BD gave a significant reduction in tumor growth, comparable to the higher single dose per day. Overall, this series of compounds appears to be highly promising as the compounds have excellent potency and reasonable pharmaceutical properties.

Other Patented Inhibitors

A number of other structural types (e.g. **89–92**) have been claimed as MDM2–p53 inhibitors in the patent literature [72,73]. Some inhibitors appear to have been based on variations of the spirooxindole chemotype, such as the simple oxindole (**89**), the ring-expanded spiro(indoline-3,3′-piperidin)-2-one (**90**), and the 4-cyanopyrrolidine (**91**).

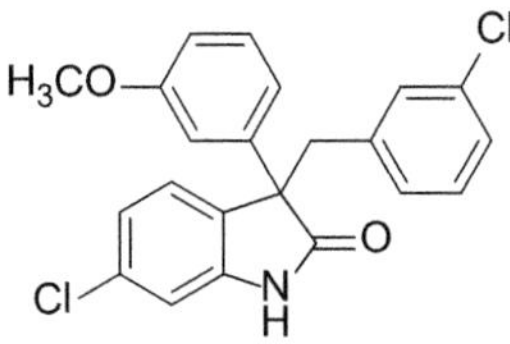

89

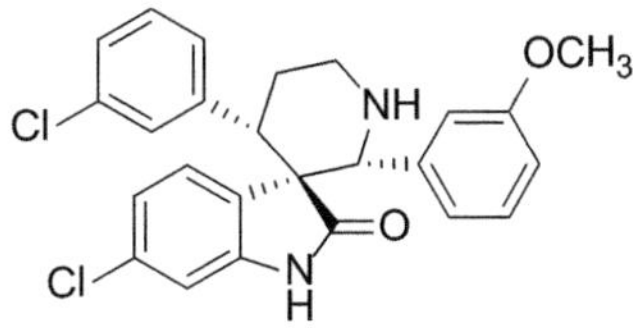

90

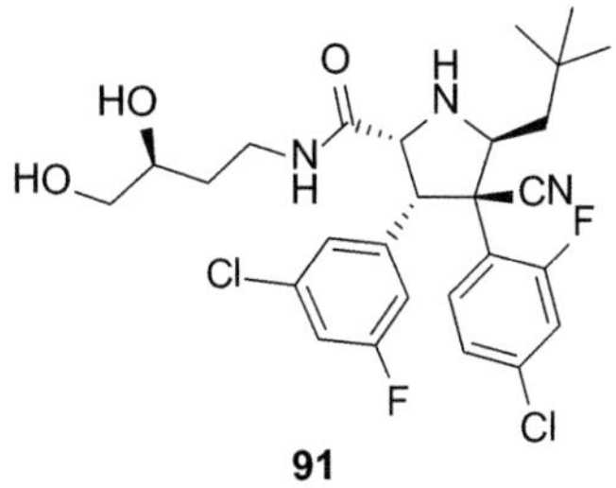

91

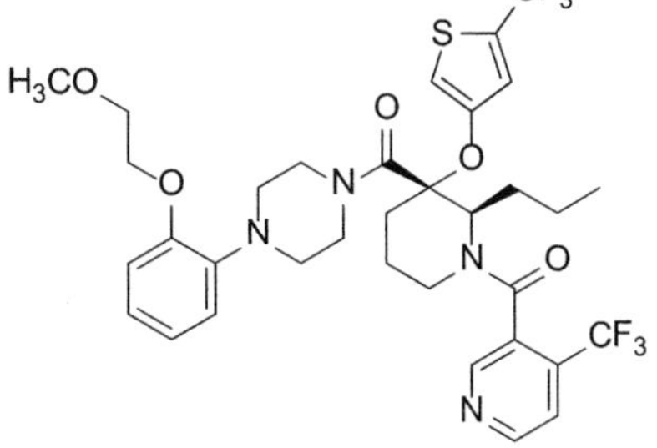

92

MDMX–p53 INHIBITORS

The rationale for the development of either selective MDMX–p53 inhibitors or compounds with mixed MDM2 and MDMX activities is similar to that proposed for MDM2–p53 inhibitors. MDMX acts as a central regulator of p53 activity, and overexpression or gene amplification has been observed in a number of tumor types. MDMX overexpression has been linked with resistance in cell lines to MDM2–p53 inhibition. The potent inhibitors described here that were optimized for the MDM2–p53 interaction show minimal inhibition of MDMX–p53, so normal or elevated MDMX levels may result in an attenuated p53 response to MDM2 inhibition. Analysis of the peptide-bound X-ray structures of MDM2 and MDMX reveals that, although the same three residues of p53 are bound, significant differences in the binding interaction result from differences in the amino acid sequences between MDM2 and MDMX [97].

Compound (**93**) has been reported as a selective MDMX inhibitor identified from an FP assay–based HTS campaign (IC_{50} = 0.9 µM) coupled with a differential cytotoxicity screen using *MDMX*-amplified cells [98]. Initial experiments suggested that **93** binds reversibly, and docking showed the compound occupying the p53-binding pocket on MDMX. In combination with Nutlin-3a (**30a**), inhibitor **93** showed additive cytotoxicity with p53 (wt) cells. However, further studies into the mechanism of action of **93** using mass spectrometry and SPR show evidence of covalent but reversible modification of the MDMX protein, via reaction of a cysteine thiol with the vinyl group, which fixes the protein in a conformation that is less able to bind p53 [99]. The reactivity of **93** makes it an unattractive candidate for further development.

93

Indolyl hydantions (e.g., **94**) were identified as hits from an HTS screen for MDMX–p53 inhibitors [100]. Modifications introduced to improve water solubility resulted in analog **95**. The compounds display potent inhibition of both MDM2–p53 and MDMX–p53 interactions (Table 13.12). NMR experiments confirmed that **95** bound to the p53 pocket of MDMX. Interestingly, size exclusion chromatography suggested that the inhibitor formed a dimeric complex with the protein, but isothermal calorimetry gave results consistent with a 1:1 or 2:2 inhibitor:protein complex. The crystal structure of **95** bound to MDMX (PDB ID: 3U15, Fig. 13.15) shows an unusual binding mode in which a dimer of **95** occupies the p53 pockets of two MDMX molecules. The 3,4-difluorophenyl moiety of one molecule of **95** occupies the Trp^{23} pocket, and the Phe^{19} pocket of the same MDMX is overlaid by the indole heterocycle of the other molecule of **95**. Similarly, the second MDMX is occupied by the alternative groups of both **95** molecules. The X-ray structure of MDM2 with **95** bound (PDB ID: 3VBG) showed a similar dimeric structure and binding mode. Interestingly, the Leu^{26} pocket is not occupied in these structures.

TABLE 13.12   Indolyl Hydantoins

Compound	MDM2 IC$_{50}$ (nM)	MDMX IC$_{50}$ (nM)
94	33	41
95	17	25

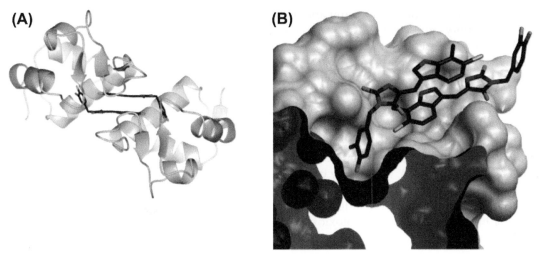

FIGURE 13.15 X-ray structure of MDMX and **95** (PDB ID: 3UI5). (A): Ribbon view showing dimer; and (B): surface showing binding interaction. (This figure is reproduced in color in the color plate section.)

The more water-soluble derivative **96** showed dose-dependent activation of p53, measuring p21 and MDM2 levels in MCF7 cells (overexpressing MDMX). Induction of apoptosis was demonstrated in SJSA-1 cells and the engineered MDMX-overexpressing line SJSA-X, which is resistant to Nutlin-3a (**30a**). In a panel of nine cancer cell lines, enhanced apoptosis was seen where MDMX levels were elevated, showing the utility of dual inhibition of MDM2 and MDMX.

CLINICAL STATUS OF MDM2–p53 INHIBITORS

A number of clinical trial candidates have been declared from different chemotypes. The most advanced series stem from Nutlin-3a (**30a**), including RG7112 (**36**). Another phase I candidate, RG7388, from the same company has been declared (structure undisclosed). A candidate from the spirooxindole series, SAR-405838, is under clinical evaluation. Other compound series are believed to be in advanced preclinical development.

RG7112

A phase I clinical study with the Nutlin analog RG7112 (**36**) has been recently reported [74]. The trial was conducted in 20 liposarcoma patients, of whom 14 had MDM2 amplification and two had *TP53* missense mutations, and it aimed to provide proof-of-mechanism for MDM2–p53 inhibition. The primary endpoint of the study was proof-of-concept by assessment of biomarker modulation. Patients received the maximum tolerated dose of 1440 mg/m^2 of RG7112 daily for 10 days on a 28-day cycle, followed by surgical removal of the tumor (where operable) or a biopsy; patients with stable disease were given up to three cycles of the drug. Tumor levels of p53; p21; Ki-67, a marker for proliferation; and TUNEL, a marker for apoptosis, were measured before and after treatment. Additionally, the blood levels of macrophage inhibitory cytokine-1 (MIC-1), a marker for p53 activation, were monitored.

The best responses prior to surgery were one partial response, 14 with stable disease, and five with progressive disease; also, following surgery, eight patients had no evidence of disease. Biomarkers were assessed, and changes seen for p53, p21, MDM2, and Ki-67 levels in evaluable patients. The variable pharmacokinetics observed in the patients allowed the TUNEL and MIC-1 biomarkers to be compared with drug exposure, showing an exposure-dependent effect on both parameters.

Toxicities to RG7112 that were observed included gastrointestinal toxicity, which was partly attributed to the large oral dose of the drug, and hematological toxicities such as thrombocytopenia and neutropenia, which may be due to p53 activation in normal tissues. It remains to be seen if these toxicities are compound specific or result from the mechanism of action of the drug. Overall, the authors conclude that RG7112 is worthy of further investigation as a single agent or in combination with cytotoxic or targeted agents.

CONCLUSIONS

Two decades after the identification of MDM2 as an oncoprotein, we now have a detailed knowledge of many facets of the interplay between MDM2 and p53 and other proteins. Understanding at a structural level of the protein–protein interaction has prompted the search for novel therapies based on the reactivation of p53 by inhibition of its binding to MDM2 in tumors. The first clinical results for the MDM2–p53 inhibitor RG7112 show great promise, and the expected clinical results from other structural classes of inhibitor will enable a profile of activity to be established and the differentiation of on- and off-target toxicities. The challenge for the medicinal chemist in this field is to design an inhibitor with the optimal shape and lipophilicity for potent MDM2 binding, whilst simultaneously optimizing the properties required for oral activity and good pharmacokinetics. The diverse range of scaffolds explored thus far for this purpose demonstrates both the challenge and the promise of the target.

Acknowledgments

Roger Griffin, John Lunec, Herbie Newell, and Martin Noble are thanked for helpful discussions. I thank Cancer Research UK for funding.

References

[1] Bogan AA, Thorn KS. Anatomy of hot spots in protein interfaces. J Mol Biol 1998;280:1–9.
[2] Moreira IS, Fernandes PA, Ramos MJ. Hot spots—a review of the protein–protein interface determinant amino-acid residues. Proteins Struct Funct Bioinf 2007;68:803–12.
[3] Wells JA, McClendon CL. Reaching for high-hanging fruit in drug discovery at protein–protein interfaces. Nature 2007;450:1001–9.
[4] Junttila MR, Evan GI. p53—a jack of all trades but master of none. Nat Rev Cancer 2009;9:821–9.
[5] Lane DP. Cancer. p53, guardian of the genome. Nature 1992;358:15–6.
[6] Bode AM, Dong Z. Post-translational modification of p53 in tumorigenesis. Nat Rev Cancer 2004;4:793–805.
[7] Murray-Zmijewski F, Slee EA, Lu X. A complex barcode underlies the heterogeneous response of p53 to stress. Nat Rev Mol Cell Biol 2008;9:702–12.

[8] MacCallum DE, Hupp TR, Midgley CA, Stuart D, Campbell SJ, Harper A, et al. The p53 response to ionising radiation in adult and developing murine tissues. Oncogene 1996;13:2575–87.

[9] Alvarez S, Drané P, Meiller A, Bras M, Deguin-Chambon V, Bouvard V, et al. A comprehensive study of p53 transcriptional activity in thymus and spleen of γ irradiated mouse: high sensitivity of genes involved in the two main apoptotic pathways. Int J Radiat Biol 2006;82:761–70.

[10] Hollstein M, Sidransky D, Vogelstein B, Harris C. p53 mutations in human cancers. Science 1991;253:49–53.

[11] Cho Y, Gorina S, Jeffrey P, Pavletich N. Crystal structure of a p53 tumor suppressor-DNA complex: understanding tumorigenic mutations. Science 1994;265:346–55.

[12] Chan WM, Siu WY, Lau A, Poon RYC. How many mutant p53 molecules are needed to inactivate a tetramer? Mol Cell Biol 2004;24:3536–51.

[13] Jõers A, Kristjuhan A, Kadaja L, Maimets T. Tumour associated mutants of p53 can inhibit transcriptional activity of p53 without heterooligomerization. Oncogene 1998;17:2351–8.

[14] Cahilly-Snyder L, Yang-Feng T, Francke U, George DL. Molecular analysis and chromosomal mapping of amplified genes isolated from a transformed mouse 3T3 cell line. Somat Cell Mol Genet 1987;13:235–44.

[15] Oliner JD, Kinzler KW, Meltzer PS, George DL, Vogelstein B. Amplification of a gene encoding a p53-associated protein in human sarcomas. Nature 1992;358:80–3.

[16] Oliner JD, Pietenpol JA, Thiagalingam S, Gyuris J, Kinzler KW, Vogelstein B. Oncoprotein MDM2 conceals the activation domain of tumor suppressor p53. Nature 1993;362:857–60.

[17] Shvarts A, Steegenga WT, Riteco N, van Laar T, Dekker P, Bazuine M, et al. MDMX: a novel p53-binding protein with some functional properties of MDM2. EMBO J 1996;15:5349–69.

[18] Shvarts A, Bazuine M, Dekker P, Ramos YFM, Steegenga WT, Merckx G, et al. Isolation and identification of the human homolog of a new p53-binding protein, MDMX. Genomics 1997;43:34–42.

[19] Jones SN, Roe AE, Donehower LA, Bradley A. Rescue of embryonic lethality in Mdm2-deficient mice by absence of p53. Nature 1995;378:206–8.

[20] Montes de Oca Luna R, Wagner DS, Lozano G. Rescue of early embryonic lethality in MDM2-deficient mice by deletion of p53. Nature 1995;378:203–6.

[21] Parant J, Chavez-Reyes A, Little NA, Yan W, Reinke V, Jochemsen AG, et al. Rescue of embryonic lethality in Mdm4-null mice by loss of Trp[53] suggests a nonoverlapping pathway with MDM2 to regulate p53. Nat Genet 2001;29:92–5.

[22] Finch RA, Donoviel DB, Potter D, Shi M, Fan A, Freed DD, et al. MDMX is a negative regulator of p53 activity in vivo. Cancer Res 2002;62:3221–5.

[23] Steinman HA, Hoover KM, Keeler ML, Sands AT, Jones SN. Rescue of Mdm4-deficient mice by Mdm2 reveals functional overlap of Mdm2 and Mdm4 in development. Oncogene 2005;24:7935–40.

[24] Momand J, Zambetti GP, Olson DC, George D, Levine A. The *mdm-2* oncogene product forms a complex with p53 protein and inhibits p53-mediated transactivation. Cell 1992;69:1237–45.

[25] Momand J, Wu H-H, Dasgupta G. MDM2—master regulator of the p53 tumor suppressor protein. Gene 2000;242:15–29.

[26] Toledo F, Wahl GM. Regulating the p53 pathway: in vitro hypotheses, in vivo veritas. Nat Rev Cancer 2006;6:909–23.

[27] Marine J-C, Jochemsen AG. MDMX as an essential regulator of p53 activity. Biochem Biophys Res Commun 2005;331:750–60.

[28] Zhang Y, Xiong Y, Yarbrough WG. ARF promotes MDM2 degradation and stabilizes p53: ARF-INK4a locus deletion impairs both the Rb and p53 tumor suppression pathways. Cell 1998;92:725–34.

[29] Honda R, Yasuda H. Association of p19(ARF) with Mdm2 inhibits ubiquitin ligase activity of Mdm2 for tumor suppressor p53. EMBO J 1999;18:22–7.

[30] Tao W, Levine AJ. P19ARF stabilizes p53 by blocking nucleo-cytoplasmic shuttling of Mdm2. Proc Natl Acad Sci U S A 1999;96:6937–41.

[31] Danovi D, Meulmeester E, Pasini D, Migliorini D, Capra M, Frenk R, et al. Amplification of Mdmx (or Mdm4) directly contributes to tumor formation by inhibiting p53 tumor suppressor activity. Mol Cell Biol 2004;24:5835–43.

[32] Gembarska A, Luciani F, Fedele C, Russell EA, Dewaele M, Villar S, et al. MDM4 is a key therapeutic target in cutaneous melanoma. Nat Med 2012;18:1239–47.

[33] Chen L, Agrawal S, Zhou W, Zhang R, Chen J. Synergistic activation of p53 by inhibition of MDM2 expression and DNA damage. Proc Natl Acad Sci U S A 1998;95:195–200.

[34] Geiger T, Husken D, Weiler J, Natt F, Woods-Cook KA, Hall J, et al. Consequences of the inhibition of Hdm2 expression in human osteosarcoma cells using antisense oligonucleotides. Anticancer Drug Des 2000;15:423–30.

[35] Kussie PH, Gorina S, Marechal V, Elenbaas B, Moreau J, Levine AJ, et al. Structure of the MDM2 oncoprotein bound to the p53 tumor suppressor transactivation domain. Science 1996;274:948–53.

[36] Uhrinova S, Uhrin D, Powers H, Watt K, Zheleva D, Fischer P, et al. Structure of free MDM2 N-terminal domain reveals conformational adjustments that accompany p53-binding. J Mol Biol 2005;350:587–98.

[37] McCoy MA, Gesell JJ, Senior MM, Wyss DF. Flexible lid to the p53-binding domain of human Mdm2: implications for p53 regulation. PNAS 2003;100:1645–8.

[38] Schon O, Friedler A, Bycroft M, Freund SMV, Fersht AR. Molecular mechanism of the interaction between MDM2 and p53. J Mol Biol 2002;323:491–501.

[39] Carotti A, Macchiarulo A, Giacchè N, Pellicciari R. Targeting the conformational transitions of MDM2 and MDMX: insights into key residues affecting p53 recognition. Proteins Struct Funct Bioinf 2009;77:524–35.

[40] Chen HF, Luo R. Binding induced folding in p53-MDM2 complex. J Am Chem Soc 2007;129:2930–7.

[41] Picksley SM, Vojtesek B, Sparks A, Lane DP. Immunochemical analysis of the interaction of p53 with MDM2—fine mapping of the MDM2 binding site on p53 using synthetic peptides. Oncogene 1994;9:2523–9.

[42] Böttger V, Böttger A, Howard SF, Picksley SM, Chene P, Garcia-Echeverria C, et al. Identification of novel MDM2 binding peptides by phage display. Oncogene 1996;13:2141–7.

[43] Wasylyk C, Salvi R, Argentini M, Dureuil C, Delumeau I, Abecassis J, et al. p53 mediated death of cells overexpressing MDM2 by an inhibitor of MDM2 interaction with p53. Oncogene 1999;18:1921–34.

[44] Garcia-Echeverria C, Chene P, Blommers MJJ, Furet P. Discovery of potent antagonists of the interaction between human double minute 2 and tumor suppressor p53. J Med Chem 2000;43:3205–8.

[45] Chene P, Fuchs J, Bohn J, Garcia-Echeverria C, Furet P, Fabbro D. A small synthetic peptide, which inhibits the p53-hdm2 interaction, stimulates the p53 pathway in tumour cell lines. J Mol Biol 2000;299:245–53.

[46] Garcia-Echeverria C, Furet P, Chene P. Coupling of the Antennapedia third helix to a potent antagonist of the p53/hdm2 protein-protein interaction. Bioorg Med Chem Lett 2001;11:2161–4.

[47] Schafmeister CE, Po J, Verdine GL. An all-hydrocarbon cross-linking system for enhancing the helicity and metabolic stability of peptides. J Am Chem Soc 2000;122:5891–2.

[48] Bernal F, Wade M, Godes M, Davis TN, Whitehead DG, Kung AL. A stapled p53 helix overcomes HDMX-mediated suppression of p53. Cancer Cell 2010;18:411–22.

[49] Baek S, Kutchukian PS, Verdine GL, Huber R, Holak TA, Lee KW, et al. Structure of the stapled p53 peptide bound to Mdm2. J Am Chem Soc 2011;134:103–6.

[50] Hu B, Gilkes DM, Chen J. Efficient p53 activation and apoptosis by simultaneous disruption of binding to MDM2 and MDMX. Cancer Res 2007;67:8810–7.

[51] Madden MM, Muppidi A, Li Z, Li X, Chen J, Lin Q. Synthesis of cell-permeable stapled peptide dual inhibitors of the p53-Mdm2/Mdmx interactions via photoinduced cycloaddition. Bioorg Med Chem Lett 2011;21:1472–5.

[52] Sakurai K, Chung HS, Kahne D. Use of a retroinverso p53 peptide as an inhibitor of MDM2. J Am Chem Soc 2004;126:16288–9.

[53] Liu M, Pazgier M, Li C, Yuan W, Li C, Lu W. A left-handed solution to peptide inhibition of the p53–MDM2 interaction. Angew Chem Int Ed 2010;49:3649–52.

[54] Liu M, Li C, Pazgier M, Li C, Mao Y, Lv Y, et al. D-peptide inhibitors of the p53–MDM2 interaction for targeted molecular therapy of malignant neoplasms. Proc Natl Acad Sci U S A 2010.

[55] Zhan C, Zhao L, Wei X, Wu X, Chen X, Yuan W, et al. An ultrahigh affinity d-peptide antagonist of MDM2. J Med Chem 2012;55:6237–41.

[56] Kritzer JA, Lear JD, Hodsdon ME, Schepartz A. Helical β-peptide inhibitors of the p53-hDM2 interaction. J Am Chem Soc 2004;126:9468–9.

[57] Michel J, Harker EA, Tirado-Rives J, Jorgensen WL, Schepartz A. In silico improvement of β3-peptide inhibitors of p53•hDM2 and p53•hDMX. J Am Chem Soc 2009;131:6356–7.

[58] Fasan R, Dias RLA, Moehle K, Zerbe O, Vrijbloed JW, Obrecht D. Using a β-hairpin to mimic an α-helix: cyclic peptidomimetic inhibitors of the p53-HDM2 protein-protein interaction. Angew Chem Int Ed 2004;43:2109–12.

[59] Fasan R, Dias RLA, Moehle K, Zerbe O, Obrecht D, Mittl PRE, et al. Structure-activity studies in a family of β-hairpin protein epitope mimetic inhibitors of the p53-HDM2 protein-protein interaction. Chem Bio Chem 2006;7:515–26.

[60] Hara T, Durell SR, Myers MC, Appella DH. Probing the structural requirements of peptoids that inhibit HDM2-p53 interactions. J Am Chem Soc 2006;128:1995–2004.

[61] Yin H, Lee GI, Park HS, Payne GA, Rodriguez JM, Sebti SM, et al. Terphenyl-based helical mimetics that disrupt the p53/HDM2 interaction. Angew Chem Int Ed 2005;44:2704–7.

[62] Shaginian A, Whitby LR, Hong S, Hwang I, Farooqi B, Searcey M, et al. Design, synthesis, and evaluation of an α-helix mimetic library targeting protein–protein interactions. J Am Chem Soc 2009;131:5564–72.

[63] Plante JP, Burnley T, Malkova B, Webb ME, Warriner SL, Edwards TA, et al. Oligobenzamide proteomimetic inhibitors of the p53-hDM2 protein–protein interaction. Chem Commun 2009:5091–3.

[64] Campbell F, Plante JP, Edwards TA, Warriner SL, Wilson AJ. N-alkylated oligoamide α-helical proteomimetics. Org Biomol Chem 2010;8:2344–51.

[65] Lee JH, Zhang Q, Jo S, Chai SC, Oh M, Im W, et al. Novel pyrrolopyrimidine-based α-helix mimetics: cell-permeable inhibitors of protein–protein interactions. J Am Chem Soc 2010;133:676–9.

[66] Sakurai K, Kahne D. Design and synthesis of functionalized trisaccharides as p53-peptide mimics. Tetrahedron Lett 2010;51:3724–7.

[67] Vassilev LT, Vu BT, Graves B, Carvajal D, Podlaski F, Filipovic Z, et al. In vivo activation of the p53 pathway by small-molecule antagonists of MDM2. Science 2004;303:844–8.

[68] Fry DC, Emerson SD, Palmeb S, Vua BT, Liua CM, Podlaskia F. NMR structure of a complex between MDM2 and a small molecule inhibitor. J Biomol NMR 2004;30:163–73.

[69] Tovar C, Rosinski J, Filipovic Z, Higgins B, Kolinsky K, Hilton H, et al. Small-molecule MDM2 antagonists reveal aberrant p53 signaling in cancer: implications for therapy. Proc Natl Acad Sci U S A 2006;103:1888–93.

[70] Workman P, Collins I. Probing the probes: fitness factors for small molecule tools. Chem Biol 2010;17:561–77.

[71] Fotouhi N, Haley GJ, Simonsen KB, Vu BT, Webber SE. Cis-2,4,5-triaryl-imidazolines and their use as anticancer medicaments, US 2006 WO/2006/097261

[72] Weber L. Patented inhibitors of p53–MDM2 interaction (2006–2008). Exp Opin Ther Pat 2010;20:179–91.

[73] Khoury K, Popowicz GM, Holak TA, Domling A. The p53-MDM2/MDMX axis: a chemotype perspective. MedChemComm 2011;2:246–60.

[74] Ray-Coquard I, Blay J-Y, Italiano A, Le Cesne A, Penel N, Zhi J, et al. Effect of the MDM2 antagonist RG7112 on the p53 pathway in patients with MDM2-amplified, well-differentiated or dedifferentiated liposarcoma: an exploratory proof-of-mechanism study. Lancet Oncol 2012;13:1133–40.

[75] Parks DJ, LaFrance LV, Calvo RR, Milkiewicz KL, Gupta V, Lattanze J, et al. 1,4-benzodiazepine-2,5-diones as small molecule antagonists of the HDM2-p53 interaction: discovery and SAR. Bioorg Med Chem Lett 2005;15:765–70.

[76] Grasberger BL, Lu TB, Schubert C, Parks DJ, Carver TE, Koblish HK, et al. Discovery and cocrystal structure of benzodiazepinedione HDM2 antagonists that activate p53 in cells. J Med Chem 2005;48:909–12.

[77] Parks DJ, LaFrance LV, Calvo RR, Milkiewicz KL, Marugan JJ, Raboisson P, et al. Enhanced pharmacokinetic properties of 1,4-benzodiazepine-2,5-dione antagonists of the HDM2-p53 protein-protein interaction through structure-based drug design. Bioorg Med Chem Lett 2006;16:3310–4.

[78] Marugan JJ, Leonard K, Raboisson P, Gushue JM, Calvo R, Koblish HK, et al. Enantiomerically pure 1,4-benzodiazepine-2,5-diones as Hdm2 antagonists. Bioorg Med Chem Lett 2006;16:3115–20.

[79] Koblish HK, Zhao SY, Franks CF, Donatelli RR, Tominovich RM, LaFrance LV, et al. Benzodiazepinedione inhibitors of the Hdm2:p53 complex suppress human tumor cell proliferation in vitro and sensitize tumors to doxorubicin in vivo. Mol Cancer Ther 2006;5:160–9.

[80] Ding K, Lu Y, Nikolovska-Coleska Z, Qiu S, Ding Y, Gao W, et al. Structure-based design of potent non-peptide MDM2 inhibitors. J Am Chem Soc 2005;127:10130–1.

[81] Ding K, Lu Y, Nikolovska-Coleska Z, Wang G, Qiu S, Shangary S, et al. Structure-based design of spiro-oxindoles as potent, specific small-molecule inhibitors of the MDM2-p53 interaction. J Med Chem 2006;49:3432–5.

[82] Shangary S, Ding K, Qiu S, Nikolovska-Coleska Z, Bauer JA, Liu M, et al. Reactivation of p53 by a specific MDM2 antagonist (MI-43) leads to p21-mediated cell cycle arrest and selective cell death in colon cancer. Mol Cancer Ther 2008;7:1533–42.

[83] Yu S, Qin D, Shangary S, Chen J, Wang G, Ding K, et al. Potent and orally active small-molecule inhibitors of the MDM2a-p53 interaction. J Med Chem 2009;52:7970–3.

[84] Mohammad RM, Wu J, Azmi AS, Aboukameel A, Sosin A, Wu S, et al. An MDM2 antagonist (MI-319) restores p53 functions and increases the life span of orally treated follicular lymphoma bearing animals. Mol Cancer 2009;8:115.

[85] Shangary S, Qin D, McEachern D, Liu M, Miller RS, Qiu S, et al. Temporal activation of p53 by a specific MDM2 inhibitor is selectively toxic to tumors and leads to complete tumor growth inhibition. Proc Natl Acad Sci U S A 2008;105:3933–8.

[86] Hardcastle IR, Ahmed SU, Atkins H, Farnie G, Golding BT, Griffin RJ, et al. Isoindolinone based inhibitors of the MDM2-p53 protein-protein interaction. Bioorg Med Chem Lett 2005;15:1515–20.

[87] Hardcastle IR, Ahmed SU, Atkins H, Farnie G, Golding BT, Griffin RJ, et al. Small-molecule inhibitors of the MDM2-p53 protein-protein interaction based on an isoindolinone scaffold. J Med Chem 2006;49:6209–21.

[88] Riedinger C, Endicott JA, Kemp SJ, Smyth LA, Watson A, Valeur E, et al. Analysis of chemical shift changes reveals the binding modes of isoindolinone inhibitors of the MDM2-p53 interaction. J Am Chem Soc 2008;130:16038–44.

[89] Riedinger C, Noble ME, Wright DJ, Mulks F, Hardcastle IR, Endicott JA, et al. Understanding small-molecule binding to MDM2: insights into structural effects of isoindolinone inhibitors from NMR spectroscopy. Chem Biol Drug Des 2011;77:301–8.

[90] Rothweiler U, Czarna A, Krajewski M, Ciombor J, Kalinski C, Khazak V, et al. Isoquinolin-1-one inhibitors of the MDM2–p53 interaction. Chem Med Chem 2008;3:1118–28.

[91] Allen JG, Bourbeau MP, Wohlhieter GE, Bartberger MD, Michelsen K, Hungate R, et al. Discovery and optimization of chromenotriazolopyrimidines as potent inhibitors of the mouse double minute 2-tumor protein 53 protein–protein interaction. J Med Chem 2009;52:7044–53.

[92] Beck HP, DeGraffenreid M, Fox B, Allen JG, Rew Y, Schneider S, et al. Improvement of the synthesis and pharmacokinetic properties of chromenotriazolopyrimidine MDM2-p53 protein–protein inhibitors. Bioorg Med Chem Lett 2011;21:2752–5.

[93] Furet P, Chène P, De Pover A, Valat TS, Lisztwan JH, Kallen J, et al. The central valine concept provides an entry in a new class of non peptide inhibitors of the p53–MDM2 interaction. Bioorg Med Chem Lett 2012;22:3498–502.

[94] Popowicz GM, Czarna A, Wolf S, Wang K, Wang W, Dömling A, et al. Structures of low molecular weight inhibitors bound to MDMX and MDM2 reveal new approaches for p53-MDMX/MDM2 antagonist drug discovery. Cell Cycle 2010;9:1104–11.

[95] Rew Y, Sun D, Gonzalez-Lopez De Turiso F, Bartberger MD, Beck HP, Canon J, et al. Structure-based design of novel inhibitors of the MDM2–p53 interaction. J Med Chem 2012;55:4936–54.

[96] Michelsen K, Jordan JB, Lewis J, Long AM, Yang E, Rew Y, et al. Ordering of the N-terminus of human MDM2 by small molecule inhibitors. J Am Chem Soc 2012;134:17059–67.

[97] Popowicz GM, Czarna A, Rothweiler U, Szwagierczak A, Krajewski M, Weber L, et al. Molecular basis for the inhibition of p53 by MDMS. Cell Cycle 2007;6:2386–92.

[98] Reed D, Shen Y, Shelat AA, Arnold LA, Ferreira AM, Zhu F, et al. Identification and characterization of the first small molecule inhibitor of MDMX. J Biol Chem 2010;285:10786–96.

[99] Bista M, Smithson D, Pecak A, Salinas G, Pustelny K, Min J, et al. On the mechanism of action of SJ-172550 in inhibiting the interaction of MDM4 and p53. PLoS ONE 2012;7:e37518.

[100] Graves B, Thompson T, Xia M, Janson C, Lukacs C, Deo D, et al. Activation of the p53 pathway by small-molecule-induced MDM2 and MDMX dimerization. Proc Natl Acad Sci U S A 2012;109:11788–93.

Targeting Altered Metabolism— Emerging Cancer Therapeutic Strategies

Minsuh Seo, Robert Blake Crochet, Yong-Hwan Lee

Department of Biological Sciences, Louisiana State University, Baton Rouge, LA, USA

METABOLIC ALTERATIONS IN CANCER

Cells have to constantly produce energy for their biological functions and survival [1–3]. To satisfy these energy needs, cells maintain optimal metabolic conditions by continuously adjusting their metabolism to ongoing physiological conditions; cancer cells are not exempt from such a stress [4]. In fact, cancer cells may be the most successful cells to carry out such metabolic adaptations for their survival and rapid growth [5,6]. Oxidation of nutrients, such as glucose, fatty acids, and amino acids, generates cellular energy in the form of adenosine triphosphate (ATP), the major energy currency of all cells [7]. However, cancer cells in rapid growth phases typically experience an insufficient oxygen supply and have limited symbiotic nutrient exchanges with neighboring cells [8]. To survive and grow under such harsh conditions, cancer cells reprogram their metabolic patterns to depend less on oxygen supplies and neighbors [5,9].

For example, glycolysis is a central carbon metabolic pathway in nearly all organisms, through which cellular energy is generated by the degradation of glucose into pyruvate (Fig. 14.1) [10]. In an aerobic environment, pyruvate is transported into mitochondria and is completely oxidized to carbon dioxide and water through the citric acid cycle and the respiratory chain, ultimately generating up to 36 ATP molecules. Under anaerobic conditions, however, pyruvate is converted to lactate and concomitantly regenerates oxidized nicotinamide adenine dinucleotide (NAD^+) for the continuous performance of glycolysis with no oxygen. In addition to energy production, glycolysis provides vitally important precursors for the synthesis of amino acids, fatty acids, and nucleotides, which are required for macromolecular synthesis and, ultimately, cell proliferation. Because of this advantage, cancer cells depend

Cancer Drug Design and Discovery, Second Edition
http://dx.doi.org/10.1016/B978-0-12-396521-9.00014-0

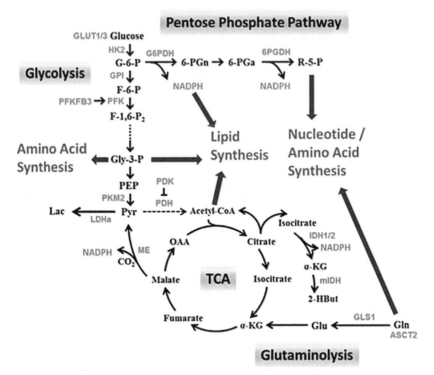

FIGURE 14.1   Pathways involved in cancer metabolism. The metabolic pathways known to be related to cancer, including the enzymes and transporters whose gene expressions are known to be activated by c-myc and HIF-1, are shown. Sources of biosynthetic intermediates and oxidative stress homeostasis regulation (NADPH) are accordingly represented with arrows or different fonts. All acronyms are as defined in text. (For color version of this figure, the reader is referred to the online version of this book.)

more on glycolysis than oxidative phosphorylation, which results in the complete oxidation of glucose to CO_2 and water [11,12]. These tumorigenic metabolic adaptations usually require metabolic enzymes and nutrient transporters that are different from those used by normal cells. Consequently, oncogenic metabolic adaptations necessarily involve the activation of gene expressions in proteins associated with adaptation. This process is performed by transcriptional regulators, whose activities are regulated by other oncogenic signal transduction molecules and/or physiological environmental factors.

Adaptive Alterations in Gene Expression Patterns

Studies have not clearly resolved the ambiguous causes and effects of altered metabolism in cancer [13]. However, it has been demonstrated that cancer is commonly related to impaired mitochondrial respiration, activation of key oncogenes, and hypoxic tumor microenvironments—alterations that are likely to be the major causes of metabolic adaptation in cancer. Tumorigenic mitochondrial impairment inevitably involves disorders in the electron transport complex system and the systems involved in apoptosis. However, the ability to perform the tricarboxylic acid (TCA) cycle seems to persist in many cases [9,14]. Although the rapid three-dimensional growth of a tumor cell mass induces the formation of new blood vessels, these vessels are inadequate. As a result, creation of a hypoxic microenvironment around the cells at the center of the tumor mass is unavoidable [15,16]. Such a condition leads to activation of hypoxia-inducible factor-1 (HIF-1), a transcriptional activator that plays a key role in the activation of glycolysis in cells under anaerobic conditions [16,17] (see also Chapters 10 and 14). Although HIF-1 is constantly degraded in normal cells with a sufficient oxygen supply, HIF-1α is stabilized in tumors, even under nonhypoxic conditions; the stabilized HIF-1α induces gene expression of nearly all proteins necessary for aerobic glycolysis, including glucose transporters, and thus leads to the Warburg phenotype [17,18]. This transcriptional activation by HIF-1 is strengthened by the oncogenes *c-myc* and *c-ras* [19].

Oncogenic activation of *c-myc*, *c-ras*, and *c-src* induces upregulation of the expression of glycolysis rate-regulating proteins, such as glucose transporter 1 and 3 (GLUT1/3), hexokinase 2 (HK2), 6-phosphofructo-2-kinase/fructose-2,6-bisphosphatase 3 and 4 (PFKFB3/4), pyruvate kinase M2 (PKM2), and lactate dehydrogenase (LDH) [20]. Numerous observations suggest that these oncogenes also strengthen the effect of HIF-1. Hence, as a result of mitochondrial defects, activation of oncogenes, and HIF-1 stabilization, cancer cells rely heavily on enhanced aerobic glycolysis for their energy production [21]. Compared to HIF-1, which mainly activates glycolysis through transcriptional activation of the glycolysis-related genes, *c-myc* activates expressions of genes involved in glutaminolysis as well as those involved in glycolysis [22]. Consequently, activation of *c-myc* results in transcriptional activation of the glutamine transporter (ASCT2) and kidney-type glutaminase (GLS1), as well as a set of genes related to the TCA cycle [23]. Aside from transcriptionally activating genes, *c-myc* has also been shown to indirectly increase gene expression through the production of miR23a and miR23b [23]. Under normal circumstances, these microRNAs bind the 3'-untranslated region of GLS1 and block translation. However, *c-myc* activation suppresses the expression of these microRNAs and, in turn, promotes translation of the GLS1 [42].

The Warburg Effect

Cancer is a disease caused by uncontrolled growth of cells that have the ability to migrate and spread to other surrounding tissues and organs [24]. To support the requirements of unrestricted cell growth and proliferation, cancer cells display dramatic changes in energy metabolism, as first noted by Warburg [14]. Among the many metabolic alterations, a dramatic increase in glucose uptake and glycolysis are the most prominent metabolic features for the majority of tumor cell types. Compared to their normal counterparts, cancer cells show enhanced conversion of glucose to lactate instead of full respiration [5,6]. A large number of tumor cells, including lung, colon, breast, skin, and leukemia, exhibit a high rate of glycolysis followed by lactic fermentation, even in the presence of abundant oxygen [11,12]. Nearly a century ago, Otto Warburg first documented and theorized that tumorigenic cells demonstrate a metabolic profile that is altered from that of their normal counterparts [14]. He proposed that tumor cells show a much higher rate of glycolysis followed by lactate fermentation due to a mitochondrial respiratory defect. This phenomenon of high glycolysis in cancer cells, which provides an integrated understanding of cancer metabolism and metabolic markers of cancer prognosis, has been termed the Warburg effect [9].

A metabolic shift toward aerobic glycolysis is likely to confer a series of advantages to cancer cells. Firstly, despite the lower net energy yield, the energy production from aerobic glycolysis is much faster and safer than aerobic respiration when compared to oxidative phosphorylation. Oxidative phosphorylation that is mediated by the TCA cycle produces reactive oxygen species (ROS). ROS production is increased when mitochondria are impaired, as in the majority of cancer cells [26,27]. A decreased reliance on oxygen for energy generation ensures cancer cell survival and growth under oxygen-limited conditions. Second, accelerated glycolytic processes provide the necessary precursors for the biosynthesis of nucleotides and lipids that are essential for cell division and proliferation [28]. Third, lower intracellular and extracellular pH levels of tumor tissues, which are established by enhanced lactate production, cause apoptosis of neighboring normal cells, enhance tumor invasion, provide the tumor with protection and resistance from the immune system and cancer drugs [29], and enable cancer cells to outcompete neighboring normal cells for nutrients needed for survival and growth by consuming the majority of substrates [30].

Accordingly, the Warburg effect has been a popular target in therapeutic development. A good clinical application of the Warburg effect is diagnosis and monitoring of cancers by positron emission tomography with [2-^{18}F]2-deoxyglucose (a radioactive glucose analog) as the probe, which allows for locating sites of high glucose uptake and glycolysis [9]. However, the significant therapeutics have only begun to be developed recently. Although glycolysis is one of the most commonly shared pathways between cells (regardless of their abnormalities), finding a reasonable therapeutic drug target became possible only after the molecular mechanisms underlying the Warburg effect began to be unraveled [13,31].

Glutaminolysis

A growing body of evidence suggests that tumorigenic metabolic adaptation tends to cause cells to favor autonomous metabolism, although a symbiotic dependence on stromal cells still remains at a limited level. In that regard, activated glycolysis is necessary but not sufficient enough to meet the anabolic demands of proliferating cells. Glycolysis can supply only carbon; however, cellular anabolic pathways, such as synthesis of amino acids and nucleotides, desperately need nitrogen. Therefore, investigators aimed to find mechanisms complimentary to glycolysis. Evidence has shown that glutamine is also actively consumed in cancer cells through the TCA cycle, a pathway called glutaminolysis [3,25]. This observation is supported by findings that the O_2 consumption of certain cancer cells living within aerobic environments is not significantly less than that of the normal cells. The TCA cycle persists, even though other mitochondrial functions are impaired. As such, results from the latest studies suggest that both glycolysis and glutaminolysis are uniquely active in cancer cells as the sources of production of both energy and precursors for anabolic metabolism [32].

Glutamine is the most abundant free amino acid in mammals and is an essential nitrogen donor for many anabolic processes [33]. It has traditionally been viewed as a nonessential amino acid whose primary functions revolve around nitrogen metabolism, storage, and transport. Over the past few decades, however, it has become clear that the significance of glutamine is not only as a precursor for nucleotides, amino acids, and other biologically important metabolites; rather, it appears that glutamine metabolism also serves as a source of energy production for rapidly growing cells [32]. Studies have demonstrated that highly prolific cells, such as those in cancer, exhibit increased dependence on glutamine for growth and proliferation [33]. More recently, it has been suggested that glutamine, in addition to its role as a biosynthetic precursor and metabolic fuel, also plays a significant role in the regulation of gene expression of metabolic proteins, signal transduction, cellular maintenance, and intracellular signaling pathways [34,35].

Glutaminolysis is a mitochondrial pathway process that is responsible for generating cellular energy from the degradation of glutamine (Fig. 14.1) [32]. For this process, glutamine is imported into cells via a high-affinity glutamine transport protein (ASCT2) [22,36]. ASCT2, although important for normal levels of glutamine uptake, is transcriptionally activated by *c-myc* and thus upregulated in many cancers [22,37,38]. Such a change in ASCT2 expression facilitates glutamine uptake and ensures its abundance within cancer cells. Once glutamine is inside the cell, a multistep process begins that uses proteins from the TCA cycle and the malate-aspartate shuttle to degrade glutamine. This process begins in the cytosol or mitochondria, depending on the glutaminase isoform, with the initial deamination of the γ-nitrogen of glutamine by glutaminase, yielding glutamate and ammonia [39]. The mitochondrial glutaminase isoform (GLS1), which was previously known as the kidney form, is especially important to cancer cells. This phosphate-activated glutaminase isoform is commonly overexpressed in cancer cells, allowing for higher levels of glutamine metabolism [40].

In the mitochondria, the glutamate generated from deamination of glutamine by GLS1 has two possible fates. It can be used to generate glutathione by glutathione cysteine ligase to combat oxidative stress from ROSs or, alternatively, it can be converted to α-ketoglutarate to serve as a substrate for the TCA cycle [37,41]. It is worth mentioning that isocitrate dehydrogenase (IDH) catalyzes the conversion of isocitrate to α-ketoglutarate in the TCA cycle, producing nicotinamide adenine dinucleotide (NADH) as a byproduct of decarboxylation. Compared to that, IDH1 and 2 (residing in cytosol) produce nicotinamide adenine dinucleotide phosphate (NADPH) instead of NADH, catalyzing the same reaction but using substrate from citrate transported to cytosol from mitochondria [37a]. This cytosolic IDH-catalyzed reaction serves as a source of NADPH, which is an important reductant in fatty acid synthesis and oxidative stress homeostasis. Moreover, cytosolic IDH is often mutated in cancer (represented as mIDH in Fig. 14.1) and catalyzes the conversion of α-ketoglutarate to 2-hydroxybutyrate instead of the normal reaction. An additional source of NADPH from glutaminolysis is decarboxylation of malate to pyruvate, a reaction catalyzed by malic enzyme (Fig. 14.1). Further reactions involving α-ketoglutarate focus either on generating energy equivalents, of which there are six ATPs and one pyruvate molecule made from each glutamine, or on making metabolic intermediates for both the TCA cycle and other metabolic pathways.

Metabolic Adaptation and Oxidative Stress

Studies have revealed that cancer cells, compared to normal cells, have higher levels of ROS, suggesting an association of ROS and oxidative stress with cancer [42,43]. However, it remains unclear whether an increase in ROS is a cause or a consequence of cancer progression [44,45]. Tumorigenic conditions, including abnormal metabolic shift, mitochondrial dysfunction, hypoxia, matrix detachment, and inflammation, have all been linked to enhanced ROS production [46,47]. Chronic increases in ROS contribute to genetic instability by causing strand breaks, alterations in guanine and thymine bases, and sister chromatid exchanges, and thus increase the malignant potential of cancer cells [48,49]. Recently, it was shown that ROS promotes cancer cell proliferation and tumor initiation and progression. Cancer cell proliferation in response to ROS is believed to be due to the ROS-induced activation of c-Jun amino-terminal kinase/stress-activated protein kinase, Rac1, NADPH-oxidase, and mitogen-activated protein kinases pathways [50,51].

Moreover, increases in ROS production have been shown to induce cell cycle progression, especially by promoting the G1/S phase transition [52–54]. Chronic oxidative stress leads to adaptive responses within cancer cells that result in an increased resistance to chemotherapy by upregulating expression of the multidrug-resistance efflux pump, P-glycoprotein. Oxidative stress also increases the blood supply to tumor cells by stimulating angiogenic factors interleukin-8, vascular endothelial growth factor, and matrix metalloproteinase-1 for vessel growth [49,55]. Moreover, ROS have been shown to facilitate invasion and metastasis by activating p38 MAP kinase and Rac1, which, in turn, alter arrangements and recognition of the actin cytoskeleton. ROS within the cancer microenvironment can directly damage endothelial cells to promote vascular invasion [56]. Although it appears to support tumor progression [49], ROS can cause detrimental oxidative stress that results in damaged cellular components, leading to cell death, when its levels are excessive. p53, a tumor suppressor protein, and pro-apoptotic signaling molecules, such as ASK1, JNK, and p38, are known to play roles in the ROS-induced apoptosis [49,57,58].

REGULATION OF OXIDATIVE STRESS HOMEOSTASIS IN CANCER

In the traditional definition, the Warburg effect can be simply defined as abnormally increased glycolysis in neoplastic cells. However, studies have extended it to overall metabolic alterations in tumor cells, including activated glutaminolysis [42,43]. The levels of ROS in cancer cells are shown to be higher than those of normal cells, largely due to the persistent TCA cycle following glutaminolysis in the impaired mitochondria. Nonetheless, they are exquisitely regulated to remain below the detrimental levels [44,45]. One of the main questions in the latest studies has been the mechanism underlying regulation of the ROS homeostasis in cancer. Tumorigenic transformation of cells is accompanied by mitochondrial dysfunction, which causes a failure in apoptotic processes and, ultimately, confers immortality to tumorigenic cells [46,47]. Mitochondrial dysfunction is believed to be at least one reason for overproduced ROS in cancer cells [59,60]. Although the majority of glucose is metabolized to lactate after glycolysis, a small fraction of pyruvate is transferred to the dysfunctional mitochondria as a form of pyruvate to perform the TCA cycle and the subsequent oxidative phosphorylation. Most of the glutaminolysis products, such as α-ketoglutarate, go into the TCA cycle. However, the dysfunctional mitochondria can carry out only impaired oxidative phosphorylation and, as a result, produce ROS [59]. Recent studies have shown that enhanced glycolysis provides cancer cells with an additional advantage to those described above. The first step of glycolysis is to generate glucose-6-phosphate (G-6-P) from glucose by hexokinase. As shown in Fig. 14.1, G-6-P is not only a glycolysis intermediate but also the entry substrate for the pentose phosphate pathway (PPP), which has an overall rate that is governed by substrate levels. In this way, glucose can go into either glycolysis or the PPP, and the pathways are mutually regulated because the PPP is the major source of NADPH. The most important cellular antioxidant, glutathione, can be regenerated using only NADPH inside the cell.

Oxidative Stress, Glutathione, and the Pentose Phosphate Pathway

Although it appears to support tumor progression, ROS production must be tightly regulated at a certain level, even in cancer cells, so that the cells are able to avoid the detrimental effects associated with excessive oxidative stress [61]. The biological mechanisms by which antioxidants are produced have evolved to protect cells from the toxic effects of ROS and to maintain the redox balance [62,63]. Antioxidants function to quench free radicals and interrupt cascades of uncontrolled oxidation. One of the most regenerable cellular antioxidants is glutathione (γ-glutamyl-cysteine-glycine; GSH), in which the sulfhydryl (thiol) group (–SH) on the cysteine residue serves as a proton donor and plays an important role in ROS scavenging [64–67]. GSH is ubiquitously found in most tissues at a millimolar range of concentrations (1–10 mM), allowing it to function as the most highly concentrated intracellular antioxidant and as an important cofactor for various antioxidant enzymes [67]. Glutathione can exist in two interchangeable redox states: reduced (GSH) and oxidized (glutathione disulfide; GSSG). In the oxidized state, glutathione forms a stable disulfide-linked complex. The ROS protective mechanism of GSH is achieved by the formation of mixed disulfides (GSSG), which is called a thiol/disulfide exchange reaction (RS–SR + R'SH ↔ R'S–SR + RSH), by donating an electron to ROS [67]. As shown in Fig. 14.2, the regeneration of GSH from GSSG is catalyzed by the enzyme glutathione reductase (GR) at the expense of reduced NADPH, which is produced at the initial steps of the PPP and at the reactions following glutaminolysis (Fig. 14.1) [68]. GSH can detoxify heavy metals, organic xenobiotics, and many other toxic metabolites that are produced as side products of cellular metabolism [69]. Thus, the ratio of GSH to GSSG within cells is often used as a sensitive indicator of oxidative stress [70].

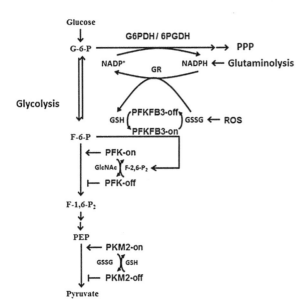

FIGURE 14.2 Mutual regulation of glycolysis and the pentose phosphate pathway. Mechanisms for covalent modifications for the two glycolysis rate-limiting enzymes and PFKFB3 are shown. The two activity states are represented by "on" and "off", which are attached to the protein names to symbolize the active and inactive states, respectively. Modification by S-glutathionylation and O-GlcNAcylation are represented by GSSG and GlcNAc, respectively. Note that the conversion between G-6-P and F-6-P is a reversible reaction whose favored direction is decided by the concentrations of the two metabolites.

In addition to its function as an accumulator of precursors for macromolecule synthesis, over 65% of the cellular need of GSH depends on the PPP, although the TCA cycle after glutaminolysis makes minor contributions through the functions of cytosolic isocitrate dehydrogenase and malic enzyme (Figs 14.1 and 14.2) [71]. The first step and third step of the PPP catalyzed by glucose-6-phosphate dehydrogenase (G6PDH) and 6-phosphogluconate dehydrogenase (6PGDH), respectively, produce NADPH used for regeneration of GSH from GSSG by glutathione reductase (GR) [67]. As a consequence, the enhanced PPP results in increased production of GSH (Fig. 14.2). In other words, periodic interruptions of glycolysis in cancer cells are necessary to activate the PPP for regeneration of GSH to neutralize the ROS that was increased by glycolysis or some other respiratory oxidation [72]. Thus, the Warburg effect must be redefined as enhanced glycolysis with regulation of ROS homeostasis by the PPP [7].

ROS Sensing and S-Glutathionylation

Aside from its primary role as a cellular antioxidant, glutathione also plays an important role in the posttranslational covalent modifications of proteins via a process called S-glutathionylation. Similarly to the protein–protein disulfide linkages that are formed under oxidizing conditions, disulfide linkages are formed between a cysteine residue of a protein and one from GSH under oxidizing conditions. As a result, the subjected proteins are covalently labeled with glutathione (PSSG) [73,74]. Glutathione covalently attached to proteins affects the functions of the proteins by hindering the entry of the substrate into the catalytic pockets and/or by conformational changes in proteins, depending on the positions of the modified cysteine residues in proteins [74–76]. S-glutathionylation is involved in diverse physiological processes, such as cell growth, cell cycle progression, differentiation, transcriptional activity, cytoskeletal functions, and metabolism [74,77]. In addition, the effects can be simply reversed in increased reducing conditions, which promote removal of glutathione from protein through mechanisms involving direct thiol/disulfide exchange reactions with reduced GSH or through reductive enzyme-mediated reactions. Because of its sensitivity to the redox conditions, this regulatory mechanism is able to operate in response to sudden changes in ROS levels. A number of proteins have been shown to undergo glutathionylation, including several metabolic enzymes (enolase, aldolase, 6-phosphoglucolactonase, adenylate kinase, phosphoglycerate kinase, triose phosphate isomerase, and pyrophosphatase), cytoskeletal proteins (myosin, tropomyosin, profilin, and actin), redox enzymes, stress proteins (HSP70 and HSP60), and fatty acid-binding proteins [74,78,79].

Studies have revealed that the rate-limiting enzymes of glycolysis are subject to an ROS-dependent regulatory mechanism. A better understanding of the underlying mechanism is very important for development of cancer therapeutics targeting the Warburg effect. In this regard, it is noteworthy to mention that the ROS-dependent regulatory mechanism is exerted in two different rate-limiting enzymes of cancer-specific glycolysis: pyruvate kinase M2 (PKM2) and PFKFB3 (Fig. 14.2) [80,81]. PKM2 is a tumor-specific isoform of muscle-type pyruvate kinase (PKM), which catalyzes the last step of glycolysis using phosphoenol pyruvate and ADP to produce pyruvate and ATP. Unlike a normal PKM, which is active as a homotetramer, PKM2 is a dimer with lower enzymatic activity. It was shown that PKM2 is S-glutathionylated at the residue Cys358 upon the increase of cellular ROS levels [81].

S-glutathionylation of PFKFB3 and PKM causes inhibition of glycolysis and activation of the PPP. This posttranslational modification is recovered by the activated PPP, suggesting a cyclic regulation of glycolysis and the PPP. As shown in Fig. 14.2, S-glutathionylation of PFKFB3 at the residue Cys206 by the same process also inhibits its ability to produce F-2,6-P$_2$, the allosteric 6-phosphofructo-1-kinase (PFK) activator, resulting in decreased glycolysis [81a]. The net metabolic results from ROS-dependent regulation of PFKFB3 and PKM are the same: a decrease in glycolysis and an increase in the PPP. The only difference is that S-glutathionylation of PFKFB3 inhibits the first glycolysis-committed step, whereas that of PKM2 inhibits the last glycolysis-committed step. Having two switch systems in a 10-enzyme pathway might be advantageous. The rerouting of glucose metabolic flux from glycolysis to the PPP and restarting of glycolysis would be much smoother than having a one-switch system; all the glycolytic intermediates between the two steps would function as a reserve for the rapid restart of glycolysis and for precursors of anabolic metabolism.

Metabolic Sensing and O-GlcNAcylation

A recent report has suggested O-linked β-N-acetyl glucosamine (O-GlcNAcylation) as an additional mechanism for regulation of glucose metabolism [82], although regulation of other proteins by glycosylation is not uncommon. It has been demonstrated that O-GlcNAcylation was made on Ser529 of the glycolysis rate-liming enzyme, 6-phosphofructo-1-kinase (PFK), in response to hypoxia (Fig. 14.2). This glycosylation decreased PFK activity by inhibiting binding of its allosteric activator fructose-2,6-bisphosphate (F-2,6-P$_2$). As a consequence, fructose-6-phosphate (F-6-P) accumulates and glucose flux is rerouted from glycolysis to the PPP. This mechanism also gives cancer cells the ability to control ROS by dually regulating glycolysis and the PPP (Fig. 14.2). The O-GlcNAcylation of proteins is catalyzed by O-GlcNAc transferase, which transfers N-acetyl glucosamine from uridine diphospho-N-acetyl glucosamine (UDP-GlcNAc) to serine or threonine residues of proteins [82a]. The significance of this mechanism is concentrated on the dynamically changing cellular level of UDP-GlcNAc, which is determined by the cellular availabilities of key metabolites such as glucose, glutamine, acetyl-CoA, uridine, and ATP. In other words, the cellular availability of UDP-GlcNAc reflects the overall status of various metabolic pathways. Compared to S-glutathionylation, which is directly induced and recovered in response to the ROS level, O-GlcNAcylation involves a number of enzymatic reactions and therefore is likely to function as a regulatory mechanism suitable for the long-term control of overall metabolism in cancer.

DEVELOPMENT OF THERAPEUTICS TARGETING CANCER METABOLISM

To date, all studies of the Warburg effect and altered cell metabolism have unequivocally suggested that specific isotypes of several metabolic proteins are selectively activated in most types of cancer. Many such cancer-specific isoforms have recently become the subject of intense investigation because of their unique potential as drug targets. In this section, we review the most promising drug targets associated with the Warburg effect and briefly describe the current stage of drug development for each. Inhibitors in clinical or

TABLE 14.1   Inhibitors Targeting Cancer Glycolysis

Molecular target	Compound	Indication	Status	Biological functions
GLUT1/3	STF-31	Renal cell carcinoma	Preclinical	Blocks glucose uptake
	Phloretin	Melanoma, leukemia, hepatocellular carcinoma, breast cancer	Preclinical	
HKII	2-Deoxyglucose	Prostate cancer	Phase II	Slows production of glucose-6-phosphate; forces HKII dissociation from mitochondrial membrane and voltage-dependent anion channels
	3-Bromopyruvate	Colorectal cancer, breast cancer, hepatocellular carcinoma	Preclinical	
	Lonidamine	Breast cancer	Phase II	
PFKFB3	3PO	Colorectal cancer, breast cancer, hepatocellular carcinoma, prostate cancer, stomach cancer	Preclinical	Inhibits $F-2,6-P_2$ production, blocking allosteric activation of PFK1
	N4A and derivatives		Preclinical	
Pyruvate dehydrogenase kinase (PDK)	DCA	Glioblastoma multiform, breast cancer	Phase 2	Prevents inactivation of PDH, favoring acetyl-CoA formation
Pyruvate dehydrogenase (PDH)	CPI-613	Pancreatic cancer	Phase 1	Inhibits PDH, disallowing acetyl-CoA formation
PKM2	TLN-232 peptide	Melanoma, renal cell carcinoma	Phase 2	Blocks the formation of pyruvate via glycolysis
LDHA	FX11	Lymphoma, pancreatic cancer	Preclinical	Inhibits lactate production and NAD^+ regeneration
	Oxamate	Hereditary leiomyomatosis and renal cell cancer, B-cell non-Hodgkin lymphoma	Preclinical	

Adapted from Ref. [37a].

developmental stages are listed in Tables 14.1 and 14.2, including descriptions of their targets and expected results.

Inhibitors Targeting Cancer Glycolysis

Glucose Transporters (GLUT1 and GLUT3)

   To meet the increased energetic demands of cancer cells, glucose must be rapidly acquired from the cellular environment. In cancer cells, obtaining large quantities of glucose is made possible by the overexpression of specific glucose transport proteins (GLUTs) [83]. Among the numerous GLUT isoforms, the gene expressions of GLUT1 and GLUT3 are commonly upregulated in cancers via the functions of the HIF-1 and *c-myc* transcription factors, as well as the serine–threonine kinase Akt/PKB [84]. By contrast, many cancers act to downregulate the insulin-sensitive GLUT4 isoform, thus promoting insulin resistance in many forms of cancer.

TABLE 14.2 Inhibitors Targeting Oxidative Stress Homeostasis and Glutaminolysis in Cancer

Molecular target	Compound	Mechanism of action	Current status
Thioredoxin reductase	Arsenic trioxide (As_2O_3)	Inhibits the function of the mitochondrial respiratory chain; enhances reactive oxygen species (ROS) generation	Approved (leukemia)
Electron transport complex	Elescolomol (STA-4783)	Induces acute ROS accumulation	Phase III
Glutathione (GSH)	Benzyl isothiocyanate	Depletes the GSH pool by binding GSH	Preclinical studies
	Phenethyl isothiocyanate	Depletes the GSH pool by binding GSH	Preclinical studies
	Aziridine derivatives	Depletes the GSH pool by binding GSH	Phase I/II
Gamma-glutamylcysteine synthetase	Buthionine sulphoximine	Inhibits GSH synthesis	Phase I/II
Glutathione S-transferase	Sulphasalazine	Inhibits GSH synthesis	Phase III
SLC6A14 (unselective amino acid transporter)	Alpha-methyl-DL-tryptophan	Decreases amino acid availability	Preclinical studies
ASCT2	1,2,3-dithiazoles	Decreases glutamine transport and availability	Preclinical studies
Glutaminase 1	6-Diazo-5-oxo-L-norleucine	Inhibits glutaminolysis	Preclinical studies
	BPTES (bis-2-(5-phenylacetamido-1,2,4-thiadiazol-2-yl)ethyl sulfide)	Inhibits glutaminolysis	Preclinical studies

STF-31

STF-31 and its related analogs are the first class of inhibitors to demonstrate selective inhibition among GLUT isoforms [85]. Studies have shown that this group of cell-permeable sulfonamides competitively and selectively bind GLUT1 in renal cell carcinomas (RCCs), effectively blocking glucose uptake and concomitantly causing cell death via necrosis. It is believed that STF-31 selectively kills RCCs by exploiting the rigidity of cancer cell metabolism. Unlike cancer cells, which require abundant levels of glucose to maintain sufficient ATP levels, normal cells remain viable during GLUT1 inhibition by using other glucose transporters and shifting energy metabolism to favor oxidative phosphorylation. Such flexibility in normal cells is possible due to the specificity of STF-31 inhibitor for GLUT1 [85].

Phloretin

Phloretin, a hydrogenated natural product, is a derivative of chalcone that inhibits the glucose transport activity of the GLUT1 and GLUT2. Treatment of human leukemia cells with Phloretin revealed that Phloretin exhibits antitumorigenesis effects through growth inhibition and apoptotic activation. Additional studies on cancers from bladder and mammary cells revealed similar antitumorigenesis properties [86,87].

Hexokinase 2

Elevated levels of glucose uptake from cancer-specific GLUT proteins are supported by the rapid conversion of glucose to glucose-6-phosphate, a process catalyzed by the enzyme hexokinase. Cancer cells upregulate this process through increased expression of hexokinase 2 (HKI2), which is bound to the mitochondrial membrane via the porin-like protein voltage-dependent anion channel (VDAC), unlike other isoforms [88]. Comparatively, levels of HK2 in cancer cells have been shown to be more than 500 times greater than those present in normal liver cells. Such dramatic elevations in HK2 expression serve to drive the vigorous levels of glycolysis necessary for cancer cells to survive; however, HK2 also serves a secondary function in promoting tumorigenesis through interactions with the mitochondria. It has been shown that the elevated levels of HK2 can interfere with the ability of cancer cells to undergo mitochondria-initiated apoptosis, contributing to the immortalization of cancer cells. Because of its dual role in promoting cancer, HK2 has been highly regarded as a potential drug target for cancer metabolism. Currently, several compounds, including 2-deoxyglucose, 3-bromopyruvate, and lonidamine, are being tested in clinical trials for HK2 [89].

2-Deoxyglucose

2-Deoxyglucose (2-DG), a derivative of glucose, is able to be phosphorylated by hexokinase, resulting in the formation of 2-deoxyglucose-phosphate (2-DG-P) [89]. The product of this reaction is trapped within the cell and cannot be used by subsequent steps of glycolysis, resulting in the accumulation of 2-DG-P and causing product inhibition of HK2 [90]. In vitro studies on 2-deoxyglucose have demonstrated HK2 inhibition as well as subsequent ATP depletion; however, in vivo studies using xerographs have been disappointing, showing that 2-deoxyglucose as a single agent does not inhibit tumor growth. However, new evidence suggests that this compound does offer some benefit when used in combination with other drugs that target tumor metabolism.

3-Bromopyruvate

3-bromopyruvate (3-BrP) is a pyruvate analog that acts as an alkylating agent and strong inhibitor of HK2. This compound inhibits HK2 (and possibly other glycolytic enzymes) by covalently modifying sulfhydryl groups through a sort of dead-end inhibition. In the case of HK2, such modifications cause the dissociation of HK2 from the mitochondria and, in turn, prevent HK2 from blocking apoptosis. This stems from the observation that mitochondria-bound hexokinase is essential for the prevention of initiating apoptosis; hence, agents that promote dissociation of the membrane-bound hexokinase may trigger apoptotic death of cancer cells [89,91].

Lonidamine (TH-070)

Lonidamine is a derivative of indazole-3-carboxilic acid and is known for its ability to inhibit aerobic glycolysis in cancer cells [92]. Under hypoxic conditions, as is common with cancers, lonidamine reduces ATP levels by interfering with membrane-bound HK2, as is also the case with 3-BrP. Studies using in vitro models show that cells treated with lonidamine exhibit the hallmarks of apoptosis. Lonidamine has also been shown to have synergistic effects when used in combination with alkylating agents such as cisplatin, melphalan, and BCNU (bis-chloronitro-sourea) [93].

Glucose-6-phosphate Isomerase

Glucose-6-phosphate isomerase (GPI), the second enzyme in the glycolytic pathway, is a dimeric enzyme that catalyzes the conversion of glucose-6-phosphate to fructose-6-phosphate. This enzyme has been linked to the proliferation and motility of cancer cells via its control over glucose-6-phosphate levels [72]. Aside from being a glycolytic intermediate, it has been seen that in certain cancers glucose-6-phosphate can act as a tumor secreted-cytokine as well as an angiogenesis-promoting factor. Moreover, evidence suggests that glucose-6-phosphate isomerase induces the expression of a matrix metalloproteinase-3 protein in some cancer cells, which subsequently increases tumor invasiveness. However, the development of therapeutics targeting GPI is not active [89].

6-Phosphofructo-2-kinase/fructose-2,6-bisphosphatase 3

6-Phosphofructo-1-kinase (PFK) catalyzes the first glycolysis-committed and irreversible step, fructose-6-phosphate to fructose-1,6-bisphosphate. As such, PFK is one of the most prominent rate-limiting enzymes in the glycolytic pathway and regulation of its activity is an important means of control in regulating glycolytic flux within cells. Typically in most eukaryotic cells, this enzyme experiences strong inhibition by cellular concentrations of ATP, thus limiting glycolysis. To overcome this inhibition, four tissue-specific isoforms of 6-phosphofructo-2-kinase/fructose-2,6-bisphosphatase (PFKFB) exist that are capable of generating fructose-2,6-bisphosphate ($F\text{-}2,6\text{-}P_2$), the most potent allosteric activator of PFK [94,95]. However, unlike normal cells, cancer cells constitutively express high levels of a rarely expressed but highly active isoform of 6-phosphofructo-2-kinase/fructose-2,6-bisphosphatase (PFKFB3), otherwise known as the inducible or cancer isoform [96,97]. This elevation of PFKFB3 results in abnormally high cellular concentrations of $F\text{-}2,6\text{-}P_2$, causing PFK to be perennially activated. Multiple studies have revealed that the $F\text{-}2,6\text{-}P_2$ levels are elevated in various cancer cell lines and often are accompanied by a high proliferative rate, cell cycle progression, and transformation. Indeed, PFKFB3 that elevates cellular $F\text{-}2,6\text{-}P_2$ concentration has been found to be overexpressed in rapidly proliferating cells and tumors, including breast cancer, leukemia, and colon adenocarcinoma, suggesting a possible correlation between PFKFB3 and the Warburg effect [98,99].

3-(3-Pyridinyl)-1-(4-pyridinyl)-2-propen-1-one

3-(3-pyridinyl)-1-(4-pyridinyl)-2-propen-1-one (3PO) was developed based on the structure derived from another isoform, PFKFB4 [100]. It blocks fructose-6-phosphate from entering the active site of the kinase domain. Cancer cells are particularly vulnerable to suppression of glycolytic flux. In vivo studies on neoplastic cells have confirmed that 3PO does suppress glycolysis. Moreover, in studies with melanoma cell lines, it was quantitatively determined that the concentrations of Fru-2, $6\text{-}P_2$, ATP, lactate, NAD^+, and NADH are reduced upon 3PO introduction. The isoform selectivity of 3PO is not yet known.

N4A and N4A Derivatives

Compared to 3PO, N4A (5,6,7,8-tetrahydroxy-2-(4-hydroxyphenyl)chromen-4-one) is a PFKFB3 inhibitor based on the crystal structure of PFKFB3. Its derivatives are suggested to be improved from the subsequent structure-guided optimization [101]. They bind to the F-6-P pocket of PFKFB3 and inhibit its $F\text{-}2,6\text{-}P_2$ synthesis, leading to low glycolysis and, ultimately, death of cultured cancer cells with no random toxicity. N4A and its derivatives are functionally selective to PFKFB3, although somewhat limited. They have been shown to induce death of cultured HeLa and T47D cancer cells by efficiently blocking glycolysis.

Pyruvate Dehydrogenase and Pyruvate Dehydrogenase Kinase

Pyruvate dehydrogenase (PDH) is one of the two component enzymes of a huge pyruvate dehydrogenase complex, which is located in mitochondria to catalyze conversion of pyruvate to acetyl-CoA, the entry substrate for the TCA cycle [102]. PDH performs a decarboxylation of pyruvate and a reductive acetylation of lipoate, which is covalently bound to the second enzyme component. PDH is regulated by pyruvate dehydrogenase kinase (PDK), which phosphorylates PDH, and phosphorylated PDH is not active. Because the activity of PDH is critical for the oxidative phosphorylation of glucose, it has been a general assumption that PDH activity is compromised, but PDK is active, in cancer cells in which the majority of pyruvate has to be converted to lactate. This notion creates a paradoxical situation in which PDH inhibition is a valid strategy for cancer therapy. Nonetheless, PDH inhibition has been shown to be very effective.

CPI-613

CPI-613 induces cancer-specific regulatory hyperphosphorylation of PDH of cancer cells, resulting in the inhibition of PDH function [103]. These effects and related cancer-specific consequences of the drug lead to catastrophic disruption of tumor mitochondrial metabolism. Tumor cells are thereby starved of energy and biosynthetic intermediates, resulting in cell death. CPI-613 is a nonredox-active lipoate derivative that disrupts mitochondrial metabolism. CPI-613 strongly inhibits tumor growth in non-small cell human lung cancer, as well as in a human pancreatic cancer preclinical mouse tumor model [104].

Dichloroacetate

Dichloroacetate (DCA) inhibition of PDK is a key step that leads to reestablishment of the mitochondrial oxidative phosphorylation pathway as the main source for cell energy. DCA inhibition of PDK frees up the mitochondrial gatekeeping enzyme PDH, which is then able to convert pyruvate to acetyl-CoA and initiate normal oxidative phosphorylation via the TCA cycle [104].

Reactivation of the Krebs cycle generates ROS and H^+ ions. Release of ROS into the cell cytoplasm regulates the opening of plasma membrane ion channels and stabilizes calcium sensitive nuclear transcription factors [105]. Efflux of H^+ ions helps to reestablish a negative mitochondrial membrane potential and thereby aids in the synthesis of ATP. Maintenance of a negative membrane potential also opens mitochondrial transition pores, thus permitting efflux of cytochrome c and apoptosis-inducing factor into the cytoplasm. Cytochrome c and ROS act to open the plasma membrane redox-sensitive K^+ channel Kv1.5, which results in cell hyperpolarization and inhibition of voltage-dependent calcium ion movement into the cell. Decreased intracellular concentration of Ca^{+2} suppresses tonic activation of the nuclear factor of activated T-lymphocytes, thus resulting in its efflux from the nucleus and further expression of Kv1.5 membrane channels. This added efflux of K^+ from the cell decreases tonic inhibition of $[K^+]$ on caspase 3 and caspase 9 and leads to enhancement of apoptosis.

Pyruvate Kinase M2

Pyruvate kinase (PK), the last enzyme in glycolysis, has long been studied for its role in the Warburg effect [3,80]. However, unlike PFKFB3, whose expression is activated by oncogenic signals to stimulate earlier stages of glycolysis, pyruvate kinase is presumed to promote tumor growth and proliferation via additional regulation of pyruvate production. This seemingly paradoxical phenomenon has been described as a "cancer-specific metabolic budgeting system", in which the ATP-generating step of forming pyruvate is downregulated in favor of producing glycolytic intermediates for use in anabolic metabolism [106].

The association of pyruvate kinase with the Warburg effect is primarily attributed to the M-type isoforms of pyruvate kinase, which are splice variants of the PKM gene that differ by 23 amino acids over a small region (amino acid residues 378–484) of the carboxyl terminus, encoding an allosteric site on the M2 isoform that is capable of binding fructose-1,6-bisphosphate (F-1,6-P$_2$) [107]. Unlike the M1 isoform, which is associated with normal cellular metabolism, the M2 isoform is widely regarded as a tumorigenesis-promoting form of the enzyme. Such regulation of pyruvate kinase by cancer cells has been shown to be key regulator of antioxidative cellular metabolism in combination with ROS-dependent regulation of PFKFB3, as mentioned earlier. By reducing pyruvate production, causing a buildup of glycolytic intermediates, cancer cells protect against ROS by generating NADPH, an essential component for reducing oxidized glutathione, and by stimulating genes regulated by the pentose phosphate pathway that are responsible for adaption to oxidative stress [106].

TLN-232

TLN-232 is a cyclic seven-amino-acid peptide developed by Thallion Pharmaceuticals that targets overexpressed PKM2, which is common in many cancers. TLN-232 was shown to be effective in in vitro animal models for treating pancreatic, melanoma, liver, sarcoma, and other types of cancers. Currently, TLN-232 has finished phase II clinical trials [104].

Lactate Dehydrogenase

Lactate dehydrogenase catalyzes the final step in anaerobic glycolysis through the conversion of pyruvate to lactate via coupled oxidation of NADH to NAD$^+$. In tumor cells, this process is facilitated by the cancer-specific LDH-A isoform that is controlled by the *c-myc* and HIF-1 transcription factors [108,109]. This increased expression of LDH-A in cancer cells results in increased pyruvate to lactate production, leaving less pyruvate available for generating acetyl-CoA. Such a shift in the branch of converting pyruvate to lactate rather than acetyl-CoA is understandable considering Warburg's observations [110]. Hence, LDH-A has long been viewed as a potential drug target for cancer metabolism. The idea behind this thinking is that if an inhibitor for LDH-A could be found, one could force the conversion of pyruvate to acetyl-CoA rather than lactate, effectively eliminating the regeneration of NAD$^+$ that is necessary for maintaining glycolysis.

FX11

FX11 has served as a proof of concept for targeting lactate dehydrogenase by demonstrating tumor regression in both models of human lymphoma and pancreatic cancer upon treatment. Additionally, certain antiprotozoal agents are showing promise as potential LDH inhibitors, such as oxalate and oxamate [104].

Inhibitors Targeting ROS Regulation and Glutaminolysis in Cancer

Increased generation of ROS and an altered redox status in cancer cells provide a rationale for two opposite therapeutic approaches to cancer. One approach is to modulate ROS levels or to upregulate antioxidant capacity in cancer, thereby overcoming the drug resistance associated with redox adaptation and suppressing cancer progression. However, studies show that several antioxidants have not yet been successfully exploited for cancer therapy in the clinic. Further characterization of underlying mechanisms for ROS-modulating cancer treatment would shed more light on expanding the therapeutic potential on ROS-targeting therapy. As severe oxidative stress can induce cell death, approaches to further increase ROS generation are likely to show toxicity in cancer cells. Interestingly, some agents that increase the production of ROS seem to exert its cytotoxic effect against cancer cells. Nevertheless, strategies to interfere with the cellular ROS scavenging system seem to be an effective approach in targeting cancer through the depletion of the GSH pool and inhibition of redox modulating enzymes, peroxidases, peroxiredoxins, superoxide dismutase, catalase, and thiol reductases.

Arsenic Trioxide

Despite the toxicity of arsenic, arsenic trioxide (As_2O_3) seems to induce apoptosis of cancer cells by inhibiting thioredoxin reductase (TR) [111,112]. Using NADPH as a reductant, TR functions to maintain a reduced condition of thioredoxin, which prevents random formation of disulfide linkage between cytosolic proteins.

Elesclomol (STA-4783)

STA-4783 is a potent oxidative stress inducer and, as a result, triggers apoptosis in cancer cells, showing therapeutic activity in malignant melanoma [113,114]. This drug is believed to interrupt the electron transport complex.

Isothiocyanate, Phenethyl Isothiocyanate, and Aziridine Derivatives

Several agents that cause GSH depletion exhibit anticancer activity in various types of cancer cells. Compounds such as benzyl isothiocyanate, phenethyl isothiocyanate, and aziridine derivatives have been found to have potent anticancer activities [115–117]. They deplete the GSH pool by binding to thiols.

Sulphasalazine

Sulphasalazine has been used in the treatment of inflammatory diseases. Because of its antiinflammatory effect, long-term therapy protects against cancer. Although phenotypic decreases in GSH synthesis are observed, the molecular mechanism is as yet unknown [117a].

Buthionine Sulphoximine

Buthionine sulphoximine is an inhibitor targeting GSH synthesis, especially the rate-limiting enzyme glutamylcysteine synthetase (γ-GCS) [118]. Buthionine sulphoximine also inhibits GSH synthesis by inhibiting the uptake of cystine, the precursor of cysteine [46,119].

Alpha-methyl-DL-tryptophan

Alpha-methyl-DL-tryptophan (α-MT) is a selective blocker of the sodium- and chloride-dependent neutral and basic amino acid transporter (SLC6A14). The inhibitor α-MT on human estrogen receptor-positive breast cancer cells caused cell death both in vitro and in vivo. Unlike ASCT2, which is upregulated by *c-myc* in most cancers, SLC6A14 upregulation is far less common. This lack of ubiquity in SLCA14 limits the chemotherapeutic potential of α-MT [119a].

1,2,3-Dithiazoles

1,2,3-Dithiazoles is one of the newly synthesized compounds to inhibit ASCT2 [119b]. Based on the observation that the inhibitory effect is released by addition of 1,4-dithiothreitol, this compound appears to cause a redox reaction onto the cysteine residues of ASCT2. Biological tests are yet to be made.

6-Diazo-5-oxo-L-norleucine and Bis-2-(5-phenylacetamido-1,2,4-thiadiazol-2-yl) ethyl Sulfide

6-Diazo-5-oxo-L-norleucine (DON) is a water-soluble glutamine analog. Studies have shown that DON binds to the glutamine pocket of GLS1 [120]. Compared to DON, bis-2-(5-phenylacetamido-1,2,4-thiadiazol-2-yl)ethyl sulfide binds to the allosteric pocket formed by the GLS1 dimeric interface according to the structural studies [121]. The two compounds ultimately act to decrease glutaminolysis in cancer cells by inhibiting the first enzyme, glutaminase 1.

PERSPECTIVE

There has recently been rapid progress in the study of cancer metabolism. It has been revealed that not only glycolysis, but also glutaminolysis, is significantly activated in cancer cells. Such metabolic changes concomitantly cause alterations in redox metabolism and ROS homeostasis. As a result, a number of proteins have emerged as potential targets for cancer therapy; their inhibitors are currently being developed. However, it is likely that studies of cancer metabolism would be more fruitful if combined with the fast-growing fields of epigenetics and metabolic profiling.

Epigenetic modifications of nucleic acids have to be linked to cellular metabolic status. Altered metabolism in cancer cells is suspected to cause changes in patterns of epigenetic modifications, just as the different metabolic needs of cancer cells cause changes in patterns of their metabolism. It is believed that an integrated approach between cancer metabolism and associated epigenetic modifications will make a valuable contribution to the understanding of cancer from viewpoints that are diversified yet unified.

Such comprehensive approaches are likely necessary to develop effective therapeutics. Cancer is not a single disease, but rather it is a group of diseases that stem from various causes resulting in unregulated cell growth. Ongoing research efforts with an additional focus on this integrated approach have the potential to lead to great discoveries in this exciting field. These efforts will also likely lead to significant contributions for other metabolic diseases, such as diabetes, stroke, and myocardial ischemia.

References

[1] Rolland F, Winderickx J, Thevelein JM. Glucose-sensing mechanisms in eukaryotic cells. Trends Biochem Sci 2001;26:310–7.

[2] McCord JM. Superoxide dismutase in aging and disease: an overview. Methods Enzymol 2002;349:331–41.

[3] Hsu PP, Sabatini DM. Cancer cell metabolism: Warburg and beyond. Cell 2008;134:703–7.

[4] Bergareche AM, Ruiz-Mirazo K. Metabolism and the problem of its universalization. Biosystems 1999;49:45–61.

[5] DeBerardinis RJ, Lum JJ, Hatzivassiliou G, Thompson CB. The biology of cancer: metabolic reprogramming fuels cell growth and proliferation. Cell Metab 2008;7:11–20.

[6] Bauer DE, Harris MH, Plas DR, Lum JJ, Hammerman PS, Rathmell JC, et al. Cytokine stimulation of aerobic glycolysis in hematopoietic cells exceeds proliferative demand. FASEB J 2004;18:1303–5.

[7] Vander Heiden MG, Cantley LC, Thompson CB. Understanding the Warburg effect: the metabolic requirements of cell proliferation. Science 2009;324:1029–33.

[8] Dirkx AE, Oude Egbrink MG, Wagstaff J, Griffioen AW. Monocyte/macrophage infiltration in tumors: modulators of angiogenesis. J Leukoc Biol 2006;80:1183–96.

[9] Wechalekar K, Sharma B, Cook G. PET/CT in oncology–a major advance. Clin Radiol 2005;60:1143–55.

[10] Welberg L. Metabolism: Spotlight on aerobic glycolysis. Nat Rev Neurosci 2010;11:729.

[11] Gatenby RA, Gillies RJ. Why do cancers have high aerobic glycolysis? Nat Rev Cancer 2004;4:891–9.

[12] Moreno-Sanchez R, Rodriguez-Enriquez S, Marin-Hernandez A, Saavedra E. Energy metabolism in tumor cells. FEBS J 2007;274:1393–418.

[13] Xu RH, Pelicano H, Zhou Y, Carew JS, Feng L, Bhalla KN, et al. Inhibition of glycolysis in cancer cells: a novel strategy to overcome drug resistance associated with mitochondrial respiratory defect and hypoxia. Cancer Res 2005;65:613–21.

[14] Warburg O. On the origin of cancer cells. Science 1956;123:309–14.

[15] Caro J. Hypoxia regulation of gene transcription. High Alt Med Biol 2001;2:145–54.

[16] Brahimi-Horn C, Pouyssegur J. The role of the hypoxia-inducible factor in tumor metabolism growth and invasion. Bull Cancer 2006;93:E73–80.

[17] Dang CV, Semenza GL. Oncogenic alterations of metabolism. Trends Biochem Sci 1999;24:68–72.

[18] Minchenko A, Leshchinsky I, Opentanova I, Sang N, Srinivas V, Armstead V, et al. Hypoxia-inducible factor-1-mediated expression of the 6-phosphofructo-2-kinase/fructose-2,6-bisphosphatase-3 (PFKFB3) gene. Its possible role in the Warburg effect. J Biol Chem 2002;277:6183–7.

[19] Ravi R, Mookerjee B, Bhujwalla ZM, Sutter CH, Artemov D, Zeng Q, et al. Regulation of tumor angiogenesis by p.53-induced degradation of hypoxia-inducible factor 1alpha. Genes Dev 2000;14:34–44.

[20] Levine AJ, Puzio-Kuter AM. The control of the metabolic switch in cancers by oncogenes and tumor suppressor genes. Science 2010;330:1340–4.

[21] Obach M, Navarro-Sabate A, Caro J, Kong X, Duran J, Gomez M, et al. 6-Phosphofructo-2-kinase (pfkfb3) gene promoter contains hypoxia-inducible factor-1 binding sites necessary for transactivation in response to hypoxia. J Biol Chem 2004;279:53562–70.

[22] Wise DR, DeBerardinis RJ, Mancuso A, Sayed N, Zhang XY, Pfeiffer HK, et al. Myc regulates a transcriptional program that stimulates mitochondrial glutaminolysis and leads to glutamine addiction. Proc Natl Acad Sci U S A 2008;105:18782–7.

[23] Gao P, Tchernyshyov I, Chang TC, Lee YS, Kita K, Ochi T, et al. c-Myc suppression of miR-23a/b enhances mitochondrial glutaminase expression and glutamine metabolism. Nature 2009;458:762–5.

[24] Dang CV, Le A, Gao P. MYC-induced cancer cell energy metabolism and therapeutic opportunities. Clin Cancer Res 2009;15:6479–83.

[25] Jones RG, Thompson CB. Tumor suppressors and cell metabolism: a recipe for cancer growth. Genes Dev 2009;23:537–48.

[26] Bui T, Thompson CB. Cancer's sweet tooth. Cancer Cell 2006;9:419–20.

[27] Holley AK, Dhar SK, St Clair DK. Curbing cancer's sweet tooth: is there a role for MnSOD in regulation of the Warburg effect? Mitochondrion 2012; [Epub ahead of print].

[28] Pfeiffer T, Schuster S, Bonhoeffer S. Cooperation and competition in the evolution of ATP-producing pathways. Science 2001;292:504–7.

[29] Williams AC, Collard TJ, Paraskeva C. An acidic environment leads to p53 dependent induction of apoptosis in human adenoma and carcinoma cell lines: implications for clonal selection during colorectal carcinogenesis. Oncogene 1999;18:3199–204.

[30] DeBerardinis RJ. Good neighbours in the tumour stroma reduce oxidative stress. Nat Cell Biol 2012;14:235–6.

[31] Pelicano H, Martin DS, Xu RH, Huang P. Glycolysis inhibition for anticancer treatment. Oncogene 2006;25:4633–46.

[32] Dang CV. Glutaminolysis: supplying carbon or nitrogen or both for cancer cells? Cell Cycle 2010;9:3884–6.

[33] Meng M, Chen S, Lao T, Liang D, Sang N. Nitrogen anabolism underlies the importance of glutaminolysis in proliferating cells. Cell Cycle 2010;9:3921–32.

[34] Feron O. Pyruvate into lactate and back: from the Warburg effect to symbiotic energy fuel exchange in cancer cells. Radiother Oncol 2009;92:329–33.

[35] Chen JQ, Russo J. Dysregulation of glucose transport, glycolysis, TCA cycle and glutaminolysis by oncogenes and tumor suppressors in cancer cells. Biochim Biophys Acta 2012;1826:370–84.

[36] Wise DR, Thompson CB. Glutamine addiction: a new therapeutic target in cancer. Trends Biochem Sci 2010;35:427–33.

[37] Wang JB, Erickson JW, Fuji R, Ramachandran S, Gao P, Dinavahi R, et al. Targeting mitochondrial glutaminase activity inhibits oncogenic transformation. Cancer Cell 2010;18:207–19.

[37a] Jones NP, Sculze A. Targeting cancer metabolism – aiming at a tumour's sweet-spot. Drug Discovery Today 2012;17:232–41.

[38] Dang CV. Rethinking the Warburg effect with Myc micromanaging glutamine metabolism. Cancer Res 2010;70:859–62.

[39] Elgadi KM, Meguid RA, Qian M, Souba WW, Abcouwer SF. Cloning and analysis of unique human glutaminase isoforms generated by tissue-specific alternative splicing. Physiol Genomics 1999;1:51–62.

[40] Erickson JW, Cerione RA. Glutaminase: a hot spot for regulation of cancer cell metabolism? Oncotarget 2010;1:734–40.

[41] Board M, Humm S, Newsholme EA. Maximum activities of key enzymes of glycolysis, glutaminolysis, pentose phosphate pathway and tricarboxylic acid cycle in normal, neoplastic and suppressed cells. Biochem J 1990;265:503–9.

[42] Lawless MW, O'Byrne KJ, Gray SG. Targeting oxidative stress in cancer. Expert Opin Ther Targets 2010;14:1225–45.

[43] Visconti R, Grieco D. New insights on oxidative stress in cancer. Curr Opin Drug Discov Dev 2009;12:240–5.

[44] Benz CC, Yau C. Ageing, oxidative stress and cancer: paradigms in parallax. Nat Rev Cancer 2008;8:875–9.

[45] Dreher D, Junod AF. Role of oxygen free radicals in cancer development. Eur J Cancer 1996;32A:30–8.

[46] Trachootham D, Alexandre J, Huang P. Targeting cancer cells by ROS-mediated mechanisms: a radical therapeutic approach? Nat Rev Drug Discov 2009;8:579–91.

[47] Valko M, Rhodes CJ, Moncol J, Izakovic M, Mazur M. Free radicals, metals and antioxidants in oxidative stress-induced cancer. Chem Biol Interact 2006;160:1–40.

[48] Perera RM, Bardeesy N. Cancer: when antioxidants are bad. Nature 2011;475:43–4.

[49] Wu WS. The signaling mechanism of ROS in tumor progression. Cancer Metastasis Rev 2006;25:695–705.

[50] Benhar M, Engelberg D, Levitzki A. ROS, stress-activated kinases and stress signaling in cancer. EMBO Rep 2002;3:420–5.

[51] Ushio-Fukai M. Compartmentalization of redox signaling through NADPH oxidase-derived ROS. Antioxid Redox Signal 2009;11:1289–99.

[52] Shackelford RE, Kaufmann WK, Paules RS. Oxidative stress and cell cycle checkpoint function. Free Radic Biol Med 2000;28:1387–404.

[53] Kopnin PB, Kravchenko IV, Furalyov VA, Pylev LN, Kopnin BP. Cell type-specific effects of asbestos on intracellular ROS levels, DNA oxidation and G1 cell cycle checkpoint. Oncogene 2004;23:8834–40.

[54] Deng X, Gao F, May Jr WS. Bcl2 retards G1/S cell cycle transition by regulating intracellular ROS. Blood 2003;102:3179–85.

[55] Chen J, Liu B, Yuan J, Yang J, Zhang J, An Y, et al. Atorvastatin reduces vascular endothelial growth factor (VEGF) expression in human non-small cell lung carcinomas (NSCLCs) via inhibition of reactive oxygen species (ROS) production. Mol Oncol 2012;6:62–72.

[56] Ishikawa K, Takenaga K, Akimoto M, Koshikawa N, Yamaguchi A, Imanishi H, et al. ROS-generating mitochondrial DNA mutations can regulate tumor cell metastasis. Science 2008;320:661–4.

[57] Simon HU, Haj-Yehia A, Levi-Schaffer F. Role of reactive oxygen species (ROS) in apoptosis induction. Apoptosis 2000;5:415–8.

[58] Tanaka H, Matsumura I, Ezoe S, Satoh Y, Sakamaki T, Albanese C, et al. E2F1 and c-Myc potentiate apoptosis through inhibition of NF-κB activity that facilitates MnSOD-mediated ROS elimination. Mol Cell 2002;9:1017–29.

[59] Singh KK. Mitochondrial dysfunction is a common phenotype in aging and cancer. Ann N Y Acad Sci 2004;1019:260–4.

[60] Modica-Napolitano JS, Singh KK. Mitochondrial dysfunction in cancer. Mitochondrion 2004;4:755–62.

[61] Finkel T, Holbrook NJ. Oxidants, oxidative stress and the biology of ageing. Nature 2000;408:239–47.

[62] Di Pietro G, Magno LA, Rios-Santos F. Glutathione S-transferases: an overview in cancer research. Expert Opin Drug Metab Toxicol 2010;6:153–70.

[63] Balendiran GK, Dabur R, Fraser D. The role of glutathione in cancer. Cell Biochem Funct 2004;22:343–52.

[64] Valko M, Leibfritz D, Moncol J, Cronin MT, Mazur M, Telser J. Free radicals and antioxidants in normal physiological functions and human disease. Int J Biochem Cell Biol 2007;39:44–84.

[65] Fridovich I. Superoxide radical and superoxide dismutases. Annu Rev Biochem 1995;64:97–112.

[66] Meister A, Anderson ME. Glutathione. Annu Rev Biochem 1983;52:711–60.

[67] Lushchak VI. Glutathione homeostasis and functions: potential targets for medical interventions. J Amino Acids 2012;2012:736837.

[68] Pastore A, Federici G, Bertini E, Piemonte F. Analysis of glutathione: implication in redox and detoxification. Clin Chim Acta 2003;333:19–39.

[69] Cooper AJ, Kristal BS. Multiple roles of glutathione in the central nervous system. J Biol Chem 1997;378:793–802.

[70] Franco R, Schoneveld OJ, Pappa A, Panayiotidis MI. The central role of glutathione in the pathophysiology of human diseases. Arch Physiol Biochem 2007;113:234–58.

[71] Schafer FQ, Buettner GR. Redox environment of the cell as viewed through the redox state of the glutathione disulfide/glutathione couple. Free Radic Biol Med 2001;30:1191–212.

[72] Cairns RA, Harris IS, Mak TW. Regulation of cancer cell metabolism. Nat Rev Cancer 2011;11:85–95.

[73] Dalle-Donne I, Rossi R, Giustarini D, Colombo R, Milzani A. S-glutathionylation in protein redox regulation. Free Radic Biol Med 2007;43:883–98.

[74] Dalle-Donne I, Rossi R, Colombo G, Giustarini D, Milzani A. Protein S-glutathionylation: a regulatory device from bacteria to humans. Trends Biochem Sci 2009;34:85–96.

[75] Shelton MD, Mieyal JJ. Regulation by reversible S-glutathionylation: molecular targets implicated in inflammatory diseases. Mol Cells 2008;25:332–46.

[76] Dulce RA, Schulman IH, Hare JM. S-glutathionylation: a redox-sensitive switch participating in nitroso-redox balance. Circ Res 2011;108:531–3.

[77] Mieyal JJ, Gallogly MM, Qanungo S, Sabens EA, Shelton MD. Molecular mechanisms and clinical implications of reversible protein S-glutathionylation. Antioxid Redox Signal 2008;10:1941–88.

[78] Cotgreave IA, Gerdes R, Schuppe-Koistinen I, Lind C. S-glutathionylation of glyceraldehyde-3-phosphate dehydrogenase: role of thiol oxidation and catalysis by glutaredoxin. Methods Enzymol 2002;348:175–82.

[79] Shenton D, Perrone G, Quinn KA, Dawes IW, Grant CM. Regulation of protein S-thiolation by glutaredoxin 5 in the yeast *Saccharomyces cerevisiae*. J Biol Chem 2002;277:16853–9.

[80] Luo W, Semenza GL. Emerging roles of PKM2 in cell metabolism and cancer progression. Trends Endocrinol Metab 2012;23:560–6.

[81] Anastasiou D, Poulogiannis G, Asara JM, Boxer MB, Jiang JK, Shen M, et al. Inhibition of pyruvate kinase M2 by reactive oxygen species contributes to cellular antioxidant responses. Science 2011;334:1278–83.

[81a] Seo M, Lee YH. PFKFB3 regulates oxidative stress homeostasis via its S-glutathionylation in cancer. Submitted for publication.

[82] Yi W, Clark PM, Mason DE, Keenan MC, Hill C, Goddard 3rd WA, et al. Phosphofructokinase 1 glycosylation regulates cell growth and metabolism. Science 2012;337:975–80.

[82a] Slawson C, Hart GW. Alterations in O-GlcNAc signaling: implications for cancer cell biology. Nature Reviews Cancer 2011;11:678–84.

[83] Medina RA, Owen GI. Glucose transporters: expression, regulation and cancer. Biol Res 2002;35:9–26.

[84] Smith TA. Facilitative glucose transporter expression in human cancer tissue. Br J Biomed Sci 1999;56:285–92.

[85] Chan DA, Sutphin PD, Nguyen P, Turcotte S, Lai EW, Banh A, et al. Targeting GLUT1 and the Warburg effect in renal cell carcinoma by chemical synthetic lethality. Sci Transl Med 2011;3; 94ra70.

[86] Chan SS, Lotspeich WD. Comparative effects of phlorizin and phloretin on glucose transport in the cat kidney. Am J Physiol 1962;203:975–9.

[87] Wu CH, Ho YS, Tsai CY, Wang YJ, Tseng H, Wei PL, et al. In vitro and in vivo study of phloretin-induced apoptosis in human liver cancer cells involving inhibition of type II glucose transporter. Int J Cancer 2009;124:2210–9.

[88] Mathupala SP, Rempel A, Pedersen PL. Glucose catabolism in cancer cells: identification and characterization of a marked activation response of the type II hexokinase gene to hypoxic conditions. J Biol Chem 2001;276:43407–12.

[89] Porporato PE, Dhup S, Dadhich RK, Copetti T, Sonveaux P. Anticancer targets in the glycolytic metabolism of tumors: a comprehensive review. Front Pharmacol 2011;2:49.

[90] Ben Sahra I, Laurent K, Giuliano S, Larbret F, Ponzio G, Gounon P, et al. Targeting cancer cell metabolism: the combination of metformin and 2-deoxyglucose induces p53-dependent apoptosis in prostate cancer cells. Cancer Res 2010;70:2465–75.

[91] Ganapathy-Kanniappan S, Vali M, Kunjithapatham R, Buijs M, Syed LH, Rao PP, et al. 3-bromopyruvate: a new targeted antiglycolytic agent and a promise for cancer therapy. Curr Pharm Biotechnol 2010;11:510–7.

[92] Miyato Y, Ando K. Apoptosis of human melanoma cells by a combination of lonidamine and radiation. J Radiat Res 2004;45:189–94.

[93] Calvino E, Estan MC, Simon GP, Sancho P, Boyano-Adanez Mdel C, de Blas E, et al. Increased apoptotic efficacy of lonidamine plus arsenic trioxide combination in human leukemia cells. Reactive oxygen species generation and defensive protein kinase (MEK/ERK, Akt/mTOR) modulation. Biochem Pharmacol 2011;82:1619–29.

[94] Reinhart GD, Lardy HA. Rat liver phosphofructokinase: kinetic activity under near-physiological conditions. Biochemistry 1980;19:1477–84.

[95] Furuya E, Uyeda K. An activation factor of liver phosphofructokinase. Proc Natl Acad Sci U S A 1980;77:5861–4.

[96] Manzano A, Rosa JL, Ventura F, Perez JX, Nadal M, Estivill X, et al. Molecular cloning, expression, and chromosomal localization of a ubiquitously expressed human 6-phosphofructo-2-kinase/fructose-2, 6-bisphosphatase gene (PFKFB3). Cytogenet Cell Genet 1998;83:214–7.

[97] Sakakibara R, Okudaira T, Fujiwara K, Kato M, Hirata T, Yamanaka S, et al. Tissue distribution of placenta-type 6-phosphofructo- 2-kinase/fructose-2,6-bisphosphatase. Biochem Biophys Res Commun 1999;257:177–81.

[98] Hamilton JA, Callaghan MJ, Sutherland RL, Watts CK. Identification of PRG1, a novel progestin-responsive gene with sequence homology to 6-phosphofructo-2-kinase/fructose-2,6-bisphosphatase. Mol Endocrinol 1997;11:490–502.

[99] Chesney J, Mitchell R, Benigni F, Bacher M, Spiegel L, Al-Abed Y, et al. An inducible gene product for 6-phosphofructo-2-kinase with an AU-rich instability element: role in tumor cell glycolysis and the Warburg effect. Proc Natl Acad Sci U S A 1999;96:3047–52.

[100] Clem B, Telang S, Clem A, Yalcin A, Meier J, Simmons A, et al. Small-molecule inhibition of 6-phosphofructo-2-kinase activity suppresses glycolytic flux and tumor growth. Mol Cancer Ther 2008;7:110–20.

[101] Seo M, Kim JD, Neau D, Sehgal I, Lee YH. Structure-based development of small molecule PFKFB3 inhibitors: a framework for potential cancer therapeutic agents targeting the Warburg effect. PLoS One 2011;6:e24179.

[102] Lee KC, Shorr R, Rodriguez R, Maturo C, Boteju LW, Sheldon A. Formation and anti-tumor activity of uncommon in vitro and in vivo metabolites of CPI-613, a novel anti-tumor compound that selectively alters tumor energy metabolism. Drug Metab Lett 2011;5:163–82.

[103] Zachar Z, Marecek J, Maturo C, Gupta S, Stuart SD, Howell K, et al. Non-redox-active lipoate derivates disrupt cancer cell mitochondrial metabolism and are potent anticancer agents in vivo. J Mol Med (Berl) 2011;89:1137–48.

[104] Cheong H, Lu C, Lindsten T, Thompson CB. Therapeutic targets in cancer cell metabolism and autophagy. Nat Biotechnol 2012;30:671–8.

[105] Bonnet S, Archer SL, Allalunis-Turner J, Haromy A, Beaulieu C, Thompson R, et al. A mitochondria-K$^+$ channel axis is suppressed in cancer and its normalization promotes apoptosis and inhibits cancer growth. Cancer Cell 2007;11:37–51.

[106] Mazurek S, Boschek CB, Hugo F, Eigenbrodt E. Pyruvate kinase type M2 and its role in tumor growth and spreading. Semin Cancer Biol 2005;15:300–8.

[107] Gupta V, Bamezai RN. Human pyruvate kinase M2: a multifunctional protein. Protein Sci 2010;19:2031–44.

[108] Shim H, Dolde C, Lewis BC, Wu CS, Dang G, Jungmann RA, et al. c-Myc transactivation of LDH-A: implications for tumor metabolism and growth. Proc Natl Acad Sci U S A 1997;94:6658–63.

[109] Qing G, Skuli N, Mayes PA, Pawel B, Martinez D, Maris JM, et al. Combinatorial regulation of neuroblastoma tumor progression by N-Myc and hypoxia inducible factor HIF-1alpha. Cancer Res 2010;70:10351–61.

[110] Fantin VR, St-Pierre J, Leder P. Attenuation of LDH-A expression uncovers a link between glycolysis, mitochondrial physiology, and tumor maintenance. Cancer Cell 2006;9:425–34.

[111] Hour TC, Huang CY, Lin CC, Chen J, Guan JY, Lee JM, et al. Characterization of molecular events in a series of bladder urothelial carcinoma cell lines with progressive resistance to arsenic trioxide. Anticancer Drugs 2004;15:779–85.

[112] Zhou P, Kalakonda N, Comenzo RL. Changes in gene expression profiles of multiple myeloma cells induced by arsenic trioxide (ATO): possible mechanisms to explain ATO resistance in vivo. Br J Haematol 2005;128:636–44.

[113] Tuma RS. Reactive oxygen species may have antitumor activity in metastatic melanoma. J Natl Cancer Inst 2008;100:11–2.

[114] Kirshner JR, He S, Balasubramanyam V, Kepros J, Yang CY, Zhang M, et al. Elesclomol induces cancer cell apoptosis through oxidative stress. Mol Cancer Ther 2008;7:2319–27.

[115] Dvorakova K, Payne CM, Tome ME, Briehl MM, McClure T, Dorr RT. Induction of oxidative stress and apoptosis in myeloma cells by the aziridine-containing agent imexon. Biochem Pharmacol 2000;60:749–58.

[116] Xu K, Thornalley PJ. Involvement of glutathione metabolism in the cytotoxicity of the phenethyl isothiocyanate and its cysteine conjugate to human leukaemia cells in vitro. Biochem Pharmacol 2001;61:165–77.

[117] Zhang Y, Talalay P. Anticarcinogenic activities of organic isothiocyanates: chemistry and mechanisms. Cancer Res 1994;54:1976s–81s.

[117a] Narang VS, Pauletti GM, Gout PW, Buckley DJ, Buckley AR. Sulfasalazine-induced reduction of glutathione levels in breast cancer cells: enhancement of growth-inhibitory activity of doxorubicin. Chemotherapy 2007;53:210–7.

[118] Griffith OW, Meister A. Potent and specific inhibition of glutathione synthesis by buthionine sulfoximine (S-n-butyl homocysteine sulfoximine). J Biol Chem 1979;254:7558–60.

[119] Lo M, Wang YZ, Gout PW. The x(c)-cystine/glutamate antiporter: a potential target for therapy of cancer and other diseases. J Cell Physiol 2008;215:593–602.

[119a] Karunakaran S, Ramachandran S, Coothankandaswamy V, Elangovan S, Babu E, Periyasamy-Thandavan S, et al. SLC6A14 (ATB0,+) protein, a highly concentrative and broad specific amino acid transporter, is a novel and effective drug target for treatment of estrogen receptor-positive breast cancer. J Biol Chem 2011;286:31830–8.

[119b] Oppedisano F, Catto M, Koutentis PA, Nicolotti O, Pochini L, Koyioni M, et al. Inactivation of the glutamine/amino acid transporter ASCT2 by 1,2,3-dithiazoles: proteoliposomes as a tool to gain insights in the molecular mechanism of action and of antitumor activity. Toxicol Appl Pharmacol 2012;265:93–102.

[120] Shapiro RA, Clark VM, Curthoys NP. Inactivation of rat renal phosphate-dependent glutaminase with 6-diazo-5-oxo-L-norleucine. Evidence for interaction at the glutamine binding site. J Biol Chem 1979;254:2835–8.

[121] Thangavelu K, Pan CQ, Karlberg T, Balaji G, Uttamchandani M, Suresh V, et al. Structural basis for the allosteric inhibitory mechanism of human kidney-type glutaminase (KGA) and its regulation by Raf-Mek-Erk signaling in cancer cell metabolism. Proc Natl Acad Sci U S A 2012;109:7705–10.

CHAPTER

15

Inhibitors of the Phosphatidylinositol 3-Kinase Pathway

William A. Denny, Gordon W. Rewcastle

Auckland Cancer Society Research Centre, School of Medical Sciences, University of Auckland, New Zealand

INTRODUCTION

The class 1A phosphatidylinositol 3-kinases (PI3Ks) catalyze the 3′-phosphorylation of phosphatidylinositol 4,5-diphosphate (PIP2) to produce primarily the important "second messenger" lipid phosphatidylinositol 3,4,5-triphosphate (PIP3) (Fig. 15.1). They exist as heterodimers of one of two regulatory subunits (p85 or p55) linked to one of three catalytic p110 subunits (α, β, or δ). The regulatory subunits are encoded by the genes PIKR1, PIKR2, and PIKR3 and respond primarily to signals from transmembrane receptor tyrosine kinases, while the p110 catalytic subunits are encoded by the genes PIK3CA, PIK3CB, and PIK3CD, respectively. The related class 1B PI3K consists of the catalytic subunit p110γ associated with regulatory subunits p84–p87 and p101, and responds primarily to signals from G protein-coupled receptors (GPCRs) [1]. The p110α and p110β isoforms occur

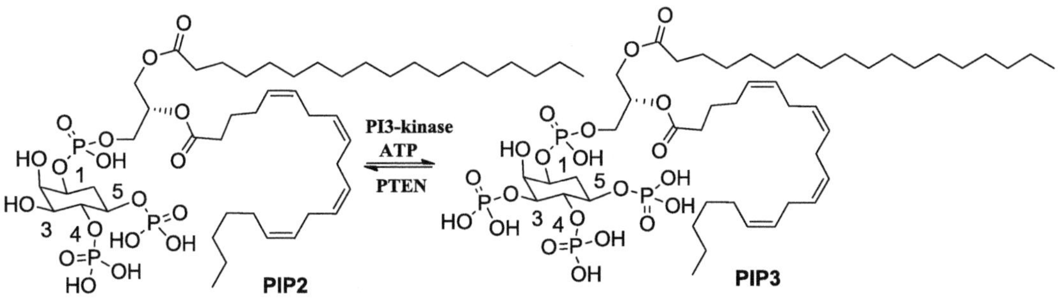

FIGURE 15.1 Function of phosphatidylinositol 3-kinase (PI3K).

Cancer Drug Design and Discovery, Second Edition
http://dx.doi.org/10.1016/B978-0-12-396521-9.00015-2

ubiquitously, whereas p110γ and p110δ are found primarily in leucocytes [2]. The class II (PI3K-C2α, PI3K-C2β, and PI3K-C2γ) [3] and class III [4] PI3Ks have roles in regulating membrane and vesicle trafficking, respectively, but have not to date been targets for inhibitor design. The class I and II PI3Ks control many signaling pathways that regulate cell growth, proliferation, survival, and migration, primarily through their generation of PIP3, which recruits the serine–threonine kinase protein kinase B (PKB/Akt) via binding to its pleckstrin-homology domain [5,6], allowing activating phosphorylations on Thr308 and Ser473 of Akt [7,8]. The action of PI3K is regulated by the phosphatase PTEN, which converts PIP_3 back to PIP_2, thereby suppressing excessive growth due to PIP_3 recruitment of AKT to the membrane [9].

To date, the primary target for the development of inhibitors has been p110α (typically called PI3Kα). This is because it alone among the isoforms is known to be frequently mutated in a significant proportion of many human cancers, notably ovarian, breast, gastric, brain, and colon (up to 30% in some types) [10–12]. Although mutations occur at many positions, the vast majority are at only two sites: in the helical domain (E542K and E545K) and the kinase domain (H1047R). While such mutants do show modest increases in catalytic efficiency, it is not entirely clear what their oncogenic potential is. While the other isoforms do not show mutations, p110β is overexpressed in colon and bladder cancers, and p110δ in acute myeloid leukemia and several other cancers [13].

MECHANISM OF INHIBITION

In common with the vast majority of the small-molecule inhibitors of protein kinases, PI3K inhibitors target the ATP site, binding competitively with ATP. This is not surprising, since they share many structural motifs with the protein kinases, including an overall two-lobe architecture, a DFG (asp–phe–gly) loop for magnesium ion coordination [14], and similar motifs for the process phosphate transfer from ATP. A crystal structure of ATP bound to p110γ [15] shows that the N1 of ATP accepts an H-bond from Val882, with the NH_2 donating to Glu880. It is thus not surprising that many crystal structures of PI3K–inhibitor complexes show H-bonding to Val882 as a key binding component.

EVOLUTION OF THE MAJOR CLASSES OF PI3K INHIBITORS

In comparison to the large family of inhibitors of the erbB receptor tyrosine kinases, which are dominated by a single 4-anilinoquinazoline motif, overall the PI3K kinase inhibitors are surprisingly structurally diverse. This is likely due to a somewhat more open ATP-binding site, as well as the search for selective inhibitors of each of the four isoforms, due to their distinct biological roles (in contrast, in erbB the search has mainly been for pan-inhibitors). Despite this diversity, some major structural classes of the different isoforms of PI3K, and their evolution, can be discerned. The main focus of the following discussion is compounds that reached clinical trial, together with some experimental compounds of particular interest.

PAN-INHIBITORS OF PI3K AND MTOR

Although selectivity for p110α was an early driving force (and remains one) behind PI3K inhibitor development, many of the early precursor compounds were not very isoform selective, but they are included on structural grounds.

LY294002 and Related Morpholino Compounds (Fig. 15.2)

The 2-morpholino-8-phenyl-4H-chromen-4-one LY294002 (**1**), from a library of Lilly synthetic compounds, is not a very potent or selective PI3K inhibitor [16,17], but it was the first widely studied one. Structure–activity relationship (SAR) studies showed that the morpholine was essential for inhibitory activity, and a crystal structure of a complex with 110γ showed the morpholine oxygen was an H-bond acceptor from the NH of Val882 [15]. In efforts to improve the short half-life of LY294002, the chromenone oxygen was alkylated through attachment of an integrin-targeted CH_2O–succinyl–Arg–Gly–Asp–Ser–CO_2H tetrapeptide unit to give SF1126 (**2**) [18,19]. In a panel of aggressive B-NHL tumor cell lines, SF1126 showed $IC_{50}s < 4\,\mu M$; decreased phosphorylation of Akt and GSK-3β, confirming the mechanism of action of a PI3K inhibitor; and induced dose-dependent apoptosis [20]. In a phase I clinical study in CD20+ B-cell malignancies, the maximum dose given was $1110\,mg/m^2$, with no dose-limiting toxicity. Stable disease was seen in 19 out of 33 (58%) of the evaluable patients [21].

In an alternative approach, attachment of a cleavable peptide linker at the 4-position of the LY294002 phenyl ring produced a prodrug that is a substrate for the prostate-specific antigen (PSA) protease [22]. The result is a water-soluble and latent PI3K inhibitor prodrug (**3**) whose activation is dependent on PSA cleavage. Once activated, the resulting leucine–O–CH_2–LY294002 (**4**) can specifically inhibit PI3K in PSA-secreting prostate cancer cells and induce apoptosis with a potency comparable to that of LY294002 itself [22].

The structural lead provided by LY294002 has been followed by numerous morpholine-containing pan-PI3K and mTOR (mammalian Target Of Rapamycin) inhibitors. The tricyclic analog PI-103 (**5**) showed much more potent broad-spectrum inhibition across the PI3K isoforms and the downstream kinase mTOR [23–25], but it had a relatively short plasma half-life (0.7 h in mice), via glucuronidation of the phenol, and was insoluble [26]; however, it was an influential compound due to its good cellular and in vivo activity. Thus, several other related inhibitors containing phenol substituents have also been investigated subsequently, but none has advanced further due to the glucuronidation problem [27–31].

Further modification of PI-103 led to the thienopyrimidine series, of which GDC-0941 (**6**) was an important member. In this compound, the half-life was improved by replacement of the phenol with an indazole, and solubility and oral bioavailability were improved with a piperazinesulfonamide [32]. X-ray analysis of a co-crystal of GDC-0941 with p110γ again showed the morpholine oxygen H-bonded to Val882, with the indazole H-bonded (NH to Asp841 and the adjacent C=N to Tyr867) and with the core thiopyrimidine located in the adenine-binding site [32,33]. Combination treatment of GDC-0941 and the MEK inhibitor GDC-0973 in animal models showed that intermittent inhibition of the PI3K and MAPK pathway is efficacious in BRAF and KRAS mutant tumors, inducing apoptosis [34]. Preclinical pharmacokinetic studies of GDC-0941 in animal models showed extensive plasma protein

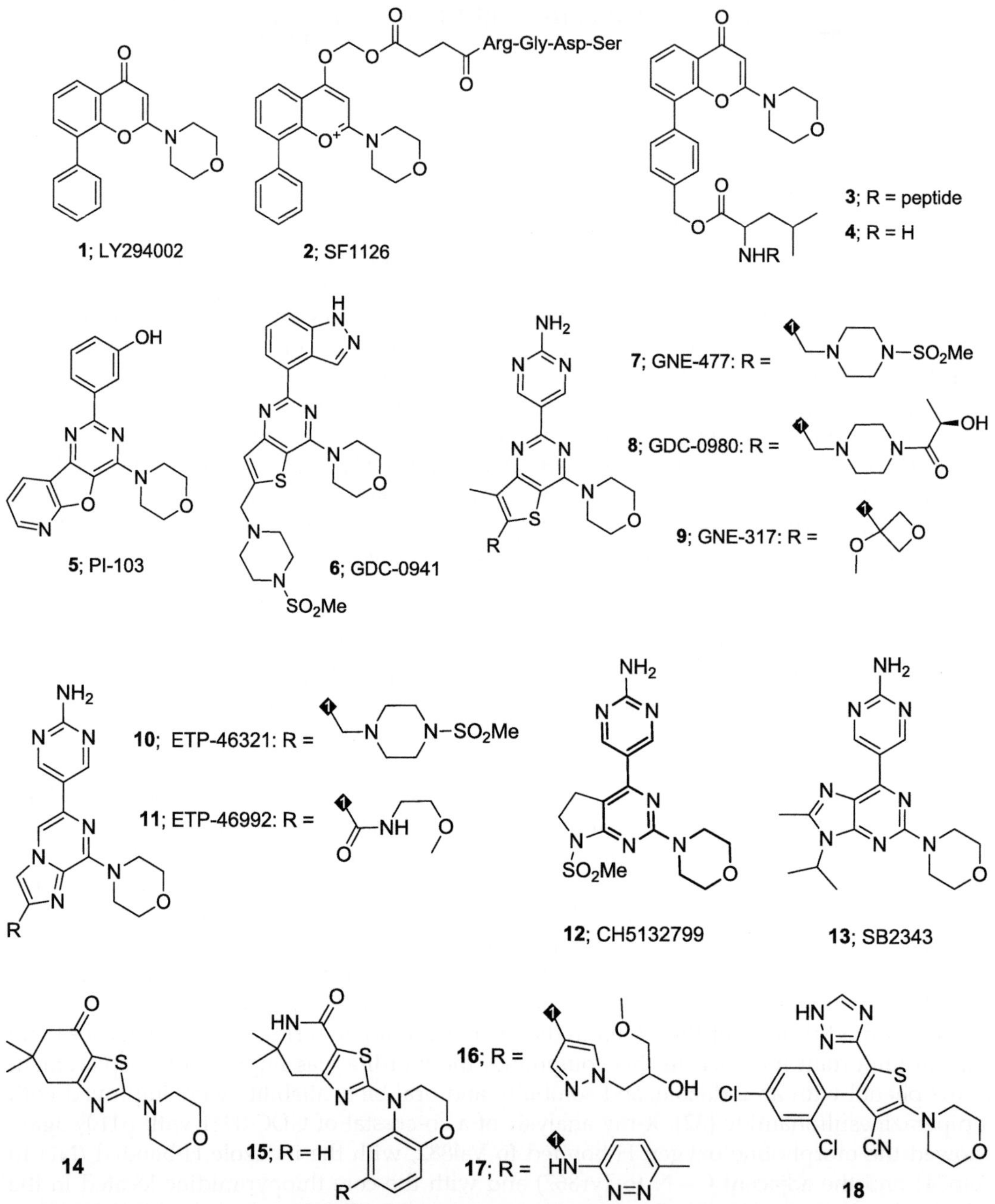

FIGURE 15.2 LY294002 and related morpholino compounds.

binding, with predicted moderate human hepatic clearance. GDC-0941 is in phase II clinical trials [35,36].

The analogs GNE-477 (**7**) and GDC-0980 (**8**) have been developed more recently, and they are both potent dual PI3K–mTOR inhibitors [37,38]. GNE-477 showed excellent growth inhibition in PC3 prostate tumor xenografts at 20 mg/kg/day [37]. Substitution of the indazole in GDC-0941 with a 2-aminopyrimidine group provided the analog GDC-0980, which is also a broad-spectrum PI3K kinase inhibitor with added mTOR potency [38]. It was selected for clinical trials on the basis of good potency in cancer cell lines, low clearance and high free fraction in mice, and good efficacy in xenograft assays [38]. It is a potent inhibitor of signal transduction downstream of both PI3K and mTOR; induced both G1 cell cycle arrest and apoptosis in cancer cell lines; inhibited tumor growth in xenograft models, including those with activated PI3K, or loss of LKB1 or PTEN; and has entered clinical trials [39]. Crystal structure studies with p110γ show that the morpholine oxygen is again H-bonded to Val882, with Asp836 and Asp841 in these cases interacting with the 2-NH_2 and N2, respectively, of the aminopyrimidine moiety [38]. GDC-0980 had low plasma protein binding and hepatic clearance, but was a P-glycoprotein and breast cancer resistance protein substrate. It is in phase II clinical trials [40].

Replacing the piperazine units of GDC-0941, GDC-0980, and GNE-477 with an oxetane group gave GNE-317 (**9**), which was optimized to cross the blood–brain barrier [41,42]. Changing the thiopyrimidine core to imidazo[1,2-*a*]pyrazine gave inhibitors such as ETP-46321 (**10**) and ETP-46992 (**11**), which are dual p110α/δ inhibitors with good selectivity against the other two isoforms and mTOR [43–45]. Other examples of morpholino derivatives also containing a 2-aminopyrimidine group include pyridylamino-pyrimidines [46], imidazolyl-pyrimidines [47], and the dihydropyrrolopyrimidine CH5132799 (**12**), which is currently in clinical trials [48,49]. CH5132799 is a selective Class I PI3K inhibitor with potent antitumor activity against tumors harboring PIK3CA mutations, but only low potency against mTOR [48,49]. In contrast, the planar purine derivative SB2343 (**13**), which also contains both the 2-aminopyrimidine and morpholino substituents, is reported to be a dual pan-inhibitor of PI3K and mTOR [50]. Other examples of morpholino-substituted bicyclic heterocycles to be investigated include pyrazolo[3,4-*d*]pyrimidines [51], imidazo[4,5-*d*]pyrimidines (purines) [52], pyrrolo[2,3-*d*]- and [3,2-*d*]pyrimidines [53], and 1,2,3-triazolo[4,5-*d*]pyrimidines [54].

Although its precise chemical structure is still classified, the dual p110α–mTOR inhibitor PWT33597 also fits within the general class of morpholino-substituted PI3K inhibitors [55]. PWT33597 inhibits p110α and mTOR with IC_{50} values of 19 and 14 nM, respectively, and is approximately 10-fold selective with respect to p110γ and p110δ. PWT33597 has good pharmacokinetic properties in multiple preclinical species, and showed durable inhibition of PI3K and mTOR pathway signaling in xenograft tumors [55]. PWT33597 entered clinical trials in July 2011.

Morpholino-substituted PI3K inhibitors are not restricted to six-membered-ring examples, and a series of 2-morpholino-thiazole derivatives have also been investigated. Thus, starting with the "virtual screening hit" **14** [56], SAR development led to the lactam **15** [57] and subsequently to multiisoform inhibitors **16** and **17**, which were optimized for cellular and pharmacological activity [58]. Finally, the tetra-substituted morpholino-thiophene **18** displayed subnanomolar potency against p110α and greater than 7000-fold selectivity against mTOR [59].

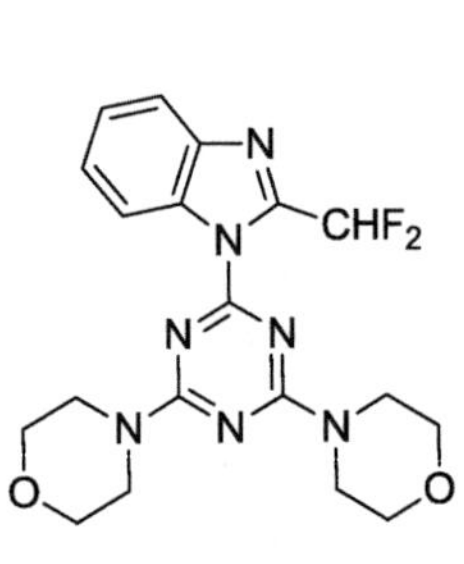

19; ZSTK474 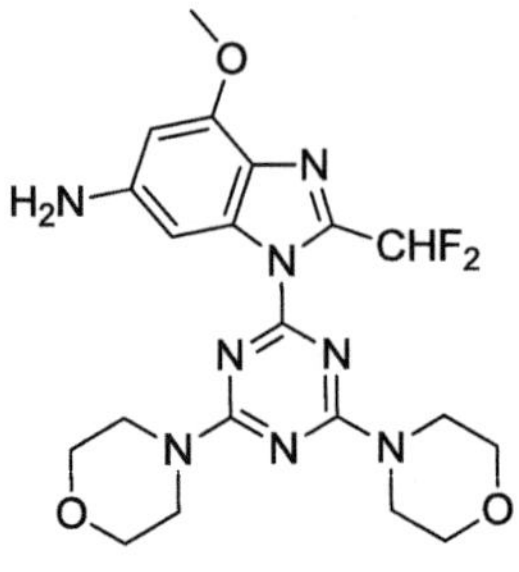   **20** 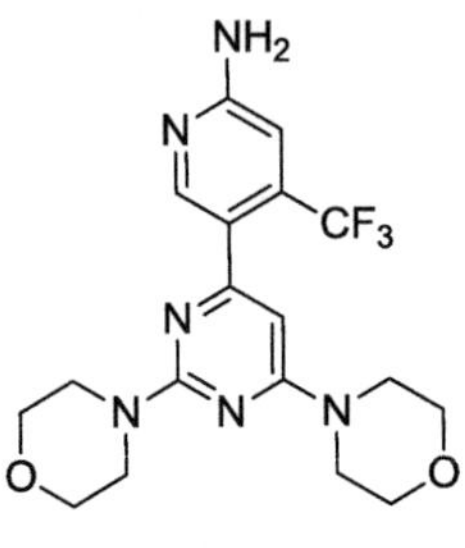   **21**; BKM120

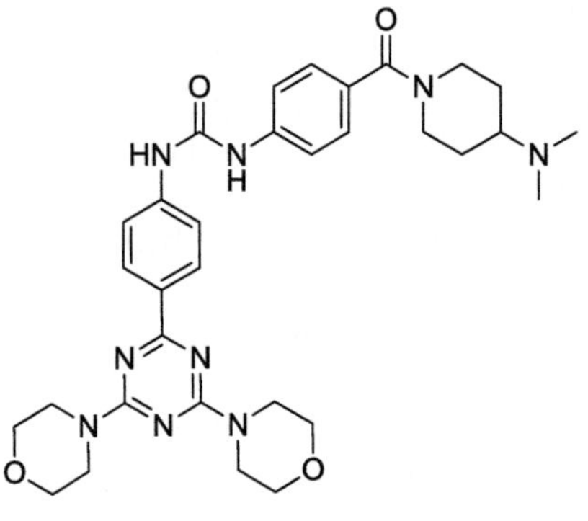

22; PKI-587/PF-05212384 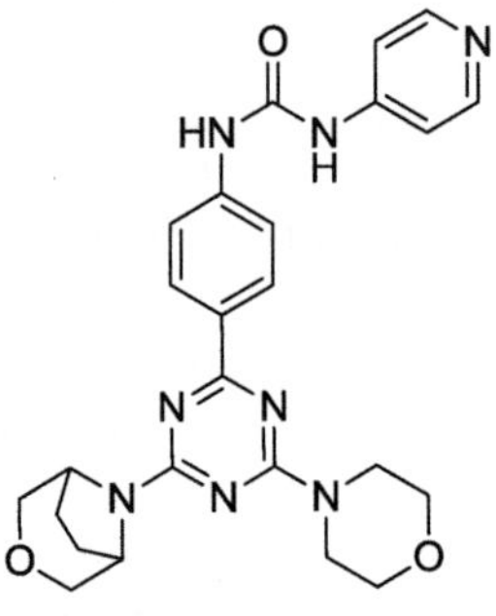   **23**; PKI-179

FIGURE 15.3   Dimorpholinopyrimidines and triazines.

Dimorpholinopyrimidines and Triazines (Fig. 15.3)

ZSTK474 (**19**) is an early triazine-based compound that was found from a screen evaluating compounds for antiproliferative activity in cancer cell lines; it is a moderately potent but relatively nonselective inhibitor of PI3 kinases [60], although it is selective for the class I PI3K isoforms over mTOR [61]. A recent crystal structure of ZSTK474 bound in the p110δ active site has shown that it binds in the same way as other morpholine-containing inhibitors [62], with one of the morpholine oxygen atoms making a critical H-bond to the hinge region Val828 residue (equivalent to Val882 in p110γ), and the benzimidazole N3 making another H-bond to Lys779 (Lys833 in p110γ). The important CHF_2 group forms a hydrogen bond contact to Pro758 in the hydrophobic affinity pocket. ZSTK474 is reported to be in phase I clinical trials [63]. The 6-amino-4-methoxy analog **20** is 15- to 75-fold more potent than ZSTK474 against the isolated PI3K enzymes (Table 15.1) and showed good inhibitory activity in a U87MG human glioblastoma xenograft [64].

The dimorpholinopyrimidine derivative NVP-BKM120 (**21**) is a moderately potent PI3K inhibitor, showing IC_{50} values from 50 to 250nM across the isoforms and 4600nM for mTOR (Table 15.1), and good in vivo efficacy in tumor xenograft models with PI3K pathway deregulation (A2780 ovarian and U87MG glioma) [66]. The loss of mTOR activity compared to NVP-BEZ235 (see next section) is considered due to the loss of a key interaction with the Ser774 residue of PI3K that was proposed to also be important for mTOR inhibition [66]. In a broad tumor cell line panel, BKM120 preferentially inhibited cells bearing PIK3CA rather

TABLE 15.1 Inhibition of PI3K Isoforms and mTOR by Inhibitors

| Inhibitor | IC$_{50}$ (nM)[a] | | | | | |
	p110α	p1I0β	p110δ	p110γ	mTOR	Ref.
PI3K and PI3K–mTOR						
1 (LY294002)	720	306	1330	7260		[65]
5 (PI-103)	2	3	3	15	<500	[26]
6 (GDC-0941)	3	33	3	75	580[b]	[32]
7 (GNE-477)	4	86	6	15	21	[37]
8 (GDC-0980)	5	27	7	14	17	[38]
9 (GNE-317)	2[b]				9[b]	[41]
10 (ETP-46321)	2.3[b]	170[b]	14[b]	179[b]	4880	[44]
11 (ETP-46992)	2.4[b]	94[b]	8[b]	63[b]	>3000	[45]
12 (CH5132799)	14	120	500	36	1600	[48]
13 (SB2343)	16	68	42	25	37	[50]
PWT33597	19		337	167	14	[55]
14	1333	693	701	3453		[56]
15		1226	1631	959		[57]
16			14	52		[58]
17			4	20		[58]
18	0.35[b]				2470[b]	[59]
19 (ZSTK474)	17	53	6			[60]
20	0.2	1.4	0.4			[64]
21 (NVP-BKM120)	52	166	116	262	4600	[66]
22 (PKI-587/ PF-05212384)	0.4	6	6	8	1.6	[67]
23 (PKI-179)	8	24	74	77	0.42	[68]
24 (NVP-BEZ235)	4	75	7	5	21	[69]
26 (PF-04979064)	0.13[b]		0.12[b]	0.11[b]	1.4[b]	[70]
27 (PIK-90)	11	350	58	18	1050	[25]
28 (BAY 80–6946)	0.5	3.7	0.7	6.4	45	[71]
29 (PF-04691502)	0.6[b]				16[b]	[72]
33 (GSK1059615)	0.4[b]	0.6[b]	1.7[b]	4.7[b]		[73]
34 (GSK2126458)	0.04	0.13[b]	0.024[b]	0.06[b]		[74]
35	4.6	13	4.3	8.1	3.9	[75]

(Continued)

TABLE 15.1   Inhibition of PI3K Isoforms and mTOR by Inhibitors   (cont'd)

Inhibitor	IC$_{50}$ (nM)[a]					
	p110α	p1I0β	p110δ	p110γ	mTOR	Ref.
38	1.2[b]	2.0[b]	1.2[b]	4.7[b]	2.0	[76]
39	1.4[b]	3.5[b]	0.8[b]	1.9[b]	0.4	[77]
41	7.7[b]	0.6[b]	0.4[b]	1.0[b]	163	[78]
43	25					[79]
44 (AMG 511)	4[b]	6[b]	2[b]	1[b]	>10^4	[80]
45 (GNE-614)	5	60	2	5	530	[81]
Alpha						
46	670					[82]
47	1.8					[82]
48	2.8	170		230		[82]
49 (PIK75)	6	1300	510	76	>1000	[25]
50	3.8	230	150			[83]
51	0.9	46	49			[83]
52 (NVP-BYL719)	5	1200	290			[84]
53 (NVS-PI3-1)	5[b]	2000[b]	220[b]	530[b]	>9100[b]	[85]
54 (A66)	32	>12,500	>1250	3480	>5000	[86]
Beta						
55 (TGX221)	5000	5	100	>10^4		[87]
56 (AZD6482/KIN-193)	136	0.69	14	48	3930	[88]
59 (GSK2636771)	>5800	5.2	58	>12,600	>50,000	[89]
60	2000	1	8	1000	32	[90]
61	320	0.3	4	60	6.3	[91]
62	2500	0.6	20	790		[92]
64	27,200	38	168	97		[93]
65	2138	42	118	>10^4		[94]
66	>10^4	99	1395	>10^4		[95]
Delta						
67 (IC87114)	>10^5	75,000	500	29,000		[96]
68 (PIK39)	>10^5	11,000	180	17,000	>10^5	[25]
69 (SW13)	1300	220	0.7	33		[62]

TABLE 15.1 Inhibition of PI3K Isoforms and mTOR by Inhibitors (cont'd)

| Inhibitor | IC$_{50}$ (nM)[a] | | | | | |
	p110α	p1I0β	p110δ	p110γ	mTOR	Ref.
70 (CAL-101/GS-1101)	820	565	2.5	89	>10^3	[97]
71	1290	760	3.8	1560	>10^3	[98]
72	78	680	2.7	630		[99]
73	168	547	2	>10^4		[100]
Gamma						
74 (AS-605240)	60	270	300	8		[101]
75 (AS-604850)	4500	>10^4	>10^4	250		[101]
76 (AS-252424)	940	20,000	20,000	30		[65]
77 (CZC24832)	>10^4	1100	>10^6	27		[102]
78	435	2059	690	18	623	[103]
79		15		3		[104]
Delta/gamma						
80 (TG100-115)	1300	1200	235	83		[105]
81	411	391	22	5		[105]
82 (IPI-145)	1602	85	2.5	27		[106]
Beta/delta						
83	41,000	60	360	18,000		[107]
Irreversible						
86 (wortmannin)	4	0.7	4.1	9		[108]
88 (PX-866)	5.5	>300	2.7	9		[108]

[a] Note variability in assay conditions.
[b] K_i values

than KRAS or PTEN mutations, was active (i.e., showed significant inhibition of p-Akt and tumor growth) in a range of xenograft models, and was synergistic in combination with MEK inhibitors [109]. A phase I study of once-daily (qd) dosing of BKM120 showed a maximum tolerated dose (MTD) of 100 mg/day, and concluded that the drug was well tolerated, with a favorable pharmacokinetic profile and clear evidence of target inhibition (phosphorylated ribosomal protein S6) [110]. BKM120 is currently in phase II clinical trial.

The triazine analog PKI-587 (PF-05212384) (**22**) is also a dual p110α–mTOR inhibitor, with IC$_{50}$ values of 0.4 nM and 1.6 nM, respectively (Table 15.1) [67]. In cell lines, growth inhibition in MDA-361 tumor cells by PKI-587 correlated with suppression of the PI3K–mTOR signaling pathway, and suppression of Akt phosphorylation at S473. It had a long half-life (14 h) in mice and pronounced regression of large (~900 mm^3) MDA-361 tumors at 20 mg/kg (intravenous (IV)) on a qd 1, 5, and 9 schedule [67]. In vivo, PKI-587 inhibited tumor growth in breast (MDA-MB-361 and BT474), colon (HCT116), lung (H1975), and glioma (U87MG) xenograft models, with regression correlating with suppression of phosphorylated Akt. Efficacy was enhanced in combination with MEK, topo I, or topo II inhibitors. PKI-587 is in phase I clinical trials [111], but had to be administered via IV because of its poor plasma levels when given orally. The analog PKI-179 (**23**) was developed to address this issue, by simplifying the solubilizing side chain to a pyridine and bridging one of the morpholines to increase lipophilicity [68]. Oral administration of PKI-179 in a mouse MDA-361 tumor xenograft model showed inhibition of PI3K and mTORC1signaling (loss of Akt T308 phosphorylation) but was primarily metabolized by hydroxylation at the ethylene bridge on the bridged morpholine group. Only one of the two morpholine groups is needed for activity with PKI-587 and analogs, and this was confirmed when replacement of the second morpholine group by a 3-oxyexetanyl group gave compounds of comparable activity [112].

Imidazo[4,5-c]quinoline NVP-BEZ235 and Related Compounds (Fig. 15.4)

The dual PI3K–mTOR inhibitor NVP-BEZ235 (**24**) originated from a series of imidazo[4,5-c]quinoline-based inhibitors of PDK1 that were found to also have low nM IC$_{50}$ values against the PI3K isoforms [69,113]. Structure-based drug design allowed development of the optimized analog NVP-BEZ235 as a dual PI3K–mTOR kinase inhibitor [69].

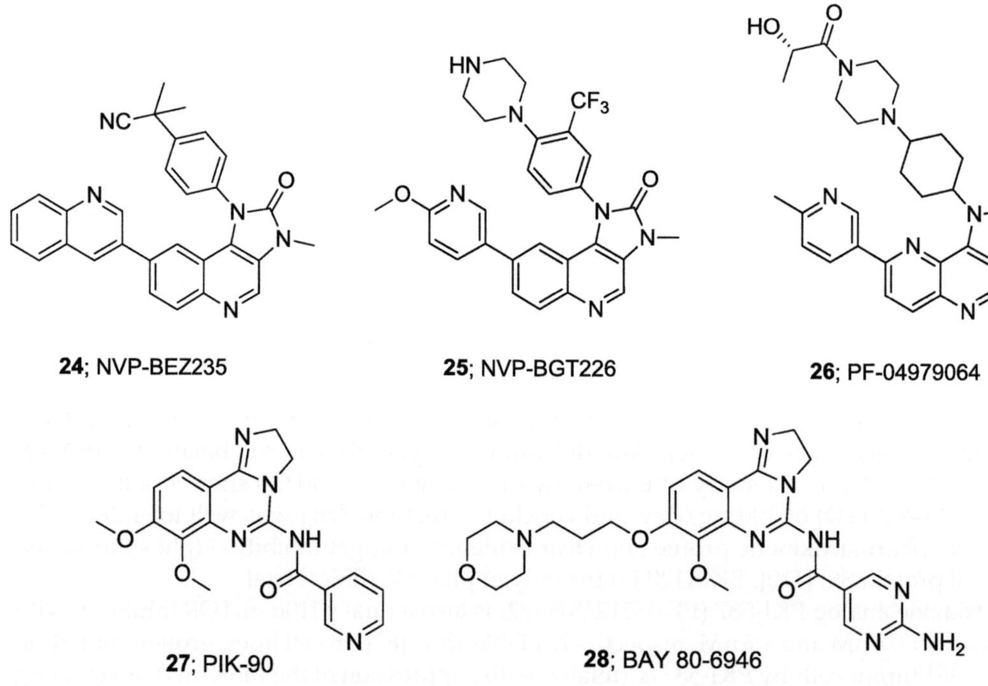

24; NVP-BEZ235　　25; NVP-BGT226　　26; PF-04979064

27; PIK-90　　28; BAY 80-6946

FIGURE 15.4 Imidazo[4,5-c]quinolones, imidazo[1,2-c]quinazolines, and related compounds.

A study of NVP-BEZ235 docked into a homology model of p110α (derived from the p110γ crystal structure) suggested it binds with the core quinoline NH-bonded with the backbone Val851 (Val882 in p110γ), as observed for many PI3K structures. Other H-bonded interactions are with the cyano group and Ser774 (Ser806 in PI3Kγ), and the peripheral quinoline N and Asp933 (Asp964 in PI3Kg), along with van der Waals contacts with conserved hydrophobic residues in the ATP site [69]. It was shown to reverse hyperactivation of the PI3K–mTOR pathway caused by E545K and H1047R mutants of p110α, had potent antitumor activity in xenograft models [114], and is in phase II clinical trial. The related imidazo[4,5-c]quinolinone NVP-BGT226 (25) is a dual PI3K–mTOR inhibitor that has also been investigated clinically in patients with advanced solid tumors [115,116], while the imidazo[4,5-c][1,5]naphthyridinone PF-04979063 (26) is also a potent dual PI3K–mTOR inhibitor that was designed as a backup clinical candidate to PF-04691502 (see Section on Pyrido[2,3-d]pyrimidinones) [70].

Imidazo[1,2-c]quinazolines (Fig. 15.4)

The imidazo[1,2-c]quinazoline derivative PIK-90 (27) is a broad-based pan-PI3K inhibitor with lesser but detectable activity against mTOR [25]. It has been quite widely used as a tool PI3K inhibitor to explore the biological effects of experimental combination therapies [23,25,117]. In a crystal structure of PIK-90 with p110γ, the PIK-90 makes one H-bond between the dihydroimidazole nitrogen and the amide nitrogen of Val882, one to the backbone carbonyl of Val882, and a third between the side chain of Asp964 and the sulfonamide, with the pyridine ring likely also H-bonded to Lys833 [25]. The elaborated analog BAY 80-6946 is much more potent, showing IC_{50}s of 0.5 nM and 45 nM against p110α and mTOR, respectively [71]. It potently blocked cell proliferation in 60 out of 140 tumor cell lines at IC_{50} values of 1–100 nM, inducing substantial apoptosis in a subset of PIK3CA-mutant breast tumors, and was efficacious in multiple tumor xenograft models with PI3CA mutations or PTEN deletions [118].

Pyrido[2,3-d]pyrimidinones (Fig. 15.5)

A high-throughput screen (HTS) led to the development of the pyrido[2,3-d]pyrimidinone PF-04691502 (29), which is a potent dual p110α–mTOR inhibitor (Ki values of 0.6 nM and

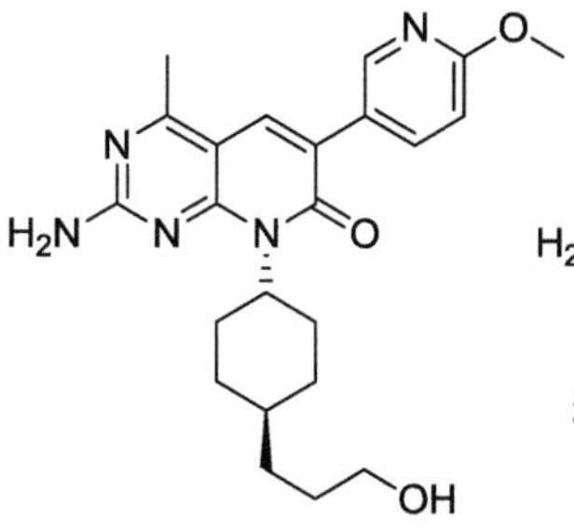

29; PF-04691502 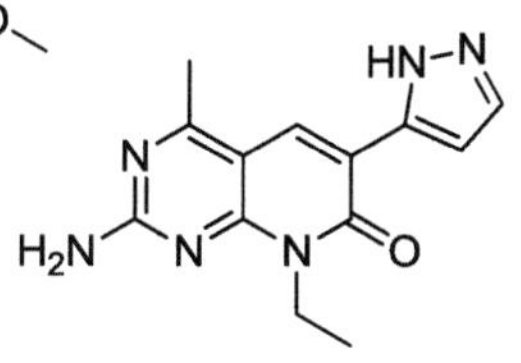   **30**; XL765/SAR245409 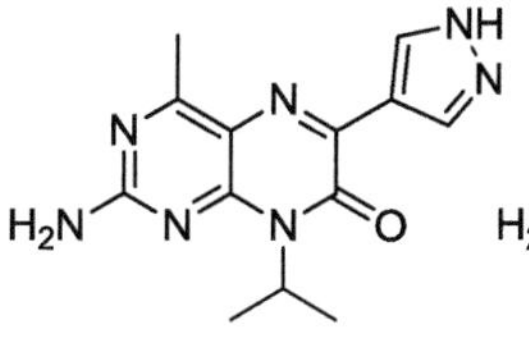   **31** 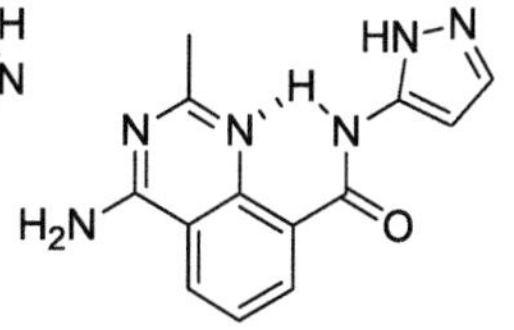   **32**

FIGURE 15.5   Pyrido[2,3-d]pyrimidinones and related compounds.

16 nM, respectively) [72,119]. A co-crystal structure of PF-04691502 with p110γ showed typical H-bonds between Val882 and the 2-amino and 3-ring nitrogens of the aminopyrimidine, with the ring nitrogen on the methoxypyridine forming a key H-bond with a conserved water molecule in the selectivity pocket. The terminal alcohol of the hydroxyethyl formed an intramolecular hydrogen bond with the oxygen atom off the cyclohexyl ring, which reduced the effective number of hydrogen bond donors. In PIK3CA-mutant and PTEN-deleted cancer cell lines, PF-04691502 reduced phosphorylation of AKT T308 and AKT S473 at IC_{50} values below 50 and 20 nM, respectively, and was active in U87MG (PTEN null), SKOV3 (PIK3CA mutation), and gefitinib- and erlotinib-resistant non-small-cell lung carcinoma (NSCLC) xenografts. It is currently in clinical trials [120].

XL765 (SAR245409) (**30**), which is a dual PI3K–mTOR inhibitor [121], and which is also reported to be in phase II trials for breast cancer [122], has the same 4-methylpyrido[2,3-*d*] pyrimidinone scaffold as PF-04691502 [123]. Similar activity has been reported for the analogous 4-methylpteridinones (e.g., **31**) [124], while quinazoline derivatives with an intramolecular hydrogen-bonding scaffold (iMHBS) (e.g., **32**) also behave similarly [125]. These compounds achieve their selectivity for PI3Ks over regular protein kinases by accessing an additional small binding pocket with the C-4 methyl group. This unique PI3K–mTOR binding pocket is large enough to accept the 4-methyl group, but not a 4-methoxy group [124].

Sulfonamidopyridines (Fig. 15.6)

The quinolinyl-thiazolidinedione GSK1059615 (**33**) is a potent pan-PI3K inhibitor that briefly entered clinical trials in patients with refractory malignancies [73,74]. In follow-up studies, designed to identify a second inhibitor with improved potency, selectivity, and pharmacokinetic profiles, the co-crystal structure of GSK1059615 with p110γ was obtained [74]. This indicated that the thiazolidinedione ring formed an interaction with the catalytic lysine (Lys833) within the ATP-binding pocket, while the quinoline nitrogen formed an H-bond with Val882 [74]. However, the structure also showed that larger groups could potentially be accommodated adjacent to the quinoline 6-position. Filling this space with an (ionizable) difluorophenylsulfonamide led to GSK2126458 (**34**), which showed a large increase in potency (p110α IC_{50} of 0.04 nM versus 2 nM for GSK1059615) [74]. The crystal structure showed the same interactions, this time between the ionized sulfonamide and Lys833, with the pyridyl nitrogen forming a key H-bond with a conserved water molecule [74]. It is reported to be in clinical trials for solid tumors and lymphomas [122]. GSK2126458 actually shows high potency against all of the PI3K isoforms and mTOR, due to the strong charged sulfonamide interaction with the conserved lysine residue (Lys833 in p110γ is equivalent to Lys802 in p110α, Lys805 in p110β, and Lys779 in p110δ). This has led to several groups investigating new inhibitors that retain the ionizable sulphonamidopyridine portion of GSK2126485, but with other heterocyclic replacements for the pyridazinyl–quinoline group.

Replacement of the pyridazinyl group of GSK2126458 by morpholine gave **35**, which is a potent inhibitor of all class I PI3K isoforms, mTOR, and hVPS34, a class III PI3K [75]. It is also a potent inhibitor of DNA-PK, although it is selective against other protein kinases [75]. Replacement of the quinoline group by other heterocycles has been the main route of investigation, with a series of imidazo[1,2-*a*]pyridines (e.g., HS-104 [**36**]), and pyrrolo[2,3-*b*]pyridines (e.g., HS-116 [**37**]) all showing potent pan-activity against all Class I PI3K isoforms and mTOR

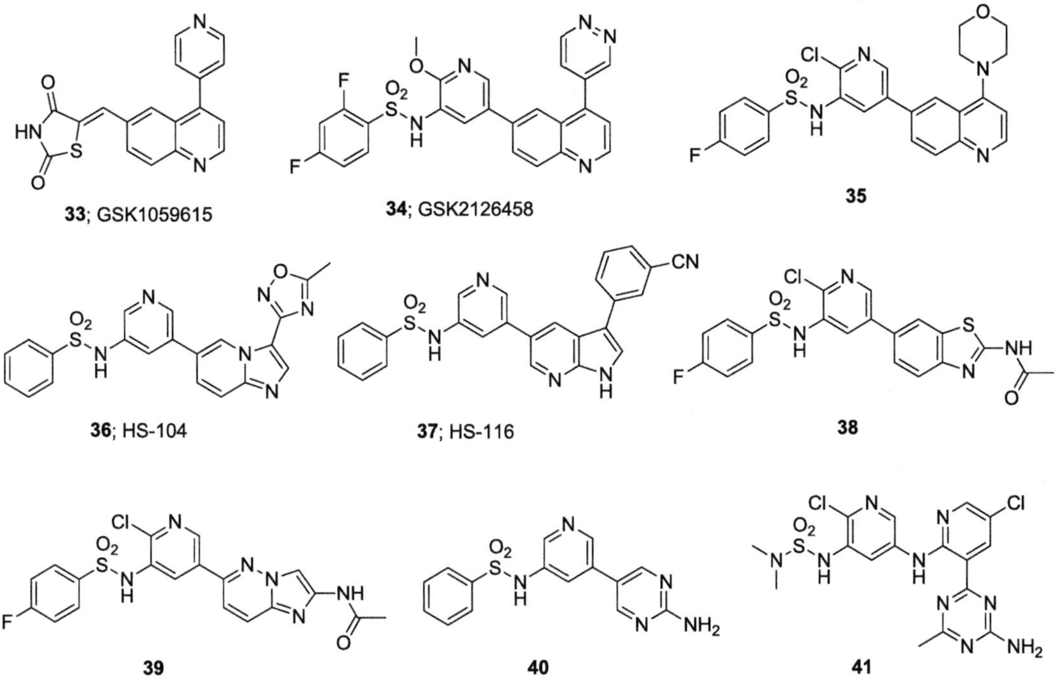

FIGURE 15.6 Sulfonamidopyridines.

[126–130]. These compounds were also found to induce apoptosis of cancer cells, and suppress angiogenesis, by targeting the PI3K–AKT–mTOR pathway [126–133].

The benzo[*d*]thiazole- and imidazo[1,2-*b*]pyridazine-acetamides **38** and **39** are both reported to be potent dual p110α–mTOR inhibitors [76,77], although comparative data for the other PI3K isoforms were not provided. The aminopyrimidine derivative **40** does show some selectivity for p110β over p110α, p110γ, and mTOR, although its selectivity over p110δ is only threefold [134]. Finally, the aminotriazine **41** is a potent pan-PI3K inhibitor with some selectivity over mTOR [78], while further examples of potent sulfonamidopyridine derivatives can be found in the patent literature (e.g., [135]).

Miscellaneous Pan-PI3K Inhibitors (Fig. 15.7)

A series of quinoxaline benzenesulfonamides, including XL147 (SAR245408) (**42**), have been reported [123,136] and shown to be PI3K inhibitors with some selectivity over mTOR [137]. XL147 is reported to be in phase II trials for endometrial and breast cancer [122], although its single-agent activity is reported to be modest against pediatric cancers [138]. Replacement of the sulfonamide group of XL147 by sulfonyl led to compounds such as WR23 (**43**), which is reported to be a p110α inhibitor (25 nM), although no comparative data for the other isoforms were provided [79,139].

The clinical candidate AMG 511 (**44**) was derived from an initial aminotriazine HTS hit [140], and is a potent pan-inhibitor of class I PI3Ks, with a superior pharmacokinetic profile

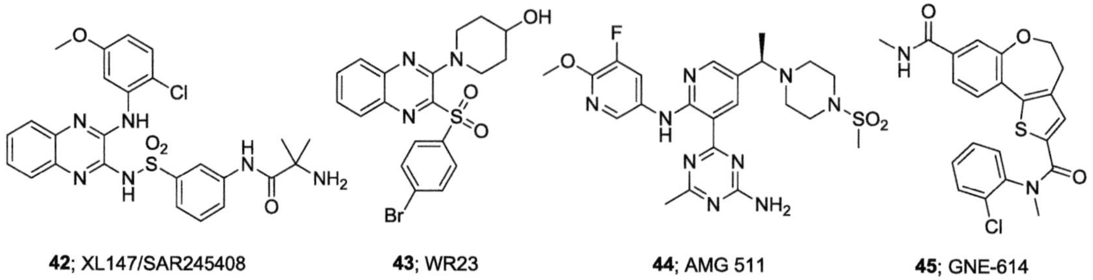

42; XL147/SAR245408   **43**; WR23   **44**; AMG 511   **45**; GNE-614

FIGURE 15.7   Miscellaneous pan-PI3K inhibitors.

[80]. An X-ray co-crystal structure of AMG 511 bound to p110γ showed that the aminotriazine group forms two hydrogen bonds to Val882 in the hinge region, and that the methoxypyridine nitrogen atom makes a hydrogen bond to an ordered water molecule sitting between Tyr867 and Asp841 [80]. The methoxy oxygen atom and the additional 3-fluoro substituent both form favorable interactions with Lys833 within the affinity pocket. The nitrogen in the pyridine central core forms a hydrogen bond to a water molecule that is associated with Asp964, and the methyl group on the benzylic position effectively fills the hydrophobic pocket formed by Thr887, Ile963, and Asp950 residues on the floor of the enzyme, while the methylsulfonamide oxygens engage in hydrogen bonds to Lys802 and Ala805 [80].

Finally, the thienobenzoxepin GNE-614 (**45**) displays moderate selectivity for the p110α, δ, and γ isoforms (IC$_{50}$ 2–5 nM) over p110β (IC$_{50}$ 60 nM) [81], although with the appropriate substituent manipulation the p110α–β ratio was able to be increased to >100-fold [141]. GNE-614 was relatively inactive against mTOR (530 nM), although it was a potent inhibitor of DNA-PK (6 nM) [81].

SELECTIVE INHIBITORS OF PI3K

Selective Inhibitors of p110α (Fig. 15.8)

The imidazo[1,5-*a*]pyridines were first identified from HTS as a novel class of potent and quite p110α-selective compounds in isolated enzyme assays [82]. Development of an initial hit (**46**) (p110α IC$_{50}$ 630 nM), primarily by substitutions on the pyridine ring, led to the much more potent analog 47 (p110α IC$_{50}$ 1.8 nM) [82] (Table 15.1). Instability of the pyrazolesulfone precluded animal studies, but further work showed this could be replaced by a more stable thiazolesulfone (**48**), which retained enzyme potency (although p110α selectivity was lost; Table 15.1) and showed cellular activity. To improve solubility, the thiazole was later replaced by a sulfonylhydrazone linker, and the pyridine ring was substituted by an electron-donating Br group, to give the analog PIK75 (PI-387) (**49**) [25,142,143]. This showed restored selectivity for p110α over the other isoforms (Table 15.1), and although it also shows potent activity against DNA-PK (IC$_{50}$ 2 nM), it has been very widely used in the literature as a tool compound [25,117]. However, instability remained, precluding its further development.

A later study reported that the imidazo[1,2-*a*]pyridine chromophore could be replaced by others [144], and showed in the process that the N1 on the chromophore was critical for

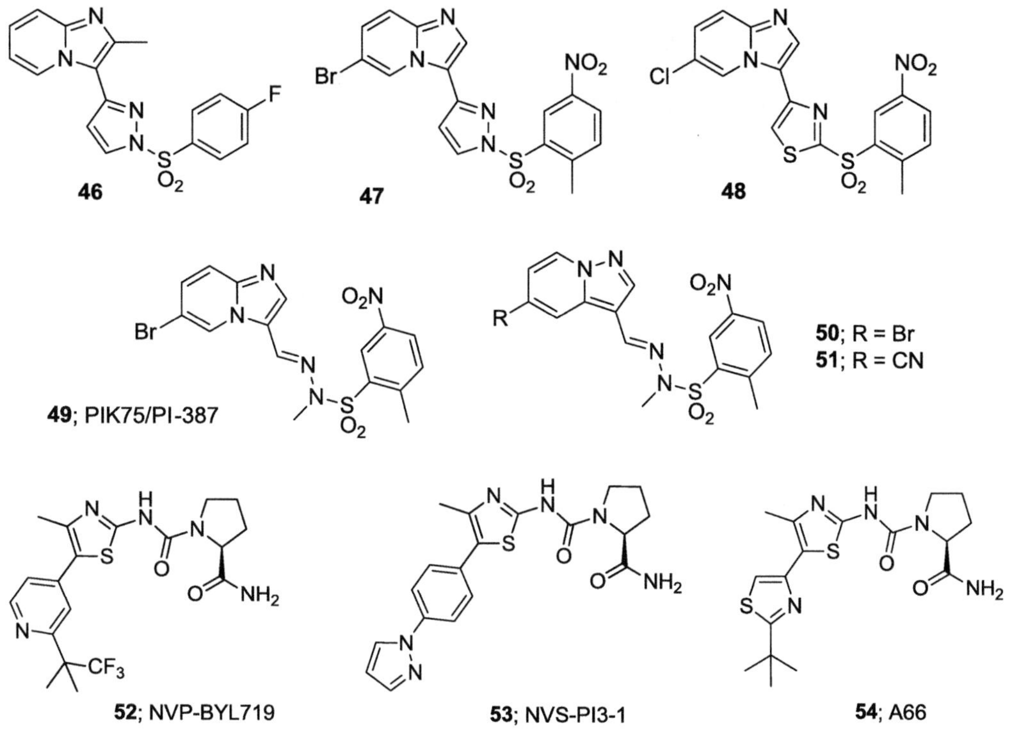

FIGURE 15.8 Imidazo[1,2-*a*]pyridines, thiazolyl-pyrrolidine-2-carboxamides, and related compounds.

binding (to NH of Val882 in the enzyme) and for biological activity. Thus, the corresponding pyrazolo[1,5-*a*]pyridines **50** (5-bromo) and especially **51** (5-cyano) were more potent inhibitors than PIK-75 [83] (Table 15.1). Other SAR studies showed that substitution of the hydrazone nitrogen and replacement of the sulfonyl linker both resulted in a loss of p110α activity, but that substitutions were tolerated around the phenyl ring, providing suggestions for the design of more soluble analogs [145].

A more recent class of p110α-specific inhibitors are the thiazolyl-pyrrolidine-2-carboxamides, exemplified by the clinical candidate NVP-BYL719 (**52**), in which selectivity is achieved by a specific H-bonding interaction between the *S*-enantiomer carboxamide group and the nonconserved residue Gln859 [84]. The development of NVP-BYL719 came from an initial HTS screen using a p110γ biochemical assay, which identified a 2-acetamidothiazole as a suitable lead compound [85]. Addition of the *S*-pyrrolidine-carboxamide unit led to p110α-selective compounds such as NVS-PI3-1 (**53**) [85], and further development then produced the more potent NVP-BYL719 [84], which is currently in clinical trials with patients whose tumors contain a mutation in the PIK3CA gene [146].

Work with the tool compound A66 (**54**) confirmed that Gln859 was the critical residue targeted by this series of compounds, and showed that the analogous *R*-enantiomer, or the related compound without the carboxamide, was >30-fold less active than A66 [86,147]. In fact, not only was Gln859 critical to binding, but also it was critical for isoform selectivity, as shown by the reciprocal mutation in p110β recovering the affinity of the A66 *S*-enantiomer [147].

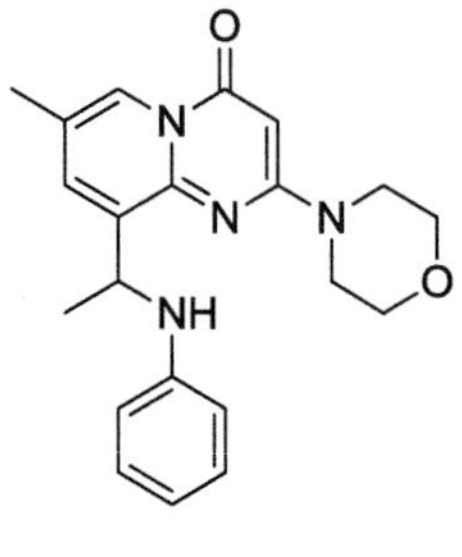

55; TGX221

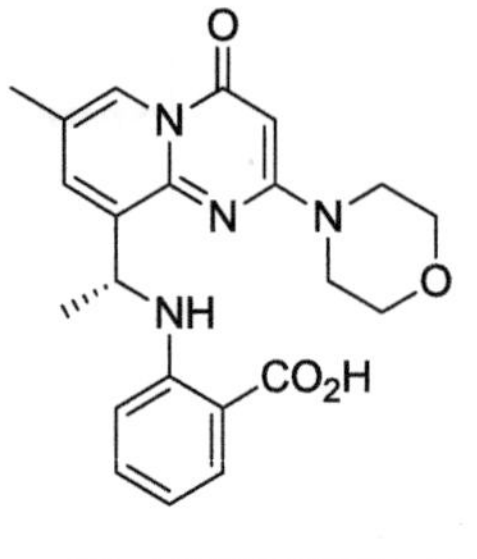

56; AZD6482/KIN-193

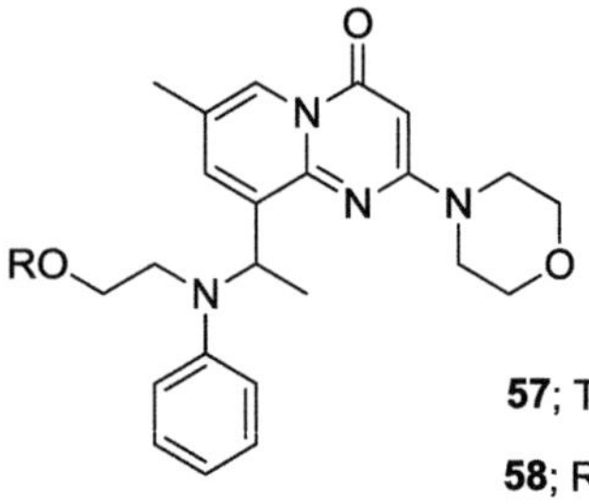

57; TGX-D1: R = H

58; R = peptide

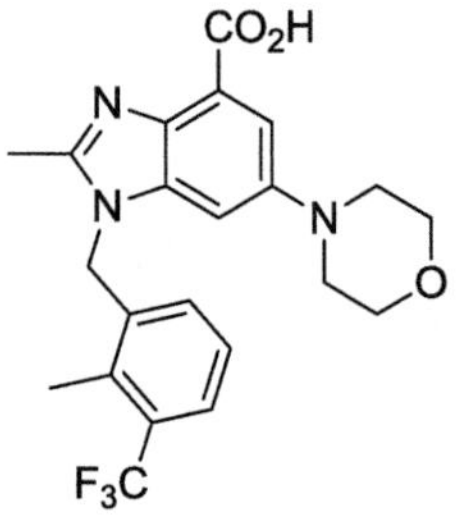

59: GSK2636771

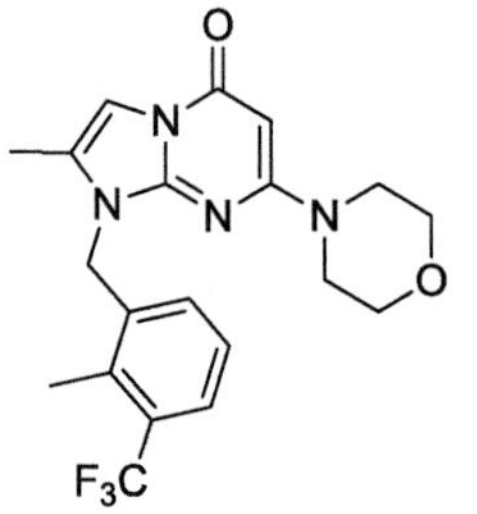

60

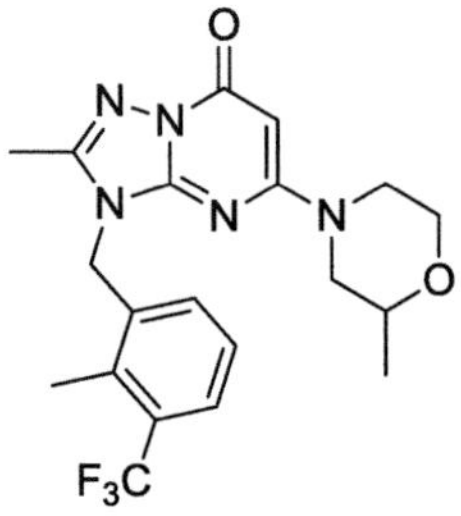

61

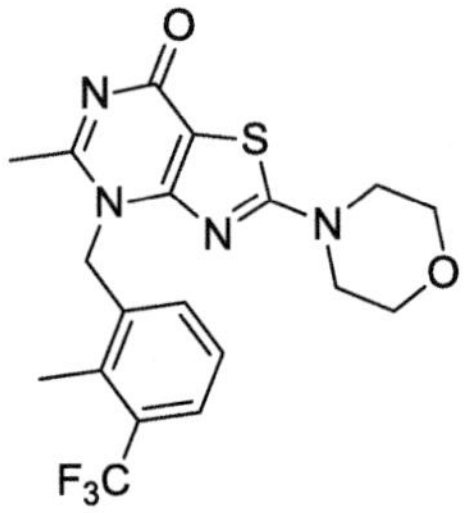

62

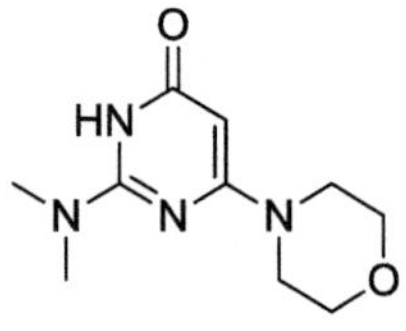

63

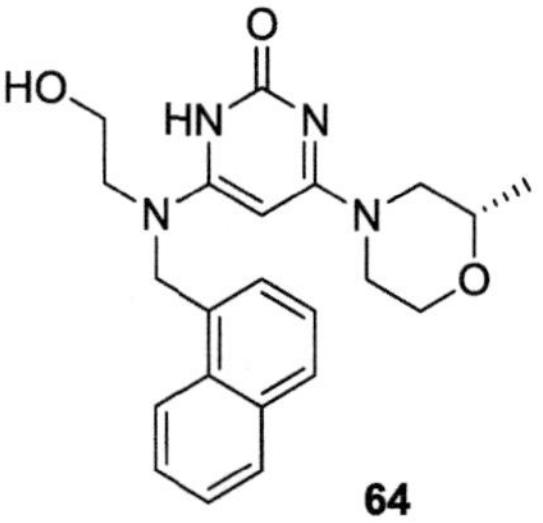

64

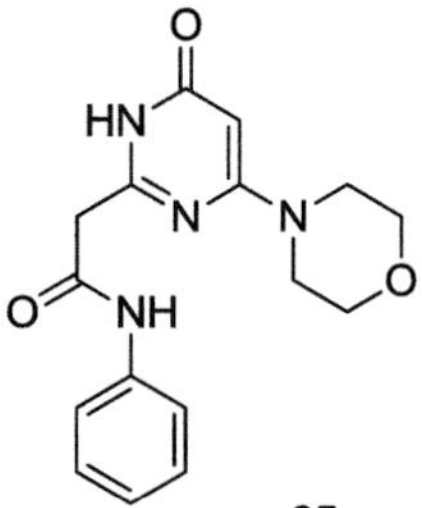

65

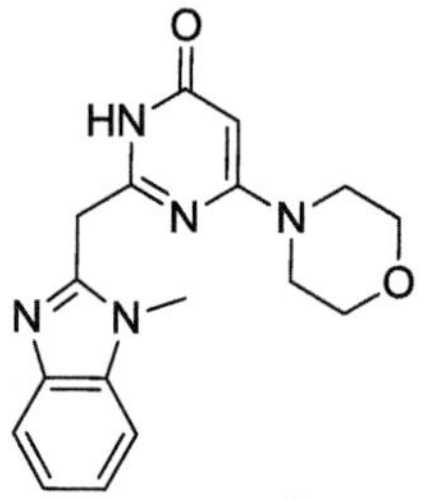

66

FIGURE 15.9 TGX221 and related compounds.

Selective Inhibitors of p110β (Fig. 15.9)

Conversion of the 2-morpholinochromenone structure of LY294002 (**1**) to the corresponding pyridopyrimidin-4-one and studies of its SAR gave rise to a series of 9-substituted compounds with a unique selectivity for p110β [148]. The most well-studied of these is TGX221 (**55**), which has a selectivity of >200-fold for p110β over p110α, and is of interest as an antithrombotic drug [149], being able to prevent integrin-mediated adhesion in platelets at the site of vascular injury [87]. TGX221 and its analogs also show some p110β–p110δ selectivity [25,87], which is considered to be due to them exploiting differences in the plasticity of the residues that form the entrance to the ATP-binding site [25].

The discovery of the importance of the p110β isoform in PTEN-deficient tumors [150,151] has led to significant recent interest in the development of p110β inhibitors as anticancer agents. It has been shown that the *R*-enantiomer of TGX-221 is the active form [90], and the *R*-carboxy analog AZD6482/KIN-193 (**56**) is also highly p110β selective (Table 15.1), and its antiproliferative activity in a large (422-member) cancer cell line panel broadly correlated with mutations in PTEN [88]. It also showed good in vivo activity in tumors derived from cell lines deficient in PTEN. This is interesting, since in vivo–active antiproliferative p110β-selective inhibitors could potentially minimize the side effects caused by pan-PI3K inhibitors and p110α-selective inhibitors [152]. This compound has also been investigated clinically as an antithrombotic agent [153].

Attachment of a HER2-targeted peptide prodrug linker to TGX-D1 (**57**), the *N*-hydroxy-ethyl derivative of TGX-221, which exhibits a similar biological profile, gave peptide–drug conjugate **58**, which was proven to be gradually cleaved by PSA to release TGX-D1 [154]. Cellular uptake of the peptide–drug conjugate **58** was significantly higher in prostate cancer cells compared to the parent drug. A related prodrug strategy to develop an encapsulation system for parenterally delivering TGX-D1 (also called BL05) to the target tissue through a prostate-specific membrane aptamer has also been investigated, with little or no side effects [155].

In a search for new p110β-selective inhibitors that might be efficacious in the treatment of PTEN-deficient tumors, a number of different structural classes have been investigated, using TGX-221 as a starting point [90]. This has culminated in the development of the benz-imidazole-4-carboxylic acid derivative GSK2636771 (**59**), which is currently in clinical trials in subjects with advanced solid tumors with PTEN deficiency [89]. GSK2636771 is an orally available, potent (5 nM) inhibitor of p110β with a 12-fold selectivity over p110δ and >1000-fold selectivity over p110α, p110γ, and mTOR [89]. Other compounds that were investigated on the route from TGX-221 to GSK2636771 include the imidazo[1,2-*a*]pyrimidinone **60** [90], the 1,2,4-triazolo[1,5-*a*]pyrimidinone **61** [91], and the thiazolo[4,5-*d*]pyrimidinone **62** [92].

Monocyclic p110β inhibitors have also been investigated, and starting with the virtual screening-derived fragment hit **63** [156], investigation of a series of 2- and 4-pyrimidinone derivatives led to the potent (38 nM) p110β-selective 2*S*-2-methylmorpholinyl derivative **64**, which displayed fourfold selectivity over p110δ and >700-fold selectivity over p110α and p110γ [93]. This compound displayed a favorable in vivo antiplatelet effect, but despite this did not significantly increase bleeding time in dogs. Additionally, due to its enhanced selectivity over p110α, it did not induce any insulin resistance in rats [93].

An alternative HTS approach identified a series of 2-pyrimidinone derivatives such as **65** [94], which was then optimized to give the benzimidazole derivative **66**, which showed significant activity and selectivity for PI3Kβ and adequate in vitro pharmacokinetic properties [95]. This compound achieved sustained target modulation and tumor growth delay at well-tolerated doses when administered orally to severe combined immunodeficiency mice implanted with PTEN-deficient human tumor xenografts [95].

Selective Inhibitors of p110δ (Fig. 15.10)

The purinylmethylquinazoline IC87114 (**67**) was the first selective p110δ inhibitor reported [96]. A crystal structure of the related PIK-39 (**68**) with p110γ showed the phenomenon of enzyme plasticity [25], where the inhibitor forms H-bonds between the purine and Val882

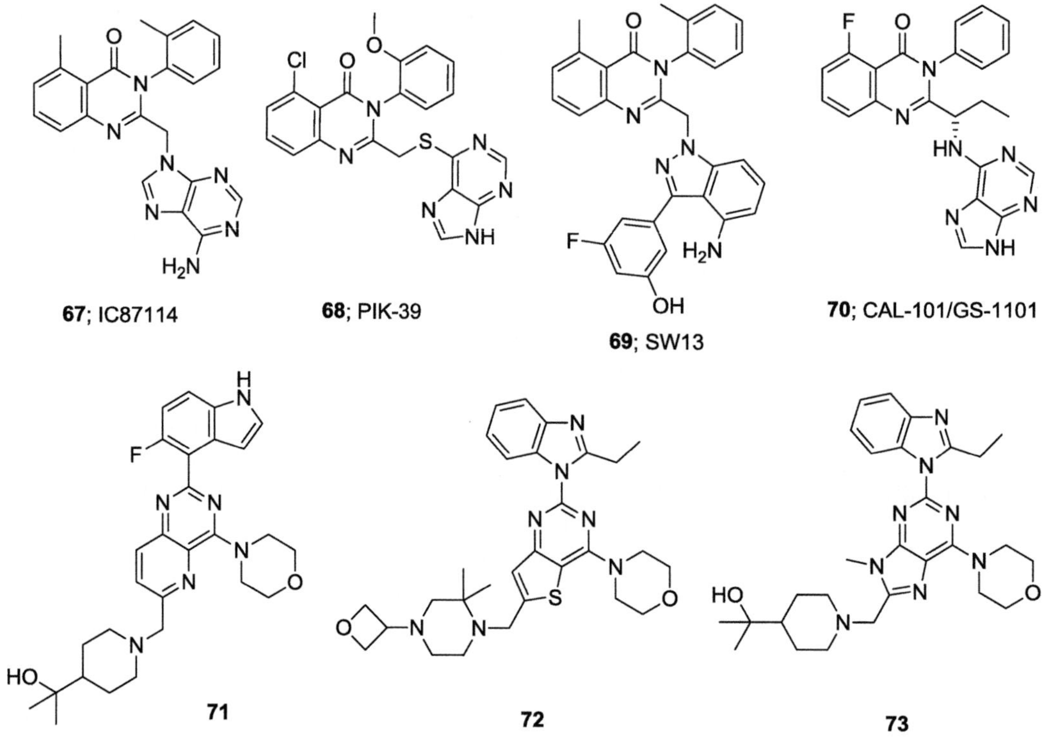

FIGURE 15.10   Selective inhibitors of p110δ.

and Glu880, and the Met804 residue moves on inhibitor binding to generate a new "selectivity pocket" that the quinazolinone ring of PIK-39 (and the related compound IC87114) occupies. This latter is considered to be the main reason for the p110δ (and, to a lesser extent, p110γ) selectivity of this class, since p110α and p110β cannot make this change. This was shown by the inability of the drugs to inhibit mutant p110δ with Met804 mutated to isoleucine or valine. A more recent crystal structure of PIK-39 with the catalytic subunit of p110δ shows a similar movement of Met804 and H-binding of the purine to the hinge region [62]. An indazole analog of IC87114 (SW13) (**69**) proved to be a much more potent p110δ inhibitor, while retaining high selectivity against p110α and p110β [157].

Another derivative of IC87114 (CAL-101, or GS-1101) (**70**) had better pharmacological properties and is in clinical trials for the treatment of B-cell cancers [97]. While the first clinical study of CAL-101 was in allergic rhinitis, reflecting the expectation that p110δ inhibitors would be primarily antiinflammatory, the recent excitement has been over its effects on a range of B-cell malignancies, including chronic lymphocytic leukemia (CLL), non-Hodgkin lymphoma (NHL), acute myeloid leukemia, and multiple myeloma [158]. The best results published so far have been in CLL, where an early phase I trial achieved a 25% overall response rate [159], and in subtypes of NHL. Studies of CAL-101 in combination with rituximab (anti-CD20) and bendamustine (a DNA alkylator) in CLL and indolent NHL also look very promising [160]. Other selective inhibitors of p110δ, such as AMG-319, are reported to

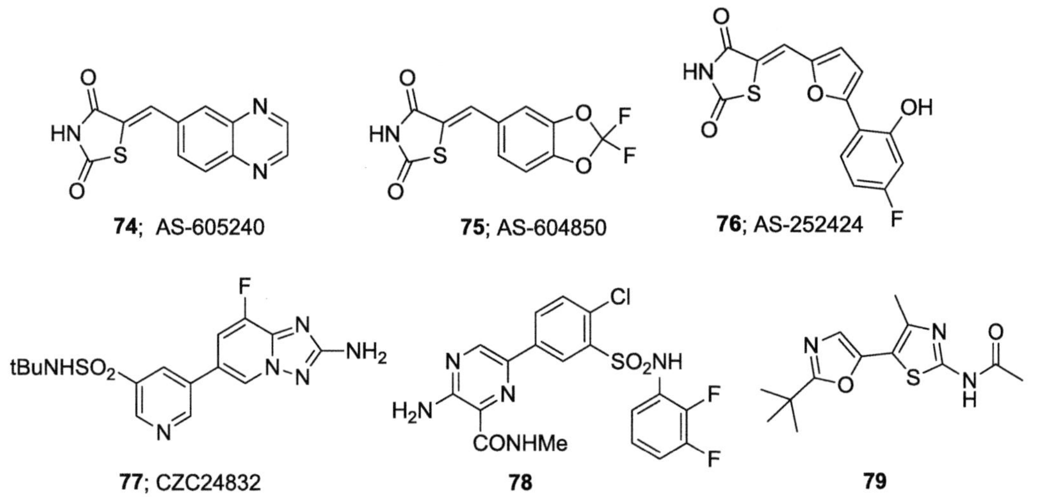

FIGURE 15.11　Selective inhibitors of p110γ.

be in clinical trials [158], although its structure has not been disclosed. Numerous other examples exist in the patent literature [161].

A totally different class of p110δ inhibitors (e.g., **71**, **72**, and **73**) has been described more recently [98–100]. Thus, while compounds such as IC87114 and CAL-101 adopt a "propeller shape" and induce an allosteric "specificity pocket", these new inhibitors bind in the affinity pocket, are derived from the morpholinyl thienopyrimidine scaffold of the Class I PI3K inhibitor GDC-0941 and the Class I PI3K–mTOR kinase inhibitor GDC-0980 that inhibit all four PI3K isoforms, and are currently in oncology clinical trials. These compounds take advantage of a shallow dimple [62], or "tryptophan shelf" formed between Met752, the small side chain of Thr750, and Trp760, which is accessed by piperidine or piperazine substituents [98–100]. In other p110 isotypes, the residue equivalent to Thr750 is a larger lysine or arginine. Initial work identified the indole derivative **71** [98], but a search for more metabolically stable inhibitors led to the benzimidazole derivatives **72** and **73**, which are both potent and highly selective inhibitors of p110δ [99,100].

Selective Inhibitors of p110γ (Fig. 15.11)

The Class 1B kinase p110γ was the easiest (and thus the first) to be crystallized. Thus, many of the early inhibitors, of varying isoform selectivity, were co-crystallized with it to obtain structural information. However, the first substantially p110γ-selective inhibitor, AS-605240 (**74**), was not reported until 2005 [101]. This compound and the related AS-604850 (**75**) were aimed at rheumatoid arthritis, a chronic inflammatory disorder of the joints mediated by neutrophils, the activation of chemotaxis for which is known to be mediated by p110γ. Both compounds are reasonably potent and modestly selective inhibitors of p110γ (Table 15.1). Crystallographic studies show that both AS-605240 and AS-604850 have been solved in complex with p110γ [101]. Both compounds form stabilizing H-bonds between the nitrogen of the quinoxaline ring or the oxygen of the benzodioxolone ring, respectively, to Val882, while the

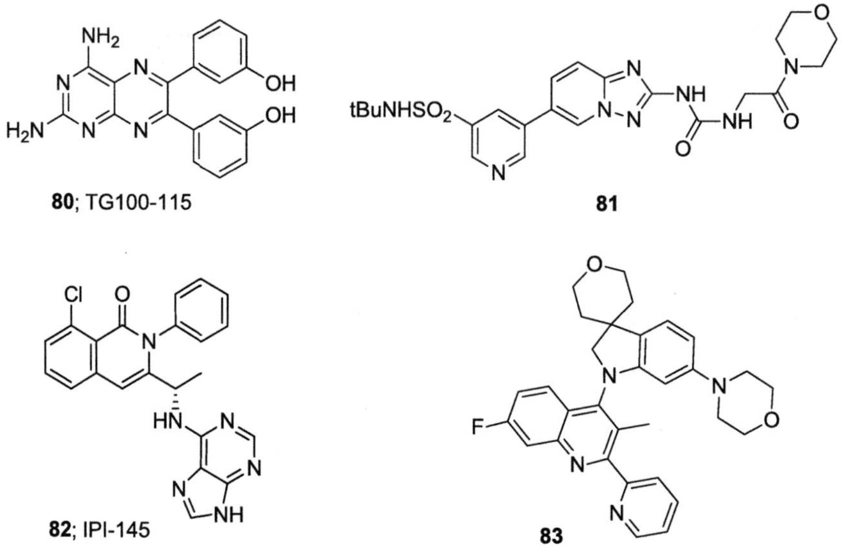

80; TG100-115

81

82; IPI-145

83

FIGURE 15.12   Dual delta–gamma and beta–delta inhibitors.

ionized thiazolidine-2,3-dione nitrogen forms a salt bridge to Lys833 and Asp964 [101]. At about the same time, the furan analog AS-252424 (**76**) was also reported as a p110γ-selective compound (IC$_{50}$ 33 nM), and the same H-bond to Val882 and salt bridge to Lys833 were observed in the crystal structure with p110γ [65].

A different class of p110γ inhibitor is represented by the amino-triazolopyridine CZC24843 (**77**), which is a potent and selective p110γ inhibitor that shows efficacy in both in vitro and in vivo models of inflammation [102,162]. The 6-aryl-2-amino-1,2,4-triazolo[1,5-*a*]pyridine core was identified by chemoproteomic screening of a kinase-focused library, and the series was then optimized to afford CZC24843 [102,162].

Other examples of selective p110γ inhibitors to have been reported include the 3-amino-pyrazine derivative **78** [103] and the oxazole derivative **79** [104].

Dual Inhibitors of p110β/δ and p110γ/δ (Fig. 15.12)

Dual inhibitors of p110γ and p110δ are of interest because of their potential in autoimmune and inflammatory diseases [157,163–165]. The diphenyl pteridine derivative TG100-115 (**80**) was the first selective dual p110γ/δ inhibitor to be reported [105]. Modeling of TG100-115 with p110γ showed strong H-bonds formed between the pteridine N3 nitrogen and the backbone NH of Val882, and from the 4-NH$_2$ to the Val backbone carbonyl. A pocket at the back of the ATP-binding site accommodates the phenol, where the OH groups may H-bond to Asp841 and/or Tyr867 [105]. TG100-115 showed activity in a rat model of myocardial infarction [166]. A study of aerosolized formulations in mouse models of asthma and chronic obstructive pulmonary disease (COPD) showed that TG100-115 markedly reduced pulmonary eosinophilia, airway hyperresponsiveness, and pulmonary inflammation, with activity profiles favorable for further development as a therapy for both asthma and COPD [167].

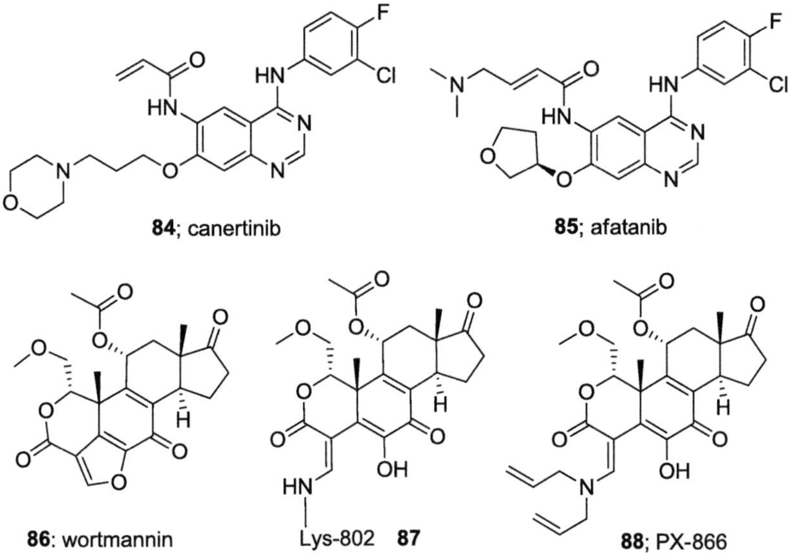

FIGURE 15.13 Wortmannin and other irreversible inhibitors.

A more recent example of a selective dual p110γ/δ inhibitor is the 1,2,4-triazolo[1,5-*a*]pyridine **81**, which is based on the p110γ selective inhibitor CZC24843 [168]. This compound showed excellent selectivity over the other PI3K isoforms and showed significant efficacy in an acute model of lung inflammation [168]. However, the most advanced dual p110γ/δ inhibitor is the quinolone IPI-145 (**82**), which is in clinical trials for the treatment of both arthritis and advanced hematological malignancies [106,169].

Selective dual inhibitors of p110β/δ also offer potential in the treatment of a number of inflammatory diseases, and the quinoline derivative **83** was found to be efficacious in animal models of inflammation, including a keyhole limpet hemocyanin study and a collagen-induced arthritis disease model of rheumatoid arthritis [107].

IRREVERSIBLE PI3K INHIBITORS (FIG. 15.13)

The concept of irreversible inhibition of kinases was first proven clinically with the erbB inhibitor canertinib (**84**), which targeted a free cysteine residue adjacent to the ATP-binding site [170], and which received phase II trials for NSCLC and ovarian cancer [171]. Since reversible inhibitors compete with high levels of ATP, it was considered that such irreversible inhibition would give a longer lived and more complete enzyme shutdown, which might translate to a lesser dependence on pharmacokinetics and thus less frequent dosing. Later related analogs such as Afatinib (**85**) are in phase III trials [172].

The discovery that the fungal metabolite wortmannin (**86**) was an ATP-noncompetitive inhibitor of PI3K isoforms was followed by mechanistic studies showing that it was alkylated on the furan ring by Lys802 (in the binding site of p110α), forming an enamine (**87**) that was stable at physiological pH but underwent hydrolysis below pH 6 [173]. SAR studies showed that the cyclopentanone D-ring, while remote from the alkylation site, was crucial for the initial binding [174]. While wortmannin proved too toxic to be used as a drug, analogs where the furan was masked in an open form by Schiff base adducts were less toxic and more stable. PX-866 (**88**) was the most stable of a number of semisynthetic viridian analogs prepared from wortmannin, and showed similar potency to wortmannin for inhibition of isolated PI3K isoforms and for shutdown of AKT (IC$_{50}$ 20 nM as measured by inhibition of phospho-Ser473-Akt) [175]. It was active in OvCar-3 human ovarian cancer and A-549 human lung cancer xenografts [175]. It acts as a prodrug, with an MTD (19.5 mg/kg) six times higher than that of wortmannin and alkylates p110α, p110γ, and p110δ but not p110β [176]. PX-866 was shown to potentiate the antitumor activity of gefitinib against large A-549 NSCLC xenografts, the combination resulting in complete tumor growth control, suggesting a potential clinical use in increasing the response to epidermal growth factor receptor inhibitors in patients with NSCLC [108]. A phase I trial of PX-866 given orally daily on either an intermittent (days 1–5 and 8–12) or continuous (days 1–28) schedule determined MTDs of 12 and 8 mg/day, respectively. Stable disease was seen in 22% and 53% of evaluable patients, respectively [177].

SUMMARY AND CONCLUSIONS

The work summarized here has shown that the early work on relatively nonspecific inhibitors evolved first into the broad class of alpha–mTOR dual inhibitors that were the first to reach the clinic. Following that, much chemistry effort, guided by an increasing body of structural biology information about the different isoforms, has allowed the generation of potent and highly selective inhibitors. Examples include compounds **52–54** for alpha; compounds **55**, **56**, and **59** for beta; compounds **69–73** for delta; and compounds **74** and **77** for gamma. These, and "dual" compounds such as **82** for delta and gamma and **83** for beta and delta, offer a range of tools for further dissection of the cellular roles that the different isoforms play.

The broad "first-generation" of alpha–mTOR dual inhibitors has shown activity in the clinic, and current studies in conjunction with standard cytotoxic chemotherapy or other kinase inhibitors such as MEK inhibitors continue. However, much of the current excitement has moved to the delta-selective inhibitors such as CAL-101 (**70**), which has shown good effects in a range of B-cell malignancies, including chronic lymphocytic leukemia, non-Hodgkin lymphoma, acute myeloid leukemia, and multiple myeloma. Overall, this field appears to hold much promise for the future.

References

[1] Fruman DA, Meyers RE, Cantley LC. Phosphoinositide kinases. Ann Rev Biochem 1998;67:481–507.
[2] Vogt PK, Bader AG, Kang S. PI 3-kinases—hidden potentials revealed. Cell Cycle 2006;5:946–9.
[3] Misawa H, Ohtsubo M, Copeland NG, Gilbert DJ, Jenkins NA, Yoshimura A. Cloning and characterization of a novel class II phosphoinositide 3-kinase containing C2 domain. Biochem Biophys Res Commun 1998;244:531–9.
[4] Schu PV, Takegawa K, Fry MJ, Stack JH, Waterfield MD, Emr SD. Phosphatidylinositol 3-kinase encoded by yeast VPS34 gene essential for protein sorting. Science 1993;260:88–91.
[5] James SR, Downes CP, Gigg R, Grove SJA, Holmes AB, Alessi DR. Specific binding of the Akt-1 protein kinase to phosphatidylinositol 3,4,5-trisphosphate without subsequent activation. Biochem J 1996;315:709–13.
[6] Kavran JM, Klein DE, Lee A, Falasca M, Isakoff SJ, Skolnik EY, et al. Specificity and promiscuity in phosphoinositide binding by pleckstrin homology domains. J Biol Chem 1998;273:30497–508.

[7] Stephens L, Anderson K, Stokoe D, Erdjument-Bromage H, Painter GF, Holmes AB, et al. Protein kinase B kinases that mediate phosphatidylinositol 3,4,5-trisphosphate-dependent activation of protein kinase B. Science 1998;279:710–4.

[8] Manning BD, Cantley LC. AKT/PKB signaling: navigating downstream. Cell 2007;129:1261–74.

[9] Cully M, You H, Levine AJ, Mak TW. Beyond PTEN mutations: the PI3K pathway as an integrator of multiple inputs during tumorigenesis. Nat Rev Cancer 2006;6:184–92.

[10] Downward J. PI 3-kinase, Akt and cell survival. Sem Cell Dev Biol 2004;15:177–82.

[11] Parsons R, Simpson L. PTEN and cancer. Methods Mol Biol 2003;222:147–66.

[12] Samuels Y, Ericson K. Oncogenic PI3K and its role in cancer. Curr Opin Oncol 2006;18:77–82.

[13] Kang S, Bader AG, Vogt PK. Phosphatidylinositol 3-kinase mutations identified in human cancer are oncogenic. Proc Natl Acad Sci U S A 2005;102:802–7.

[14] Walker EH, Perisic O, Ried C, Stephens L, Williams RL. Structural insights into phosphoinositide 3-kinase catalysis and signalling. Nature 1999;402:313–20.

[15] Walker EH, Pacold ME, Perisic O, Stephens L, Hawkins PT, Wymann MP, et al. Structural determinants of phosphoinositide 3-kinase inhibition by wortmannin, LY294002, quercetin, myricetin, and staurosporine. Mol Cell 2000;6:909–19.

[16] Vlahos CJ, Matter WF, Hui KY, Brown RF. A specific inhibitor of phosphatidylinositol 3-kinase, 2-(4-morpholinyl)-8-phenyl-4H-1-benzopyran-4-one (LY294002). J Biol Chem 1994;269:5241–8.

[17] Matter WF, Brown RF, Vlahos CJ. The inhibition of phosphatidylinositol 3-kinase by quercetin and analogs. Biochem Biophys Res Commun 1992;186:624–31.

[18] Garlich JR, De P, Dey N, Jing DS, Peng X, Miller A, et al. A vascular targeted pan phosphoinositide 3-kinase inhibitor prodrug, SF1126, with antitumor and antiangiogenic activity. Cancer Res 2008;68:206–15.

[19] Peirce SK, Findley HW, Prince C, Dasgupta A, Cooper T, Durden DL. The PI-3 kinase-Akt-MDM2-survivin signaling axis in high-risk neuroblastoma: a target for PI-3 kinase inhibitor intervention. Cancer Chemother Pharmacol 2011;68:325–35.

[20] Qi W, Stejskal A, Morales C, Cooke LS, Garlich JR, Durden D, et al. SF1126, a pan-PI3K inhibitor has potent pre-clinical activity in aggressive B-cell non-Hodgkin lymphomas by inducing cell cycle arrest and apoptosis. J Cancer Sci Ther 2012;4:207–13.

[21] Mahadevan D, Chiorean EG, Harris WB, Von Hoff DD, Stejskal-Barnett A, Qi W, et al. Phase I pharmacokinetic and pharmacodynamic study of the pan-PI3K/mTORC vascular targeted pro-drug SF1126 in patients with advanced solid tumours and B-cell malignancies. Eur J Cancer 2012;48:3319–27.

[22] Baiz D, Pinder TA, Hassan S, Karpova Y, Salsbury F, Welker ME, et al. Synthesis and characterization of a novel prostate cancer-targeted phosphatidylinositol-3-kinase inhibitor prodrug. J Med Chem 2012;55:8038–46.

[23] Fan QW, Cheng CK, Nicolaides TP, Hackett CS, Knight ZA, Shokat KM, et al. A dual phosphoinositide-3-kinase alpha/mTOR inhibitor cooperates with blockade of epidermal growth factor receptor in PTEN-mutant glioma. Cancer Res 2007;67:7960–5.

[24] Hayakawa M, Kaizawa H, Moritomo H, Koizumi T, Ohishi T, Yamano M, et al. Synthesis and biological evaluation of pyrido[3',2':4,5]furo[3,2-d]pyrimidine derivatives as novel PI3 kinase p110α inhibitors. Bioorg Med Chem 2007;15:2438–42.

[25] Knight ZA, Gonzalez B, Feldman ME, Zunder ER, Goldenberg DD, Williams O, et al. A pharmacological map of the PI3-K family defines a role for p110α in insulin signaling. Cell 2006;125:733–47.

[26] Raynaud FI, Eccles S, Clarke PA, Hayes A, Nutley B, Alix S, et al. Pharmacologic characterization of a potent inhibitor of class I phosphatidylinositide 3-kinases. Cancer Res 2007;67:5840–50.

[27] Pecchi S, Renhowe PA, Taylor C, Kaufman S, Merritt H, Wiesmann M, et al. Identification and structure-activity relationship of 2-morpholino-6-(3-hydroxyphenyl)pyrimidines, a class of potent and selective PI3 kinase inhibitors. Bioorg Med Chem Lett 2010;20:6895–8.

[28] Wang J, Wang X, Chen Y, Chen S, Chen G, Tong L, et al. Discovery and bioactivity of 4-(2-arylpyrido[3',2':3,4]pyrrolo[1,2-f][1,2,4]triazin-4-yl) morpholine derivatives as novel PI3K inhibitors. Bioorg Med Chem Lett 2012;22:339–42.

[29] Large JM, Torr JE, Raynaud FI, Clarke PA, Hayes A, di Stefano F, et al. Preparation and evaluation of trisubstituted pyrimidines as phosphatidylinositol 3-kinase inhibitors. 3-Hydroxyphenol analogues and bioisosteric replacements. Bioorg Med Chem 2011;19:836–51.

[30] Hayakawa M, Kaizawa H, Moritomo H, Koizumi T, Ohishi T, Okada M, et al. Synthesis and biological evaluation of 4-morpholino-2-phenylquinazolines and related derivatives as novel PI3 kinase p110α inhibitors. Bioorg Med Chem 2006;14:6847–58.

[31] Li T, Wang J, Wang X, Yang N, Chen S-m, Tong L-j, et al. WJD008, a dual phosphatidylinositol 3-kinase (PI3K)/ mammalian target of rapamycin inhibitor, prevents PI3K signaling and inhibits the proliferation of transformed cells with oncogenic PI3K mutant. J Pharmacol Exp Ther 2010;334:830–8.

[32] Folkes AJ, Ahmadi K, Alderton WK, Alix S, Baker SJ, Box G, et al. The identification of 2-(1H-indazol-4-yl)-6-(4-methanesulfonyl-piperazin-1-ylmethyl)-4-morpholin-4-yl-thieno[3,2-d]pyrimidine (GDC-0941) as a potent, selective, orally bioavailable inhibitor of class I PI3 kinase for the treatment of cancer. J Med Chem 2008;51:5522–32.

[33] Sutherlin DP, Sampath D, Berry M, Castanedo G, Chang Z, Chuckowree I, et al. Discovery of (thienopyrimidin-2-yl)aminopyrimidines as potent, selective, and orally available pan-PI3-kinase and dual pan-PI3-kinase/mTOR inhibitors for the treatment of cancer. J Med Chem 2010;53:1086–97.

[34] Hoeflich KP, Merchant M, Orr C, Chan J, Den Otter D, Berry L, et al. Intermittent administration of MEK inhibitor GDC-0973 plus PI3K inhibitor GDC-0941 triggers robust apoptosis and tumor growth inhibition. Cancer Res 2012;72:210–9.

[35] Raynaud FI, Eccles SA, Patel S, Alix S, Box G, Chuckowree I, et al. Biological properties of potent inhibitors of class I phosphatidylinositide 3-kinases: from PI-103 through PI-540, PI-620 to the oral agent GDC-0941. Mol Cancer Ther 2009;8:1725–38.

[36] Salphati L, Pang J, Plise EG, Chou B, Halladay JS, Olivero AG, et al. Preclinical pharmacokinetics of the novel PI3K inhibitor GDC-0941 and prediction of its pharmacokinetics and efficacy in human. Xenobiotica 2011;41:1088–99.

[37] Heffron T, Berry G, Castanedo G, Chang I, Chuckowree J, Dotson A, et al. Identification of GNE-477, a potent and efficacious dual PI3K/mTOR inhibitor. Bioorg Med Chem Lett 2010;20:2408–11.

[38] Sutherlin DP, Bao L, Berry M, Castanedo G, Chuckowree I, Dotson J, et al. Discovery of a potent, selective, and orally available class I phosphatidylinositol 3-kinase (PI3K)/mammalian target of rapamycin (mTOR) kinase inhibitor (GDC-0980) for the treatment of cancer. J Med Chem 2011;54:7579–758.

[39] Wallin JJ, Edgar KA, Guan J, Berry M, Prior WW, Lee L, et al. GDC-0980 is a novel class I PI3K/mTOR kinase inhibitor with robust activity in cancer models driven by the PI3K pathway. Mol Cancer Ther 2011;10:2426–36.

[40] Salphati L, Pang J, Plise EG, Lee LB, Olivero AG, Prior WW, et al. Preclinical assessment of the absorption and disposition of the phosphatidylinositol 3-kinase/mammalian target of rapamycin inhibitor GDC-0980 and prediction of its pharmacokinetics and efficacy in human. Drug Metab Dispos 2012;40:1785–96.

[41] Heffron TP, Salphati L, Alicke B, Cheong J, Dotson J, Edgar K, et al. The design and identification of brain penetrant inhibitors of phosphoinositide 3-kinase α. J Med Chem 2012;55:8007–20.

[42] Salphati L, Heffron TP, Alicke B, Nishimura M, Barck K, Carano RA, et al. Targeting the PI3K pathway in the brain-efficacy of a PI3K inhibitor optimized to cross the blood-brain barrier. Clin Cancer Res 2012;18:6239–48.

[43] Martinez Gonzalez S, Hernandez AI, Varela C, Rodriguez-Aristegui S, Alvarez RM, Garcia AB, et al. Imidazo[1,2-a]pyrazines as novel PI3K inhibitors. Bioorg Med Chem Lett 2012;22:1874–8.

[44] Martinez Gonzalez S, Hernandez AI, Varela C, Rodriguez-Aristegui S, Lorenzo M, Rodriguez A, et al. Identification of ETP-46321, a potent and orally bioavailable PI3K α, δ inhibitor. Bioorg Med Chem Lett 2012;22:3460–6.

[45] Martinez Gonzalez S, Hernandez AI, Varela C, Lorenzo M, Ramos-Lima F, Cendon E, et al. Rapid identification of ETP-46992, orally bioavailable PI3K inhibitor, selective versus mTOR. Bioorg Med Chem Lett 2012;22:5208–14.

[46] Burger MT, Knapp M, Wagman A, Ni Z-J, Hendrickson T, Atallah G, et al. Synthesis and in vitro and in vivo evaluation of phosphoinositide-3-kinase inhibitors. ACS Med Chem Lett 2011;2:34–8.

[47] Poulsen A, Williams M, Nagaraj HM, William AD, Wang H, Soh CK, et al. Structure-based optimization of morpholino-triazines as PI3K and mTOR inhibitors. Bioorg Med Chem Lett 2012;22:1009–13.

[48] Ohwada J, Ebiike H, Kawada H, Tsukazaki M, Nakamura M, Miyazaki T, et al. Discovery and biological activity of a novel class I PI3K inhibitor, CH5132799. Bioorg Med Chem Lett 2011;21:1767–72.

[49] Tanaka H, Yoshida M, Tanimura H, Fujii T, Sakata K, Tachibana Y, et al. The selective class I PI3K inhibitor CH5132799 targets human cancers harboring oncogenic PIK3CA mutations. Clin Cancer Res 2011;17:3272–81.

[50] Hart S, Novotny-Diermayr V, Goh KC, Williams M, Tan YC, Ong LC, et al. VS-5584, a novel and highly selective PI3K/mTOR kinase inhibitor for the treatment of cancer. Mol Cancer Ther 2013;12:151–61.

[51] Gilbert A, Nowak P, Brooijmans N, Bursavich MG, Dehnhardt C, Santos ED, et al. Novel purine and pyrazolo[3,4-d]pyrimidine inhibitors of PI3 kinase-α: hit to lead studies. Bioorg Med Chem Lett 2010;20:636–9.

[52] Venkatesan AM, Dehnhardt CM, Chen Z, Santos ED, Dos Santos O, Bursavich M, et al. Novel imidazolopyrimidines as dual PI3-kinase/mTOR inhibitors. Bioorg Med Chem Lett 2010;20:653–6.

[53] Chen Z, Venkatesan AM, Dehnhardt CM, Ayral-Kaloustian S, Brooijmans N, Mallon R, et al. Synthesis and SAR of novel 4-morpholinopyrrolopyrimidine derivatives as potent phosphatidylinositol 3-kinase inhibitors. J Med Chem 2010;53:3169–82.

[54] Dehnhardt CM, Venkatesan AM, Delos Santos E, Chen Z, Santos O, Ayral-Kaloustian S, et al. Lead optimization of N-3-substituted 7-morpholinotriazolopyrimidines as dual phosphoinositide 3-kinase/mammalian target of rapamycin inhibitors: discovery of PKI-402. J Med Chem 2010;53:798–810.

[55] Matthews DJ, O'Farrell M, James J, Stott G, Giddens AC, Rewcastle GW, et al. Preclinical characterization of PWT33597, a dual inhibitor of PI3-kinase alpha and mTOR. Proceedings of the 102nd Annual Meeting of the American Association for Cancer Research, Apr 2–6, 2011, Orlando, FL., Cancer Res. 71 (Suppl.), Abstract 4485.

[56] Alexander R, Balasundaram A, Batchelor M, Brookings D, Crepy K, Crabbe T, et al. 4-(1,3-Thiazol-2-yl)morpholine derivatives as inhibitors of phosphoinositide 3-kinase. Bioorg Med Chem Lett 2008;18:4316–20.

[57] Perry B, Alexander R, Bennett G, Buckley G, Ceska T, Crabbe T, et al. Achieving multi-isoform PI3K inhibition in a series of substituted 3,4-dihydro-2H-benzo[1,4]oxazines. Bioorg Med Chem Lett 2008;18:4700–4.

[58] Perry B, Beevers R, Bennett G, Buckley G, Crabbe T, Gowers L, et al. Optimization of a series of multi-isoform PI3 kinase inhibitors. Bioorg Med Chem Lett 2008;18:5299–302.

[59] Liu KK-C, Zhu JJ, Smith GL, Yin M-J, Bailey S, Chen JH, et al. Highly selective and potent thiophenes as PI3K inhibitors with oral antitumor activity. ACS Med Chem Lett 2011;2:809–13.

[60] Yaguchi SI, Fukui Y, Koshimizu I, Yoshimi H, Matsuno T, Gouda H, et al. Antitumor activity of ZSTK474, a new phosphatidylinositol 3-kinase inhibitor. J Natl Cancer Inst 2006;98:545–56.

[61] Kong D, Yamori T. ZSTK474 is an ATP-competitive inhibitor of class I, phosphatidylinositol 3 kinase isoforms. Cancer Sci 2007;98:1638–42.

[62] Berndt A, Miller S, Williams O, Le DD, Houseman BT, Pacold JI, et al. The p110δ structure: mechanisms for selectivity and potency of new PI(3)K inhibitors. Nature Chem Biol 2010;6:117–24.

[63] Dan S, Okamura M, Mukai Y, Yoshimi H, Inoue Y, Hanyu A, et al. ZSTK474, a specific phosphatidylinositol 3-kinase inhibitor, induces G1 arrest of the cell cycle in vivo. Eur J Cancer 2012;48:936–43.

[64] Rewcastle GW, Gamage SA, Flanagan JU, Frederick R, Denny WA, Baguley BC, et al. Synthesis and biological evaluation of novel analogues of the pan class I phosphatidylinositol 3-kinase (PI3K) inhibitor 2-(difluoromethyl)-1-[4,6-di(4-morpholinyl)-1,3,5-triazin-2-yl]-1H-benzimidazole (ZSTK474). J Med Chem 2011;54:7105–26.

[65] Pomel V, Klicic J, Covini D, Church DD, Shaw JP, Roulin K, et al. Furan-2-ylmethylene thiazolidinediones as novel, potent, and selective inhibitors of phosphoinositide 3-kinase γ. J Med Chem 2006;49:3857–71.

[66] Burger MT, Pecchi S, Wagman A, Ni Z-J, Knapp M, Hendrickson T, et al. Identification of NVP-BKM120 as a potent, selective, orally bioavailable class I PI3 kinase inhibitor for treating cancer. ACS Med Chem Lett 2011;2:774–9.

[67] Venkatesan AM, Dehnhardt CM, Delos Santos E, Chen Z, Dos Santos O, Ayral-Kaloustian S, et al. Bis(morpholino-1,3,5-triazine) derivatives: potent adenosine 5-triphosphate competitive phosphatidylinositol-3-kinase/mammalian target of rapamycin inhibitors: discovery of compound 26 (PKI-587), a highly efficacious dual inhibitor. J Med Chem 2010;53:2636–45.

[68] Venkatesan AM, Chen Z, Dos Santos O, Dehnhardt C, Santos ED, Ayral-Kaloustian S, et al. PKI-179: an orally efficacious dual phosphatidylinositol-3-kinase (PI3K)/mammalian target of rapamycin (mTOR) inhibitor. Bioorg Med Chem Lett 2010;20:5869–73.

[69] Maira SM, Stauffer F, Brueggen J, Furet P, Schnell C, Fritsch C, et al. Identification and characterization of NVP-BEZ235, a new orally available dual phosphatidylinositol 3-kinase/mammalian target of rapamycin inhibitor with potent in vivo antitumor activity. Mol Cancer Ther 2008;7:1851–63.

[70] Cheng H, Li C, Bailey S, Baxi SM, Goulet L, Guo L, et al. Discovery of the highly potent PI3K/mTOR dual inhibitor PF-04979064 through structure based drug design. ACS Med Chem Lett 2013;4:91–7.

[71] Scott WJ, Hentemann M, Rowley B, Bull C, Jenkins S, Bullion AM, et al. Novel 2,3-dihydroimidazo[1,2-c]quinazoline PI3K inhibitors: discovery and structure-activity relationship. 22nd EORTC-NCI-AACR symposium, Berlin, 2010, Abstract 444, poster 185.

[72] Cheng H-M, Bagrodia S, Bailey S, Edwards M, Hoffman J, Hu Q-Y, et al. Discovery of the highly potent PI3K/mTOR dual inhibitor PF-04691502 through structure based drug design. Med Chem Commun 2010;1:139–44.

[73] Auger KR, Luo L, Knight SD, Van Aller G, Tummino PJ, Copeland RA, et al. GSK1059615: a novel inhibitor of phosphoinositide 3-kinase for the treatment of cancer. EORTC-NCI-AACR International Conference on Molecular Targets and Cancer, Geneva, Switzerland, October, 2008.

[74] Knight SD, Adams ND, Burgess JL, Chaudhari AM, Darcy MG, Donatelli CA, et al. Discovery of GSK2126458, a highly potent inhibitor of PI3K and the mammalian target of rapamycin. ACS Med Chem Lett 2010;1:39–43.

[75] Nishimura N, Siegmund A, Liu L, Yang K, Bryan MC, Andrews KL, et al. Phosphoinositide 3-kinase (PI3K)/mammalian target of rapamycin (mTOR) dual inhibitors: discovery and structure-activity relationships of a series of quinoline and quinoxaline derivatives. J Med Chem 2011;54:4735–51.

[76] D'Angelo ND, Kim T-S, Andrews K, Booker SK, Caenepeel S, Chen K, et al. Discovery and optimization of a series of benzothiazole phosphoinositide 3-kinase (PI3K)/mammalian target of rapamycin (mTOR) dual inhibitors. J Med Chem 2011;54:1789–811.

[77] Stec MM, Andrews KL, Booker SK, Caenepeel S, Freeman DJ, Jiang J, et al. Structure-activity relationships of phosphoinositide 3-kinase (PI3K)/mammalian target of rapamycin (mTOR) dual inhibitors: investigations of various 6,5-heterocycles to improve metabolic stability. J Med Chem 2011;54:5174–84.

[78] Wurz RP, Liu L, Yang K, Nishimura N, Bo Y, Pettus LH, et al. Synthesis and structure-activity relationships of dual PI3K/mTOR inhibitors based on a 4-amino-6-methyl-1,3,5-triazine sulfonamide scaffold. Bioorg Med Chem Lett 2012;22:5714–20.

[79] Wu P, Su Y, Liu X, Zhang L, Ye Y, Xu J, et al. Synthesis and biological evaluation of novel 2-arylamino-3-(arylsulfonyl)quinoxalines as PI3Kα inhibitors. Eur J Med Chem 2011;46:5540–8.

[80] Norman MH, Andrews KL, Bo YY, Booker SK, Caenepeel S, Cee VJ, et al. Selective class I phosphoinositide 3-kinase inhibitors: optimization of a series of pyridyltriazines leading to the identification of a clinical candidate, AMG 511. J Med Chem 2012;55:7796–816.

[81] Staben ST, Siu M, Goldsmith R, Olivero AG, Do S, Burdick DJ, et al. Structure-based design of thienobenzoxepin inhibitors of PI3-kinase. Bioorg Med Chem Lett 2011;21:4054–8.

[82] Hayakawa M, Kaizawa H, Kawaguchi KI, Ishikawa N, Koizumi T, Ohishi T, et al. Synthesis and biological evaluation of imidazo[1,2-a]pyridine derivatives as novel PI3 kinase p110α inhibitors. Bioorg Med Chem 2007;15:403–12.

[83] Kendall JD, O'Connor P, Marshall A, Frederick R, Flanagan JU, Rewcastle GW, et al. Discovery of pyrazolo [1,5-a]pyridines as p110α-selective PI3 kinase inhibitors. Bioorg Med Chem 2012;20:69–85.

[84] Caravatti G, Guagnano V, Fairhurst R, Imbach P, Bruce I, Knapp M, et al. 2-Aminothiazoles as potent and selective PI3K alpha inhibitors: discovery of NVP-BYL719 and structural basis for the isoform selectivity. Proceedings of the 103rd Annual Meeting of the American Association for Cancer Research, Mar 31–Apr 4, 2012, Chicago, IL. Cancer Res. 72(Suppl.), Abstract 1922.

[85] Bruce I, Akhlaq M, Bloomfield GC, Budd E, Cox B, Cuenoud B, et al. Development of isoform selective PI3-kinase inhibitors as pharmacological tools for elucidating the PI3K pathway. Bioorg Med Chem Lett 2012;22:5445–50.

[86] Jamieson S, Flanagan JU, Kolekar S, Buchanan C, Kendall JD, Lee W-J, et al. A drug targeting only p110α can block phosphoinositide 3-kinase signalling and tumour growth in certain cell types. Biochem J 2011;438:53–62.

[87] Jackson SP, Schoenwaelder SM, Goncalves I, Nesbitt WS, Yap CL, Wright CE, et al. PI 3-kinase p110β: A new target for antithrombotic therapy. Nat Med 2005;11:507–14.

[88] Ni J, Liu Q, Xie S, Carlson CB, Von T, Vogel KW, et al. Functional characterization of an isoform-selective inhibitor of PI3K–p110β as a potential anticancer agent. Cancer Discovery 2012;2:425–33.

[89] Blackman SC, Gainer SD, Suttle BB, Skordos KW, Greshock JD, Motwani M, et al. A phase I/IIa, first time in human, open-label dose-escalation study of GSK2636771 in subjects with advanced solid tumors with PTEN deficiency. Proceedings of the 103rd Annual Meeting of the American Association for Cancer Research, Mar 31–Apr 4, 2012, Chicago, IL. Cancer Res. 72(Suppl.), Abstract 1752.

[90] Lin H, Erhard K, Hardwicke MA, Luengo JI, Mack JF, McSurdy-Freed J, et al. Synthesis and structure–activity relationships of imidazo[1,2-a]pyrimidin-5(1H)-ones as a novel series of beta isoform selective phosphatidylinositol 3-kinase inhibitors. Bioorg Med Chem Lett 2012;22:2230–4.

[91] Sanchez RM, Erhard K, Hardwicke MA, Lin H, McSurdy-Freed J, Plant R, et al. Synthesis and structure-activity relationships of 1,2,4-triazolo[1,5-a]pyrimidin-7(3H)-ones as novel series of potent β isoform selective phosphatidylinositol 3-kinase inhibitors. Bioorg Med Chem Lett 2012;22:3198–202.

[92] Lin H, Schulz MJ, Xie R, Zeng J, Luengo JI, Squire MD, et al. Rational design, synthesis, and SAR of a novel thiazolopyrimidinone series of selective PI3K-beta inhibitors. ACS Med Chem Lett 2012;3:524–9.

[93] Giordanetto F, Waallberg A, Ghosal S, Iliefski T, Cassel J, Yuan Z-Q, et al. Discovery of phosphoinositide 3-kinases (PI3K) p110β isoform inhibitor 4-[2-hydroxyethyl(1-naphthylmethyl)amino]-6-[(2S)-2-methylmorpholin-4-yl]-1H-pyrimidin-2-one, an effective antithrombotic agent without associated bleeding and insulin resistance. Bioorg Med Chem Lett 2012;22:6671–6.

[94] Certal V, Halley F, Virone-Oddos A, Thompson F, Filoche-Romme B, El-Ahmad Y, et al. Preparation and optimization of new 4-(morpholin-4-yl)-(6-oxo-1,6-dihydropyrimidin-2-yl)amide derivatives as PI3Kβ inhibitors. Bioorg Med Chem Lett 2012;22:6381–4.

[95] Certal V, Halley F, Virone-Oddos A, Delorme C, Karlsson A, Rak A, et al. Discovery and optimization of new benzimidazole- and benzoxazole-pyrimidone selective PI3Kβ inhibitors for the treatment of phosphatase and TENsin homologue (PTEN)-deficient cancers. J Med Chem 2012;55:4788–805.

[96] Sadhu C, Masinovsky B, Dick K, Sowell CG, Staunton DE. Essential role of phosphoinositide 3-kinase δ in neutrophil directional movement. J Immunol 2003;170:2647–54.

[97] Lannutti BJ, Meadows SA, Herman SEM, Kashishian A, Steiner B, Johnson AJ, et al. CAL-101, a p110δ selective phosphatidylinositol-3-kinase inhibitor for the treatment of B-cell malignancies, inhibits PI3K signaling and cellular viability. Blood 2011;117:591–4.

[98] Sutherlin DP, Baker S, Bisconte A, Blaney PM, Brown A, Chan BK, et al. Potent and selective inhibitors of PI3Kδ: obtaining isoform selectivity from the affinity pocket and tryptophan shelf. Bioorg Med Chem Lett 2012;22:4296–302.

[99] Safina BS, Baker S, Baumgardner M, Blaney PM, Chan BK, Chen Y-H, et al. Discovery of novel PI3-kinase δ specific inhibitors for the treatment of rheumatoid arthritis: taming CYP3A4 time-dependent inhibition. J Med Chem 2012;55:5887–900.

[100] Murray JM, Sweeney ZK, Chan BK, Balazs M, Bradley E, Castanedo G, et al. Potent and highly selective benzimidazole inhibitors of PI3-kinase delta. J Med Chem 2012;55:7686–95.

[101] Camps M, Ruckle T, Ji H, Ardissone V, Rintelen F, Shaw J, et al. Blockade of PI3K gamma suppresses joint inflammation and damage in mouse models of rheumatoid arthritis. Nat Med 2005;11:936–43.

[102] Bergamini G, Bell K, Shimamura S, Werner T, Cansfield A, Mueller K, et al. A selective inhibitor reveals PI3Kγ dependence of TH17 cell differentiation. Nat Chem Biol 2012;8:576–82.

[103] Leahy JW, Buhr CA, Johnson HWB, Kim BG, Baik T, Cannoy J, et al. Discovery of a novel series of potent and orally bioavailable phosphoinositide 3-kinase γ inhibitors. J Med Chem 2012;55:5467–82.

[104] Oka Y, Yabuuchi T, Fujii Y, Ohtake H, Wakahara S, Matsumoto K, et al. Discovery and optimization of a series of 2-aminothiazole-oxazoles as potent phosphoinositide 3-kinase γ inhibitors. Bioorg Med Chem Lett 2012;22:7534–8.

[105] Palanki MSS, Dneprovskaia E, Doukas J, Fine RM, Hood J, Kang X, et al. Discovery of 3,3′-(2,4-diaminopteridine-6,7-diyl)diphenol as an isozyme-selective inhibitor of PI3K for the treatment of ischemia reperfusion injury associated with myocardial infarction. J Med Chem 2007;50:4279–94.

[106] Porter JR, Ali J, DiNitto JP, Dunbar J, Faia K, Hoyt J, et al. The potent phosphoinositide-3-kinase-(δ,γ) inhibitor IPI-145 is active in preclinical models of arthritis and well tolerated in healthy adult subjects. American College of Rheumatology (ACR)/Association of Rheumatology Health Professionals (ARHP); 2012, 2012 Annual Meeting, Washington, D.C., November 9–14, 2012. Abstract 338.

[107] Gonzalez-Lopez de Turiso F, Shin Y, Brown M, Cardozo M, Chen Y, Fong D, et al. Discovery and in vivo evaluation of dual PI3Kβ/δ inhibitors. J Med Chem 2012;55:7667–85.

[108] Ihle NT, Paine-Murrieta G, Berggren MI, Baker A, Tate WR, Wipf P, et al. The phosphatidylinositol-3-kinase inhibitor PX-866 overcomes resistance to the epidermal growth factor receptor inhibitor gefitinib in A-549 human non-small cell lung cancer xenografts. Mol Cancer Ther 2005;4:1349–57.

[109] Maira S-M, Pecchi S, Huang A, Burger M, Knapp M, Sterker D, et al. Identification and characterization of NVP-BKM120, an orally available pan-class I PI3-kinase inhibitor. Mol Cancer Ther 2012;11:317–28.

[110] Bendell JC, Rodon J, Burris HA, de Jonge M, Verweij J, Birle D, et al. Phase I, dose-escalation study of BKM120, an oral pan-class I PI3K inhibitor, in patients with advanced solid tumors. J Clin Oncol 2012;30:282–90.

[111] Mallon R, Feldberg LR, Lucas J, Chaudhary I, Dehnhardt C, Santos ED, et al. Antitumor efficacy of PKI-587, a highly potent dual PI3K/mTOR kinase inhibitor. Clin Cancer Res 2011;17:3193–203.

[112] Dehnhardt CM, Venkatesan AM, Chen Z, Delos-Santos E, Ayral-Kaloustian S, Brooijmans N, et al. Identification of 2-oxatriazines as highly potent pan-PI3K/mTOR dual inhibitors. Bioorg Med Chem Lett 2011;21:4773–8.

[113] Stauffer F, Sauveur-Michel M, Furet P, García-Echeverría C. Imidazo[4,5-c]quinolines as inhibitors of the PI3K/PKB-pathway. Bioorg Med Chem Lett 2008;18:1027–30.

[114] Serra V, Markman B, Scaltriti M, Eichhorn PJA, Valero V, Guzman M, et al. NVP-BEZ235, a dual PI3K/mTOR inhibitor, prevents PI3K signaling and inhibits the growth of cancer cells with activating PI3K mutations. Cancer Res 2008;68:8022–30.

[115] Chang K-W, Tsai SY, Wu C-M, Yen C-J, Chuang B-F, Chang J-Y. Novel phosphoinositide 3-kinase/mTOR dual inhibitor, NVP-BGT226, displays potent growth-inhibitory activity against human head and neck cancer cells in vitro and in vivo. Clin Cancer Res 2011;17:7116–26.

[116] Markman B, Tabernero J, Krop I, Shapiro GI, Siu L, Chen LC, et al. Phase I safety, pharmacokinetic, and pharmacodynamic study of the oral phosphatidylinositol-3-kinase and mTOR inhibitor BGT226 in patients with advanced solid tumors. Ann Oncol 2012;23:2399–408.

[117] Chen JS, Zhou LJ, Entin-Meer M, Yang X, Donker M, Knight ZA, et al. Characterization of structurally distinct, isoform-selective phosphoinositide 3′-kinase inhibitors in combination with radiation in the treatment of glioblastoma. Mol Cancer Ther 2008;7:841–50.

[118] Liu N, Rowley B, Schneider C, Bull C, Hoffmann J, Kaekoenen S, et al. BAY 80-6946, a highly selective and potent pan class I PI3K inhibitor induces tumor apoptosis in vitro and tumor regression in vivo in a sub-set of tumor models. Proceedings of the 101st Annual Meeting of the American Association for Cancer Research, Apr 17–21, 2010, Washington, DC. Cancer Res. 70(8 Suppl.): Abstract 4476.

[119] Le PT, Cheng H, Ninkovic S, Plewe M, Huang X, Wang H, et al. Design and synthesis of a novel pyrrolidinyl pyrido pyrimidinone derivative as a potent inhibitor of PI3Kα and mTOR. Bioorg Med Chem Lett 2012;22:5098–103.

[120] Yuan J, Mehta PP, Yin M-J, Sun S, Zou A, Chen J, et al. PF-0469502, a potent and selective oral inhibitor of PI3K and mTOR kinases with antitumor activity. Mol Cancer Ther 2011;10:2189–99.

[121] LoRusso P, Markman B, Tabarnero J, Shazer R, Nguyen L, Heath E, et al. A phase I dose-escalation study of the safety, pharmacokinetics (PK), and pharmacodynamics of XL765, a PI3K/TORC1/TORC2 inhibitor administered orally to patients (pts) with advanced solid tumors. American Society of Clinical Oncology, 2009 Annual Meeting, Orlando, FL, Abstract 3502.

[122] Verheijen JC, Richard DJ, Zask DJ. Non-protein kinases as therapeutic targets. RSC Drug Discovery Series, 19(Kinase Drug Discovery), 161–217; 2012.

[123] Debussche L, Garcia-Echeverria C, Ma J, McMillan S, Ogden JAM, Vincent L. Compositions comprising a PI3K inhibitor and a MEK inhibitor and their use for treating cancer. WO 2012/078832, published 14th June, 2012.

[124] Liu KK-C, Bagrodia S, Bailey S, Cheng H, Chen H, Gao L. 4-Methylpteridinones as orally active and selective PI3K/mTOR dual inhibitors. Bioorg Med Chem Lett 2010;20:6096–9.

[125] Liu KKC, Huang X, Bagrodia S, Chen JH, Greasley S, Cheng H, et al. Quinazolines with intra-molecular hydrogen bonding scaffold (iMHBS) as PI3K/mTOR dual inhibitors. Bioorg Med Chem Lett 2011;21:1270–4.

[126] Kim O, Jeong Y, Lee H, Hong S-S, Hong S. Design and synthesis of imidazopyridine analogues as inhibitors of phosphoinositide 3-kinase signaling and angiogenesis. J Med Chem 2011;54:2455–66.

[127] Lee H, Li G-Y, Jeong Y, Jung KH, Lee J-H, Hamb K, et al. A novel imidazopyridine analogue as a phosphatidylinositol 3-kinase inhibitor against human breast cancer. Cancer Lett 2012;318:68–75.

[128] Li G-Y, Jung KH, Lee H, Son MK, Seo J-H, Hong S-W, et al. A novel imidazopyridine derivative, HS-106, induces apoptosis of breast cancer cells and represses angiogenesis by targeting the PI3K/mTOR pathway. Cancer Lett 2013;329:59–67.

[129] Lee H, Jung KH, Jeong Y, Hong S, Hong S-S. HS-173, a novel phosphatidylinositol 3-kinase (PI3K) inhibitor, has anti-tumor activity through promoting apoptosis and inhibiting angiogenesis. Cancer Lett 2013;328:152–9.

[130] Jung KH, Choi M-J, Hong S, Lee H, Hong S-W, Zheng H-M, et al. HS-116, a novel phosphatidylinositol 3-kinase inhibitor induces apoptosis and suppresses angiogenesis of hepatocellular carcinoma through inhibition of the PI3K/AKT/mTOR pathway. Cancer Lett 2012;316:187–95.

[131] Jung KH, Zheng H-M, Jeong Y, Choi M-J, Lee H, Hong S-W, et al. Suppression of tumor proliferation and angiogenesis of hepatocellular carcinoma by HS-104, a novel phosphoinositide 3-kinase inhibitor. Cancer Lett 2013;328:176–87.

[132] Lee J-H, Lee H, Yun S-M, Jung KH, Jeong Y, Yan HH, et al. IPD-196, a novel phosphatidylinositol 3-kinase inhibitor with potent anticancer activity against hepatocellular carcinoma. Cancer Lett 2013;329:99–108.

[133] Hong S, Lee S, Kim B, Lee H, Hong S-S, Hong S. Discovery of new azaindole-based PI3Kα inhibitors: apoptotic and antiangiogenic effect on cancer cells. Bioorg Med Chem Lett 2010;20:7212–5.

[134] Kim J, Hong S, Hong S. Discovery of new aminopyrimidine-based phosphoinositide 3-kinase beta (PI3Kβ) inhibitors with selectivity over PI3Kα. Bioorg Med Chem Lett 2011;21:6977–81.

[135] Adams ND, Darcy MG, Johnson NW, Kasparec J, Knight SD, Newlander KA, et al. Pyridosulfonamide derivatives as PI3 kinase inhibitors. WO 2009/055418, published 30th April, 2009.

[136] Aftab DT, Decillis A. Phosphatidylinositol 3-kinase inhibitors and methods of their use. WO 2012/065057, published 18th May, 2012.

[137] Foster PG. Potentiating the antitumor effects of chemotherapy with the selective PI3K inhibitor XL147. AACR-NCI-EORTC International Conference on Molecular Targets and Cancer Therapeutics, San Francisco, CA, October 22–26, 2007, Abstract C199.

[138] Reynolds CP, Kang MH, Carol H, Lock R, Gorlick R, Kolb EA, et al. Initial testing (stage 1) of the phosphatidylinositol 3′ kinase inhibitor, SAR245408 (XL147) by the pediatric preclinical testing program. Pediatr Blood Cancer 2013;60:791–8.

[139] Wu P, Su Y, Liu X, Yang B, He Q, Hu Y. Discovery of novel 2-piperidinol-3-(arylsulfonyl)quinoxalines as phosphoinositide 3-kinase α (PI3Kα) inhibitors. Bioorg Med Chem 2012;20:2837–44.

[140] Smith AL, D'Angelo ND, Bo YY, Booker SK, Cee VJ, Herberich B, et al. Structure-based design of a novel series of potent, selective inhibitors of the class I phosphatidylinositol 3-kinases. J Med Chem 2012;55:5188–219.

[141] Heffron TP, Wei BQ, Olivero A, Staben ST, Tsui V, Do S, et al. Rational design of phosphoinositide 3-kinase α inhibitors that exhibit selectivity over the phosphoinositide 3-kinase β isoform. J Med Chem 2011;54:7815–33.

[142] Hayakawa M, Kawaguchi KI, Kaizawa H, Koizumi T, Ohishi T, Yamano M, et al. Synthesis and biological evaluation of sulfonylhydrazone-substituted imidazo[1,2-a]pyridines as novel PI3 kinase p110α inhibitors. Bioorg Med Chem 2007;15:5837–44.

[143] Guillard S, Clarke PA, te Poele R, Mohri Z, Bjerke L, Valenti M, et al. Molecular pharmacology of phosphatidylinositol 3-kinase inhibition in human glioma. Cell Cycle 2009;8:443–53.

[144] Kendall JD, Rewcastle GW, Frederick R, Mawson C, Denny WA, Marshall ES, et al. Synthesis, biological evaluation and molecular modeling of sulfonohydrazides as selective PI3 kinase p110α inhibitors. Bioorg Med Chem 2007;15:7677–87.

[145] Kendall JD, Giddens A, Tsang S, Frederick R, Flanagan JU, Rewcastle GW, et al. Novel pyrazolo[1,5-a]pyridines as p110α-selective PI3 kinase inhibitors: exploring the benzenesulfonohydrazide SAR. Bioorg Med Chem 2012;20:58–68.

[146] Fritsch CM, Schnell C, Chatenay-Rivauday C, Guthy DA, De Pover A, Wartmann M, et al. NVP-BYL719, a novel PI3K alpha selective inhibitor with all the characteristics required for clinical development as an anticancer agent. Proceedings of the 103rd Annual Meeting of the American Association for Cancer Research, Mar 31–Apr 4, 2012, Chicago, IL. Cancer Res. 72(8 Suppl.), Abstract 3748.

[147] Zheng Z, Amran SI, Zhu J, Schmidt-Kittler O, Kinzler KW, Vogelstein B, et al. Definition of the binding mode of a new class of phosphoinositide 3-kinase α-selective inhibitors using in vitro mutagenesis of non-conserved amino acids and kinetic analysis. Biochem J 2012;444:529–35.

[148] Robertson AD, Jackson S, Kenche V, Yaip C, Parbaharan H, Thompson P. Therapeutic morpholino-substituted compounds. WO 2001/53266, published 26th July; 2001.

[149] Sturgeon SA, Jones C, Angus JA, Wright CE. Advantages of a selective β-isoform phosphoinositide 3-kinase antagonist, an anti-thrombotic agent devoid of other cardiovascular actions in the rat. Eur J Pharmacol 2008;587:209–15.

[150] Wee S, Wiederschain D, Maira S-M, Loo A, Miller C, de Beaumont R, et al. PTEN-deficient cancers depend on PIK3CB. Proc Natl Acad Sci U S A 2008;105:13057–62.

[151] Jia S, Liu Z, Zhang S, Liu P, Zhang L, Lee SH, et al. Essential roles of PI(3)K-p110β in cell growth, metabolism and tumorigenesis. Nature 2008;454:776–9.

[152] Smith GC, Ong WK, Rewcastle GW, Kendall JD, Han W, Shepherd PR. Effects of acutely inhibiting PI3K isoforms and mTOR on regulation of glucose metabolism in vivo. Biochem J 2012;442:161–9.

[153] Nylander S, Kull B, Bjorkman JA, Ulvinge JC, Oakes N, Emanuelsson BM. Human target validation of phosphoinositide 3-kinase (PI3K)β: effects on platelets and insulin sensitivity, using AZD6482 a novel PI3Kβ inhibitor. J Thromb Haemost 2012;10:2127–36.

[154] Tai W, Shukla RS, Qin B, Li B, Cheng K. Development of a peptide-drug conjugate for prostate cancer therapy. Mol Pharmaceutics 2011;8:901–12.

[155] Zhao Y, Duan S, Zeng X, Liu C, Davies N, Li B. Prodrug strategy for PSMA-targeted delivery of TGX-221 to prostate cancer cells. Mol Pharmaceutics 2012;9:1705–16.

[156] Giordanetto F, Waallberg A, Cassel J, Ghosal S, Kossenjans M, Yuan Z-Q. Discovery of 4-morpholino-pyrimidin-6-one and 4-morpholino-pyrimidin-2-one-containing phosphoinositide 3-kinase (PI3K) p110β isoform inhibitors through structure-based fragment optimisation. Bioorg Med Chem Lett 2012;22:6665–70.

[157] Williams O, Houseman BT, Kunkel EJ, Aizenstein B, Hoffman R, Knight ZA. Discovery of dual inhibitors of the immune cell PI3Ks p110δ and p110γ: a prototype for new anti-inflammatory drugs. Chem Biol 2010;17:123–34.

[158] Fruman DA, Rommel C. PI3Kδ inhibitors in cancer: rationale and serendipity merge in the clinic. Cancer Discovery 2011;1:562–72.

[159] Furman RR, Byrd JC, Brown JR, Coutre SE, Benson DM, Wagner-Johnston ND, et al. CAL-101, an isoform-selective inhibitor of phosphatidylinositol 3-kinase p.110δ, demonstrates clinical activity and pharmaco-dynamic effects in patients with relapsed or refractory chronic lymphocytic leukemia. Blood (ASH Annual Meeting Abstracts) 116, Abstract 55; 2010.

[160] Courtney KD, Corcoran RB, Engelman JA. The PI3K pathway as drug target in human cancer. J Clin Oncol 2010;28:1075–83.

[161] Norman P. Selective PI3Kδ inhibitors: a review of the patent literature. Expert Opin Ther Pat 2011;21:1773–90.

[162] Bell K, Sunose M, Ellard K, Cansfield A, Taylor J, Miller W, et al. SAR studies around a series of triazolopyridines as potent and selective PI3Kγ inhibitors. Bioorg Med Chem Lett 2012;22:5257–63.

[163] Cushing TD, Metz DP, Whittington DA, McGee LR. PI3Kδ and PI3Kγ as targets for autoimmune and inflammatory diseases. J Med Chem 2012;55:8559–81.

[164] Foster JG, Blunt MD, Carter E, Ward SG. Inhibition of PI3K signaling spurs new therapeutic opportunities in inflammatory/autoimmune diseases and hematological malignancies. Pharmacol Rev 2012;64:1027–54.

[165] Rommel C, Camps M, Ji H. PI3K delta and PI3K gamma: partners in crime in inflammation in rheumatoid arthritis and beyond? Nat Rev Immunol 2007;7:191–201.

[166] Doukas J, Wrasidlo W, Noronha G, Dneprovskaia E, Fine R, Weis S, et al. Phosphoinositide 3-kinase γ/δ inhibition limits infarct size after myocardial ischemia/reperfusion injury. Proc Natl Acad Sci U S A 2006;103:19866–71.

[167] Doukas J, Eide L, Stebbins K, Racanelli-Layton A, Dellamary L, Martin M, et al. Aerosolized phosphoinositide 3-kinase γ/δ inhibitor TG100-115 [3-[2,4-diamino-6-(3-hydroxyphenyl)pteridin-7-yl]phenol] as a therapeutic candidate for asthma and chronic obstructive pulmonary disease. J Pharmacol Exp Ther 2009;328:758–65.

[168] Ellard K, Sunose M, Bell K, Ramsden N, Bergamini G, Neubauer G. Discovery of novel PI3Kγ/δ inhibitors as potential agents for inflammation. Bioorg Med Chem Lett 2012;22:4546–9.

[169] Flinn IW, Horwitz SM, Patel M, Younes A, Porter JR, Sweeney J, et al. Clinical safety and activity in a phase 1 trial of IPI-145, a potent inhibitor of phosphoinositide-3-kinase (PI3K)-δ,γ in patients with advanced hematologic malignancies. 54th American Society of Hematology (ASH) Annual Meeting, Atlanta, GA, December 8–11, 2012. Abstract 3663.

[170] Smaill JB, Rewcastle GW, Loo JA, Greis KD, Chan OH, Reyner EL, et al. Tyrosine kinase inhibitors. 17. Irreversible inhibitors of the epidermal growth factor receptor: 4-(phenylamino)quinazoline- and 4-(phenylamino)pyrido[3,2-d]pyrimidine-6-acrylamides bearing additional solubilizing functions. J Med Chem 2000;43:1380–97.

[171] Srivastava SK, Jha A, Agarwal SK, Mukherjee R, Burman AC. Synthesis and structure–activity relationships of potent antitumor active quinoline and naphthyridine derivatives. Anticancer Agents Med Chem 2007;7:685–709.

[172] Hirsh V. Afatinib (BIBW 2992) development in non-small-cell lung cancer. Future Oncol 2011;7:817–25.

[173] Wymann MP, Bulgarelli-Leva G, Zvelebil MJ, Pirola L, Vanhaesebroeck B, Waterfield MD, et al. Wortmannin inactivates phosphoinositide 3-kinase by covalent modification of Lys-802, a residue involved in the phosphate transfer reaction. Mol Cell Biol 1996;16:1722–33.

[174] Norman BH, Shih C, Toth JE, Ray JE, Dodge JA, Johnson DW, et al. Studies on the mechanism of phosphatidylinositol 3-kinase inhibition by wortmannin and related analogs. J Med Chem 1996;39:1106–11.

[175] Ihle NT, Williams R, Chow S, Chew W, Berggren MI, Paine-Murrieta G, et al. Molecular pharmacology and antitumor activity of PX-866, a novel inhibitor of phosphoinositide-3-kinase signalling. Mol Cancer Ther 2004;3:763–72.

[176] Howes AL, Chiang GG, Lang ES, Ho CB, Powis G, Vuori K, et al. The phosphatidylinositol 3-kinase inhibitor, PX-866, is a potent inhibitor of cancer cell motility and growth in three-dimensional cultures. Mol Cancer Ther 2007;6:2505–14.

[177] Hong DS, Bowles DW, Falchook GS, Messersmith WA, George GC, O'Bryant CL, et al. A multicenter phase I trial of PX-866, an oral irreversible phosphatidylinositol 3-kinase inhibitor, in patients with advanced solid tumors. Clin Cancer Res 2012;18:4173–82.

16

Antibody–Drug Conjugates Delivering DNA Cytotoxics

John A. Hartley

Cancer Research UK Drug-DNA Interactions Research Group, UCL Cancer Institute, London, UK

INTRODUCTION

It was Paul Ehrlich who pioneered the use of cytotoxic chemotherapy and who also pointed to the future of antibodies as "magic bullets". These two classes of therapeutic agents are today the most successful in oncology, but they have largely developed independently. Naked antibodies have great specificity but, as single agents, often have limited antitumor activity, particularly against solid tumors. Because of their favorable safety profile, antibodies can be combined successfully with chemotherapy, which alone often suffers from lack of tumor specificity and significant systemic toxicity.

Development of the new class of therapeutics called antibody–drug conjugates (ADCs) has the aim of achieving potent and selective target cell killing by taking advantage of the exquisite selectivity of a monoclonal antibody combined with the potent cell-killing activity of a small-molecule cytotoxic. If successful, the limitations of the two major components should be overcome. Although simple in concept, developing clinically effective ADCs has proven to be highly challenging in practice. The idea of ADCs has been around for over 30 years [1,2], but it is only recently that they are emerging as an important and rapidly growing class of therapeutic agent against both hematological malignancies and solid tumors [3–6]. In particular, the field has been boosted by the approval in 2011 of brentuximab vedotin (Adcetris®) to treat Hodgkin lymphoma and anaplastic large-cell lymphoma [7,8], and in 2013 of trastuzumab emtansine (T-DM1, Kadcyla®) to treat HER2-positive breast cancer [9].

COMPOSITION OF ANTIBODY–DRUG CONJUGATES

ADCs are highly complex molecular entities. The three components of an ADC—antibody, linker, and drug (Fig. 16.1)—all need careful optimization, and the bench-to-bedside

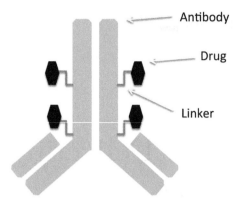

FIGURE 16.1 Schematic representation of an antibody–drug conjugate (ADC) showing the three components: antibody, linker, and drug.

translation of ADCs requires a quantitative mechanistic understanding. In addition, the choice of target antigen is critical to the activity and tolerability of an ADC. The ideal antigen should have high and relatively homogeneous tumor expression, with little or no expression on normal tissue to ensure the maximum therapeutic index, and it should not be downregulated during therapy. The target antigen, necessarily present on the cell surface, should be internalizing to enable the ADC, following binding, to be efficiently transported into the cell through receptor-mediated endocytosis prior to active drug release in, for example, the lysosome (Fig. 16.2). If the antigen is noninternalizing, the toxic agent would need to be locally released extracellularly and then be able to diffuse into target cells. This approach, however, may be more applicable to agents that do not require internalization (or release) to kill cells, such as radioisotopes [10]. Clearly, target antigen expression level is important in determining the potency of an ADC [11], although effective therapy of a tumor with a relatively low expression level can be achieved if an exquisitely potent cyto-toxic "warhead" is utilized.

To date, the most frequently used targeting component for an ADC is a whole antibody, although smaller fragments and nonantibody scaffolds, down to simple peptides, are potential delivery vehicles that are being widely evaluated. The development of human-ized, deimmunized, or fully human antibodies derived from transgenic or phage display techniques has been an important factor in ADC evolution, and only whole antibodies, mostly the immunoglobulin-G 1 (IgG1) isotype, have so far undergone clinical evaluation as ADCs. Such antibodies exceed the size limit for renal clearance and have a long clini-cal half-life. Pharmacokinetics, however, may not necessarily be optimal because studies with radiolabeled antibodies indicate that less than 0.1% of the injected dose of an IgG is delivered per gram of solid tumor [12]. Interaction with Fc receptors is also possible, which would add immune effector functions to the ADC. This could potentially con-tribute to the effectiveness of the ADC or, conversely, contribute to unwanted systemic side effects due to internalization of the ADC into Fc receptor–expressing immune cells. Although few clinical studies have directly compared an ADC with its corresponding unconjugated antibody, ADCs demonstrate better response rates as single agents than naked antibodies targeting the same cell surface antigen when similar patient popula-tions are compared.

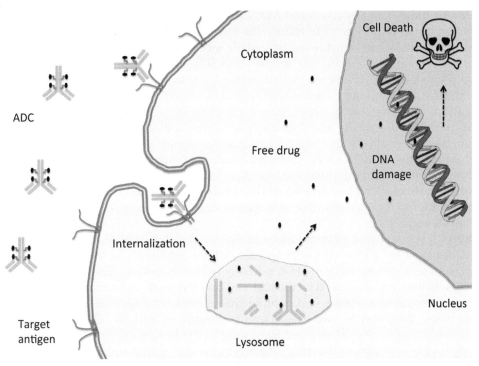

FIGURE 16.2 Mechanism of action of ADCs delivering DNA cytotoxics. The ADC binds to the target antigen on the cell surface, and the ADC–antigen complex is internalized through receptor-mediated endocytosis. Release of the active drug can occur in the lysosome either by direct cleavage of the linker or by proteolysis of the antibody. The released cytotoxic warhead is free to traffic to the nucleus to deliver DNA damage, leading to cell death.

The linkage between the antibody and the cytotoxic payload is a critical component of an ADC and requires careful design and development. It must attach to the antibody without affecting antibody–antigen binding function, and to the drug in a way that enables efficient release from the antibody only after internalization in the target cell. Stability of the linker during storage and in the blood circulation is essential to avoid release of free drug and the potential for off-target nonspecific toxicity while maximizing exposure to the tumor [13].

The mode of attachment of the drug–linker to the antibody can influence both activity and tolerability. Chemical conjugation is generally to either lysine or thiol groups, the latter offering the possibility for more controlled or site-specific attachment. A consequence of conjugation to random reactive groups on an antibody (e.g., the abundant lysine residues or resulting from partial reduction of interchain disulfides) is a heterogeneous drug-loading stoichiometry. For example, trastuzumab emtansine has an average drug:antibody ratio (DAR) of 3.5 with a distribution of 1–7 modified lysines per antibody, and brentuximab vedotin has a DAR of approximately 4 with a distribution of 0–8 modified thiols on the chimeric antibody. The DAR can influence a number of important biophysical and biological properties, including aggregation, antigen binding, pharmacokinetics, potency, and toxicity. Specifically, the conjugation of too many drug molecules can lead to a reduced half-life in circulation and increased toxicity [14]. As indicated here, the optimum average

DAR for the most clinically advanced ADCs appears to be around 4. This may, however, be a reflection of the requirement to reduce the DAR 0 component of the ADC mixture. Site-specific conjugation can be achieved by genetic modification to introduce, for example, an unpaired cysteine at a specific surface location [15], an unpaired selenocysteine [16], or pacetyl phenylalanine [17] as sites of attachment. An example of the engineered cysteine is the THIOMAB technology from Genentech [18], which results in a more homogeneous conjugation, and therefore a more uniform distribution of the drug, a property that has relevance for manufacturing and regulatory approval. A direct comparison of anti-MUC16 ADCs in the thio-engineered versus nonengineered formats gave similar efficacy but better tolerability for the THIOMAB ADC. Interestingly, a comparison of different locations for attachment, however, highlighted the in vivo sensitivity of ADCs to conjugation site quality and, in particular, the importance of the susceptibility of the maleimide-coupled ADC reaction in highly exposed cysteine attachment sites to exchange onto cysteines on other serum proteins [19].

Release of active drug can be achieved using either a cleavable or a noncleavable linker. Linkers designed to be cleaved under specific cellular conditions include acid-labile hydrazone linkers sensitive to the low-pH conditions in the endosome and lysosome, disulfide-based linkers that can be reduced by the high (millimolar) levels of reduced glutathione in the cell cytosol compared to serum, or dipeptide linkers cleaved by specific lysosomal proteases. In some cases, there may be two release events through an initially released prodrug form. Noncleavable linkers rely on efficient trafficking to the lysosome, where proteolysis of the antibody results in release of the drug attached to the conjugated amino acid. This can therefore be effective only in cases where nuclear transport and activity of the cytotoxic agent can tolerate the additional group. The nature of the linker influences not only the potential for extracellular release but also the drug pharmacodynamics, including bystander effects, which could be to both tumor and normal cells.

The final important component of the ADC is the cytotoxic drug, or "warhead". Although early ADCs utilized conventional clinically used chemotherapeutic agents such as doxorubicin, methotrexate, or chlorambucil [1,20], it became clear that much more potent agents were required, particularly if the DARs were to be kept low. Plant toxins, such as ricin [21], and microbial toxins, such as *Pseudomonas* endotoxin [22], have been evaluated, but were found to have limitations, including immunogenicity. The current clinical-stage ADCs employ highly potent cytotoxic agents that are, in most cases, too toxic to be used in an untargeted manner. These fall into two main mechanistic classes. The first are tubulin inhibitors, which act on dividing cells by binding to tubulin, thereby inhibiting polymerization, resulting in cell cycle arrest and apoptosis. They are exemplified by the auristatins, based on the naturally occurring dolastatin-10, and derivatives of maytansine, originally isolated from the bark of the African shrub *Maytenus ovatus*. Monomethyl auristatin E is the cytotoxic component of brentuximab vedotin, and a maytansine derivative is the cytotoxic component of trastuzumab emtansine. The majority of current clinical-stage ADCs utilize one of these two classes of tubulin-binding agent, although there are some tumor types that are inherently resistant to this type of agent (e.g., colon and pancreatic cancers). The other main mechanistic class of drugs used as ADC warheads are agents that target cellular DNA, and this is the focus of the remainder of this chapter.

ANTIBODY–DRUG CONJUGATES CONTAINING CONVENTIONAL DNA-INTERACTING AGENTS

The first clinical use of an ADC used the conventional DNA cross-linking agent chlorambucil [1]. Cell-surface localizing heterologous antibodies against a human melanoma bound with chlorambucil retained both the alkylating activity of the drug and the antibody binding. In a patient with disseminated malignant melanoma, injection of the conjugate locally into metastatic nodules, or intravenously, resulted in regression of disease. Two decades later, the DNA-intercalating anthracycline drug doxorubicin conjugated to the chimeric human–mouse antibody BR96, directed against the Lewis-Y antigen, was shown to display impressive activity against human carcinoma xenografts in vivo [23]. Subsequent clinical trials of this conjugate, which had a DAR of approximately 8, in patients with metastatic breast cancer, however, showed limited clinical antitumor activity with significant gastrointestinal toxicity [24]. More recently, a humanized anti-CD74 antibody–doxorubicin conjugate (milatuzumab-Dox), again with a DAR of 8, has shown efficacy in vivo [25] and is currently in clinical phase I/II trials against multiple myeloma (Table 16.1). The only other ADC that is undergoing clinical evaluation and that contains a conventional DNA-interacting chemotherapeutic drug warhead is a CEACAM5-targeted humanized antibody conjugated to SN-38, the active metabolite form of the topoisomerase I inhibitor camptothecin. This ADC (labetuzumab-SN-38) with a DAR of 6–7 showed activity against colon and pancreatic cancer xenografts in vivo [26] and is currently undergoing phase I trial against colorectal cancer (Table 16.1).

ANTIBODY–DRUG CONJUGATES CONTAINING DNA-CLEAVING AGENTS

The first ADC to gain approval was gemtuzumab ozogamicin (Mylotarg®). It was approved in 2000 under the US Food and Drug Administration's accelerated approval program for the treatment of CD33-positive acute myeloid leukemia (AML) patients in first relapse who are 60 years of age or older and who are not considered suitable for other cytotoxic chemotherapy [27]. It consists of a humanized IgG4 antibody directed against CD33 conjugated via an acid-labile hydrazine linker to the potent warhead calicheamicin (Fig. 16.3). Calicheamicins are naturally occurring antitumor antibiotics isolated from the soil bacterium *Micromonospora echinospora* subsp. *calichensis*. The mechanism of action of calicheamicin is through binding in the minor groove of DNA. When activated by glutathione, it generates a diradical species that cleaves the DNA backbone, resulting in cell death. Several potent members of this class have undergone evaluation as stand-alone agents but have not succeeded clinically due to delayed toxicity and a narrow therapeutic index.

Approval of gemtuzumab ozogamicin was based on results from a total of 142 AML patients in first relapse from three open-label single-arm phase II studies in which patients receiving $9\,mg/m^2$ every two weeks obtained an overall remission rate of 30% (complete remission or complete remission with incomplete platelet recovery) [28]. Significant hepatotoxicity was reported in some patients. A post-approval randomized phase III trial (SWOG 106) in first-line patients, comparing standard induction therapy ($60\,mg/m^2$ daunorubicin plus cytosine arabinoside) versus $45\,mg/m^2$ daunorubicin plus cytosine arabinoside with the addition of

TABLE 16.1 Antibody–Drug Conjugates that contain DNA Cytotoxic Warheads and are Currently in Clinical Development

Antibody–drug conjugate	Molecular target	Clinical indication(s)	Clinical phase	Linker type	Cytotoxic warhead
Gemtuzumab ozogamycin (Mylotarg®)	CD33	AML	Accelerated approval (United States) 2000, withdrawn 2010	Hydrazone, acid cleavable	Calicheamicin (DNA strand cleavage)
Inotuzumab ozogamicin	CD22	Relapsed refractory non-Hodgkin lymphoma (NHL), all	III	Hydrazone, acid cleavable	Calicheamicin (DNA strand cleavage)
Milatuzumab-Dox (IMMU-110)	CD74	Multiple myeloma	I/II	MCC thioether, noncleavable	Doxorubicin (DNA intercalator and topoisomerase II inhibitor)
MDX-1203	CD70	Renal cell carcinoma, NHL	I	Val-cit, peptide cleavable	Duocarmycin/ CC1065 analog (DNA minor groove alkylator)
Labetuzumab-SN-38 (IMMU-130)	CEACAM5	Colorectal cancer	I	CL2A, acid cleavable	SN-38, active form of camptothecin (DNA topoisomerase I inhibitor)

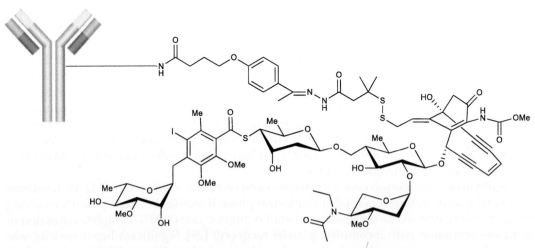

FIGURE 16.3 ADC gemtuzumab ozogamicin consists of a humanized IgG4 antibody directed against CD33 conjugated through a lysine on the antibody via an acid-labile hydrazone linker to the potent warhead calicheamicin. (For color version of this figure, the reader is referred to the online version of this book.)

$6\,mg/m^2$ gemtuzumab ozogamicin, failed to show any benefit of adding gemtuzumab ozo-gamicin. Furthermore, patients in the gemtuzumab ozogamicin–containing arm had a higher induction death rate. The drug was voluntarily withdrawn from the market by Pfizer in 2010.

More recent trials, however, suggest that gemtuzumab ozogamicin may benefit defined subpopulations of patients. The MRC AML15 trial showed a significant benefit for gemtu-zumab ozogamicin–containing induction therapy ($3\,mg/m^2$ single dose) in younger AML patients (<60 years) who have favorable cytogenetics [29]. Subsequently, the NCRI AML16 trial showed in older patients (age range 51–84) a statistically significant survival advan-tage for those who received gemtuzumab ozogamicin [30]. In this case, the benefit was not restricted to any subgroup. These studies randomized over 2000 patients, and the addition of gemtuzumab ozogamicin was found to be well tolerated. In the ALFA-0701 phase III study, the addition of fractionated doses of gemtuzumab ozogamicin ($3\,mg/m^2$ on days 1,4, and 7) when added to standard chemotherapy significantly improved event-free survival and overall survival in AML patients aged 50–70 years [31]. As in AML15, benefit was limited to patients with cytogenetically favorable and intermediate-risk disease. Taken together, these studies suggest that gemtuzumab ozogamicin may have a clinical role, particularly in patients with good or intermediate risk, and highlight the importance of appropriate clinical trial design and personalization of therapy [32].

The other calicheamicin-containing ADC undergoing clinical evaluation is inotuzumab ozogamicin (Table 16.1). This drug consists of a humanized anti-CD22 IgG4 antibody conju-gated to the warhead using the same acetyl butyrate acid-labile linker used in gemtuzumab ozogamicin. CD22 is a B-cell surface antigen expressed widely on non-Hodgkin lymphomas (NHLs) and acute lymphoblastic leukemias. Preclinical models supported the development of inotuzumab ozogamicin either alone or in combination with rituximab [33,34]. Several sin-gle-arm trials have been performed, providing evidence of clinical activity. A dose escalation study in multiple-relapsed or treatment-refractory lymphoma patients defined the maximum tolerated dose as $1.8\,mg/m^2$ when administered every four weeks, which was much lower than that for gemtuzumab ozogamicin. The dose-limiting toxicities were thrombocytopenia and neutropenia, and the objective response rate across the various lymphoma subtypes and dose levels was 39% [35]. A phase II study in refractory and relapsed acute lymphocytic leu-kemia gave an overall response rate of 57% [36].

ANTIBODY–DRUG CONJUGATES CONTAINING DNA MINOR GROOVE–ALKYLATING AND CROSS-LINKING AGENTS

Another ADC in clinical development containing a DNA-interactive warhead is MDX-1203 (Table 16.1). In this case, an antibody to CD70 is conjugated via a maleimide-containing cleavable peptide-based linker to a duocarmycin analog (Fig. 16.4). The duocarmycins, which include CC1065, are derived from *Streptomyces* species. Similar to calicheamicin, the mem-bers of this family of naturally occurring antitumor antibiotics are potent, but they cannot be used clinically on their own because of delayed toxicity, in this case hepatotoxicity. They are DNA minor groove–binding agents, forming sequence-selective covalent linkages to the N3-position of specific adenine bases. MDX-1203 was found to be highly active against CD70-expressing human tumor xenograft models [37] and is currently being evaluated in

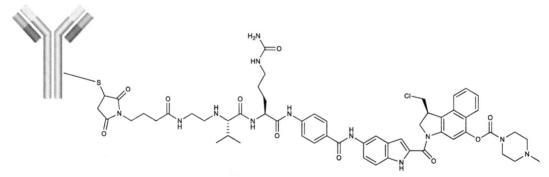

FIGURE 16.4 ADC MDX-1203 consists of an antibody to CD70 conjugated through a cysteine sulfhydryl group on the antibody via a maleimide-containing cleavable peptide-based valine-citrulline linker to a duocarmycin analog. Following cleavage of the linker by protease, further processing by carboxyesterases results in removal of the protecting carbamate to generate the active drug. (For color version of this figure, the reader is referred to the online version of this book.)

early-phase trials against renal cell carcinoma and NHL, two cancers in which CD70 is highly overexpressed. It is of note that the activity of the duocarmycin derivative in MDX-1203 not only is dependent on the cleavage of the linker by lysosomal proteases but also requires activation by carboxyesterases to remove a protecting carbamate group, potentially giving an additional level of safety.

Another group of agents that are rapidly emerging as next-generation warheads in the ADC space are the pyrrolobenzodiazepines (PBDs) [38]. They are another class of naturally occurring antitumor antibiotics found in *Streptomyces*. PBD monomers bind in the DNA minor groove and form single covalent aminal linkage to the exocyclic N2 amino group of guanine within purine–guanine–purine sequences. Joining two PBD monomers together via an appropriate polymethylene tether produces PBD dimers that have the ability to produce two covalent bonds forming highly cytotoxic DNA interstrand cross-links. The cross-links formed are relatively nondistorting of the DNA structure, making them hidden to repair mechanisms, which often contributes to the acquired resistance of tumors to conventional cross-linking drugs. A PBD dimer, SG2000, is currently in phase II clinical trials for the treatment of cisplatin-refractory ovarian cancer and hematological malignancies.

An important feature of the PBD dimers is that rational structural modification can modulate cross-linking ability and cytotoxic potency over a large range from the nanomolar to the subpicomolar [38]. In addition, they can be readily functionalized with linkers in either cleavable or noncleavable formats for attachment to antibodies. For example, linkers at the N10 position or on C2-anilino substituents (e.g., SGD-1910; Fig. 16.5) must be fully cleavable to liberate an active PBD, whereas an aromatic tether can accommodate either a cleavable or a noncleavable linker. The synthetic PBD dimers are therefore ideally suited for a role as DNA cytotoxic warheads in an ADC approach, combining exquisite potency with a demonstrated therapeutic index (unlike calicheamycin and the duocarmycins), and lack of cross-resistance to widely used chemotherapy agents. Another advantage of PBD-containing ADCs is the ability to monitor, by a modification of the comet assay [39], the DNA cross-links produced in cells following release of the drug. Such a pharmacodynamic readout is not possible with other ADC warheads.

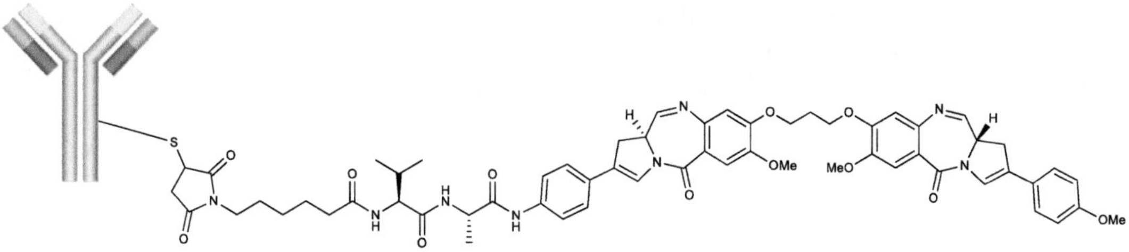

FIGURE 16.5 ADC resulting from attachment via maleimide conjugation of a valine–alanine protease-cleavable linker to a highly potent pyrrolobenzodiazepine dimer (SGD-1919). (For color version of this figure, the reader is referred to the online version of this book.)

Recently, the utility of PBD-containing ADCs has been demonstrated against both solid tumors and hematological malignancies. For example, an anti-CD70 ADC with a uniform DAR of 2 resulting from attachment of SGD-1919 (Fig. 16.5) via maleimide conjugation to a single engineered heavy-chain cysteine residue displayed selective antitumor activity in CD70-expressing renal cell carcinoma xenograft models at well-tolerated doses as low as 0.1 mg/kg [40]. In a second study, an ADC employing the same drug linker attached to a CD33 antibody (SGN-CD33A) exhibited antitumor activity against a broad panel of primary AML samples and durable remissions in preclinical models of AML (including multidrug resistant-positive AML) that are characteristically resistant to conventional chemotherapy and to the calicheamicin-containing CD33 ADC gemtuzumab ozogamicin [41]. Forthcoming clinical trials will determine the clinical utility of PBD-containing ADCs.

FUTURE DEVELOPMENT OF ANTIBODY–DRUG CONJUGATES

The approvals of Adcetris® and Kadcyla® have highlighted the significant potential of ADCs as targeted treatments for cancer. The field is rapidly expanding, with over 20 ADCs currently in clinical trials and many more in preclinical development. The ability to profile patients for target expression is critical for success in the clinic. ADCs continue to be optimized for clinical use by careful consideration of the appropriate tumor target, and by exploiting innovations in antibody engineering, conjugation chemistry, linker technology, and design of the cytotoxic warhead. In addition, novel antigens on hematological and solid tumors, with optimal internalization and intracellular trafficking properties, are being discovered and exploited as targets for ADCs.

Some cell surface antigens expressed on hematological tumors are present at a higher copy number compared to therapeutic antigens on solid tumors. They can also have more optimal internalization kinetics. In addition, target antigens on hematological malignancies are often more homogeneously expressed within the tumor cell population (and more easily quantifiable), are more accessible to therapy, and have more limited expression on healthy tissue. For these reasons, and the fact that hematological tumor cells are often inherently very sensitive to DNA-damaging agents, hematological malignancies are an obvious choice for ADC therapies delivering DNA cytotoxics. Nevertheless, with the identification of optimal tumor antigens and appropriate drug design, ADCs should also have an important role in treating solid tumors, as is being demonstrated for trastuzumab emtansine. One approach in solid tumors may be to target tumor-initiating (or cancer stem) cells that are inherently resistant to conventional chemotherapy but that may succumb to highly potent, non–cell cycle specific ADC warheads such as DNA-cleaving or cross-linking agents.

Further studies will be likely to establish the importance of site-specific drug attachment and may also confirm the potential of antibody fragments and nonantibody scaffolds. A reduction in the molecular size of the targeting moiety could result in increased ADC penetration into solid tumors. Although the majority of current clinical-stage ADCs utilize tubulin-binding agents as the cytotoxic warhead, the clinical results with gemtuzumab ozogamicin and the impressive preclinical data emerging with ADCs targeting drugs such as the PBD dimers suggest that ADCs delivering DNA cytotoxics will be major contributors to the next generation of this important, rapidly emerging class of cancer therapeutic.

References

[1] Ghose T, Norvell ST, Guclu A, Cameron D, Bodurtha A, MacDonald AS. Immunochemotherapy of cancer with chlorambucil-carrying antibody. Br Med J 1972;3:495–9.

[2] Rowland GF, O'Neill GJ, Davies DA. Suppression of tumour growth in mice by a drug-antibody conjugate using a novel approach to linkage. Nature 1975;255:487–91.

[3] Polson AG, Ho WY, Ramakrishnan V. Investigational antibody-drug conjugates for hematological malignancies. Expert Opin Investig Drugs 2011;20:75–85.

[4] Sapra P, Hooper AT, O'Donnell CJ, Gerber HP. Investigational antibody drug conjugates for solid tumors. Expert Opin Investig Drugs 2011;20:1131–49.

[5] Adair JR, Howard PW, Hartley JA, Williams DG, Chester KA. Antibody drug conjugates—a perfect synergy. Expert Opin Biol Ther 2012;12:1191–206.

[6] Sievers EL, Senter PD. Antibody-drug conjugates in cancer therapy. Annu Rev Med 2012; [Epub ahead of print].

[7] Younes A, Bartlett NL, Leonard JP, Kennedy DA, Lynch CM, Sievers EL, et al. Brentuximab vedotin (SGN-35) for relapsed CD30-positive lymphomas. N Engl J Med 2010;363:1812–21.

[8] Gualberto A. Brentuximab vedotin (SGN-35), an antibody-drug conjugate for the treatment of CD30-positive malignancies. Expert Opin Investig Drugs 2012;21:205–16.

[9] Verma S, Miles D, Gianni L, Krop IE, Welslau M, Baselga J, et al. EMILIA Study Group. Trastuzumab emtansine for HER2-positive advanced breast cancer. N Engl J Med 2012;367:1783–9.

[10] Dancey G, Violet J, Malaroda A, Green AJ, Sharma SK, Francis R, et al. A phase I clinical trial of CHT-25, a 131I-labeled chimeric anti-CD25 antibody showing efficacy in patients with refractory lymphoma. Clin Cancer Res 2009;15:7701–10.

[11] Mao W, Luis E, Ross S, Silva J, Tan C, Crowley C, et al. EphB2 as a therapeutic antibody drug target for the treatment of colorectal cancer. Cancer Res 2004;64:781–8.

[12] Sharkey RM, Goldenberg DM. Targeted therapy of cancer: new prospects for antibodies and immunoconjugates. CA Cancer J Clin 2006;56:226–43.

[13] Teicher BA, Chari RV. Antibody conjugate therapeutics: challenges and potential. Clin Cancer Res 2011;17:6389–97.

[14] Hamblett KJ, Senter PD, Chace DF, Sun MM, Lenox J, Cerveny CG, et al. Effects of drug loading on the antitumor activity of a monoclonal antibody drug conjugate. Clin Cancer Res 2004;10:7063–70.

[15] Lyons A, King DJ, Owens RJ, Yarranton GT, Millican A, Whittle NR, et al. Site-specific attachment to recombinant antibodies via introduced surface cysteine residues. Protein Eng 1990;3:703–8.

[16] Hofer T, Thomas JD, Burke Jr TR, Rader C. An engineered selenocysteine defines a unique class of antibody derivatives. Proc Natl Acad Sci U S A 2008;105:12451–6.

[17] Hutchins BM, Kazane SA, Staflin K, Forsyth JS, Felding-Habermann B, Smider VV, et al. Selective formation of covalent protein heterodimers with an unnatural amino acid. Chem Biol 2011;18:299–303.

[18] Junutula JR, Raab H, Clark S, Bhakta S, Leipold DD, Weir S, et al. Site-specific conjugation of a cytotoxic drug to an antibody improves the therapeutic index. Nat Biotechnol 2008;26:925–32.

[19] Shen BQ, Xu K, Liu L, Raab H, Bhakta S, Kenrick M, et al. Conjugation site modulates the in vivo stability and therapeutic activity of antibody-drug conjugates. Nat Biotechnol 2012;30:184–9.

[20] Senter PD. Potent antibody drug conjugates for cancer therapy. Curr Opin Chem Biol 2009;13:235–44.

[21] Tsukazaki K, Hayman EG, Ruoslahti E. Effects of ricin A chain conjugates of monoclonal antibodies to human alpha-fetoprotein and placental alkaline phosphatase on antigen-producing tumor cells in culture. Cancer Res 1985;45:1834–8.

[22] Pirker R, FitzGerald DJ, Hamilton TC, Ozols RF, Willingham MC, Pastan I. Anti-transferrin receptor antibody linked to *Pseudomonas exotoxin* as a model immunotoxin in human ovarian carcinoma cell lines. Cancer Res 1986;45:751–7.

[23] Trail PA, Willner D, Lasch SJ, Henderson AJ, Hofstead S, Casazza AM, et al. Cure of xenografted human carcinomas by BR96-doxorubicin immunoconjugates. Science 1993;261:212–5.

[24] Tolcher AW, Sugarman S, Gelmon KA, Cohen R, Saleh M, Isaacs C, et al. Randomized phase II study of BR96-doxorubicin conjugate in patients with metastatic breast cancer. J Clin Oncol 1999;17:478–84.

[25] Sapra P, Stein R, Pickett J, Qu Z, Govindan SV, Cardillo TM, et al. Anti-CD74 antibody-doxorubicin conjugate, IMMU-110, in a human multiple myeloma xenograft and in monkeys. Clin Cancer Res 2005;11:5257–64.

[26] Govindan SV, Cardillo TM, Moon SJ, Hansen HJ, Goldenberg DM. CEACAM5-targeted therapy of human colonic and pancreatic cancer xenografts with potent labetuzumab-SN-38 immunoconjugates. Clin Cancer Res 2009;15:6052–61.

[27] Trail PA, Willner D, Lasch SJ, Henderson AJ, Hofstead S, Casazza AM, et al. Approval summary: gemtuzumab ozogamicin in relapsed acute myeloid leukemia. Clin Cancer Res 2001;7:1490–6.

[28] Sievers EL, Larson RA, Stadtmauer EA, Estey E, Löwenberg B, Dombret H, et al. Mylotarg Study Group. Efficacy and safety of gemtuzumab ozogamicin in patients with CD33-positive acute myeloid leukemia in first relapse. J Clin Oncol 2001;19:3244–54.

[29] Burnett AK, Hills RK, Milligan D, Kjeldsen L, Kell J, Russell NH, et al. Identification of patients with acute myeloblastic leukemia who benefit from the addition of gemtuzumab ozogamicin: results of the MRC AML15 trial. J Clin Oncol 2011;29:369–77.

[30] Burnett AK, Russell NH, Hills RK, Kell J, Freeman S, Kjeldsen L, et al. Addition of gemtuzumab ozogamicin to induction chemotherapy improves survival in older patients with acute myeloid leukemia. J Clin Oncol 2012;30:3924–31.

[31] Castaigne S, Pautas C, Terré C, Raffoux E, Bordessoule D, Bastie JN, et al. Acute Leukemia French Association. Effect of gemtuzumab ozogamicin on survival of adult patients with de-novo acute myeloid leukaemia (ALFA-0701): a randomised, open-label, phase 3 study. Lancet 2012;379:1508–16.

[32] Ravandi F, Estey EH, Appelbaum FR, Lo-Coco F, Schiffer CA, Larson RA, et al. Gemtuzumab ozogamicin: time to resurrect? J Clin Oncol 2012;30:3921–3.

[33] DiJoseph JF, Goad ME, Dougher MM, Boghaert ER, Kunz A, Hamann PR, et al. Potent and specific antitumor efficacy of CMC-544, a CD22-targeted immunoconjugate of calicheamicin, against systemically disseminated B-cell lymphoma. Clin Cancer Res 2004;10:8620–9.

[34] DiJoseph JF, Dougher MM, Kalyandrug LB, Armellino DC, Boghaert ER, Hamann PR, et al. Antitumor efficacy of a combination of CMC-544 (inotuzumab ozogamicin), a CD22-targeted cytotoxic immunoconjugate of calicheamicin, and rituximab against non-Hodgkin's B-cell lymphoma. Clin Cancer Res 2006;12:242–9.

[35] Advani A, Coiffier B, Czuczman MS, Dreyling M, Foran J, Gine E, et al. Safety, pharmacokinetics, and preliminary clinical activity of inotuzumab ozogamicin, a novel immunoconjugate for the treatment of B-cell non-Hodgkin's lymphoma: results of a phase I study. J Clin Oncol 2010;28:2085–93.

[36] Kantarjian H, Thomas D, Jorgensen J, Jabbour E, Kebriaei P, Rytting M, et al. Inotuzumab ozogamicin, an anti-CD22-calecheamicin conjugate, for refractory and relapsed acute lymphocytic leukaemia: a phase 2 study. Lancet Oncol 2012;13:403–11.

[37] Cardarelli P, King D, Terrett J, Gangwar S, Cohen L, Pan C, et al. Efficacy and safety of a human anti-CD70 antibody-MGBA conjugate. Proceedings American Association for Cancer Research Annual Meeting 49 Abstract 4061; 2008.

[38] Hartley JA. The development of pyrrolobenzodiazepines as antitumour agents. Expert Opin Investig Drugs 2011;20:733–44.

[39] Spanswick VJ, Hartley JM, Hartley JA. Measurement of DNA interstrand crosslinking in individual cells using the single cell gel electrophoresis (Comet) assay. Methods Mol Biol 2010;613:267–82.

[40] Jeffrey S, Burke P, Meyer D, Lyon R, Miyamoto J, Anderson M, et al. Anti-CD70 antibody-drug conjugates containing pyrrolobenzodiazepine dimers demonstrate robust antitumor activity. Proceedings American Association Cancer Research 2012; 53, abstract 4631.

[41] Sutherland MSK, RB Walter, SC Jeffrey, Burke PJ, Yu C, Harrington KH, et al. SGN-CD33A: a novel CD33-directed antibody-drug conjugate, utilizing pyrrolobenzodiazepine dimers, demonstrates preclinical antitumor activity against multi-drug resistant human AML. Proceedings American Society Haematology 2012, abstract 3589.

17

Inhibition of Telomerase: Promise, Progress, and Potential Pitfalls

Christopher G. Tomlinson[1,2], *Scott B. Cohen*[1,2],
Tracy M. Bryan[1,2]

[1]Children's Medical Research Institute, Westmead, NSW, Australia
[2]University of Sydney, Sydney, NSW, Australia

INTRODUCTION

Telomeres are repetitive DNA–protein structures located at the termini of linear chromosomes. With each cycle of cell division and DNA replication, telomeres gradually shorten until a critical threshold is reached, resulting in replicative senescence. Telomerase is the enzyme that catalyzes the elongation of telomeres via nucleotide addition, thereby counteracting telomere shortening and allowing for unlimited cell proliferation. Approximately 85–90% of all human cancers require telomerase for growth. Therefore, inhibition of telomerase provides a promising avenue for the development of anticancer treatments expected to be effective against a broad range of cancers. Furthermore, treatment by telomerase inhibitors is expected to be less toxic than current therapeutics due to most normal cells having undetectable or very low levels of telomerase. This chapter provides a brief overview of telomere biology and telomerase, and reviews current telomerase inhibitors and potential caveats in their effectiveness. We cover both direct enzymatic inhibition of telomerase, as well as indirect targeting of the telomeric substrate. Note that there are other promising telomerase-based cancer therapeutics in the clinical pipeline, including immunotherapy against cells expressing telomerase components and gene therapy using telomerase promoter-driven expression of a "suicide gene"; these strategies have recently been reviewed elsewhere [1,2].

Telomeres

Human telomeres are located at the ends of chromosomes and are composed of the repeating DNA sequence 5′-TTAGGG-3′ [3,4], typically ~5–15 kilobasepairs (kbp). This is terminated with ~300–500 nucleotides of single-stranded TTAGGG repeats to provide a 3'-overhang [5,6]. Telomeric DNA is protected by a specialized group of proteins collectively called *shelterin* [7]. The human shelterin complex consists of six proteins: telomere repeat binding factor 1 (TRF1; [8]), TRF2 [9,10], repressor–activator protein 1 (RAP1) [11], TRF1-interacting nuclear protein 2 (TIN2) [12], TIN2-interacting protein TPP1 [13–15], and protection of telomeres 1 (POT1) [16]. The combination of sufficiently long telomere length and intact shelterin components is essential for chromosome stability and telomeric protection against DNA damage repair [17–19].

The ends of linear DNA molecules cannot be fully replicated by the semiconservative DNA replication machinery. During cell division, the parental DNA is unwound at the replication fork into two single strands of DNA, the lagging and leading strands. Due to the 5'→3' directionality of DNA synthesis, the leading strand is created continuously, forming blunt-ended DNA at the end of the telomere, whereas the lagging strand is generated discontinuously through individually synthesized Okazaki fragments [20]. At the completion of lagging-strand synthesis, the RNA primer is not replaced with DNA as there is no incoming 5'→3' DNA polymerase δ to displace it. This RNA primer is then degraded, which recreates the pre-existing 3' single-stranded overhang. However, as the leading strand remains blunt-ended, regeneration of a 3'-overhang can only be achieved through exonuclease action of the *template* DNA strand, resulting in net telomere loss. This is termed the "end replication problem" [21–23] (Fig. 17.1), and in normal human somatic cells telomeres shorten by ~50–200 bp with every cell division [24]. Eventually a threshold of telomere length is reached which results in cell replication being arrested. This is sometimes termed the "mortality 1" (M1) stage and is caused by the shortening of a few telomeres to a size that leads to a growth arrest called *cellular senescence* (Fig. 17.2) [25,26]. Senescence is not cell death, but a stable nondividing state that can be bypassed by abrogation of the function of the p53 and pRB human tumor suppressor genes [27]. Cells are then able to replicate until the telomeres become critically shortened, which produces the M2, or crisis stage [26]. When most of the telomeres are extremely short, end-to end fusions and chromosome breakage–fusion–bridge cycles cause marked lethal chromosomal abnormalities and apoptosis [28]. Telomere shortening can therefore be seen as an intrinsic counting mechanism in the cellular aging process. The limited replicative capacity of normal human cells is a major tumor suppressor mechanism; conversely, escape from the senescence barrier (immortalization) is a critically important aspect of tumorigenesis [25].

Escaping Senescence and Achieving Immortality

There are two known telomere maintenance mechanisms by which cells can achieve immortality (Fig. 17.2). The first pathway, which will be the focus of this chapter, is through the action of the ribonucleoprotein enzyme complex telomerase. Telomerase mediates the elongation of telomeres via nucleotide addition by catalyzing the de novo synthesis of TTAGGG repeats, thereby counteracting shortening and allowing for unlimited cell proliferation [29]. Although active in rapidly dividing cells and a wide variety of tissues during embryonic development [30], levels of telomerase are low or undetectable in most somatic tissues [31,32]. In contrast, telomerase is present at high levels in approximately 85–90% of all human cancers and is necessary for their unlimited proliferation [32–35]. This makes telomerase a highly specific target for both cancer diagnosis and the development of novel therapeutic agents. Inhibiting the

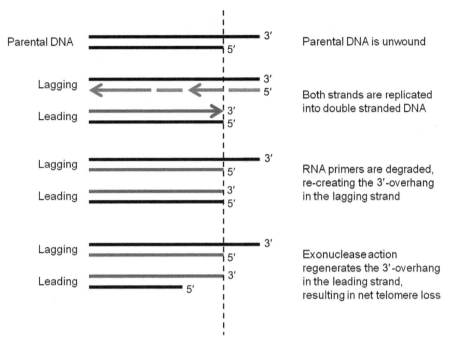

Parental DNA — Parental DNA is unwound

Lagging / Leading — Both strands are replicated into double stranded DNA

Lagging / Leading — RNA primers are degraded, re-creating the 3'-overhang in the lagging strand

Lagging / Leading — Exonuclease action regenerates the 3'-overhang in the leading strand, resulting in net telomere loss

FIGURE 17.1 The "end replication problem". Loss of telomeric DNA through each cycle of DNA replication occurs, at least partly, through exonuclease degradation of the leading template DNA strand, so as to regenerate the requisite 3' overhang at the telomere. (This figure is reproduced in color in the color plate section.)

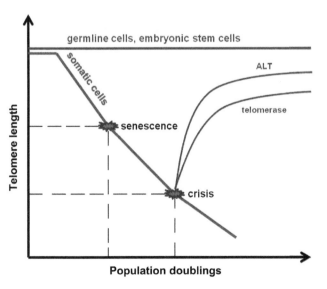

FIGURE 17.2 Telomere dynamics in human biology. Telomere shortening is the cell's "counting mechanism", activating the nonproliferative state of cellular senescence, considered a major tumor suppressor mechanism. Inactivation of tumor suppressor genes may allow a cell to bypass senescence and continue proliferating until the telomeres reach a critical length (crisis), resulting in genomic instability and cell death. Activation of a telomere maintenance mechanism (telomerase or ALT) will allow a cell to resume proliferation and confer immortality. (This figure is reproduced in color in the color plate section.)

activity of telomerase will provide potential treatment for the majority of cancers. Furthermore, treatment by telomerase inhibitors is expected to be less toxic than current therapeutics due to most normal cells having low or undetectable levels of telomerase.

The second route a cell can use to escape senescence is the alternative lengthening of telomeres (ALT) pathway [36]. Approximately 4–15% of human cancers use the ALT pathway to overcome telomere shortening [37–39]. The ALT mechanism involves telomere recombination [40] and cells that utilize it have unusual characteristics, including heterogeneous telomere lengths (relative to telomerase-positive cells) [36] and abundant extrachromosal telomeric DNA (reviewed in Ref. [38]). ALT occurs in a wide range of tumors but is relatively rare in the most common types of cancers, carcinomas, which are derived from epithelia [39,41].

Telomerase Components

The core active human telomerase complex has been purified and was found to consist of three components: human telomerase reverse transcriptase (hTERT), an RNA component (hTR), and the protein dyskerin [42]. Genetic mutations in any of the three telomerase genes—hTERT [43], hTR [44], or dyskerin [45]—or other telomerase-associated proteins, result in low levels of telomerase or an enzyme with compromised activity, resulting in insufficient telomere maintenance from embryogenesis through development. This can manifest in one of a number of telomere syndromes such as dyskeratosis congenita (DC) and idiopathic pulmonary fibrosis (IPF) (reviewed in Ref. [46]). The dyskerin gene, an X-linked gene, was first identified through familial linkage analysis in patients with DC [47], a disease characterized by the premature failure of proliferative tissues, notably bone marrow failure. Mutations in dyskerin lead to the most severe cases of DC, with patients having a life expectancy of less than 20 years [48]. Mutations in hTERT or hTR lead to autosomal dominant DC, indicating that even partly reduced levels of telomerase during development are deleterious [43,44,49]. IPF is a devastating fibrotic lung disease with late adult onset. A buildup of excess scar tissue in the lungs results in a reduced lung volume and symptoms include a chronic cough and shortness of breath. Some familial cases of IPF are caused by mutations in the genes that encode hTR and hTERT [50]. Patients with DC and IPF have significantly shorter telomeres compared to the mean of healthy aged matched individuals [48,51,52].

Telomerase Mechanism

Telomerase-mediated elongation of telomeres is initiated by the binding of hTR to the 3′ end of the telomere (Fig. 17.3). Once bound, hTERT catalyzes the addition of nucleotides to the telomere complementary to the hTR template. Once the 3′ boundary of the hTR template is reached, one of two mechanisms for further nucleotide addition occurs:

1. Dissociation; the telomere simply dissociates and reassociates with another telomerase molecule.
2. Repeat addition processivity; involves separation of the DNA–RNA duplex and a 6-nt translocation of the DNA relative to the enzyme active site, such that multiple copies of telomeric DNA repeats can be added to the same molecule without dissociation.

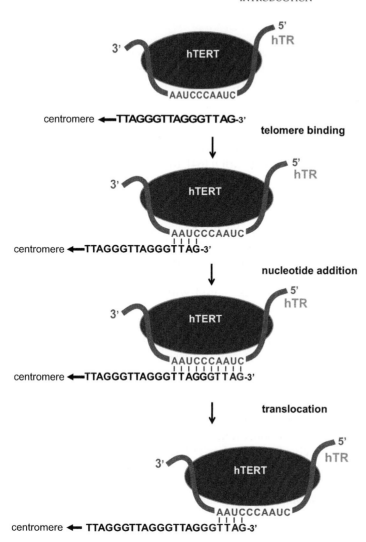

FIGURE 17.3 Schematic representation of the human telomerase telomere-lengthening mechanism. Telomerase binds to the 3' end of the telomere. Once bound, nucleotides complementary to the hTR template are added to the DNA. Once the template boundary is reached, hTR translocates while telomerase remains bound to the telomere. (This figure is reproduced in color in the color plate section.)

The details of the latter mechanism have not been fully elucidated, but likely require a major conformational change of the enzyme. It is well established that an interaction between telomerase and the 5' region of the DNA primer (two to three repeats from the 3' end), which is distinct from the RNA–DNA hybrid, is required for translocation [53–57]. This "anchor site" allows telomerase to remain bound to DNA during translocation when the DNA unpairs from the RNA prior to realignment. Formation of the stable hTR–hTERT complex and repeat addition processivity are two unique properties of telomerase that distinguish its mechanism of action from that of other reverse transcriptases. Dyskerin is the least characterized of the three components. Its primary function is thought to be stabilization of hTR, as a reduction in dyskerin expression or mutation of the protein have been shown to lead to substantially reduced hTR levels [45,58,59].

Telomerase Structure

Although the structure of the entire telomerase complex has yet to be solved, structures of TERT and TR subdomains have increased our understanding of its organization and the mechanism of its unique reverse transcriptase activity.

Telomerase Reverse Transcriptase

The human telomerase reverse transcriptase (TERT) protein (1132 amino acids, 127 kDa) [60–62] contains four conserved structural domains: the telomerase essential N-terminal (TEN) domain [63], the telomerase RNA binding domain (TRBD) [64], the reverse transcriptase (RT) domain [65] and the C-terminal extension (CTE) domain (Fig. 17.4). Structures of regions of TERT from the ciliated protozoan *Tetrahymena thermophilia* (TRBD and TEN) [63,66] and the full-length, albeit truncated, TERT from the beetle *Triboleum castaneum* [67] have been solved. TcTERT lacks the TEN domain and consists of only 596 amino acids; as yet the RNA component has not been identified [68]. However, the RT domain is relatively well conserved, so the TcTERT crystal structure provides a useful guide to the possible architecture of the RT domain of higher eukaryotes.

The RT domain contains seven conserved motifs shared with conventional RTs: motifs 1, 2, and A, B′, C, D, and E. The protein conformation observed in TcTERT is similar to the palm and finger domain of retroviral RT, with the fingers adopting a similar open conformation in the absence of DNA substrate [67,69,70]. Motifs A and C contain a catalytic triad of universally conserved aspartate residues; mutating any of these residues abolishes telomerase activity [65]. This supports a mechanism in which telomerase coordinates metal ions to stabilize developing negative charge during nucleotide addition, a mechanism common to conventional reverse transcriptases. A unique feature of the RT domain is the insertion between fingers domain (IFD) which lies between motifs A and B. The IFD is thought to mediate in part the ability of telomerase to stabilize short RNA–DNA hybrids which is crucial for translocation and telomerase function in vivo [71]. Another TERT-specific motif within the RT domain, known as motif 3, is also involved in separation and realignment of the RNA–DNA hybrid during translocation [72,73].

Structures of the TRBD from *T. thermophilia* and *T. castaneum* are very similar despite the large phylogenetic diversity between the two species. The highly conserved TRBD is essential for activity in vitro and in vivo and confers the specialized RNA-binding activity of TERT

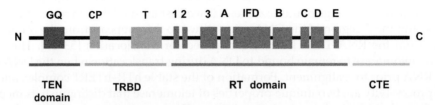

FIGURE 17.4 Linear representation of the hTERT protein. The telomerase essential N-terminal (TEN) domain, the telomerase RNA binding domain (TRBD), the reverse transcriptase (RT) domain, and the C-terminal extension (CTE) domain are shown with their conserved functional motifs highlighted. (This figure is reproduced in color in the color plate section.)

[64,74–76]. The T and CP motifs of the TRBD are critical for RNA binding [64,77], and the QFP motif has also been shown to have an effect on binding [75,77].

The TEN domain exists at the N-terminus of TERT. Its main function is believed to be stabilization of the binding of DNA primer to telomerase (i.e., it constitutes the telomerase "anchor site") (reviewed in Ref. [78]). It is also proposed to facilitate a conformational change in telomerase, orientating the 3′ end of the primer into the active site for nucleotide addition [79]. It is therefore not surprising that deletion of the TEN domain significantly reduces telomerase activity and abolishes repeat addition processivity [63,76].

The role of the C terminal domain is largely unknown; however, studies have shown an importance for in vivo and in vitro telomerase activity, low-affinity DNA binding, and processivity [80,81].

Telomerase RNA

In contrast to the conserved nature of TERT, the RNA component of telomerase varies considerably in both size and sequence across species. However, telomerase RNAs (TR) nonetheless contain a number of conserved motifs [82–84] that support the existence of a common mechanism in telomerase-mediated telomere elongation. Most telomerase RNAs contain a template sequence that is flanked on the 5′ side by a template boundary element (TBE) [85,86] and on the 3′ side by a stretch of single-stranded RNA followed by a pseudoknot [87–89]. Covalent connectivity between the template and the sequences flanking it is required for efficient translocation and may be involved in template positioning in *T. thermophilia* telomerase [90,91]. A model for involvement of the telomerase RNA in translocation has been proposed, in which single-stranded regions of RNA on either side of the template undergo reciprocal compression and expansion to accommodate movement of the template RNA during the catalytic cycle [92]. This has been termed *the RNA accordion model*.

POTENTIAL CAVEATS OF TELOMERASE INHIBITORS

Telomerase is expressed in the great majority of malignant tumors [31,32]. The use of telomerase inhibitors in the treatment of cancer holds much promise as a highly specific therapy but any success is far from assured. There are several considerations about telomerase as an anticancer target that need to be addressed.

The Lag Phase

Several different approaches to inhibit the activity of telomerase have been developed. The basic premise of these strategies is that direct or indirect telomerase inhibition will result in telomere shortening and ultimately cell growth arrest or cell death. However, due to the requirement for extensive telomere shortening over many population doublings (PDs), there will be an expected *lag phase* between the time telomerase is inhibited and the time when the telomeres of cancer cells are sufficiently short to signal senescence and/or cell death. This lag phase will vary depending on the initial tumor telomere length and would result in sustained inhibition being required. Indeed, tumors with initially long telomeres showed no growth defect despite telomere shortening over a year in culture with the telomerase inhibitor BIBR1532 (see Section "BIBR1532, a Nonnucleosidic Telomerase-Specific Inhibitor") [93]. This long treatment time has the potential to result in toxicity in some proliferative tissues of patients. As a result, any antitelomerase drug would need to be potent, nontoxic, and ideally be able to act synergistically with existing therapeutics. Combinations of telomerase inhibition and some anticancer drugs have been used to reduce this lag phase and induce cell death more rapidly [94–100]. This effect has been suggested to be specific to DNA damaging agents that are toxic in the S/G2 phase of the cell cycle, implicating telomerase in protection against DNA damage [101]. In some cases combination therapy was still dependent on telomere shortening [98,99], but in other cases, rapid apoptosis occurred in the absence of apparent telomere shortening [97,100]. This may be due to a telomere capping function of telomerase, and has particularly been observed using strategies to reduce levels of hTERT or hTR such as ribozymes or silencing RNA [102–106]. Further research into the mechanism of telomerase-mediated telomere capping is ongoing in many laboratories, and is likely to lead to novel ways of overcoming the lag phase of telomerase inhibition.

Effect on Somatic Cells that Express Telomerase

Along with cancer cells, telomerase is expressed in hematopoietic stem cells, germline cells, and rapidly dividing cells such as cells of the basal layer of the epidermis and intestinal crypts [30,107,108]. Inhibitors of telomerase could potentially affect the function of these cells. Given that the telomeres of normal (nondiseased) cells have been observed to be longer than telomeres of the corresponding cancerous cells in many tumor types (see e.g., Fig. 17.6) [109–113], it is hoped that any telomere shortening resulting from temporary telomerase inhibition would have negligible effect on normal cells. For some solid tumors such as prostate cancer, this difference in telomere length appears to be marginal [111], so careful selection of tumor types for initial clinical trials is warranted, and has been applied in the case of the inhibitor GRN163L (see Section "GRN163L, an Oligonucleotide-Based Antisense Inhibitor") [1].

Further to this, the deepest stem cells only proliferate intermittently and when quiescent, telomere shortening does not occur and telomerase activity is negligible (reviewed in Ref. [115]). These differences in telomerase expression, telomere length, and predicted stem cell kinetics in normal versus tumor cells make telomerase potentially the safest cancer target to date. However, even though any effects are expected to be minor, one cannot assume that normal tissues would not be affected by telomerase inhibitors. The most informative test of the safety of telomerase inhibitors will be phase I clinical trials; the drug GRN163L (see Section "GRN163L, an Oligonucleotide-Based Antisense Inhibitor") is the only telomerase inhibitor to have reached this stage, but is reportedly well tolerated to date [1].

Resistance to Telomerase Inhibitors

Cancer cells essentially have unlimited ability to evolve, and the possibility that cancer cells might become resistant to telomerase inhibitors must be considered. Regardless of the therapeutic approach, preexisting or new refractory cancers are likely to be found in some patients.

Antitelomerase therapies would not be expected to be effective against the 4–15% of human cancers that use the ALT pathway and lack detectable telomerase activity. Furthermore, malignancies that initially have only telomerase activity could become resistant to telomerase inhibitors by activating the ALT mechanism. A switch of mechanism is relatively uncommon in in vitro experiments using human cancer cell lines [116], but as the number of cells in typical cell culture experiments is orders of magnitude lower than in clinically important tumors, this mechanism cannot be dismissed. A recent study has shown that a switch between the telomerase and ALT pathways is possible in mice [117]. Mice with telomeres of limiting length were engineered with inducible TERT expression such that the effects of telomerase reactivation and subsequent extinction in telomerase-positive T-cell lymphomas could be monitored. Telomerase activation enabled full malignant progression and prevented telomere dysfunction-induced checkpoints. When telomerase expression was halted, tumor growth eventually slowed; however, growth subsequently resumed via the ALT pathway. How relevant these observations are to human tumor biology cannot be ascertained at this time.

Some tumors may utilize both telomerase and ALT activity [37,38], at least in part due to intratumoral heterogeneity. However, it is not known whether both telomere-lengthening mechanisms can spontaneously be activated within the same cell. Certainly, if the tumor growth was in part dependent on ALT-positive cells, these tumors would become rapidly resistant to telomerase inhibitors.

The precise molecular details about how the ALT pathway operates are not yet known; however, as more studies focus on ALT, specific molecular targets and vulnerabilities may be identified that lead to the development of ALT inhibitors. One way to tackle any resistance to telomerase inhibitors afforded by the ALT pathway would therefore be to use an approach that combined inhibitors to both telomerase and ALT. The same approach could also be used in the treatment of ALT-positive tumors, such that using a combination of telomerase and ALT inhibitors could prove to be a powerful tool in the treatment of the vast majority of cancers [118].

A common mechanism mediating tumor drug resistance is the expression of transporter molecules that remove the drug from the cell, such as P-glycoprotein [119]. It has been suggested that oligonucleotide telomerase inhibitors such as GRN163L (see Section "GRN163L, an Oligonucleotide-Based Antisense Inhibitor") are unlikely to be substrates for such drug efflux pathways, reducing the likelihood of this mode of resistance, at least for this type of inhibitor. Targeted cancer therapies are also prone to the development of resistance due to mutations in the protein being targeted [120]. For this reason, it is essential that research into the structure and mechanism of telomerase function is continued in parallel with the effort to find inhibitors, so we can rationally design inhibitors targeting many parts of the enzyme and aspects of its function.

DIRECT ENZYMATIC INHIBITION OF TELOMERASE BY SMALL-MOLECULE DRUGS

The use of small-molecule drugs to directly inhibit telomerase enzymatic activity has as yet seen only modest success, with just a few compounds demonstrating high enzyme affinity and specificity, and phenotypic effects at the cellular level. At the time of this writing, only *one* compound has proceeded to clinical trials. Major challenges to progress in this endeavor have been, and still are, (1) the extremely low cellular abundance of human telomerase, even in immortal cell lines that display "robust" telomerase activity, measured at ~50 molecules per cell [42]; (2) the inability to generate large amounts of pure enzyme for the development of a high-throughput *direct* activity assay, applicable to large (>10^6) compound libraries; and (3) the lack of structural data for the complete enzyme complex to guide structure-based drug design. To date, there are no structural data for hTERT, and just a few small segments of hTR have been solved by nuclear magnetic resonance (NMR) (see e.g., [121–123]); the overall architecture of the complete six-molecule enzyme complex is unknown.

This section will first describe some of the standard in vitro and cell-based assays applied to the study of telomerase activity and telomere length dynamics. This will be followed by a discussion of the most promising and well-characterized drug candidates, including their biochemical mechanisms of inhibition and biological effects in cell-based assays and in vivo tumor models.

Assays for Telomerase Activity and Telomere Length Dynamics

There are three established in vitro assays to measure telomerase activity, defined here as the enzyme's ability to catalyze addition of 5'-TTAGGG-3' repeats onto a synthetic DNA substrate. The telomere repeat amplification protocol (TRAP) is a PCR-based assay that exploits the enzyme's ability to utilize a specific nontelomeric DNA as its substrate, to which it readily adds TTAGGG repeats in the presence of dTTP, dATP, and dGTP [31]. The nontelomeric sequence allows the use of distinct PCR primers (the other being complementary to TTAGGG) to amplify the extension products, making TRAP extraordinarily sensitive, routinely detecting telomerase from as few as 100 tumor cells. Amplification also allows easy detection following electrophoresis of the products, visible as a ladder of bands, each differing in length by one TTAGGG repeat. Development of the TRAP was instrumental in establishing the strong correlation between human cancer and dysregulated telomerase activity [31]. It should be noted that, as a PCR-based assay, TRAP displays only modest quantitativeness and is susceptible to inhibitors of *Taq* DNA polymerase present in crude cell lysates. In fact, the presence of such inhibitors can even lead to an *inverse* relationship between sample input and signal output (i.e., less sample → less inhibitors → greater PCR amplification) [124,125].

Simply referred to as the "direct assay", treating a solution of telomerase with a saturating concentration (~1 µM) of the synthetic DNA substrate 5'-(TTAGGG)$_3$-3' and deoxynucleoside triphosphates (dNTPs) will lead to the addition of TTAGGG repeats onto the DNA substrate [56]. As the name implies, this assay format does not use PCR and thus does not display the sensitivity of TRAP. Typically, the reaction is supplemented with α-^{32}P-dGTP, which is incorporated into the products for visualization by autoradiography or phosphorimaging, appearing as a ladder of products differing in size by six nucleotides (one TTAGGG repeat) (Fig. 17.5). Because of its lower sensitivity, combined with the low cellular abundance of telomerase, the direct assay is rarely effective on crude cell lysates; rather, some form of enrichment and/or chromatography of the enzyme is usually required [114,126,127]. Nonetheless, the direct assay is the method of choice when quantitative analyses of activity are required, for example when evaluating potential telomerase inhibitors.

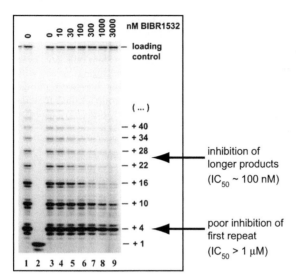

FIGURE 17.5 Inhibition of telomerase activity by BIBR1532. BIBR1532 specifically inhibits the translocation step of telomerase, resulting in a marked inhibition of longer products compared to generation of the first repeat. *Reproduced with permission from Ref. [114].*

A moderately high-throughput version of the direct assay, known as Telospot, visualizes telomerase products by spotting the DNA on a nylon membrane and hybridizing with an oligonucleotide probe, obviating the need for gel electrophoresis [128]. The assay may be scaled with the use of 96- or 386-well format automated liquid handlers. Once hits are identified, they can then be verified and their mechanism of action determined using a gel-based direct assay [128].

The length of telomeres in a cell is directly linked to its telomere maintenance mechanism (or lack thereof). The terminal restriction fragment (TRF; unrelated to TRF1/2) analysis provides a measurement of the distribution of all telomeres within a population of cells [129]. The TRF analysis is most informative when looking at cells over many PDs, when changes may occur. Treating the genomic DNA with a cocktail of restriction endonucleases that do not recognize $(TTAGGG)_n$ fragments the DNA while leaving the telomeres intact. The products are separated by electrophoresis, and the telomeric DNA is detected by Southern hybridization with a radiolabeled DNA complementary to TTAGGG, as illustrated in Fig. 17.6. The "smear" down the lane illustrates the heterogeneity of telomere lengths within a population of cells.

Quantitative measurement of the rate of PDs of a cell culture over time can reflect the dynamics of telomere maintenance. For an immortal cell line with a telomere maintenance mechanism (TMM), not limited by media or space in culture, plotting the number of PDs (*y*-axis) against time in culture (*x*-axis) yields essentially a linear relationship indefinitely. However, disruption of the TMM, such as with a telomerase inhibitor, may eventually lead to deviation from this linear relationship and reaching of a plateau as critically short telomeres induce cellular senescence.

Inhibition of Telomerase by Classical Nucleoside-Based RT Inhibitors

Upon recognition that telomerase functions as an RT [65], classical retroviral RT inhibitors (Chart 1) were promptly evaluated for their ability to inhibit telomerase [130]. To test

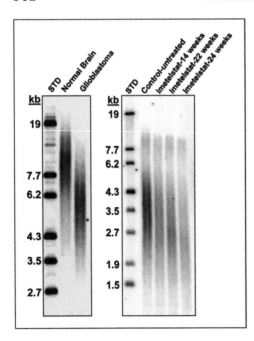

FIGURE 17.6 Terminal restriction fragment (TRF) analysis of telomeres from normal and diseased brain cells. Left: the shorter telomere length of glioblastoma cells compared to normal brain cells. Right: glioblastoma stem cells have even shorter telomeres, which then shorten during culture with GRN163L. This differential telomere length between normal and diseased cells provides a safety margin for the long-term administration of telomerase inhibitors. *Reproduced with permission from Ref. [113].*

inhibition of telomerase in an in vitro direct activity assay, Strahl and Blackburn evaluated the corresponding 5′-triphosphates of 2′,3′-dideoxyguanosine (ddG) and 3′-azidothymidine (AZT), both chain terminators. AZT was found to be a weak inhibitor of telomerase, requiring high micromolar (~100 μM) concentrations; competition against dTTP was achieved only with equimolar or greater concentrations of AZT. More effective inhibition was observed with ddGTP, wherein 1 μM was sufficient to reduce activity by 50% in a direct assay, even in the presence of 5 μM dGTP. This difference may partly reflect the greater affinity of guanosine derivatives over thymidine. As chain terminators, it could be expected that telomerase would incorporate these derivatives into the growing DNA product, thus terminating the reaction and affording a change in distribution to shorter products; however, this was not observed, suggesting that the inhibitory effect of ddGTP is competitively reversible in nature rather than a result of irreversible incorporation into the DNA product.

Addition of 10 μM ddG to the culture medium of immortalized B-cell lines resulted in significant telomere shortening over the first ~50 PDs; however, telomere length then remained stable with continued culturing up to 200 PDs (~1 year), during which time there was no change in the doubling rate of the cell lines. This is longer than the aforementioned "lag phase" for the onset of telomere-induced senescence. To determine if the telomerase of the later cultures had acquired resistance to ddG through mutation and selection, the authors measured—and confirmed—the ability of ddGTP to inhibit in vitro telomerase activity. Thus, the authors concluded that although the activity of telomerase in these cell lines was diminished, the extent of inhibition was insufficient to induce senescence [130].

A variety of synthetic nucleotide analogs, bearing modification of the base, have since been evaluated. For example, 7-deaza-dATP and 7-deaza-dGTP were found to inhibit telomerase in a direct assay with IC_{50}s of 8 μM and 11 μM, respectively [131]. By far, the most potent

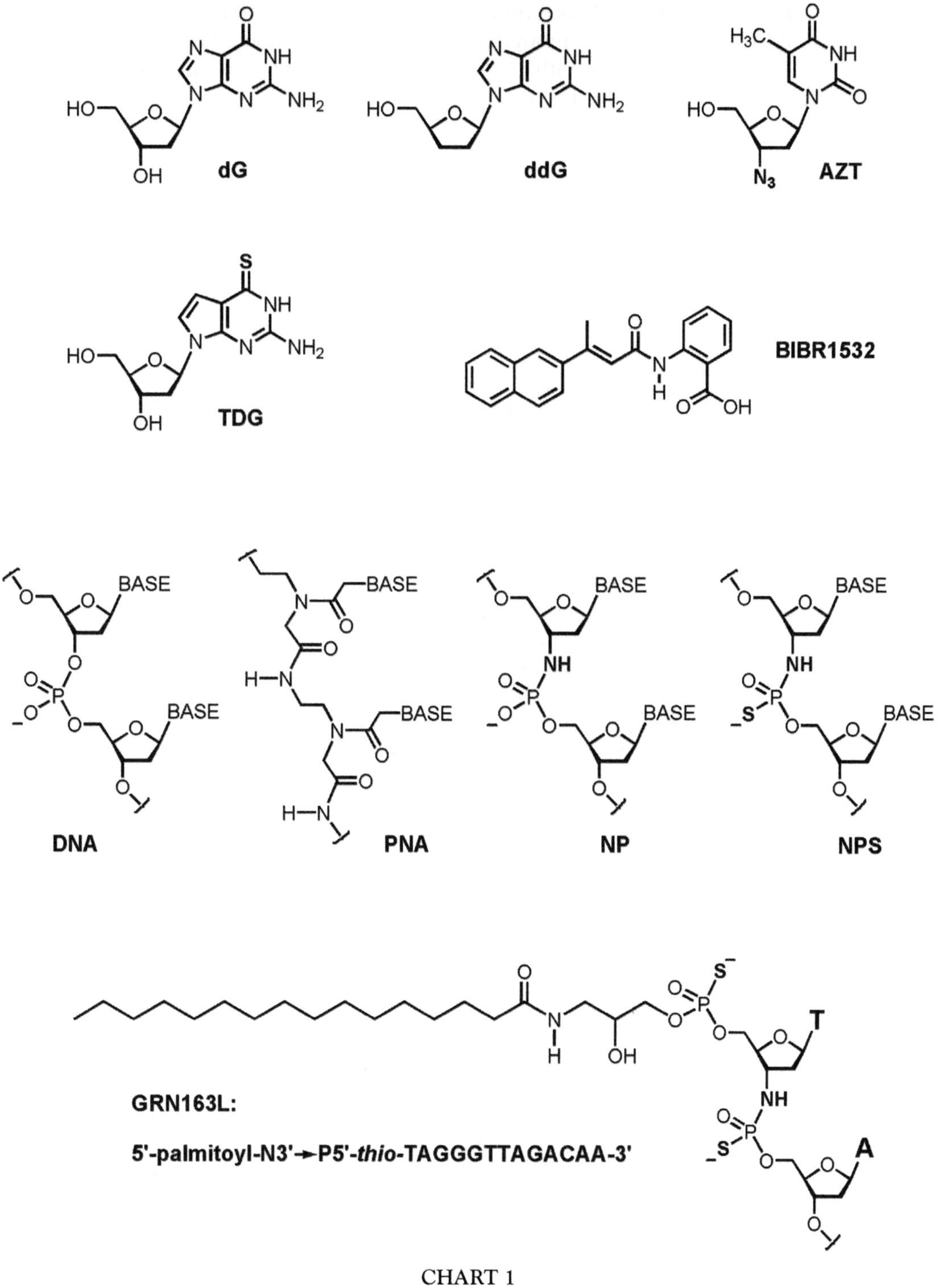

dG   ddG   AZT

TDG   BIBR1532

DNA   PNA   NP   NPS

GRN163L:

5'-palmitoyl-N3'→P5'-*thio*-TAGGGTTAGACAA-3'

CHART 1

II. DRUGS IN THE LABORATORY AND CLINIC

nucleotide analog described to date is 6-thio-7-deaza-dGTP (TDG, Chart 1) [132], displaying an IC_{50} of 60 nM in a direct assay, compared to an IC_{50} of 2.5 μM against DNA polymerase α. Unfortunately, further experiments with TDG in cell culture were not performed, and studies with this analog appear to have not been continued.

BIBR1532, a Nonnucleosidic Telomerase-Specific Inhibitor

In 2001, scientists from Boehringer Ingelheim Pharma reported the first nonnucleosidic inhibitor of human telomerase, designated BIBR1532 (Chart 1) [133]. The scope and size of the compound library were not revealed; however, the authors had previously developed a method for ~1000-fold enrichment of human telomerase from cell lysates [134], enabling at least a limited screening program using a direct assay. BIBR1532 was found to inhibit telomerase from HeLa cell lysate with an IC_{50} of ~90 nM, a factor of 100–1000 more potent than some of the nucleoside-based RT inhibitors described in this chapter. This same IC_{50} was observed when using recombinant, in vitro reconstituted telomerase, demonstrating that BIBR1532 indeed targets the telomerase enzyme directly rather than through an indirect mechanism, such as an enzyme cofactor or associated protein that could conceivably be present in a cell-based system. Perhaps not surprisingly, the specificity of BIBR1532 for telomerase over other nucleic acid polymerases is far superior compared to the nucleoside-based RT inhibitors; none of the enzymes in Table 17.1 was inhibited in the presence of <50 μM BIBR1532.

Close examination of the profile of DNA extension products upon titration of BIBR1532 immediately suggested an unexpected mode of enzymatic inhibition [114]. As illustrated in Fig. 17.5, synthesis of *longer* DNA extension products, corresponding to three or more cycles of nucleotide addition and translocation, is preferentially inhibited with lower concentrations of BIBR1532 than is synthesis of the first nucleotide addition cycle; the product corresponding to the first round of nucleotide addition is only slightly inhibited, even at 3 μM BIBR1532. Another feature of BIBR1532 inhibition is that the six-nucleotide product profile is conserved: BIBR1532 does not impede reverse transcription along the RNA template, which

TABLE 17.1   Inhibition of Nucleic Acid Polymerases by BIBR1532

Enzyme	IC_{50} (μM)
Human telomerase	0.09
Taq DNA polymerase	–
Human DNA polymerase α, β, γ	–
Calf thymus DNA polymerase α	–
Human RNA polymerase I, II, and III	>100 μM
In vitro translation	–
Bacterial DNA helicase	–
HIV-1 reverse transcriptase	–

(–): No Effect at 50 μM.
Data from Ref. [133].

would generate products of intermediate lengths. These observations suggest that BIBR1532 exerts its effect at the point of translocation, when reverse transcription has reached the end of the template (the addition of 5′-GGTTAG-3′). Mechanistically, this could occur through (1) an *increase* in the rate of dissociation between the enzyme and DNA product, and/or (2) a *decrease* in the rate of conformational change that defines translocation. Kinetic experiments aimed at determining the precise mode of enzymatic inhibition revealed a decrease in V_{max} without a change in the K_m for the DNA substrate, indicating that the BIBR1532 does not compete for the DNA binding site; for the dNTPs, a weak (~two- to threefold) allosteric inhibition with BIBR1532 was observed, wherein BIBR1532 displayed greater affinity for the dNTP-free enzyme, and dNTPs a greater affinity for the BIBR1532-free enzyme. The authors conclude that BIBR1532 behaves as a mixed-type noncompetitive inhibitor [114].

Addition of 10 µM BIBR1532 to the culture media of immortal human cell lines resulted in dramatic effects on telomere dynamics and cellular growth properties. Cell lines derived from cancers of the lung, breast, and prostate all displayed significant telomere shortening over ~100–140 PDs, from ~4 to 5 kb (typical for a telomerase-positive cell line) to ~1.5 kb [133]. The doubling rates of these cell lines were essentially unchanged for at least 100 PDs, despite constant culture with BIBR1532 and telomere shortening. This represents the *lag phase* described in this chapter: the proliferative potential that must be exhausted before doubling rates are affected. However, by PD ~120, a clear decrease in doubling rate ensued, followed by an almost complete cessation of proliferation by PD ~140. This was accompanied by morphological changes consistent with a senescent phenotype.

Two subsequent studies examined the effect of BIBR1532 on hematopoietic disorders: chronic lymphocytic leukemia (CCL), acute myeloid leukemia (AML) [135], and T-cell prolymphocytic leukemia (T-PLL) [112]. In these studies, BIBR1532 was applied at much higher concentrations, in the range of 50–100 µM; presumably, telomerase activity was completely inhibited, although this was not confirmed experimentally. Whereas cells treated with 10 µM BIBR1532 continued doubling until their proliferative potential was exhausted through gradual telomere shortening, the high levels of BIBR1532 resulted in *immediate* cytotoxic effects, with <10% cell viability within just 10 days of culture. Furthermore, this cytotoxicity was *independent* of telomerase activity, because some of the CCL and AML cells (patient-derived samples) tested negative for telomerase activity. The cytotoxicity is likely a consequence of a telomere-capping defect induced by BIBR1532; the telomere-binding protein TRF2 was depleted, and chromosomal end-to-end fusions, a hallmark of telomere dysfunction, were present [135]. In contrast, normal cells from healthy donors did not display this short-term sensitivity to BIBR1532; unstimulated T-cells and progenitor cells from cord blood were resistant up to 100 and 120 µM, respectively. The molecular mechanism responsible for the telomere uncapping by BIBR1532 is not understood at this time.

The fate of BIBR1532 is unclear. Despite the compound displaying impressive enzymatic inhibition and specificity, it appears not to have progressed to clinical trials.

GRN163L, an Oligonucleotide-Based Antisense Inhibitor

To the best of our knowledge, only one direct enzymatic inhibitor of telomerase has progressed to clinical trials: the synthetic antisense oligonucleotide GRN163L, developed by Geron Corporation (Menlo Park, CA, USA). The approach of using antisense oligomers complementary to the template region of the telomerase RNA (hTR) through complementary base pairing became readily apparent with the realization that, biochemically, telomerase is a reverse transcriptase. As part of functionally characterizing the hTR gene, the authors demonstrated inhibition of telomerase with an antisense RNA [136]. DNA or RNA oligomers are not ideal as either research tools for in vitro analyses of cell lysates or as drug candidates in vivo due to their rapid degradation by nucleases. The first report of targeted antisense inhibition of telomerase using a chemically modified oligonucleotide—a collaboration between scientists at the University of Texas Southwestern Medical Center and Geron—applied peptide nucleic acids (PNAs, Chart 1) [137]. As determined by the telomere repeat amplification protocol (TRAP) assay, the 13-mer PNA TAGGGTTAGACAA inhibited telomerase with an IC_{50} of 0.9 nM. Note that only eight of the PNA "bases" (underlined) pair with the template region of hTR, while the other four extend into the 5′ distal region of the RNA. As a demonstration of specificity, the noncomplementary 13-mer PNA TGTAAGGAACTAG (same base composition) did not show any inhibition.

Using the optimized sequence TAGGGTTAGACAA, two other chemically modified and nuclease-resistant phosphate linkages, N3′→P5′ phosphoramidates (NPs) and N3′→P5′ *thio*-phosphoramidates (NPSs, Chart 1), were evaluated for enzymatic inhibition and specificity. These NP and NPS oligonucleotides displayed high duplex stability with hTR, with melting temperatures (T_m) of 72.4 and 70.5 °C, respectively [138]. In practical terms, such stability would translate to essentially irreversible inhibition of telomerase once the duplex is formed; this is supported by the fact that a complex of telomerase and NPS-TAGGGTTAGACAA was observed as a discrete band on a native polyacrylamide gel, attesting to its stability. In contrast, the noncomplementary TAGGTGTAAGCAA NP and NPS compounds did not form stable duplexes with hTR (T_ms ~ 20 °C). The in vitro TRAP and T_m analyses indicated that the NP and NPS compound displayed similar properties. However, in cell culture experiments with an epithelial breast cancer cell line, a striking difference was observed. The NP compound, in the presence of a cationic lipid carrier (FuGENE6) to promote cellular uptake, displayed an IC_{50} of ~1 μM. The NPS compound, differing only in the uniform substitution of a nonbridging oxygen with a sulfur, was ~200-fold more potent, with an IC_{50} of ~5 nM. The presence of the sulfur is speculated to afford a "softer" molecule that can penetrate cells more efficiently (i.e., it has greater bioavailability) compared to the "harder" oxygen. NPS-TAGGGTTAGA-CAA, hereafter designated GRN163, was then taken on for further development.

GRN163 added to culture medium demonstrated telomerase inhibition against a variety of immortal cell lines derived from tumors of the breast, prostate, lung, colon, and others. In the absence of lipid uptake enhancers, IC_{50} values were generally ~0.5–1.0 μM, as determined by TRAP [139]. Long-term culture of A431 epidermoid tumor cells with GRN163 displayed a growth profile consistent with telomere attrition due to lack of TMM: doubling time continued at a near linear rate for ~100 PDs, at which time the culture entered crisis at day 162. TRF analysis confirmed telomere attrition, from ~4.5 kb at the start of the experiment to ~1.8 kb at crisis. Similar trends were observed in multiple myeloma cell lines and patient samples [140,141].

A consistent observation with cell lines was that applying GRN163 in conjunction with a lipid uptake enhancer reduced IC_{50}s to ~1 nM. The increased bioavailability conferred by lipid enhancers led to the final evolution of GRN163L: addition of a lipid (palmitoyl) to the 5′ end (Chart 1) [142]. The increase in cellular uptake upon lipid modification of GRN163 was assessed in a panel of 12 immortal cell lines representing eight tissue types. Measurement of telomerase activity after culturing with either GRN163 or GRN163L—without lipid uptake enhancer—demonstrated a clear decrease in the $IC_{50}s$, by a factor of up to 40 depending on the cell line. Consistent with telomerase being a target of broad scope, GRN163L has demonstrated antitumor efficacy in preclinical studies of in vivo mouse xenograft models for a range of human cancers, including cancers of the lung [143], liver [144], breast [145], and others.

More recently, GRN163L has shown efficacy against *cancer stem cells*, which are rare cells within a tumor that can self-renew and initiate the formation of a new tumor. Cancer stem cells may bear greater resistance to treatment, and their residual presence is believed to be largely responsible for the recurrence of some types of tumors. For example, in glioblastoma, a lethal cancer of the brain with a median survival of ~1 year, recurrence occurs due to the presence of cancer stem cells that are resistant to ionizing radiation by virtue of their increased DNA repair capacity [146]. Long-term culture of glioblastoma stem cells in the presence of 2 µM GRN163L resulted in a decrease in their rate of proliferation and also in their ability to initiate nonadherent growth of a new cell (tumor) mass when plated at low density [113]. Telomere length analysis further supports telomerase inhibition as a viable approach against glioblastoma. Normal (mortal) brain cells displayed an average telomere length of ~12 kb, compared to ~6 kb for glioblastoma cells, consistent with the general idea that tumor cells have shorter telomeres than normal cells. The stem cells had even shorter telomeres of ~3.5 kb, which progressively shortened to <2 kb over a period of 24 weeks (~20 PDs) of continuous culture with 2 µM GRN163L (Fig. 17.6) [113]. Another challenge of treating brain tumors is the delivery of drugs across the blood–brain barrier. GRN163L reduced telomerase activity by ~70% in a xenograft model of human glioblastoma stem cells injected into the brains of mice, a significant attribute likely conferred by the palmitoyl modification [113].

Furthermore, GRN163L caused *preferential* telomere shortening and reduced proliferation in stem cells from prostate, multiple myeloma, breast, and pancreatic cancer cell lines compared to the bulk tumor cells, leading to a depletion of cancer stem cells from the total population [147–149]. The mechanism for this effect is unknown, since in some of these studies initial telomere length did not differ between the two populations, but it provides hope that telomerase inhibition will result in less tumor recurrence than other types of therapy.

The promising preclinical data across a range of tumor types provided the foundation for Geron Corporation to proceed to clinical trials of GRN163L (referred to in the clinic as "imetelstat"). By the end of 2011, phase I trials of GRN163L had been completed for the blood disorders chronic lymphocytic leukemia and multiple myeloma and for solid tumors of the breast and lung. The principal aim was to establish a maximum tolerated dose and demonstrate safety, which was considered sufficient to advance to targeted phase II studies in 2012. GRN163L is currently being evaluated as a single agent for multiple myeloma, one of several myeloproliferative diseases (blood disorders); these disorders may be well suited for telomerase therapy as the cells responsible have distinctly *short* telomeres [150]. Preliminary data are reported to be encouraging (http://www.geron.com/imetelstat), with a rapid decrease in the cell count of progenitor cells observed in most patients. In contrast, another phase II trial, GRN163L in combination with paclitaxel in patients with metastatic breast cancer, did not afford improved outcome, and this trial was discontinued. These outcomes illustrate the heterogeneity of cancer at the molecular, cellular, and physiological levels, and the long road to a successful therapy. Despite this recent setback, direct inhibition of telomerase is still considered a promising avenue for cancer therapy.

INDIRECT TELOMERASE INHIBITION WITH G-QUADRUPLEX-STABILIZING MOLECULES

An alternative strategy to achieve telomere shortening in cancer cells involves targeting the in vivo substrate of telomerase, the telomere, rather than telomerase itself. Telomeres are one of several guanine-rich areas of the genome that have a well-characterized tendency in vitro for the four guanines to hydrogen-bond with each other in a planar cyclical arrangement called a G-quartet; the cavity at the core is the binding site for monovalent cations (e.g., Na$^+$, K$^+$) that stabilize this structure [151]. Multiple layers of G-quartets stack to form G-quadruplexes, in which the DNA strands assemble together in either *intra*molecular or *inter*molecular configuration. G-quadruplexes exhibit extensive structural polymorphism. The 5′ to 3′ orientation of the DNA backbone may be antiparallel (Fig. 17.7(A)), parallel (Fig. 17.7(B)), or a mixture of both (known as a "hybrid" conformation; Fig. 17.7(C)), and the length and topology of the loops connecting the G-quartets can vary widely [152].

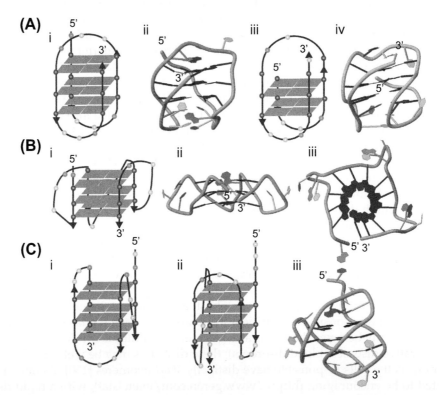

FIGURE 17.7 Human telomeric intramolecular G-quadruplexes. (A) Topology and NMR structure of oligonucleotide AGGG(TTAGGG)$_3$ in sodium solution (i,ii; [153]) or oligonucleotide GGG(TTAGGG)$_3$T in potassium solution (iii,iv; [154]), demonstrating two different antiparallel conformations. (B) Topology (i) and crystal structure (ii, iii) of oligonucleotide AGGG(TTAGGG)$_3$ in potassium, showing a parallel "propeller" structure [155]. The crystal structure is shown as a side view (ii) and a top view (iii). (C) Hybrid conformations in potassium solution. Hybrid 1 (i) and hybrid 2 (ii) topologies illustrate differences in loop structures [156,157]. The NMR structure of hybrid 2 is shown in (iii) [157]. (This figure is reproduced in color in the color plate section.)

The functions of telomeric G-quadruplex structures in human cells are unknown. Different conformations may carry out distinct roles. Intermolecular G-quadruplexes could facilitate telomere–telomere associations; such interactions have been observed in the telomere-rich macronuclei of ciliated protozoa, and there is evidence that they are mediated by G-quadruplexes [158,159]. Direct evidence for these G-quadruplexes was provided by their detection with an anti-G-quadruplex antibody [159]. Telomere-binding proteins were involved in the formation of these G-quadruplexes and their resolution during DNA replication [160]. It has also been postulated that intermolecular parallel G-quadruplexes may be involved in the alignment of sister chromatids during meiosis [161]. Hybrid intramolecular forms of the human telomeric sequence have the potential to stack end to end in long arrays, which may accomplish compaction of telomeric DNA [156,157,162]. A very large number of proteins have been demonstrated to bind, promote, resolve, or cleave G-quadruplexes, which supports the in vivo relevance of such structures [163]. A labeled small molecule that specifically recognizes G-quadruplexes (pyridostatin; discussed further in this chapter) bound to sites throughout the genome in fixed cells, providing evidence for the existence of G-quadruplexes in the human genome prior to fixation [164]. Recently, it was found that in the absence of natural telomere capping, G-quadruplexes can fulfill capping functions at telomeres in vivo in *Saccharomyces cerevisiae* [165]. G-quadruplexes at the telomeres and throughout the genome of human cells have been directly visualized using a G-quadruplex-specific antibody, confirming the existence of these structures in vivo [166].

A seminal paper in 1991 demonstrated that G-quadruplexes formed from the telomeric sequence of the ciliate *Oxytricha nova* could not be extended by telomerase [167]. This suggested the possibility that small molecules that stabilize such telomeric G-quadruplexes in vivo could block telomerase action. In the intervening two decades, there has been a flurry of activity to develop G-quadruplex-stabilizing ligands as potential cancer therapeutics (reviewed in Ref. [168]). There are now hundreds, or possibly thousands, of such molecules described in the literature; we will not attempt to comprehensively review them all, but will discuss here the exciting recent trends toward greater specificity and biological effectiveness of these molecules.

In recent years, our expanding knowledge of telomerase and telomeres has revealed that this strategy may be more complicated than originally envisaged. For example, our laboratory has demonstrated that telomerase from ciliated protozoa and humans, while indeed unable to extend intramolecular antiparallel G-quadruplexes, has the ability to extend telomeric G-quadruplexes that are intermolecular and parallel (see Refs [169,170] and K. Porter and T. Bryan, unpublished data). It remains likely that this activity can be blocked by G-quadruplex-stabilizing ligands, since partial unwinding of the 3′ end of the G-quadruplex is necessary for hybridization of the telomerase template RNA, and many ligands have been shown to end-stack on the terminal G-quartet [171–174]. Nevertheless, such inhibition remains to be demonstrated, and the finding also illustrates the need to be aware of different biological functions of various G-quadruplex conformations. Furthermore, many recent studies have demonstrated that G-quadruplex-stabilizing ligands have both telomeric and nontelomeric in vivo effects that go well beyond simple telomerase inhibition (discussed further in this chapter). Nevertheless, it is becoming apparent that many of these effects converge on the specific death of cancer cells, making G-quadruplex ligands a very promising emerging group of therapeutic agents.

Affinity and Specificity of G-quadruplex Ligands

A key property for effective in vivo use with low toxicity is the specificity of the compound for G-quadruplex structures over the abundant duplex DNA in the genome. Early efforts focused on flat aromatic molecules that could stack on the external G-quartet and would be too large to intercalate into duplex DNA. Porphyrins, as aromatic planar macrocycles, are good candidates, although early examples such as TMPyP4 were found to possess very poor G-quadruplex specificity [175–177]. The addition of bulky side arms greatly improved specificity, with porphyrins such as N-methyl mesoporphyrin X (NMM, Chart 2), a pentacationic manganese (III) porphyrin, or protoporphyrin IX reported to have 500- to 1000-fold G-quadruplex-to-duplex specificity [176–181]. A recent re-examination of the specificity of TMPyP4 revealed that even this porphyrin possesses ~100-fold specificity for particular subtypes of human telomeric G-quadruplexes over duplex DNA [182].

The bisquinolium family emerged as a group of compounds with both excellent affinity and selectivity for G-quadruplexes. For example, the well-studied molecule 360A and the more recent PhenDC3 (Chart 2) have selectivities over duplex of 50–100 [183–185]. The similarly flat and aromatic molecule pyridostatin (Chart 2) shows even higher affinity for G-quadruplexes with comparable specificity [186]. A classic example of a flat, aromatic ligand is an extensively studied natural-product macrocycle, telomestatin (Chart 2) [187], which shows ~70-fold specificity over duplex DNA [188] and promising biological properties (discussed further in this chapter), but it is not easy to obtain due to the complexity of its synthesis [189]. A more accessible family of macrocycles are the cyclo-bis-intercalators (for example, see **structure 1,** Chart 2), which differ from the above classes of molecules in that they are nonplanar and somewhat flexible. A two-stage screening process—first, screening a large number of such molecules for affinity for a human telomeric G-quadruplex and, second,

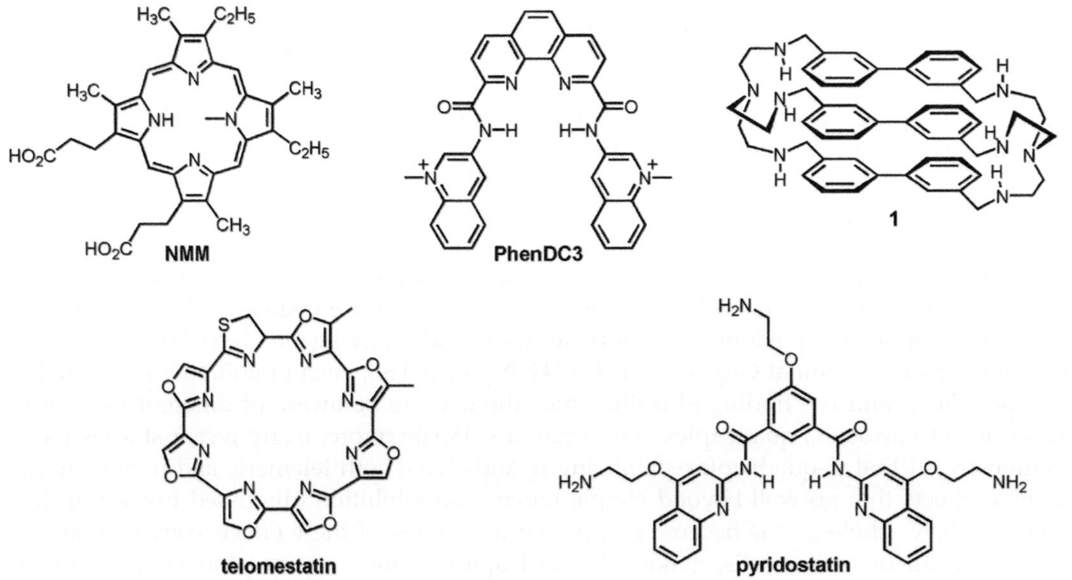

CHART 2

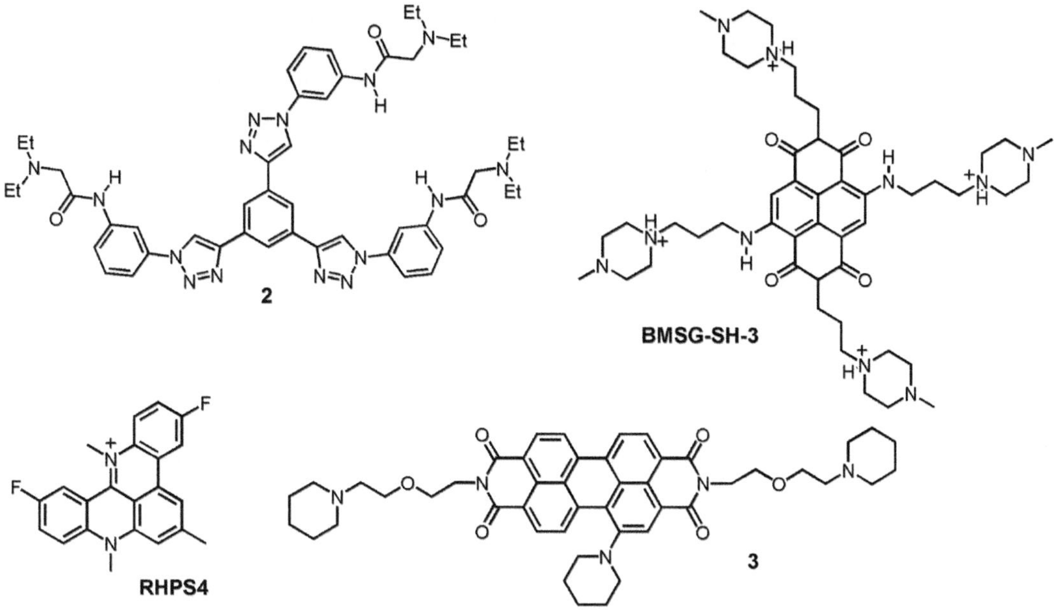

CHART 3

testing the selectivity of high-affinity hits—uncovered two macrocycles with excellent affinity and >50-fold selectivity [190]. Indeed, it is becoming apparent that some flexibility in the molecule is desirable, probably to target the loops and grooves of the G-quadruplex rather than just the face of the G-quartet. Good examples of this concept are a series of bis-indole carboxamides with 300- to 2000-fold selectivity for G-quadruplex over duplex [191], and a series of triarylpyridines [192]. Among the latter group of compounds, there was a trend for those compounds with exceptionally high G-quadruplex-stabilizing ability to have lower selectivity against duplex DNA than the compounds with more modest affinity [192], indicating that it may not always be desirable to select for the highest-affinity compounds.

With the increasing availability of crystal and NMR structures of different G-quadruplexes [193], structure-based drug design and molecular modeling are playing an increasing role in the design of G-quadruplex-specific compounds. For example, the crystal structure of parallel human telomeric DNA complexed with the tri-substituted acridine BRACO19 was used as a starting point for structure-based design of improved mimetics of this compound, resulting in a series of tri-substituted triazoles with G-quadruplex-to-duplex selectivities of >1000 (**structure 2**, Chart 3) [194], which is much higher than the 30- to 40-fold selectivity of BRACO19 itself [195].

Telomerase Inhibition and Telomere Shortening

The original premise for developing G-quadruplex-stabilizing molecules was the inhibition of telomerase, and many of these compounds have proven to be very effective inhibitors. The extent of inhibition of many of the compounds, however, may be overestimated, due to the widespread use of the TRAP assay to measure telomerase activity in the presence of G-quadruplex ligands. It has been unambiguously demonstrated that the TRAP assay is inappropriate for this purpose, since the ligand can stabilize G-quadruplexes in the extended telomerase products and block their amplification by *Taq* polymerase [196]. An improvement on the standard TRAP assay involves removal of the ligand after the telomerase extension step (i.e., prior to the PCR step), and this technique (known as TRAP-LIG [197]) is becoming more widely used. Use of this assay or the direct telomerase activity assay has demonstrated that many G-quadruplex compounds inhibit telomerase with low micromolar or submicromolar IC_{50}s, including BRACO19, telomestatin, TMPyP4, PhenDC3, 360A, a tetrasubstituted naphthalene diimide (BMSG-SH-3, Chart 3), 2-phenyl-benzopyranopyrimidine derivatives, platinum(II) dipyridophenazine compounds, and a series of perylene diimides (for example, see **structure 3**, Chart 3) [175,196,198–201].

A direct telomerase activity assay is the method of choice, however, since it can also provide valuable information regarding the mechanism of telomerase inhibition. Use of a four-repeat telomeric primer substrate provides a direct measure of the degree of inhibition due to locking of the substrate primer in a folded conformation; telomestatin, PhenDC3, and 360A all have IC_{50} values in the tens-of-nanomolar range for this mode of inhibition [196]. A three-repeat telomeric primer or nontelomeric primer, on the other hand, is unable to form into intramolecular G-quadruplexes; inhibition of *initial* extension of these substrates is indicative of a direct inhibitory effect on the telomerase enzyme or non-G-quadruplex-related interactions of ligand with primer, which occurred at relatively high concentrations for all ligands examined [196]. Once a nontelomeric or three-repeat telomeric primer has been extended by four or one repeats, respectively, the telomerase product may form into an intramolecular G-quadruplex. As was elegantly demonstrated in the first description of telomerase inhibition by a G-quadruplex ligand [202], the compound can stabilize this product G-quadruplex and cause dissociation of telomerase from the DNA, leading to a decrease in processivity with a characteristic four-repeat periodicity. This effect has been subsequently demonstrated to occur in the presence of a variety of different compounds [175,196,201]. Interestingly, however, not all G-quadruplex-stabilizing molecules have this ability; telomestatin caused a slight *increase* in telomerase processivity [196], despite its exceptional affinity for G-quadruplexes [188]. Telomestatin specifically binds antiparallel G-quadruplexes [188], which may indicate that G-quadruplexes forming in telomerase products are parallel or hybrid structures; it will be interesting to correlate the effects on telomerase processivity with specificity for particular structures as these are becoming better characterized (discussed further in this chapter).

When incubated with telomerase-positive immortal cells at subcytotoxic concentrations, many of the G-quadruplex ligands that were demonstrated to inhibit telomerase cause gradual telomere shortening and eventual senescence or apoptosis [99,200,203–209]. This demonstrates the principle that these compounds could be used as anticancer agents by virtue of their telomerase inhibition, albeit with the aforementioned lag period.

Telomere Uncapping Caused by G-quadruplex Ligands

It has recently become apparent, however, that G-quadruplex-stabilizing compounds may also have much more rapid effects on cancer cell viability. Some of the same compounds known to inhibit telomerase and induce telomere shortening (e.g., BRACO19, 360A, and the pentacyclic acridine **RHPS4**, Chart 3) also caused a rapid cessation of cell proliferation in the absence of telomere shortening when used at slightly higher concentrations [183,206,210]. Reduction of the length of the 3′ telomere overhang was observed, along with telomere end-to-end fusions [183,206,210–213] and telomere aggregations in the nucleus, which are known to precede chromosomal fusions in transformed cells [214,215]. Telomere levels of the protective shelterin proteins POT1 and TRF2 were reduced by many G-quadruplex ligands [186,211,212,216–218], and proteins associated with the DNA damage response, such as γH2AX, accumulated at telomeres [186,212,217–219]. These DNA damage foci, known as telomere-damage induced foci (TIFs), are a hallmark of uncapped telomeres. G-quadruplex-induced TIFs were suppressed by the overexpression of POT1 and TRF2, confirming that removal of these proteins from the telomere plays a role in this telomere uncapping [217]. Many G-quadruplex ligands, including telomestatin, BRACO19, RHPS4, 360A, pyridostatin, perylene **3**, and BMSG-SH-3, have now been demonstrated to cause telomere uncapping [183,206,210,211,213,214,218].

Several lines of evidence suggest that G-quadruplex-induced TIFs result from difficulties during the replication of telomeric DNA. The TIFs can arise in S phase [164,218,219] and are dependent on the kinase ATR (ataxia telangiectasia and Rad3-related), which plays a key role in the response to replication fork stalling throughout the genome [217,220]. The ligands RHPS4 and 360A have both been shown to induce duplicated telomeres, known as "telomere doublets" or "fragile telomeres", which are known to arise due to replication fork stalling [219,221,222]; those induced by 360A occur primarily on the lagging (G-rich) strand [221,223]. These data are consistent with a model in which G-quadruplex ligands induce excessive stabilization of G-quadruplexes on the G-rich telomeric strand during replication, which blocks replication, causing recruitment of ATR and a DNA damage response. Interestingly, loss of either ATR or the DNA damage response kinase ATM (ataxia telangiectasia, mutated) in the presence of 360A causes an increased number of telomere aberrations such as telomere losses and fusions [221,224], suggesting that the DNA damage response is an attempt to protect the telomeres from undergoing these aberrations and thereby causing massive genome instability. The mechanism for this is unknown, but it may involve recruitment by ATR of the helicases WRN and BLM, which are enriched at telomeres after treatment with RHPS4, are phosphorylated by ATR, and are known to unwind G-quadruplex structures [219,225–227].

Overexpression of POT1 or TRF2 suppresses both the telomeric DNA damage response and the rapid cell death caused by RHPS4 [217], indicating that telomere uncapping and telomere aberrations are causally related to the rapid cell death induced by many of these ligands. Although unexpected, these effects have two promising implications for cancer treatment: (1) they overcome the lag period while waiting for telomeres to shorten after telomerase inhibition, and (2) they predict that cancer cells that use ALT rather than telomerase may also be susceptible to G-quadruplex-mediated cell death. Indeed, many G-quadruplex ligands have been shown to induce telomere dysfunction and cell death in ALT cell lines, including telomestatin, 360A, RHPS4, TMPyP4, and an anthracene derivative [183,188,228–231]. This may not be universal, however, since neither pyridostatin nor the triazine 12459 was able to kill ALT cells [213,232]. Only a small number of ALT cell lines have been treated with G-quadruplex ligands to date; to establish the generality of the response, a much bigger panel of cell lines needs to be examined.

Specificity for Cancer Cells over Normal Cells

A general effect on telomere capping and stability implies that G-quadruplex ligands will also have detrimental effects on normal cells. Empirically, it seems that this is not necessarily the case; many of the ligands discussed in this chapter have been demonstrated to show specificity, to varying extents, for causing cell death of cancer cells. Some compounds, particularly telomestatin and a series of 4,5-disubstituted acridones, show excellent differential IC_{50} values between cancer cell lines and normal cells [198,199,211,233–236]. Several G-quadruplex ligands cause TIFs in transformed cell lines but not in normal cells [211,217,218,237]. The molecular basis for this discrimination is unknown; it is possible that telomere architecture differs between normal cells and those that have an active TMM, or the absence of intact cell cycle checkpoints in transformed cells may result in a different response to telomeric damage. Again, only one or two cell strains have been tested with each compound (typically the fibroblasts WI38, IMR90, or BJ-hTERT), so a much wider range of different cell types should be tested to establish the generality of this discrimination.

Other compounds display more modest or no specificity for cancer cell lines, despite having excellent ability to discriminate between G-quadruplexes and duplex DNA [200,213,238,239]. This emphasizes the need to test the cell line specificity for each compound before proceeding with preclinical studies.

Specificity for Different Conformations of G-quadruplexes

G-quadruplexes formed in vitro from human telomeric sequences are highly polymorphic; a four-repeat telomeric oligonucleotide can fold into at least five different conformations, including parallel, antiparallel, and hybrid forms, depending on the conditions and oligonucleotide used (reviewed in Ref. [152]; Fig. 17.7). It is likely that all of these conformations exist at telomeres in vivo under different circumstances, but we do not yet know which conformation is predominant under which cellular circumstance. Given that telomerase can extend parallel but not antiparallel telomeric G-quadruplexes [169,170], it is likely that different conformations carry out different biological functions. Furthermore, telomeres are by no means the only G-rich portion of the genome; bioinformatic analysis has identified ~375,000 candidate sequences within the human genome that could form G-quadruplex structures [240,241]. Putative G-quadruplex-forming sequences are concentrated in promoter regions; nearly one-half of all known genes in the human genome harbor such sequences within 1000 nucleotides upstream of the transcription start site [242]. For several genes, it has been experimentally confirmed that the G-quadruplex-forming region plays a critical role in regulating expression of the gene (reviewed in Ref. [243]). A single point mutation that destabilizes the G-quadruplex found in the c-*MYC* promoter resulted in a threefold increase in basal transcriptional activity of this gene; conversely, TMPyP4 was able to suppress c-*MYC* activation [244]. Other G-quadruplex ligands modulate expression of the genes for hTERT and c-*KIT*, which also harbor G-quadruplex-forming regions in their promoters [245,246]. G-quadruplex-forming sequences are also enriched in the 5′ untranslated regions of many genes, and formation of a G-quadruplex in the mRNA of these genes has been shown to modulate translation (reviewed in Ref. [247]).

In order to specifically target telomeric G-quadruplexes, it is therefore desirable to design or select for compounds that have the ability to discriminate between different conformations.

Many compounds described thus far show little selectivity for different conformations [185], but structure-specific ligands are starting to appear. An early example was telomestatin; among the known conformations of intramolecular human telomeric G-quadruplexes, it is specific for the antiparallel "basket" form [188,248], although it has also been shown to bind to the G-quadruplex found in the hTERT promoter [249]. Other compounds that favor binding to antiparallel over parallel human telomeric G-quadruplexes include RHPS4, an acyclic oligoheteroaryle known as TOxaPy, and a series of phenanthrolines [250–252], while a particular enantiomer of a chiral metallo-helical compound showed strong specificity for the hybrid human telomeric G-quadruplex over all other tested telomeric or promoter conformations [209,253]. A number of compounds bind to the parallel rather than antiparallel or hybrid telomeric G-quadruplex [178,254–257], but a consideration for these compounds is that many promoter G-quadruplexes are also parallel. Recently, structure-based drug design using the crystal structure of the parallel human telomeric G-quadruplex has yielded both naphthalene diimides and triazole–acridine conjugates that do show high specificity for human telomeric G-quadruplexes over that in the c-*KIT* promoter [198,236]. Conversely, a bisaryldiketene derivative demonstrated ~200-fold specificity for the c-*MYC* promoter G-quadruplex over human telomeric conformations [258]. The possibility of specifically targeting different G-quadruplexes for different clinical purposes is therefore becoming closer to reality.

The genomic location of sites of DNA damage, visualized by immunofluorescence against γH2AX, can provide some clues regarding the in vivo propensity for different compounds to specifically target telomeres. Perylene **3** induced γH2AX foci throughout the nucleus, only a small proportion of which colocalized with telomeres [218], whereas it was reported that 70% of RHPS4-induced DNA damage sites were telomeric [217]. For both telomestatin and pyridostatin, DNA damage sites are mostly nontelomeric at low doses of the compound, with telomere localization increasing at higher doses [164,212]. No ligand has yet been reported to cause exclusively telomeric γH2AX foci.

Intriguingly, however, the frequency at which potentially G-quadruplex-forming sequences are found within transcribed regions displays a propitious correlation with cancer gene function. They are frequently found in proto-oncogenes, including c-*MYC*, *VEGF*, c-*KIT*, *HIF-1a*, and *BCL2*, but are significantly underrepresented in tumor suppressor genes [259]. This raises the possibility that even G-quadruplex stabilizers with broad affinity for many G-quadruplex types may result in anticancer effects through multiple pathways. Pyridostatin, which causes robust telomere uncapping [186], has also been demonstrated to downregulate oncogenes, particularly *SRC* [164]. The effects on telomerase activity and telomere integrity of telomestatin are well established, and this compound also downregulates the oncogene c-*MYB* in glioma cells [234]. Caution should be exercised with this approach, however, since G-quadruplex ligands certainly target genes other than oncogenes; microarray analysis of HeLa cells after treatment with PhenDC3 or 360A revealed changes in the expression of many metabolic genes [260], and pyridostatin downregulated some tumor suppressor genes in addition to oncogenes [164].

Preclinical Studies with Telomere G-quadruplex-Targeting Compounds

Promising data are emerging from preclinical studies with several of the aforementioned compounds. BRACO19, telomestatin, RHPS4, and BMSG-SH-3 have all caused impressive reductions in tumor volumes in mouse xenograft models [205,217,229,233,234,261,262]. BRACO19 augmented the antitumor effect of the drug paclitaxel [263], and RHPS4 showed a dramatic synergism with several topoisomerase I (TopoI) inhibitors [229,261,264]. Examination of the mechanism for the latter effect revealed that RHPS4, when used alone, causes an increase in TopoI at telomeres, leading to the hypothesis that TopoI is involved in repairing the telomeric damage caused by G-quadruplex stabilization. RHPS4 also induced high levels of γH2AX in xenograft tumors; both the γH2AX and the reduction in tumor volume were abolished by overexpression of TRF2 or POT1, providing good evidence that the antitumor effect of this compound was mediated by telomere uncapping.

CONCLUSIONS AND FUTURE PROSPECTS

The inhibition of telomerase, either directly or indirectly, is extremely promising as a future cancer therapeutic strategy, but there remains a great deal of work to be done to achieve this goal. In our opinion, the most pressing areas in which to concentrate current research efforts include the following:

1. Determination of a high-resolution structure of the active human telomerase complex, to enable structure-based drug design
2. Elucidation of the mechanism of "telomere uncapping", which is induced by enzymatic inhibitors of telomerase, reduction of telomerase components, or G-quadruplex-stabilizing molecules, in order to harness this effect to overcome the "lag phase" of telomerase inhibition
3. Testing the approaches discussed in this chapter against a wider range of normal human cells, including stem cells, in order to establish the specificity of the treatments for cancer cells
4. Continuation of biochemical structure–function analyses of the human telomerase enzyme, in order to rationally design alternative ways of blocking in vivo function
5. Identification of telomere-specific G-quadruplex-stabilizing molecules, or stabilizers specific to the promoter G-quadruplexes of particular oncogenes

References

[1] Harley CB. Telomerase and cancer therapeutics. Nat Rev Cancer 2008;8:167–79.
[2] Ruden M, Puri N. Novel anticancer therapeutics targeting telomerase. Cancer Treat Rev 2012.
[3] Moyzis RK, Buckingham JM, Cram LS, Dani M, Deaven LL, Jones MD, et al. A highly conserved repetitive DNA sequence, $(TTAGGG)_n$, present at the telomeres of human chromosomes. Proc Natl Acad Sci U S A 1988;85:6622–6.
[4] McEachern MJ, Krauskopf A, Blackburn EH. Telomeres and their control. Annu Rev Genet 2000;34:331–58.
[5] Makarov VL, Hirose Y, Langmore JP. Long G tails at both ends of human chromosomes suggest a C strand degradation mechanism for telomere shortening. Cell 1997;88:657–66.
[6] Wright WE, Tesmer VM, Huffman KE, Levene SD, Shay JW. Normal human chromosomes have long G-rich telomeric overhangs at one end. Genes Dev 1997;11:2801–9.
[7] de Lange T. Shelterin: the protein complex that shapes and safeguards human telomeres. Genes Dev 2005;19:2100–10.
[8] Zhong Z, Shiue L, Kaplan S, de Lange T. A mammalian factor that binds telomeric TTAGGG repeats in vitro. Mol Cell Biol 1992;12:4834–43.

[9] Broccoli D, Smogorzewska A, Chong L, de Lange T. Human telomeres contain two distinct Myb-related proteins, TRF1 and TRF2. Nat Genet 1997;17:231–5.

[10] Bilaud T, Brun C, Ancelin K, Koering CE, Laroche T, Gilson E. Telomeric localization of TRF2, a novel human telobox protein. Nat Genet 1997;17:236–9.

[11] Li B, Oestreich S, de Lange T. Identification of human Rap1: implications for telomere evolution. Cell 2000;101:471–83.

[12] Kim SH, Kaminker P, Campisi J. TIN2, a new regulator of telomere length in human cells. Nat Genet 1999;23:405–12.

[13] Houghtaling BR, Cuttonaro L, Chang W, Smith S. A dynamic molecular link between the telomere length regulator TRF1 and the chromosome end protector TRF2. Curr Biol 2004;14:1621–31.

[14] Liu D, Safari A, O'Connor MS, Chan DW, Laegeler A, Qin J, et al. PTOP interacts with POT1 and regulates its localization to telomeres. Nat Cell Biol 2004;6:673–80.

[15] Ye JZ, Hockemeyer D, Krutchinsky AN, Loayza D, Hooper SM, Chait BT, et al. POT1-interacting protein PIP1: a telomere length regulator that recruits POT1 to the TIN2/TRF1 complex. Genes Dev 2004;18:1649–54.

[16] Baumann P, Cech TR. Pot1, the putative telomere end-binding protein in fission yeast and humans. Science 2001;292:1171–5.

[17] d'Adda di Fagagna F, Reaper PM, Clay-Farrace L, Fiegler H, Carr P, von Zglinicki T, et al. A DNA damage checkpoint response in telomere-initiated senescence. Nature 2003;426:194–8.

[18] Palm W, de Lange T. How shelterin protects mammalian telomeres. Annu Rev Genet 2008;42:301–34.

[19] Sfeir A, de Lange T. Removal of shelterin reveals the telomere end-protection problem. Science 2012;336: 593–7.

[20] Ogawa T, Okazaki T. Discontinuous DNA replication. Annu Rev Biochem 1980;49:421–57.

[21] Watson JD. Origin of concatemeric T7 DNA. Nat New Biol 1972;239:197–201.

[22] Olovnikov AM. A theory of marginotomy. The incomplete copying of template margin in enzymic synthesis of polynucleotides and biological significance of the phenomenon. J Theor Biol 1973;41:181–90.

[23] Lingner J, Cooper JP, Cech TR. Telomerase and DNA end replication: no longer a lagging strand problem? Science 1995;269:1533–4.

[24] Harley CB, Futcher AB, Greider CW. Telomeres shorten during ageing of human fibroblasts. Nature 1990;345:458–60.

[25] Reddel RR. The role of senescence and immortalization in carcinogenesis. Carcinogenesis 2000;21:477–84.

[26] Wright WE, Shay JW. The two-stage mechanism controlling cellular senescence and immortalization. Exp Gerontol 1992;27:383–9.

[27] Shay JW, Pereira-Smith OM, Wright WE. A role for both RB and p53 in the regulation of human cellular senescence. Exp Cell Res 1991;196:33–9.

[28] Counter CM, Avilion AA, LeFeuvre CE, Stewart NG, Greider CW, Harley CB, et al. Telomere shortening associated with chromosome instability is arrested in immortal cells which express telomerase activity. EMBO J 1992;11:1921–9.

[29] Greider CW, Blackburn EH. Identification of a specific telomere terminal transferase activity in *Tetrahymena* extracts. Cell 1985;43:405–13.

[30] Wright WE, Piatyszek MA, Rainey WE, Byrd W, Shay JW. Telomerase activity in human germline and embryonic tissues and cells. Dev Genet 1996;18:173–9.

[31] Kim NW, Piatyszek MA, Prowse KR, Harley CB, West MD, Ho PL, et al. Specific association of human telomerase activity with immortal cells and cancer. Science 1994;266:2011–5.

[32] Shay JW, Bacchetti S. A survey of telomerase activity in human cancer. Eur J Cancer 1997;33:787–91.

[33] Hiyama E, Hiyama K. Clinical utility of telomerase in cancer. Oncogene 2002;21:643–9.

[34] Herbert BS, Pitts AE, Baker SI, Hamilton SE, Wright WE, Shay JW, et al. Inhibition of human telomerase in immortal human cells leads to progressive telomere shortening and cell death. Proc Natl Acad Sci U S A 1999;96:14276–81.

[35] Zhang X, Mar V, Zhou W, Harrington L, Robinson MO. Telomere shortening and apoptosis in telomerase-inhibited human tumor cells. Genes Dev 1999;13:2388–99.

[36] Bryan TM, Englezou A, Gupta J, Bacchetti S, Reddel RR. Telomere elongation in immortal human cells without detectable telomerase activity. EMBO J 1995;14:4240–8.

[37] Bryan TM, Englezou A, Dalla-Pozza L, Dunham MA, Reddel RR. Evidence for an alternative mechanism for maintaining telomere length in human tumors and tumor-derived cell lines. Nat Med 1997;3:1271–4.

[38] Henson JD, Reddel RR. Assaying and investigating alternative lengthening of telomeres activity in human cells and cancers. FEBS Lett 2010;584:3800–11.

[39] Heaphy CM, Subhawong AP, Hong SM, Goggins MG, Montgomery EA, Gabrielson E, et al. Prevalence of the alternative lengthening of telomeres telomere maintenance mechanism in human cancer subtypes. Am J Pathol 2011;179:1608–15.

[40] Dunham MA, Neumann AA, Fasching CL, Reddel RR. Telomere maintenance by recombination in human cells. Nat Genet 2000;26:447–50.

[41] Durant ST. Telomerase-independent paths to immortality in predictable cancer subtypes. J Cancer 2012;3: 67–82.

[42] Cohen SB, Graham ME, Lovrecz GO, Bache N, Robinson PJ, Reddel RR. Protein composition of catalytically active human telomerase from immortal cells. Science 2007;315:1850–3.

[43] Armanios M, Chen JL, Chang YP, Brodsky RA, Hawkins A, Griffin CA, et al. Haploinsufficiency of telomerase reverse transcriptase leads to anticipation in autosomal dominant dyskeratosis congenita. Proc Natl Acad Sci U S A 2005;102:15960–4.

[44] Vulliamy T, Marrone A, Goldman F, Dearlove A, Bessler M, Mason PJ, et al. The RNA component of telomerase is mutated in autosomal dominant dyskeratosis congenita. Nature 2001;413:432–5.

[45] Mitchell JR, Wood E, Collins K. A telomerase component is defective in the human disease dyskeratosis congenita. Nature 1999;402:551–5.

[46] Armanios M, Blackburn EH. The telomere syndromes. Nat Rev Genet 2012;13:693–704.

[47] Heiss NS, Knight SW, Vulliamy TJ, Klauck SM, Wiemann S, Mason PJ, et al. X-linked dyskeratosis congenita is caused by mutations in a highly conserved gene with putative nucleolar functions. Nat Genet 1998;19:32–8.

[48] Vulliamy TJ, Kirwan MJ, Beswick R, Hossain U, Baqai C, Ratcliffe A, et al. Differences in disease severity but similar telomere lengths in genetic subgroups of patients with telomerase and shelterin mutations. PLoS One 2011;6:e24383.

[49] Vulliamy TJ, Walne A, Baskaradas A, Mason PJ, Marrone A, Dokal I. Mutations in the reverse transcriptase component of telomerase (TERT) in patients with bone marrow failure. Blood Cells Mol Dis 2005;34:257–63.

[50] Armanios MY, Chen JJ, Cogan JD, Alder JK, Ingersoll RG, Markin C, et al. Telomerase mutations in families with idiopathic pulmonary fibrosis. N Engl J Med 2007;356:1317–26.

[51] Vulliamy T, Marrone A, Szydlo R, Walne A, Mason PJ, Dokal I. Disease anticipation is associated with progressive telomere shortening in families with dyskeratosis congenita due to mutations in TERC. Nat Genet 2004;36:447–9.

[52] Goldman F, Bouarich R, Kulkarni S, Freeman S, Du HY, Harrington L, et al. The effect of TERC haploinsufficiency on the inheritance of telomere length. Proc Natl Acad Sci U S A 2005;102:17119–24.

[53] Lee MS, Gallagher RC, Bradley J, Blackburn EH. In vivo and in vitro studies of telomeres and telomerase. Cold Spring Harb Symp Quant Biol 1993;58:707–18.

[54] Finger SN, Bryan TM. Multiple DNA-binding sites in *Tetrahymena* telomerase. Nucleic Acids Res 2008;36: 1260–72.

[55] Lue NF, Peng Y. Negative regulation of yeast telomerase activity through an interaction with an upstream region of the DNA primer. Nucleic Acids Res 1998;26:1487–94.

[56] Morin GB. The human telomere terminal transferase enzyme is a ribonucleoprotein that synthesizes TTAGGG repeats. Cell 1989;59:521–9.

[57] Harrington LA, Greider CW. Telomerase primer specificity and chromosome healing. Nature 1991;353:451–4.

[58] Montanaro L, Brigotti M, Clohessy J, Barbieri S, Ceccarelli C, Santini D, et al. Dyskerin expression influences the level of ribosomal RNA pseudo-uridylation and telomerase RNA component in human breast cancer. J Pathol 2006;210:10–8.

[59] Wong JM, Collins K. Telomerase RNA level limits telomere maintenance in X-linked dyskeratosis congenita. Genes Dev 2006;20:2848–58.

[60] Nakamura TM, Morin GB, Chapman KB, Weinrich SL, Andrews WH, Lingner J, et al. Telomerase catalytic subunit homologs from fission yeast and human. Science 1997;277:955–9.

[61] Kilian A, Bowtell DD, Abud HE, Hime GR, Venter DJ, Keese PK, et al. Isolation of a candidate human telomerase catalytic subunit gene, which reveals complex splicing patterns in different cell types. Hum Mol Genet 1997;6:2011–9.

[62] Meyerson M, Counter CM, Eaton EN, Ellisen LW, Steiner P, Dickinson Caddle S, et al. hEST2, the putative human telomerase catalytic subunit gene, is up-regulated in tumor cells and during immortalization. Cell 1997;90:785–95.

[63] Jacobs SA, Podell ER, Cech TR. Crystal structure of the essential N-terminal domain of telomerase reverse transcriptase. Nat Struct Mol Biol 2006;13:218–25.

[64] Bryan TM, Goodrich KJ, Cech TR. Telomerase RNA bound by protein motifs specific to telomerase reverse transcriptase. Mol Cell 2000;6:493–9.

[65] Lingner J, Hughes TR, Shevchenko A, Mann M, Lundblad V, Cech TR. Reverse transcriptase motifs in the catalytic subunit of telomerase. Science 1997;276:561–7.

[66] Rouda S, Skordalakes E. Structure of the RNA-binding domain of telomerase: implications for RNA recognition and binding. Structure 2007;15:1403–12.

[67] Gillis AJ, Schuller AP, Skordalakes E. Structure of the *Tribolium castaneum* telomerase catalytic subunit TERT. Nature 2008;455:633–7.

[68] Osanai M, Kojima KK, Futahashi R, Yaguchi S, Fujiwara H. Identification and characterization of the telomerase reverse transcriptase of *Bombyx mori* (silkworm) and *Tribolium castaneum* (flour beetle). Gene 2006;376: 281–9.

[69] Ding J, Das K, Hsiou Y, Sarafianos SG, Clark Jr AD, Jacobo-Molina A, et al. Structure and functional implications of the polymerase active site region in a complex of HIV-1 RT with a double-stranded DNA template-primer and an antibody Fab fragment at 2.8 Å resolution. J Mol Biol 1998;284:1095–111.

[70] Rodgers DW, Gamblin SJ, Harris BA, Ray S, Culp JS, Hellmig B, et al. The structure of unliganded reverse transcriptase from the human immunodeficiency virus type 1. Proc Natl Acad Sci U S A 1995;92:1222–6.

[71] Lue NF, Lin YC, Mian IS. A conserved telomerase motif within the catalytic domain of telomerase reverse transcriptase is specifically required for repeat addition processivity. Mol Cell Biol 2003;23:8440–9.

[72] Qi X, Xie M, Brown AF, Bley CJ, Podlevsky JD, Chen JJ. RNA/DNA hybrid binding affinity determines telomerase template-translocation efficiency. EMBO J 2011;31:150–61.

[73] Xie M, Podlevsky JD, Qi X, Bley CJ, Chen JJ. A novel motif in telomerase reverse transcriptase regulates telomere repeat addition rate and processivity. Nucleic Acids Res 2010;38:1982–96.

[74] Friedman KL, Cech TR. Essential functions of amino-terminal domains in the yeast telomerase catalytic subunit revealed by selection for viable mutants. Genes Dev 1999;13:2863–74.

[75] Moriarty TJ, Huard S, Dupuis S, Autexier C. Functional multimerization of human telomerase requires an RNA interaction domain in the N terminus of the catalytic subunit. Mol Cell Biol 2002;22:1253–65.

[76] Lai CK, Mitchell JR, Collins K. RNA binding domain of telomerase reverse transcriptase. Mol Cell Biol 2001;21:990–1000.

[77] Bosoy D, Peng Y, Mian IS, Lue NF. Conserved N-terminal motifs of telomerase reverse transcriptase required for ribonucleoprotein assembly in vivo. J Biol Chem 2003;278:3882–90.

[78] Collins K. Single-stranded DNA repeat synthesis by telomerase. Curr Opin Chem Biol 2011;15:643–8.

[79] Jurczyluk J, Nouwens AS, Holien JK, Adams TE, Lovrecz GO, Parker MW, et al. Direct involvement of the TEN domain at the active site of human telomerase. Nucleic Acids Res 2011;39:1774–88.

[80] Huard S, Moriarty TJ, Autexier C. The C terminus of the human telomerase reverse transcriptase is a determinant of enzyme processivity. Nucleic Acids Res 2003;31:4059–70.

[81] Banik SS, Guo C, Smith AC, Margolis SS, Richardson DA, Tirado CA, et al. C-terminal regions of the human telomerase catalytic subunit essential for in vivo enzyme activity. Mol Cell Biol 2002;22:6234–46.

[82] Chen JL, Greider CW. An emerging consensus for telomerase RNA structure. Proc Natl Acad Sci U S A 2004;101:14683–4.

[83] Lin J, Ly H, Hussain A, Abraham M, Pearl S, Tzfati Y, et al. A universal telomerase RNA core structure includes structured motifs required for binding the telomerase reverse transcriptase protein. Proc Natl Acad Sci U S A 2004;101:14713–8.

[84] Lingner J, Hendrick LL, Cech TR. Telomerase RNAs of different ciliates have a common secondary structure and a permuted template. Genes Dev 1994;8:1984–98.

[85] Lai CK, Miller MC, Collins K. Template boundary definition in *Tetrahymena* telomerase. Genes Dev 2002;16:415–20.

[86] Chen JL, Greider CW. Template boundary definition in mammalian telomerase. Genes Dev 2003;17:2747–52.

[87] ten Dam E, van Belkum A, Pleij K. A conserved pseudoknot in telomerase RNA. Nucleic Acids Res 1991;19:6951.

[88] Romero DP, Blackburn EH. A conserved secondary structure for telomerase RNA. Cell 1991;67:343–53.

[89] Chen JL, Blasco MA, Greider CW. Secondary structure of vertebrate telomerase RNA. Cell 2000;100:503–14.

[90] Mason DX, Goneska E, Greider CW. Stem-loop IV of *Tetrahymena* telomerase RNA stimulates processivity in trans. Mol Cell Biol 2003;23:5606–13.

[91] Miller MC, Collins K. Telomerase recognizes its template by using an adjacent RNA motif. Proc Natl Acad Sci U S A 2002;99:6585–90.

[92] Berman AJ, Akiyama BM, Stone MD, Cech TR. The RNA accordion model for template positioning by telomerase RNA during telomeric DNA synthesis. Nat Struct Mol Biol 2011;18:1371–5.

[93] Mueller S, Hartmann U, Mayer F, Balabanov S, Hartmann JT, Brummendorf TH, et al. Targeting telomerase activity by BIBR1532 as a therapeutic approach in germ cell tumors. Invest New Drugs 2007;25:519–24.

[94] Misawa M, Tauchi T, Sashida G, Nakajima A, Abe K, Ohyashiki JH, et al. Inhibition of human telomerase enhances the effect of chemotherapeutic agents in lung cancer cells. Int J Oncol 2002;21:1087–92.

[95] Tentori L, Portarena I, Barbarino M, Balduzzi A, Levati L, Vergati M, et al. Inhibition of telomerase increases resistance of melanoma cells to temozolomide, but not to temozolomide combined with poly (adp-ribose) polymerase inhibitor. Mol Pharmacol 2003;63:192–202.

[96] Kondo Y, Kondo S, Tanaka Y, Haqqi T, Barna BP, Cowell JK. Inhibition of telomerase increases the susceptibility of human malignant glioblastoma cells to cisplatin-induced apoptosis. Oncogene 1998;16:2243–8.

[97] Ludwig A, Saretzki G, Holm PS, Tiemann F, Lorenz M, Emrich T, et al. Ribozyme cleavage of telomerase mRNA sensitizes breast epithelial cells to inhibitors of topoisomerase. Cancer Res 2001;61:3053–61.

[98] Chen Z, Koeneman KS, Corey DR. Consequences of telomerase inhibition and combination treatments for the proliferation of cancer cells. Cancer Res 2003;63:5917–25.

[99] Cookson JC, Dai F, Smith V, Heald RA, Laughton CA, Stevens MF, et al. Pharmacodynamics of the G-quadruplex-stabilizing telomerase inhibitor 3,11-difluoro-6,8,13-trimethyl-8H-quino[4,3,2-kl]acridinium methosulfate (RHPS4) in vitro: activity in human tumor cells correlates with telomere length and can be enhanced, or antagonized, with cytotoxic agents. Mol Pharmacol 2005;68:1551–8.

[100] Massard C, Zermati Y, Pauleau AL, Larochette N, Metivier D, Sabatier L, et al. hTERT: a novel endogenous inhibitor of the mitochondrial cell death pathway. Oncogene 2006;25:4505–14.

[101] Tamakawa RA, Fleisig HB, Wong JM. Telomerase inhibition potentiates the effects of genotoxic agents in breast and colorectal cancer cells in a cell cycle specific manner. Cancer Res 2010;70:8684–94.

[102] Saretzki G, Ludwig A, von Zglinicki T, Runnebaum IB. Ribozyme-mediated telomerase inhibition induces immediate cell loss but not telomere shortening in ovarian cancer cells. Cancer Gene Ther 2001;8:827–34.

[103] Li S, Rosenberg JE, Donjacour AA, Botchkina IL, Hom YK, Cunha GR, et al. Rapid inhibition of cancer cell growth induced by lentiviral delivery and expression of mutant-template telomerase RNA and anti-telomerase short-interfering RNA. Cancer Res 2004;64:4833–40.

[104] Kedde M, Sage CL, Duursma A, Zlotorynski E, Leeuwen BV, Nijkamp W, et al. Telomerase independent regulation of ATR by human telomerase RNA. J Biol Chem 2006;281:40503–14.

[105] Lai SR, Cunningham AP, Huynh VQ, Andrews LG, Tollefsbol TO. Evidence of extra-telomeric effects of hTERT and its regulation involving a feedback loop. Exp Cell Res 2007;313:322–30.

[106] Folini M, Bandiera R, Millo E, Gandellini P, Sozzi G, Gasparini P, et al. Photochemically enhanced delivery of a cell-penetrating peptide nucleic acid conjugate targeting human telomerase reverse transcriptase: effects on telomere status and proliferative potential of human prostate cancer cells. Cell Prolif 2007;40:905–20.

[107] Blasco MA. Telomere length, stem cells and aging. Nat Chem Biol 2007;3:640–9.

[108] Roth A, Yssel H, Pene J, Chavez EA, Schertzer M, Lansdorp PM, et al. Telomerase levels control the lifespan of human T lymphocytes. Blood 2003;102:849–57.

[109] Engelhardt M, Drullinsky P, Guillem J, Moore MA. Telomerase and telomere length in the development and progression of premalignant lesions to colorectal cancer. Clin Cancer Res 1997;3:1931–41.

[110] Damle RN, Batliwalla FM, Ghiotto F, Valetto A, Albesiano E, Sison C, et al. Telomere length and telomerase activity delineate distinctive replicative features of the B-CLL subgroups defined by Ig V gene mutations. Blood 2003;103:375–82.

[111] Engelhardt M, Albanell J, Drullinsky P, Han W, Guillem J, Scher HI, et al. Relative contribution of normal and neoplastic cells determines telomerase activity and telomere length in primary cancers of the prostate, colon, and sarcoma. Clin Cancer Res 1997;3:1849–57.

[112] Roth A, Durig J, Himmelreich H, Bug S, Siebert R, Duhrsen U. Short telomeres and high telomerase activity in T-cell prolymphocytic leukemia. Leukemia 2007;21:2456–62.

[113] Marian CO, Cho SK, McEllin BM, Maher EA, Hatanpaa KJ, Madden CJ, et al. The telomerase antagonist, imetelstat, efficiently targets glioblastoma tumor-initiating cells leading to decreased proliferation and tumor growth. Clin Cancer Res 2010;16:154–63.

[114] Pascolo E, Wenz C, Lingner J, Hauel N, Priepke H, Kauffmann I, et al. Mechanism of human telomerase inhibition by BIBR1532, a synthetic, non-nucleosidic drug candidate. J Biol Chem 2002;277:15566–72.

[115] Allen ND, Baird DM. Telomere length maintenance in stem cell populations. Biochim Biophys Acta 2009;1792:324–8.

[116] Bechter OE, Zou Y, Walker W, Wright WE, Shay JW. Telomeric recombination in mismatch repair deficient human colon cancer cells after telomerase inhibition. Cancer Res 2004;64:3444–51.

[117] Hu J, Hwang SS, Liesa M, Gan B, Sahin E, Jaskelioff M, et al. Antitelomerase therapy provokes ALT and mitochondrial adaptive mechanisms in cancer. Cell 2012;148:651–63.

[118] Shay JW, Reddel RR, Wright WE. Cancer and telomeres—an ALTernative to telomerase. Science 2012;336: 1388–90.

[119] Xia CQ, Smith PG. Drug efflux transporters and multidrug resistance in acute leukemia: therapeutic impact and novel approaches to mediation. Mol Pharmacol 2012;82:1008–21.

[120] Reddy EP, Aggarwal AK. The ins and outs of BCR-ABL inhibition. Genes Cancer 2012;3:447–54.

[121] Theimer CA, Finger LD, Trantirek L, Feigon J. Mutations linked to dyskeratosis congenita cause changes in the structural equilibrium in telomerase RNA. Proc Natl Acad Sci U S A 2003;100:449–54.

[122] Leeper T, Leulliot N, Varani G. The solution structure of an essential stem-loop of human telomerase RNA. Nucleic Acids Res 2003;31:2614–21.

[123] Zhang Q, Kim NK, Peterson RD, Wang Z, Feigon J. Structurally conserved five nucleotide bulge determines the overall topology of the core domain of human telomerase RNA. Proc Natl Acad Sci U S A 2010;107: 18761–8.

[124] Wright WE, Shay JW, Piatyszek MA. Modifications of a telomeric repeat amplification protocol (TRAP) result in increased reliability, linearity and sensitivity. Nucleic Acids Res 1995;23:3794–5.

[125] Au AY, Hackl T, Yeager TR, Cohen SB, Pass HI, Harris CC, et al. Telomerase activity in pleural malignant mesotheliomas. Lung Cancer 2011;73:283–8.

[126] Cristofari G, Lingner J. Telomere length homeostasis requires that telomerase levels are limiting. EMBO J 2006;25:565–74.

[127] Cohen SB, Reddel RR. A sensitive direct human telomerase activity assay. Nat Methods 2008;5:355–60.

[128] Cristofari G, Reichenbach P, Regamey PO, Banfi D, Chambon M, Turcatti G, et al. Low- to high-throughput analysis of telomerase modulators with Telospot. Nat. Methods 2007;4:851–3.

[129] de Lange T, Shiue L, Myers RM, Cox DR, Naylor SL, Killery AM, et al. Structure and variability of human chromosome ends. Mol Cell Biol 1990;10:518–27.

[130] Strahl C, Blackburn EH. Effects of reverse transcriptase inhibitors on telomere length and telomerase activity in two immortalized human cell lines. Mol Cell Biol 1996;16:53–65.

[131] Fletcher TM, Salazar M, Chen SF. Human telomerase inhibition by 7-deaza-2′-deoxypurine nucleoside triphosphates. Biochemistry 1996;35:15611–7.

[132] Fletcher TM, Cathers BE, Ravikumar KS, Mamiya BM, Kerwin SM. Inhibition of human telomerase by 7-deaza-2′-deoxyguanosine nucleoside triphosphate analogs: potent inhibition by 6-thio-7-deaza-2′-deoxyguanosine 5′-triphosphate. Bioorg Chem 2001;29:36–55.

[133] Damm K, Hemmann U, Garin-Chesa P, Hauel N, Kauffmann I, Priepke H, et al. A highly selective telomerase inhibitor limiting human cancer cell proliferation. EMBO J 2001;20:6958–68.

[134] Schnapp G, Rodi HP, Rettig WJ, Schnapp A, Damm K. One-step affinity purification protocol for human telomerase. Nucleic Acids Res 1998;26:3311–3.

[135] El-Daly H, Kull M, Zimmermann S, Pantic M, Waller CF, Martens UM. Selective cytotoxicity and telomere damage in leukemia cells using the telomerase inhibitor BIBR1532. Blood 2005;105:1742–9.

[136] Feng J, Funk WD, Wang SS, Weinrich SL, Avilion AA, Chiu CP, et al. The RNA component of human telomerase. Science 1995;269:1236–41.

[137] Norton JC, Piatyszek MA, Wright WE, Shay JW, Corey DR. Inhibition of human telomerase activity by peptide nucleic acids. Nat Biotechnol 1996;14:615–9.

[138] Shea-Herbert B, Pongracz K, Shay JW, Gryaznov SM. Oligonucleotide N3′→P5′ phosphoramidates as efficient telomerase inhibitors. Oncogene 2002;21:638–42.

[139] Asai A, Oshima Y, Yamamoto Y, Uochi TA, Kusaka H, Akinaga S, et al. A novel telomerase template antagonist (GRN163) as a potential anticancer agent. Cancer Res 2003;63:3931–9.

[140] Akiyama M, Hideshima T, Shammas MA, Hayashi T, Hamasaki M, Tai YT, et al. Effects of oligonucleotide N3′→P5′ thio-phosphoramidate (GRN163) targeting telomerase RNA in human multiple myeloma cells. Cancer Res 2003;63:6187–94.

[141] Wang ES, Wu K, Chin AC, Chen-Kiang S, Pongracz K, Gryaznov S, et al. Telomerase inhibition with an oligonucleotide telomerase template antagonist: in vitro and in vivo studies in multiple myeloma and lymphoma. Blood 2003;103:258–66.

[142] Herbert BS, Gellert GC, Hochreiter A, Pongracz K, Wright WE, Zielinska D, et al. Lipid modification of GRN163, an N3′→P5′ thio-phosphoramidate oligonucleotide, enhances the potency of telomerase inhibition. Oncogene 2005;24:5262–8.

[143] Dikmen ZG, Gellert GC, Jackson S, Gryaznov S, Tressler R, Dogan P, et al. In vivo inhibition of lung cancer by GRN163L: a novel human telomerase inhibitor. Cancer Res 2005;65:7866–73.

[144] Djojosubroto MW, Chin AC, Go N, Schaetzlein S, Manns MP, Gryaznov S, et al. Telomerase antagonists GRN163 and GRN163L inhibit tumor growth and increase chemosensitivity of human hepatoma. Hepatology 2005;42:1127–36.

[145] Hochreiter AE, Xiao H, Goldblatt EM, Gryaznov SM, Miller KD, Badve S, et al. Telomerase template antagonist GRN163L disrupts telomere maintenance, tumor growth, and metastasis of breast cancer. Clin Cancer Res 2006;12:3184–92.

[146] Bao S, Wu Q, McLendon RE, Hao Y, Shi Q, Hjelmeland AB, et al. Glioma stem cells promote radioresistance by preferential activation of the DNA damage response. Nature 2006;444:756–60.

[147] Marian CO, Wright WE, Shay JW. The effects of telomerase inhibition on prostate tumor-initiating cells. Int J Cancer 2010;127:321–31.

[148] Joseph I, Tressler R, Bassett E, Harley C, Buseman CM, Pattamatta P, et al. The telomerase inhibitor imetelstat depletes cancer stem cells in breast and pancreatic cancer cell lines. Cancer Res 2010;70:9494–504.

[149] Brennan SK, Wang Q, Tressler R, Harley C, Go N, Bassett E, et al. Telomerase inhibition targets clonogenic multiple myeloma cells through telomere length-dependent and independent mechanisms. PLoS One 2010;5:e12487.

[150] Wu KD, Orme LM, Shaughnessy J, Jacobson J, Barlogie B, Moore MA. Telomerase and telomere length in multiple myeloma: correlations with disease heterogeneity, cytogenetic status and overall survival. Blood 2003;101:4982–9.

[151] Williamson JR, Raghuraman MK, Cech TR. Monovalent cation-induced structure of telomeric DNA: the G-quartet model. Cell 1989;59:871–80.

[152] Phan AT. Human telomeric G-quadruplex: structures of DNA and RNA sequences. FEBS J 2010;277:1107–17.

[153] Wang Y, Patel DJ. Solution structure of the human telomeric repeat d[AG3(T2AG3)3] G-tetraplex. Structure 1993;1:263–82.

[154] Lim KW, Amrane S, Bouaziz S, Xu W, Mu Y, Patel DJ, et al. Structure of the human telomere in K+ solution: a stable basket-type G-quadruplex with only two G-tetrad layers. J Am Chem Soc 2009;131:4301–9.

[155] Parkinson GN, Lee MP, Neidle S. Crystal structure of parallel quadruplexes from human telomeric DNA. Nature 2002;417:876–80.

[156] Phan AT, Kuryavyi V, Luu KN, Patel DJ. Structure of two intramolecular G-quadruplexes formed by natural human telomere sequences in K+ solution. Nucleic Acids Res 2007;35:6517–25.

[157] Dai J, Carver M, Punchihewa C, Jones RA, Yang D. Structure of the Hybrid-2 type intramolecular human telomeric G-quadruplex in K+ solution: insights into structure polymorphism of the human telomeric sequence. Nucleic Acids Res 2007;35:4927–40.

[158] Lipps HJ. In vitro aggregation of the gene-sized DNA molecules of the ciliate *Stylonychia mytilus*. Proc Natl Acad Sci U S A 1980;77:4104–7.

[159] Schaffitzel C, Berger I, Postberg J, Hanes J, Lipps HJ, Pluckthun A. *In vitro* generated antibodies specific for telomeric guanine-quadruplex DNA react with *Stylonychia lemnae* macronuclei. Proc Natl Acad Sci U S A 2001;98:8572–7.

[160] Paeschke K, Simonsson T, Postberg J, Rhodes D, Lipps HJ. Telomere end-binding proteins control the formation of G-quadruplex DNA structures in vivo. Nat Struct Mol Biol 2005;12:847–54.

[161] Sen D, Gilbert W. Formation of parallel four-stranded complexes by guanine-rich motifs in DNA and its implications for meiosis. Nature 1988;334:364–6.

[162] Yu HQ, Miyoshi D, Sugimoto N. Properties of long human telomeric DNAs under cell-mimicking conditions. Nucleic Acids Symp Ser (Oxf) 2006;50:207–8.

[163] Oganesian L, Bryan TM. Physiological relevance of telomeric G-quadruplex formation: a potential drug target. BioEssays 2007;29:155–65.

[164] Rodriguez R, Miller KM, Forment JV, Bradshaw CR, Nikan M, Britton S, et al. Small-molecule-induced DNA damage identifies alternative DNA structures in human genes. Nat Chem Biol 2012;8:301–10.

[165] Smith JS, Chen Q, Yatsunyk LA, Nicoludis JM, Garcia MS, Kranaster R, et al. Rudimentary G-quadruplex-based telomere capping in *Saccharomyces cerevisiae*. Nat Struct Mol Biol 2011;18:478–85.

[166] Biffi G, Tannahill D, McCafferty J, Balasubramanian S. Quantitative visualization of DNA G-quadruplex structures in human cells. Nat Chem 2013.

[167] Zahler AM, Williamson JR, Cech TR, Prescott DM. Inhibition of telomerase by G-quartet DNA structures. Nature 1991;350:718–20.

[168] Monchaud D, Teulade-Fichou MP. A hitchhiker's guide to G-quadruplex ligands. Org Biomol Chem 2008;6:627–36.

[169] Oganesian L, Moon IK, Bryan TM, Jarstfer MB. Extension of G-quadruplex DNA by ciliate telomerase. EMBO J 2006;25:1148–59.

[170] Oganesian L, Graham ME, Robinson PJ, Bryan TM. Telomerase recognizes G-quadruplex and linear DNA as distinct substrates. Biochemistry 2007;46:11279–90.

[171] Gavathiotis E, Heald RA, Stevens MF, Searle MS. Drug recognition and stabilisation of the parallel-stranded DNA quadruplex d(TTAGGGT)(4) containing the human telomeric repeat. J Mol Biol 2003;334:25–36.

[172] Gabelica V, Baker ES, Teulade-Fichou MP, De Pauw E, Bowers MT. Stabilization and structure of telomeric and c-myc region intramolecular G-quadruplexes: the role of central cations and small planar ligands. J Am Chem Soc 2007;129:895–904.

[173] Campbell NH, Parkinson GN, Reszka AP, Neidle S. Structural basis of DNA quadruplex recognition by an acridine drug. J Am Chem Soc 2008;130:6722–4.

[174] Parkinson GN, Cuenca F, Neidle S. Topology conservation and loop flexibility in quadruplex-drug recognition: crystal structures of inter- and intramolecular telomeric DNA quadruplex-drug complexes. J Mol Biol 2008;381:1145–56.

[175] Wheelhouse RT, Sun DK, Han HY, Han FX, Hurley LH. Cationic porphyrins as telomerase inhibitors: the interaction of tetra-(*N*-methyl-4-pyridyl)porphine with quadruplex DNA. J Am Chem Soc 1998;120:3261–2.

[176] Ren J, Chaires JB. Sequence and structural selectivity of nucleic acid binding ligands. Biochemistry 1999;38:16067–75.

[177] Arthanari H, Basu S, Kawano TL, Bolton PH. Fluorescent dyes specific for quadruplex DNA. Nucleic Acids Res 1998;26:3724–8.

[178] Nicoludis JM, Barrett SP, Mergny JL, Yatsunyk LA. Interaction of human telomeric DNA with *N*-methyl mesoporphyrin IX. Nucleic Acids Res 2012;40:5432–47.

[179] Dixon IM, Lopez F, Tejera AM, Esteve JP, Blasco MA, Pratviel G, et al. A G-quadruplex ligand with 10000-fold selectivity over duplex DNA. J Am Chem Soc 2007;129:1502–3.

[180] Romera C, Bombarde O, Bonnet R, Gomez D, Dumy P, Calsou P, et al. Improvement of porphyrins for G-quadruplex DNA targeting. Biochimie 2011;93:1310–7.

[181] Li T, Wang E, Dong S. Parallel G-quadruplex-specific fluorescent probe for monitoring DNA structural changes and label-free detection of potassium ion. Anal Chem 2010;82:7576–80.

[182] Martino L, Pagano B, Fotticchia I, Neidle S, Giancola C. Shedding light on the interaction between TMPyP4 and human telomeric quadruplexes. J Phys Chem B 2009;113:14779–86.

[183] Pennarun G, Granotier C, Gauthier LR, Gomez D, Hoffschir F, Mandine E, et al. Apoptosis related to telomere instability and cell cycle alterations in human glioma cells treated by new highly selective G-quadruplex ligands. Oncogene 2005;24:2917–28.

[184] De Cian A, Delemos E, Mergny JL, Teulade-Fichou MP, Monchaud D. Highly efficient G-quadruplex recognition by bisquinolinium compounds. J Am Chem Soc 2007;129:1856–7.

[185] Tran PL, Largy E, Hamon F, Teulade-Fichou MP, Mergny JL. Fluorescence intercalator displacement assay for screening G4 ligands towards a variety of G-quadruplex structures. Biochimie 2011;93:1288–96.

[186] Rodriguez R, Muller S, Yeoman JA, Trentesaux C, Riou JF, Balasubramanian S. A novel small molecule that alters shelterin integrity and triggers a DNA-damage response at telomeres. J Am Chem Soc 2008;130:15758–9.

[187] Shin-Ya K, Wierzba K, Matsuo K, Ohtani T, Yamada Y, Furihata K, et al. Telomestatin, a novel telomerase inhibitor from *Streptomyces anulatus*. J Am Chem Soc 2001;123:1262–3.

[188] Kim MY, Gleason-Guzman M, Izbicka E, Nishioka D, Hurley LH. The different biological effects of telomestatin and TMPyP4 can be attributed to their selectivity for interaction with intramolecular or intermolecular G-quadruplex structures. Cancer Res 2003;63:3247–56.

[189] Linder J, Garner TP, Williams HE, Searle MS, Moody CJ. Telomestatin: formal total synthesis and cation-mediated interaction of its *seco*-derivatives with G-quadruplexes. J Am Chem Soc 2011;133:1044–51.

[190] Granzhan A, Monchaud D, Saettel N, Guedin A, Mergny JL, Teulade-Fichou MP. "One ring to bind them all" – part II: identification of promising G-quadruplex ligands by screening of cyclophane-type macrocycles. J Nucleic Acids 2010; pii: 460561.

[191] Dash J, Nath Das R, Hegde N, Pantos GD, Shirude PS, Balasubramanian S. Synthesis of bis-indole carboxamides as G-quadruplex stabilizing and inducing ligands. Chemistry 2012;18:554–64.

[192] Smith NM, Labrunie G, Corry B, Tran PL, Norret M, Djavaheri-Mergny M, et al. Unraveling the relationship between structure and stabilization of triarylpyridines as G-quadruplex binding ligands. Org Biomol Chem 2011;9:6154–62.

[193] Haider SM, Neidle S, Parkinson GN. A structural analysis of G-quadruplex/ligand interactions. Biochimie 2011;93:1239–51.

[194] Lombardo CM, Martinez IS, Haider S, Gabelica V, De Pauw E, Moses JE, et al. Structure-based design of selective high-affinity telomeric quadruplex-binding ligands. Chem Commun (Camb) 2010;46:9116–8.

[195] Read M, Harrison RJ, Romagnoli B, Tanious FA, Gowan SH, Reszka AP, et al. Structure-based design of selective and potent G quadruplex-mediated telomerase inhibitors. Proc Natl Acad Sci U S A 2001;98:4844–9.

[196] De Cian A, Cristofari G, Reichenbach P, De Lemos E, Monchaud D, Teulade-Fichou MP, et al. Reevaluation of telomerase inhibition by quadruplex ligands and their mechanisms of action. Proc Natl Acad Sci U S A 2007;104:17347–52.

[197] Reed J, Gunaratnam M, Beltran M, Reszka AP, Vilar R, Neidle S. TRAP-LIG, a modified telomere repeat amplification protocol assay to quantitate telomerase inhibition by small molecules. Anal Biochem 2008;380:99–105.

[198] Hampel SM, Sidibe A, Gunaratnam M, Riou JF, Neidle S. Tetrasubstituted naphthalene diimide ligands with selectivity for telomeric G-quadruplexes and cancer cells. Bioorg Med Chem Lett 2010;20:6459–63.

[199] Ma DL, Che CM, Yan SC. Platinum(II) complexes with dipyridophenazine ligands as human telomerase inhibitors and luminescent probes for G-quadruplex DNA. J Am Chem Soc 2009;131:1835–46.

[200] Wu WB, Chen SH, Hou JQ, Tan JH, Ou TM, Huang SL, et al. Disubstituted 2-phenyl-benzopyranopyrimidine derivatives as a new type of highly selective ligands for telomeric G-quadruplex DNA. Org Biomol Chem 2011;9:2975–86.

[201] D'Ambrosio D, Reichenbach P, Micheli E, Alvino A, Franceschin M, Savino M, et al. Specific binding of telomeric G-quadruplexes by hydrosoluble perylene derivatives inhibits repeat addition processivity of human telomerase. Biochimie 2012;94:854–63.

[202] Sun D, Thompson B, Cathers BE, Salazar M, Kerwin SM, Trent JO, et al. Inhibition of human telomerase by a G-quadruplex-interactive compound. J Med Chem 1997;40:2113–6.

[203] Tauchi T, Shin-Ya K, Sashida G, Sumi M, Nakajima A, Shimamoto T, et al. Activity of a novel G-quadruplex-interactive telomerase inhibitor, telomestatin (SOT-095), against human leukemia cells: involvement of ATM-dependent DNA damage response pathways. Oncogene 2003;22:5338–47.

[204] Gunaratnam M, Greciano O, Martins C, Reszka AP, Schultes CM, Morjani H, et al. Mechanism of acridine-based telomerase inhibition and telomere shortening. Biochem Pharmacol 2007;74:679–89.

[205] Burger AM, Dai F, Schultes CM, Reszka AP, Moore MJ, Double JA, et al. The G-quadruplex-interactive molecule BRACO-19 inhibits tumor growth, consistent with telomere targeting and interference with telomerase function. Cancer Res 2005;65:1489–96.

[206] Leonetti C, Amodei S, D'Angelo C, Rizzo A, Benassi B, Antonelli A, et al. Biological activity of the G-quadruplex ligand RHPS4 (3,11-difluoro-6,8,13-trimethyl-8H-quino[4,3,2-kl]acridinium methosulfate) is associated with telomere capping alteration. Mol Pharmacol 2004;66:1138–46.

[207] Zhou JM, Zhu XF, Lu YJ, Deng R, Huang ZS, Mei YP, et al. Senescence and telomere shortening induced by novel potent G-quadruplex interactive agents, quindoline derivatives, in human cancer cell lines. Oncogene 2006;25:503–11.

[208] Li Z, Tan JH, He JH, Long Y, Ou TM, Li D, et al. Disubstituted quinazoline derivatives as a new type of highly selective ligands for telomeric G-quadruplex DNA. Eur J Med Chem 2012;47:299–311.

[209] Yu H, Zhao C, Chen Y, Fu M, Ren J, Qu X. DNA loop sequence as the determinant for chiral supramolecular compound G-quadruplex selectivity. J Med Chem 2010;53:492–8.

[210] Incles CM, Schultes CM, Kempski H, Koehler H, Kelland LR, Neidle S. A G-quadruplex telomere targeting agent produces p16-associated senescence and chromosomal fusions in human prostate cancer cells. Mol Cancer Ther 2004;3:1201–6.

[211] Tahara H, Shin-Ya K, Seimiya H, Yamada H, Tsuruo T, Ide T. G-quadruplex stabilization by telomestatin induces TRF2 protein dissociation from telomeres and anaphase bridge formation accompanied by loss of the 3′ telomeric overhang in cancer cells. Oncogene 2006;25:1955–66.

[212] Gomez D, Wenner T, Brassart B, Douarre C, O'Donohue MF, El Khoury V, et al. Telomestatin induced telomere uncapping is modulated by POT1 through G-overhang extension in HT1080 human tumor cells. J Biol Chem 2006;281:38721–729.

[213] Muller S, Sanders DA, Di Antonio M, Matsis S, Riou JF, Rodriguez R, et al. Pyridostatin analogues promote telomere dysfunction and long-term growth inhibition in human cancer cells. Org Biomol Chem 2012;10: 6537–46.

[214] Hampel SM, Pepe A, Greulich-Bode KM, Malhotra SV, Reszka AP, Veith S, et al. Mechanism of the anti-proliferative activity of some naphthalene diimide G-quadruplex ligands. Mol Pharmacol 2013;83:470–80.

[215] Louis SF, Vermolen BJ, Garini Y, Young IT, Guffei A, Lichtensztejn Z, et al. c-Myc induces chromosomal rearrangements through telomere and chromosome remodeling in the interphase nucleus. Proc Natl Acad Sci U S A 2005;102:9613–8.

[216] Gomez D, O'Donohue MF, Wenner T, Douarre C, Macadre J, Koebel P, et al. The G-quadruplex ligand telomestatin inhibits POT1 binding to telomeric sequences in vitro and induces GFP-POT1 dissociation from telomeres in human cells. Cancer Res 2006;66:6908–12.

[217] Salvati E, Leonetti C, Rizzo A, Scarsella M, Mottolese M, Galati R, et al. Telomere damage induced by the G-quadruplex ligand RHPS4 has an antitumor effect. J Clin Invest 2007;117:3236–47.

[218] Casagrande V, Salvati E, Alvino A, Bianco A, Ciammaichella A, D'Angelo C, et al. N-cyclic bay-substituted perylene G-quadruplex ligands have selective antiproliferative effects on cancer cells and induce telomere damage. J Med Chem 2011;54:1140–56.

[219] Rizzo A, Salvati E, Porru M, D'Angelo C, Stevens MF, D'Incalci M, et al. Stabilization of quadruplex DNA perturbs telomere replication leading to the activation of an ATR-dependent ATM signaling pathway. Nucleic Acids Res 2009;37:5353–64.

[220] Dart DA, Adams KE, Akerman I, Lakin ND. Recruitment of the cell cycle checkpoint kinase ATR to chromatin during S-phase. J Biol Chem 2004;279:16433–40.

[221] Pennarun G, Hoffschir F, Revaud D, Granotier C, Gauthier LR, Mailliet P, et al. ATR contributes to telomere maintenance in human cells. Nucleic Acids Res 2010;38:2955–63.

[222] Sfeir A, Kosiyatrakul ST, Hockemeyer D, MacRae SL, Karlseder J, Schildkraut CL, et al. Mammalian telomeres resemble fragile sites and require TRF1 for efficient replication. Cell 2009;138:90–103.

[223] Gauthier LR, Granotier C, Hoffschir F, Etienne O, Ayouaz A, Desmaze C, et al. Rad51 and DNA-PKcs are involved in the generation of specific telomere aberrations induced by the quadruplex ligand 360A that impair mitotic cell progression and lead to cell death. Cell Mol Life Sci 2012;69:629–40.

[224] Pennarun G, Granotier C, Hoffschir F, Mandine E, Biard D, Gauthier LR, et al. Role of ATM in the telomere response to the G-quadruplex ligand 360A. Nucleic Acids Res 2008;36:1741–54.

[225] Pichierri P, Franchitto A. Werner syndrome protein, the MRE11 complex and ATR: menage-à-trois in guarding genome stability during DNA replication? BioEssays 2004;26:306–13.

[226] Mohaghegh P, Karow JK, Brosh Jr RM, Bohr VA, Hickson ID. The Bloom's and Werner's syndrome proteins are DNA structure-specific helicases. Nucleic Acids Res 2001;29:2843–9.

[227] Sun H, Karow JK, Hickson ID, Maizels N. The Bloom's syndrome helicase unwinds G4 DNA. J Biol Chem 1998;273:27587–92.

[228] Temime-Smaali N, Guittat L, Sidibe A, Shin-Ya K, Trentesaux C, Riou JF. The G-quadruplex ligand telomestatin impairs binding of topoisomerase IIIα to G-quadruplex-forming oligonucleotides and uncaps telomeres in ALT cells. PLoS One 2009;4:e6919.

[229] Salvati E, Scarsella M, Porru M, Rizzo A, Iachettini S, Tentori L, et al. PARP1 is activated at telomeres upon G4 stabilization: possible target for telomere-based therapy. Oncogene 2010;29:6280–93.

[230] Folini M, Pivetta C, Zagotto G, De Marco C, Palumbo M, Zaffaroni N, et al. Remarkable interference with telomeric function by a G-quadruplex selective bisantrene regioisomer. Biochem Pharmacol 2010;79:1781–90.

[231] Fujimori J, Matsuo T, Shimose S, Kubo T, Ishikawa M, Yasunaga Y, et al. Antitumor effects of telomerase inhibitor TMPyP4 in osteosarcoma cell lines. J Orthop Res 2011;29:1707–11.

[232] Riou JF, Guittat L, Mailliet P, Laoui A, Renou E, Petitgenet O, et al. Cell senescence and telomere shortening induced by a new series of specific G-quadruplex DNA ligands. Proc Natl Acad Sci U S A 2002;99:2672–7.

[233] Tauchi T, Shin-Ya K, Sashida G, Sumi M, Okabe S, Ohyashiki JH, et al. Telomerase inhibition with a novel G-quadruplex-interactive agent, telomestatin: in vitro and in vivo studies in acute leukemia. Oncogene 2006;25:5719–25.

[234] Miyazaki T, Pan Y, Joshi K, Purohit D, Hu B, Demir H, et al. Telomestatin impairs glioma stem cell survival and growth through the disruption of telomeric G-quadruplex and inhibition of the proto-oncogene, c-Myb. Clin Cancer Res 2012;18:1268–80.

[235] Cuenca F, Moore MJ, Johnson K, Guyen B, De Cian A, Neidle S. Design, synthesis and evaluation of 4,5-di-substituted acridone ligands with high G-quadruplex affinity and selectivity, together with low toxicity to normal cells. Bioorg Med Chem Lett 2009;19:5109–13.

[236] Sparapani S, Haider SM, Doria F, Gunaratnam M, Neidle S. Rational design of acridine-based ligands with selectivity for human telomeric quadruplexes. J Am Chem Soc 2010;132:12263–72.

[237] Franceschin M, Rizzo A, Casagrande V, Salvati E, Alvino A, Altieri A, et al. Aromatic core extension in the series of N-cyclic bay-substituted perylene G-quadruplex ligands: increased telomere damage, antitumor activity, and strong selectivity for neoplastic over healthy cells. Chem Med Chem 2012;7:2144–54.

[238] Campbell NH, Karim N, Parkinson GN, Gunaratnam M, Petrucci V, Todd AK, et al. Molecular basis of structure-activity relationships between salphen metal complexes and human telomeric DNA quadruplexes. J Med Chem 2012;55:209–22.

[239] Drewe WC, Nanjunda R, Gunaratnam M, Beltran M, Parkinson GN, Reszka AP, et al. Rational design of substituted diarylureas: a scaffold for binding to G-quadruplex motifs. J Med Chem 2008;51:7751–67.

[240] Huppert JL, Balasubramanian S. Prevalence of quadruplexes in the human genome. Nucleic Acids Res 2005;33:2908–16.

[241] Todd AK, Johnston M, Neidle S. Highly prevalent putative quadruplex sequence motifs in human DNA. Nucleic Acids Res 2005;33:2901–7.

[242] Huppert JL, Balasubramanian S. G-quadruplexes in promoters throughout the human genome. Nucleic Acids Res 2007;35:406–13.

[243] Balasubramanian S, Hurley LH, Neidle S. Targeting G-quadruplexes in gene promoters: a novel anticancer strategy? Nat Rev Drug Discov 2011;10:261–75.

[244] Siddiqui-Jain A, Grand CL, Bearss DJ, Hurley LH. Direct evidence for a G-quadruplex in a promoter region and its targeting with a small molecule to repress c-MYC transcription. Proc Natl Acad Sci U S A 2002;99: 11593–8.

[245] Shalaby T, von Bueren AO, Hurlimann ML, Fiaschetti G, Castelletti D, Masayuki T, et al. Disabling c-Myc in childhood medulloblastoma and atypical teratoid/rhabdoid tumor cells by the potent G-quadruplex interactive agent S2T1-6OTD. Mol Cancer Ther 2010;9:167–79.

[246] Gunaratnam M, Swank S, Haider SM, Galesa K, Reszka AP, Beltran M, et al. Targeting human gastrointestinal stromal tumor cells with a quadruplex-binding small molecule. J Med Chem 2009;52:3774–83.

[247] Bryan TM, Baumann P. G-quadruplexes: from guanine gels to chemotherapeutics. Mol Biotechnol 2011;49: 198–208.

[248] Rezler EM, Seenisamy J, Bashyam S, Kim MY, White E, Wilson WD, et al. Telomestatin and diseleno sapphyrin bind selectively to two different forms of the human telomeric G-quadruplex structure. J Am Chem Soc 2005;127:9439–47.

[249] Palumbo SL, Ebbinghaus SW, Hurley LH. Formation of a unique end-to-end stacked pair of G-quadruplexes in the hTERT core promoter with implications for inhibition of telomerase by G-quadruplex-interactive ligands. J Am Chem Soc 2009;131:10878–91.

[250] Garner TP, Williams HE, Gluszyk KI, Roe S, Oldham NJ, Stevens MF, et al. Selectivity of small molecule ligands for parallel and anti-parallel DNA G-quadruplex structures. Org Biomol Chem 2009;7:4194–200.

[251] Wang L, Wen Y, Liu J, Zhou J, Li C, Wei C. Promoting the formation and stabilization of human telomeric G-quadruplex DNA, inhibition of telomerase and cytotoxicity by phenanthroline derivatives. Org Biomol Chem 2011;9:2648–53.

[252] Hamon F, Largy E, Guedin-Beaurepaire A, Rouchon-Dagois M, Sidibe A, Monchaud D, et al. An acyclic oligoheteroaryle that discriminates strongly between diverse G-quadruplex topologies. Angew Chem Int Ed Engl 2011;50:8745–9.

[253] Yu H, Wang X, Fu M, Ren J, Qu X. Chiral metallo-supramolecular complexes selectively recognize human telomeric G-quadruplex DNA. Nucleic Acids Res 2008;36:5695–703.

[254] Manet I, Manoli F, Donzello MP, Viola E, Andreano G, Masi A, et al. A cationic Zn^{II} porphyrazine induces a stable parallel G-quadruplex conformation in human telomeric DNA. Org Biomol Chem 2011;9:684–8.

[255] Chen M, Song G, Wang C, Hu D, Ren J, Qu X. Small-molecule selectively recognizes human telomeric G-quadruplex DNA and regulates its conformational switch. Biophys J 2009;97:2014–23.

[256] Li Q, Xiang J, Li X, Xu X, Tang Y, Zhou Q, et al. Stabilizing parallel G-quadruplex DNA by a new class of ligands: two non-planar alkaloids through interaction in lateral grooves. Biochimie 2009;91:811–9.

[257] Gornall KC, Samosorn S, Tanwirat B, Suksamrarn A, Bremner JB, Kelso MJ, et al. A mass spectrometric investigation of novel quadruplex DNA-selective berberine derivatives. Chem Commun (Camb) 2010;46:6602–4.

[258] Peng D, Tan JH, Chen SB, Ou TM, Gu LQ, Huang ZS. Bisaryldiketene derivatives: a new class of selective ligands for *c-myc* G-quadruplex DNA. Bioorg Med Chem 2010;18:8235–42.

[259] Eddy J, Maizels N. Gene function correlates with potential for G4 DNA formation in the human genome. Nucleic Acids Res 2006;34:3887–96.

[260] Halder R, Riou JF, Teulade-Fichou MP, Frickey T, Hartig JS. Bisquinolinium compounds induce quadruplex-specific transcriptome changes in HeLa S3 cell lines. BMC Res Notes 2012;5:138.

[261] Biroccio A, Porru M, Rizzo A, Salvati E, D'Angelo C, Orlandi A, et al. DNA damage persistence as determinant of tumor sensitivity to the combination of Topo I inhibitors and telomere-targeting agents. Clin Cancer Res 2011;17:2227–36.

[262] Gunaratnam M, de la Fuente M, Hampel SM, Todd AK, Reszka AP, Schatzlein A, et al. Targeting pancreatic cancer with a G-quadruplex ligand. Bioorg Med Chem 2011;19:7151–7.

[263] Gowan SM, Harrison JR, Patterson L, Valenti M, Read MA, Neidle S, et al. A G-quadruplex-interactive potent small-molecule inhibitor of telomerase exhibiting in vitro and in vivo antitumor activity. Mol Pharmacol 2002;61:1154–62.

[264] Leonetti C, Scarsella M, Riggio G, Rizzo A, Salvati E, D'Incalci M, et al. G-quadruplex ligand RHPS4 potentiates the antitumor activity of camptothecins in preclinical models of solid tumors. Clin Cancer Res 2008;14:7284–91.

Targeting B-RAF: The Discovery and Development of B-RAF Inhibitors

Philip A. Harris

GlaxoSmithKline, Collegeville, PA, USA

B-RAF KINASE SIGNALING

In signal transduction, extracellular signals are transduced via membrane receptor activation, with amplification and propagation involving a complex cascade of protein phosphorylation and dephosphorylation events. These signaling pathways are highly regulated, often by intermeshed kinase pathways, where each kinase may itself be regulated by one or more other kinases and protein phosphatases. The ultimate function of this is to link receptor activity at the cell membrane with modification of cytoplasmic or nuclear targets that govern cell proliferation, differentiation, and survival. Three classical mitogen-activated protein kinase (MAPK) pathways have been identified in mammalian cells that share a number of characteristics, such as activation dependent on two phosphorylation events, a three-tiered kinase cascade, and similar substrate recognition sites [1]. The c-jun kinase (JNK) pathway is primarily associated with response to cellular stress, the p38 pathway is critical for inflammatory responses, and the extracellular signal-regulated kinase (ERK) pathway plays a key role in the regulation of cell division, as illustrated in Fig. 18.1 [2].

The MAPK pathway most associated with normal and uncontrolled cell growth is the RAS–RAF–MEK–ERK pathway [3]. Binding of extracellular mitogenic ligands to tyrosine kinase receptors results in trans-autophosphorylation, which leads to recruitment of the adaptor protein Grb2. Grb2 recruits the guanine exchange factors SOS1/SOS2, which then promote RAS activation by facilitating exchange of bound guanosine diphosphate (GDP) for guanosine triphosphate (GTP). RAS–GTP then triggers the activation of RAF kinase by recruitment to the plasma membrane, where RAF undergoes a complex pattern of phosphorylation and conformational changes that promotes formation of B-RAF and C-RAF homodimers and heterodimers. Specifically, localization of RAF to the plasma membrane induces an "open" conformation, which facilitates its transphosphorylation on regulatory serine and threonine residues. Phosphorylation of RAF proteins at these regulatory sites

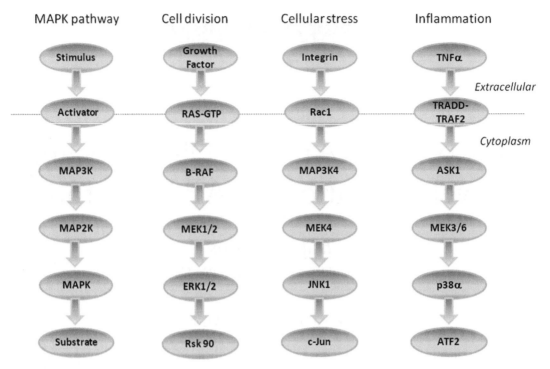

FIGURE 18.1 Classical MAPK pathways. (For color version of this figure, the reader is referred to the online version of this book.)

destabilizes the inactive conformation, resulting in kinase activation. Activated RAF kinase then phosphorylates and activates the intracellular protein kinases MEK1 and MEK2 (MAP–ERK kinase). MEK1/2 are dual-specificity protein kinases that mediate the phosphorylation of tyrosine before threonine in ERK1 or ERK2, their only substrates. This phosphorylation activates ERK1/2, which are serine and threonine protein kinases, via dimerization. Unlike RAF and MEK1/2, which have narrow substrate specificity, ERK1 and ERK2 have dozens of substrates and are capable of eliciting a complex array of biological responses throughout the cell, including translocation to the nucleus, where they have multiple roles, including regulation of nuclear transport, DNA repair, nucleosome assembly, mRNA processing, and protein translation (Fig. 18.2).

RAF belongs to the serine–threonine kinase family and is composed of three isoforms—A-RAF, B-RAF, and C-RAF—which are related to retroviral oncogenes discovered in 1983 [4]. The murine sarcoma virus 3611 enhances fibrosarcoma induction in newborn MSF/N mice, and the name RAF corresponds to rapidly accelerated fibrosarcoma. RAF-1, which was discovered in 1985, is now called C-RAF; A-RAF was discovered the following year, and B-RAF followed in 1988. BRAF residue numbering changed in 2004 owing to a prior DNA sequencing error, so residues in the original version after position 32 increased by one [5]. B-RAF exhibits higher basal kinase activity than A-RAF and C-RAF, which are rarely implicated in human cancers. Over 40 different mutations in the B-RAF kinase domain have been identified to date, in contrast to rare mutations found in A-RAF and C-RAF.

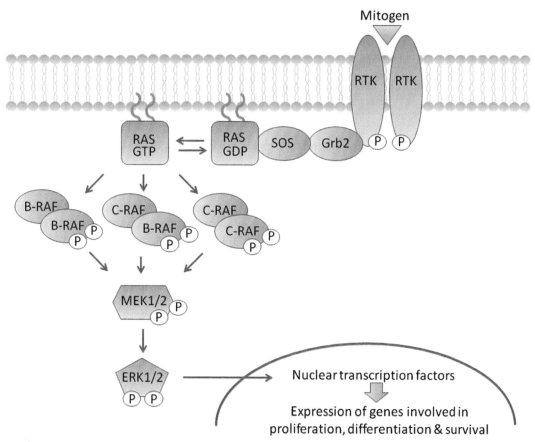

FIGURE 18.2 The RAS–RAF–MEK–ERK signaling pathway. (For color version of this figure, the reader is referred to the online version of this book.)

The RAS–RAF–MEK–ERK signal transduction cascade has been implicated in many human cancers, often resulting in constitutive activation of the ERK pathway [6]. Aberrant expression or activating somatic mutations in the upstream pathway *RAS*, *BRAF*, and *MEK* genes can result in a constitutively active ERK kinase cascade. Substantial drug discovery efforts have been made that target activated RAS, but none have met with success, suggesting that RAS is a pharmacologically intractable target. On the other hand, B-RAF has emerged as a particularly appealing target since kinases are proven tractable targets for drug discovery and the large majority of activating mutation occurs in B-RAF. A significant advance in the understanding of the role of B-RAF in cancer came in 2002, when Davies and colleagues at the Sanger Institute reported that B-RAF-activating somatic mutations occurred in about 8% of all human cancers, including 60% of melanomas, 40% of thyroid cancer, and 20% of colon and ovarian cancers. *BRAF* mutations cluster in the glycine-rich loop (exon 11) and the activation loop (exon 15) of the kinase [7]. Strikingly, a single substitution of glutamic acid to valine at codon 600 (V600E) in the activation loop accounts for approximately 90% of *BRAF* mutations. The V600E *BRAF* mutation occurs in a

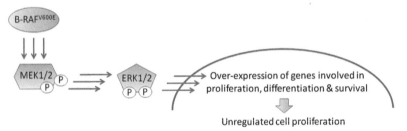

FIGURE 18.3   Unregulated signaling through B-RAF^{V600E} mutation. (For color version of this figure, the reader is referred to the online version of this book.)

nonoverlapping distribution, with mutations in RAS suggesting that the activation of either is sufficient to promote engagement of the MEK–ERK cascade. Wan et al. observed in the crystal structure of the B-RAF kinase domain that an intramolecular interaction between the glycine-rich loop and the activation segment helps maintain an inactive status of B-RAF [6]. However, phosphorylation within the activation segment or the V600E mutation breaks the intramolecular interaction to activate B-RAF. Therefore, the B-RAF^{V600E} mutation bypasses the requirement for RAS-mediated dimerization and phosphorylation activation, and is constitutively active and can thus lead to unregulated cell proliferation and tumor growth (Fig. 18.3). Tumors carrying a *BRAF* V600E allele display high MEK–ERK activity, and the growth of their xenografts is highly dependent on this pathway.

REGULATION AND STRUCTURE OF B-RAF

Of the kinase RAF's isoforms, B-RAF is the largest, comprising 766 residues and a molecular weight of 84.4 KDa. They share three highly conserved regions—CR1, CR2, and CR3—all illustrated in Fig. 18.4 [8]. The N-terminal CR1 contains the RAS–GTP binding domain (RBD), which initiates the interaction with RAS–GTP through a conserved arginine residue (R188 in B-RAF) required for recruitment and activation of RAF at the plasma membrane, and a cysteine-rich domain (CRD) that can bind two zinc ions. The CR2 is a serine-rich domain, one of which (S365) when phosphorylated can bind to 14-3-3, a negative regulatory protein [9]. A stimulatory 14-3-3-binding site occurs after the kinase domain at S729. In unstimulated cells, both S365 and S729 in B-RAF are phosphorylated, which mediates binding to a 14-3-3 protein dimer thought to tether and stabilize a closed inactive conformation. Binding to RAS–GTP results in displacement of 14-3-3 from phopsho-S365, inducing an open conformation and exposure of the kinase domain to its substrate MEK.

CR3 is the protein kinase domain located near the C-terminus. The kinase possesses the characteristic small N-terminal and large C-terminal lobes found in all protein kinases, as shown in Fig. 18.5 for the co-crystal structure of B-RAF and sorafenib [6]. The smaller N-terminal lobe has a predominantly antiparallel β-sheet structure and anchors and orients ATP or the inhibitor. It contains a glycine-rich ATP–phosphate-binding loop (G-rich loop), sometimes also called the P-loop, and the αC-helix. The activation loop of the kinase is a flexible loop that, in the unactivated state, blocks catalysis. This loop contains phosphorylation sites (threonine and serine, in the case of B-RAF) that, upon phosphorylation, cause a

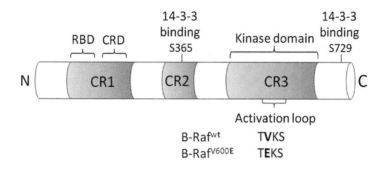

FIGURE 18.4 B-RAF conserved regions and regulatory domains. (For color version of this figure, the reader is referred to the online version of this book.)

Domain	CR1	RBD	CRD	CR2	CR3 Kinase domain	Activation Loop
Residues	150-290	155-227	234-280	360-375	451-717	594-623

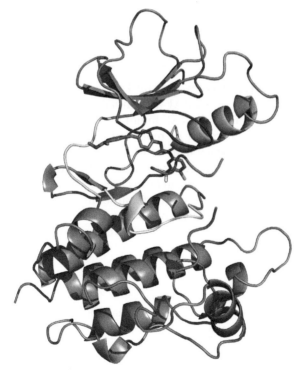

FIGURE 18.5 Co-crystal structure of B-RAF and sorafenib. (This figure is reproduced in color in the color plate section.)

conformational change in the loop to open up the catalytic pocket and correctly align conserved amino acids for the catalytic transfer of the γ-phosphate. In the crystal structure, several regions of the *activation loop* are *disordered* due to its flexibility. The larger S-terminal lobe is mainly α-helical in structure and contains the binding site for the substrates MEK1/2. The catalytic ATP-binding pocket lies in the cleft between the small and large lobes tethered together by a *hinge region*. The adenine heterocycle of ATP makes bidentate hydrogen bonds with the hinge backbone. The B-RAF kinase inhibitors are ATP competitive and, similar to ATP, make hydrogen bond interactions at the hinge via core heterocycles.

Activation of the RAK kinases requires phosphorylation events both at the N-terminal end of the kinase domain and in the activation loop [10]. In C-RAF, this involves RAS-dependent phosphorylation of S338/339 and Y340/341 in the N-terminal end; whereas in B-RAF, this corresponds to S446/447 and D448/449 [9]. With the two aspartic acids D448/449 and S446, which are constitutively phosphorylated, the N-terminal domain of B-RAF does not require additional enzyme-catalyzed modifications to become negatively charged, accounting for the high basal in vitro kinase activity of B-RAF. In the crystal structure of the B-RAF kinase domain, D448 was found to stabilize the active conformation through a salt bridge with R506 on the α-helix [6]. A second critical event for B-RAF activation is phosphorylation of T599 and S602 in the activation loop. The gain-of-function mutation in the *BRAF* gene is predominantly the glutamic acid substitution of valine 600, which mimics the conformational change induced by these two activating phosphorylations.

SORAFENIB (NEXAVAR®, OR BAY43-9006)

Sorafenib is a novel pyridyl biaryl urea multikinase inhibitor identified by Bayer and Onyx that targets both antiproliferative RAF and antiangiogenic VEGFR–PDGFRβ signaling pathways. It is the first small-molecule RAF inhibitor approved by the US Food and Drug Administration (FDA) for the treatment of renal cell carcinoma (RCC) and hepatocellular carcinoma (HCC), although its efficacy against RCC is likely due in large part to its antiangiogenic activity. Sorafenib was approved by the FDA in December 2005 and received European marketing authorization in July 2006, in both cases for use in the treatment of advanced renal cancer. The European Commission granted marketing authorization to the drug for the treatment of patients with HCC, the most common form of liver cancer, in October 2007, and FDA approval for unresectable HCC followed in November 2007. Clinical trials of sorafenib against melanoma were unsuccessful.

Discovery of Sorafenib

The initial hit discovery took place in 1995, 10 years before eventual approval, in which a phenyl-urea thiophene ester **1** was identified from a high-throughput screen of small-molecule chemical libraries employing a scintillation proximity assay against the C-RAF–MEK–ERK kinase cascade (Fig. 18.6) [11]. This hit (**1**) had moderate activity against C-RAF (IC$_{50}$ 17 μM), and a 10-fold improvement was observed by 4-methyl substitution on the phenyl ring yielding **2**. A library of bis-aryl urea analogs of the lead compound was then

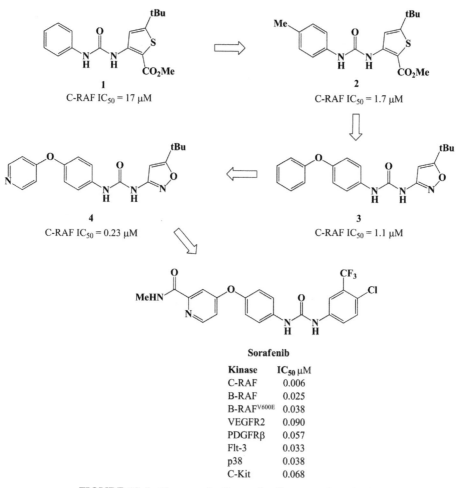

FIGURE 18.6 Key steps leading to the discovery of sorafenib.

Kinase	IC$_{50}$ μM
C-RAF	0.006
B-RAF	0.025
B-RAF^{V600E}	0.038
VEGFR2	0.090
PDGFRβ	0.057
Flt-3	0.033
p38	0.038
C-Kit	0.068

constructed to further explore the structure–activity relationship (SAR) of the series, which identified the 3-amino-isoxazole **3** with C-RAF kinase inhibition IC$_{50}$ of 1.1 μM. A fivefold increase in C-RAF activity was achieved by replacing its distal ring with a 4-pyridine **4**, which also decreased lipophilicity, improved the aqueous solubility, and imparted significant inhibitory activity against human colon carcinoma HCT116 cell proliferation, accompanied by decreased phosphorylation of MEK and ERK. This compound (**4**) possessed oral bioavailability and inhibited the growth of HCT116 xenografts in vivo, thereby providing proof of principle for this new kinase inhibitor class. Further SAR studies were then undertaken, including addition of the amide functionality adjacent to the pyridine to lead to the preparation of sorafenib with C-RAF kinase inhibition IC$_{50}$ of 6nM. Further profiling revealed sofarenib potently inhibits B-RAF, both wild type and V600E, as well as VEGFR2 and a number of other kinases.

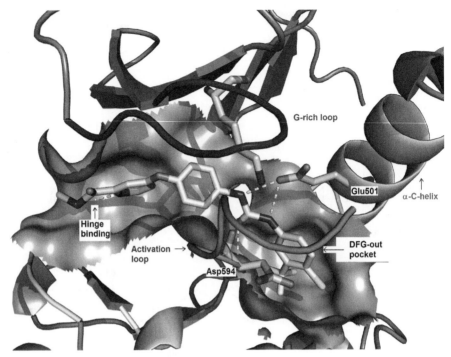

FIGURE 18.7   Sorafenib binding in the ATP-binding pocket of B-RAF. (This figure is reproduced in color in the color plate section.)

Structure of Sorafenib in B-RAF

In the co-crystal structure of sorafenib bound to the B-RAF kinase domain, the nitrogen of 4-pyridyl group of sorafenib accepts a hydrogen bond from the backbone NH of Cys532 in the hinge, whereas the methylamide NH donates a hydrogen bond to the carbonyl of Cys532, as shown in Fig. 18.7 [6]. It is interesting that the pyridyl moiety was introduced late in the lead optimization stage, meaning that the initial hit (**1**) and early leads (**2–3**) did not possess any hinge-binding motif. The inhibitor binds to the Asp–Phe–Gly (DFG)-out inactive conformation of the kinase, characterized by an almost 180° rotation of the conserved DFG motif at the start of the activation loop in the ATP-binding cleft, relative to the active form, and a shift in the α C-helix. This creates a hydrophobic pocket (DFG-out pocket) that is occupied by the aryl-urea portion of sorafenib, with the lipophilic trifluoromethyl group of sorafenib occupying an additional small hydrophobic pocket. The urea group makes a pair of hydrogen-bonding interactions, first with the backbone of Asp594 from the DFG on the activation loop and second with a bidentate interaction with the acid side chain of Glu501 located in the middle of the αC helix, respectively.

Biology of Sorafenib

In addition to inhibiting C-RAF and B-RAF, sorafenib has an inhibitory effect against several tyrosine receptor kinases, such as VEGFR-1, 2, and 3; PDGFRβ; Flt-3; and c-Kit, which are associated with the antitumorigenic and antiangiogenic activity of this compound. Wilhelm et al. demonstrated that in cellular assays using various cancer cell lines, sorafenib suppresses the proliferation of tumor cells involving colon, pancreatic, thyroid, lung, and breast cancers and melanoma [12]. Sorafenib also demonstrated complete blockage of tumor growth in xenograft mouse models inoculated with colon cancer (HT-29 and Colo-205, both of which are B-RAF^{V600E}, and DLD-1, which is *k-ras* positive) at doses of 30 and 60 mg/kg. It also achieved complete tumor stasis in a breast carcinoma xenograft model (MDA-MB-231 containing G463V *b-raf* and *k-ras* oncogenes). In addition, sorafenib inhibited the growth of a number of additional human xenografts, including ovarian (SK-OV-3), pancreatic (*k-ras*-positive Mia PaCa 2), and thyroid (containing oncogenic RET) cancers as well as melanoma (LOX, UACC 903, and 1205 Lu containing B-RAF^{V600E}), and two non-small-cell lung cancer (NSCLC) xenograft models (A549 and NCI-H460) [12].

The association between antitumor activity and inhibition of the RAF–MEK–ERK pathway was determined in HT-29 and MDA-MB-231 tumor xenografts, as measured by p-ERK levels determined by Western blot analysis and immunohistochemistry [12]. However, no significant effect on pERK1/2 phosphorylation could be observed for human colon (Colo-205) and NSCLC (A549 and NCI-H460) xenograft models, suggesting that efficacy was primarily driven in these tumors by antiangiogenic activity. Significant reductions in microvessel area and microvessel density for the Colo-205, HT-29, and MDA-MB-231 tumors were observed compared to vehicle or untreated mice, suggesting that antiangiogenic activity was a component of their efficacy, and for Colo-205, in the absence of pERK 1/2 phosphorylation, it was the main factor. Presumably, inhibition of endothelial cell VEGFR2 and pericyte PDGFRβ kinase activity by sorafenib drives the antiangiogenic effects in these models.

Clinical Efficacy of Sorafenib

In a phase I clinical trial of sorafenib in 69 patients with advanced refractory solid tumors, the maximum tolerated dose (MTD) was 400 mg twice daily (bid) given on continuous days (continuous) [13]. Dose-limiting toxicities (DLTs) were grade 3 diarrhea and fatigue at 800 mg bid and grade 3 skin toxicity at 600 mg bid. Significant decreases of ERK phosphorylation were identified at doses of 200 mg bid continuous and higher. Of 45 patients assessed for efficacy, one patient had a partial response (HCC at 400 mg bid continuous) and 25 patients had stable disease, with eight lasting >6 months and five for >12 months. Eighteen patients had progressive disease, and tumor response could not be evaluated in one patient.

Sorafenib was administered orally at a continuous dose of 400 mg bid for 12 weeks in a phase II randomized discontinuation trial of 202 patients with metastatic RCC [14]. Sixty-five patients with stable disease were then randomized to placebo or continuation of sorafenib. Twelve weeks after randomization, progression-free survival (PFS) was 24 versus six weeks in favor of sorafenib. Skin rash and desquamation, hand and foot skin reactions, and fatigue were the most common adverse events. The high rate of RCC patients who were progression-free after 12 weeks of dosing led to its approval for the treatment of advanced RCC by the FDA and other regulatory authorities and the initiation of a randomized controlled phase III study known as the Treatment Approaches in Renal Cancer Global Evaluation Trial (TARGET) [15]. Nine hundred and three previously treated patients were randomly assigned to receive sorafenib versus placebo. On demonstration of a PFS benefit with sorafenib, patients assigned to placebo were offered sorafenib. The final overall survival of patients receiving sorafenib was comparable with that of patients receiving placebo (17.8 versus 15.2 months); however, when post-cross-over placebo survival data were censored, the difference became significant (17.8 versus 14.3 months, respectively). The results of TARGET establish the efficacy and safety of sorafenib in advanced RCC.

Similarly, sorafenib was administered orally at a continuous dose of 400 mg bid for 12 weeks in a phase II randomized discontinuation trial of 37 patients with advanced melanoma [16]. One patient had over 25% tumor shrinkage after the run-in and continued on open-label sorafenib, whereas 27 patients had tumor growth over 25% and discontinued treatment. Six other patients had less than 25% tumor growth and were randomized to placebo or sorafenib, but all three patients who were randomized to sorafenib progressed by week 24. Overall, the confirmed best responses for each of the 37 melanoma patients who received sorafenib were 19% stable disease and 62% progressive disease (PD), with 19% not evaluable. In conclusion, sorafenib had little or no antitumor activity in advanced melanoma patients as a single agent at 400 mg bid. There was no relationship between V600E *BRAF* status and disease stability.

In preclinical experiments, sorafenib had antiproliferative activity in liver cancer cell lines, and it reduced tumor angiogenesis and increased tumor cell apoptosis in a mouse xenograft model of human HCC [17]. It is known that the Ras–RAF–MEK–ERK pathway plays a role in HCC, that such tumors are highly vascularized, and that vascular endothelial growth factor (VEGF) augments HCC development and metastasis. This provided a good rationale for investigating sorafenib for this indication. In a randomized phase III study, known as the Sorafenib HCC Assessment Randomized Protocol (SHARP), the median overall survival increased from 7.9 months in the placebo group to 10.7 months in the sorafenib group [18]. Sorafenib showed a significant benefit also in terms of time to progression, with a median of 5.5 months in the sorafenib group and 2.8 months in the placebo group. On the basis of these findings, sorafenib was approved for the treatment of advanced HCC treatment. The most common adverse events reported in the SHARP trial were diarrhea and hand–foot skin reactions. These findings have been replicated by a randomized controlled trial in Asia, and safety data were reproduced in a large phase IV study of sorafenib in more than 1500 patients, establishing sorafenib as the standard of care for advanced HCC [19].

RAF265

Discovery of RAF265

RAF265, also known as (CHIR-265), is an arylaminobenzimidazole-based B-RAF, C-RAF, and VEGFR2 inhibitor developed by Chiron Corporation, later acquired by Novartis. Its initial design was based on the sorafenib structure in which the urea was tied back onto the adjacent central phenyl ring to form the benzimidazole analog **5** shown in Fig. 18.8 [20]. This resulted in an initial drop in potency compared to sorafenib that was recovered through lead optimization. Methylation of the benzimidazole heterocycle, specifically the nitrogen para to the oxygen linker, significantly improved enzymatic potency from fivefold to 60-fold against both isoforms of RAF. Benzimidazole **6** was selected for evaluation in a mouse HT29 (B-RAF^{V600E}) human colon tumor xenograft model because of its improved solubility over

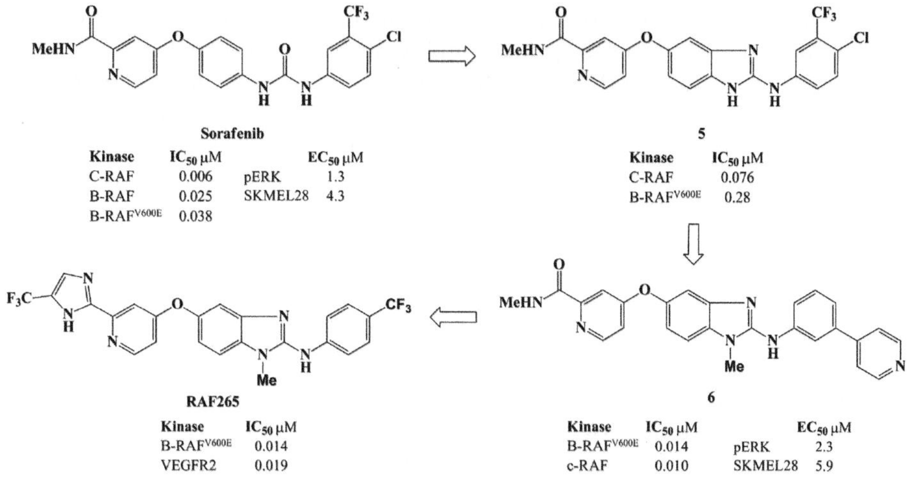

FIGURE 18.8 Key steps leading to the discovery of RAF265.

other analogs in this series, likely due to the second basic pyridine heterocycle. Dosed at 10, 30, or 100 mg/kg daily for 28 days, benzimidazole **6** demonstrates significant antitumor activity at doses of 30 mg/kg/day and 15% tumor regression at 100 mg/kg/day. The compound showed time-dependent inhibition of phosphorylated ERK (pERK) consistent with inhibition of B-Raf^{V600E} in tumors. However, since the inhibitor has similar additional activity against VEGFR and PDGFRβ kinases as sorafenib, the contribution of an antiangiogenesis mechanism to the observed efficacy cannot be discounted.

Structure of RAF265 in B-RAF

Molecular modeling of the binding of this series in the B-RAF kinase domain suggests a very similar binding mode to that of sorafenib, with the same pyridyl and methylamide group hinge interactions with the backbone of Cys532 as shown in Fig. 18.7 [20]. The inhibitor is thought to bind to the DFG-out inactive conformation of the kinase, with the three nitrogens of the aminobenzimidazole moiety mimicking the hydrogen bond network observed for the urea of sorafenib with the Asp594–Glu501 pair in the catalytic region.

Clinical Efficacy of RAF265

The most advanced inhibitor from this series is RAF265. In a preclinical study to determine the effectiveness of RAF265, advanced metastatic melanoma tumors from 17 patients were orthotopically implanted in nude mice and evaluated for response to RAF265 at a daily dose of 40 mg/kg for 30 days [21]. The relation between patient characteristics, gene mutation profile, global gene expression profile, and RAF265 effects on tumor growth, phosphorylated MEK (pMEK) and pERK phosphorylation, proliferation, and apoptosis markers was evaluated. Interestingly, of the nine tumors that were B-RAF$^{V600E/K}$, only two responded to RAF265 treatment, defined as over 50% reduction in tumor growth, whereas five of the eight that were B-RAF^{WT}

responded. Gene expression microarray data revealed that responders exhibited enriched expression of genes involved in cell growth, proliferation, development, cell signaling, gene expression, and cancer pathways. Response to RAF265 did not correlate with pERK1/2 reduction observed by Western blots. However, RAF265 responders did exhibit reduced pMEK1, and this inhibition was accompanied by reduction in phospho-cyclin D1 (Thr286) and polo-like kinase 1 (PLK1), indicating an inhibition of cell cycle progression in response to RAF265.

RAF265 was investigated in a phase I dose escalation study in 76 patients with advanced malignant melanoma with oral daily doses starting from 2 to 67 mg [22]. RAF265 was rapidly absorbed with a maximum concentration occurring about 3 h post dose and a prolonged mean half-life of 11 days. Mutations in B-RAF and NRAS were detected in 59% and 16% of 70 evaluated tumor samples, respectively. Of 71 evaluable patients, six experienced dose-limiting toxicities within the first cycle of 28 days, and dose-limiting thrombocytopenia at grades 3 and 4 occurred at the top daily dose of 67 mg, leading to an MTD of 48 mg being assigned. The overall response rate was 16% from 37 patients with mutated B-RAF and 13% from 30 patients with wild-type B-RAF. The phase II dose expansion portion of the study has reportedly been canceled (http://www.clinicaltrials.gov ID: NCT00304525). However a phase Ib dose escalation study of RAF265 combined with the MEK inhibitor MEK162, discovered by Array Biopharma and licensed to Novartis, is underway in patients with advanced solid tumors harboring RAS or B-RAF$^{V600E/K}$ mutations (http://www.clinicaltrials.gov ID: NCT01352273).

LGX818

Novartis has recently advanced another B-RAF inhibitor, LGX818, whose structure has yet to be disclosed into phase I clinical trials. It has high potency against the A375 (B-RAF^{V600E}) human melanoma cell line, suppressing both pERK ($EC_{50} = 3$ nM) and proliferation ($EC_{50} = 4$ nM), showing good selectivity against 100 measured kinases, and not inhibiting the proliferation of over 400 cell lines expressing wild-type B-RAF [23]. LGX818 is reported to have an extremely slow off-rate from B-RAF^{V600E} with a dissociation half-life over 24 h, which translated into sustained target inhibition in cells following drug washout. A single oral dose of LGX818 at 6 mg/kg in human melanoma xenograft models (B-RAF^{V600E}) showed a 75% decrease in pMEK for over 24 h, even following clearance of the drug from circulation. LGX818-induced tumor regression in multiple B-RAF mutant human tumor xenograft models at doses as low as 1 mg/kg, but no activity against B-RAF wild-type tumors at up to 300 mg/kg doses twice daily. A phase I clinical trial in patients with B-RAF^{V600E} melanoma or colorectal cancers is currently recruiting patients (http://www.clinicaltrials.gov ID: NCT01436656), and a phase Ib dose escalation study of LGX818 combined with the MEK inhibitor MEK162 is also recruiting patients with advanced solid tumors harboring the B-RAF$^{V600E/K}$ mutation (http://www.clinicaltrials.gov ID: NCT01543698).

VEMURAFENIB (ZELBORAF®, OR PLX4032)

Vemurafenib is the first-in-class small-molecule selective B-RAF inhibitor approved by the FDA in August 2011 for the treatment of patients with unresectable or metastatic melanoma with the *B-RAF*^{V600E} mutation, and in Europe in February 2012 as monotherapy in adults with *B-RAF*^{V600}-positive mutations [24]. The name "vemurafenib" comes from V600E-mutated B-RAF inhibition. It was discovered by Plexxicon, now owned by Daiichi Sankyo, and co-developed with Roche.

Discovery of Vemurafenib

The discovery of vemurafenib by Plexxikon employed a scaffold-based approach to identify the lead template as opposed to a high-throughput screen [25]. This approach screened a library of 20,000 small molecules with favorable chemical properties (i.e., low molecular weights, a low number of hydrogen bond donors and acceptors and rotatable bonds, and good solubilities). Five different kinases were screened through the library at a concentration of 200 μM, and 238 compounds, which inhibited a minimum of three kinases (PIM-1, p38, and CSK), were selected for follow-up co-crystallography in at least one of these kinases. Over 100 structures of kinases co-crystallized with inhibitors were successfully determined. PIM1 kinase provided the most robust system for co-crystallizing small low-affinity compounds. One of the PIM1 co-structures was 7-azaindole bound in the ATP-binding site, albeit in multiple binding modes consistent with a weak affinity (IC$_{50}$ > 200 μM). The 3-anilino-7-azaindole (**7**) was subsequently prepared with improved potency over PIM-1 (IC$_{50}$ ~ 100 μM), with a single observed binding mode making two hydrogen bond interactions with the kinase hinge (Fig. 18.9). Further optimization coupled with additional co-crystallography, this time with FGFR1, identified 3-(*m*-methoxybenzyl)-7-azaindole (**8**) with a substantial potency increase (IC$_{50}$ 1.9 μM), likely due to an additional hydrogen bond interaction between the methoxy oxygen and the protein. Libraries of mono- and disubstituted analogs built around the 7-azaindole core were prepared and screened that led to the identification of the difluoro-phenylsulfonamide substructural motif that gave excellent B-RAF potency. These compounds were then co-crystallized in engineered forms of B-RAF^{V600E} and wild-type B-RAF, which allowed for an additional iteration of optimization and resulted in identification of PLX4720, with excellent potency for B-RAF^{V600E} (IC$_{50}$ 0.013 μM) and about a 10-fold window over B-RAF^{WT}. Key to the success of this approach was a robust expression and crystallization system for B-RAF, and a highly soluble form of the B-RAF kinase domain was engineered by mutating surface hydrophobic residues into relatively isosteric hydrophilic amino acids. This high-throughput structural biology approach allowed the group to obtain over 100 co-crystal structures of different inhibitors bound to B-RAF, and these structures, accompanied by molecular modeling and subsequent rounds of lead optimization, allowed for rapid progress toward PXR4720 and vemurafenib, first prepared in early 2005. Vemurafenib and PLX4720 were chosen to progress over analogs with similar in vitro and in vivo activities due to their consistent pharmacokinetics in rodents. For further drug development, vemurafenib was eventually selected in preference to PLX4720 because its pharmacokinetic properties scaled more favorably in dogs and monkeys [24].

Structure of Vemurafenib in B-RAF

In the co-crystal structure of vemurafenib and the kinase domain of B-RAF^{V600E}, the protein forms a dimer in the active DFG-in conformation in which the conserved Asp–Phe–Gly

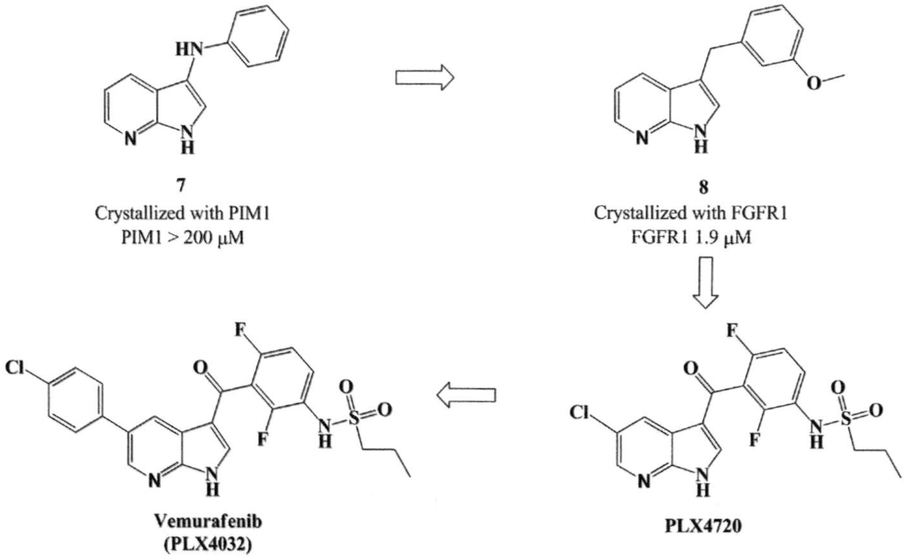

7
Crystallized with PIM1
PIM1 > 200 μM

8
Crystallized with FGFR1
FGFR1 1.9 μM

Vemurafenib
(PLX4032)

Kinase	IC$_{50}$ μM
C-RAF	0.048
B-RAF	0.100
B-RAF^{V600E}	0.031
SRMS	0.018
ACK1	0.019
MAP4K5	0.051
FGR	0.063
LCK	0.183
BRK	0.213
NEK11	0.317
BLK	0.547

PLX4720

Kinase	IC$_{50}$ μM
C-RAF*	0.007
B-RAF	0.160
B-RAF^{V600E}	0.013
BRK	0.130
FRK	1.300
CSK	1.500
SRC	1.700
VEGFR2	2.300

*C-RAF Y340D, Y341D

FIGURE 18.9 Key steps leading to the discovery of vemurafenib.

motif at the start of the activation loop is buried inside and away from the ATP-binding pocket [24]. Interestingly, vemurafenib is present in only one of the protomers. However, in the co-structure of wild-type B-RAF with PLX4720, the ligand fully occupies one ATP pocket of the protein dimer, and the other has a lower occupancy of about 60%. In the protomer with partial ligand occupancy, the B-RAF exists in the inactive DFG-out conformation, where the Asp–Phe–Gly motif makes an almost 180 °C rotation, leaving the phenylalanine residue obstructing the ATP pocket. The 7-azaindole core of the template shown in Fig. 18.10 is the hinge binder, occupying approximately the ATP adenine-binding region, making a hydrogen bond acceptor interaction to the NH of Cys532, similar to the pyridine of sorafenib, and a hydrogen bond donor interaction to the carbonyl of Gln530. The nitrogen of the arylsulfonamide moiety is depicted to bind in its deprotonated form, allowing for an additional hydrogen bond acceptor interaction with the backbone amide NH of Asp594, while the oxygen atoms of the sulfonamide form hydrogen bonds to the backbone NH of Phe595 and the side chain of Lys483. The propyl chain of the sulfonamide group fits a small lipophilic interior pocket formed by an outward shift of the regulatory αC-helix specific to the RAF family,

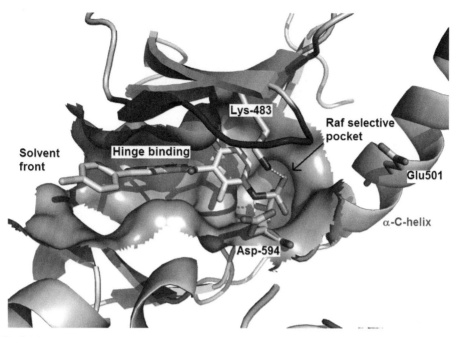

FIGURE 18.10   Vemurafenib binding in the ATP-binding pocket of B-RAF. (This figure is reproduced in color in the color plate section.)

likely accounting for its favorable kinase selectivity profile. The 5-*p*-chloro-phenyl moiety is directed toward the solvent front of the kinase.

The B-RAF^{V600E} dimer has an extensive interface between the two protomers characterized by a number of polar interactions, including 16 hydrogen bonds and seven salt bridges [24]. Arg509 on one protomer forms four hydrogen bonds with the αC helix of its dimer partner, and mutation of this residue abolishes dimer formation. Vemurafenib binding, specifically the propyl chain of the sulfonamide group into the small lipophilic pocket, causes an outward shift in the regulatory αC helix of B-RAF^{V600E}, thereby altering its interaction with Arg509 and in turn affecting RAF dimerization. Paradoxically, it is proposed that the drug upregulates downstream signaling in cells lacking B-RAF mutations through allosteric transactivation of the nondrug bound protomer in B-RAF–C-RAF heterodimers and C-RAF homodimers, as shown in Fig. 18.11. In cells harboring B-RAF^{V600E}, signaling occurs via monomers, and the inhibitor can completely block its kinase activity. This could explain both the specificity of the drug for B-RAF-mutant tumors and the complication of low-grade squamous cell carcinomas that can arise from normal skin cells in some patients being treated with vemurafenib. This can sometimes appear within just a few weeks of initiating vemurafenib therapy, and it appears likely that vemurafenib accelerates the growth of pre-existing lesions with neoplastic potential in these patients. Studies in mice add support to this hypothesis in which RAF inhibitors do not initiate or promote skin carcinogenesis, but substantially enhance the proliferation of lesions that both have *HRAS* mutations and are exposed to tumor promoters [26].

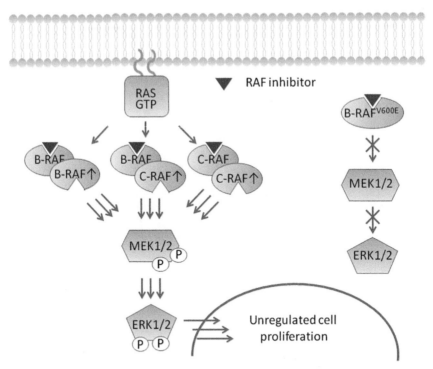

FIGURE 18.11 Model of paradoxical activation of the nonmutated RAF–MAPK pathway. (For color version of this figure, the reader is referred to the online version of this book.)

Biology of Vemurafenib

The selectivity of vemurafenib for B-RAF^{V600E} over wild type observed in biochemical assays translated to increases in cellular selectivity observed in a series of experiments evaluating the effect of vemurafenib on RAF–MEK–ERK pathway inhibition and proliferation suppression in a panel of cancer cell lines [27]. In 17 melanoma cell lines, vemurafenib was a potent inhibitor of proliferation in those cell lines expressing codon 600 *BRAF* mutations (V600E, V600R, V600D, and V600R) but not *BRAF* wild type. This increased selectivity is likely due to cells that possess B-RAF mutations being dependent on the activated MAPK pathway for cell proliferation.

Vemurafenib was reported to inhibit phosphorylation of MEK and ERK in the V600E-expressing melanoma cell lines COLO 829 and LOX as measured by Western blotting [27]. In addition, it also exhibited potent inhibitory effects on MEK and ERK phosphorylation in melanoma cell lines that expressed other mutations at the V600 positions such as WM2664 (V600D) and WM1341D (V600R). The effects of vemurafenib on MEK and ERK phosphorylation in melanoma cell lines that do not express codon 600 *BRAF* mutations were more variable.

The effects of vemurafenib on antitumor activity and survival were determined in vivo using the murine LOX melanoma xenograft model dosed at 12.5, 25, and 75 mg/kg bid [27]. Vemurafenib induced complete tumor regression at both the 25 and 75 mg/kg doses and in

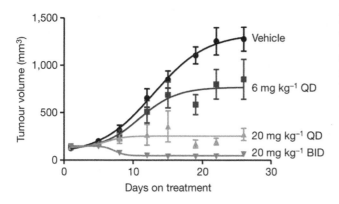

the majority (5 of 9) of mice treated at 12.5 mg/kg. Vemurafenib was also reported to significantly increase survival relative to vehicle with eight of 10 mice in the 75 mg/kg bid group considered to have been completely cured. However, tumors were reported to recur following complete regression in mice treated with lower doses. In other melanoma models, vemurafenib showed complete tumor regression against both the A-375 and COLO 829 tumors, dosed at 75 and 100 mg/kg bid, respectively. In the A-375 model, survival was prolonged by 227% compared to vehicle-treated mice after 11 days of treatment; whereas in the COLO 829 model, survival was prolonged by 61% after 21 days of treatment.

The effect of vemurafenib on antitumor activity was determined in vivo using the colorectal cancer (CRC) COLO 205 xenograft model dosing at 6 and 20 mg/kg daily and 20 mg/kg bid, as illustrated in Fig. 18.12 [28]. In this model, tumor growth inhibition was modest at 6 mg/kg daily, whereas tumor stabilization was observed at 20 mg/kg daily. Significant tumor regressions were observed at 20 mg/kg bid, corresponding to exposures in the rat of vemurafenib of about 300 µM h as determined on day 7.

Clinical Efficacy of Vemurafenib

In preclinical safety assessment, rats and dogs dosed with vemurafenib for 28 days at doses of up to 1000 mg/kg/day showed no toxicity, and tolerability was confirmed further in rats for 26 weeks and dogs for 13 weeks [28]. This safety profile was achieved in spite of very high exposures, reaching 2600 µM in rats and 820 µM in dogs. No histological changes were observed in the skin in any animal at any dose or duration of treatment.

The initial formulation of vemurafenib for oral delivery consisted of capsules of a crystalline powder, which, although adequate for initial clinical testing, were unsuitable for manufacturing and storage as the crystalline form was unstable. To improve solubility and stability, Roche reformulated vemurafenib into a stable amorphous form characterized as a microprecipitated bulk powder, formed by precipitating it into a polymer matrix. This microprecipitated bulk powder formulation was shown to yield a sixfold increase in bioavailability in humans compared to the crystalline formulation.

The phase I dose escalation study portion started in late 2006, with the crystalline form at a starting dose level of 200 mg/day increasing to 1600 mg bid [28]. The drug exposure with this initial formulation reached a saturation of exposure with a plateau of <200 µM h, which was below the targeted exposure of 300 μM h associated with tumor regression in preclinical studies. However, the reformulation of vemurafenib enabled dose escalation studies to restart, and at a dose of 240 mg bid, the exposure reached 300 μM•h and led to the first evidence of tumor shrinkage in patients as measured by computed tomography, proving a rare example of translational science in oncology where in vivo xenograft models correctly predicted human efficacy. As the dose was increased up to 720 mg bid, more consistent and pronounced tumor regressions were observed, including at metastatic sites. A total of 21 patients with metastatic melanoma, 16 of them with *BRAF* mutations, were treated at doses that achieved AUC exposures above the threshold of 300 μM h. Ten of the patients with *BRAF*-mutant melanoma achieved tumor regressions qualifying as partial responses, and one patient had a complete response, with none of the patients with melanomas lacking *BRAF* mutations achieving a partial response. Further enrollment was therefore limited to patients with *BRAF*-mutant tumors. Dose-limiting toxicities detected at the top bid dose of 1120 mg included fatigue, rash, and joint pain; therefore, a dose of 960 mg bid was chosen for future studies.

Following the dose escalation portion of the phase I study, an extension phase commenced consisting of two cohorts, one of 32 patients with metastatic melanoma and one of 21 patients with *BRAF*-mutant CRC [29]. Of the 26 of 32 patients with melanoma carrying a B-RAF^{V600E} mutation who took part in the extension phase, a remarkable 81% achieved an objective response, with two patients achieving a complete response. The duration of the tumor response and the benefit of prolonged overall survival of patients receiving this dose were compelling when compared to patients with wild-type *BRAF* or those treated with subtherapeutic doses of vemurafenib.

Positron emission tomography (PET) scanning was used to image tumors in the phase I extension study using a glucose analog, 18F-deoxyglucose, as illustrated for representative patients in Fig. 18.13 [28]. Patients were scanned before initiating therapy and after two weeks of vemurafenib treatment. All patients from this study who were evaluated showed a blockade of tumor metabolism by vemurafenib. Tumor regressions were subsequently documented for these patients: best responses were 70% for patient 45, 70% for patient 59, 68% for patient 61, and 37% for patient 69.

Of the 21 patients with *BRAF*-mutant CRC, there was some evidence of activity, including one patient who had a partial response [24]. However, the much lower response rate compared to that of melanoma suggests differences in the biology of *BRAF*-mutant metastatic CRC. Supporting this clinical observation, *BRAF*-mutant CRC cells were reported to be less sensitive to inhibition by vemurafenib and the pERK suppression was reported to be more transient compared to *BRAF*-mutant melanoma cells [30,31]. Epidermal growth factor receptor (EGFR)-mediated reactivation of the MAPK pathway was identified as contributing to this relative insensitivity. In *BRAF*-mutant CRC cell lines, co-treatment of vemurafenib with the EGFR inhibitor gefitinib or with the dual EGFR–ErbB2 inhibitor lapatinib led to more complete suppression of pERK and inhibition of proliferation. An RNA interference–based screen in human cells reported that blockade of EGFR shows strong synergy with B-RAF^{V600E} inhibition [31]. *BRAF*-mutant CRC xenografts derived from HT-29, WiDr, and VACO432 CRC cells were also much more sensitive to a combination of vemurafenib and an EGFR inhibitor, either the antibody drug cetuximab or one of the small-molecule drugs gefitinib or erlotinib, leading to tumor regressions in mice, compared to any of those agents dosed alone. B-RAF^{V600E} inhibition causes a rapid feedback activation of EGFR, which supports continued

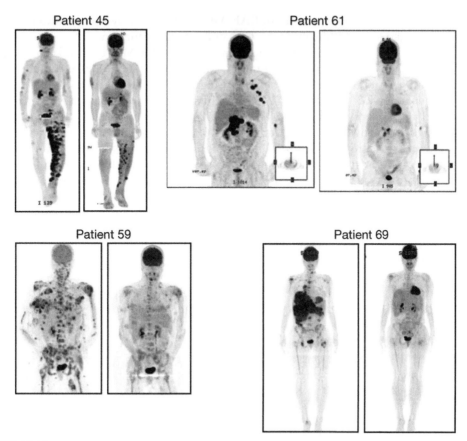

FIGURE 18.13 Representative PET scans for patients before and following 2 weeks of dosing with vemurafenib. *Images reproduced with permission from Ref. [28] © (2010) Macmillan Publishers Ltd. All rights reserved.*

proliferation in the presence of B-RAF^{V600E} inhibition. Melanoma cells express low levels of EGFR and are therefore not subject to this feedback activation. This suggests that reactivation of the MAPK pathway can occur through EGFR-mediated activation of RAS and C-RAF, and supports the evaluation of combined BRAF and EGFR inhibitors in patients with *BRAF*-mutant CRC.

Based on the unprecedented responses in the phase I trial, Plexxikon and Roche committed to initiating the large randomized phase III study concurrently with a phase II trial to expedite the time to registration. The phase II study evaluated the efficacy and safety of vemurafenib in a larger population of patients with previously treated metastatic melanoma bearing a B-RAF^{V600} mutation [32]. Of a total of 132 patients in the study, the confirmed overall response rate was 53%, including 6% complete responses. The median duration of response was 6.7 months. The median overall survival was 15.9 months, compared to 6–10 months previously observed in patients with metastatic melanoma. The most common adverse events were grade 1 or grade 2 joint pain, rash, photosensitivity, fatigue, and alopecia. Cutaneous squamous cell carcinomas (the majority of which were of the keratoacanthoma type) were found in 26% of patients, likely a result of RAF–MEK–ERK pathway upregulation in predisposed sun-damaged skin, within about 8 weeks of treatment initiation.

In 2010, a randomized phase III registration trial (known as BRIM-3) enrolled 675 melanoma patients with the activating B-RAF^{V600} mutation, comparing vemurafenib as a monotherapy to the alkylating agent dacarbazine in treatment-naïve patients with unresectable stage IIIc or stage IV melanoma [33]. By early 2011, an interim analysis of overall survival rates clearly demonstrated the superior efficacy of vemurafenib, and the dacarbazine-treated patients were allowed to switch over to receive vemurafenib. Analysis of data from the phase III clinical trial showed that there was a clinically meaningful and statistically significant improvement in the duration of survival in patients who received vemurafenib compared to those who received dacarbazine, with a 63% reduction in the risk of death. Longer follow-up of the patients from the phase III trial will be necessary to provide reliable estimates of median overall survival. Despite the remarkable success of vemurafenib, a number of challenges remain that should not be underestimated. These include addressing the melanoma patients with wild-type B-RAF who are not treatable with vemurafenib and those with mutant B-RAF who don't respond to treatment because of intrinsic resistance. Additionally, nearly all patients relapse with time despite ongoing treatment due to acquired resistance, so understanding the underlying mechanisms that drive resistance and developing combination therapy options to overcome this are currently under intensive investigation and are reviewed in this chapter.

DABRAFENIB (TAFINLAR® or GSK2118436)

Discovery of SB-590885

Research into developing a B-RAF inhibitor began at SmithKline Beecham during the late 1990s initially as a neuroprotective therapy for the treatment of stroke, based on the observation that increased activation of ERK was observed in in vitro models of neuronal death [34]. The initial lead identified from screening was the trisubstituted imidazole **9** with moderate B-RAF activity, prepared initially as a p38 kinase inhibitor (Fig. 18.14). A related triaryl imidazole, L-779450, disclosed by Merck in 1998, showed that a significant increase in B-RAF activity was obtained by replacement of the 4-fluorophenyl with a chlorophenol moiety. This led the team to explore the SAR around this triaryl imidazole template, from which the triaryl imidazole **10** was identified with an indane-oxime functioning as a bioisostere of the chlorophenol, giving similar potency to L-779450. Attachment of a basic amine linker to improve aqueous solubility resulted in SB-590885, with excellent potency against B-RAF and an approximately 10-fold selectivity over C-RAF. Strikingly, SB-590885 displayed remarkable specificity for B-RAF inhibition, with minimal off-target kinase activity, making it an excellent tool molecule to further investigate the biological role of B-RAF. SB-590885 demonstrated neuroprotective activity in vitro by protection of rat hippocampal slice cultures from death induced by oxygen and glucose deprivation. However, despite its impressive in vitro profile, SB-590885 showed moderate blood clearance and poor central nervous system penetration, making it suboptimal for this indication.

The effects of SB-590885 in the oncology setting were determined by incubating cultures of normal and malignant human cell lines [35]. Inhibition of cellular proliferation was

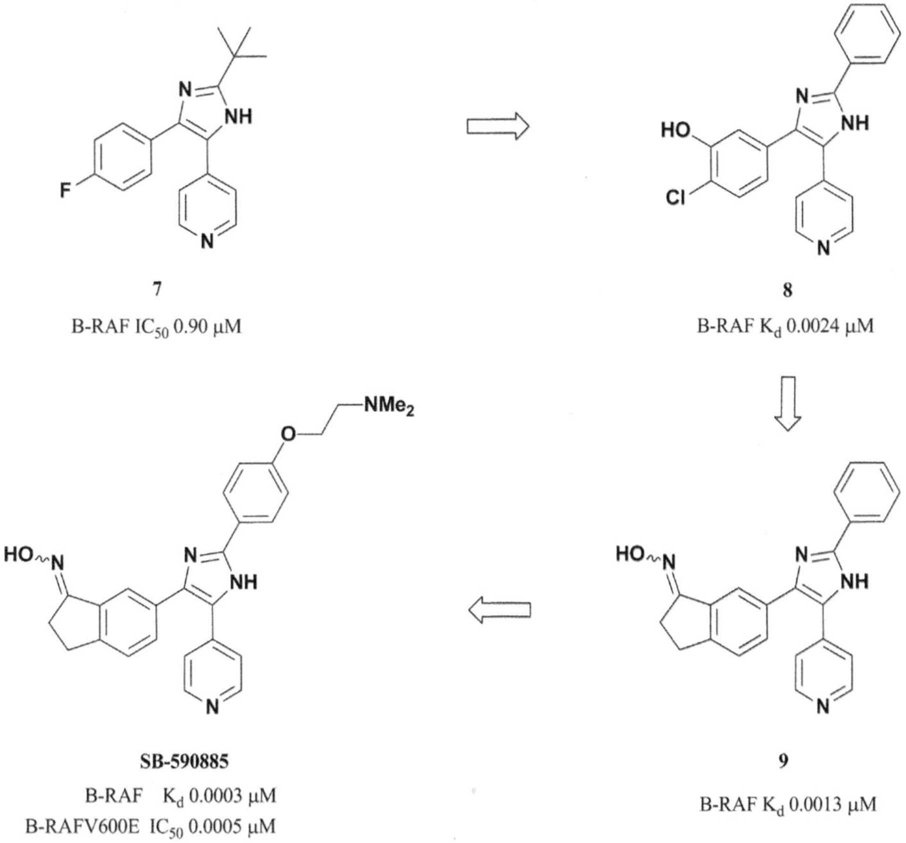

7

B-RAF IC$_{50}$ 0.90 μM

8

B-RAF K$_d$ 0.0024 μM

SB-590885

B-RAF   K$_d$ 0.0003 μM

B-RAFV600E IC$_{50}$ 0.0005 μM

9

B-RAF K$_d$ 0.0013 μM

FIGURE 18.14   Key steps leading to the discovery of SB-590885.

most apparent in established CRC (Colo-205 and HT29) and melanoma cell lines (A375P, SKMEL28, and MALME-3M) that expressed B-RAF^{V600E} following brief incubation with SB-590885, whereas normal cells (HFF, HMEC, and PREC) and malignant cells not expressing mutant B-RAF (HT-1080, HCT-116, and SKMEL2) showed intermediate sensitivity or resistance. Furthermore, prolonged incubation with SB-590885 preferentially decreased the proliferation of cells expressing oncogenic B-RAF^{V600E}. Both normal melanocytes and primary melanoma cells that express B-RAF^{WT} (WM-NCI) showed increased phosphorylated ERK levels following brief incubation with SB-590885, another example of the paradoxical activation of the nonmutated RAF MAPK pathway by a B-RAF inhibitor (Fig. 18.11). SB-590885 decreased tumorigenesis in murine xenografts established from mutant B-RAF-expressing A375P melanoma cells, although the effect on tumor growth was modest. A combination of the poor pharmacokinetics of SB-590885, the modest efficacy in xenograft models, and a low safety window in seven-day toxicology studies led to termination of its development as an anticancer agent.

Co-crystals of SB-590885 bound to the B-RAF^{V600E} kinase domain revealed that SB-590885 occupies the ATP-binding pocket and binds to an active conformation of B-RAF, as shown in

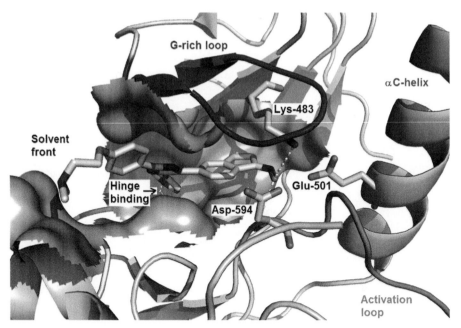

FIGURE 18.15 SB-590885 binding in the ATP-binding pocket of B-RAF. (This figure is reproduced in color in the color plate section.)

Fig. 18.15 [35]. The pyridine forms the hinge-binding interaction with the NH of Cys532. The indane-oxime crystallizes with Z-geometry, forming a strong interaction with the salt bridge of B-RAF formed between Lys403 and Glu501, as well as a hydrogen bond with a backbone amide of Asp594 in the activation loop, thus likely driving the selectivity and potency of SB-590885.

Discovery of Dabrafenib

The origin of the development of dabrafenib was a program to develop a follow-up drug to the dual EGFR–erbB2 kinase inhibitor lapatinib (Tykerb®), which in the early 2000s was progressing through clinical trials. The goal of the program during this early period was to identify an inhibitor with activity against both EGFR–erbB2 and additional kinases, such as B-RAF and IGF1R, that were thought to be involved in pathways important for proliferation in tumors that had acquired resistance to lapatinib. Screening of the kinase inhibitor collection at GlaxoSmithKline identified the pyrazolopyridine **11**, which had excellent EGFR–erbB2 inhibition plus modest activity against both B-RAF and IGF1R (Fig. 18.16). A significant increase in B-RAF potency was observed by switching the heterocycle to an imidazopyridine core and attachment of the N-methyl-tetrahydroisoquinoline to the pyrimidine amine to yield **12** [36]. However, imidazopyridine **12** had little activity in either mechanistic (pERK) or antiproliferative cell-based assays using the B-RAF^{V600E} mutant SKMEL28 cell line. Further lead optimization efforts around alternative heterocycle "cores" led to the identification of the thiazole **13**, which had the advantage over other heterocyclic analogs in demonstrating efficacy in the mechanistic pERK assay.

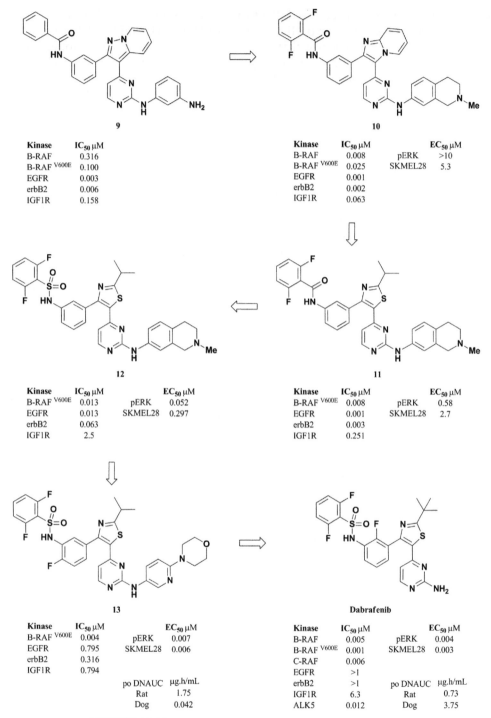

FIGURE 18.16 Key steps leading to the discovery of dabrafenib.

As the lead optimization progressed, the focus of the program morphed from looking to optimize a triple kinase inhibitor profile (EGFR–erbB2, B-RAF, and/or IGF1R) to a B-RAF stand-alone effort. The rationale was that as lapatinib successfully moved through late-stage clinical trials and its probability of being approved increased, it became clear that multikinase inhibition could be more easily evaluated as combinations of single agents instead of trying to fit the desired profile into one molecule. This had the benefit of greatly simplifying the lead optimization process for the thiazole series. Evaluation of several replacements for the aryl amide linker revealed that the arylsulfonamide thiazole **14** showed a substantial 10-fold improvement in cellular potency, specifically the pERK mechanistic and antiproliferative assays run in B-RAF^{V600E} mutant SKMEL28 cells. This 2,6-difluorinated sulfonamide provided the best combination of potency and metabolic stability, and was thus used for further SAR exploration in other regions of the molecule. Having achieved excellent potency in the enzyme and cellular assays, the focus turned to further improving the metabolic stability of the series, as it suffered from high intrinsic clearances in rat liver microsomes and poor oral exposures in the rat. In an attempt to improve the metabolic stability of the series, potential metabolic sites were targeted, and one approach was to systematically install fluorines around the phenyl ring connecting the thiazole core to the sulfonamide. Fluorination para to the thiazole as shown in thiazole **15** was found to reduce both intrinsic and intravenous clearance, providing an almost 70-fold increase in the rat oral dose-normalized AUC for compared to the nonfluronated analog. The large jump in rat oral exposure afforded by this fluorination may be the result of both an increased metabolic stability, by blocking a major metabolic site, and oral absorption, perhaps by affording an intramolecular hydrogen-bonding interaction with the sulfonamide NH, thus masking one hydrogen bond donor.

The remaining challenge was to improve the pharmacokinetics in higher species such as dog. Metabolite identification studies conducted in dog and monkey liver microsomes identified several major metabolites clustered in the isopropylthiazole core and 6-(4-morpholinyl)-3-pyridinamine regions of **15** [37]. To modify these metabolic hotspots, the isopropyl group attached to the thiazole of **15** was replaced with a *t*-butyl group, and the pyrimidine moiety was truncated to a free 2-amino-pyrimidine, which had the added benefit of substantially reducing the molecular weight by over 20%. Finally, relocation of the fluorine ortho to both the thiazole and the sulfonamide yielded dabrafenib. Dabrafenib displayed compelling nanomolar inhibitory activity in enzyme and cellular mechanistic assays, and in cell proliferation assays in B-RAF^{V600E}-driven melanoma lines. Additionally, acceptable rat and dramatically improved dog pharmacokinetic profiles were observed, in contrast to earlier analogs prepared.

Structure of Dabrafenib in B-RAF

Dabrafenib is an ATP-competitive reversible inhibitor of B-RAF and is postulated to bind to an inactive conformation of the kinase. The crystal structure of a related thiazole analog **16** (Fig. 18.17) co-crystallized in the B-RAF^{V600E} kinase domain is illustrated in Fig. 18.18 [37]. Similar to that observed in the crystal structure of vemurafenib, the αC helix "shifts out" relative to an active-like conformation, and a salt bridge between the conserved Lys483 and Glu501 is broken. While Phe595 is not in a "DFG-out" conformation, it is rotated to form the floor of a pocket similar to that observed in a reported lapatinib–EGFR co-structure. The pyrimidine N1 forms the classic hinge interaction with Cys532 in the ATP-binding

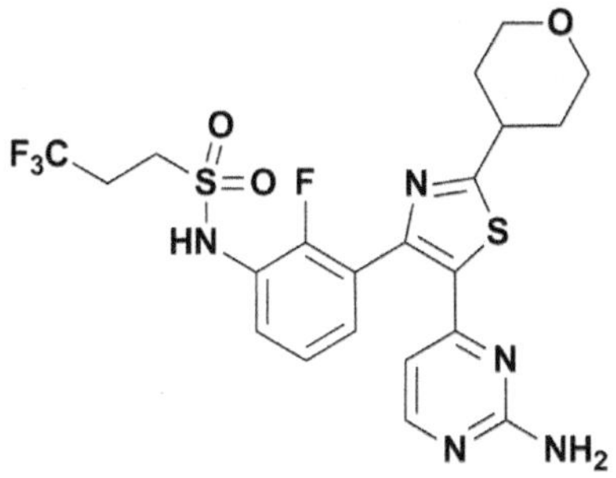

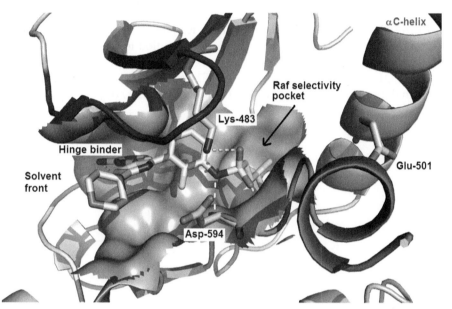

16

FIGURE 18.17 Dabrafenib analog **14**.

FIGURE 18.18 Dabrafenib analog **14** binding in the ATP-binding pocket of B-RAF. (This figure is reproduced in color in the color plate section.)

pocket of the enzyme. The *t*-butyl group and thiazole core bind underneath the P-loop, leaving only a relatively small portion of the inhibitor as solvent exposed. Analogous to vemurafenib, the arylsulfonamide binds into the "Raf selectivity pocket". The sulfonamide NH is depicted in a deprotonated form, leaving the nitrogen to participate as a hydrogen bond acceptor to the backbone NH of Asp594. This is consistent with the calculated pKa of the sulfonamide NH of around 7, while the pKa for other linkers examined such as amide or urea ranged from 10 to 12. The difference in pKa and thus the ability of the NH to ionize at cellular pH may explain the large potency gain observed with the sulfonamide linker. Finally, the ammonium ion of Lys483 is in close proximity to the sulfonamide anion, and can form a hydrogen bond with one of the sulfonamide oxygens, whereas the other sulfonamide oxygen forms a hydrogen bond with the backbone NH of Phe595. The improvement in potency observed with compounds bearing a fluorine substitution is hypothesized to be potentially a result of both modulating the pKa of the sulfonamide NH, which could allow both increased ionization at cellular pH, and allowing for a more favorable conformation for arylsulfonamide to bind.

Biology of Dabrafenib

Dabrafenib was screened against a set of 61 kinases representing broad coverage of the kinome and was found to be a potent nanomolar biochemical inhibitor of B-RAF^{V600E}, wt B-RAF, and C-RAF, with >500 fold selectivity for B-RAF compared to most kinases screened. Significant other activity (<100-fold selectivity) was observed only for Alk5 kinase in the screening panel [37]. Potent inhibitory activity was observed in the cellular mechanistic assay (pERK EC$_{50}$ 4 nM); as well as cell proliferation assays in B-RAF^{V600E}-driven melanoma lines SKMEL28 (IC$_{50}$ 3 nM) and A375P F11 (pERK IC$_{50}$ 8 nM); and the colorectal carcinoma line, Colo-205 (pERK IC$_{50}$ 7 nM). Dabrafenib was also studied in vivo and was found to dramatically reduce tumor growth in mice bearing B-Raf^{V600E} human melanoma tumors [38]. In this model, CD1 *nu/nu* mice bearing A375P F11 (B-Raf^{V600E}) tumors were dosed orally once daily with dabrafenib at doses of 0.1, 1, 10, and 100 mg/kg/day for 14 days (Fig. 18.19).

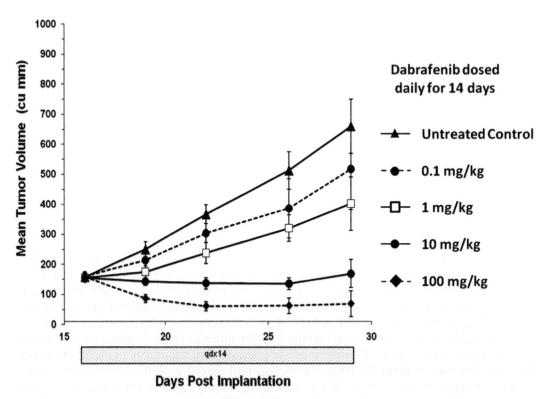

FIGURE 18.19   In vivo efficacy of dabrafenib in CD1 *nu/nu* mice bearing A375P F11 (B-Raf^{V600E}) tumors, $n = 8/$ group.

Dose-proportional reductions in tumor growth were observed. Tumor growth delay was observed at 0.1 and 1 mg/kg, tumor stasis at 10 mg/kg, and tumor regression in the 100 mg/kg dose groups. Body weight was also measured, and no significant changes were observed at all doses tested. Notably, in the 100 mg/kg group, complete tumor regression was observed in 50% of treated animals.

Additionally, dabrafenib reduced the levels of pERK in A375P F11 (B-Raf^{V600E}) tumor tissue in vivo in a dose-dependent manner after a single oral dose [37]. Tumors were collected at 2, 6, and 24 h post dose, and pERK levels in each were measured and normalized to the total ERK present. Levels of pERK and ERK were substantially reduced at 2 and 6 h post dose, with a notable pharmacodynamic effect (>50% inhibition) at doses ≥3 mg/kg in this single-dose study, which returned to untreated levels by 24 h at doses ≤30 mg/kg.

Clinical Efficacy of Dabrafenib

A phase I dose escalation trial of dabrafenib enrolled 184 patients with B-RAF mutations, of whom 156 had metastatic melanoma [39]. Doses were increased to 300 mg bid with no MTD recorded, and, on the basis of safety, pharmacokinetic, and response data, a phase II dose of 150 mg bid was chosen. The most common treatment-related adverse events of grade 2 or worse were cutaneous squamous cell carcinoma (11%), fatigue (8%), and pyrexia (6%). At the 150 mg bid dose in 36 patients with B-RAF^{V600} mutant melanoma, responses were reported in 25 patients and confirmed responses in 18 patients, with 17 patients on treatment for more than 6 months. Responses were recorded in patients with non-B-RAF^{V600E} mutations. In patients with melanoma and untreated brain metastases, remarkably, nine of 10 patients had reductions in size of brain lesions. The activity of dabrafenib against brain metastases was initially a serendipitous finding at one study site. Dabrafenib was not designed to cross the blood–brain barrier, and patients with brain metastases would not normally be included in the clinical trial as no benefit would be predicted. In one patient, a PET scan performed just before starting treatment revealed a brain metastasis, but this result was not available until after treatment began. A follow-up PET scan two weeks later showed decreased metabolic activity in the brain metastasis, and subsequent magnetic resonance imaging showed a reduction in its size. In 28 patients with B-RAF mutant nonmelanoma solid tumors, apparent antitumor activity was noted in a gastrointestinal stromal tumor, papillary thyroid cancers, NSCLC, ovarian cancer, and CRC.

In a phase II study in patients with asymptomatic active brain metastases, known as BREAK-MB, patients with histologically confirmed B-RAF^{V600E} or B-RAF^{V600K} mutant melanoma and at least one asymptomatic brain metastasis were treated with dabrafenib [40]. The study enrolled 172 patients, of whom 81% had B-RAF^{V600E} mutant melanoma. Patients were split into two cohorts: those in cohort A had not received previous local treatment for brain metastases, and those in cohort B had progressive brain metastases after previous local treatments. A total of 29 of 74 patients with B-RAF^{V600E} mutant melanoma in cohort A achieved an overall intracranial response, as did 20 of 65 in cohort B. One of 15 patients with B-RAF^{V600K} mutant melanoma achieved an overall intracranial response in cohort A, as did four of 18 such patients in cohort B. Treatment-related adverse events of grade 3 or worse occurred in 38 (22%) patients.

An open-label randomized phase III study of dabrafenib (BREAK-3) was conducted in 250 patients with B-RAF^{V600E}-mutated metastatic melanoma [41]. Patients were randomly

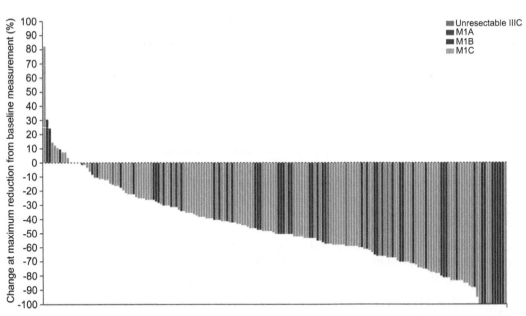

FIGURE 18.20 Maximum tumor percent change from baseline in patients treated with dabrafenib ($n = 187$). Each bar represents data for an individual patient; negative values indicate tumor shrinkage. *Figure reproduced with permission from Ref. [41] © (2012) Elsevier. All rights reserved.* (This figure is reproduced in color in the color plate section.)

assigned in a 3:1 ratio to dabrafenib at 150 mg orally bid or dacarbazine at 1000 mg/m^2 intravenously every three weeks, with patients in the dacarbazine arm allowed to cross over in cases of disease progression. Confirmed objective responses were reported in 93 (50%) of the 187 patients randomly assigned to dabrafenib, in keeping with phase I–II studies as well as with the vemurafenib BRIM-3 trial; whereas six (3%) had a complete response, as illustrated in Fig. 18.20. The median PFS (the time from randomization to the earliest date of disease progression or death due to any cause) was 5.1 months. The most common adverse events were cutaneous squamous cell cancer, pyrexia, fatigue, headache, and arthralgia. More severe toxic effects of grades 3–4 were uncommon. Although precise comparisons are not possible across trials, the toxicity profile of dabrafenib seems to be different from that of vemurafenib, with lower incidence of photosensitivity (<1% versus 12%), squamous cell cancer (6% versus 18%), joint pain (6% versus 21%), and fatigue (6% versus 13%). The more favorable profile of dabrafenib is potentially the result of the lower dose or increased potency against C-RAF or wild-type B-RAF compared to vemurafenib.

XL281 (BMS-908662)

XL281 is an ATP competitive inhibitor of B-RAF^{WT}, B-RAF^{V600E}, and C-RAF, with potencies of 4.5, 6.0, and 2.6 nM, respectively [42]. It was developed by Exelixis and licensed to Bristol Myers Squibb. The structure of XL281 has not been disclosed. XL281 is active in a range of tumor cell lines and human tumor xenograft models with mutant or wild-type B-RAF or

KRAS (A375, MDA-MB-231, HCT116, and A431), and showed potent pMEK and pERK biomarker inhibition following single oral dose administration. A phase I clinical trial of XL281 was undertaken in 2007 in 30 patients with CRC, papillary thyroid cancer (PTC), NSCLC, malignant melanoma, and other tumors [42]. XL281 was dose-escalated orally once daily on a 28-day cycle, and the oral MTD was determined to be 150 mg. Dose-limiting toxicities of fatigue, nausea, vomiting, and diarrhea were observed at the highest dose of 225 mg administered. Downregulation of both pERK and pMEK of about 70% was observed in tumor and surrogate tissues, with decreases in cell proliferation and increases in apoptosis. Ten patients each with CRC, melanoma, PTC, and NSCLC tumors were treated at the MTD of 150 mg. One patient with ocular melanoma achieved a partial remission of 4 months' duration, and 12 subjects had stable disease lasting over three months, including two PTC patients harboring B-RAF^{V600E} mutations. Subsequent to this study, a phase I study of XL281 in combination with cetuximab (Erbitux®), an EGFR monoclonal antibody, was undertaken in subjects with KRAS or B-RAF mutation–positive advanced or metastatic CRC (http://www.clinicaltrials.gov ID: NCT01086267).

RESISTANCE MECHANISMS

De Novo Resistance

Drug resistance can be divided into two general types: de novo resistance presents in patients who are resistant to therapy from the beginning of the treatment, and acquired resistance occurs in those who develop resistance during treatment. Few mechanisms of primary resistance to mutant B-RAF inhibitors have been validated to be recurrent and significant in patients. The most readily available system for such investigations is immortalized B-RAF^{V600E} melanoma-resistant cell lines exposed chronically to selective B-RAF inhibitors, but it remains to be validated that these cell lines truly represent primary melanoma resistance in the clinic. In considering the phenomenon of de novo resistance, the fact that B-RAF mutation is commonly accompanied by genetic alterations that result in activation of the PI3K–AKT and cyclin D1–CDK4 pathways is noteworthy [43]. Phosphatase and tensin homolog (PTEN) functions as a tumor suppressor by negatively regulating the PI3K–AKT signaling pathway (Fig. 18.21). Approximately half of B-RAF mutant melanomas are thought to harbor PTEN mutations or have deletions or epigenetic silencing that significantly reduces PTEN expression. In cell lines with both B-RAF^{V600E} and PTEN loss, sensitivity to B-RAF small interfering RNA knockdown or one of the selective B-RAF inhibitors is less than in B-RAF^{V600E}- and PTEN-intact cell lines. In vitro synergy has been demonstrated between inhibitors of PI3K, AKT, or mTOR in combination with B-RAF inhibitors, and it remains to be seen in the clinic how well tolerated a combined targeting of B-RAF and/or MEK inhibitors with PI3K pathway inhibitors will be [44].

Acquired Resistance

The emergence of acquired resistance with cancer drugs is an unfortunate but predictable event, and with single-agent B-RAF therapy this is evidenced by the limited duration of the

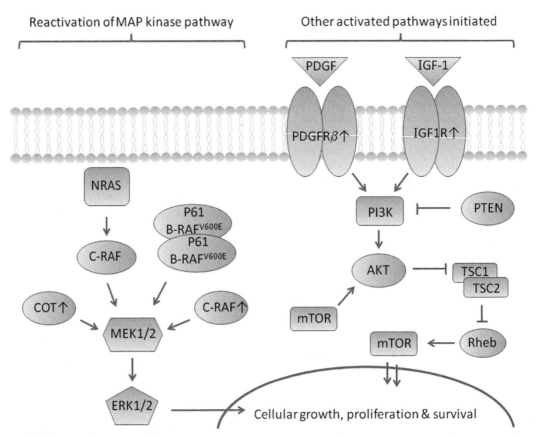

FIGURE 18.21   Potential mechanisms of B-RAF-acquired resistance. (For color version of this figure, the reader is referred to the online version of this book.)

antitumor effect observed in the clinic. Therefore, understanding the resistance mechanism to this new generation of B-RAF inhibitors is critical to providing clues both for developing improved inhibitors and for guiding the selection of appropriate drug combinations for therapy. Acquired resistance to kinase inhibitors has precedence. For example, shortly after the introduction in 2001 of imatinib (Gleevec®), the first approved small-molecule kinase inhibitor, investigators began to describe a number of in vitro–derived cell lines with acquired resistance to the drug, which was rapidly followed by clinical resistance in patients. Imatinib inhibits the Bcr–Abl tyrosine kinase, and the Bcr–Abl-dependent mechanisms include point mutations within the Bcr–Abl kinase domain that interfere with imatinib binding while retaining the kinase's full oncogenic activity. The understanding of this resistance mechanism in chronic myeloid leukemia accelerated the development of the two next-generation inhibitors, dasatinib and nilotinib, for patients with resistance or intolerance to imatinib; these were approved in 2006 and 2007, respectively. Following this precedent, secondary mutations in the B-RAF kinase domain would be the expected primary driver of acquired resistance to vemurafenib, but surprisingly this appears not to be the case. Direct sequencing of *B-RAF* exons from tumors biopsied or resected from patients with acquired resistance to vemurafenib showed no secondary B-RAF mutations, and the V600E mutation was conserved [45]. This observation is even more surprising given that engineered mutations mimicking those that confer resistance to imatinib, specifically at the threonine gatekeeper residue at the back of the ATP-binding pocket, were found to confer vemurafenib resistance to B-RAF^{V600E}-driven tumors in xenograft models [46].

Two distinct categories of resistance mechanisms have been described to date from multiple patients who have relapsed on either vemurafenib or dabrafenib, those that reactivate the MAP kinase pathway and those that have initiated other activated pathways, as shown in Fig. 18.21 [45]. Appearance of activating NRAS or MEK mutations, concurrent with B-RAF^{V600E}, has been identified in individual cases. Mutated RAS has previously been shown to preferentially signal through C-RAF as opposed to B-RAF [47]. Increased expression of COT, a kinase that also phosphorylates MEK in a B-RAF-independent manner, has also been described [45]. In addition, B-RAF^{V600E} truncation, via alternative splicing, resulting in a RAS-independent constitutively activated p61 B-RAF^{V600E} dimer has been shown to reactivate the MAPK pathway in the face of B-RAF inhibition [48]. Alternatively, receptor tyrosine kinase overexpression of platelet-derived growth factor receptor (PDGFRβ) and insulin-like growth factor receptor (IGF1-R) upregulates the PI3K–AKT pathway, serving to provide MAPK-redundant survival signaling [43].

COMBINATORIAL THERAPIES

Fully understanding the resistance mechanisms will be vital to designing combinatorial targeted treatments designed to overcome resistance in B-RAF inhibitor therapy. Patients who have acquired resistance to vemurafenib or dabrafenib by reactivation of the MAP kinase pathway and restoration of MEK activation would be expected to respond to combined therapy of a B-RAF inhibitor and MEK inhibitor to either prevent or delay resistance. In addition, this combination should prevent MEK activation in normal tissues, which could overcome the complication of low-grade squamous cell carcinomas. Dabrafenib drug-resistant clones were isolated from the A375 B-RAF^{V600E} and the YUSIT1 B-RAF^{V600K} melanoma cell lines, which also showed reduced sensitivity to the MEK inhibitor trametinib. The combination of dabrafenib and trametinib effectively inhibited cell growth, decreased ERK phosphorylation, decreased cyclin D1 protein, and increased p27kip1 protein in these resistant clones [44].

A phase I and II open-label study of combined treatment with dabrafenib and trametinib was conducted involving 247 patients with metastatic melanoma and B-RAF^{V600} mutations [49]. The pharmacokinetic activity and safety of oral dabrafenib and trametinib in 85 patients were initially evaluated; there were no drug-to-drug interactions, and both agents could be safely combined when each was administered at its full single-agent dose. In the phase II portion of the study, 162 patients were randomized into three groups that received different dose combinations: two daily 150 mg doses of dabrafenib plus one 2 mg or 1 mg trametinib dose, or treatment with dabrafenib alone. Participants receiving dabrafenib alone were able to cross over to the full-dose combination treatment if their cancer resumed progression. Patients taking dabrafenib and trametinib together delayed tumors from progressing for 9.4 months,

TABLE 18.1   Announced or active B-RAF combination clinical trials

B-RAF Inhibitor	Combination therapy	Mechanism	ClinicalTrials.gov
Vemurafenib	Everolimus (Afinitor®, Novartis)	mTOR inhibitor	NCT01596140
	Temsirolimus (Torisel®, Pfizer)	mTOR inhibitor	NCT01596140
	PX-866 (Oncothyreon)	PI3K inhibitor	NCT01616199
	BKM120 (BMS)	PI3K inhibitor	NCT01512251
	GDC-0973 (Exelixis)	MEK inhibitor	NCT01689519
	XL888 (Exelixis)	HSP90 inhibitor	NCT01657591
	Ipilimumab (Yervoy®, BMS)	CTLA-4 mAb	NCT01400451
	Bevacizumab (Avastin®, Roche)	VEGF-A mAb	NCT01495988
Dabrafenib	Trametinib (Mekinist®, GSK)	MEK inhibitor	NCT01584648 NCT01597908
	Panitumumab (Vectibix®, Amgen)	EGFR mAb	NCT01750918
	Pazopanib (Votrient®, GSK)	VEGFR inhibitor	NCT01713972
LGX818	MEK162 (Array/Novartis)	MEK inhibitor	NCT01543698
	BYL719 (Novartis)	PI3K inhibitor	NCT01719380
RAF265	MEK162 (Array/Novartis)	MEK inhibitor	NCT01352273
Sorafenib	Temsirolimus (Torisel®, Pfizer)	mTOR inhibitor	NCT00349206
	Everolimus (Afinitor®, Novartis)	mTOR inhibitor	NCT01687673

compared with 5.8 months for patients taking dabrafenib alone. After one year of treatment, 41% of those receiving the full-dose combination treatment had no progression of their cancer, compared with only 9% of those receiving one drug. Dose-limiting toxic effects were infrequently observed in patients receiving combination therapy with 150 mg of dabrafenib and 2 mg of trametinib. Cutaneous squamous cell carcinoma was seen in 7% of patients receiving combination and in 19% receiving monotherapy, whereas pyrexia was more common in the combination group than in the monotherapy group (71% versus 26%). These data confirm that the MAPK pathway plays a role in resistance to B-RAF inhibitor therapy and that the addition of an MEK inhibitor to a B-RAF inhibitor represents one strategy for delaying the emergence of this resistance mechanism.

As shown in Table 18.1, a large number of clinical trials are now underway or recruiting patients for combination studies of B-RAF inhibitors with additional agents targeted to overcome resistance seen in melanoma therapy. MEK inhibitors, which should block reactivation of the MAP kinase, are under active investigation with dabrafenib, vemurafenib, LGX818, and RAF265. Combinations with PI3K or mTOR inhibitors, which should block restoration of MEK activation via the PI3K–AKT pathway, are being studied with vemurafenib, LGX818, and sorafenib. A combination study of dabrafenib with an EGFR antibody to block EGFR-mediated reactivation of the MAPK pathway has recently been initiated specifically in CRCs.

CONCLUSIONS

For decades, stage IV metastatic melanoma was treated with chemotherapy of limited value with a low survival rate, making it one of the most lethal solid tumors unless detected early. The discovery a decade ago of *B-RAF* mutations in a large percentage of melanoma patients has provided a new therapeutic opportunity, leading to a new generation of selective B-RAF inhibitors targeting the molecular underpinnings of this cancer. Agents such as vemurafenib and dabrafenib have demonstrated very high response rates even in patients with very advanced, symptomatic, metastatic disease and have completely changed the therapeutic landscape. However, these exciting findings are tempered by the fact that these responses are typically not long-lived, and understanding and exploiting the mechanisms of resistance via combination therapy or second-generation drugs are high priorities if further advances are going to be made. One hopes that the introduction of these selective B-RAF inhibitors is the beginning of a new era in drug development targeting metastatic melanoma and other cancers driven by *B-RAF* mutations, and that one day such cancers can be considered beaten.

Acknowledgments

The author would like to thank Ami Lakdawala Shah (GlaxoSmithKline, King of Prussia, PA, USA) for creating the co-crystal structure images illustrated in Figs 18.5, 18.7, 18.15, and 18.18, which were made using PyMOL.

References

[1] Pearson G, Robinson F, Beers Gibson T, Xu BE, Karandikar M, Berman K, et al. Mitogen-activated protein (MAP) kinase pathways: regulation and physiological functions. Endocr Rev 2001;2:153–83.

[2] Cargnello M, Roux PP. Activation and function of the MAPKs and their substrates, the MAPK-activated protein kinases. Microbiol Mol Biol Rev 2011;75:50–83.

[3] Robinson MJ, Cobb MH. Mitogen-activated protein kinase pathways. Curr Opin Cell Biol 1997;9:180–6.

[4] Zebisch A, Troppmair J. Back to the roots: the remarkable RAF oncogene story. Cell Mol Life Sci 2006;63:1314–30.

[5] Wellbrock C, Karasarides M, Marais R. The RAF proteins take centre stage. Nat Rev Mol Cell Biol 2004;5:875–85.

[6] Wan PT, Garnett MJ, Roe SM, Lee S, Niculescu-Duvaz D, Good VM, et al. Mechanism of activation of the RAF–ERK signaling pathway by oncogenic mutations of B-RAF. Cell 2004;116:855–67.

[7] Davies H, Bignell GR, Cox C, Stephens P, Edkins S, Clegg S, et al. Mutations of the BRAF gene in human cancer. Nature 2002;417:949–54.

[8] Roskoski Jr R. RAF protein-serine/threonine kinases: structure and regulation. Biochem Biophys Res Commun 2010;399:313–7.

[9] Brummer T, Martin P, Herzog S, Misawa Y, Daly RJ, Reth M. Functional analysis of the regulatory requirements of B-Raf and the B-Raf$^{(V600E)}$ oncoprotein. Oncogene 2006;25:6262–76.

[10] Santarpia L, Lippman SM, El-Naggar AK. Targeting the MAPK-RAS-RAF signaling pathway in cancer therapy. Expert Opin Ther Targets 2012;16:103–19.

[11] Wilhelm S, Carter C, Lynch M, Lowinger T, Dumas J, Smith RA, et al. Discovery and development of sorafenib: a multikinase inhibitor for treating cancer. Nat Rev Drug Discov 2006;5:835–44.

[12] Wilhelm SM, Carter C, Tang L, Wilkie D, McNabola A, Rong H, et al. BAY 43-9006 exhibits broad spectrum oral antitumor activity and targets the RAF/MEK/ERK pathway and receptor tyrosine kinases involved in tumor progression and angiogenesis. Cancer Res 2004;64:7099–109.

[13] Strumberg D, Richly H, Hilger RA, Schleucher N, Korfee S, Tewes M, et al. Phase I clinical and pharmacokinetic study of the novel Raf kinase and vascular endothelial growth factor receptor inhibitor BAY 43-9006 in patients with advanced refractory solid tumors. J Clin Oncol 2005;23:965–72.

[14] Ratain MJ, Eisen T, Stadler WM, Flaherty KT, Kaye SB, Rosner GL, et al. Phase II placebo-controlled randomized discontinuation trial of sorafenib in patients with metastatic renal cell carcinoma. J Clin Oncol 2006;24:2505–12.

[15] Escudier B, Eisen T, Stadler WM, Szczylik C, Oudard S, Staehler M, et al. Sorafenib for treatment of renal cell carcinoma: final efficacy and safety results of the phase III treatment approaches in renal cancer global evaluation trial. J Clin Oncol 2009;27:3312–8.

[16] Eisen T, Ahmad T, Flaherty KT, Gore M, Kaye S, Marais R, et al. Sorafenib in advanced melanoma: a phase II randomised discontinuation trial analysis. Br J Cancer 2006;95:581–6.

[17] Liu L, Cao Y, Chen C, Zhang X, McNabola A, Wilkie D, et al. Sorafenib blocks the RAF/MEK/ERK pathway, inhibits tumor angiogenesis, and induces tumor cell apoptosis in hepatocellular carcinoma model PLC/PRF/5. Cancer Res 2006;66:11851–8.

[18] Llovet JM, Ricci S, Mazzaferro V, Hilgard P, Gane E, Blanc JF, et al. Sorafenib in advanced hepatocellular carcinoma. N Engl J Med 2008;359:378–90.

[19] Forner A, Llovet JM, Bruix J. Hepatocellular carcinoma. Lancet 2012;379:1245–55.

[20] Ramurthy S, Subramanian S, Aikawa M, Amiri P, Costales A, Dove J, et al. Design and synthesis of orally bioavailable benzimidazoles as Raf kinase inhibitors. J Med Chem 2008;51:7049–52.

[21] Su Y, Vilgelm AE, Kelley MC, Hawkins OE, Liu Y, Boyd KL, et al. RAF265 inhibits the growth of advanced human melanoma tumors. Clin Cancer Res 2012;18:2184–98.

[22] Sharfman WH, Hodi FS, Lawrence DP, Flaherty KT, Amaravadi RK, Kim KB, et al. Results from the first-in-human (FIH) phase I study of the oral RAF inhibitor RAF265 administered daily to patients with advanced cutaneous melanoma. J Clin Oncol 2011;29(Suppl.); Abstract 8508.

[23] Stuart DD, Li N, Poon DJ, Aardalen K, Kaufman S, Merritt H, et al. Preclinical profile of LGX818: a potent and selective RAF kinase inhibitor. Cancer Res 2012;72(8 Suppl); Abstract 3790.

[24] Bollag G, Tsai J, Zhang J, Zhang C, Ibrahim P, Nolop K, et al. Vemurafenib: the first drug approved for BRAF-mutant cancer. Nat Rev Drug Discov 2012;11:873–86.

[25] Tsai J, Lee JT, Wang W, Zhang J, Cho H, Mamo S, et al. Discovery of a selective inhibitor of oncogenic B-Raf kinase with potent antimelanoma activity. Proc Natl Acad Sci USA 2008;105:3041–6.

[26] Su F, Viros A, Milagre C, Trunzer K, Bollag G, Spleiss O, et al. RAS mutations in cutaneous squamous-cell carcinomas in patients treated with BRAF inhibitors. N Engl J Med 2012;366:207–15.

[27] Yang H, Higgins B, Kolinsky K, Packman K, Go Z, Iyer R, et al. RG7204 (PLX4032), a selective BRAFV600E inhibitor, displays potent antitumor activity in preclinical melanoma models. Cancer Res 2010;70:5518–27.

[28] Bollag G, Hirth P, Tsai J, Zhang J, Ibrahim PN, Cho H, et al. Clinical efficacy of a RAF inhibitor needs broad target blockade in BRAF-mutant melanoma. Nature 2010;467:596–9.

[29] Flaherty KT, Puzanov I, Kim KB, Ribas A, McArthur GA, Sosman JA, et al. Inhibition of mutated, activated BRAF in metastatic melanoma. N Engl J Med 2010;363:809–19.

[30] Corcoran RB, Ebi H, Turke AB, Coffee EM, Nishino M, Cogdill AP, et al. EGFR-mediated re-activation of MAPK signaling contributes to insensitivity of BRAF mutant colorectal cancers to RAF inhibition with vemurafenib. Cancer Discov 2012;2:227–35.

[31] Prahallad A, Sun C, Huang S, Di Nicolantonio F, Salazar R, Zecchin D, et al. Unresponsiveness of colon cancer to BRAF(V600E) inhibition through feedback activation of EGFR. Nature 2012;483:100–3.

[32] Sosman JA, Kim KB, Schuchter L, Gonzalez R, Pavlick AC, Weber JS, et al. Survival in BRAF V600-mutant advanced melanoma treated with vemurafenib. N Engl J Med 2012;366:707–14.

[33] Chapman PB, Hauschild A, Robert C, Haanen JB, Ascierto P, Larkin J, et al. Improved survival with vemurafenib in melanoma with BRAF V600E mutation. N Engl J Med 2011;364:2507–16.

[34] Takle AK, Brown MJ, Davies S, Dean DK, Francis G, Gaiba A, et al. The identification of potent and selective imidazole-based inhibitors of B-Raf kinase. Bioorg Med Chem Lett 2006;16:378–81.

[35] King AJ, Patrick DR, Batorsky RS, Ho ML, Do HT, Zhang SY, et al. Demonstration of a genetic therapeutic index for tumors expressing oncogenic BRAF by the kinase inhibitor SB-590885. Cancer Res 2006;66:11100–5.

[36] Stellwagen JC, Adjabeng GM, Arnone MR, Dickerson SH, Han C, Hornberger KR, et al. Development of potent B-RafV600E inhibitors containing an arylsulfonamide headgroup. Bioorg Med Chem Lett 2011;21:4436–40.

[37] Rheault TR, Stellwagen JC, Dickerson SH, Adjabeng GM, Hornberger KR, Petrov KG, et al. The discovery of GSK2118436 (dabrafenib): a potent and selective inhibitor of Raf kinases with anti-tumor activity against oncogenic B-Raf driven tumors. ACS Med Chem Lett 2013;4:358–62.

[38] King AJ, Arnone MR, Bleam MR, Moss KG, Yang J, Fisher KE, et al. Dabrafenib; Preclinical Characterization, Increased Efficacy when Combined with Trametinib, while BRAF/MEK Tool Combination Reduced Skin Lesions. PLoS One; 2013 in press.

[39] Falchook GS, Long GV, Kurzrock R, Kim KB, Arkenau TH, Brown MP, et al. Dabrafenib in patients with melanoma, untreated brain metastases, and other solid tumors: a phase 1 dose-escalation trial. Lancet 2012;379:1893–901.

[40] Long GV, Trefzer U, Davies MA, Kefford RF, Ascierto PA, Chapman PB, et al. Dabrafenib in patients with Val-600Glu or Val600Lys BRAF-mutant melanoma metastatic to the brain (BREAK-MB): a multicentre, open-label, phase 2 trial. Lancet Oncol 2012;13:1087–95.

[41] Hauschild A, Grob JJ, Demidov LV, Jouary T, Gutzmer R, Millward M, et al. Dabrafenib in BRAF-mutated metastatic melanoma: a multicentre, open-label, phase 3 randomised controlled trial. Lancet 2012;380:358–65.

[42] Schwartz GK, Robertson S, Shen A, Wang E, Pace L, Dials H, et al. A phase I study of XL281, a selective oral RAF kinase inhibitor, in patients (Pts) with advanced solid tumors. J Clin Oncol 2009;27(15s Suppl.); Abstract 3513.

[43] Pérez-Lorenzo R, Zheng B. Targeted inhibition of BRAF kinase: opportunities and challenges for therapeutics in melanoma. Biosci Rep 2012;32:25–33.

[44] Greger JG, Eastman SD, Zhang V, Bleam MR, Hughes AM, Smitheman KN, et al. Combinations of BRAF, MEK, and PI3K/mTOR inhibitors overcome acquired resistance to the BRAF inhibitor GSK2118436 dabrafenib, mediated by NRAS or MEK mutations. Mol Cancer Ther 2012;11:909–20.

[45] Solit D, Sawyers CL. Drug discovery: how melanomas bypass new therapy. Nature 2010;468:902–3.

[46] Whittaker S, Kirk R, Hayward R, Zambon A, Viros A, Cantarino N, et al. Gatekeeper mutations mediate resistance to BRAF-targeted therapies. Sci Transl Med 2010;2:1–0.

[47] Heidorn SJ, Milagre C, Whittaker S, Nourry A, Niculescu-Duvas I, Dhomen N, et al. Kinase-dead BRAF and oncogenic RAS cooperate to drive tumor progression through CRAF. Cell 2010;140:209–21.

[48] Molina-Arcas M, Downward J. How to fool a wonder drug: truncate and dimerize. J Cancer Cell 2012;21:7–9.

[49] Flaherty KT, Infante JR, Daud A, Gonzalez R, Kefford RF, Sosman J, et al. Combined BRAF and MEK inhibition in melanoma with BRAF V600 mutations. N Engl J Med 2012;367:1694–703.

PART III

THE REALITY OF CANCER DRUGS IN THE CLINIC

Failure Modes in Anticancer Drug Discovery and Development

Richard A. Walgren, Christopher A. Slapak

Lilly Research Laboratories, Eli Lilly and Company, Indianapolis, IN, USA

INTRODUCTION

The drug development process is highly complex, and the outcomes are difficult to predict. It involves significant risks, due in part to interactions with incompletely understood biology, the involvement of patients with serious illnesses in each phase of development, and the need to operate in a highly regulated environment. Given these challenges, it is not surprising that drug development is also lengthy and highly expensive. Recent decades have witnessed significant advances in elucidating the molecular pathogenesis of various diseases that have served to identify a markedly greater number of potential targets than had been previously available. Improved preclinical models, including more complex, engineered cell lines and animal disease models that may more closely mimic human disease, have facilitated the ability to test the contributions of these relationships and allow the prioritization of putative drug targets. High-throughput chemical-screening techniques, including advances in automation, have increased the scale with which chemical compounds can be screened against targets. This has led to the availability of more diverse chemical leads for comparisons and the optimization of biologically active compounds. The end result is that new molecular entities with biological activity can be generated more quickly than was previously possible.

Despite these enhancements in preclinical drug development, testing of new molecules in the clinical stages of development has not seen similar improvements in efficiency and remains a lengthy, high-risk process. In that regard, overall success rates in clinical development have not improved. In fact, with oncology drug development, the current success rate for new molecules first tested in humans from 1993 to 2004 was less than 10% [1].

An additional significant barrier has been the dramatic costs of developing new drugs, which has been increasing for decades. Using two different methodologies, DiMasi et al. and Vernon et al. have estimated that the average pretax cost per new molecular entity (NME) is $803–992 million (in US$ 2000 values) [2,3]. Embedded in the overall cost of development

Cancer Drug Design and Discovery, Second Edition
http://dx.doi.org/10.1016/B978-0-12-396521-9.00019-X

are the many failures inherent in the overall low success rates in clinical development. The average cost per new drug approval (where the estimated cost is calculated based on a company's research and development budget divided by the average number of NMEs over the same period of time) ranges from $3.7 to $11.8 billion [4]. An important implication with this calculation is the suggestion that reductions in the failure rates in drug development could significantly reduce costs. Alternatively, if failures are to occur, it is best that they occur as early as possible in the development process.

To minimize failure rates and maximize the opportunities for success, it is important to understand the "failure modes" in anticancer drug development. In an attempt to investigate the reasons "why drugs fail", this chapter will focus on the clinical development of drugs to treat cancer. The definition of failure will refer to the inability to satisfactorily advance a new molecular entity to the next stage of testing and ultimately to adequately satisfy the regulatory standards of safety and efficacy for new drug approval.

PROBLEMS IN CLINICAL DEVELOPMENT

There is an abundance of new insights into the biology of neoplasia, and with each new piece of the puzzle revealed, new opportunities as well as new complexities need to be considered. Indeed, given the speed and volume of new information, it is challenging for compound development plans to rapidly incorporate new findings as clinical trials may take years to plan, execute, interpret, and move to the next stage. Much of the new information relates to the genetic basis of cancer that is manifest by mutations, deletions, splice variants, overexpression, translocations, or the silencing of genes or gene products involved in the disease process. With the potential importance of these changes, patient selection based on these putative markers is becoming a critical component of trial design, but often within a limited focus as it is not possible to embrace all of the potential variables that may be associated with the underlying biology of cancer. Given the range of questions that are addressed and the conditions that should be experimentally controlled, there are a diverse number of ways to fail in clinical development. Clinical development must start with the formulation of a testable hypothesis and a series of objectives that can be explored and answered under controlled conditions that allow opportunities to systematically discharge the most important risks. There are a number of ways to categorize the sources of failures during this process. It may be useful to regard failures that may arise from one of two conditions. The first source of failure is where the clinical hypothesis is tested and the null hypothesis is confirmed. In essence, the compound was inactive in a particular disease setting. This type of failure occurs when the assumptions about the effects of target pharmacology or the clinical consequences of target engagement and/or pathway modulation do not result in improved clinical outcomes. Failures involving the clinical hypothesis may be disappointing, but if well conducted, they may still increase scientific knowledge and may help direct efforts toward future successes.

The second broad category of failure is where the clinical hypothesis was not adequately tested due to reasons of compound performance or other technical challenges. This type of failure is unfortunately too frequently encountered in the field of experimental therapeutics and may be related to problems with drug delivery as well as absorption, distribution, metabolism, and excretion (ADME properties) that hinder the ability of a molecule to engage a target. This type of failure can also be related to toxicity that may limit compound exposure.

Also included in this group are the external forces that influence the ability of a trial to operate or accrue patients, or that influence the population available for study participation.

The ultimate determination of success or failure of a new anticancer agent in development will be ascertained through the clinical trial process. Clinical development attempts to address a wide range of questions and in doing so assemble a data set that will ultimately inform researchers on the appropriate use of a pharmaceutical agent in a given patient population. These questions range from simple characterization of the compound's intrinsic features (e.g., solubility and pharmacokinetic (PK) properties) to more complex evaluation of the interaction between the experimental agent and a variety of patient features, culminating in an evaluation of efficacy in the disease of interest. It is only through the generation of sufficient, robust clinical data that a compound may ultimately receive governmental regulatory approval and become available for clinical use.

The development paradigm for new anticancer drugs was initially optimized for the introduction of new cytotoxic agents. Under that paradigm, many new agents were introduced into clinical practice that led to significant advancements in patient care such as diminished rates of cancer-related morbidity and mortality. This clinical trial methodology for objectively assessing the clinical safety and efficacy of new agents has continued to evolve over this past half-century. The progression of a novel agent through the phases of clinical trial testing—Phases I, II, and III—is similar for all therapeutic areas. However, notable exceptions for cancer drug development exist that may ultimately influence the overall success rates for the field; these will be discussed in this chapter.

PHASE I

Phase I clinical trials are the first test of a new agent in humans. From a purist viewpoint, phase I trials are those that are truly first-in-humans. However, due to the somewhat empirical nature of determining scheduling for cancer compounds, and the fact that most anticancer agents will be used and developed in combination with other anticancer compounds, most agents in development will undergo multiple phase I trials. With these considerations, phase I studies are best identified functionally via their primary objective of determining a regimen (i.e., a schedule and dose for use either alone or in a combination) that may be safely administered to patients for further efficacy-guided development. Early testing in phase I typically focuses on characterizing and gaining understanding of the clinical properties needed for the effective use of any drug, such as achieving adequate and reproducible exposures and identifying potential dose-limiting toxicities. Testing is generally limited to a small number of subjects or patients and is focused on discharging those risks that may prohibit the eventual ability to test the clinical hypothesis.

Historically, most anticancer agents proceed directly into patients with cancer—usually those who have exhausted all treatments of proven benefit. This has been justified by the fact that the narrow therapeutic window of most anticancer drugs raises safety concerns in noncancer patients. This practice of running phase I studies in patients is in contradistinction to other therapeutic areas that utilize normal subjects in controlled clinical pharmacology units.

The consequences of initiating phase I trials in patients include identifying a population that has the specified study disease(s) but also contains a representative diversity of features that will allow interpretation of study endpoints examining absorption, metabolism, exposure,

Examples	Risk Impact Range				
	Very Low	Low	Intermediate	High	Very High
Solubility and Dissolution	good / no food effect		variable / + food effect		poor
PK/PD Variability	low variability				highly variable
CYP Inhibition	none / well described				mechanism based / poorly characterized
Drug–Drug Interaction	none		involves combination unlikely to be used for target population		involves agent with narrow therapeutic index
Ease of Regimen	similar to current standards				complex / intensive
Margin of Safety	wide				narrow
Observed Toxicity	None		monitorable / reversible / amenable to mitigation		idiosyncratic / progressive / life threatening
Target Pharmacology	previously clinically validated				novel / previously unvalidated
PD Biomarker	gold standard available				unvalidated or unavailable
Endpoint Availability	final Phase 3 suitable		established surrogate		novel / undefined / exploratory endpoint(s)
Clinical Efficacy	demonstrated early in development				delayed demonstration
Clinical Response	addresses unmet medical need		similar to existing therapy		inadequate clinical response
	response as single agent				response only in combination therapy
Time to Response	short				long
Durability of Response	long				short
Target Population	prevalent or multiple indications				narrow indication(s) / very rare / dependent on prior line(s) of therapy
Tailoring Opportunity	well defined / previously validated				no opportunity / stratification necessary but unavailable
Companion Diagnostic (CDx)	approved CDx available		CDx unvalidated / unapproved		simultaneous development of novel CDx and drug

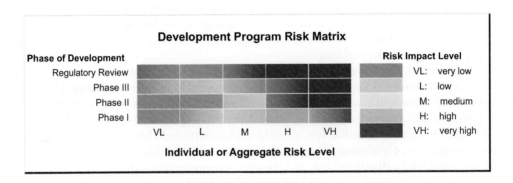

Development Program Risk Matrix

Phase of Development

- Regulatory Review
- Phase III
- Phase II
- Phase I

VL   L   M   H   VH

Individual or Aggregate Risk Level

Risk Impact Level

- VL: very low
- L: low
- M: medium
- H: high
- VH: very high

and safety. Cancer patients may have comorbidities related to their disease (organ dysfunction), latent effects due to prior lines of anticancer therapy (postsurgical, postradiation, or postchemotherapy), or illnesses from diseases unrelated to the study and/or past medical history, all of which can confound outcomes. Disease-related changes could alter absorption due to anatomic changes, metabolism due to metastatic liver involvement or injury, or distribution due to increased third-space volume due to ascites or effusions. Organ dysfunction may also have contributed to changes that predispose trial participants to enhanced sensitivity to potential toxicities. Examples include radiation recall dermatitis in patients receiving cytotoxic agents after prior radiation therapy or increased risk of cardiac toxicity after anthracycline therapy [5]. Understanding of these risks aids in the appropriate formulation of inclusion and exclusion criteria for protocol design. However, overly strict enrollment criteria may limit patient availability in early-phase trials and must be balanced against potential delays in trial enrollment (Fig. 19.1).

During a phase I oncology trial, PK parameters should be measured, pharmacodynamics assessed, toxicity monitored, and any evidence of antitumor activity ascertained. Understanding these parameters as early as possible in the development process is important to the ultimate success of determining an optimal phase II dose. The cohort dose escalation format used to ascertain a maximally tolerated dose has been a useful paradigm for cytotoxic agents [6]. Less established are paradigms for determining an optimal phase II dose for targeted agents. It is clear that experimental agents that proceed into late-stage clinical trials without a thorough exploration of the dose range and subsequent understanding of the most appropriate dose and schedule risk a negative outcome [7].

The efficiency of phase I investigations is closely related to the number of patients per cohort required for evaluation and the number of cohorts required to establish the recommended phase II dose and schedule. Increasing the number of patients evaluated per cohort adds reliability to the assessment of toxicity and better estimates the true frequency of observed adverse events. However, this may inadvertently increase the risk to trial participants by exposing a larger number to an intolerable dose level. Dose escalation typically continues up to a level that defines the maximum tolerated dose, which generally is defined only after exposing some patients to "unacceptable toxicity".

Prior to the availability of the International Conference on Harmonisation of Technical Requirements for Registration of Pharmaceuticals for Human Use (ICH) S9 Guidance, most ICH S guidances and the ICH M3 guidance had excluded cancer therapies from their recommendations. Lack of a unified guidance created uncertainty and differences in development requirements between Europe, the United States, and Japan. The new S9 guidance provides recommendations for nonclinical evaluations to aid in identifying pharmacologic properties,

FIGURE 19.1 Sources of risk and their contribution to failures in clinical development. Clinical development must start with the formulation of a testable clinical hypothesis and a series of objectives that can be explored and answered under controlled conditions that allow opportunities to systematically discharge the most important risks. Optimally, the development of experimental therapeutics must be tailored to the risk specific to that program, seeking a balance between early discharges of risk from the clinical hypothesis versus other potential program risks that could prevent testing that hypothesis. A failure to discharge risks early in development may result in an aggregated risk of failure in the later stages of clinical development, where there is less tolerance of risk. (This figure is reproduced in color in the color plate section.)

identifying a safe initial dose level for humans, and increasing the understanding of the toxicological profile for agents intended for cancer patients. Due to the life-threatening nature of malignancy, the S9 requirements were developed with the intention to facilitate timely anticancer development. Applying S9 to preclinical testing results in describing "minimal considerations for initial clinical trials in patients with advanced cancer", and the resulting data package is less comprehensive than that required by the M3 guideline. For example, S9 requires nonclinical data from one-month studies to support phase I in advanced cancer. Under S9, clinical phase I data are typically sufficient to move to phase II and into second- or front-line therapy. Nonclinical repeat-dose studies of three months' duration are expected prior to phase II and are "considered sufficient to support marketing". A recognized trade-off of this reduction in requirements is the potential for toxicities associated with chronic administration to go undetected until later in clinical development, and thus potentially delay the discharge of program risks. Somewhat paradoxically, as more tyrosine kinase inhibitors are moving to incorporate healthy-volunteer studies in their regulatory submissions, a lack of a more comprehensive toxicology data package may delay timelines for relative bioavailability assessments.

Phase I dose-finding studies are typically undertaken with very simple formulations such as drug-in-capsule formulations. This simplicity is favorable on initial timelines and accepted based on the premise that it allows exploration of the absorption of the "native" properties of the experimental drug. It is important to note that most of these simple formulations may include apparently inert ingredients or excipients that aid in manufacturing and allow for consistent drug loading of the test article. Excipients may be included as diluents (e.g., lactulose and dibasic calcium phosphate), disintegrants and diluents (e.g., starch and microcrystalline cellulose), lubricants (e.g., magnesium stearate, steric acid, hydrogenated vegetable oil, and talc), granulating agents (e.g., sucrose and polyvinyl pyrrolidone), or coating agents or a capsule (e.g., gelatin, methylcellulose, and cellulose acetate phthalate). Some of these excipients may in fact alter drug absorption characteristics to increase the rate of drug absorption or prolong retention time in the gastrointestinal tract and in so doing increase the amount of drug absorbed. Other excipients may retard drug dissolution or shorten residence time in the intestine and thus reduce drug absorption. Excipients or concomitant medications that alter pH may also alter absorption characteristics. The relative amounts of these excipients also typically increase as more test articles are administered with each dose escalation.

Additionally, most agents undergo formulation changes such that phase I and phase III test articles differ markedly in excipient content. This has the potential to result in differences in maximum blood concentrations (C_{max}), time to C_{max}, blood area under the concentration–time curve (AUC), and parameters such as time above target concentration such that initial dose finding and efficacy testing in phases I and II may become less accurate predictors of phase III outcomes.

Pharmacokinetic variability may also be significantly impacted by the fed state (i.e., whether a drug is administered with food or after the patient has fasted) via the chemical and physiologic influence of food [8]. This may be of significant importance for many kinase inhibitors, which, as a class, tend to have low solubility and high permeability. Agents with low solubility and high permeability, which are termed Class II according to the Biopharmaceutics and Classification System [9], are also susceptible to changes in absorption based on pH effects that can occur independently of the fed state, especially due to antacids or proton pump inhibitors [10,11]. Lapatinib is a 4-anilinoquinazoline competitive inhibitor of both ErbB1 and ErbB2 tyrosine kinases and is approved for use in combination with capecitabine for the management of advanced metastatic breast cancer. Interestingly, while capecitabine is indicated for use in the fed state, lapatinib is indicated for use in a fasted state. Like many kinase inhibitors, clinical testing of lapatinib primarily focused on exposures in a fasted state. However, a comparison of pharmacokinetics between fed and fasted states gives cause for concern [12]. When compared with the fasted state, administration of lapatinib with a low-fat breakfast produced a 2.67-fold increase in mean AUC and a 2.42-fold increase in the mean C_{max}. When administered with a high-fat breakfast, these increases were magnified further, with a 4.25-fold increase in lapatinib AUC and a 3.03-fold increase in C_{max}. Importantly, this increased bioavailability in the fed state did not significantly decrease relative variability, but rather the absolute variability in systemic exposure was increased. Generalizing beyond this example, changes in exposure of this magnitude are sufficient to potentially cause differences in safety or efficacy outcomes. Indeed, if identified earlier in development, the influence of the fed state could have been a significant contributor to study design and interpretation of outcomes or may have led to the development and testing of different formulations.

The ABL kinase inhibitor nilotinib illustrates how risk of exposure variability may be compounded from different potential sources. Nilotinib is approved for use in patients with chronic-phase and accelerated-phase chronic myeloid leukemia who are resistant or intolerant to prior therapy, including imatinib [13]. Nilotinib is labeled for administration in a fasted state and has also been shown to have increased absorption when taken with food [14]. With fasted administration, nilotinib demonstrates solubility-limited absorption at doses greater than 400 mg. In healthy subjects, administration of nilotinib with a high-fat meal was found to delay T_{max} by 4–5 h and was associated with a 2.12-fold increase in C_{max} and a 1.82-fold increase in AUC. Nilotinib is also subject to potential drug–drug interactions involving inducers or inhibitors of CYP3A4 [15]. In healthy subjects, CYP3A4 induction by rifampin resulted in an average decrease of 64% in C_{max} and 80% in AUC, while CYP3A4 inhibition by ketoconazole resulted in an average 1.84-fold increase in C_{max} and a 3.01-fold increase in AUC.

One design feature that may be contributing to the delay in understanding potential PK variability is the sole reliance on blood testing done in the clinic. In current clinical studies, it is routine to have serial testing of blood levels drawn over a monitored but limited duration of time following administration. Due to clinic schedules and patient inconvenience, this results in sparse testing generally not exceeding 24 h and on a very limited number of days. Moreover, administration of an oral dose in the clinic is relatively controlled and may not accurately represent the variability observed when a patient takes a dose at home. Recently, there has been an increasing interest in the use of dried blood sample testing (DBS) for PK assessments [16,17]. DBS is an extension of the screening method used for decades for the neonatal metabolic disorder phenylketonuria. The approach has gained interest due to its use of small sample volume, simplified sample handling, and cost-effective shipping and storage. As a result, this method is being piloted as a replacement for standard PK measurement of plasma or whole blood. However, due to its less invasive nature and it ease of collection and handling, the DBS approach may also lend itself to be used by patients at home as an adjunct source for PK monitoring in addition to standard in-clinic blood draws. The routine use of home glucose monitoring suggests that patients should have few problems collecting serial samples for DBS from in-home finger sticks at prescribed or random times. DBS cards are available with coated materials that can deactivate bacteria and viruses and have suitable stability such that patients could return or mail the cards, allowing less sparse and more chronic assessment of PK performance.

The application of pharmacological-based biomarkers, particularly when coupled with pharmacokinetics to establish a formal pharmacokinetic-pharmacodynamic (PK-PD) relationship, has been argued to be the most appropriate manner for determining a phase II dose for targeted agents [18]. Although sound in principle, the application of biomarkers to the clinical development of targeted agents in oncology continues to be a process in evolution. Several systematic reviews of recent agents in development suggest that few targeted agents have actually relied on biomarkers for important decision making or dose selection, demonstrating the difficulty in execution of this approach [7,19]. Goulart et al. [19] have reported that over the period from 1991 to 2002, 20% of American Society of Clinical Oncology Phase I abstracts (503 of 2458) included biomarkers, and this proportion was increasing over time (14% in 1991 compared with 26% in 2002; $P < 0.02$). From these abstracts, 87 studies had phase I trial data published in peer-reviewed literature. Whereas 11 (13%) utilized biomarkers to support dose selection for phase II studies, the primary determinants of phase II dose and schedule were toxicity and/or efficacy in all but one of these trials. In contrast, biomarker studies did provided evidence supporting the proposed mechanism of action in 34 (39%) of the 87 published trials.

In the era of targeted therapy with well-defined patient populations, there may be a necessity for co-development of a pharmacodynamic or patient selection biomarker with the experimental therapeutic, adding to the technical challenges as well as trial and regulatory complexities. The development of biomarker assays often lags behind the development of an experimental therapeutic for a number of reasons. Often, there are difficulties in quantitative assessment and performance of the assays. These challenges are further accentuated by the presence of significant interpatient and intrapatient variability. In the end, early-phase studies using biomarkers must not only answer the question of the right dose but also determine "What is a significant result coming from an unvalidated assay?" Faced with the challenges of incorporating biomarkers, there may be a reliance on the paradigm that the highest tolerated dose should be the one taken forward. Clearly, phase I studies benefit from earlier progress in the development and validation of pharmacodynamic biomarker assays capable of aiding in dose selection. In the absence of a biomarker, a default to the highest safe dose tested (that may or may not be the optimal dose for a target) is often used. Thus, better biomarkers may be able to inform this scenario and allow discharge of risks earlier.

The ability to gain hints of efficacy within the phase I oncology population is an important distinction between cancer drug development and other therapeutic areas. The question of whether evidence of efficacy must be demonstrated before investing in further development has been debated [20,21]. Given the high attrition rates in the development of oncologic therapeutics, there is a great desire to identify promising drug candidates early on to expedite their advancement and also to avoid additional development costs on those molecules that have been evaluated to have a higher risk of eventual failure. From a patient standpoint, there is a more compelling reason to avoid enrollment to trials that will eventually fail due to a lack of efficacy. In the era of cytotoxic drug development, retrospective analysis suggested that demonstration of tumor shrinkage, even in a minority of patients (10%), should be seen or the compound may be doomed to failure [22]. In the molecularly targeting era, many phase I trials have been conducted with the goal of generating preliminary evidence of clinical activity.

Analyses that have included targeted agents have suggested that overall response rates in phase I have declined with time, perhaps as a result of the differing populations now available for phase I clinical trials [23,24]. However, agents that ultimately were successful in phase III trials had a higher average response rate compared to those that failed (8% versus 3%) [24]. It is also noteworthy that examples exist for both cytotoxic and targeted agents that demonstrated a bona fide 0% response rate but were ultimately successful in phase III trials [25].

Enrichment of a trial's enrolled population to include a specific and targetable oncogenic lesion or pathway appears to be an ideal situation to discharge risk early and potentially stop development if the result is negative. In practice, it has not been common for a phase I trial to include a design where a targeted agent can be appropriately paired with a population of patients whose tumors are driven predominantly by the target of interest. Implementation of an enrichment strategy can face a number of challenges. Given that most advanced human malignancies have complex molecular compositions and given the limited availability of validated biomarker assays for such molecular signals, interrogation of a single or even a few of the relevant pathways in a small number of patients in a phase I trial, without the presence of controls, is at best exploratory and can hinder enrollment rates. When enrichment is used, the scientific rationale for selection of a target patient population should be strong and extend beyond retrospective clinicopathological associations between target expression and clinical outcomes. Several phase I trials have successfully been enriched for specific target patient populations, including patients with advanced basal cell carcinoma treated with the Hedgehog inhibitor GDC-0449 [26], patients with non-small-cell lung cancer (NSCLC) harboring the *EML4-ALK* translocation treated with the oral c-MET and ALK inhibitor crizotinib (PF-02341066) [27], and patients with malignant melanoma harboring the *BRAF* V600E mutation treated with the BRAF inhibitor PLX4032 [28]. Enrollment in these enriched phase I trials was not limited to these populations, and patients with other advanced solid tumor types were enrolled. This ensures that patients can be enrolled regardless of the performance of the biomarker assay, and this facilitates the primary goal of phase I trials to recommend a dose and schedule that are safe for subsequent disease-specific evaluations not limited to the target patient groups first tested.

PHASE II

While phase I studies have the potential to identify hints of clinical activity of an experimental therapeutic agent, phase II studies are specifically designed to explore clinical activity and serve as the first test of the clinical hypothesis for an agent. Ideally, the risk of failure to demonstrate clinical efficacy should be discharged early in phase II and preferably not in phase III. The high failure rate of oncology phase III trials has been ascribed to the poor predictive value of phase II trials to ultimately identify active compounds. Traditionally, phase II studies have enrolled relatively small groups (i.e., 20–50 patients), with a histologically defined tumor type, who have received a specified number of prior lines of cancer therapy. Historically, many phase II studies have not included controls, and the endpoint, such as response rate, has been compared with that of historical controls. This approach suffers from an inability to equate historical response rates to current response rates as these may shift over time due to changes in diagnostic or supportive care measures. The predictive value of phase II results for phase III outcomes is dependent on the confidence interval associated with the sample size and the treatment effect size. In reality, many experimental therapies have a modest treatment effect. Although in aggregate these modest treatment advances can lead to significant improvements in patient care, a modest magnitude of effect results in greater uncertainty in the prediction of phase III outcomes [29]. The predictive value of phase II results for phase III outcomes is also influenced by differences in molecular characteristics or pathway phenotypes. In diseases where a variety of different low-frequency mutation events are present but not included in study stratification schemes, it is highly possible that there will be differences in enrollment rates for these markers across trials. Within this setting, it is difficult to tease out what is a "treatment effect" and what is a "trial effect" [30], and the success of phase III studies is subject to influence from differences stemming from changes in endpoints between phases II and III (i.e., response rates vs. survival), patient and tumor heterogeneity, and a strong sampling bias [31,32].

A variety of improvements to phase II study designs have been proposed [33]. The application of two-stage designs may allow earlier termination of inactive agents, and two-stage designs may spare patients exposure to such compounds. However, this design has not been demonstrated to ultimately improve outcomes in phase III.

The use of randomized phase II trials, where an active comparator is used rather than historical controls, has gained favor in the development of targeted agents. Notable successes have been reported with this randomized approach. A three-arm randomized phase II trial of flurouracil and leucovorin with or without bevacizumab in approximately 100 patients with advanced colorectal cancer provided a sufficiently strong signal to guide clinical testing to the ultimately successful phase III trial [34]. These data not only guided the go/no-go decision in this indication but also provided guidelines for the ultimate size of the phase III trial that would be required for success [35]. However, opponents to this approach argue that these designs are underpowered phase III trials with lowered α and β values whose ultimate predictive value is limited by the wide confidence intervals.

In situations where less is known about the target and a given disease setting, exploration of biology may be more relevant than confirmation of an effect, and thus the use of adaptive design trials may be more rewarding and efficient. Adaptive trials are those studies that allow the use of modifications to the trial or statistical plan based on the data accrued to that point in the study. Adaptive clinical trials may allow changes in sample size, inclusion or exclusion criteria, dose, regimen, or study endpoints that are intended to enhance the trial and potential benefit to the patient. The ability of a trial to react in "real time" to emerging results has clear efficiency benefits and has potential ethical merits by controlling enrollment based on a dynamic schedule of safety evaluation. Less clear is the amount of flexibility that will be allowed by regulatory reviewers or other competent authorities. Trial adaptations can introduce bias, but the introduction of bias may be minimized by the limitation of ad hoc adaptation in favor of prospective adaptation. During the course of a trial, it is possible for an adaptive trial to change in a manner such that the final study population is significantly different from the original target population. Depending on the tumor type and final population, this may result in a failure of the trial to achieve its intended purpose. Also inherent is the risk that extensive changes may affect the reliability of statistical inferences, such as the confidence interval for the treatment effect under study, resulting in an inability to generate reproducible results.

No one trial design is ideal for phase II testing, and in practice trial designs range widely. In large part, the selection of a design depends on the existing knowledge of an experimental agent, its intended target(s), and the prior state of validation of the target(s). Trial designs are also heavily influenced by the existence and effectiveness of current therapies. In the absence of an effective therapy, it may be reasonable for cancer patients to enroll in a phase II trial with a single arm that tests an experimental therapy. However, a similar design is less likely to be acceptable for a disease where active but not curative agents exist. In this setting, trials may need a design that compares two therapies and allows cross-over or allows for the comparison of standard of care plus or minus the experimental agent.

PHASE III

Ultimately, phase II trials must aid in assessments of whether to advance a molecule into phase III trials and must provide insights into the appropriate design for phase III study. Regulatory approval of a novel oncology compound requires pivotal trial(s) that are "adequate and well controlled". Typically, FDA approval is based on "end points that demonstrate that the drug provides a longer life, a better life, or a favorable effect on an established surrogate for a longer or better life" [36]. These requirements generally dictate the use of randomized prospective trials that are adequately powered for a chosen endpoint, and they include testing against an active comparator, usually a clinically accepted standard of care in that indication [37].

It has been suggested that the high attrition rates in oncology phase III trials are in part due to the demands of the regulatory authorities in this area [38]. Whereas the demonstration of a survival advantage is the ultimate test of efficacy, it is a hurdle not generally required in other therapeutic areas. Within oncology clinical trials, the use of "non-inferiority" endpoints is generally discouraged on the basis that they are viewed as not advancing the field in an area of large unmet medical need. Under this construct, it is easy to see how an experimental therapeutic that demonstrates an improvement in overall survival offers an advantage. However, avoidance of "non-inferiority" endpoints may hinder competition and, together with the reliance on survival as an endpoint, may slow the development of agents offering significant reductions in costs, morbidity, or health care utilization.

To some extent, the use of overall survival as an ultimate measure of efficacy may be hampered by the availability of additional lines of therapy or the use of cross-over designs. This situation may limit the ability to show a potential overall survival advantage absent subsequent therapy. Agents that have biological activity and offer clinically meaningful effects may not be able to demonstrate an overall survival advantage because of factors such as tumor heterogeneity. A number of tyrosine kinase inhibitors have been able to demonstrate positive progression-free survival effects in solid tumors by RECIST criteria in phase II but have failed to demonstrate similar effects on overall survival. Selection of drug targets may play a role, but most cancers do not appear to be directly dependent on one aberrant signaling molecule in the way that chronic myelogenous leukemia (CML) is dependent on *BCR–ABL*. Indeed, the responses to targeted therapies in many other tumor types have been less durable. This may in part be due to the emergence of preexisting or de novo resistance stemming from other molecular targets. The complexity of tumor heterogeneity makes this a predictable outcome and suggests that future success will be dependent on the use of appropriate combinations of targeted agents. If successes in phases II and III are based solely on overall survival advantages, there will be significant development challenges to the introduction of effective combinations.

The anticipated clinical outcome of an experimental agent is a key input for the selection of an endpoint. Trials with endpoints that involve prevention of an illness or complications of an illness will be different in size and duration than those studies that focus on disease progression or improving overall survival. Prior successful examples of development for cancer prevention include the approval of tamoxifen for the reduction of the risk of breast cancer in patients deemed to be at high risk. In December 1999, the FDA approved the use of celecoxib for prevention of adenomatous colorectal polyps in patients with familial adenomatous polyposis. However, the burden of proof in prevention studies may require large numbers of patients and substantial longitudinal observation. If successful, confirmation of these findings can prove challenging, as demonstrated in the case of celecoxib where the sponsor voluntarily withdrew marketing authorization in Europe, citing slow clinical trial enrollment as the reason for being unable to provide confirmatory clinical benefit data [39].

While the demonstration of an overall survival benefit is a standard endpoint for phase III studies, clinical development may also focus on endpoints that modulate the complications and symptoms of a disease that are recognized as unmet needs. The JAK2 inhibitor ruxolitinib received FDA approval in 2011 for use in the treatment of myelofibrosis without a demonstration of overall survival or progression-free survival benefit [40]. Full approval was granted on the basis of two randomized clinical trials with a primary endpoint of percentage of patients with a ≥35% spleen volume reduction and a key secondary endpoint of percentage of patients who achieve ≥50% reduction in Total Symptom Score on a patient-reported outcome instrument (changes in disease-related symptoms were not assessed in the supporting trial) [41,42].

The inability to properly select patients who are most likely to benefit from a given therapy remains one of the largest hurdles to successful outcome in pivotal trials for oncology. Patient selection or segmentation biomarkers aimed at enrolling those most likely to benefit hold the promise to diminish sample sizes and increase the probability of success. Examples of success stemming from the use of this approach have emerged. One of the most notable was in the development of trastuzumab in patients with metastatic breast cancer. The pivotal trial for trastuzumab employed an immunohistochemistry assay that selected for those patients with the highest levels of expression of the target, HER2 [43]. Subsequent analysis has suggested that without the patient selection, the pivotal trial, which enrolled 469 patients, would have required over 23,500 patients to achieve the same outcome [44].

The most common cause of treatment failure of metastatic cancer is drug resistance [45]. In a very real sense, this fact underscores the failure of established drugs and remains a challenge to the discovery and development of novel therapies. Since the mechanisms of drug resistance for many classes of drugs have been determined [45–47], it should be possible to incorporate these considerations in the advancement of drugs that follow these resistance paradigms, but how is it possible to account for unanticipated resistance mechanisms in the discovery of novel drugs?

Resistance mechanisms remain an obstacle to the successful discovery and development of novel targeted therapies. The genomic instability that is a hallmark of cancer contributes to the ability of tumors to develop resistance during therapy (acquired resistance), and the intrapatient heterogeneity of most advanced solid tumors invariably leads to the selection of resistant clones (intrinsic resistance). This has been clearly demonstrated in the development of targeted kinase inhibitors. For example, the kinase inhibitor imatinib demonstrates remarkable clinical efficacy in the treatment of CML via inhibition of the constitutively active kinase BCR-ABL. Imatinib is also remarkably efficacious in the treatment of gastrointestinal stromal tumors (GISTs) via inhibition of the kinase c-KIT. Resistance mechanisms to imatinib have been identified in the treatment of both of these diseases due to mutations in the binding site the drug shares with the endogenous ligand adenosine triphosphate [48,49].

Intrinsic drug resistance may mask the efficacy of targeted therapy in patient populations wherein the majority of patients present with a less sensitive variant of the drug's target. Treatment of NSCLC with the tyrosine kinase inhibitors gefitnib or erlotinib is complicated by virtue of a mutation in the target that renders the tumor especially sensitive to these drugs [50]. This is due to a somatic mutation in the drugs' target, the epidermal growth factor receptor. As a result, clinical trials that failed to select for patients expressing this sensitizing alteration were seriously compromised in their ability to achieve their efficacy endpoints for the treatment of first-line NSCLC. Thus, patient selection will become an even more important determinant in the successful development of new drugs, and the elaboration of predictive biomarkers and pharmacogenomic determinants will become a necessary component of drug discovery [18,51–54].

CONCLUSIONS

The drug development process, from a first-in-humans study to regulatory approval in multiple geographies, remains high risk, with the majority of compounds ultimately failing. Despite dramatic strides toward understanding the fundamental biology of cancer, oncology drug development continues to have among the highest levels of attrition, with overall success rates estimated to be less than 10%. Compounding the high rate of failures is the staggering cost of successfully launching a new molecular entity, which is now estimated by multiple sources to far exceed US$1 billion dollars. The generally held view is that this paradigm of enormous cost with high rates of failure is not sustainable.

Understanding why drugs fail along the development path is critical if this trend is to be altered. Drug development is a continuum of data collection and risk discharge. A properly designed series of clinical trials should assess, by phase, important questions that allow risks to be discharged and development to proceed. Failure to address fundamental issues in early development, such as basic pharmacology, the ability to modulate the pathway of interest, or the establishing of patient safety in the targeted population, leads to carrying additional risk into late-stage development, increasing the likelihood of ultimate failure.

Project termination, or failures, in the early stages of development is often a difficult decision informed with only limited data sets. The desire not to abandon prematurely a potential new anticancer drug must be balanced against continued resource utilization and exposing patients to a compound of unproven safety and efficacy. Conversely, many recently approved oncology drugs have encountered major challenges that were overcome during their successful passage from early development to regulatory approval. Understanding the risks and challenges that may be encountered will potentially enable investigators and development teams to better negotiate the complex path to regulatory approval.

References

[1] DiMasi JA, Feldman L, Seckler A, Wilson A. Trends in risks associated with new drug development: success rates for investigational drugs. Clin Pharmacol Ther 2010;87:272–7.

[2] DiMasi JA, Hansen RW, Grabowski HG. The price of innovation: new estimates of drug development costs. J Health Econ 2003;22:151–85.

[3] Vernon JA, Golec JH, Dimasi JA. Drug development costs when financial risk is measured using the Fama–French three-factor model. Health Econ 2010;19:1002–5.

[4] Herper M. The truly staggering cost of inventing new drugs. Forbes 2012.

[5] Morris PG, Hudis CA. Trastuzumab-related cardiotoxicity following anthracycline-based adjuvant chemotherapy: how worried should we be? J Clin Oncol 2010;28:3407–10.

[6] Decoster G, Stein G, Holdener EE. Responses and toxic deaths in phase I clinical trials. Ann Oncol 1990;1:175–81.

[7] Parulekar WR, Eisenhauer EA. Phase I trial design for solid tumor studies of targeted, non-cytotoxic agents: theory and practice. J Natl Cancer Inst 2004;96:990–7.

[8] Singh BN, Malhotra BK. Effects of food on the clinical pharmacokinetics of anticancer agents: underlying mechanisms and implications for oral chemotherapy. Clin Pharm 2004;43:1127–56.

[9] Custodio JM, Wu CY, Benet LZ. Predicting drug disposition, absorption/elimination/transporter interplay and the role of food on drug absorption. Adv Drug Deliv Rev 2008;60:717–33.

[10] Budha NR, Benet LZ, Ware JA. Response to "Drug interactions produced by proton pump inhibitors: not simply a pH effect". Clin Pharmacol Ther 2012.

[11] Budha NR, Frymoyer A, Smelick GS, Jin JY, Yago MR, Dresser MJ, et al. Drug absorption interactions between oral targeted anticancer agents and PPIs: is pH-dependent solubility the Achilles heel of targeted therapy? Clin Pharmacol Ther 2012;92:203–13.

[12] Koch KM, Reddy NJ, Cohen RB, Lewis NL, Whitehead B, Mackay K, et al. Effects of food on the relative bioavailability of lapatinib in cancer patients. J Clin Oncol 2009;27:1191–6.

[13] Kim TD, le Coutre P, Schwarz M, Grille P, Levitin M, Fateh-Moghadam S, et al. Clinical cardiac safety profile of nilotinib. Haematologica 2012;97:883–9.

[14] Tanaka C, Yin OQ, Sethuraman V, Smith T, Wang X, Grouss K, et al. Clinical pharmacokinetics of the BCR-ABL tyrosine kinase inhibitor nilotinib. Clin Pharmacol Ther 2010;87:197–203.

[15] Tanaka C, Yin OQ, Smith T, Sethuraman V, Grouss K, Galitz L, et al. Effects of rifampin and ketoconazole on the pharmacokinetics of nilotinib in healthy participants. J Clin Pharmacol 2011;51:75–83.

[16] Edelbroek PM, van der Heijden J, Stolk LML. Dried blood spot methods in therapeutic drug monitoring: methods, assays, and pitfalls. Ther Drug Monit 2009;31:327–36. 10.1097/FTD.0b013e31819e91ce.

[17] Xu Y, Fang W, Zeng W, Leijen S, Woolf E. Evaluation of dried blood spot (DBS) technology versus plasma analysis for the determination of MK-1775 by HILIC-MS/MS in support of clinical studies. Anal Bioanal Chem 2012;404:3037–48.

[18] Woude GF, Kelloff GJ, Ruddon RW, Koo HM, Sigman CC, Barrett JC, et al. Reanalysis of cancer drugs: old drugs, new tricks. Clin Cancer Res 2004;10:3897–907.

[19] Goulart BHL, Clark JW, Pien HH, Roberts TG, Finkelstein SN, Chabner BA. Trends in the use and role of biomarkers in phase I oncology trials. Clin Cancer Res 2007;13:6719–26.

[20] Horstmann E, McCabe MS, Grochow L, Yamamoto S, Rubinstein L, Budd T, et al. Risks and benefits of phase 1 oncology trials, 1991 through 2002. N Engl J Med 2005;352:895–904.

[21] Kurzrock R, Benjamin RS. Risks and benefits of phase 1 oncology trials, revisited. N Engl J Med 2005;352:930–2.

[22] Estey E, Hoth D, Simon R, Marsoni S, Leyland-Jones B, Wittes R. Therapeutic response in phase I trials of antineoplastic agents. Cancer Treat Rep 1986;70:1105–15.

[23] Chen EX, Tannock IF. Risks and benefits of phase 1 clinical trials evaluating new anticancer agents: a case for more innovation. J Am Med Assoc 2004;292:2150–1.

[24] Roberts Jr TG, Goulart BH, Squitieri L, Stallings SC, Halpern EF, Chabner BA, et al. Trends in the risks and benefits to patients with cancer participating in phase 1 clinical trials. J Am Med Assoc 2004;292:2130–40.

[25] Sekine I, Yamamoto N, Kunitoh H, Ohe Y, Tamura T, Kodama T, et al. Relationship between objective responses in phase I trials and potential efficacy of non-specific cytotoxic investigational new drugs. Ann Oncol 2002;13:1300–6.

[26] Von Hoff DD, LoRusso PM, Rudin CM, Reddy JC, Yauch RL, Tibes R, et al. Inhibition of the hedgehog pathway in advanced basal-cell carcinoma. N Engl J Med 2009;361:1164–72.

[27] Kwak EL, Camidge DR, Clark J, Shapiro GI, Maki RG, Ratain MJ, et al. Clinical activity observed in a phase I dose escalation trial of an oral c-met and ALK inhibitor, PF-02341066. ASCO Meeting Abstracts 2009;27:3509.

[28] Flaherty K, Puzanov I, Sosman J, Kim K, Ribas A, McArthur G, et al. Phase I study of PLX4032: proof of concept for V600E BRAF mutation as a therapeutic target in human cancer. ASCO Meeting Abstracts 2009;27:9000.

[29] Berry D. Statistical innovations in cancer research. In: Kufe DW, Pollock RE, Weichselbaum RR, Bast RC, Gansler TS, Holland JF, editors. Holland-Frei Cancer Medicine. 6th ed. London: BC Decker; 2003. p. 465–87.

[30] Estey EH, Thall PF. New designs for phase 2 clinical trials. Blood 2003;102:442–8.

[31] Ratain MJ, Karrison TG. Testing the wrong hypothesis in phase II oncology trials: there is a better alternative. Clin Cancer Res 2007;13:781–2.

[32] Vickers AJ, Ballen V, Scher HI. Setting the bar in phase II trials: the use of historical data for determining " go/no go" decision for definitive phase III testing. Clin Cancer Res 2007;13:972–6.

[33] Dent S, Zee B, Dancey J, Hanauske A, Wanders J, Eisenhauer E. Application of a new multinomial phase II stopping rule using response and early progression. J Clin Oncol 2001;19:785–91.

[34] Ferrara N, Hillan KJ, Gerber HP, Novotny W. Discovery and development of bevacizumab, an anti-VEGF antibody for treating cancer. Nat Rev Drug Discov 2004;3:391–400.

[35] Hurwitz H, Fehrenbacher L, Novotny W, Cartwright T, Hainsworth J, Heim W, et al. Bevacizumab plus irinotecan, fluorouracil, and leucovorin for metastatic colorectal cancer. N Engl J Med 2004;350:2335–42.

[36] Johnson JR, Williams G, Pazdur R. End points and United States Food and Drug Administration approval of oncology drugs. J Clin Oncol 2003;21:1404–11.

[37] Schilsky RL. End points in cancer clinical trials and the drug approval process. Clin Cancer Res 2002;8:935–8.

[38] Booth B, Glassman R, Ma P. Oncology's trials. Nat Rev Drug Discov 2003;2:609–10.

[39] Agency EM, editor. European Medicines Agency concludes on use of celecoxib in familial adenomatous polyposis. 2011.

[40] Summary Review Application Number 202192Orig1s000 (CDER, ed.).

[41] Harrison C, Kiladjian J-J, Al-Ali HK, Gisslinger H, Waltzman R, Stalbovskaya V, et al. JAK inhibition with ruxolitinib versus best available therapy for myelofibrosis. N Engl J Med 2012;366:787–98.

[42] Verstovsek S, Mesa RA, Gotlib J, Levy RS, Gupta V, DiPersio JF, et al. A double-blind, placebo-controlled trial of ruxolitinib for myelofibrosis. N Engl J Med 2012;366:799–807.

[43] Slamon DJ, Leyland-Jones B, Shak S, Fuchs H, Paton V, Bajamonde A, et al. Use of chemotherapy plus a monoclonal antibody against HER2 for metastatic breast cancer that overexpresses HER2. N Engl J Med 2001;344: 783–92.

[44] Simon R, Maitournam A. Evaluating the efficiency of targeted designs for randomized clinical trials. Clin Cancer Res 2004;10:6759–63.

[45] Gottesman MM. Mechanisms of cancer drug resistance. Annu Rev Med 2002;53:615–27.

[46] Chen S, Masri S, Wang X, Phung S, Yuan YC, Wu X. What do we know about the mechanisms of aromatase inhibitor resistance? J Steroid Biochem Mol Biol 2006;102:232–40.

[47] Wang, Guo Z. The role of sulfur in platinum anticancer chemotherapy. Anticancer Agents Med Chem 2007;7: 19–34.

[48] Fletcher JA, Rubin BP. KIT mutations in GIST. Curr Opin Genet Dev 2007;17:3–7.

[49] Ritchie E, Nichols G. Mechanisms of resistance to imatinib in CML patients: a paradigm for the advantages and pitfalls of molecularly targeted therapy. Curr Cancer Drug Targets 2006;6:645–57.

[50] Riely GJ, Politi KA, Miller VA, Pao W. Update on epidermal growth factor receptor mutations in non-small cell lung cancer. Clin Cancer Res 2006;12:7232–41.

[51] Park JW, Kerbel RS, Kelloff GJ, Barrett JC, Chabner BA, Parkinson DR, et al. Rationale for biomarkers and surrogate end points in mechanism-driven oncology drug development. Clin Cancer Res 2004;10:3885–96.

[52] Baker M. In biomarkers we trust? Nat Biotechnol 2005;23:297–304.

[53] Lenz HJ. Pharmacogenomics and colorectal cancer. Adv Exp Med Biol 2006;587:211–31.

[54] Longley DB, Allen WL, Johnston PG. Drug resistance, predictive markers and pharmacogenomics in colorectal cancer. Biochim Biophys Acta 2006;1766:184–96.

Anticancer Drug Registration and Regulation: Current Challenges and Possible Solutions

Erling Donnelly[1], Silvia Chioato[2], David Taylor[3]

[1]Pfizer Inc, Cambridge, MA, USA [2]Pfizer Srl, Milan, Italy [3]UCL School of
Pharmacy, London, UK

INTRODUCTION

The twentieth century saw the development of a wide range of effective treatments for many of the infectious and noncommunicable conditions that affect children and working-age populations. Yet, as communities have grown older and age-specific death rates from causes such as myocardial infarction and stroke have also fallen, cancer has emerged as a leading cause of morbidity and mortality among middle-age and older individuals. As a result, when satisfactory licensed treatments are not available, there is growing demand for early access to unlicensed anticancer therapies [1], even when these therapies may not provide significant survival and/or quality-of-life advantages.

The agencies responsible for regulating the safety of medicine and controlling its entry to market are therefore coming under pressure to amend their policies. In addition to concerns expressed by consumer groups, the agencies may be exposed to conflicting demands from, for example, pharmaceutical companies and other research funders seeking to maintain their incomes (and capacities to fund future innovations) and allow consumers the chance of benefit on the one hand and health service funders seeking to limit service costs and protect public interests in service affordability on the other. A sometimes unspoken dimension of the political and allied controversies surrounding the issues at the heart of this chapter is the desire of some health care funders to extend clinical trial periods—during which external bodies such as pharmaceutical companies are responsible for meeting treatment costs—for as long as possible, whereas research funding agencies wish to "normalize" treatment funding as early as possible in an intellectual property's protected lifetime.

Cancer Drug Design and Discovery, Second Edition
http://dx.doi.org/10.1016/B978-0-12-396521-9.00020-6

Beyond Europe and North America, changing patterns of cancer care needs and demands are becoming discernible in China, India, Brazil, and other emergent economies (see, for instance, Ref. [2]). As people living in these settings develop higher expectations for health care, concerns about whether or not they can be assured of timely and affordable access to oncology-related diagnostic services and anticancer therapies of all types tend to increase. This situation creates tension that may have been reflected in, for instance, decisions in India to issue compulsory licenses that permit local companies to produce and sell alternative versions of patented medicines, such as Bayer's Nexavar (sorafenib tosylate), which is primarily used for patients with late-stage kidney and liver cancer. Access to such modern anticancer drugs is not normally life saving, particularly if other (in aggregate terms, much more costly) elements of the health service infrastructures needed to treat cancer effectively are lacking. However, members of the public do not necessarily have the information required to understand this reality, particularly in countries with less developed educational and health care systems. From a policy analysis and political economy perspective, high-profile disputes about cancer drug pricing can sometimes serve to draw attention away from more fundamentally challenging questions relating to the availability of preventive and early-stage cancer care.

In fact, the extent to which access to anticancer medicines per se is linked to markedly better health outcomes is presently questionable [3,4]. In overall terms, age-standardized mortality rates from cancer as a whole have not (as yet) fallen to a major extent in either affluent nations or anywhere else in the world, even though the number of people living with diagnosed cancers and/or the unwanted sequelae of current radiotherapeutic, drug, and surgical interventions are increasing [5]. For specific disorders, such as acute lymphoblastic leukemia in childhood and breast, testicular, prostate, and colon cancers in adulthood, improved early-stage detection and better surgical, pharmacological, and other treatments have started to reduce age-standardized death rates in more developed communities. In addition, declines in lung and other tobacco-linked (for instance, bladder) cancer incidence and mortality rates, along with benefits in areas such as cardiovascular health, have been noted in populations with reductions in smoking rates (see, for example, Ref. [6]).

The view taken here is that valuable, cost-effective [7] progress has been achieved since Richard Nixon signed the US National Cancer Act in 1971. Milestone events have included the launch of the first major hormone treatment for advanced breast cancer, tamoxifen, in 1972 and the approval of imatinib mesylate, initially for the treatment of chronic myeloid leukemia, in 2001. Nevertheless, there remains a pressing unmet need for more effective and less toxic anticancer treatments.

Despite, for example, the recent survival improvements seen in patients with breast cancer [8], this disease is still a major cause of premature mortality and human suffering. In poorer settings, such as sub-Saharan Africa and rural India, even young women often do not present until their disease is well advanced and they are in considerable distress. In many less affluent nations (and in some relatively wealthy ones), even access to pain-reducing therapies such as morphine can be seriously unsatisfactory.

There is evidence (in part described elsewhere in this book) that members of the global oncology research community—working in commercially, publicly, and charitably funded institutions—are responding to the challenges outlined above [9]. As the twenty-first century unfolds, a significantly increased number of new pharmaceutical treatments for neoplastic disorders is set to enter the world market. However, it may well be the case that costly innovative efforts will need to be sustained until the middle of the twenty-first century before we can achieve the goal of reliably and safely preventing or successfully managing all (or nearly all) cancer cases.

Against this background, this chapter explores the concerns and opportunities relating to the registration and regulation of anticancer medicines in the United States and Europe. In addition to describing provisions such as the orphan drug and pediatric medicine development incentives in each market, it offers a discussion of the regulatory advantages and disadvantages of the common endpoints used in oncology drug development. This chapter also analyzes three other topics of growing interest in the oncology drug regulatory field, namely adaptive licensing, the codevelopment of therapeutic agents and companion diagnostics, and the testing and licensing for use of combinations of two or more investigational oncology products.

THE REGULATORY FRAMEWORK IN THE UNITED STATES

In the United States, anticancer (and other) drug sponsors must provide the US Food and Drug Administration (FDA) with substantial evidence of effectiveness (i.e., clinical benefit) from adequate and well-controlled investigations in order to gain drug approval. Clinical benefit has typically been defined as a prolongation of survival or an improvement in quality of life through the prevention or amelioration of cancer-related symptoms. In some disease settings, such as renal cell carcinoma (RCC), breast cancer, and non-small cell lung cancer (NSCLC), extended progression-free survival durations have been viewed as evidence of clinical benefit.

Under the accelerated approval regulations introduced in 1992,[1] the FDA may permit the supply of a product that is intended to treat serious or life-threatening diseases and that either demonstrates an improvement over available therapy or offers treatment where none has previously existed. Under these regulations, the FDA may grant approval based on an effect on a *surrogate* endpoint that is *reasonably likely* to predict clinical benefit. Such surrogates are less well established than the endpoints in regular use. A drug is licensed under accelerated approval on the condition that the sponsor conducts clinical studies to verify and describe the actual clinical benefit. If postmarketing studies fail to demonstrate clinical benefit or if the applicant does not demonstrate due diligence in conducting the required studies, the drug may be removed from the market under an expedited process [10]. In the period between

---

[1] See 21 Code of Federal Regulations, Part 314.510 and 21 Code of Federal Regulations, Part 601.41. Another US regulatory provision that can positively support oncology drug development is termed Fast Track, which is "designed to facilitate the development and expedite the review of drugs to treat serious diseases and fill an unmet medical need". The FDA is required to make a decision of granting a Fast Track status within 60 days of the NDA's submission. It involves early and frequent verbal and written communication between the FDA and the applicant throughout the drug development and review process, and allows companies to submit completed sections of their responses to questions as they become available. A drug that is granted Fast Track status (of which there were 248 between 1998 and 2011) is expected to have an impact on survival rate, quality of life, or disease progression and have advantages over existing therapies. The latter can include superior effectiveness, reduced side effects, improved diagnosis or decreased toxicity. Drugs selected for Fast Track are also eligible for other accelerating measures.

December 1992 and July 2010, the FDA granted accelerated approval to 35 oncology products for 47 new indications [11].

The FDA normally requires at least two adequate and well-controlled clinical trials. However, evidence from a single trial can be sufficient in certain instances, such as cases in which a single multicenter study provides highly reliable and statistically robust evidence of an important clinical benefit (such as an extension of survival) and in which confirmation of the result in a second trial would be practically or ethically impossible. For drugs approved for the treatment of patients with a specific stage of a particular malignancy, evidence from one trial may also be sufficient to support an efficacy supplement for treatment of a different stage of the same cancer.[2]

The Advisory Process in United States

If questions arise during the review of an oncology product's New Drug Application (NDA) or Biologic License Application, the FDA can convene an Oncologic Drugs Advisory Committee (ODAC) to obtain independent expert advice. ODACs are typically comprised of physician scientists, statisticians, a patient advocate or consumer representative, and an industry representative. These committee meetings, which are open to the public, are held on an as-needed basis, typically four to five times a year. In addition to investigating product-specific questions about an NDA under review, the FDA can also use the ODAC to address matters such as the endpoints used to support approval in a given tumor setting or other key development issues.

As a result of the 2012 prescription drug user-fee amendment reauthorization process (which led in July 2012 to the signing into US law of the Food and Drug Administration Safety and Innovation Act, or FDASIA), sponsors are now notified of the need for an advisory committee when they receive their filing determination letter—a key step in the NDA submission and review process. The first Prescription Drug User Fee Act (PDUFA) was enacted by Congress in 1992. It authorized the FDA to collect fees from companies that produce human drug and biological products. Since the passage of PDUFA, user fees have played an important (if sometimes controversial) role in expediting the drug approval process. The relevant legislation must be reauthorized every 5 years.

Orphan Drugs in the United States

Upon the request of a sponsor, the Orphan Drug Act (ODA) grants a special status, called an Orphan Drug Designation, to a product for the treatment of a rare disease or condition. Sponsors must demonstrate that the disease or condition for which the medicine or other pharmaceutical product is intended affects fewer than 200,000 people in the United States (which implied a prevalence of approximately 10 per 10,000 people when this option was originally established). Orphan designation qualifies the sponsor of the product for a tax credit and marketing incentives specified in the ODA. For example, a marketing application for a prescription drug product that has been designated as a drug for a rare disease

---

[2] See http://www.fda.gov/ForIndustry/UserFees/PrescriptionDrugUserFee/ucm144411.htm.

or condition is not subject to a prescription drug user fee unless the application includes an indication for something other than a rare disease or condition.

In oncology, products for many rare or uncommon tumor types fall under the orphan drug designation. In addition, products for small subsets (based on molecular status) of large tumor types can also receive orphan drug designation status. This status is becoming increasingly relevant in oncology as the molecular-level understanding of oncogenesis and associated biological mechanisms increases.

Breakthrough Therapy Designation

Another result of the FDASIA is that Breakthrough Therapy Designations will become applicable to compounds for which authorizations are being sought. The exact terms and benefits are (at the time of writing) still being addressed by FDA and will be described in future guidance. The two main requirements are that a drug is intended, alone or in combination with one or more other drugs, to treat a serious or life-threatening disease or condition, and that there is preliminary clinical evidence indicating that the drug represents a substantial improvement over existing therapies on one or more clinically significant endpoints. This may, for instance, include situations such as substantial new treatment effects being observed early in a product's clinical development.

In theory, a Breakthrough Therapy Designation will lead the FDA to at least:

- Hold meetings between the sponsor and the review team throughout the development of the drug;
- Provide timely advice to the sponsor regarding development of the drug, to ensure that the nonclinical and clinical development program is as efficient and practicable as possible; and
- Take steps to ensure that the design of the required clinical trials is also as efficient and practicable as possible through, for instance, minimizing the number of patients exposed to a potentially less efficacious treatment.

Pediatrics

In the United States, two pieces of legislation are aimed at promoting investments in pediatric drug development, namely the Best Pharmaceuticals for Children Act (BPCA) and the Pediatric Research Equity Act (PREA). The FDASIA made these pieces of legislation permanent. Previously, the BPCA had to be renewed every 5 years.

PREA provides incentives to drug developers to perform pediatric studies in order to improve the efficacy and safety data available for products used in children and infants. It allows sponsors to qualify for an additional 6 months of marketing exclusivity for the drug (added to the end of the patent life) if specific studies addressing relevant indications are completed and submitted to FDA. A Written Request is a document issued by the FDA that outlines the type of studies to be conducted, including their design and objectives and the age groups to be studied.

Because the pediatric exclusivity provision is voluntary, the drug sponsor may decline a Written Request, although the process of producing one can be initiated by either the sponsor or the FDA. A sponsor may submit a Proposed Pediatric Study Request to the FDA to conduct pediatric studies. If the FDA determines that there is a public health need for such research, it will issue a Written Request. The studies specified may or may not include those proposed by the sponsor and can include both nonclinical and clinical investigations. As already noted, the FDA may in addition issue a Written Request on its own initiative, as and when it identifies a need for pediatric data.

In contrast to BPCA, which provides incentives for drug developers to voluntarily perform pediatric studies, PREA requires such investigations to be performed. However, this only applies to the specific indications for which the sponsor is seeking approval for their oncology product. PREA is triggered when an application (or supplemental application) is submitted for a new indication, new dosing regimen, new active ingredient, new dosage form, and/or a new route of administration.

Under PREA, the FDA may require that the sponsor develop age-appropriate formulations for use in pediatric studies that must generate data to inform pediatric dosing and administration. However, most oncology products are exempt from PREA. This can be because their indications fall under orphan drug designation, and/or the fact that oncology drug indications tend to differ markedly between the adult and pediatric settings.

THE REGULATORY FRAMEWORK IN THE EUROPEAN UNION

The European Medicines Agency (EMA) is a relatively autonomous body within the European Union (EU) structure; its headquarters is in London. The EMA is responsible for the protection and promotion of public and animal health through the evaluation and supervision of medicines for human and veterinary use. The EMA brings together the scientific resources of over 40 Member State level competent authorities in 30 EU and European Economic Area (EEA)–European Free Trade Agreement countries via a network of over 4500 European experts. It contributes to international and regional activities through its work with global committees and initiatives, such as The International Conference on Harmonisation of Technical Requirements for Registration of Pharmaceuticals for Human Use (the ICH).

The EMA is responsible for the scientific evaluation of applications for EU marketing authorizations for human and veterinary medicines through the centralized procedure. By this procedure, pharmaceutical companies submit a single marketing authorization application. Once granted by the European Commission on the basis of the EMA's scientific committee recommendations, such authorizations are valid in all EU Member States as well as in the EEA countries of Iceland, Liechtenstein, and Norway. A company can only start to market a medicine in the EU after it has received a marketing authorization. The centralized procedure is compulsory for:

- Human medicines for the treatment of human immunodeficiency virus (HIV)/acquired immunodeficiency syndrome, cancer, diabetes, neurodegenerative diseases, autoimmune and other immune dysfunctions, and viral diseases;
- Medicines derived from biotechnology processes, such as genetic engineering;
- Advanced-therapy medicines, such as gene therapy, somatic cell therapy, or tissue-engineered medicines; and
- Officially designated orphan medicines (medicines used for rare human diseases).

For medicines that do not fall within these categories (unlike oncology drugs), companies also have the option of submitting an application for a centralized marketing authorization to the EMA, as long as the medicine concerned is regarded as a significant therapeutic, scientific, or technical innovation or if its authorization would be in the interest of public health. Applications made through the centralized procedure are submitted directly to the EMA. A Rapporteur and a Corapporteur are designated by the competent EMA scientific committee, the Committee for Medicinal Products for Human Use (CHMP). The CHMP coordinates the Rapporteurs' assessment of the medicinal product for which authorization is being sought and prepares draft reports. Once these are available, the CHMP's comments or objections are communicated to the applicant. The Rapporteur is the privileged interlocutor of the applicant and continues to play this role even after marketing authorization has been granted.

The CHMP may deem it necessary to seek the opinion of the Scientific Advisory Group on Oncology (SAG-O). The SAG-O is a core group of independent European experts selected according to their specific expertise and other individual experts who may be called upon to participate in given meetings and bring additional expertise in specific domains [12]. The CHMP, while taking into account the position expressed by the SAG-O, remains ultimately responsible for its own opinions.

The applicant's replies to the questions raised by the Rapporteur and Corapporteur are received, assessed, and then submitted for discussion to the CHMP. Taking into account the conclusions of the CHMP's debate, a final assessment report is prepared. Once the evaluation process is completed, the CHMP gives an opinion on whether or not to grant the requested authorization. When the opinion is favorable, it includes a draft of the Summary of Product Characteristics (SmPC), which is the package leaflet and text proposed for the various packaging materials, and is transmitted to the European Commission. The European Commission has the ultimate authority for granting marketing authorizations in the EU.

Evaluation by the EMA takes up to 210 days, plus additional time for "clock stoppages" that take place while the applicant is preparing responses to the queries received during the procedure. However, on an applicant's request, "an accelerated assessment" may be granted. An accelerated assessment requires the EMA to ensure that the CHMP's opinion is given within 150 days; however, at any time during such an assessment, the CHMP may decide to revoke its decision and continue the process within the standard timelines described above.

Approval Schemes in European Union

Three types of marketing authorizations can be granted by the EMA: normal approval, conditional approval, and exceptional circumstances.

Normal Approval

Normal approval is granted for products for which the comprehensive data needed for assessing the risk-benefit balance (that is, a "full dossier") have been provided. In accordance with Article 14 [1–3] of Regulation (EC) No. 726/2004, such a marketing authorization (MA) is initially valid for 5 years. It may be renewed upon application by the MA holder at least 9 months before its expiry. On the basis of an overall reevaluation of the risk-benefit balance, the CHMP may recommend to grant unlimited validity to the MA or to require an additional 5-year renewal before making a final decision.

Conditional Approval[3]

Conditional marketing authorizations may be granted for products such as new anticancer medicines when, although comprehensive clinical data have not been provided, all of the following requirements are met:

- There is evidence that the benefit/risk balance is likely to be positive;
- It is likely that comprehensive clinical data will become available;
- Unmet medical needs will be addressed by supplying the product for which a marketing authorization is being sought; and
- It can be reasonably concluded that the public health benefits derived from immediate availability will outweigh the risks associated with the need for additional evidence.

As with accelerated approvals in the United States, conditional marketing authorizations are subject to specific obligations to complete ongoing studies or conduct new studies, with a view to confirming the positive benefit-risk balance that the regulatory body has assumed. Such temporary authorizations are not intended to remain conditional. They are reviewed and can be renewed once a year, but once the full data required for confirming the positive benefit-risk relationship are provided, they are converted to normal marketing authorizations.

Conditional approvals were sanctioned by the European Parliament in 2006, over a decade after the initial US legislation in this area. The first oncology compound to receive conditional approval was sunitinib, which was developed by Pfizer as an orphan medicinal product. It was initially used in the treatment of unresectable and/or metastatic malignant gastro-intestinal stromal tumors after the failure of imatinib mesylate treatment due to resistance or intolerance, as well as the treatment of advanced and/or metastatic RCC after the failure of cytokine-based therapy. Conditional approval for this product was converted to normal approval in early 2007 upon the provision of the results of a randomized phase 3 trial in which sunitinib was employed as a first-line treatment for RCC.

In 2012, crizotinib received conditional approval from the EC for the treatment of adults with previously treated anaplastic lymphoma kinase-positive advanced NSCLC. Bren-tuximab, an orphan medicinal product developed by the Japanese company Takeda, also received a conditional approval in 2012. This drug can be used for the treatment of adults with relapsed or refractory CD30+ Hodgkin lymphoma after autologous stem cell transplant (ASCT) or after at least two prior therapies when ASCT or multiagent chemotherapy is not a treatment option.

A list of medicinal products approved under the conditional schema as of January 2013 is reported in Table 20.1. The focus of pharmaceutical and medical research continues to shift toward treatments aimed to target genetic and other molecular-level disease mechanisms, which is taking place alongside the developing social and economic forces alluded to in the introduction to this chapter; therefore, it seems inevitable that drug regulation and registration will increasingly involve incremental forms of licensing approval.

Although the EU conditional marketing authorization process is similar to the US Subpart H accelerated approval mechanism, the qualifying criteria are slightly different (Table 20.2).

---

[3] See Regulation (EC) THE EUROPEAN PARLIAMENT AND OF THE COUNCIL No 507/2006 and also EMEA/419,127/05 GUIDELINE ON THE PROCEDURE FOR ACCELERATED ASSESSMENT PURSUANT TO ARTICLE 14 (9) OF REGULATION (EC) No 726/2004.

Moreover, a conditional marketing authorization can be granted only to the original MAA (Marketing Authorization Application) and not to subsequent efficacy variations; in contrast, accelerated approval in the US can be granted more than once to the same oncology product. Such variations are likely to raise globally relevant questions as to the future of pharmaceutical licensing approaches, especially if (in areas such as oncology) the molecular-level targeting of medicines leads to a growing number of differing specifically licensed applications for given active moieties.

Exceptional Circumstances[4]

Article 14(8) of Regulation (EC) 726/2004 states that "in exceptional circumstances and following consultation with the applicant, the authorisation may be granted subject to a requirement for the applicant to introduce specific procedures, in particular concerning the safety of the medicinal product, notification to the competent authorities of any incident relating to its use, and action to be taken". This authorization may be granted when the applicant is unable to provide comprehensive data because of:

- The rarity of the disease;
- Limitations in the present state of scientific knowledge;
- Ethical constraints; and
- The existence of an opportunity to fulfill an as-yet-unmet medical need.

The capacity to grant marketing authorizations under the exceptional circumstance provisions can be seen as complementing the flexibilities and incentives existing elsewhere in the European regulatory legislation. Such authorizations are subject to annual reassessments of the benefit/risk balance by the CHMP. A list of the medicines that received an exceptional circumstances-based marketing authorization as of January 2013 is provided in Table 20.3.

Orphan Drugs in the European Union

Orphan medicinal product designation is based on the criteria laid down in Regulation (EC) No 141/2000. To qualify for orphan designation, a medicine must meet one or both of the following criteria:

- It is intended for the diagnosis, prevention, or treatment of a life-threatening or chronically debilitating condition affecting no more than 5 in 10,000 people in the EU (that is, up to about 250,000 individuals in the EU's overall population) at the time of submission of the designation application; or
- It is intended for the diagnosis, prevention, or treatment of a life-threatening, seriously debilitating, or serious and chronic condition in a situation such that, without the incentives orphan designation offers, it is unlikely that the revenue after marketing of the medicinal product would cover the investment needed for its development.

In both cases, there must also be either no satisfactory (i.e., previously authorized) method of diagnosis, prevention, or treatment for the condition concerned or, if such a method does exist, the medicine must be intended to offer significant additional benefits to those affected by the condition.

[4] Parliament and Council Regulation (EC) No 726/2004 of 30 April 2004.

TABLE 20.1   Medicinal Products Approved Via the European Conditional Authorization Arrangements, as of January 2013

Trade name	Active substance	Indication	Approval date	Orphan
Adcetris	Brentuximab vedotin	Hodgkin disease, non-Hodgkin lymphoma	October 25, 2012	Yes
Arepanrix	Split influenza virus, inactivated, containing antigen[1]: A/California/7/2009 (H1N1)v like strain (X-179A)	Disease outbreaks and immunization for human influenza	March 23, 2010	No
Arzerra	Ofatumumab	Leukemia, lymphocytic, chronic, B-cell	April 19, 2010	Yes
Caprelsa	Vandetanib	Thyroid neoplasms	February 17, 2012	No
Diacomit	Stiripentol	Myoclonic epilepsy, Juvenile	January 4, 2007	Yes
Fampyra	Fampridine	Multiple sclerosis	July 20, 2011	No
Humenza	Split influenza virus, inactivated, containing antigen[1]: A/California/7/2009 (H1N1)v like strain (X-179A)	Disease outbreaks and immunization of human influenza	June 8, 2010	No
Intelence	Etravirine	HIV infections	August 28, 2008	No
Pixuvri	Pixantrone dimaleate	Lymphoma, non-Hodgkin	May 10, 2012	No
Tyverb	Lapatinib	Breast neoplasms	June 10, 2008	No
Vectibix	Panitumumab	Colorectal neoplasms	December 3, 2007	No
Votrient	Pazopanib	Carcinoma, renal cell	June 14, 2010	No
Votubia	Everolimus	Astrocytoma	September 2, 2011	Yes
Xalkori	Crizotinib	Carcinoma, non-small cell lung	October 23, 2012	No

[1] *Produced in eggs.*

Once the application is complete, the sponsor should submit it to the EMA, where the Committee for Orphan Medicinal Products is charged with reviewing designation applications from persons or companies seeking to develop medicines for rare diseases (so-called orphan drugs). Sponsors with medicines designated as orphan medicines by the European Commission can benefit from a range of incentives, including:

- Protocol assistance: The EMA provides a form of scientific advice specifically for orphan medicines called protocol assistance, which allows sponsors to obtain answers to technical questions regarding the types and design of studies needed adequately to demonstrate the medicine's benefit-risk balance. These may concern product quality issues, as well as nonclinical and clinical aspects of a medicine's use. Protocol assistance is free of charge for both initial and subsequent requests;
- Access to the centralized authorization procedure;

TABLE 20.2   Qualifying Criteria for EU Conditional Marketing Authorizations compared to US Accelerated Approval

EU conditional marketing authorization	US accelerated approval
Benefit-risk balance is positive	Drug product has effect on surrogate endpoint that is likely to predict clinical benefit
It is likely that the applicant can provide comprehensive clinical data within an agreed-upon timeframe	Approval is based on condition that sponsor conducts clinical studies to verify and describe the actual clinical benefit
Unmet medical needs will be fulfilled	Drug will treat serious and/or life-threatening disease and fill an unmet medical need
Benefit of immediate access for public health outweighs any risk inherent in the fact that additional data are still required	

- 10 years of market exclusivity for the use of the medicine concerned in the orphan indication setting; and
- 2 years of marketing exclusivity if the orphan product is compliant with the EU's pediatric medicines regulation (see below).

In the EU, orphan medicinal products eligible for these incentives should have a separate trademark from that applying to other presentations of the same drug to allow for easy and unequivocal identification. Unlike the situation in the US, orphan and nonorphan indications cannot be covered by the same marketing authorization. Thus, it is not possible in Europe to extend an existing marketing authorization for a nonorphan indication to cover a new orphan indication, and vice versa.

Pediatric Medicines

The pediatric regulation came into force in January 2007. Its main objective is to contribute to improving the health of children (<18 years of age) in Europe without subjecting them to unnecessary trials or delaying the authorization of medicinal products for use in adults. A key component of these reforms was the establishment of the Paediatric Committee (PDCO), which is responsible for coordinating EMA's work on medicines for children. Its main role is to specify the studies that companies must carry out on children as part of the Pediatric Investigation Plans (PIPs) that the regulation requires.

All applications for marketing authorization for new medicines that were not granted in the EU before January 26, 2007 have to include the results of studies carried out in children of different ages. This requirement also applies when a company wants to add a new indication, pharmaceutical form, or route of administration for a patented medicine that is already authorized for marketing. The PDCO may, however, grant deferrals (which allow applicants to delay development of medicines in children until there is enough information to demonstrate their safety and effectiveness in adults) or waivers. Waivers apply when the development of a medicine in children is not needed or is not appropriate, such as when the relevant indication only affects the elderly population.

TABLE 20.3   Medicinal Products Approved under the European Exceptional Circumstances Regulations as of January 2013

Name	Active substance	Indication	Date of authorization	Orphan
AlduRazyme	Laronidase	Mucopolysaccharidosis I	June 10, 2003	Yes
Atriance	Nelarabine	Precursor T-cell lymphoblastic leukemia-lymphoma	August 22, 2007	Yes
ATryn	Antithrombin alfa	Antithrombin III deficiency	July 28, 2006	No
Ceplene	Histamine dihydrochloride	Leukemia, myeloid, acute	October 7, 2008	Yes
Daronrix	Whole virion, inactivated, containing antigen[1]: A/Vietnam/1194/2004 (H5N1)	Disease outbreaks and immunization of human influenza	March 21, 2007	No
Elaprase	Idursulfase	Mucopolysaccharidosis II	January 8, 2007	Yes
Evoltra	Clofarabine	Precursor cell lymphoblastic leukemia-lymphoma	May 29, 2006	Yes
Firdapse (previously Zenas)	Amifampridine	Lambert-Eaton myasthenic syndrome	December 23, 2009	Yes
Foclivia	Influenza virus surface antigens, inactivated: A/Viet Nam/1194/2004 (H5N1)	Disease outbreaks and immunization for human influenza	October 19, 2009	
Glybera	Alipogene tiparvovec	Hyperlipoproteinemia type I		Yes
Ilaris	Canakinumab	Cryopyrin-associated periodic syndromes	October 23, 2009	No
Increlex	Mecasermin	Laron syndrome	August 3, 2007	Yes
Naglazyme	Galsulfase	Mucopolysaccharidosis VI	January 24, 2006	Yes
Pandemic influenza vaccine (H5N1) (split virion, inactivated, adjuvanted) GlaxoSmithKline biologicals	Split influenza virus, inactivated, containing antigen[1]: A/VietNam/1194/2004 (H5N1) like strain used (NIBRG-14)	Disease outbreaks and immunization for human influenza	October 19, 2009	No
Pandemic influenza vaccine H5N1 Baxter	Whole virion inactivated containing antigen of pandemic strain: A/Vietnam/1203/2004 (H5N1) 7.5 µg per 0.5 ml dose	Disease outbreaks and immunization for human influenza	October 16, 2009	No
Prialt	Ziconotide	Injections, spinal pain	February 21, 2005	Yes

TABLE 20.3 Medicinal Products Approved under the European Exceptional Circumstances Regulations as of January 2013 (*cont'd*)

Name	Active substance	Indication	Date of authorization	Orphan
Replagal	Agalsidase alfa	Fabry disease	August 3, 2001	Yes
Vedrop	Tocofersolan	Cholestasis vitamin E deficiency	July 24, 2009	No
Ventavis	Iloprost	Hypertension, pulmonary	September 16, 2003	Yes
Vyndaqel	Tafamidis	Amyloidosis	November 16, 2011	Yes
Xagrid	Anagrelide	Thrombocythemia, essential	November 16, 2004	Yes
Yondelis	Trabectedin	Ovarian neoplasms sarcoma	September 17, 2007	Yes

[1] *Produced in eggs.*

Medicines that have been authorized across the EU with the results of PIP studies included in the product information are eligible for an extension of their overall patent term of 6 months, even when the results of studies are negative. As noted, orphan medicines compliant with the Pediatric Regulation receive an additional 2 years of marketing exclusivity. Other incentives to develop better medicines for children in Europe include the provision of scientific advice and protocol assistance by the EMA, which is free of charge for questions relating to the development of pediatric drugs.

Medicines developed specifically for children that are already authorized but not protected by a patent or supplementary protection certificate can apply for a pediatric-use marketing authorization (PUMA). When a PUMA is granted, the product will benefit from 10 years of market protection, even if it is already widely available in Europe as a generic medicine for use in the treatment of adults.

This last provision may occasionally be challenged, and sometimes even evaded, by care providers and/or funders and questioned by generic medicine manufacturers whose financial interests are affected. Nevertheless, it is a legally defined part of the implicit social contract associated with all forms of pharmaceutical regulation aimed at protecting public interests—not only for the safety and affordability of existing treatments but also for the quality and continuing viability of research and development aimed at generating new opportunities for future benefit.

CURRENT ISSUES AND FUTURE DIRECTIONS IN ANTICANCER DRUG REGULATION

The overall regulatory frameworks outlined previously, along with additional controls applying in areas such as the design and conduct of preclinical and clinical trials (Box 20.1), mean that both the US and the EU have established robust and largely complementary systems for licensing medicines and regulating their development, safety, production, and sale since the thalidomide tragedy of the late 1950s and early 1960s. Despite some continuing concerns regarding factors such as publication transparency [13], this positive achievement

BOX 20.1

PRECLINICAL AND CLINICAL TRIALS

The human medicine preclinical and clinical development and trials process that has evolved in developed nations since the thalidomide event at the start of the 1960s is not static. It also has a number of special oncology-related characteristics (see, for example, Refs [14,15]) However, in essence, it involves the following stages:

- **Preclinical development and testing**. During this stage, new chemical (or molecular) entities (NCEs or NMEs) identified as being potentially active against a defined biological target are evaluated (typically in animal models, but also increasingly in in vitro systems) with regard to their likely (cellular and organ) toxicity and pharmacokinetics in humans. Other preclinical investigations are aimed at elucidating the chemical and allied characteristics of the substances under investigation, so that appropriate manufacturing arrangements can be made as required and suitable formulations produced. Conventional estimates suggest that up to a quarter of all drug development costs may (at least until recently) be associated with preclinical research and development of various types.
- **Phase 1 human trials**. These "first-in-man" investigations typically take place among limited numbers of healthy volunteers. They address basic safety and dosing issues. However, potential anticancer treatments for which suitable activity biomarkers exist can now on occasions be used first in selected patient volunteers. Such "phase 0" studies involve small doses of new drugs being given to small numbers of people for limited periods, such as a week, in order to generate initial

data on a new drug entity's impacts in, and pathway through, the body [16]. Investigations of this type can help speed a product's development or save costs by showing at the earliest possible moment that an NCE is unlikely to be suitable for medicinal usage.

- **Phase 2 human trials**. These trials take place in limited numbers of patients with the condition for which the treatment is being developed. They serve to define and refine the treatment protocol to be applied in subsequent large-scale therapeutic trials.
- **Phase 3 human trials**. These trials involve greater numbers of patients in what are normally randomized design-based tests of the new treatment's effects against relevant comparators. In traditional licensing processes, they provide the evidence required for a new medicine to be judged safe (or not safe) for use and hence to be approved by agencies such as the FDA in the US or the EMA in the European Union, albeit that in many countries anticancer medicines are commonly used "off-label" once licensed. The true cost of developing a new medicine is a controversial question, especially because of disputes as to the extent to which outlays on failed drug candidate research should be allocated to successfully marketed products and how the true cost of risk capital can best be calculated. Nevertheless, it is has been claimed that one effective way for innovators to reduce their costs and speed approvals would be to enhance phase 1 and 2 evaluations, to permit savings at the phase 3 stage [17]. Established sources suggest that phase 3 trials account for around a third of all premarketing

---

BOX 20.1 *(cont'd)*

drug research and development costs [18,19], although they may in fact account for over half of all such investments.

- **Phase 4 postmarketing pharmacovigilance studies**. These studies classically take place after medicines have been marketed and are being supplied for normal use. It is at this stage that, as patient numbers build, relatively infrequent side effects may be identified. A common unwanted side effect with an incidence rate of 1 in 500 against a similar natural background occurrence rate of 1 in 500 can be expected to be revealed via trials involving around 20,000 patients. However, in the case of a side effect with an incidence of 1 in 5000 with a higher background rate of 1 in 200, for example, the number of patients using the drug would have to be in excess of a million before there is a mathematical likelihood of the side effect being detected within the normally applied (95%) limits of probability [20].

---

deserves appropriate recognition. However, as the challenges facing researchers and medicine suppliers working in areas such as oncology in both developed and developing countries continue to evolve, further developments in certain areas—such as balancing the need to speed patient access to new drugs for potentially fatal conditions against the desirability of prudent testing—will be needed.

The remainder of this chapter therefore explores a number of related fields, starting with a consideration of the endpoints used in trials for conducted for regulatory purposes. These endpoints should normally be discussed with the FDA, EMA, and other authorities prior to the initiation of clinical trials to ensure that they will accurately assess the efficacy of the drug being evaluated with a minimum of potential bias or other error [21] while also respecting stakeholder interests in timeliness and economic efficiency.

Traditionally, overall survival has been viewed as the gold standard endpoint for demonstrating clinical benefit in areas such as cancer care. As an endpoint, overall survival is normally relatively easy to measure without bias because it can be documented by the date of death. Yet such advantages should not draw attention away from the reality that symptomatically based improvements in patient-reported outcomes can also be indicative of important forms of clinical benefit that may not be reflected in mortality-based data.

The regulatory precedence for approvals in oncology using health-related quality-of-life measures as primary endpoints is so far very limited. Ruxolitinib was authorized in both the US and EU for the treatment of myelofibrosis, in large part on the basis of its effects as measured via an health-related quality-of-life instrument called the Myelofibrosis Symptom Assessment Form Diary (http://www.proqolid.org/instruments/myelofibrosis_symptom_assessment_form_mfsaf). Other endpoints, such as progression-free survival, objective response rate, and durable complete responses have also on occasions been used to support approvals.

The latter tumor assessment endpoints are often based on indirect assessments, calculations, and estimates. As such, for studies that have one of these measures as a primary endpoint, global regulators have to decide whether or not the results should be used as the basis for a regular/normal approval or for an accelerated/conditional approval. For accelerated/conditional approval, the ongoing authorization process will, as already described, require subsequent confirmation of benefit in a further trial or trials.

It is normally agreed that the use of such endpoints for registration purposes should be verified by blinded central reviewers. However, in July 2012, the FDA's Oncologic Drugs Advisory Committee supported easing the requirement for blinded, independent, central review of all patient scans in studies using progression-free survival as the primary endpoint. Members also indicated that the FDA should retain the right to require full case audits in certain circumstances, depending upon the tumor type and study size. Table 20.4 (which is adapted from an FDA guidance document—FDA, 2007) provides further information on the strengths and weaknesses of the alternative endpoints that are potentially suitable for use in anticancer drug studies.

Adaptive Licensing

Traditional drug licensing approaches can be described as having been based on binary decisions. These decisions imply that, at the moment of licensing, an experimental therapy is presumptively transformed into a fully vetted, safe and efficacious therapy for given disease or physiological site-based indications. However, this has always been a questionable assumption, which is increasingly being seen as inappropriate in areas such as oncology.

Recently, a wave of proposals for planned adaptive approaches to drug licensing and supply has emerged under various labels, including staggered approval, managed entry, adaptive approval, progressive authorization, and coverage with evidence development. Such proposals vary in detail, but all are based on acceptance of the fact that knowledge of drug safety and application is not in fact binary but continues to evolve over time. Adaptive licensing has, for instance, been defined [20] as "a prospectively planned, flexible approach to regulation of drugs and biologics. Through iterative phases of evidence gathering to reduce uncertainties followed by regulatory evaluation and license adaptation, adaptive licensing seeks to maximize the positive impact of new drugs on public health by balancing timely access for patients with the need to assess and to provide adequate evolving information on benefits and risks so that better informed patient-care decisions can be made."

In essence, the further introduction of such approaches to authorizing the use of medicines will mean that the "magic moment" between nonapproval and drug approval is replaced with progressive management and reduction of uncertainty. In an era of personalized and better targeted medicine use, such progress is likely to be welcomed. It may have the potential to help curb the increasing costs and apparently falling productivity of medicine development in areas such as cancer care, without sacrificing public interests in safeguarding therapeutic safety. However, a number of caveats should be added to this conclusion, including the following:

- Without clear central guidelines, there may be continuing disputes in any conditional approval process between the providers of innovative treatments on the one hand and health care providers and funders on the other regarding the borderline points at which drug costs are normally funded, as opposed to being met by the product sponsor; and

- However precisely drugs are targeted at the molecular level, there will always a risk of unpredictable and/or otherwise unwanted side effects, such as the initially unexpected cardiovascular consequences of using trastuzumab for the treatment of breast cancer. The rhetoric of personalized care should not be allowed to obscure the continuing need for informed caution when employing all new or existing therapies, based on rational and systematic evaluations of risk and benefit for populations as well as individuals.

Therapeutic Agent and Companion Diagnostic Codevelopments

The FDA and other regulatory agencies are increasingly requiring coordinated therapeutic and companion diagnostic codevelopment programs [22]. The FDA defines an in vitro diagnostic (IVD) companion diagnostic device as one that provides information that is essential for the safe and effective use of a corresponding therapeutic product. The use of an IVD companion diagnostic device with a particular therapeutic product should be stipulated in the instructions for use in the labeling of both the diagnostic device and the corresponding therapeutic product. These instructions should be developed and approved contemporaneously on order to support the therapeutic product's safe and effective use, at least from the normally assumed regulatory perspective. However, if inappropriately imposed, such a requirement may be seen as undesirably delaying patient access to potentially effective treatments.

When planning a global therapeutic and companion diagnostic development program, a number of key items should be considered. First and foremost, regulators are likely to want the clinical utility of a novel diagnostic product to be demonstrated in the trials supporting registration of the therapeutic agent. This requires advanced planning as well as analytical validation and verification of the companion diagnostic prior to its use for the selection of the patients to be included in pivotal therapeutic trials. In addition, in markets such as the United States, regulatory filings must be made to allow the use of an investigational IVD companion diagnostic to prospectively select patients for trial enrollment. This can currently be done in the United States either by filing for an Investigational Device Exemption (IDE) or by submitting required diagnostic information via the Investigational New Drug (IND) application.

In the United States, Presubmission (formerly known as Pre-IDE) meetings can be requested at any time during the codevelopment of an IVD to seek advice from the FDA's Center for Devices and Radiological Health (CDRH) for issues concerning development and registration. In particular, a Presubmission meeting should be held with CDRH along with representatives from the therapeutic review division prior to the initiation of pivotal trials designed to support the registration of the therapeutic and companion diagnostic. In the light of the long lead times needed to address analytical validation and other technical requirements, it is advisable for sponsors to meet with the CDRH as early as possible in the development cycle. There is no limit to the number of Presubmission meetings that can be held. The planning of and preparation for the meetings are usually led by the IVD company, with input and participation from the pharmaceutical/biotech company involved. Close coordination between such partners is critically important.

There is much to consider from clinical and clinical operations perspectives when developing a codevelopment program. For instance, the location and number of central laboratories used for diagnostic testing is important. To meet US FDA requirements, at least three laboratories must be involved. In addition, a diagnostic reproducibility study demonstrating

TABLE 20.4 Oncology Approval Endpoints

Endpoint	Regulatory evidence	Study design	Advantages	Disadvantages
Overall survival	Clinical benefit for regular/normal approval	• Randomized studies essential • Blinding not essential	• Universally accepted direct measure of benefit • Easily measured • Precisely measured	• May involve longer studies • May be affected by crossover therapy and sequential therapy
Symptom endpoints (patient-reported outcomes)	Clinical benefit for regular/normal approval	• Randomized studies • Blinding preferred	• Patient perspective of direct clinical benefit	• Blinding is often difficult • Data are frequently missing or incomplete • Clinical significance of small changes is unknown • Multiple analyses
Disease-free survival	Surrogate for accelerated/conditional approval or regular/normal approval[1]	• Randomized studies essential • Blinding preferred • Blinded review recommended	• Smaller sample size and shorter follow-up necessary compared with survival studies	• Not statistically validated as surrogate for survival in all settings • Not precisely measured, subject to assessment bias (particularly in open-label studies), • Definitions vary among studies
Objective response rate	Surrogate for accelerated/conditional approval or regular/normal approval[1]	• Single-arm or randomized studies can be used • Blinding preferred in comparative studies • Blinded review recommended	• Can be assessed in single-arm studies • Assessed earlier and in smaller studies compared with survival studies • Effect attributable to drug (not natural history)	• Not a direct measure of benefit • Not a comprehensive measure of drug activity

Endpoint	Regulatory use	Study design	Advantages	Limitations
Complete response	Surrogate for accelerated/conditional approval or regular/normal approval[1]	• Single-arm or randomized studies can be used • Blinding preferred in comparative studies • Blinded review recommended	• Can be assessed in single-arm studies • Durable complete responses can represent clinical benefit • Assessed earlier and in smaller studies compared with survival studies	• Not a direct measure of benefit • Not a comprehensive measure of drug activity
Progression-free survival (includes all deaths) or Time to progression (deaths before progression censored)	Surrogate for accelerated/conditional approval or regular/normal approval[1]	• Randomized studies essential • Blinding preferred • Blinded review recommended	• Smaller sample size and shorter follow-up necessary compared with survival studies • Measurement of stable disease included • Not affected by crossover or subsequent therapies • Generally based on objective and quantitative assessment	• Not statistically validated as surrogate for survival in all settings • Not precisely measured, subject to assessment bias (particularly in open-label studies) • Definitions vary among studies • Frequent radiological or other assessments • Involves balanced timing of assessments among treatment arms

[1] *Adequacy as a surrogate endpoint for accelerated/conditional approval or regular/normal approval is highly dependent upon other factors, such as effect size, effect duration, and benefits of other available therapy.*

III. THE REALITY OF CANCER DRUGS IN THE CLINIC

that the assay generates consistent results across the different laboratories and other study participants must be conducted prior to approval. The design of case report forms and subsequently the clinical database must be tailored to capture information specific to the use of the diagnostic in patient screening and trial enrollment. Early and frequent regulatory interactions with FDA and EMA are always critical, but even more so with therapeutics that have a focused patient selection or companion diagnostic component.

Another important priority for therapeutic and companion diagnostic codevelopment programs is to ensure the capture of information on biomarker-negative patients treated with the candidate therapeutic agent. Data from these patients are needed to demonstrate that the diagnostic test in question is indeed needed and adds value. If the response rate in biomarker-positive and biomarker-negative patients are equal, then an IVD companion diagnostic obviously lacks clinical utility. Conversely, if a new therapeutic agent were to be shown to only be safe and effective in the biomarker-positive patient population, then the IVD companion diagnostic would be defined as essential to the safe and effective its use. Gathering clinical data on biomarker-negative patients can be challenging late in a therapeutic agent's lifecycle, so advance consideration of how such information will be gathered is important.

Outside the US, there is less specific guidance regarding the codevelopment of new medicines and companion diagnostics, but there are growing expectations that the latter ought to be available in the form of CE-marked or locally approved or required products in order to identify patients for whom the therapeutic agent on trial has a positive benefit-risk profile. The EMA is not presently directly involved in the approval process for companion diagnostics. However, there is no restriction on the provision of scientific advice for questions related to the codevelopment of drugs and allied diagnostics.

As in the United States, feedback from the medical device branches of health authorities regarding the development and registration of IVDs can be very valuable during the planning stages of global pivotal trials. There is also an ongoing need to keep alert to changes in this area of the regulatory landscape in regions such as Japan, China, and Europe, where a proposed new regulation on in vitro diagnostic medical devices is presently under discussion.

The current diversity of diagnostic regulations and lack of precedents for therapeutic and companion diagnostic codevelopment globally can be seen as problematic; in general, however, meeting the FDA's approval requirements should help position would-be applicants for regulatory success globally. Although there are opportunities for the accelerated or conditional approval of therapeutic products for use in oncology or elsewhere, advance consideration and scenario planning relating to the impacts on companion diagnostic development, registration, and commercialization processes should be considered.

Finally, looking to the future, as molecularly defined subsets of tumors (such as lung cancer) become better, smaller, and more precisely demarcated, the paradigm of a single therapeutic agent plus a single companion diagnostic might prove to be unsustainable. Very small patient populations inevitably make it more difficult to screen for and enroll sufficient numbers of participants in clinical trials. It can be difficult to obtain enough tumor tissue to perform sequential testing for several biomarkers. Such difficulties add to the challenges of detecting rare and complex tumor types. As a result, there is an emergent need for new platforms and technologies (for example, multiplex assays or next-generation sequencing) to allow the identification of multiple biomarkers using a single tissue specimen. The introduction of new approaches for resolving such challenges will in turn raise new issues for industry, regulators, and academic and other stakeholders to work through as collaboratively as possible.

Investigational Combinations of Two or More Oncology Products

Combination therapy is established as an important modality in many settings, including some blood and other cancers, cardiovascular disease prevention and treatment, and the control of a wider variety of infectious conditions. The availability of fixed-dose combination products incorporating drugs with complementary actions has already transformed the effectiveness of anti-HIV programs. Hopefully, the further use of such strategies will achieve similar gains in oncology.

Current regulatory models tend to focus primarily on assessing the effectiveness and safety of single new investigational drugs acting alone or in combination with an already approved drug. However, from a public interest viewpoint, these models should be flexible enough to allow and even facilitate the introduction of more radical alternatives. As a result of constantly improved understandings of the mechanisms underpinning oncogenesis and phenomena such as anticancer drug resistance, there is an emerging trend toward using combinations of two or more investigational oncology products not previously developed for any purpose in clinical development programs, in the hope of achieving increased efficacy and/or inhibiting the development of resistance.

However, this trend is creating a need for more sophisticated approaches in a number of areas linked to regulatory processes, such as the identification and agreed employment of statistical techniques capable of accurately assessing the contributions (or lack thereof) of individual combination therapy components along with the impacts of the combination as a whole. One goal should be to specify phase 3 trials in ways that avoid needlessly large, complex, and costly designs.

In recognition of the challenges and possible public health gains associated with investigational combinations of oncology products, the FDA has recently issued draft guidance intended to assist sponsors working toward the codevelopment of two or more novel (not previously marketed) drugs.[5] The FDA argues that codevelopment should ordinarily be reserved for situations in which:

- The combination is intended to treat a serious disease or condition;
- There is a compelling biological rationale for its use (for instance, when the agents employed inhibit distinct targets in the same molecular pathway, provide inhibition of both a primary and compensatory pathway, or inhibit the same target at different binding sites in order to decrease resistance or allow use of doses that minimize toxicity);
- A preclinical model (in vivo or in vitro) or short-term clinical study on an established biomarker suggests that the combination has substantial activity and provides a greater than simply additive effect or a more durable response (as through delayed resistance) as compared to the single use of the individual agents alone; and

[5] Draft Guidance for Industry: Codevelopment of Two or More Unmarketed Investigational Drugs for Use in Combination. US Food and Drug Administration. December 2012.

- There is a compelling reason why the agents cannot be developed individually (for example, when monotherapy for the disease of interest leads to resistance and/or one or both of the agents is expected to have very limited activity when used as monotherapy).

As these conditions suggest, the codevelopment of novel therapeutic agents is most appropriately pursued in circumstances in which the biology of the disease, pathogen, or tumor type in question is understood sufficiently to permit the development of a plausible biological rationale for the use of combination therapy to treat the disease or condition. The FDA recommends that sponsors should gather evidence to support the posited biological rationale for the combination in an in vivo or in vitro model. When developing nonclinical safety characterizations for two or more investigational drugs to be used in combination, the FDA further advises that sponsors should consult the recently revised International Conference on Harmonisation Guidance on Nonclinical Safety Studies.[6]

Current guidance suggests that, whenever possible, the safety profile of each individual drug should be characterized in phase 1 studies in the same manner as would be done for the development of a single drug, including determination of the maximum tolerated dose, the nature of the dose-limiting toxicity, and pharmacokinetic parameters. For initial human effectiveness studies of the combination, the starting dose, dosing escalation intervals, and doses to be used in dose–response studies should be determined on the basis of phase 1 safety data for the individual components, if and as available.

As for clinical pharmacology, the expectation is that the same clinical pharmacology studies will be conducted for each of the individual drugs in the combination as would be done if the drugs were being developed separately. They ought to cover variables such as bioavailability and the relevant mass balances. Exposure responses should also be evaluated, as should the effects of intrinsic factors (such as renal and hepatic impairments) and extrinsic factors (such as food effects and drug interactions) on each medicinal substance's pharmacokinetics and pharmacodynamics; these studies may be conducted with the combination instead of the individual drugs.

In terms of phase 2 proof-of-concept studies, the testing involved should:

- Demonstrate the contribution of each component of the combination to the extent possible and needed, given available nonclinical and pharmacological data;
- Provide evidence of the effectiveness of the combination; and
- Optimize the dose or doses of the combination for use in phase 3 trials.

The study design chosen will depend on the nature of the combination being developed and the disease for which treatment is being developed, along with other factors such as the magnitude of benefit expected. If the findings from the in vivo or in vitro models and/or the phase 2 trials conducted adequately demonstrate the contribution of each component to the combination under investigation, phase 3 trials comparing the combination with standard care or placebo will generally be sufficient to establish effectiveness. If the contribution of the individual components is not clear and it is ethically feasible to use a component

---

[6] Guidance for Industry: M3(R2) Nonclinical Safety Studies for the Conduct of Human Clinical Trials and Marketing Authorization, January 2010 (this guidance is a revision of 1997 ICH guidance M3: Nonclinical Safety Studies for the Conduct of Human Clinical Trials for Pharmaceuticals).

or components of the combination as monotherapy in a study arm, it may be necessary to demonstrate the contribution of the components in phase 3 studies via the employment of a factorial design.

However, despite the availability of much comprehensive guidance, some regulatory questions remain open. For example, it is anticipated that the level of statistical rigor needed to demonstrate the contribution of each of an investigational combination's components will vary with its treatment effect size versus that of standard care. This will probably have to be decided on a case-by-case basis, taking into consideration the overall benefits and risks of the investigational combination.

Furthermore, in some cases it may not be ethical to test each agent separately. Another key question is whether or not the contribution of each combination component (or lack thereof) will have to be demonstrated using the same endpoint as that used in the pivotal phase 3 trials, or whether alternative surrogate endpoints (such as, for instance, the overall response rates) might be used. It may be argued that unless such contributions can be demonstrated with earlier endpoints and/or less stringent levels of evidence than are currently anticipated, the feasibility of developing therapeutic combinations will be significantly impaired. Lastly, the level of preclinical and clinical data required prior to initiating investigational combination is also still to be determined.

CONCLUSIONS

This is an unprecedented time in oncology. Against the background of an exponential expansion in fundamental scientific understanding of the molecular drivers of cancer, there are (alongside advances in surgery and radiotherapy) increasing opportunities to use a growing array of pharmaceutical treatment types—from small molecule-based medicines to monoclonal antibodies, antibody-drug conjugates, therapeutic vaccines, and innovative combination treatments, with or without companion diagnostics—in the care of people living with cancer. Taking such advances together, there is every reason to hope that in the next few decades major improvements in both cancer prevention and survival will become achievable on a global basis.

Nevertheless, the rate at which technical and allied advances will in practice become available to, and be employed to benefit, people living in the different communities of the world will almost certainly vary according to factors ranging from the affordability of new medicines to levels of access to diagnostic services, as well as the availability of good-quality medical, pharmaceutical and nursing care that is needed to ensure that therapies can be used optimum effect. Rates of investment in innovation will also be influenced by the incomes that research funders are able to draw from their products. This will in large part be determined (especially in circumstances where the numbers of patients qualifying for each individually licensed treatment are relatively small) by the extent of the effective intellectual property protection available to drug discoverers for initially registered indications as well as second and subsequent uses of both new and maturing medicines.

The nature of the regulatory systems, which are in place to both prevent the marketing of unduly hazardous therapies and facilitate the supply of innovative treatments with risk-benefit balances acceptable to the people for whom they are intended, will also be an important influence on the future economic viability of anticancer medicines research. This chapter has not attempted to explore in depth the effects of changing regulatory requirements on the costs and productivity of research programs. The interactions between oncology drug marketing authorization and allied procedures and other important factors, such as the mechanisms in place for treatment funding across the world, were not discussed. Also, it did not investigate detailed aspects of anticancer drug registration and regulation in particular national settings, such as those of the United Kingdom or India.

In the United Kingdom, for instance, the Medicines and Healthcare Products Regulatory Agency [23] recently held a consultation on permitting patients to have early access to some drugs before they have been formally licensed. In India, by contrast, the use of compulsory licensing powers for patented anticancer treatments is relevant to not only medicine access issues, but also to industrial policy and anticancer research funding strategies worldwide.

However, despite its limitations, this chapter outlined the main regulatory provisions in place in the European Union and the United States, and indicated the types of provisions that are being introduced to address the challenges resulting from the changing nature of anticancer drug research in the early twenty-first century.

It would be foolhardy to suggest that current arrangements for the approval and licensing of new oncology treatments are optimal, either technically or in financial terms. Yet, the need for new flexibilities and an approach that is genuinely patient- and public interest-centered has been recognized by many of the individuals responsible for leading agencies, such as the FDA and the EMA. It can reasonably be concluded that active efforts are being made to both help assure the ongoing viability of anticancer medicines research in industrial, academic, and voluntarily funded settings, as well as to ensure that regulatory procedures do not fail to protect patient safety nor counterproductively impede access to treatments that can represent a last hope for individuals and families living with cancer.

References

[1] Eichler HG, Pignatti F, Flamion B, Leufkens H, Breckenridge A. Balancing early market access to new drugs with the need for benefit/risk data: a mounting dilemma. Nat Rev Drug Discov 2008;7(10):818–26.
[2] Boyle P, Howell A. The globalisation of breast cancer. Breast Cancer Res 2010;12(Suppl. 4):S7.
[3] Jonsson B, Wilking N. A global comparison regarding patient access to cancer drugs. Karolinska Institutet and the Stockholm School of Economics Ann Oncol 2007;18(Suppl. 3):1–74.
[4] Coleman MP. Not credible: a subversion of science by the pharmaceutical industry. Ann Oncol 2007;18:1433–5.
[5] Maher, J. Personal communication with DGT. 2012.
[6] US Department of Health and Human Services. The health consequences of smoking: a report of the Surgeon General. US Department of Health and Human Services, Centers for Disease Control and Prevention, National Center for Chronic Disease Prevention and Health Promotion, Office on Smoking and Health; 2004.
[7] Lichtenberg F. The impact of new drug launches on longevity: evidence from longitudinal. Disease-Level Data from 52 Countries, 1982–2001 Int J Health Care Finance Econ 2001;5:47.
[8] Peto, R. Harveian Oration, http://www.rcplondon.ac.uk/webstreamed-events/harveian-oration-2012-halving-premature-death-sir-richard-peto; 2012 [accessed February 2013].
[9] Kanavos P, Sullivan R, Lewison G, Schurer W, Eckhouse S, Vlachopioti Z. The role of funding and policies on innovation in cancer drug development. London: The London School of Economics and Political Science; 2010.
[10] US FDA. Guidance for industry: clinical trial endpoints the approval of cancer drugs and biologics: clinical trial endpoints for the approval of cancer drugs and biologics. US Food and Drug Administration; 2007.
[11] Johnson JR, Ning YM, Farrell A, Justice R, Keegan P, Pazdur R. Accelerated approval of oncology products: the food and drug administration experience. J Natl Cancer Inst 2011;103(8):636–44.

[12] EMA. Human Medicines Development and Evaluation Mandate, objectives and rules of procedure for the scientific advisory groups (SAGs) and ad-hoc experts groups. 2010 (EMA/117014/2010)

[13] Goldacre, B. Bad pharma: how drug companies mislead doctors and harm patients. 2012, Fourth Estate.

[14] Booth CM, Cescon DW, Wang L, Tannock IF, Krzyzanowska MK. Evolution of the randomized controlled trial (RCT) in oncology over three decades. J Clin Oncol 2008;26:5458–64.

[15] Davies JE, Neidle S, Taylor DG. Developing and paying for medicines for orphan indications in oncology: utilitarian regulation versus equitable care? Br J Cancer 2012;106(1):14–7.

[16] Lancet. Phase 0 trials: a platform for drug development? Lancet 2009;374:176.

[17] Paul SM, Mytelka DS, Dunwiddie CT, Persinger CC, Munos BH, Lindborg SR, et al. How to improve R&D productivity: the pharmaceutical industry's grand challenge. Nat Rev Drug Discov 2010;9:203–14.

[18] Di Masi JA, Hansen RW, Grabowski HG. The price of innovation: new estimates of drug development costs. J Health Econ 2003;22:151–85.

[19] Kaitin K. Deconstructing the drug development process: the new face of innovation. Clin Pharmacol Ther 2010;87(3):356–61.

[20] Eichler HG, Oye K, Baird LG, Abadie E, Brown J, Drum CL, et al. Adaptive licensing: taking the next step in the evolution of drug approval. Clin Pharmacol Ther 2012(3):426–37.

[21] Pazdur R. Endpoints for assessing drug activity in clinical trials. Oncologist 2008;13(2):19–21.

[22] Pourkavoos N. Unique risks, benefits and challenges of developing drug–drug combination products in a pharmaceutical industrial setting. Comb Prod Ther 2012; 10.1007/s13556-012-0002-2.

[23] MHRA. Consultation on a proposal to introduce an early access to medicines scheme in the UK (MLX 376). London: the Medicines and Healthcare Products Regulatory Agency; 2012.

Glossary

ABC adenosine triphosphate binding cassette

ACTH adrenocortico-tropic hormone

ADCC antibody-dependent cell-mediated cytotoxicity

ADT androgen deprivation therapy

AFF2 AF4/FMR2 family, member 2

AGT O^6-alkylguanine DNA alkyltransferase, the protein which removes alkyl groups from the O^6-position of guanine

AKT v-akt murine thymoma viral oncogene homolog 1

ALK anaplastic lymphoma receptor tyrosine kinase

Alkylating agent chemical that alkylates cellular molecules, especially DNA

APC 7-ethyl-10-[4-N-(5-aminopentanoic acid)-1-piperidino]-carbonyloxy-camptothecin

AR androgen receptor

ARID1A AT-rich interactive domain 1A (SWI-like)

ATP adenosine-5′-triphosphate

AUC area under the curve

BER/SSBR base excision repair/single-strand break repair, a DNA repair pathway that repairs single base damage or nicks in DNA

BRAF v-raf murine sarcoma viral oncogene homolog B1

BSA body surface area

CAB combined androgen blockade

CBFB core-binding factor, beta subunit

CCDC6 coiled-coil domain containing 6

CCND3 cyclin D3

CDKN2A cyclin-dependent kinase inhibitor 2A

CFTR cystic fibrosis transmembrane conductance regulator

C_{max} maximal concentration

CPY19 aromatase, estrogen synthase

CRH corticotropin-releasing hormone

CRPC castration-resistant prostate cancer

CYP cytochrome P450

CYP11A1 P450scc, cholesterol side-chain cleavage enzyme

CYP11B1 11β-hydroxylase

CYP11B2 aldosterone synthase

CYP17 17α-hydroxylase-17,20-lyase

DACH1 dachshund homolog 1

DDR2 discoidin domain receptor tyrosine kinase 2

DHEA dehydroepiandrosterone

DHEA-S dehydroepiandrostenedione sulfate

DHT dihydrotestosterone

DNA DSB DNA double strand break

DNA SSB DNA single-strand break

DNA deoxyribonucleic acid

DOC 11-deoxycorticosterone

DPD dihydropyrimidine dehydrogenase

DPYD dihydropyrimidine dehydrogenase gene

DRE digital rectal examination

EGF epidermal growth factor

EGFR epidermal growth factor receptor

EM extensive metabolizer

EML4   echinoderm microtubule-associated protein-like 4
FDA   US Food and Drug Administration
FdUMP   fluorodeoxyuridine monophosphate
FdUTP   fluorodeoxyuridine triphosphate
FGFR   fibroblast growth factor receptor
FISH   fluorescence in situ hybridization
FoxA1   forkhead box transcription factor A
FSH   follicle-stimulating hormone
5-FU   5-fluorouracil
FUTP   fluorouridine triphosphate
G6PD   glucose-6-phosphate dehydrogenase
GIST   gastrointestinal stromal tumor
GnRH   gonadotropin-releasing hormone
GWAS   genome-wide association study
hCE   carboxylesterase
HER   v-erb-b2 erythroblastic leukemia viral oncogene homolog
HR   hazard ratio
HRAS   v-Ha-ras Harvey rat sarcoma viral oncogene homolog
HRR   homologous recombination repair, a DNA DSB repair pathway involving use of the sister chromatid as a template for repair of the damaged DNA
IC$_{50}$ the concentration of a drug that inhibits the activity of its target by 50%
IGF   insulin-like growth factor
IHC   immunohistochemistry
IM   intermediate metabolizer
IR   ionizing radiation, such as X-rays
Isogenic   of the same genetic background
JAK   Janus kinase
Ki   inhibition constant
KIF5B   kinesin family member 5B
KIT   v-kit Hardy–Zuckerman 4 feline sarcoma viral oncogene homolog
KM   Michaelis constant
KRAS   v-Ki-ras2 Kirsten rat sarcoma viral oncogene homolog
LH   luteinizing hormone
LHRH   hypothalamic luteinizing hormone–releasing hormone
Ligation   joining DNA ends
M phase   cell division or mitosis phase of the cell cycle
MAPK   mitogen-activated protein kinase
MET   hepatocyte growth factor receptor
MMR   DNA mismatch repair
6-MP   6-mercaptopurine
MSI   microsatellite instability
NAD$^+$ nicotinamide adenine dinucleotide
NF1   neurofibromin 1
NHEJ   nonhomologous end joining, a DNA DSB repair pathway where the DNA ends are brought together and religated
NPC   7-ethyl-10-(4-amino-1-piperidino)-carbonyloxy-camptothecin
NPM   nucleophosmin
NRAS   neuroblastoma RAS viral (v-ras) oncogene homolog
NSCLC   non-small-cell lung cancer
ORR   overall response rate
OS   overall survival
PARP   poly(ADP-ribose) polymerase, an enzyme involved in signaling DNA SSB to the BER/SSBR pathway
PARPi   PARP inhibitor
PCa   prostate cancer

PDGFRA   platelet-derived growth factor receptor-a
PFS   progression-free survival
PI3K   phosphatidylinositol 3 kinase
PIK3R1   phosphoinositide-3-kinase, regulatory subunit 1 (alpha)
PM   poor metabolizer
PREX2   phosphatidylinositol-3,4,5-trisphosphate-dependent Rac exchange factor 2
PSA   prostate-specific antigen
PTPN22   protein tyrosine phosphatase, nonreceptor type 22
PTPRD   protein tyrosine phosphatase, receptor type, D
5α-R   5-reductase
RAF   v-raf murine sarcoma viral oncogene homolog
RBM10   RNA-binding motif protein 10
RECIST   response evaluation criteria in solid tumors
RELN   reelin
RET   ret proto-oncogene
ROS1   c-ros oncogene 1, receptor tyrosine kinase
RUNX1   runt-related transcription factor 1
S phase   DNA replication or synthesis-phase of the cell cycle
SAR   structure–activity relationship, where the chemical structure of inhibitors with a range of potency is compared to determine the structural features that confer potency
SCF   stem cell factor
SF3B1   splicing factor 3b, subunit 1
SLCO   solute carrier organic anion transporter family
SN-38G   SN-38 glucuronide
STAT   signal transducer and activator of transcription
Synapsis   bringing together of DNA molecules
TBX3   T-box 3
T-DM1   trastuzumab–emtansine
TGF-α   transforming growth factor-alpha
TK   tyrosine kinase
TKI   tyrosine kinase inhibitor
TMZ   temozolomide
TPM   tropomyosin
TPMT   thiopurine methyltransferase
TS   thymidylate synthase
Tumor xenograft   tumor material or cells from one species (usually human) implanted into an immunocompromized host (usually mouse)
TYMS   thymidylate synthase gene
U2AF1   U2 small nuclear RNA auxiliary factor 1
UGT   uridine 5′-diphospho-glucuronosyltransferase
UM   ultrarapid metabolizer
UTR   untranslated enhancer region
VNTR   variable-number tandem repeat
WNT   wingless-type MMTV integration site family

Index

Note: Page numbers with "f" denote figures; "t" tables; and "b" boxes.

Color Plates

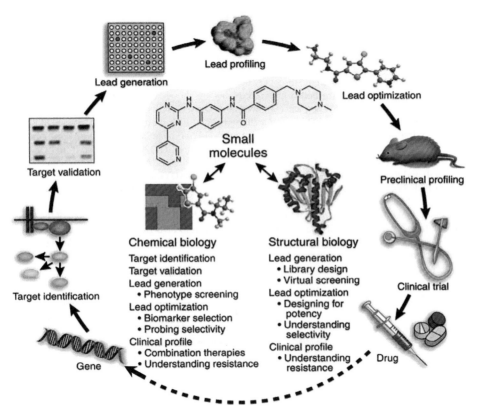

FIGURE 1.2 The integrated and nonlinear way in which modern drug discovery often occurs. Structural biology and the various approaches collectively referred to as "chemical biology" link together the multiple elements of the drug discovery process. *Reproduced with permission from [3].*

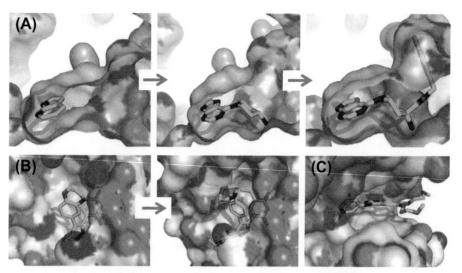

FIGURE 1.6 Structure-based design in the discovery of new targeted treatments. Ligands are shown as stick models colored according to atom type (carbon = green). Proteins are shown as transparent surfaces colored according to atom type (carbon = gray). (A) Sequence showing the X-ray crystal structure of the fragment 7-azaindole bound to the adenosine triphosphate (ATP) site of a chimeric PKA–PKB protein (adapted from PDB 2UVX [172]), its elaboration by fragment growing into a more potent and selective pyrrolopyrimidine PKB inhibitor (adapted from PDB 2VNY [173]), and subsequently into the orally active inhibitor CCT129254 (adapted from PDB 2X39 [174]). (B) Sequence showing the X-ray crystal structure of CCT018159 bound to the HSP90 ATPase domain (adapted from PDB 2BRC [176]) and its elaboration into the clinical candidate NVP-AUY922 bound to the HSP90 ATPase domain (adapted from PDB 2VCI [177]). The resorcinol group in CCT018159 that interacts with protein-bound water molecules is retained, while additional potency is gained from new interactions to the additional amide substituent. The morpholine group that modulates pharmacokinetic behavior extends out into solvent. (C) Detail of the X-ray crystal structure of erlotinib bound to the EGFR kinase domain (adapted from PDB 1M17 [178]) showing the separation of the functionality-mediating target binding, buried in the binding pocket, and the group-modulating solubility and pharmacokinetic properties, which are exposed to solvent.

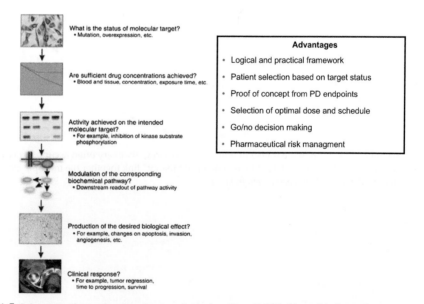

FIGURE 1.7 Schematic illustrating the pharmacological audit trail. This hierarchical set of parameters provides a conceptual and practical framework to aid decision making in preclinical and clinical drug development. The audit trail links the status of the molecular target (through pharmacokinetic exposures and pharmacodynamic effects on the target), pathway, and biological effect to therapeutic and toxic responses. It is also useful to help select the optimal drug dose and schedule. *Modified with permission from Ref. [3].*

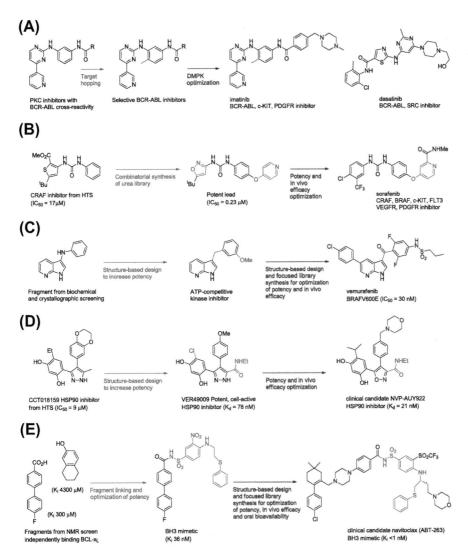

SCHEME 1.1 Selected case histories of lead generation and lead optimization for small-molecule targeted molecular cancer therapeutics. (A) The phenylaminopyrimidine core of imatinib emerged from screening of protein kinase C inhibitors and was rendered selective for BCR–ABL by addition of a single methyl substituent (red). Lead optimization focused on improving DMPK properties (blue). The second-generation BCR–ABL inhibitor dasatinib has activity against some imatinib-resistant BCR–ABL mutant kinases. (B) The starting point for the discovery of the multitargeted kinase inhibitor sorafenib came from high-throughput screening (HTS) of a large compound collection against CRAF. Combinatorial variation of the two substituents on the central urea generated a potent lead (red). Lead optimization focused on improving potency and in vivo antitumor activity (blue). (C) The 3-anilino-7-azaindole core of vemurafenib was identified as a low-molecular-weight drug fragment binding to the ATP-binding site of kinases, including BRAF, by a combined biochemical and crystallographic screening approach. Elaboration of the fragment generated more active 3-benzyl-7-azaindole inhibitors (red). A focused library approach combined with structure-based design led to the optimized compound vemurafenib (PLX4720) (blue). (D) HTS against the HSP90 ATPase identified the novel resorcinylic pyrazole inhibitor CCT018159, which was co-crystallized with the enzyme. Structure-based design guided the positioning of extra lipophilic and hydrogen-bonding functional groups to generate the potent cell active inhibitor VER-49009 (red). Further optimization of potency and of pharmacokinetic and pharmacodynamic properties (blue) gave the isoxazole clinical candidate NVP-AUY922. (E) Screening using NMR identified fragments binding weakly to two adjacent subsites on the BCL-X_L protein. Linking of the fragments to retain their orientations and further substitution gave a potent inhibitor of BH3 binding to Bcl-X_L that occupies the whole binding site (red). Structure-based design to optimize potency and in vivo efficacy, and subsequently oral pharmacokinetic properties, led to the clinical candidate navitoclax (blue).

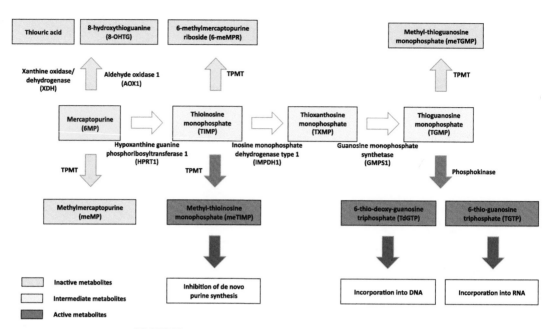

FIGURE 2.1 The metabolic pathways of 6-MP in humans.

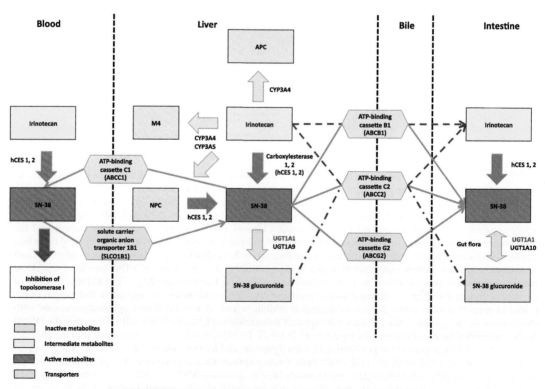

FIGURE 2.2 The metabolic pathways of irinotecan in humans.

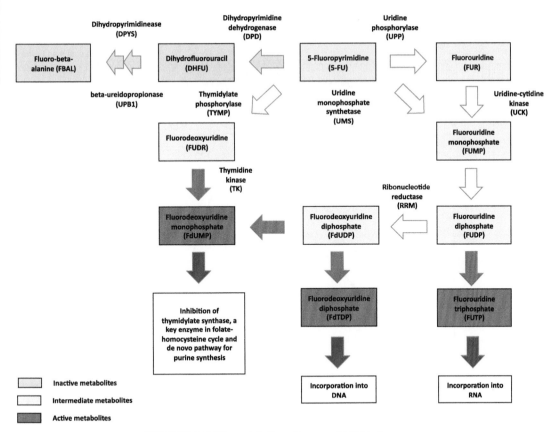

FIGURE 2.3 The metabolic pathways of 5-FU in humans.

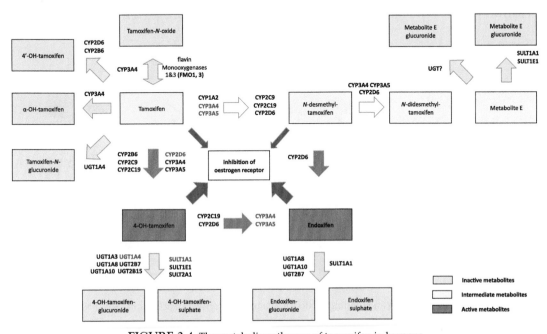

FIGURE 2.4 The metabolic pathways of tamoxifen in humans.

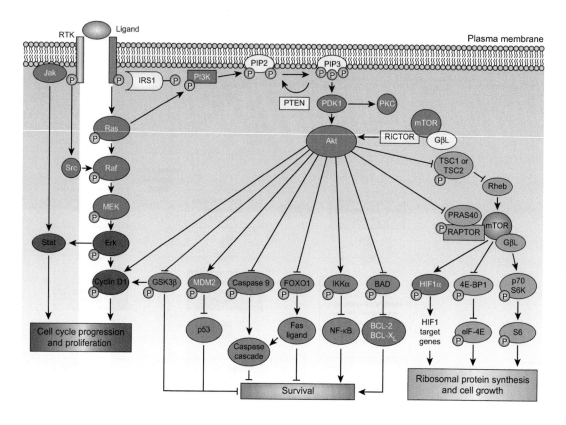

FIGURE 4.1 The role of PKB in cell signaling. *Source: Reproduced from Yap TA et al., Nature Reviews Cancer 2009.*

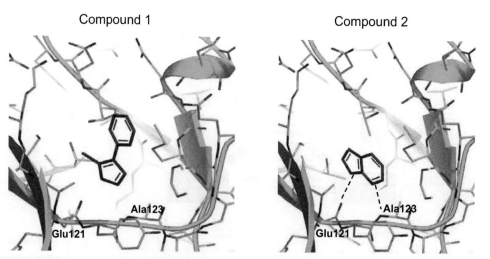

FIGURE 4.2 Fragment hits and binding modes shown by X-ray crystal structures in PKA–PKB chimera.

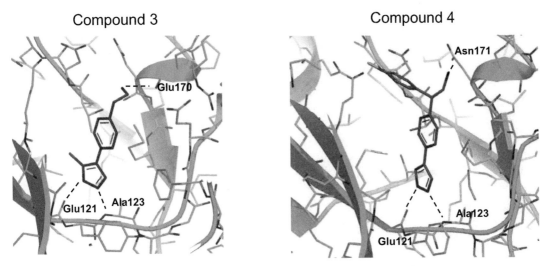

FIGURE 4.4 X-ray structures of **3** and **4** bound to PKA–PKB chimera.

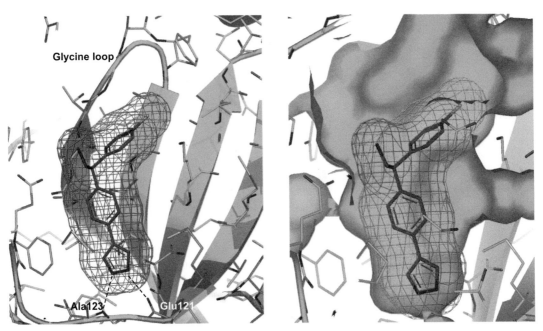

FIGURE 4.5 X-ray structure of **4** rotated by 180° (cf. Fig. 4.4) showing interactions on the left and space filling with surfaces of ligand and protein on the right.

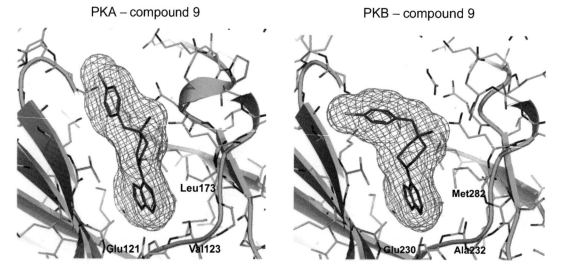

FIGURE 4.8 X-ray structure and comparison of binding modes of **9** in PKA and PKB. Orientation of the ligand in PKB offers better space-filling and surface contact, resulting in higher affinity.

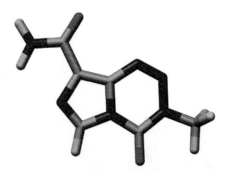

FIGURE 5.1 Structure of temozolomide. *Source: Thanks to Dr Mark Beardsall for this image.*

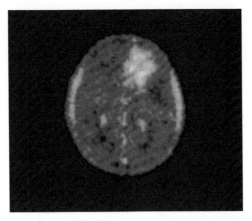

FIGURE 5.8 Positron emission tomography (PET) image of a patient with a glioblastoma tumor treated with temozolomide labeled in the C-4 position with ^{11}C isotope.

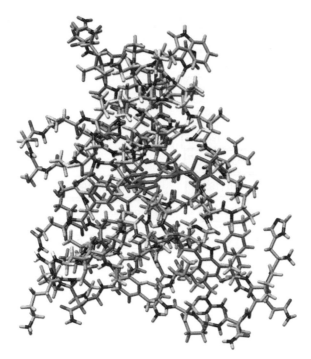

FIGURE 5.10 The inhibitor Patrin 2 in noncovalent association at the active site of MGMT. Source: *Thanks to Dr Mark Beardsall for this image.*

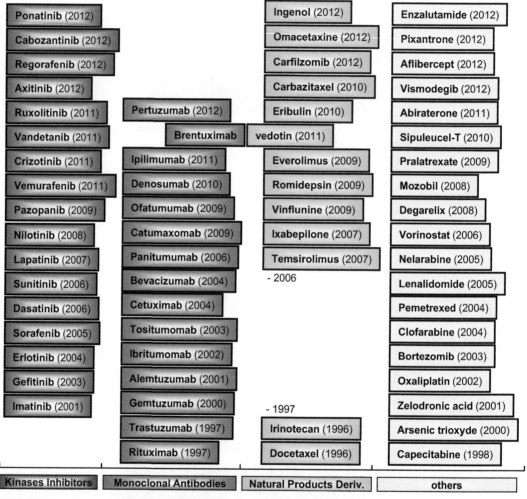

FIGURE 7.1 Four categories of drugs recently approved for the treatment of cancers (year of first US Food and Drug Administration or European Medicines Agency approval). For the sake of clarity, all small molecules are not mentioned.

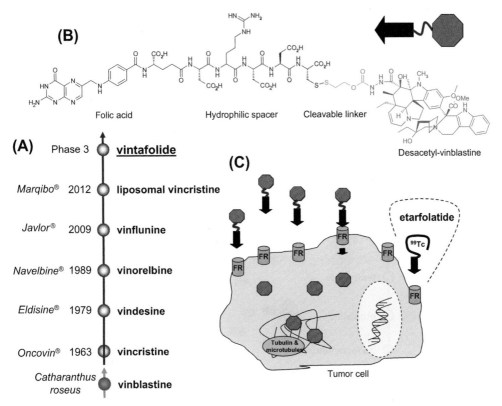

(B)

Folic acid   Hydrophilic spacer   Cleavable linker

Desacetyl-vinblastine

(A)

Phase 3	**vintafolide**
Marqibo® 2012	**liposomal vincristine**
Javlor® 2009	**vinflunine**
Navelbine® 1989	**vinorelbine**
Eldisine® 1979	**vindesine**
Oncovin® 1963	**vincristine**
Catharanthus roseus	**vinblastine**

(C)

etarfolatide

^{99}Tc

FR

Tubulin & microtubules

Tumor cell

FIGURE 7.2 (A) *Vinca* alkaloids approved for cancer treatments: vinblastine extracted from the Madagascan periwinkle, *Catharanthus roseus*; vincristine (Oncovin®), for leukemia, 1963; vindesine (Eldisine®), for leukemia, 1979; vinorelbine (Navelbine), for NSCLC, 1989, and for breast cancer, 1991; vinflunine (Javlor), for bladder cancer, 2009; liposomal vincristine (Marqibo®), for acute lymphoblastic leukemia, 2012; and vintafolide, currently in phase III for the treatment of ovarian cancer. (B) Structure of vintafolide with its subunits. (C) Illustration of the mode of action of vintafolide: Uptake via the folate receptor (FR) and, after cleavage of the linker, release of the cytotoxic tubulin binder inside the cell to inhibit tubulin polymerization into microtubules and mitotic progression. The technecium (^{99m}Tc)-containing companion imaging agent etarfolatide serves to identify FR-positive tumors by single-photon emission computed tomography.

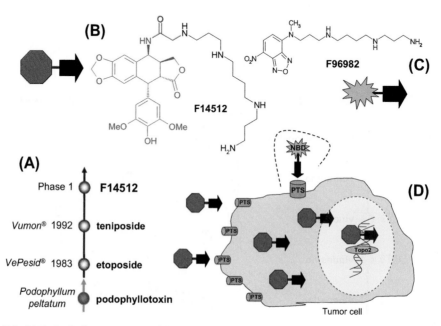

FIGURE 7.3 (A) Podophyllotoxin extracted from *Podophyllum peltatum* is at the origin of the epipodophyllotoxin derivatives etoposide and teniposide, and the new drug candidate F14512. (B) and (C) Structures of F14512 and the probe F96982 containing an NBD fluorescent moiety. (D) Illustration of the cell delivery mechanism and mode of action of F14512: Uptake via the polyamine transport system (PTS) and accumulation into cell nuclei to poison topoisomerase II–DNA complexes, leading to DNA damage and cell death. The fluorescent probe F96982 is used to analyze the PTS activity in leukemic cells.

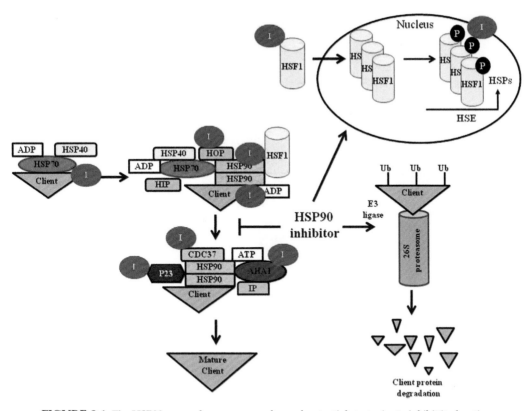

FIGURE 9.1 The HSP90 super-chaperone complex and potential strategies to inhibit its function.

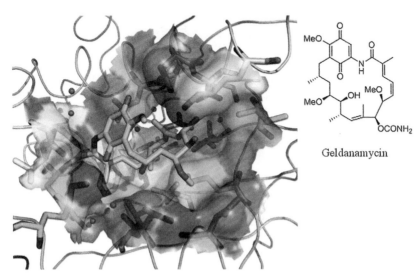

Geldanamycin

FIGURE 9.3 Geldanamycin bound to the N-terminal domain of human HSP90 (PDB code: 1YET).

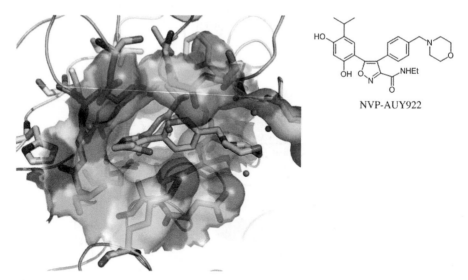

NVP-AUY922

FIGURE 9.4 NVP-AUY922 bound to the N-terminal domain of human HSP90 (PDB code: 2VCI).

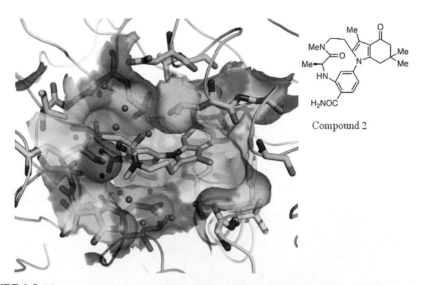

Compound 2

FIGURE 9.5 Pfizer macrocycle 2 bound to the N-terminal domain of human HSP90 (PDB code: 3R91).

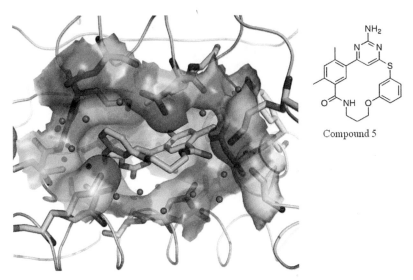

Compound 5

FIGURE 9.6 Chugai macrocycle 5 bound to the N-terminal domain of human HSP90 (PDB code: 3VHC).

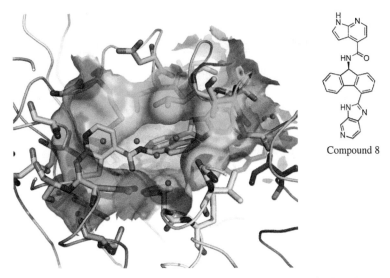

Compound 8

FIGURE 9.7 Sanofi-Aventis compound 6 bound to the N-terminal domain of HSP90 (PDB code: 2YKI).

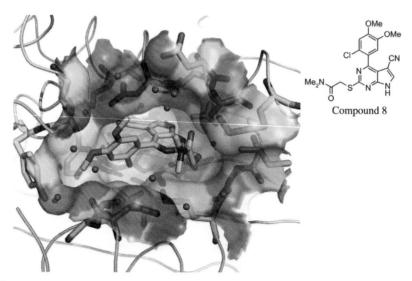

Compound 8

FIGURE 9.8 Vernalis–Novartis compound (compound 8) bound to the N-terminal domain of human HSP90 (PDB code: 4FCR).

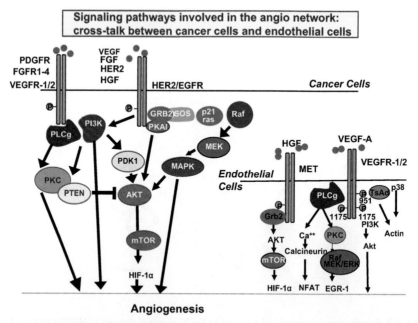

FIGURE 10.1 The angio-network: cross-talk between cancer cells and endothelial cells. ERK, extracellular signal-regulated kinase; MAPK, mitogen-activated protein kinase; PI3K, phosphatidylinositol 3′ kinase; PKB, protein kinase B.

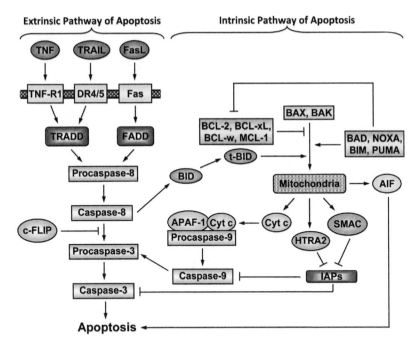

FIGURE 12.1 Extrinsic and intrinsic pathways of apoptosis. The two pathways are independent but connected through BID, and they share caspase-3 as the common effector protease.

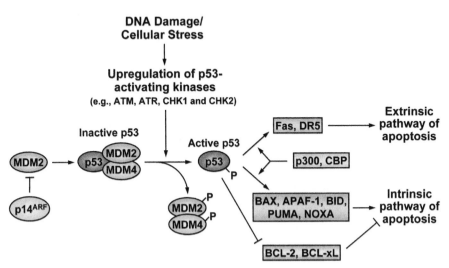

FIGURE 12.2 Induction of apoptosis by the tumor suppressor p53. Binding to MDM2 and MDM4 inactivates p53, but posttranslational phosphorylation releases p53 to transactivate downstream target genes and induce apoptosis via the extrinsic and intrinsic pathways.

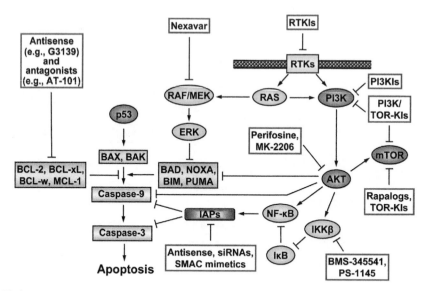

FIGURE 12.4 Activating the intrinsic pathway of apoptosis by targeting antiapoptotic proteins. The antitumor agents, shown in the red box, induce apoptosis by downregulating antiapoptotic BCL-2 family members or inhibitor of apoptosis proteins (IAPs), or via inhibition of receptor tyrosine kinases (RTKs) and the PI3K–AKT–mTOR, IKKβ–IκB–NF-κB, or RAS–RAF–MEK–ERK pathway.

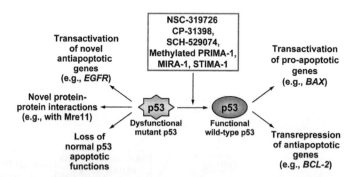

FIGURE 12.5 Rescuing mutant p53. Mutation in p53 can cause loss of normal p53 functions, but may also enable mutant p53 to acquire novel functions. Small-molecule modifiers, as exemplified in the red box, interact with mutant p53, alter the conformational structure, and restore wild-type p53 apoptotic functions.

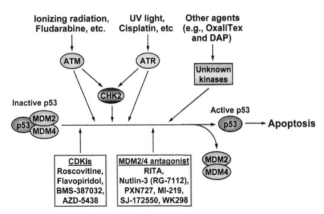

FIGURE 12.6 Activating wild-type p53 by disrupting its binding to MDM2/MDM4. Wild-type p53 is kept inactive by its interaction with MDM2/MDM4 proteins. The CDK inhibitors (CDKIs) and MDM2/4 antagonists, shown in their respective red boxes, interfere with p53 binding and thereby release and activate wild-type p53 to induce apoptosis. Also, p53 may be activated by agents activating independent DNA damage pathways. Thus, inactive wild-type p53, by virtue of loss of a posttranslational modifying kinase (e.g. ATM), can be reactivated by another agent inducing an alternative kinase (e.g. ATR).

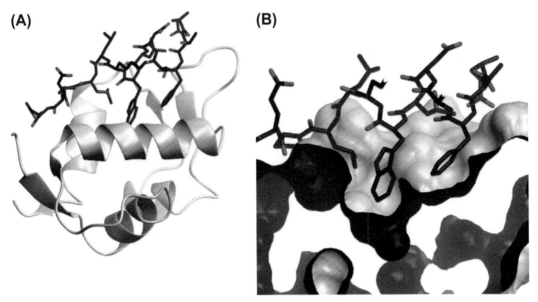

FIGURE 13.3 X-ray structure of MDM2 and p53 peptide (PDB ID: 1YCR). (A): Ribbon view; and (B): Surface showing the binding interaction.

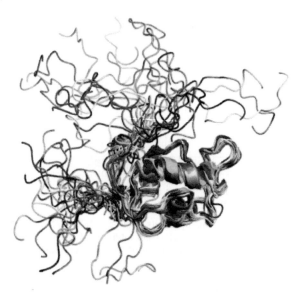

FIGURE 13.4 NMR structure of MDM2 (PDB ID: 1Z1M).

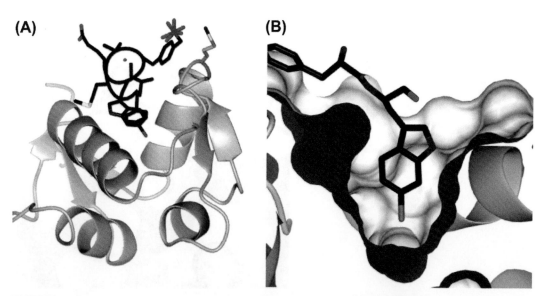

FIGURE 13.5 X-ray structure of MDM2 and AP peptide (PDB ID: 2GV2). (A): End on ribbon view; (B): Surface showing Trp[23] binding pocket.

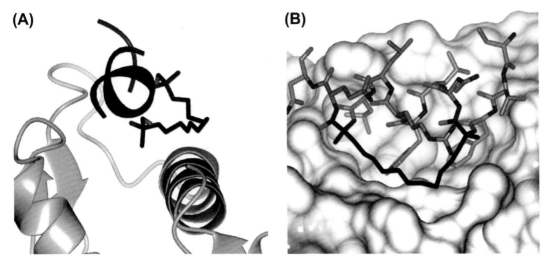

FIGURE 13.6 X-ray structure of MDM2 and stapled peptide **10** (PDB ID: 3V3B). (A): End on ribbon view; and (B): surface showing interaction of hydrocarbon staple.

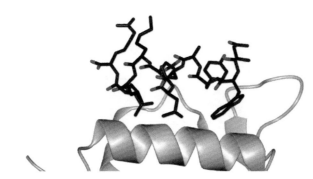

FIGURE 13.7 X-ray structure of MDM2 and ᴰPMI-α (**15**) (PDB ID: 3LNJ).

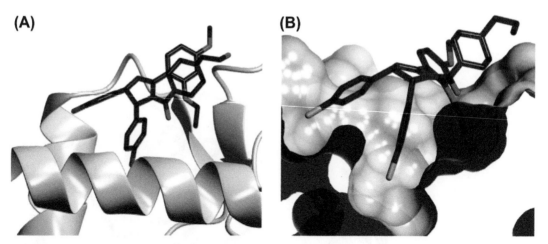

FIGURE 13.8 X-ray structure of MDM2 and Nutlin-2 (**29**) (PDB ID: 1RV1). (A): Ribbon view; and (B): surface showing binding interaction.

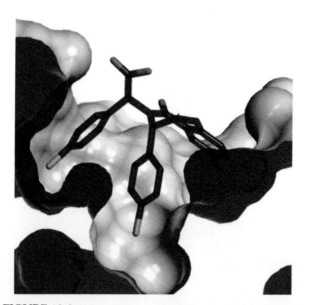

FIGURE 13.9 X-ray structure of MDM2 and **39** (PDB ID: 1T4E).

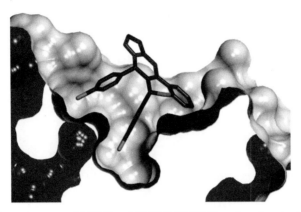

FIGURE 13.10 X-ray structure of MDM2 and **63** (PDB ID: 3JZK) surface showing binding interaction.

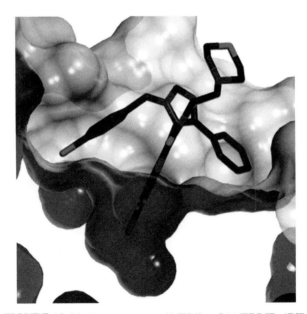

FIGURE 13.11 X-ray structure of MDM2 and **74** (PDB ID: 4DIJ).

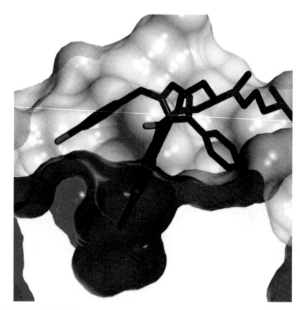

FIGURE 13.12 X-ray structure of MDMX and **76** (PDB ID: 4LBJ).

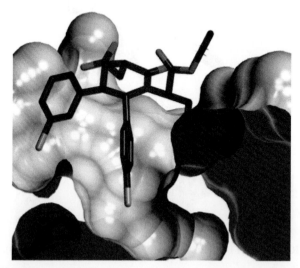

FIGURE 13.13 X-ray structure of MDM2 and **87** (PDB ID: 4ERF).

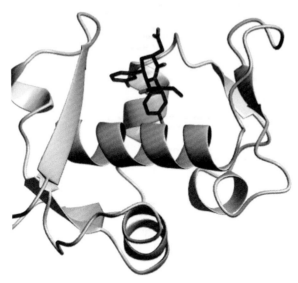

FIGURE 13.14 X-ray structure of MDM2 (amino acids 6–125) and **88** (PDB ID: 4HBM).

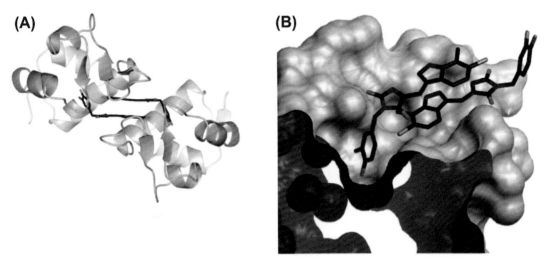

FIGURE 13.15 X-ray structure of MDMX and **95** (PDB ID: 3UI5). (A): Ribbon view showing dimer; and (B): surface showing binding interaction.

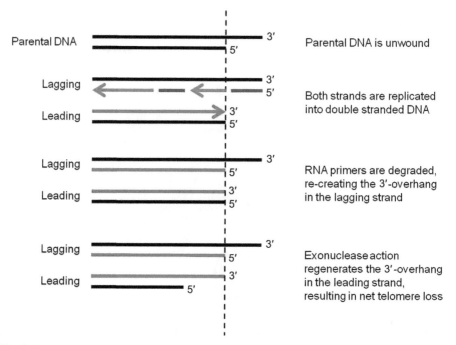

FIGURE 17.1 The "end replication problem". Loss of telomeric DNA through each cycle of DNA replication occurs, at least partly, through exonuclease degradation of the leading template DNA strand, so as to regenerate the requisite 3′ overhang at the telomere.

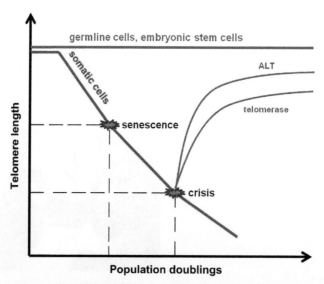

FIGURE 17.2 Telomere dynamics in human biology. Telomere shortening is the cell's "counting mechanism", activating the nonproliferative state of cellular senescence, considered a major tumor suppressor mechanism. Inactivation of tumor suppressor genes may allow a cell to bypass senescence and continue proliferating until the telomeres reach a critical length (crisis), resulting in genomic instability and cell death. Activation of a telomere maintenance mechanism (telomerase or ALT) will allow a cell to resume proliferation and confer immortality.

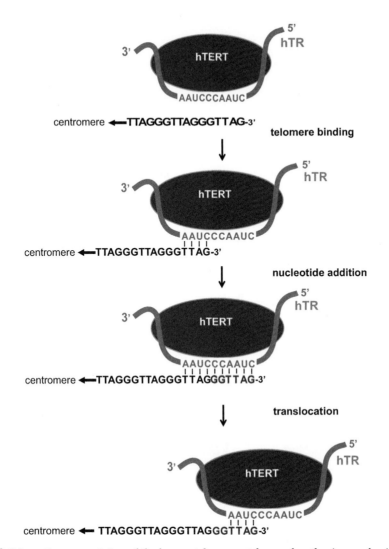

FIGURE 17.3 Schematic representation of the human telomerase telomere-lengthening mechanism. Telomerase binds to the 3′ end of the telomere. Once bound, nucleotides complementary to the hTR template are added to the DNA. Once the template boundary is reached, hTR translocates while telomerase remains bound to the telomere.

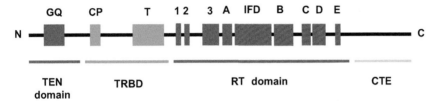

FIGURE 17.4 Linear representation of the hTERT protein. The telomerase essential N-terminal (10) domain, the telomerase RNA binding domain (TRBD), the reverse transcriptase (RT) domain, and the C-terminal extension (CTE) domain are shown with their conserved functional motifs highlighted.

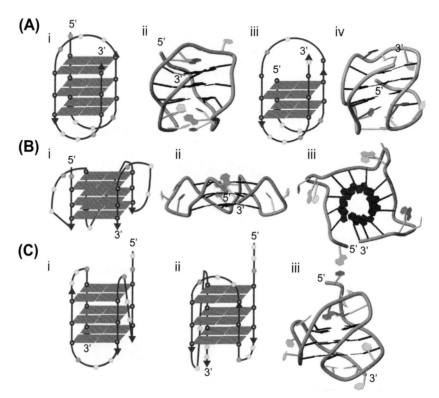

FIGURE 17.7 Human telomeric intramolecular G-quadruplexes. (A) Topology and NMR structure of oligonucleotide AGGG(TTAGGG)$_3$ in sodium solution (i,ii; [153]) or oligonucleotide GGG(TTAGGG)$_3$T in potassium solution (iii,iv; [154]), demonstrating two different antiparallel conformations. (B) Topology (i) and crystal structure (ii, iii) of oligonucleotide AGGG(TTAGGG)$_3$ in potassium, showing a parallel "propeller" structure [155]. The crystal structure is shown as a side view (ii) and a top view (iii). (C) Hybrid conformations in potassium solution. Hybrid 1 (i) and hybrid 2 (ii) topologies illustrate differences in loop structures [156,157]. The NMR structure of hybrid 2 is shown in (iii) [157].

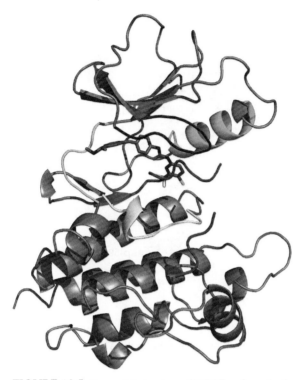

FIGURE 18.5 Co-crystal structure of B-RAF and sorafenib.

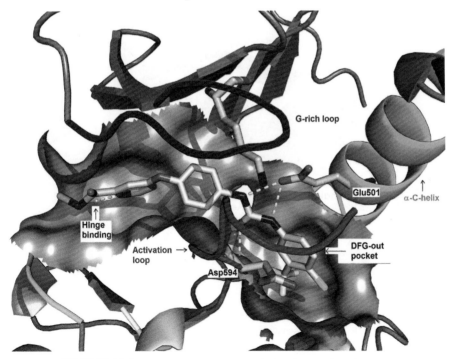

FIGURE 18.7 Sorafenib binding in the ATP-binding pocket of B-RAF.

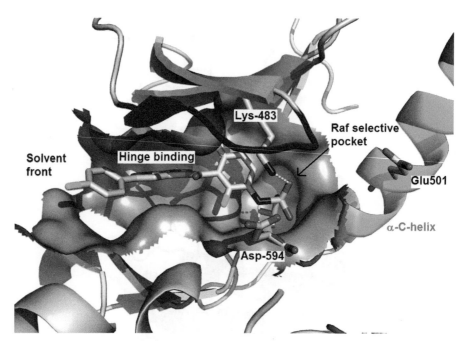

FIGURE 18.10 Vemurafenib binding in the ATP-binding pocket of B-RAF.

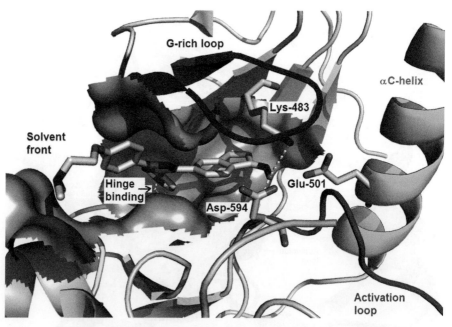

FIGURE 18.15 SB-590885 binding in the ATP-binding pocket of B-RAF.

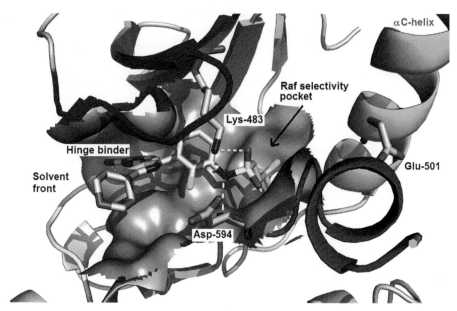

FIGURE 18.18 Dabrafenib analog **14** binding in the ATP-binding pocket of B-RAF.

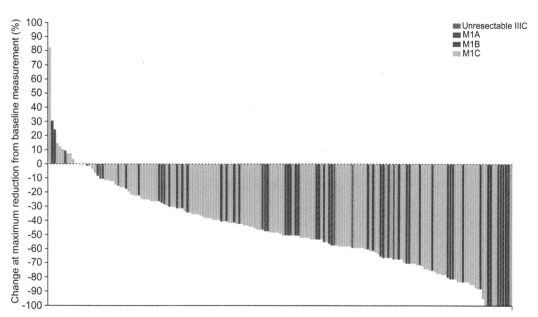

FIGURE 18.20 Maximum tumor percent change from baseline in patients treated with dabrafenib (*n* = 187). Each bar represents data for an individual patient; negative values indicate tumor shrinkage. *Figure reproduced with permission from Ref. [41] © (2012) Elsevier. All rights reserved.*

Examples	Risk Impact Range				
	Very Low	Low	Intermediate	High	Very High
Solubility and Dissolution	good / no food effect		variable / + food effect		poor
PK/PD Variability	low variability				highly variable
CYP Inhibition	none / well described				mechanism based / poorly characterized
Drug–Drug Interaction	none		involves combination unlikely to be used for target population		involves agent with narrow therapeutic index
Ease of Regimen	similar to current standards				complex / intensive
Margin of Safety	wide				narrow
Observed Toxicity	None		monitorable / reversible / amenable to mitigation		idiosyncratic / progressive / life threatening
Target Pharmacology	previously clinically validated				novel / previously unvalidated
PD Biomarker	gold standard available				unvalidated or unavailable
Endpoint Availability	final Phase 3 suitable		established surrogate		novel / undefined / exploratory endpoint(s)
Clinical Efficacy	demonstrated early in development				delayed demonstration
Clinical Response	addresses unmet medical need		similar to existing therapy		inadequate clinical response
	response as single agent				response only in combination therapy
Time to Response	short				long
Durability of Response	long				short
Target Population	prevalent or multiple indications				narrow indication(s) / very rare / dependent on prior line(s) of therapy
Tailoring Opportunity	well defined / previously validated				no opportunity / stratification necessary but unavailable
Companion Diagnostic (CDx)	approved CDx available		CDx unvalidated / unapproved		simultaneous development of novel CDx and drug

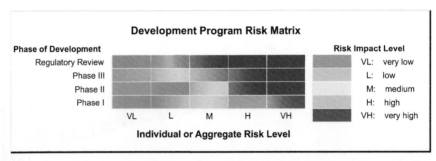

Development Program Risk Matrix

Phase of Development: Regulatory Review, Phase III, Phase II, Phase I

Individual or Aggregate Risk Level: VL, L, M, H, VH

Risk Impact Level
VL: very low
L: low
M: medium
H: high
VH: very high

FIGURE 19.1 Sources of risk and their contribution to failures in clinical development. Clinical development must start with the formulation of a testable clinical hypothesis and a series of objectives that can be explored and answered under controlled conditions that allow opportunities to systematically discharge the most important risks. Optimally, the development of experimental therapeutics must be tailored to the risk specific to that program, seeking a balance between early discharges of risk from the clinical hypothesis versus other potential program risks that could prevent testing that hypothesis. A failure to discharge risks early in development may result in an aggregated risk of failure in the later stages of clinical development, where there is less tolerance of risk.

Printed and bound by CPI Group (UK) Ltd, Croydon, CR0 4YY

08/05/2025

01864978-0001